ENDOSCOPY

ENDOSCOPY

EDITED BY

GEORGE BERCI, M.D., F.C.S.H.

Director, Department of Endoscopy, Cedars-Sinai Medical Center, Los Angeles; Attending Surgeon, Veterans Administration Hospital, Wadsworth, Los Angeles; Clinical Associate Professor, Department of Surgery, UCLA School of Medicine, Los Angeles, California

with 58 coauthors

FOREWORD BY

Maurice R. Ewing, M.Sc., M.B., Ch.B.,
F.R.C.S. (Ed), F.R.C.S. (Eng), F.R.A.C.S.,
F.A.C.S. (Hon), M.D. (Hon)

*Stewart Professor of Surgery,
University of Melbourne, Melbourne, Australia*

APPLETON-CENTURY-CROFTS/New York

Library of Congress Cataloging in Publication Data
Main entry under title:

Endoscopy.

   Includes bibliographies and indexes.
   1. Endoscope and endoscopy. I. Berci, George,
1921–
RC78.7.E5E53   616.07′54   76-18700
ISBN 0-8385-2216-5

Copyright © 1976 by APPLETON-CENTURY-CROFTS
A Publishing Division of Prentice-Hall, Inc.

76 77 78 79 80/10 9 8 7 6 5 4 3 2 1

*Prentice-Hall International, Inc., London
Prentice-Hall of Australia, Pty. Ltd., Sydney
Prentice-Hall of India Private Limited, New Delhi
Prentice-Hall of Japan, Inc., Tokyo
Prentice-Hall of Southeast Asia (Pte.) Ltd., Singapore*

Printed in the United States of America

This book is dedicated to my wife Suzie
and to my children
Katherine, Winton, and Ninette

Contributors

Daniel L. Anderson, Lt. Col., MC
Assistant Chief, Gastroenterology Service, Walter Reed Army Medical Center, Washington, D.C.

George Berci, M.D., F.C.S.H.
Director, Department of Endoscopy, Cedars-Sinai Medical Center, Los Angeles; Attending Surgeon, Veterans Administration Hospital, Wadsworth, Los Angeles; Clinical Associate Professor, Department of Surgery, UCLA School of Medicine, Los Angeles, California

H. Worth Boyce, Jr., Col., MC
Chief, Gastroenterology Service, Walter Reed Army Medical Center, Washington, D.C.

Thomas C. Calcaterra, M.D., F.A.C.S.
Associate Professor, Division of Head and Neck Surgery, UCLA School of Medicine, Los Angeles, California

Richard C. Cammerer, Maj., MC
Gastroenterology Staff, Walter Reed Army Medical Center, Washington, D.C.

Angelo E. Dagradi, M.D., F.A.C.P.
Chief, Gastroenterology Section, Veterans Administration Hospital, Long Beach, California; Associate Clinical Professor of Medicine, University of California at Irvine, Irvine, California

Joachim W. Dudenhausen, M.D.
Research Fellow, Department of Perinatal Medicine, Free University, Berlin, West Germany

L. Penfield Faber, M.D., F.A.C.S.
Professor of Surgery, Associate Dean, Surgical Sciences and Service, Rush-Presbyterian, St. Luke's Medical Center, Chicago, Illinois

Jon K. Fitzgerald, M.B.A.
Electro-Medical Systems, Inc., Denver, Colorado

Eugene Flaum, M.D., F.A.C.S.
Clinical Instructor, Department of Oto-Laryngology, University of Southern California, Los Angeles; Assistant Attending Surgeon, Department of Oto-Laryngology, Childrens Hospital, Los Angeles, California

Hans Frangenheim, M.D.
Chief, Department of Obstetrics and Gynecology, Municipal Hospital, Konstanz, West Germany

Walter D. Gaisford, M.D., F.A.C.S.
Associate Professor in Surgery, College of Medicine, University of Utah, Salt Lake City, Utah

Stephen L. Gans, M.D., F.A.C.S.
Chief, Pediatric Surgery Service, Department of Surgery, Cedars-Sinai Medical Center, Los Angeles; Associate Clinical Professor, Department of Surgery, UCLA School of Medicine, Los Angeles, California

Jan Gillquist, M.D.
Assistant Professor, Department of Surgery, University of Linkoping, Linkoping, Sweden

Ruben F. Gittes, M.D., F.A.C.S.
Professor of Surgery/Urology, University of California at San Diego, School of Medicine, San Diego, California

Gino Hasler
Research Assistant, Department of Surgical Endoscopy, Cedars of Lebanon Hospital, Los Angeles, California

James G. Helmuth, E.E., M.S.
Chadwick-Helmuth Electronics, Inc., Monrovia, California

Basil I. Hirschowitz, M.D., M.R.C.P., F.A.C.P., F.R.C.P. (Ed)
Professor of Medicine, University of Alabama Medical Center, Director, Division of Gastroenterology, Birmingham, Alabama

John C. Hobbins, M.D.
Assistant Professor, Department of Obstetrics and Gynecology, Yale University, School of Medicine, New Haven, Connecticut

Harold H. Hopkins, F.R.S.
Professor of Applied Optics, Department of Physics, University of Reading, Reading, Whiteknights, England

Johannes H. Iizuka, M.D., D.M.Ch., F.I.C.S.
Assistant Neuro-Surgeon, Chief, Section of Stereotaxic Neuro-Surgery, Neurosurgical University Hospital, Bonn, West Germany

Peter Illum, M.D.
Assistant Professor, Department of Otolaryngology, St. Joseph Hospital, Aalborg, Denmark

T. T. Irvin, Ch.M., F.R.C.S.E.
Senior Lecturer, University Surgical Unit, University of Sheffield, Sheffield, England

Dale G. Johnson, M.D., F.A.C.S.
Chairman, Department of Surgery, Primary Children's Medical Center, University of Utah, College of Medicine, Salt Lake City, Utah

Joseph J. Kaufman, M.D., F.A.C.S.
Professor and Chief, Department of Urology, UCLA School of Medicine, Los Angeles, California

Horst R. Konrad, M.D., F.A.C.S.
Assistant Professor, Division of Head and Neck Surgery, UCLA School of Medicine, Los Angeles, California

Sten-Otto Liljedahl, M.D.
Professor of Surgery, Department of Surgery, University of Linkoping, Linkoping, Sweden

Hans Joachim Lindemann, M.D.
Chief, Department of Obstetrics and Gynecology, Elisabeth Hospital, Hamburg, West Germany

Wolfgang Lutzeyer, M.D.
Professor and Chairman, Department of Urology, Medical Faculty, Rhein.-Westf. Technical University, Aachen, West Germany

Margaret McQueen, R.N.
Associate Director, Department of Nursing, Cedars of Lebanon Hospital, Los Angeles, California

Maurice J. Mahoney, M.D.
Associate Professor, Department of Human Genetics and Pediatrics, Yale University, School of Medicine, New Haven, Connecticut

W. J. Mautner, B.A., M.A.
Consultant Biophysicist, Los Angeles, California

W. Messerklinger, M.D.
Professor and Chairman, Department Ear, Nose and Throat, University of Graz, Graz, Austria

J. Meyer-Burg, M.D.
Dozent, Klinikum Steglitz, Free University, Berlin, West Germany

Leon Morgenstern, M.D., F.A.C.S.
Director, Division of Surgery, Cedars-Sinai Medical Center, Los Angeles; Clinical Professor, Department of Surgery, UCLA School of Medicine, Los Angeles, California

Gabriella Nemethy
Instructor, Department of Surgical Endoscopy, Cedars of Lebanon Hospital, Los Angeles, California

Valerie Olson, B.A., M.S.
Consulting Physicist, Los Angeles, California

Joel F. Panish, M.D., F.A.C.P.
Clinical Chief, Department of Gastroenterology, Cedars-Sinai Medical Center, Los Angeles; Associate Clinical Professor, Department of Medicine, UCLA School of Medicine, Los Angeles, California

Alan D. Perlmutter, M.D., F.A.C.S.
Professor of Urology, Department of Pediatric Urology, Wayne State University, School of Medicine, Children's Hospital of Michigan, Detroit, Michigan

Thomas G. Polanyi, Ph.D.
Gas Laser Research, American Optical Corporation, Framington, Massachusetts

Werner Prott, M.D.
Dozent, Department Ear, Nose, Throat, University of Wurzburg, Wurzburg, West Germany

John E. Rayl, M.D., F.A.C.S.
Associate Chief of Staff, Veterans Administration Hospital, Lake City, Florida; Associate Professor in Surgery, Department of Surgery, University of Florida, Gainesville, Florida

Jack Robertson, M.D., F.A.C.O.G.
Clinical Associate Professor, Department of Obstetrics and Gynecology, University of Southern California School of Medicine, Los Angeles, California

László Sáfrány, M.D.
Dozent, Chirurgische Universitätsklinik, Münster, West Germany

Erich Saling, M.D.
Professor of Obstetrics and Gynecology, Head of Department of Perinatal Medicine, Free University, Berlin, West Germany

Melvin Schapiro, M.D., F.A.C.P.
Chief of Gastroenterology, Valley Presbyterian Hospital, Encino, California; Assistant Clinical Professor of Medicine, UCLA School of Medicine, Los Angeles, California

J. Manny Shore, M.D., F.A.C.S.
Attending Surgeon, Cedars-Sinai Medical Center, Los Angeles, California

W. Rex Sittner, Ph.D.
Electro-Medical Systems, Inc., Denver, Colorado

Irving J. Slotnick, Ph.D., F.A.M.
Chief, Section of Microbiology; Cedars-Sinai Medical Center, Los Angeles; Lecturer, Department of Bacteriology, UCLA School of Medicine, Los Angeles, California

Robert Smith, M.D., F.A.C.S.

Assistant Professor of Surgery-Urology, UCLA School of Medicine; Chief, Department of Urology, Veterans Administration Wadsworth Hospital, Los Angeles, California

Henning Sorensen, M.D.

Director, Department of Ear, Nose and Throat, Municipal Hospital, Copenhagen, Professor, Department of Oto-Laryngology, University of Copenhagen, Copenhagen, Denmark

Patrick C. Steptoe, M.D., F.R.C.O.G.

Consultant in Gynecology, Oldham, Lancershire, Oldham, England

M. Stuart Strong, M.D., F.A.C.S.

Chief of Otolaryngology, University Hospital and Boston Veterans Administration Hospital; Professor of Otolaryngology, B.U.S.M., Boston, Massachusetts

Jacob Swierenga, M.D.

Chief, Department of Lung Diseases, St. Antonius Hospital, Utrecht, Holland

Bodo Terhorst, M.D.

Privat-Dozent, Department of Urology, Medical Faculty, Rhein.-Westf. Technical University, Aachen, West Germany

Duane E. Townsend, M.D., F.A.C.O.G.

Associate Professor and Chief, Section of Gynecologic Oncology, University of Southern California School of Medicine, Los Angeles, California

Paul H. Ward, M.D., F.A.C.S.

Professor and Chief, Division of Head and Neck Surgery, UCLA School of Medicine, Los Angeles, California

J. L. Williams, S.T.

Division of Urology, Department of Surgery, University of California at San Diego, School of Medicine, San Diego, California

R. Wittmoser, M.D.

Director, Institute of Neuro-vegetative Surgery, Dusseldorf, West Germany

Preface

At the turn of the century endoscopic procedures and doctors interested in performing those techniques of examination were relatively few in number. Urologists led, followed by thoracic, ear, nose, and throat surgeons, and a few internists. The main reason for such restricted participation was the lack of perfection in instrumentation that resulted in limited diagnostic accuracy and relatively high complication and risk. Outstanding skills were required to maneuver huge tubes through the various orifices, down into the organ. Many enthusiasts turned to other areas after their initial attempts were unsuccessful.

The invention of the rod-lens system, flexible fiber light transmission, and flexible fiber endoscopes opened new chapters of application in endoscopic diagnosis and treatment. Exceedingly good results consequently widened the narrow field of indications, and today it is estimated that 10 million endoscopic examinations are performed each year in the United States alone.

The sophistication of the instruments now in use has increased the need for explanation. The complexity of these tools and their application to other areas, such as electrosurgery, radiology, television, filming, ultrasound, and laser, have required the development of a comprehensive textbook where the investigator could obtain data without taking a course in physics or other disciplines. Steadily growing knowledge and depth in every subspecialty has made it otherwise impossible for the individual investigator to familiarize himself with every facet of examination and the new tools needed.

At one time Benedict's *Endoscopy* (1951) was "the manual" of the available American literature, but unfortunately it became outdated. In 1957 Turell introduced the *Symposium in Endoscopy* with a citation from Goethe: "What one knows one sees." I think we can modify that thought to "What one sees should become known and documented."

We are now at the beginning of an interesting epoch when the abundant technologic achievements need coordination to be employed successfully in medicine. Despite the wide acceptance of endoscopy today, it is interesting to note that basic research in this field is seldom reflected in literature. Research groups should be established to promote further advancement. *"Tempora mutantur et nos mutamur in illis"*: Times are changing and we are changing with the times. Kussmaul used a sword swallower to get his first open tube esophagoscope down into the gullet. At this stage it is a bedside procedure. Would Nitze not be shocked at the sight of a transurethral resection of an enlarged prostate on a color television monitor?

Over the past 20 years I have had the opportunity to become more familiar with basic parameters, to conduct research in many technical and clinical fields, and to initiate new developments. I realize that progress in medicine and technology is so rapid and continuous that some chapters in this volume are perhaps outdated even at this time. Others have been omitted because recent developments have cast uncertainty on their clinical value. We hope to issue supplements to this text periodically in an effort to keep pace with clinical and technologic advancements.

The enormity of the field to be covered has made it impossible for us to achieve the same depth in each area. However, we have attempted to present an overall picture of the current state of the art. Areas, such as adult urology, that have already been very well covered by monographs have been treated here only in those aspects that are new or of special interest.

I believe that this book will close the information gap that has been created by the rapid developments of this century. I do hope that it will be of value to the endoscopist, to guide him with data of performance and knowledge in his and adjacent areas; to the general practitioner, to help him become quickly acquainted with new procedures and their results; and to the fellow in training, for an overall view and references.

I would like to take this opportunity to express my gratitude to Professor M. R. Ewing, Chairman of the Department of Surgery at the University of Melbourne (Australia), for his continuous help and encouragement during my 12 years of activity in his department, when the first research section in endoscopy was established; to my former research assistant, Leslie Kont, who provided me with invaluable help over the years; and, to my present coauthors who made it possible for this book to cover authoritatively every area of endoscopy, as well as physics and optics.

I appreciate the generosity of my publisher, who supported this work and included so many color illustrations, and extend special thanks to Ms. Hilary Evans for her outstanding coordinating abilities and efforts in compiling this book. I would like to acknowledge the large number of photographic illustrations provided by my research assistant, Gino Hasler. I am indebted to my secretary, Mrs. A. Wasser, for her administrative help.

George Berci

Contents

COLORPLATES

Plate A

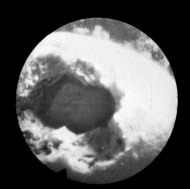

Chap. 12, Fig. 5

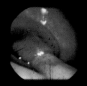   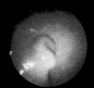   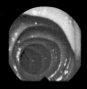

Chap. 21, Fig. 1   Chap. 21, Fig. 2   Chap. 21, Fig. 3

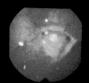   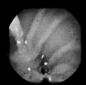   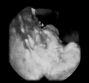

Chap. 22, Fig. 1   Chap. 22, Fig. 2   Chap. 22, Fig. 3

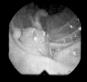   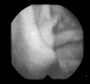

Chap. 22, Fig. 5   Chap. 22, Fig. 6   Chap. 22, Fig. 8

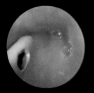   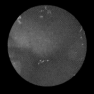   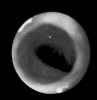

Chap. 24, Fig. 1   Chap. 24, Fig. 2   Chap. 24, Fig. 3

Plate B

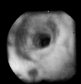
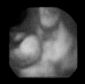
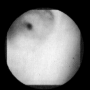

Chap. 26, Fig. 2   Chap. 26, Fig. 3   Chap. 26, Fig. 4

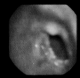
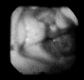
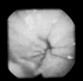

Chap. 26, Fig. 5   Chap. 26, Fig. 6   Chap. 26, Fig. 7

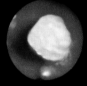
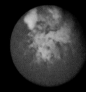
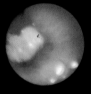

Chap. 28, Fig. 1   Chap. 28, Fig. 2   Chap. 28, Fig. 3

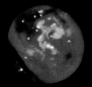
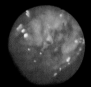
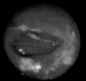

Chap. 28, Fig. 4   Chap. 28, Fig. 5   Chap. 28, Fig. 6

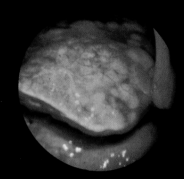
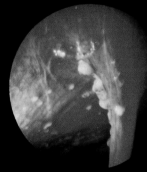
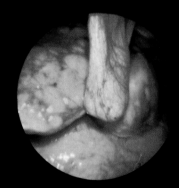

Chap. 29, Fig. 10   Chap. 29, Fig. 11   Chap. 29, Fig. 12

Chapter 30

FIG. 2. Macronodular cirrhosis in a patient with advanced chronic active hepatitis. Multiple regenerative nodules of varying sizes are present.

FIG. 3. Micronodular cirrhosis in a patient with alcoholic liver disease. The falciform ligament is deviated laterally by a typically enlarged left hepatic lobe. Multiple highlights are produced by reflections from micronodules.

FIG. 4. Right hepatic lobe with irregular surface changes associated with collagen deposition in a patient with advancing chronic active hepatitis.

FIG. 5. Greenish black discoloration of the right hepatic lobe and a Courvoisier gallbladder in a patient with neoplastic obstruction of the common duct.

FIG. 6. Enlarged, pale yellow hepatic lobes representing fatty metamorphosis in a patient with alcoholic liver disease. Fat accumulation in the falciform is also shown.

FIG. 7. Engorgement and apparent proliferation of vascular channels throughout the round and falciform ligaments are indicative of portal hypertension.

Chapter 31

FIG. 2. **A.** Gaucher's disease. Note the characteristic yellow, mottled appearance of the enlarged liver with rounded edges. **B.** Liver after biopsy has been taken. (A and B enlarged from one 16-mm movie frame.) **C.** Right inguinal hernia seen from the abdominal cavity through the laparoscope.

Plate C

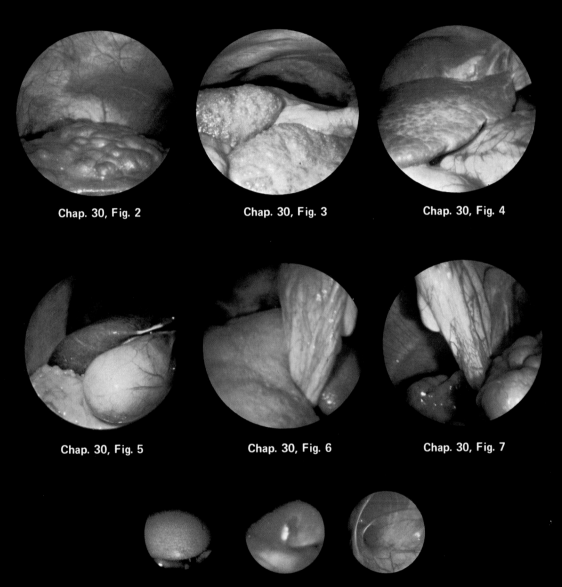

Chap. 30, Fig. 2   Chap. 30, Fig. 3   Chap. 30, Fig. 4

Chap. 30, Fig. 5   Chap. 30, Fig. 6   Chap. 30, Fig. 7

Chap. 31, Fig. 2A   Chap. 31, Fig. 2B   Chap. 31, Fig. 2C

Plate D

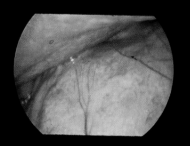 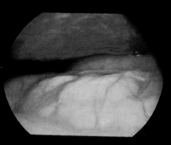 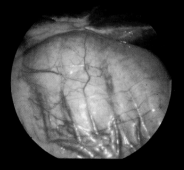

Chap. 33, Fig. 3   Chap. 33, Fig. 4   Chap. 33, Fig. 5

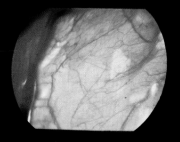 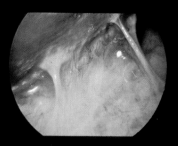

Chap. 33, Fig. 6   Chap. 33, Fig. 7

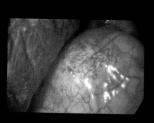 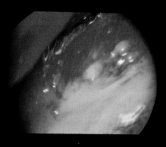

Chap. 33, Fig. 8   Chap. 33, Fig. 9

FIG. 3. Normal pancreas (body). The glandular structure of the organ is well seen; it is yellowish but is clearly distinguished from the discrete fatty structure present in the lesser omentum. The visible vessels are in the lesser omentum. The pink and red structure at the top of the picture is the undersurface of the left lobe of the liver.

FIG. 4. Normal pancreas (body). Slightly nodular, normal-appearing organ with discrete blood vessels in the lesser omentum. Top, Dark-appearing undersurface of the left lobe of the liver.

FIG. 5. Head of the normal pancreas. Part of the gallbladder and the right lobe of the liver are seen (at top left). The duodenal curve is evident below that. Within the duodenal curve the head of the pancreas is seen as a half moon covered by vessels belonging to the greater omentum.

FIG. 6. Resolving acute pancreatitis seen by supragastric pancreoscopy. Calcifications following fatty necrosis are discovered. The pancreas itself is markedly erythematous and under palpation seemed to have a hard consistency.

FIG. 7. Chronic pancreatitis seen by supragastric pancreoscopy. The lesser omentum is thickened and shows inflammatory adhesions to the undersurface of the left lobe of the liver. This area was definitely indurated when palpated with a probe.

FIG. 8. Pancreatic carcinoma in the region of the body. Distinct tumor protrusion as a whitish gray hard mass. The vessels are irregular. Carcinoma of the body of the pancreas was proved by biopsy.

FIG. 9. Extensive pancreatic carcinoma seen by supragastric pancreoscopy. Tumor protrusions manifest as whitish gray, partially cicatricial-like masses. Metastases appeared in the lower omentum.

Plate E

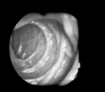 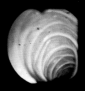 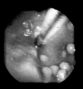

Chap. 34, Fig. 4A   Chap. 34, Fig. 4B   Chap. 34, Fig. 4C

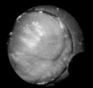 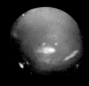

Chap. 35, Fig. 1   Chap. 35, Fig. 2

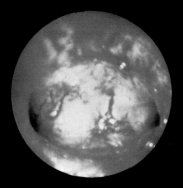 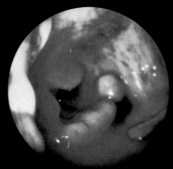 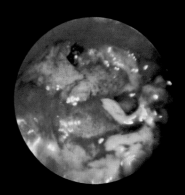

Chap. 38, Fig. 1   Chap. 38, Fig. 2   Chap. 38, Fig. 3

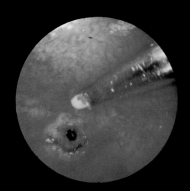 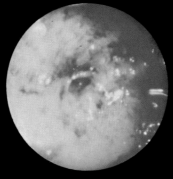 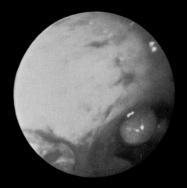

Chap. 38, Fig. 4   Chap. 38, Fig. 5   Chap. 38, Fig. 6

Plate F

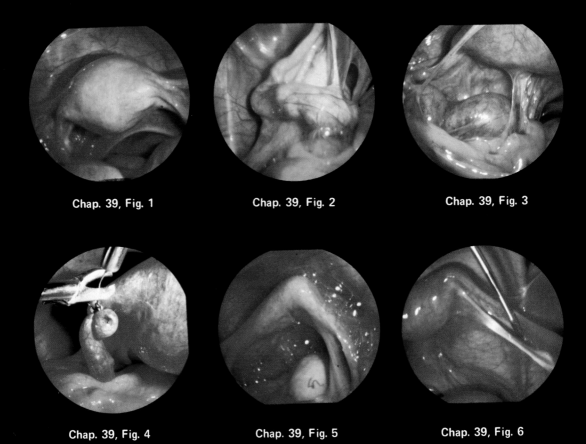

Chap. 39, Fig. 1

Chap. 39, Fig. 2

Chap. 39, Fig. 3

Chap. 39, Fig. 4

Chap. 39, Fig. 5

Chap. 39, Fig. 6

FIG. 1. Mobilization of the uterus, adnexae, and intestine allows the detection of pathology which otherwise would not be accessible by either palpation, pertubation, hysterosalpingography, pneumography.

FIG. 2. Laparoscopy is superior to all other diagnostic measures for evaluating primary and secondary sterility. It gives definite information about the anatomic situation of the adnexae. Laparoscopic findings can indicate the most advantageous operation for the sterility and give the best results for assessing the chances for fertility.

FIG. 3. Intact tubal pregnancy, seventh week of gestation. In suspected ectopic pregnancies considerably more intact tubal pregnancies are found by laparoscopy compared to palpation or puncture of the pouch of Douglas. The patient can be operated on at an early stage, before great blood loss produces a life-threatening situation.

FIG. 4. Laparoscopic tubal sterilization by ligation is a modification of the old Madlener technique. Large portions of the tubes remain intact, which is valuable for the increasing number of younger women asking for sterilization. There are good chances for recanalization if required.

FIG. 5. Extreme hypoplasia of the uterus. The ovaries and tubes are normal.

FIG. 6. Turner's syndrome. There is ovarian aplasia and extreme hypoplasia of both uterus and tubes. The anatomic situation should be corrected shortly after puberty in order to start suitable hormonal therapy. Laparascopy does not replace chromosomal analysis.

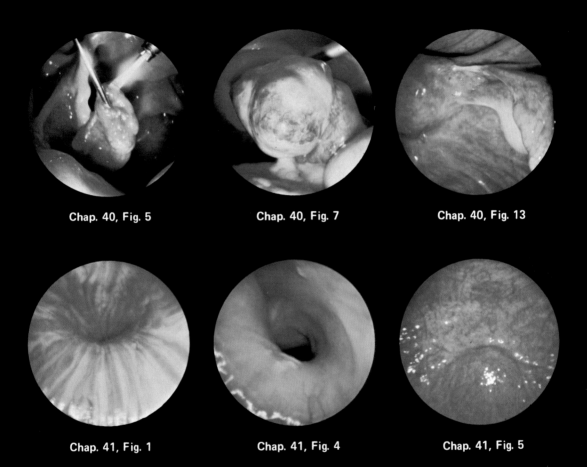

Chap. 40, Fig. 5   Chap. 40, Fig. 7   Chap. 40, Fig. 13

Chap. 41, Fig. 1   Chap. 41, Fig. 4   Chap. 41, Fig. 5

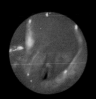

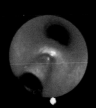

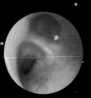

Chap. 42, Fig. 1   Chap. 42, Fig. 2   Chap. 42, Fig. 3

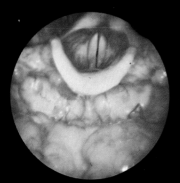

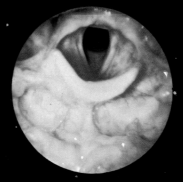

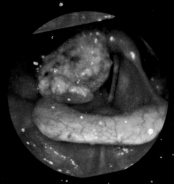

Chap. 45, Fig. 7A   Chap. 45, Fig. 7B   Chap. 45, Fig. 7C

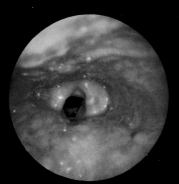

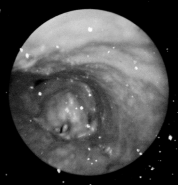

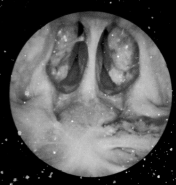

Chap. 45, Fig. 7D   Chap. 45, Fig. 7E   Chap. 45, Fig. 7F

Chapter 42

FIG. 1. View through the miniature bronchoscope used in newborns. Epiglottis (top) is lifted up with the beak of the sheath, and the vocal cords are well visualized.

FIG. 2. H-type TEF. Ureteral catheter introduced into opening of fistula. (Enlarged from a 16-mm movie frame.)

FIG. 3. Right upper lobe orifices as seen through the telescope.

Chapter 45

FIG. 7. **A** and **B.** Vallecula and base of tongue during phonation (**A**) and inspiration (**B**). **C.** Supraglottic lesion involving the aryepiglottic fold without involving the vocal cords. **D** and **E.** Appearance of the healed larynx following supraglottic laryngectomy during inspiration (**D**) and phonation (**E**). Note how the arytenoids pull inward and forward toward the base of the tongue, opening up pyriform sinuses and the hypopharynx superiorly in the figure. **F.** The Hopkins rod telescope allows thorough visualization of the entire nasopharynx, including the septum choanae, turbinates, eustachian cushions, vault area, and Rosenmüller's fossae. (**A** through **F**, from 16-mm movie frames.)

Chapter 48

FIG. 5. Normal right maxillary sinus. The ostium is relatively large.

FIG. 6. Chronic maxillary sinusitis. Edema, polypoid changes, and fibrosis alternate. Streaks of mucopus are scattered over the surface.

FIG. 8. Left sinus during a hay fever attack. Small edematous papules are present. The color is pale "peach-like."

FIG. 10. Typical mucosal cyst.

FIG. 11. Edema of the floor of the sinus caused by a periapical dental infection.

FIG. 12. Small benign tumor in the bottom of the right sinus. The mucosa covering the tumor is normal.

FIG. 15. Six weeks after a Caldwell-Luc operation. Newly formed thin mucosal membrane with easily distinguished blood vessels. Note the commencing fibrous scar formation in the central area.

Plate I

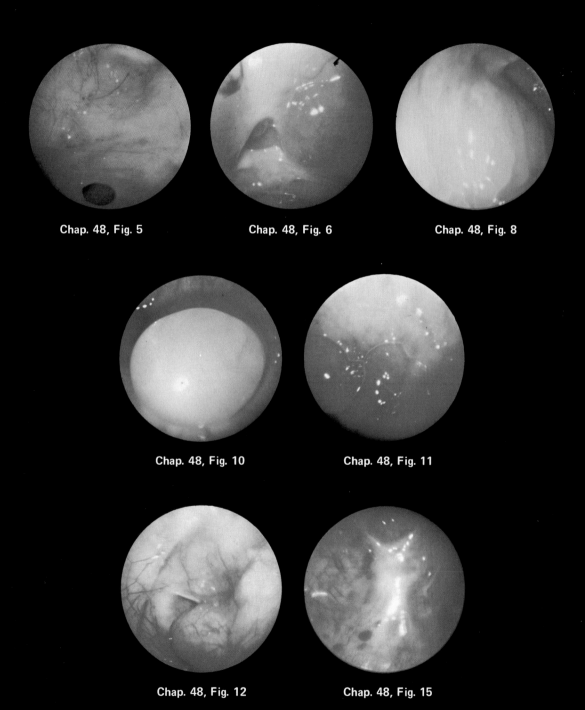

Chap. 48, Fig. 5   Chap. 48, Fig. 6   Chap. 48, Fig. 8

Chap. 48, Fig. 10   Chap. 48, Fig. 11

Chap. 48, Fig. 12   Chap. 48, Fig. 15

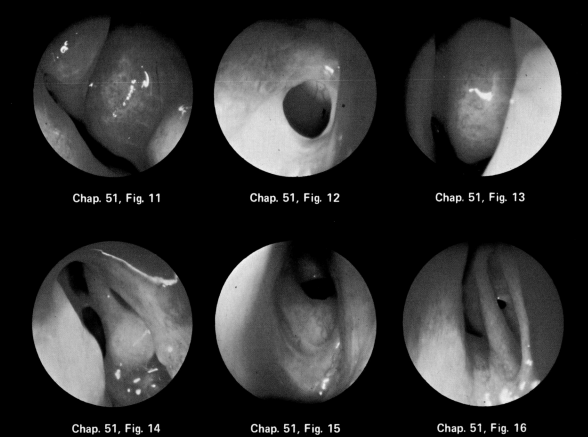

Chap. 51, Fig. 11   Chap. 51, Fig. 12   Chap. 51, Fig. 13

Chap. 51, Fig. 14   Chap. 51, Fig. 15   Chap. 51, Fig. 16

FIG. 11. The left inferior fontanelle is swollen to such an extent that the middle nasal meatus is obstructed.

FIG. 12. Left maxillary ostium at the end of the hiatus semilunaris with a view into the maxillary sinus.

FIG. 13. Left bulla ethmoidalis, which protrudes like a mushroom from the lateral nasal wall and reaches the conchal sinus.

FIG. 14. Left middle meatus: a small bulla ethmoidalis surrounded by openings of ethmoidal cells. Left, Middle nasal concha. Right, Processus uncinatus.

FIG. 15. Normal left sphenoid ostium.

FIG. 16. Left superior concha, concha suprema with operculum, and ostium in the superior nasal meatus.

Chapter 52

Plate K

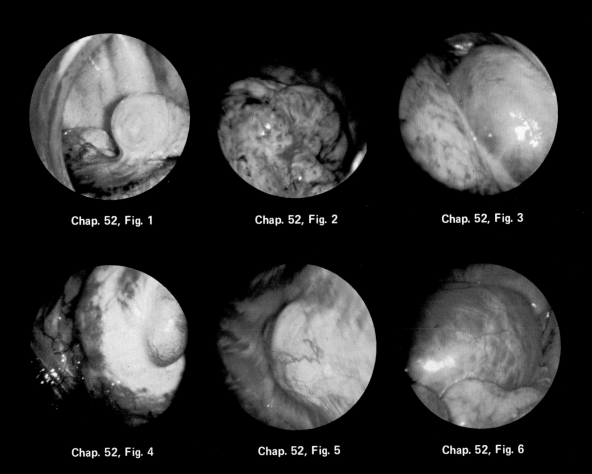

Chap. 52, Fig. 1

Chap. 52, Fig. 2

Chap. 52, Fig. 3

Chap. 52, Fig. 4

Chap. 52, Fig. 5

Chap. 52, Fig. 6

Plate L

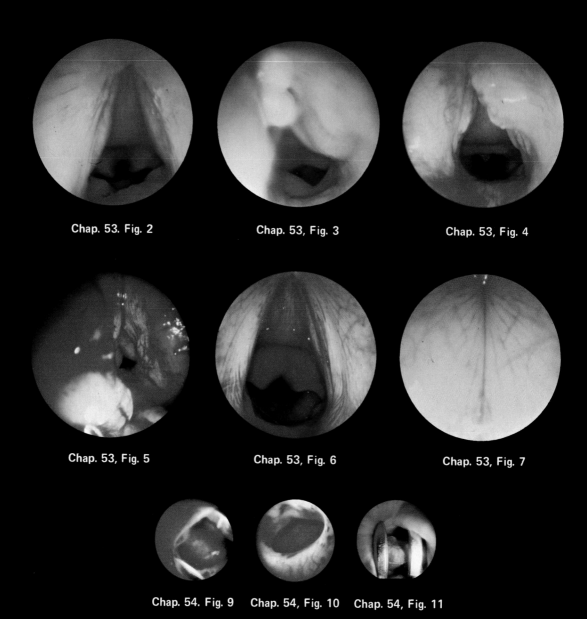

Chap. 53. Fig. 2   Chap. 53, Fig. 3   Chap. 53, Fig. 4

Chap. 53, Fig. 5   Chap. 53, Fig. 6   Chap. 53, Fig. 7

Chap. 54. Fig. 9   Chap. 54, Fig. 10   Chap. 54, Fig. 11

Chapter 55

FIG. 9. Midportion of the anterior cruciate ligament. The synovial vessels are well identified as the twisted fibers of the ligament.

FIG. 11. Hook inserted to test the lateral meniscus.

FIG. 14. Old rupture of the anterior cruciate ligament. Only a small remnant is seen. The posterior cruciate ligament is well identified.

FIG. 15. Partial rupture of posterior cruciate ligament. Loose part is caught with a hook.

FIG. 17. Arthroscopy 1 year after reconstruction of the anterior cruciate ligament with a strip from the patellar tendon. The patient's knee joint became unstable after a new accident. The main part of the transposed tendon is well vascularized and functioning. However, about one-third of the strip has ruptured at the upper end and is floating in the injected saline.

FIG. 18. A piece of nonresorbed suture material has torn loose in the femuropatellar joint. It was extracted by the biopsy instrument, and the synovitis disappeared.

Chapter 56

FIG. 2. Prostatic fossa (BPH).

FIG. 3. Ureteral orifice (normal).

FIG. 4. Bladder tumor.

Plate M

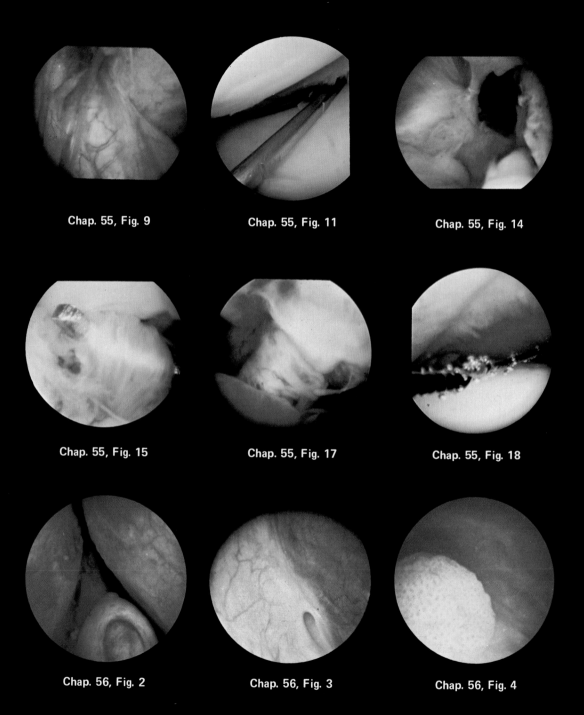

Chap. 55, Fig. 9

Chap. 55, Fig. 11

Chap. 55, Fig. 14

Chap. 55, Fig. 15

Chap. 55, Fig. 17

Chap. 55, Fig. 18

Chap. 56, Fig. 2

Chap. 56, Fig. 3

Chap. 56, Fig. 4

Plate N

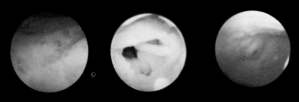

Chap. 57, Fig. 1   Chap. 56, Fig. 2A   Chap. 57, Fig. 2B

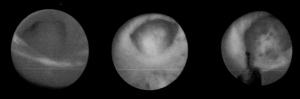

Chap. 57, Fig. 11A   Chap. 57, Fig. 11B   Chap. 57, Fig. 11C

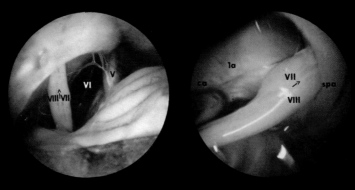

Chap. 58, Fig. 6   Chap. 58, Fig. 7

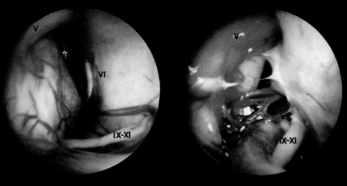

Chap. 58, Fig. 17   Chap. 58, Fig. 18

Chapter 57

FIG. 1. Cystoscopic view of severe chronic cystitis cystica in 9-year-old girl. Note multiple cystic lesions, almost confluent, covering the trigone and bladder base, and the increased vascularity of the mucosa. Some lesions are hemorrhagic.

FIG. 2. **A** and **B.** Cystoscopic views of cloacal malformation in a 13-year-old pubertal girl. Abdominoperineal anoplasty for imperforate anus had been performed in infancy. A congenital rectal fistula had entered the proximal urogenital sinus, which presented as single perineal opening. A double vagina and cervix are present. The urogenital anomaly has not yet been corrected. **A.** View of cloaca, with the objective lens of the telescope at 3 cm, within the upper urogenital sinus at the level of the hymen. Hymeneal tags are seen at the edges. Openings to the double vagina are slightly eccentric and separated by an oblique mucosal fold. Larger orifice is on the patient's right, near middle of the field. A stump of rectal fistula is just below the vaginal openings. The urethral opening is poorly seen and is represented by an upper transverse fissure near margin of the field. **B.** View into left hemivagina showing vertical septum (left), normal ballooning of upper vagina, and pubertal cervix at the apex. Similar, mirror-image findings were present on the right side.

FIG. 11. **A–C.** Urethral views of posterior urethral valves distal to the colliculus, mildly obstructing, in a 10-year-old male. A 70-mm lens and a miniature forward-oblique telescope was used. The objective lens was in the region of the external sphincter. **B.** Diaphragmatic appearance of the valve, with a fold radiating outward on each side. The colliculus bulges above the valve. **C.** Right leaflet of the valve is pulled downward by an electrode fashioned from a No. 3 uretheral catheter with a wire stylet bent into a tiny loop. Attachment of the valve commissure to the crista urethralis (inferior extension of the colliculus) is well demonstrated.

Chapter 58

FIG. 6. General view of a left cerebellopontine angle with the cranial nerves V, VI, VII, intermedius (↑), and VIII. On the left side is the porus of the inner ear canal; on the right side, the cerebellum.

FIG. 7. Right porus of the inner ear canal with the nerves VII, intermedius (↑), and VIII. ca, anterior inferior cerebellar artery; la, labyrinthine artery; spa, superior petrosal artery.

FIG. 17. Lower part of the right lateral pontine cistern with the nerves V, VI, IX, X, and XI. At the bottom is some residue of liquor.

FIG. 18. Similar situation to that in Fig. 17. As anatomic anomaly, a big inferior petrosal vein is seen instead of the inferior petrosal sinus.

Chapter 59

FIG. 16. Normal intraventricular foramen with choroid plexus overlaying it. No surgical or postmortem examination has yet revealed the site of the choroid artery and its affection in hypersecretory hydrocephalus; this is the first evidence of it. (Telescope: Lumina-Optik 180 degrees. Camera: Exakta-Varex II b. Film: Ektachrome EH 135, 160 ASA. Exposure: 1/30 second with electronic flash. Generator: type 5004, 800 watts/second.)

FIG. 17. A subependymal hemorrhage has been neither observed nor recorded in the literature until this endoscopic documentation, which clearly shows that petechial bleeding may arise on sudden surgical decompression of intracranial pressure of more than 300 to 500 mm H_2O. (Telescope: Lumina-Optik 180 degrees. Camera: Exakta-Varex II b. Film: Agfachrome 50 L, Professional. Exposure: 1/30 second with electronic flash. Generator: type 5004, 800 watts/second.)

FIG. 18. Even the extremely flexible catheter for the ventriculoatriostomy may perforate the wall or floor of the lateral ventricle in the course of a surgical implantation. Aimed endoscopy of the third ventricle can perform an endoscopic anastomosis between the third ventricle and the basal cisterna through a terminal lamina by its perforation, as is seen here. (Telescope: Lumina-Optik 120 degrees. Camera: Minox 144. Film: Agfacolor CN 14, 20 ASA. Exposure: 1/30 second with electronic flash. Generator: type 5004, 800 watts/second.)

FIG. 19. A ventricular catheter may be buried in the wall of the lateral ventricle if it has been in the cavity too long and placed close to the ventricular wall. Capillary vascularizations are shown here along the buried catheter 1 year later. (Telescope: Lumina-Optik 120 degrees. Camera: Minox 135. Film: Minochrome 13, 16 ASA. Exposure: 2 seconds at 150 watts with continuous illumination.)

FIG. 20. A major cerebral artery runs through the intraventricular cavity free from the wall, usually coated with fibrous membranes. Such secondary degeneration of the artery does not necessarily correspond with the severity of the accompanying inflammation. The fibrous coating can be scarce, as is seen here in a case of omniventricular hydrocephalus. The yellowish tint is due to the xanthochromic CSF. (Telescope: Lumina-Optik 90 degrees. Camera: Minox 144. Film: Minochrome 13, 16 ASA. Exposure: 1/30 second with electronic flash. Generator: type 5004, 800 watts/second.)

FIG. 21. A choroid cyst is not necessarily of therapeutic concern so long as it is not obstructing the CSF pathways or occupying the limited intracranial space, as it is here in a patient suffering from parkinsonism. (Telescope: Lumina-Optik 120 degrees. Camera: Minox 144. Film: Minochrome 13, 16 ASA. Exposure: 1/30 second with electronic flash. Generator: type 5004, 800 watts/second.)

Plate O

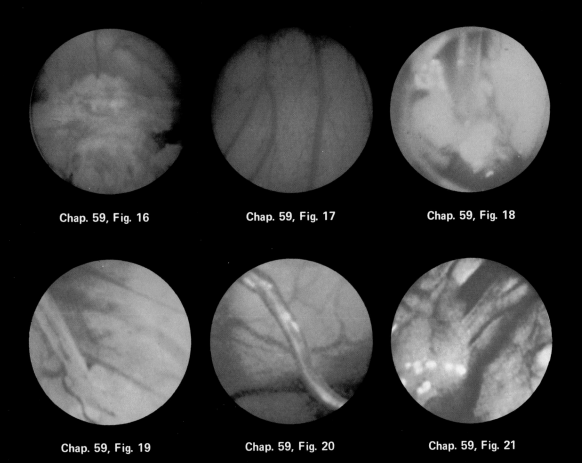

Chap. 59, Fig. 16   Chap. 59, Fig. 17   Chap. 59, Fig. 18

Chap. 59, Fig. 19   Chap. 59, Fig. 20   Chap. 59, Fig. 21

Foreword

Precision in diagnosis is an essential preliminary to rational treatment. The sooner we arrive at a diagnosis, the more promptly will proper treatment be instituted, and, in general, the sooner the appropriate therapy is offered, the greater is the expectation that illness will be cut short and disablement prevented.

But diagnosis is often a protracted and time-consuming exercise and involves the tedious and patient accumulation of evidence, much of which is of negative value only and may in the end leave us with an answer that is no more than tentative. This is especially so when the suspected pathology is at an inaccessible site. It is not so long since a physician might be heard emphasizing his own inadequacy in diagnosis by the reiterated complaint, "If only we could see what is going on inside." This has become the challenge for the endoscopist—and how very effectively he has met it within recent times!

His early incursions were, naturally enough, through the body orifices, and he has become increasingly venturesome in exploring the ultimate recesses of our hollow tubes. Success in this direction has encouraged him to make his own little openings to explore the more remote corners, and this again he has done with outstanding success.

As time has gone on, the terms of reference of the endoscopist have been drawn up with increasing insistence, and a lot is now expected of him. "Seeing is believing" we are told, but that is far from enough. He must also be able to take a biopsy and a photograph, or better still both together, and to do this with a minimum of discomfort and a minimum of risk.

In meeting these specifications with outstanding success, the endoscopist has recruited the help of the physicist and of the technologist, and there has been during the past decade or so a quite spectacular development of new equipment and of new techniques.

Surprisingly, we do not see better at the expense of wider caliber instruments, with the kind of manipulative risks and restraints that their use would necessarily impose. Quite the reverse, for the development of the Hopkins rod-lens system has made it possible to redefine the place of rigid endoscopy in the diagnosis of disease and to explore new areas even in the newborn or infant.

However it was not so long ago that the endoscopist seemed likely to be hobbled by the restraints imposed by the rigid telescopic system: These difficulties are left behind, now that the image faithfully follows the meanderings of the fiber bundle. Gone are most of his fumblings, for the darkness of even the remote recesses are now resolved by the intensity of illumination that allows him to make not only a still, but also a ciné record of what is to be seen there.

To round it off, there is the exciting potential of television, which allows us to pick up the image at the end of the telescope, to project it where we will or to store it for later analysis, if we feel so inclined.

These developments in endoscopy have been going ahead in many special areas and have involved the recruitment of persons with widely differing skills and interests. It is high time that there was a gathering together and a stock taking.

I was proud and delighted when Dr. George Berci was entrusted with the editorial direction of such a work. Much of his earlier essays in this field were done in my department, most of it on a shoestring. Like all effective initiators, he was never content. The climbing of one peak necessarily led him to make an assault on a new and higher pinnacle. He has been through the business literally from end to end, but has also enjoyed the great advantage of being able always to view the problem from the clinician's angle.

Since leaving this continent, he has continued to make a notable contribution in this field, and I can think of no one better to accept this role.

It is evident from the imposing list of contributors, that he has been able to enlist the help of the leaders in the exploitation of every new technique and we can be assured, not only of a comprehensive but also of an authoritative text.

The publishers are to be congratulated for embarking on such an ambitious task. I believe that this work is timely and that a warm reception for it is assured.

I am proud and happy to contribute the foreword and wish the publication every success.

Maurice R. Ewing, M.Sc., M.B., Ch.B., F.R.C.S. (Ed), F.R.C.S. (Eng), F.R.A.C.S., F.A.C.S. (Hon) M.D. (Hon)

History of Endoscopy

George Berci

It is always interesting to learn how pioneers conceived an idea, the motives behind and the circumstances under which a theoretical concept was transformed to a functioning unit. Sometimes we wonder at the simplicity of a particular solution, and we wonder why no one else thought about this obvious answer. Alternatively, we wonder at the ingeniousness of the inventor, to be able to complete this sophisticated design in perfect operating condition without the support of an armada of consulting specialists from various disciplines or access to data-compiling libraries linked by automatic typewriters, microfilm fiches, computers, or other technologic aids.

The discoveries at the turn of the century or even earlier needed much more individual depth because in the majority the originators were left on their own. Perhaps one great asset of those times was the availability of time for thinking. No deadlines for submission had to be met or preprogrammed phases completed. If the mood or spirit was not present, the sketch or draft was put aside, to be taken into consideration again when the inventor felt he could accomplish his task.

"Inter arma silent musae" is valid for the creative act not only during wartime but whenever pressure or tension is high and constant: the creative solution is difficult today because there is support only for the "earth-shaking" invention or preprogrammed revolutionary idea.

The word *endoscopy* was inherited from the Greek, meaning "to examine within." The term was adopted to mean the adding of a specific adjunct to a specific organ for the examination of the interior of the viscus. Later, the meaning was reinterpreted as the examination of the interior of a deep, hollow viscus that communicates with the outside through an orifice of the body by means of a channel through which an instrument can be introduced.

It is not the aim of this history to produce an accurate chronology of the various discoveries; that itself would require a decade of research in libraries. I would like simply to discuss some of the important events that in my opinion contributed to today's vast field and the large number of endoscopic areas. References are given to assist those who are interested in studying the development of endoscopy in great detail. There are likely to be inaccuracies and regrettable omissions in my presentation because of the limitation of time.

I am indebted to the librarians of the Medical Library of the Universities of Vienna and Bern for their enthusiastic support in providing me with microfilms from valuable reports dating back to the nineteenth century.

EARLY ENDOSCOPY

Bozzini (1806) recognized the need to build a direct light to facilitate the examination or operation of more deeply seated organs. He employed a wax candle enclosed in a shaped tin tube. He was also the first to use a mirror as a reflector.

Desormeaux (1867) described an open tube endoscope for the examination of the genitourinary passages. He was also the first to come up with the idea of using a small flame (light source) with a mixture of alcohol and turpentine. He found that if a lens is inserted, the beam can be condensed to a much narrower but brighter spot.

Everybody knows Kussmaul's story about the volunteer professional sword swallower employed as the first patient on whom he attempted to perform an esophagogastroscopy. Kussmaul (1870) was very fortunate that in his time written consent or malpractice insurance did not exist. He took the responsibility for experimenting and proved that a rigid tube can be passed through the mouth, pharynx, and esophagus into the stomach. With this historic step he saved thousands of human lives by giving other examiners the courage to pass tubes into the esophagus, remove foreign bodies, or diagnose diseases.

OPEN-TUBE ENDOSCOPY

With a four-inch-long and three-quarter-inch-wide tube and the use of candlelight, Bevan (1868) extracted foreign bodies and saw strictures in the esophagus. Waldenburg (1870) realized the imperfections of instrumentation and designed a longer instrument in which two tubes "telescoped" into each other for an easier introduction; if the upper portion was straight, the inner tube could be extended further distally. He used sunlight reflected by a mirror. The tubes were made of pure silver. He had no problems with insurance premiums or precautionary measures in storing pure silver.

Stoerk (1887) designed a right-angled open tube esophagoscope where one limb was used as a handle and the other (the one introduced) consisted of two tubes (similar to the Waldenburg model) that telescoped into each other. The advancing maneuver was adjusted from the handle. His esophagoscope was the first remote-control mechanism.

Rosenheim (1895) employed a flexible rubber extended obturator for safer introduction and easier finding of the lumen. He used metal tubes with an outside diameter of 11.5 to 13 mm. He already stated that an outside diameter of more than 13 to 14 mm could cause complications during introduction. The length of his scope was 40 to 50 cm. It is interesting to note that already the necessity of an articulated (flexible) esophagoscope had become apparant.

Kelling (1897) designed a flexible scope with a diameter of 13 mm, consisting of small inter-digiting metal rings on a handle that could be straightened or stiffened from the handle after introduction, according to necessity. It was covered by soft rubber, and the various shapes could be locked into position.

Killian (1898) became the father of bronchoscopy. He used local (cocaine) anesthesia and was the first to employ a head mirror; he turned later to the reflected light of an electric globe. For adults he used tubes 9 to 10 mm in outside diameter, and he used smaller tubes for children.

In the United States a few years later Jackson established a school for bronchoesophagology.

ENDOSCOPY WITH TELESCOPES

The real progress in endoscopy was the invention of an optical system to transmit the image from the deeply located organ to the surface.

Nitze (1879), with a optician, Beneche (Berlin), and an instrument maker, Leiter (Vienna), made the first cystoscope with an outside diameter of 7 mm and a deviating prism on the distal end. As illumination in his first model a platinum wire was overburned and cooled by separate water circulation. The idea of a glowing wire was taken from a dentist (Lesky, 1965).

A gastroscope with a similar optical and illumination system was also built in 1880 after the introduction of the cystoscope, but it did not gain acceptance. In 1887 Nitze introduced the first miniature electric globe (Mignon Lampchen), which was employed without separate cooling.

Mikulicz (1881) introduced the gastroscope, which was made also by Leiter. First, a number of small optical units were designed to couple them together with articulated joints. It was so complicated that a rigid telescope with an outside diameter of 13 mm was decided on instead. The first model still used a platinum wire with water cooling for illumination. The total length of the gastroscope was 650 mm; the working (distal) end, 180 mm long, was attached to the straight, rigid part in a 150-degree angulation. A cover plate protected the objective during the introduction and was withdrawn after the scope was in position. Mikulicz recommended that the patient fast and that the stomach be washed out with water before the procedure. He also distended the stomach with air insufflation and used the lateral position. The patient received morphine as premedication, and his gastroscopies were performed in narcosis (inhalation, general anesthesia). He described three physiologic movements of the stomach: peristalsis, respiration, and transmission of aorta pulsation.

Rosenheim (1896) employed cocaine and morphine as topical instead of general anesthesia. He used a three-tube technique for gastroscopy. The straight, rigid outer one of 12 mm was introduced first with a protective rubber fingertip guide at the working end. The other tube had a built-in glass window with a 16-v water-cooled electric lamp. If the outer sheath was introduced by means of a slot, the telescope, as a third tube, was advanced with a direction of view of 60 degrees. In 1896, he reported 20 successful gastroscopies and mentioned the existence of "blind spots." He built a second gastroscope with a total outside diameter of 10 mm where he eliminated the cooling (water) system of the lamp, but he could use the scope only for only 10 seconds of viewing time, with a five-second pause between illuminations, because of the heat production.

Rewidzoff (1897) was the first to introduce a rubber tube that was used in position as a guide for the rigid telescope.

Kuttner (1897) used a similar system in respect to the telescope but changed the direction of view to 90 degrees. He was first to mention the use of a distal prism that could be maneuvered by remote control or rotated 360 degrees to increase the small viewing field of the objective.

After his invention of the flexible esophagoscope (1897), Kelling invented a gastroscope (1898), the lower third of which was flexed to 45 degrees and the objective window of which could be rotated a full 360 degrees. He employed a miniature electric globe that was built together with the prism. The working tip could be bent in one plane to both sides in 135 degrees. This masterpiece of optics and mechanics was made by the instrument maker Albrecht before the turn of the century. He made a number of molds from cadaver stomachs before he designed the configuration of his instruments.

Reading the original paper, one is amazed at how many details and refinements were included by the pioneers of gastroscopy and the precision instrument makers.

Lange and Meltzing (1898) designed, used, and reported the first results with a gastro-camera in 15 patients. Exposure time was one-half to one second. The displayed size of the image on film was 4 mm. The rigid head was only 66 mm long and divided into three compartments: the film magazine (15 mm), the camera head (20 mm), and the electric globe (20 mm). A 5-mm-wide film strip 400 to 500 mm long, was pulled out from a roll of the film placed in the magazine after each exposure. Fifty exposures were made per examination. The rest of the camera consisted of a rubber tube in which the electric wires, air insufflation, and the pulling mechanism of the film was incorporated.

The blind gastro-camera, introduced 62 years later, had similar design features.

Schindler (1936) introduced the second phase of gastroscopy by designing with Wolf, an optical physicist and manufacturer in Berlin, a semiflexible instrument 77 cm long, incorporating a rubber finger at the working end. This scope was 12 mm in diameter at the flexible portion and 8.5 mm in the rigid part. An electric globe was used for illumination. A lateral view was provided. The system contained more than 48 lenses. The flexible portion consisted of a steel spiral containing lenses that were kept in place by a special spring covered by two rubber tubes through which air could be insufflated into the stomach. The upper or rigid segment was 34 cm long and contained the rest of the lenses, air channels, and electric connections, and the eyepiece (Benedict, 1951).

The third phase of gastroscopy was initiated by Hirchowitz et al (1958) with the introduction of flexible fiber glass gastroscopes.

The invention of Nitze opened a new era in endoscopy; it is interesting to note, however, that in certain applications (for instance, viewing of the esophagus and the bronchial tree) the telescope was employed only later.

In the United States Otis (1900) reported his first results with a new cystoscope consisting of a telescopic system and a distal electric globe. The instrument maker Reinhold Wappler, "a skillful electrician, acquired the art of grinding lenses and soon became far more adapted to optics than his instructors. . . . " (Otis, 1905). The instrument was smaller than the original Nitze scope and had a larger viewing field.

The telescopic system of the latest design is the invention of the Hopkin's rod-lens system (see Chapter 1), which provides transmitted images of much better quality than those of standard lenses.

DOCUMENTATION

The need for a permanent record was recognized since the invention of the endoscope and the introduction of a visual examination.

Musehold (1893) described an apparatus to photograph the larynx.

Nitze (1893) reported his experience with a photocystoscope and published a few years later the first atlas of the pathology of the urinary bladder based on a collection of pathology recorded with his photocystoscope.

Henning and Keilhack (1938) produced the first color pictures from a stomach using a rigid Schindler gastroscope.

Segal and Watson (1948) employed a semiflexible Schindler type gastroscope where the distal electric globe was overloaded to 80 v to obtain a shorter exposure time.

Lejeune (1936) reminded us of the necessity of motion picture records in assessing laryngeal lesions.

Holinger and Brubaker (1941) produced the first high-quality movie films from the bronchial tree, larynx, and esophagus. The system was later employed also for proctoscopic cinematography by Pessel et al (1942).

Fourestier (1952) and Montreynaud (1956) with their colleagues introduced a new type of illumination transmission (quartz rod) that facilitates the application of cinematography through normal-size adult endoscopes.

A number of pioneers with successful preliminary results have not been mentioned in this brief history, but a list of pertinent sources is given for further reference, and original contributions in specialized areas are mentioned in greater detail in the work that follows.

REFERENCES

History

Barnes RW: Encyclopedia of Urology. Berlin, Springer 1959 (in English)

Bevan L: The esophagoscope. Lancet 1:470, 1868

Bozzini PH: Lichtleiter, eine Erfindung zur Anschauung innerer Teile und Krankheiten. J Prak Heilk 24:107, 1806

Desormeaux AJ: Endoscope and its application to the diagnosis and treatment of affections of the genito-urinary passages. Chicago Med J, Chicago, 1867

Fourestier M, Gladu A, Vulmiere J: Étude technique de l'endoscope medical universel. Sem Med 56:13, 1956

Hacker V: Elektro-Endoskopie der Speiserohre im Allgemeinem und für die Entfernung von Fremdkorpern. Wien Klin Wochenschr 49:50, 1894

Henning N: Über ein neues Ösophagoskope. Klin Woehenschr 11:1673, 1932

Hirschowitz BI, Curtis LE, Peters CW, Pollard HM: Demonstration of a new gastroscope: "The Fiberscope." Gastroenterology 35:50, 1958

Ikeda S, Yanai N, Ishikawa S: Flexible bronchofiberscope. Keio J Med 17:1, 1968

Jackson C, Jackson CL: Bronchoscopy, Esophagoscopy and Gastroscopy, Philadelphia, Saunders, 1934

Jacobeus HC: Über die Möglichkeit die Zystoskopie bei Untersuchungen, seroser Hohlungen anzuwenden. Munch Med Wochenschr 57:2090, 1910

Kelling G: Endoscopie für Speiserohre und Magen. Munch Med Wochenschr 34:934, 1897

———: Gegliedertes, winklig streckbares Gastroskope mit rotierbarem Sehprisma. Munch Med Wochenschr 49:1556, 1898

Kuttner L: Über Gastroskopie: ein gegliedertes Gastroskope dass durch Rotation gestreckt werden kann. Klin Wochenschr 43:939, 1897

Killian G: Über direkte Bronchoskopie. Munch Med Wochenschr 27:845, 1898

Kussmaul J: Über Magenspiegelung. Verh Naturforschenden Ges Freiburg 5:112, 1870

Lamm H: Biegsame Optische Geräte. Z Instr 50:579, 1930

Lowe L: Beiträge zur Esophagoskopie. Dtsch Med Wochenschr 12:271, 1893

McCarthy JF: A new system for observation and operation in the urinary bladder. J Urol 57:575, 1947

Mikulicz J: Über Gastroskopie und Ösophagoskopie. Wien Med Presse 45:1405, 1881

Nesbit RM: An improved resectoscope in sizes Fr. 24–26. J Urol 63:191, 1950

Nitze M: Beobachtungs and Untersuchungsmethode für Harnrohre Harnblase und Rectum. Wien Med Wochenschr 24:651, 1879 (Platin)

———: Verähderungen an meinen elektro-endoskopischen Instrumenten. Ill Monat Aerztl Polytechnik 9:60, 1887

Otis WK: Concerning the new electrocystoscope. NY Med J 81:625, 1905

Rewidzoff: Zur Technik der Gastroskopie: Modifikation der Rosenheimsche Methode. Klin Wochenschr 42:893, 1897

Rosenheim T: Über Esophagoskopie. Klin Wochenschr 12:247, 1895

———: Über Gastroskopie. Klin Wochenschr 13:275, 1896

———: Über Gastroskope. Klin Wochenschr 15:325, 1896

Schindler R: Gastroscope with a flexible gastroscope Am J Dig Dis Nutr 2:656, 1936

Stoerk P: Ein neues Ösophagoskope. Wien Med Wochenschr 34:1117, 1887

Voltolini R: Report at a meeting of the Society of Scientific Medicine, Berlin, 2 July 1860. Dtsch Klinik 12:393, 1860

Waldenburg L: Esophagoskopie Klin Wochenschr 47:578, 1870

Photography-Documentation

Barrett B: Gastroscopic color photography. Bull Gastroint Endoscopy 8:13, 1961

Colcher H: Gastrophotography and cinematography. Prog Gastroent 1:97, 1968

Fourestier M, Gladu A, Vulmiere J: Perfectionnements à l'endoscopie médicale. Presse Médicale 60:1292, 1952

Henning N, Keilhack H: Farbenphotography der Magenhohle. Dtsch Med Wochenschr 64:1328, 1938

Holinger P, Brubaker PH: The larynx, bronchi and esophagus in Kodachrome. J Biol Photogr Assoc 10:83, 1941

Hull WM: Endoscopic Photography. J Biol Photogr Assoc 9:59, 1940

Jaupitre M: La cystocinématographie en couleur. Comm Congrès Fr Urol, October:128, 1955

Lange F, Meltzing: Die photography des Mageninnern. Munch Med Wochenschr 50:1585, 1898

LeJeune FE: Motion picture study of laryngeal lesions. Surg Gynecol Obstet 62:492, 1936

Maassen W: Entwicklungen auf dem Gebiete der Farbfotographie endobronchiale. Tuberkulosearzt 6:352, 1963

McCrea LE: Experimental studies in intravesical photography. J Urol 47:148, 1942

Montreynaud DJM, Edwards RJ, Gladu, AJ: A new method of bronchoscopy with cinematography and photography. Laryngoscope 66:637, 1956

Musehold A: Ein neuer Apparat zur Fotographie des Kehlkopfes. Dtsch Med Wochenschr 12:274, 1893

Nelson RS: Routine gastroscopic photography. Gastroenterology 30:661, 1956

Nitze M: Zur Photographie der menschlichen Harnblase. Med Wochenschr 2:744, 1893

Pessel JF, Garner JM, Nesselrod JF: Proctoscopic cinematography. Am J Dig Dis 9:140, 1942

Pickert H: Gastroscopic color photography. Progr Gastroenterol 2:377, 1957

Reuter HJ: Urologische Photo-, Film- und Fernsehenendoskopie. Urologe 2:187, 1963

Segal HL, Watson JS: Color photography through the flexible gastroscope. Gastroenterology 10:575, 1948

Trethowan JD: Experiments in endoscopic photography. J Photogr Sci 4:145, 1956

Monographs

Barnes RW: Encyclopedia of Urology. Berlin, Springer, 1959

Benedict EB: Endoscopy. Baltimore, Williams and Wilkins, 1951

Ikeda S: Atlas of Flexible Bronchofiberscopy. Baltimore, University Park Press, 1974

Montreynaud DJM, Bruneau Y, Jomain J: Traité pratique de photographie et de cinématographie medicales. Paris, Montel, 1960

Turell R: Endoscopy. Surg Clin North Am, Nationwide Number. Philadelphia, Saunders, October 1957

Books

Berry LH: Gastrointestinal Pan-Endoscopy. Springfield, Thomas, 1974

Engel CE: Photography for the Scientist. London–New York, Academic Press, 1968

Lesky E: Die wiener medizinische Schule im 19 Jahrhundert. Vienna, Bolau, 1965

Metler CC, Metler FA: History of Medicine. Toronto, Blakiston, 1947

Motokawa K: Physiology of Color and Pattern Vision. Berlin, Springer, 1970

Wittman I: Peritoneoscopy, vol 1 and 2. Budapest, Academic Press, 1966

ENDOSCOPY

Part I
GENERAL
PRINCIPLES

1

Optical Principles of the Endoscope

Harold H. Hopkins

The function of an endoscope is to render the interior of a cavity observable to the endoscopist exactly as if it were being viewed directly. This is illustrated in Figure 1, where the image of the object O is formed at O' and seen by an observer E_2, when using a right-angle viewing endoscope. When observed through the endoscope the image at O' must be identical, apart from a possible change of scale, with the view of an observer at E_1 looking directly at the object.

This necessary identity between the object when observed directly and the view obtained endoscopically requires not only that the image seen from E_2 be of a desired size and at such distance from E_2 that the observer may focus sharply on it, but also that the image be seen correctly in terms of top and bottom, as well as left and right, as illustrated by the letter F used in Figure 1. These aspects of the endoscope call for an understanding of the way images are formed and relayed by successive lenses, what is meant by visual magnification, and the geometric relations between an object and its image both as formed by a lens system and when a mirror or reflecting prism is used.

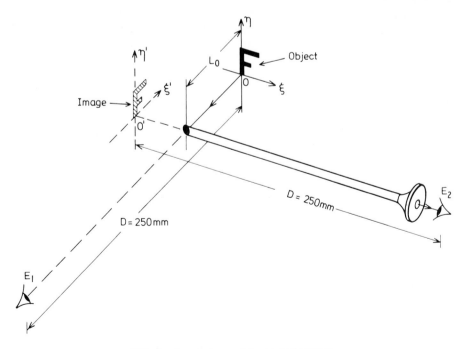

FIG. 1. Image formed by an endoscope.

THE EYE: VISUAL MAGNIFICATION

The action of the eye may be understood from the diagrams in Figure 2. Rays diverging from an object point *O,* as in the upper diagram, are brought to focus at *O'* on the retina. The larger part of the focusing occurs at the anterior surface of the cornea. The lens is responsible for accommodation, by which means the normal eye may be made to focus sharply for any distance between infinity and the near point, the latter being about 250 mm from the eye.

To find the size of the retinal image of an object of height *(OQ)* = η, as in the lower diagram of Figure 2, that ray from *Q* which passes through the front focal point *E* of the eye is considered. This ray is parallel to the axis in the eye itself and shows the size of the reduced and inverted image that is formed on the retina. The size of the retinal image depends only on the angle β, which the object subtends at *E,* and not simply on the linear size of the object. The angle β becomes greater as the distance *D* becomes smaller:

$$\beta = \frac{\eta}{D} \qquad (1)$$

The maximum detail is seen by making *D* = 250 mm, since at closer distances the advantage of the increased size of retinal image is offset by blurring of detail because of the inability of the eye to focus sharply for *D* less than this distance.

It is for the above reason that a conventional

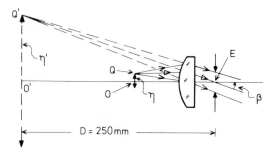

FIG. 3.   Action of a simple magnifier.

definition is adopted for the magnification of a visual instrument such as a simple magnifier, an eyepiece, or a complete endoscope. Figure 3 shows the effect of a simple magnifier. The object of height *(OQ)* = η above the axis is considered to be placed at such a distance from the lens that rays from *Q,* after being refracted to pass into the pupil of the observer's eye at *E,* appear to diverge from point *Q'* such that the image plane *Q'O'* is at a distance *D* = 250 mm from *E.* The visual magnification is then conventionally defined to be the linear magnification for this position of the image:

$$M = \frac{\eta'}{\eta} \qquad (2)$$

where η = *(O'Q')* is the image height.

In practice different observers focus the magnifier to form the image at different distances from *E.* The linear magnification between object and image is then different from Eq. (2), but the angular size of the image *(β)* is not appreciably changed. The visual magnifying effect is thus always represented by the value of *M* given by Eq. (2) and using the convention described.

As may be seen from Eq. (2) the visual magnification gives the ratio of the size of retinal image formed with the magnifier focused for *D* = 250 mm to the size of the retinal image formed when the same object is observed directly from a distance of 250 mm. The same definition is adopted for the magnification of an eyepiece or for a complete endoscope.

The smallest detail the eye can resolve depends on the pupil diameter. The optimum resolution occurs when the pupil is about 3 mm in diameter. For this pupil diameter and under the best conditions the resolution limit occurs for detail subtending an angle β = 1 minute of

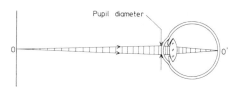

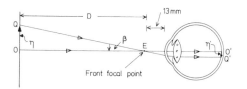

FIG. 2.   Image formation by the eye.

arc at the eye. This corresponds to a 0.075-mm detail at a distance (D) of 250 mm. A useful rule of thumb is thus to take the limit of resolution as 0.10 mm at 250 mm. This is also the limit of smallness of the size of the detail for an endoscope having a visual magnification equal to unity. For an endoscope of linear magnification (M) the limit of resolution, measured at the object, is given by

$$\eta = \left(\frac{0.10}{M} \right) \text{ mm} \qquad (3)$$

The linear magnification (M) of an endoscope is inversely proportional to the object distance. The smallest size of detail that can be resolved when measured at the object is therefore smaller in direct proportion to the closeness of the object to the distal end of the endoscope.

BASIC OPTICS OF THE ENDOSCOPE

The essential optical components of an endoscope are seen in Figure 4; a forward-viewing system is shown. The front combination of lenses constitutes the *objective*, which at I produces an inverted image of the object O_oQ_o. The central rays of the pencils from any point such as Q_o are usually arranged to be parallel to the optical axis in the image space. A *relay system*, comprising a *field lens* and objective, then forms an image of I at I_1 with unit magnification. In most endoscopes there would be several unit-magnification relay systems of this kind in succession, which would produce successive images $I_1, I_2, \ldots$ of the image I. The final of these images, which would be I_1 for the case shown in Figure 4, is then viewed with an *eyepiece*, which produces a magnified virtual image of O_oQ_o at $O'_oQ'_o$. This image is seen by the observer's eye when placed at the *exit pupil* (E').

If the endoscope is set at a distance L_o from the object O_oQ_o, such that the final image $O'_oQ'_o$ is formed at a distance (D) of 250 mm to the left of E', the overall visual magnification is, by definition, equal to the linear magnification between O_oQ_o and $O'_oQ'_o$. This magnification is given by the product of the linear magnification of the objective (m_o) and the visual magnification (m_c) of the eyepiece, since each relay stage is designed to have unit magnification, i.e.,

$$M_o = m_o m_c \qquad (4)$$

gives the (visual) magnification of the endoscope *for the object distance L_o.*

If the object is now moved to a greater distance (L) from the endoscope, the final image $O'_oQ'_o$ is formed further from E' but may still be focused by a change in accommodation of the observer's eye. The object point shown as Q is on the central ray through Q_o, and so the image of Q is at a point on the emergent central ray Q'_oE', which ray enters the observer's eye under the angle β'. The object height $\eta = OQ$ thus still subtends the same angle as the object $\eta_o = (O_oQ_o)$ at the distal end of the endoscope, and its image also still subtends the same angle (β') to the observer's eye. The retinal image of the object OQ is thus the same size as that of the original object O_oQ_o. Since the larger object size $\eta = (OQ)$ gives the same size of retinal image, the linear magnification for the object distance L is smaller and is given by

$$M = \left(\frac{\eta_o}{\eta} \right) M_o = \left(\frac{L_o}{L} \right) M_o \qquad (5)$$

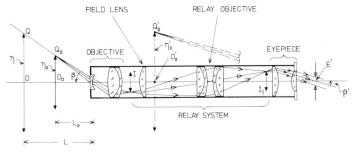

FIG. 4. Image formation by an endoscope.

The linear magnification is thus inversely proportional to the object distance.

There are several useful comments to be made in relation to the above considerations. First, the specification of an endoscope should include a statement of the magnification obtained for a stated object distance. This facilitates comparisons between different instruments, which is important because the higher the magnification the smaller is the finest object detail that can be resolved. Second, taking L_o as the object distance for which the image distance $D' = (E'O'_o) = 250$ mm gives the *near point* of the endoscope for an emmetropic eye, since any object closer to the endoscope forms its image nearer to E', i.e., at less than the shortest distance on which the observer can focus. The linear magnification between the object and the film plane of an endoscopic camera also varies inversely with the distance L of the object (*vide infra*).

Before leaving the question of magnification of an endoscope, it is desirable to consider the question of inverted and erect images. In Figure 4 the objective produces an inverted image of the object, as may been seen from the paths of the rays. The magnification of the objective is thus of negative sign. The relay system also has a negative magnification, so that the final image presented to the eyepiece is an erect one. The eyepiece has a positive magnification, and so the final image seen by the observer is also an erect one. Thus to correct for the inversion produced by the objective, it is necessary in a system such as that shown in Figure 4 to have an odd number of relay stages. An even number of relay stages would produce an inverted image. There are additional considerations in cases such as right-angle or fore-oblique viewing systems (*vide infra*).

If there were no field lens immediately following the image plane in Figure 4, the pencil of rays originating at Q_o would continue after the image plane of the objective and strike the wall of the endoscope tube. Only the points in the centre part of the image would then have all their rays transmitted, and the field of view would be severely limited. The action of the field lens is to deviate these rays so that the central ray of the pencil passes centrally through the relay objective. It is for this reason that each relay stage consists of a field lens and a relay objective. The ray paths shown leaving the final image, which is presented to the

eyepiece, would similarly also simply continue to hit the inner wall of the endoscope tube were there not a field lens as the first element of the eyepiece. A comparison of the eyepiece in Figure 4 with the simple magnifier of Figure 3 shows that this eyepiece is just a field lens plus a simple magnifier.

IMAGE INVERSIONS: USE OF REFLECTING PRISMS IN ENDOSCOPES

To obtain a right-angle or fore-oblique direction of view, the optical axis of the endoscope must be reflected at the distal end of the instrument. It is customary to use reflecting prisms for this purpose, as illustrated in Figure 5, where the reflecting prism systems are incorporated as part of the objective. The reason for using reflecting prisms instead of simple mirrors is primarily the ease of mounting, although there are other advantages: the protection of the reflecting surface; in some cases the use of total internal reflection; and the fact that after refraction at the entry face of a prism all rays are less inclined to the optical axis and thereby reduce the space occupied by the reflecting element. The function of the erecting prism in the system shown in Figure 5A is explained later.

The image produced by an endoscope must be "right side up" and must also be correct for left and right sides. Achieving this requires an un-

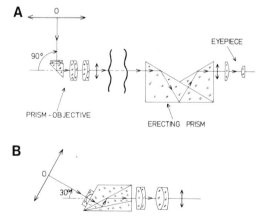

FIG. 5. Prism objectives giving different viewing directions. **A.** Ninety degrees. **B.** Thirty degrees.

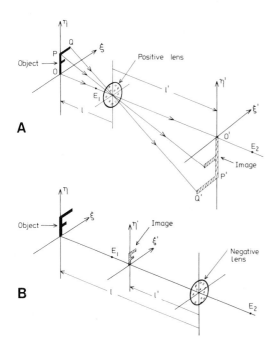

A

B

FIG. 6. Inverted (**A**) and erect (**B**) images produced by lenses.

derstanding of the different natures of the image inversions produced by lenses and mirrors.

Figure 6A shows the inverted image produced when the object and image are on opposite sides of the lens, which is usually the case with a positive lens. Apart from an enlargement of scale, the image A is simply the object F turned through an angle of 180 degrees around the optical axis. This is a lens inversion, where there is top-to-bottom as well as left-to-right inversion. If the object and image distances l and l' are measured from the lens as origin of coordinates, l is negative and l' is positive for the case shown. The magnification is given by

$$M = \frac{l'}{l} \tag{6}$$

and is of negative sign when the image is inverted. If this image is reimaged using a second system of negative magnification, the second image is correct top-to-bottom as well as left-to-right. Thus a total even number of such stages gives a correct image, while an odd number gives an inverted image.

The case shown in Figure 6B is when object and image are on the same side of the lens. The

image is then an erect image; and since l and l' are of the same sign, the magnification is of positive sign. This is more often the case with a negative lens. In the objective of Figure 4, for example, the negative lens produces an erect image, and the positive lens an inverted image.

There is an essential difference between the inversion produced by a lens and that produced by reflection in a mirror. For the lens there is an inversion around both the horizontal and vertical axes. By contrast, with the mirror there is an inversion around only one axis. In Figure 7 the observer at E_1 looks directly at the object and sees the letter F. The observer at E_2 sees the object by reflection in a plane mirror; and, as the rays show, the image seen is F, i.e., the object is inverted about the vertical axis only. The important fact is that a mirror inversion can be corrected only by introducing a second, compensating mirror inversion. After an even number of reflections the image is left with no mirror inversion, whereas any odd number of reflections produces such inversion.

Thus an endoscope must have an even number of reflections in order to produce a correct image of the object. The case of Figure 5A illustrates this. The objective has a single reflection, and the image produced by the prism objective has a mirror inversion. This image is relayed down the endoscope tube always as a mirror image, the mirror inversion being corrected by the K prism, which is here used as an inverting prism. Used as shown, the K prism merely corrects the mirror inversion of the first prism. This is the arrangement employed if there are an odd number of relay

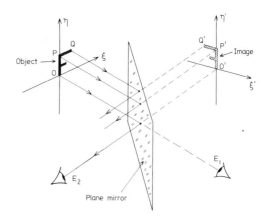

FIG. 7. Mirror inversion produced on reflection.

stages. With an even number of relay stages the K prism would be turned through an angle of 90 degrees around the optical axis, when the two mirror inversions (i.e., around a horizontal axis and then a vertical axis) are equivalent to a lens inversion.

The mirror inversion produced by a simple reflecting prism is illustrated in Figure 8A, where the observer E' sees a mirror inversion of the object as observed directly from E. Sometimes the plane hypotenusal reflecting face is replaced by a "roof," giving the Amici roof prism (Fig. 8B). The image now seen is equivalent to a lens inversion. The angle of the "roof" must be exactly 90 degrees, and the roof edge must be made very sharp. With the small size of prisms employed in endoscopes, which may be only approximately 2 mm square, this is extremely difficult to achieve, and the use of an erecting prism is recommended.

The action of the K prism is demonstrated in Figure 9. The emergent axis is a continuation of the incident axis; and since there are three reflections—at P_1, P_2, and P_3 respectively—there is a mirror inversion of any object seen through it.

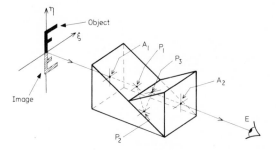

FIG. 9. Mirror inversion produced by a K prism.

ILLUMINATION SYSTEMS

Prior to the 1960s a body cavity being observed endoscopically was illuminated by means of a small tungsten filament lamp located at the distal end of the instrument. This gave a relatively low level of illumination, as well as a low colour temperature. The heat produced by such a lamp was a further disadvantage. This situation has been radically changed by the introduction of fibreoptics, where an external high-intensity light source is used, the light being conducted to the endoscope by means of a flexible light guide (Fig. 10). This guide then connects to a bundle of fibres in the endoscope (Fig. 11).

The fibreoptic light cable, as indicated in Figure 10(a), consists of a large number of glass fibres formed into a bundle, typically 4 to 5 mm in diameter. An "incoherent" bundle is used, the individual fibres having no particular order. For conveying an optical image, on the other hand, the fibre bundle must be ordered (i.e., each fibre occupies the same relative position at the exit face of the bundle as at the entry face); this is known as a "coherent bundle." With an incoherent bundle the transmitted image would be completely "scrambled" and unrecognisable.

No ordering is necessary for a light guide, which is used merely to transmit illumination. This is fortunate in that the cost of a coherent bundle can be many times that of an incoherent bundle. Each fibre of the light guide has a diameter of 25 μm or greater and consists of an inner core of high-refractive-index glass and a cladding of low-index glass. The thickness of the cladding is typically 1 μm. With any given refractive indices for the core and cladding, all the rays of light falling on the core of each fibre up to a certain angle (α) are trapped in the

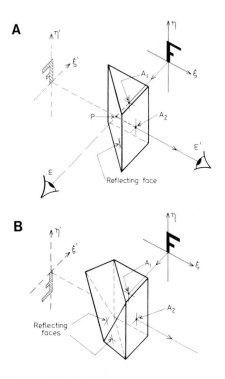

FIG. 8. Images formed by prisms. **A.** Simple reflecting prism. **B.** Amici roof prism.

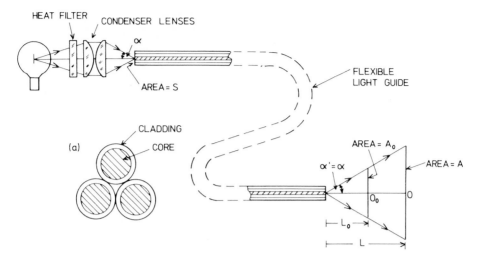

FIG. 10. Light source and fibreoptic light guide.

fibre by total internal reflection; this light travels along the core of the fibre by repeated reflections at the interface between the core and the cladding. There can be in excess of 15,000 reflections per metre in a light guide. It is consequently essential to ensure that the light is totally reflected, and it is for this reason that clad fibres are employed. With an unclad fibre, damage or contamination of the surface can impair the reflection and thereby drastically reduce the transmittance. With a clad fibre the total reflection takes place at the interface between the core and the cladding and is thus unaffected by minor imperfections of the outer surface of the cladding.

The light source is imaged on the entry face of the fibre bundle (Fig. 10). Because of aberrations in the condenser lenses it is desirable to arrange for the magnification to be such that the image of the light source is slightly greater than the entry face of the fibre bundle. The aperture angle of the light falling on the bun-

dle, shown as α in Figure 10, should also be not less than the maximum angle of aperture transmitted by the fibres of the given bundle. For a 2-metre flexible light guide, low-aperture fibres are usually employed, for which the angle α may be typically between 30 and 40 degrees.

A short length at each end of a light guide has the fibres bonded together. An epoxy resin is often used for this purpose, but for good heat resistance the two ends of the bundles are made into a solid matrix of glass by fusion of the claddings. This is necessary with very-high-intensity lamps because the heat filter does not remove all the heat. An alternative to a conventional heat filter is the cold mirror system (Fig. 12). Such a mirror has a reflecting surface that uses multilayer thin films having the resultant property of high reflection for the visible region of the spectrum and very low reflection for the infrared region. Although this is more efficient than a conventional heat

FIG. 11. Coupling of a light guide to an endoscope.

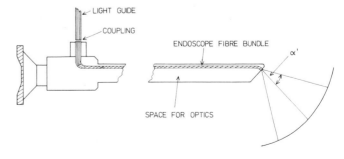

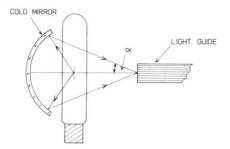

FIG. 12. Use of a dichroic (cold) mirror.

filter, the heat reflected may still be sufficient to damage the entry face of the light guide and/or to make the distal end of the bundle too hot for safety. As with the lens condenser system, it is necessary for the image of the source to cover the fibre bundle and for the angle α to be not less than the maximum aperture that is accepted by the fibres of the bundle.

With the size of the source image and the angle of aperture satisfying the above conditions, the only other factors affecting the level of the resulting illumination are (1) light losses by reflection at the air-glass surfaces of the heat filter, the condenser lenses, and the fibre end-faces; (2) the fact that only the cores of the fibres conduct light, any light falling on the cladding or interspaces not being trapped and so lost at the outer sheath of the bundle; and (3) absorption of light in the glass of the core of each fibre. The reflection losses in (1) amount to about 30 percent for six air-glass surfaces. These losses can be reduced to around 10 percent by ordinary blooming of the surfaces, and to a negligible amount by the use of multilayer antireflection coatings. It is an important factor—for both still and ciné colour photography—that all such reflection losses be kept to a minimum. The reduced transmission described in (2) depends on the "core packing fraction," i.e., the ratio of the area of cross section of the bundle that is occupied by the cores to the total area. This fraction is typically 70 percent and cannot be reduced. The reflection losses at the entry- and exit-faces of the fibre cores may also be as high as 6 percent for each surface. Because of technical difficulties it is not customary to employ antireflection coatings on the ends of the fibre bundles, and so these losses up to now have been accepted.

A more important aspect of light loss in a light guide is absorption in the glass of the

fibres. Taking into account the core packing fraction, the two reflection losses, and the absorption in the glass, for a good-quality 2-metre light guide the overall transmission is typically about 40 percent for white light. It is of course striking that such high transmission values can be obtained; but despite this there is a serious disadvantage in that the absorption losses are much greater in the blue end of the spectrum than in the yellow, green, and red parts of the spectrum. For a 1-metre fibre light guide, the transmission for the blue end of the spectrum is typically only 50 percent as great as the transmission for the yellow light in the middle of the visible spectrum. This ratio is reduced to about 34 percent for a 2-metre light guide. There is thus a serious relative depletion of blue in the spectrum of the transmitted light, the depletion increasing as the length of the light guide is increased. It is consequently essential for good colour reproduction to use a source of high colour temperature.

The higher absorption of light in the blue region of the spectrum tends to be greater as the refractive index of the glass becomes higher. High-aperture light guides require the use of high-refractive-index glass for the cores of the fibres, and hence show an even more marked absorption .of blue light. It is for this reason that low-aperture light guides are used wherever possible, and that the lengths of the high-aperture bundles are kept as short as possible.

The coupling of the flexible light guide to the fibre bundle in the endoscope is illustrated in Figure 11. In addition to reflection losses at the air-glass surfaces of the fibres, there is a loss of transmitted light arising from a mismatch between the fibres of the lightguide and those in the endoscope. This occurs because each fibre of the endoscope does not lie exactly opposite a corresponding fibre in the flexible light guide. Consequently some of the light from the flexible guide falls on the claddings and interspaces of the endoscope bundle. This light is not trapped and is lost at the containing wall of the endoscope. The effect of this mismatch is to give an effective transmittance of about 80 percent. Thus even with no reflection losses in the condenser system, the light transmittance of a 2-metre light guide (transmittance 40 percent) coupled to an endoscope is only about 32 percent, apart from losses in the endoscope fibre bundle. This transmittance can be further reduced if the abutting ends of the flexible light guide and the endoscope bundle are not almost in contact. The separation between them should not exceed a few tenths of a millimetre.

In the case of a cystoscope, or any endoscope used in water, it is usually necessary to increase the aperture of the cone of rays entering the endoscope bundle in order to illuminate the desired angle of field. The reason for this is illustrated in Figure 13. The two top diagrams show a low-aperture fibre, with an acceptance angle (α) of 38 degrees. When this fibre feeds into air (Fig. 13A) the emergent light is refracted at the exit face of the fibre to give a cone of light of angle $\alpha' = \alpha$, identical to that of the incident cone. In Figure 13B the fibre feeds into water, where there is less refraction at the exit face of the fibre, and the angle of the emergent cone (α') is reduced to 27 degrees. Thus while bundles of such fibres illuminate a field with an angle of about 76 degrees in air, it covers only about 54 degrees in water. This is

inadequate, for example, with a 70-degree cystoscope system.

A high-aperture fibre is shown in Figure 13C and D which accepts light cones with an angle (α) of 53 degrees. Feeding into air (Fig. 13C) the emergent cone has $\alpha' = \alpha$, so that the angle of field illuminated is about 106 degrees. This angle is reduced to about 74 degrees when the fibre feeds into water (Fig. 13D). To achieve this high aperture for light emerging into water, it is of course necessary to use high-aperture fibres for the endoscope bundle and also to have a high-aperture cone of light as input. In such systems it is customary to use a low-aperture bundle for the flexible light guide, thereby having smaller excess absorption in the blue region of the spectrum, and then to couple the output of the light guide to a relatively short bundle of high-aperture fibres in the endoscope by means of a "fibre cone." The latter is made from a short cylinder of fused high-aperture fibres, which are then heated to the softening point of the glass and drawn to taper in the form of a cone. The end-faces of this cone are then ground flat and polished. If the entry-face of the fibre cone is of radius r and this tapers to a smaller radius r' at the exit-face, a light cone of semiangle α entering in air emerges into air with a larger angle α'

$$\sin \alpha' = \left(\frac{r}{r'}\right) \sin \alpha \qquad (7)$$

so that the same amount of light, apart from the transmission losses normal to a fibre bundle, is concentrated in a smaller area but gives a cone of light of increased angle. From Eq. (7) the cone needed to couple a bundle of the low-aperture fibres (Fig. 13A) to a bundle of high-aperture fibres (Fig. 13D) would need to taper to a diameter approximately 0.75 times that of its entry-face.

When a fibre cone is used in the above manner there is an additional mismatch factor between the fibres at the exit-face of the cone and those of the endoscope bundle. The reflection losses at these two air-glass surfaces can usually be avoided by cementing the fibre cone to the endoscope fibre bundle. The overall mismatch factor for such a coupling between the flexible light guide and the endoscope bundle is then about $(0.80)^2$, i.e., 64 percent. This additional reduction in white light transmittance

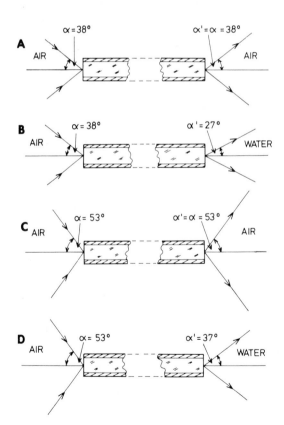

FIG. 13. Fibres feeding into air and water. **A** and **B.** Low-aperture fibre: $n = 1.64$, $n' = 1.52$. **C** and **D.** High-aperture fibre: $n = 1.72$, $n' = 1.52$.

is preferable to using a longer length of high-aperture fibres with the consequent greater relative depletion of blue in the transmitted light.

The overall illuminating system of an endoscope is illustrated in Figure 14. The semiangle of field illuminated is the angle shown as α', and this is determined by the maximum aperture of the endoscope fibre bundle, provided the aperture angle α_o of light accepted from the source is sufficiently large. The level of illumination over the illuminated area (A) depends on the luminance (B) of the source, which measures its intrinsic brightness, the transmittance factors of all the optical elements between the source S_o and the final exit-face S', the area of S', and the distance L. If T is the overall transmittance factor (i.e., the product of the fractional transmittances of all the optical elements) and B the luminance of the source, the intensity of illumination at area A is given by

$$I = \frac{BTS'}{L^2} \qquad (8)$$

where S' is the area of the final exit-face, and L is the distance from S' to the object at A. It is as if a source of the same luminance as S_o and of area S' were placed at position S' and then illuminated the object through a simple plate of transmittance T. The illumination of the object A in any given case can be increased only by increasing the transmittance or by using either a source of greater luminance or a fibre bundle of larger cross section.

Even for a good quality system the overall transmittance T is not likely to be greater than about 0.20 (20 percent) for a cystoscopic or similar system. T can be larger if no fibre cone

is needed; and in such cases an even greater improvement can be obtained by making the flexible light guide integral with the endoscope bundle. This is often useful in cases where colour television or still or ciné photography is to be used. Nevertheless it is usually necessary to use very-high-intensity sources (e.g., xenon arc lamps) and to have a source of high colour temperature in order to offset as much as possible the excess absorption in the blue end of the spectrum.

FACTORS DETERMINING THE BRIGHTNESS OF THE ENDOSCOPIC IMAGE

The level of illumination of the image seen in an endoscope depends in the first place on the level of illumination falling on the object being viewed. In accordance with Eq. (8), this is inversely proportional to the square of the object distance L. This is illustrated for the case of a single fibre in Figure 10. The cone of rays from this fibre intercepts areas A_o and A at distances L_o and L, respectively. The same total amount of light is thus spread over the larger area A, and the intensities of illumination (i.e., the light fluxes incident per unit area) are in the ratio

$$\frac{I}{I_o} = \frac{A_o}{A} = \left(\frac{L_o}{L}\right)^2 \qquad (9)$$

If the object distance is doubled, for example, the level of illumination falls by a factor of four. Again, the level of illumination at a distance $L = 40$ mm is 16 times smaller than for $L = 10$ mm, and consequently photography

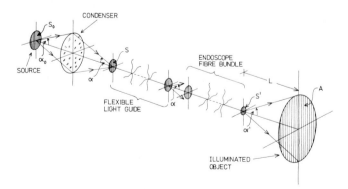

FIG. 14. Intensity of illumination of the object.

would require an exposure 16 times as long. This inverse square dependence of the level of illumination of the object usually makes automatic exposure control a necessity for satisfactory colour film and television purposes.

Part of the light emerging from the endoscope fibre bundle falls on a particular point (*O*) of the object (Fig. 15). If the object surface were perfectly smooth and reflecting, the incident light would be reflected into the endoscope viewing optics only if the object at *O* were almost perpendicular to the light incident on it from the bundle. It is usually only diffusely reflected light which enters the viewing optics, and the reflection coefficient for the light diffusely reflected to the viewing optics depends on the orientation and diffusing properties of the surface. From any element of the object, such as at *O,* the aperture diameter of the entrance pupil limits the part of this light that is accepted to a small cone of semiangle α:

$$\sin\ \alpha\ =\ \frac{h}{L} \tag{10}$$

where *h* is the radius of entrance pupil, and *L* is the distance of the object. The endoscope views a limited angle of field; if this is equal to 2β, as in Figure 4, the radius of object viewed at a distance *L* is given by

$$\eta\ =\ L\tan\beta \tag{11}$$

The total amount of light entering the endoscope from a uniformly diffuse reflecting surface whose reflection coefficient is *R* is given by

$$E\ =\ IR(\pi\eta^2)(\pi\sin^2\alpha)$$

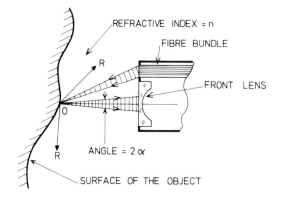

FIG. 15. Light accepted by an endoscope.

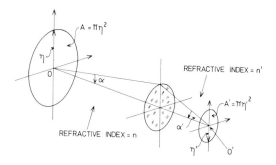

FIG. 16. Optical invariant.

where $\pi\eta^2$ is the area of the object, and $\pi\sin^2\alpha$ measures the solid angle of the cone of rays accepted by the endoscope from the points such as *O*. These are illustrated in Figure 16. This formula, which is usefully written

$$E\ =\ \pi IR(\sin\ \alpha\ \eta)^2 \tag{12}$$

is only approximate, in that the angles α and β are assumed to be not very large. Using Eq. (10) and (11), Eq. (12) becomes

$$E\ =\ \pi IR(h\tan\beta)^2 \tag{13}$$

The total light accepted by the endoscope thus depends only on the object distance through the inverse square dependence of the intensity of illumination (*I*) on this distance, as seen in Eq. (8). The viewing optics visualises a larger area of the object when this is at a greater distance from the endoscope, but it accepts a correspondingly smaller cone of light from each point of the object. These two effects exactly cancel each other, so that the total light transmitted by the endoscope depends only on the level of illumination of the object (*I*) and on the fraction *R* of this light that is reflected back in the direction of the endoscope.

Equation (13), when considered in relation to the basic laws of optical image formation, has very important consequences. It was these considerations which led to the invention of the Hopkins rod-lens systems by the author. At this point we indicate only the nature of the optical law involved.

Figure 17 shows an optical system that images an object at *O* of radius η. If the edge ray from the point *O* makes an angle α with the optical axis, and in the image space this ray

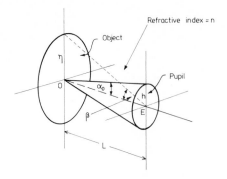

FIG. 17. Total light accepted by an endoscope.

converges to O' under an angle α', the linear magnification M is given by

$$M = \frac{\eta'}{\eta} = \frac{n \sin \alpha}{n' \sin \alpha'} \tag{14}$$

where η' is the radius of the image and n and n' are the refractive indices of the object and image spaces, respectively. From Eq. (14) it follows that the product

$$H = n \sin \alpha\eta = n' \sin \alpha'\eta' \tag{15}$$

is an invariant for the system—that is, it has the same value in every space where an image is formed, e.g., after the objective and then after each relay stage in an endoscope, as indicated in Figure 4. The above result, in the form of either Eq. (14) or (15), is variously attributed to Helmholtz, Lagrange, or Robert Smith. It is perhaps more convenient to use the term "optical magnification law" for Eq. (14), and "optical invariant" for Eq. (15).

Suppose now that $\sin \alpha$ and η in Eq. (15) refer to the object space at the distal end of an endoscope. The value of the product ($\sin \alpha\eta$) in Eq. (12) is then given by H/n, where n is the refractive index of the medium filling the object space. If this is air then $n = 1$; for water it has the value $n = 4/3$. From Eq. (12) the total amount of light entering the endoscope is now given by

$$E = \left(\frac{\pi^2 IR}{n^2}\right)H^2 \tag{16}$$

and, for given conditions of illumination and any given object distance, this depends only on the value of H^2. In turn, the value of the optical

invariant (H) depends simply on the construction employed for the viewing optics of the endoscope. The form of this dependence is discussed below.

The final image formed by the endoscope is either viewed directly by the observer or received by a film or television camera. If A' is the area of this final image, its intensity of illumination is given by

$$I' = \frac{E}{A'} \tag{17}$$

where E is the total amount of light E. This same amount of light is spread over a smaller or larger area, and the level of illumination of the final image is accordingly larger or smaller.

For visual observation of an object at a distance L millimetres and magnification M, the radius of the object viewed is $\eta = L \tan \beta$, and the radius of the image formed at a distance of 250 mm is given by $\eta' = M\eta = ML \tan \beta$, where M is the visual magnification for the object distance L. The area of the image is thus

$$A' = \pi\eta'^2 = \pi(ML)^2 \tan^2 \beta$$

or since, as in Eq. (5), $ML = M_oL_o$, this may be written

$$A' = \pi(M_oL_o)^2 \tan^2 \beta \tag{18}$$

The area of the final image, which is independent of the object distance L, may thus be calculated provided the visual magnification M_o for a stated object distance L_o is known, together with the semiangle of view in the object space.

If the focus of the eyepiece of the endoscope is set to form an image at infinity, the visual magnification is still defined as the linear magnification given when the focal setting is for an image formed at 250 mm. In either case the semiangle of field of the image, denoted by β' in Figure 4, is given by $\tan \beta' = \eta'/250$. Now, for any object distance L, we have $\eta' = M\eta = ML \tan \beta$; or since $ML = M_oL_o$, the semiangle of field for the image is given by

$$\tan \beta' = \frac{(M_oL_o) \tan \beta}{250} \tag{19}$$

where L_o is again in millimetres. For an endoscope with the image formed at infinity, the objective of the camera must also be focused on infinity; the radius of image formed is then given by $\eta'_c = F_c \tan \beta'$, where F_c is the focal length of the camera objective. Using Eq. (19) the radius of the image formed by the camera is

$$\eta'_c = \frac{(M_o L_o) \tan \beta F_c}{250} \tag{20}$$

where all lengths are in millimetres. The area of the image is thus given by

$$A'_c = \pi (M_o L_o)^2 \tan^2 \beta \left(\frac{F_c}{250}\right)^2 \tag{21}$$

This equation, used in Eq. (17), gives the level of illumination for the camera image. As expected, the radius of this image is proportional to F_c, and the level of illumination depends on F_c^2.

The considerations immediately above assume that the final endoscopic image is formed at infinity. In practice this image may fall at a finite distance and require a refocusing of the camera objective. The size of the camera image may then change slightly, but the above formula usually remains of sufficient accuracy for most practical purposes.

HOPKINS ROD-LENS SYSTEMS

The total amount of light that can be transmitted by an endoscope is limited by the value of H^2, where H is the optical invariant for the particular system. The value of H is determined by the construction adopted for the relay system of an endoscope.

Figure 18 shows the original object viewed at O by an endoscope, together with one stage of

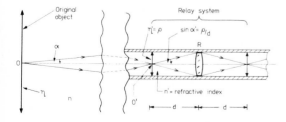

FIG. 18. Optical invariant for an endoscope.

the relay system. The latter is indicated as a relay lens at R, which picks up the intermediate image formed at O'. The objective is designed to make the image at O' of a diameter that fills the tube. Thus if ρ is the radius of the clear bore of the tube, the image at O' is of radius $\eta' = \rho$. The cone of light diverging from O' is similarly made to fill the aperture of the lens R, and is thus of semiangle α', where $\sin \alpha' = \rho/d$, if d is the distance between O' and R. The optical invariant for the system is thus given by

$$H = n' \sin \alpha' \eta' = n' \left(\frac{\rho}{d}\right)\rho \tag{22}$$

To maximise H, and therefore the light-transmitting capacity, means that both η' and $\sin \alpha'$ must be at their maximum values. Now η' is a maximum when $\eta' = \rho$; also $\sin \alpha'$ is at its maximum when d is chosen such that the cone of rays from O' fills the lens at R, i.e., when $\sin \alpha' = \rho/d$. These two conditions are assumed to have been satisfied in obtaining Eq. (22).

Suppose now that the endoscope is of total length D. Each relay stage relays the image a distance $2d$ along the tube, so that the number of relay stages required is given by

$$N = \frac{D}{2d} \tag{23}$$

Substituting for $1/d$ from Eq. (23), Eq. (22), for the optical invariant, becomes

$$H = \left(\frac{2}{D}\right) n' \rho^2 N \tag{24}$$

In accordance with Eq. (16), the total amount of light transmitted by the endoscope is thus given by

$$E = \left(\frac{\pi I R}{n}\right)\left(\frac{2}{D}\right)^2 n'^2 \rho^4 N^2 \tag{25}$$

in which the final factors are simply the value of H^2, with H of Eq. (24).

Equation (25) assumes that there are no light losses by absorption in the glass of the endoscope optics or by reflection at the air-

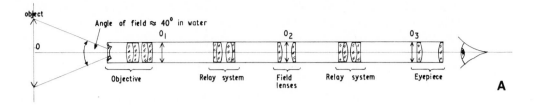

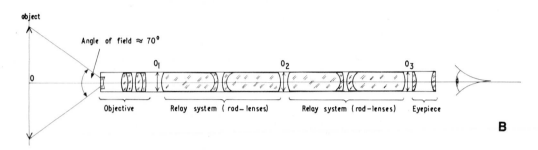

FIG. 19. Optics of a traditional cystoscope (**A**) and a rod-lens system (**B**).

glass surface. It thus gives the theoretically maximum total light that can be transmitted. In modern endoscopes these losses are in fact small *(vide infra)*.

There are two important conclusions to be drawn from Eq. (25). First, if the medium between the relay lenses is air, the refractive index has the value $n' = 1$ and the factor n'^2 in Eq. (25) also has the value unity. This is the case with earlier endoscopes, which had relay and field lenses of glass and long air spaces (Fig. 19A). In the Hopkins rod-lens system the roles of glass and air are interchanged (Fig. 19B). We now have air lenses and long glass spaces. The result is that n' is now the refractive index of the glass spaces and so has a value of approximately 1.50 to 1.60; the factor n'^2 then is 2.25 to 2.56. With the same number of relay stages the light-transmitting capacity of the endoscope is therefore increased more than twofold. This is the consideration which led to the invention of the rod-lens system.

The second conclusion to emerge from Eq. (25) is that the value of H^2, and therefore of the total light flux *(E)*, is proportional to ρ^4, i.e., to the fourth power of the radius of the inner bore of the endoscope tube. The rod-lens principle allows advantage to be taken of this strong dependence of E on the radius of the clear aperture available to the viewing optics. The reason

for this is illustrated in Figure 20, which indicates the two mechanical arrangements employed. In the traditional optical system (Fig. 20A) a series of very small lenses are assembled in a long, narrow tube. In a cystoscope, for example, there may be five relay stages in a 300-mm tube, each lens having a diameter of perhaps 3 mm. The practical difficulty of as-

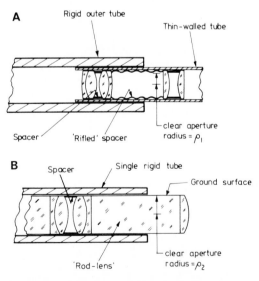

FIG. 20. Mechanical construction of the traditional endoscope (**A**) and the new system (**B**).

sembling such lenses in the bore of a long, rigid tube was overcome by assembling the lenses first in a more flexible thin-walled tube, which could then easily be inserted in the rigid outer tube (Fig. 20A). The lenses are maintained with the appropriate spacings along the axis by means of spacers in the form of tubes. The longer of these spacer tubes need to be "rifled" in order to suppress light being strongly reflected at glancing incidence on the inner surface, since such stray light can seriously impair the contrast in the final image. The result is that the clear aperture radius available to the optics, shown as ρ_1 in Figure 20A, can be appreciably smaller than the outer radius of the endoscope.

By contrast, the mounting of a rod-lens system is not only a simpler matter but also permits a radius of clear aperture (ρ_2), which can be appreciably larger than the value for a traditional system of the same outer diameter (ρ_1). Since each rod-lens is in the form of a cylinder and its length is approximately 10 times its diameter, it can be precision ground and assembled directly into a rigid but relatively thin-walled tube. The spacers, being very short, may be made thin and thus do not obtrude much into the clear aperture. Moreover, specular reflection of light at glancing incidence is avoided since the outer surface of each rod-lens is finely ground.

In the first prototype of the new rod-lens system it was possible to make the clear aperture ρ_2 equal to about 1.4 times as large as that for a typical traditional system of the same outer diameter. Thus $\rho_2 = 1.4\,\rho_1$, and the ratio of the light-transmitting capacities was thus

$$\frac{E_2}{E_1} = \left(\frac{n'_2}{n'_1}\right)^2 \left(\frac{\rho_2}{\rho_1}\right)^4$$

$$= (1.52)^2(1.4)^4 = 8.9 \qquad (26)$$

since $n'_2 = 1.52$ for the glass employed, and $n'_1 = 1.00$ for air. This is a ninefold increase.

The above advantage was exploited commercially both to reduce the outer diameter of the endoscope and at the same time to design a cystoscope giving an angle of view in water of 70 degrees compared with an angle of 40 degrees in water, which was more typical of the traditional systems.

To obtain a large angle of field in the object

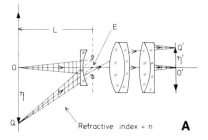

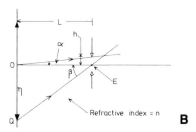

FIG. 21. Objective of a modern endoscope.

space requires the use of a suitably designed objective. A useful construction for this is shown in Figure 21. The pencils of rays are accepted from the axial object point O and from an extraaxial object point Q (Fig. 21A). If continued all pass through an imaginary circular aperture at E, which is the entrance pupil of the system. The essential optical properties of the system, so far as the object space is concerned, are shown in Figure 21B. Now, as seen above, the construction adopted for the relay system determines the value of the optical invariant H. It follows from this that for a given semiangle of field (β) the radius of the entrance pupil (h) is fixed.

Thus since H is invariant

$$H = n \sin \alpha \eta \qquad (27)$$

where η is the radius of the object, α is the semiangle of the aperture, and n is the refractive index of the object space. Sin $\alpha = h/L$, and tan $\beta = \eta/L$, so Eq. (27) may be written alternatively as

$$H = nh \tan \beta \qquad (28)$$

Given the value of H, as specified by the relay system, and the semiangle of field β, the radius h of the entrance pupil is given by Eq. (28). For a typical case $H = 0.10$ mm, and with $n = 1.33$ (for water) and $\beta = 35°$ (corresponding to a full field $2\beta = 70°$), $h = 0.11$ mm. The diameter of the entrance pupil ($2h = 0.22$ mm) is thus very small.

To obtain a system with a total field angle 2β requires the objective to have a focal length F implied by the formula

$$nF \tan \beta = \eta' = \rho \qquad (29)$$

with the image height η' being set equal to the inner radius ρ of the endoscope tube. For $2\beta = 70°$ and $\rho = 1.4$ mm, the focal length of the objective is very short: $F = 1.50$ mm. To obtain a smaller angle of field the objective has a longer focal length; and since the product $h \tan \beta$ remains constant by Eq. (28), the radius of the entrance pupil increases. The end result is that the objective accepts more light from a smaller field of view, but the total amount of light accepted remains constant.

It may be also mentioned that even for details as large as 0.25 mm to be well resolved the correction of aberrations of an endoscope and the precision needed in production are comparable with those of a good quality microscope objective. The rod-lens type of system has the further advantage that it lends itself to accurate assembly of the optical components, with each element being very precisely square to the optical axis and with no eccentricity.

ANTIREFLECTION COATINGS: ABSORPTION IN GLASS

If light falls on an untreated air-glass surface, about 4 to 7 percent is reflected, depending on the refractive index of the glass. For a glass of refractive index $n = 1.52$ the reflection coefficient is $R = 4.26$ percent; for $n = 1.67$ it rises to $R = 6.30$ percent. A typical endoscope (e.g., a cystoscope with five relay stages of rod-lenses) may have 32 air-glass surfaces. Used with a camera and a dual viewing attachment, this may rise to 40 to 50 surfaces. The transmittance of such a system when using untreated surfaces is very small, as may be seen from the curves in Figure 22. This shows the percentage transmittance, ignoring any absorption in the glass, of N surfaces for values up to $N = 50$. The curves for $R = 4.26$ percent and $R = 6.30$ percent give the transmittance that would be obtained using untreated sur-

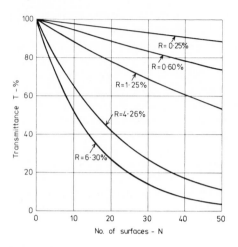

FIG. 22. Percentage transmission (T) of N surfaces for different reflection losses per surface. R is the percentage reflection coefficient for one surface.

faces for glass of refractive index $n = 1.52$ and 1.67, respectively. These curves represent the mean transmittances throughout the visible spectrum.

The reflection coefficient for an untreated glass surface is almost independent of the wavelength of the light (Fig. 23). The reflection

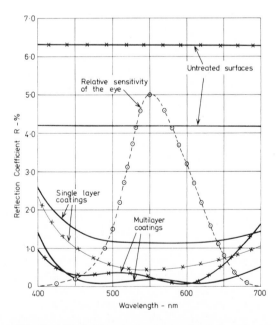

FIG. 23. Reflection from single air-glass surfaces showing the effects of different antireflection coatings. Refractive indices: for the continuous line $n = 1.52$; for the line marked with crosses $n = 1.67$.

losses when using untreated surfaces thus do not impair the colour rendering, but they do have two serious consequences. The first is of course the very poor transmittance. Taking a mean between the refractive index values $n = 1.52$ and 1.67, for which $R = 4.26$ and 6.30 percent, respectively, a typical rod-lens cystoscope having some 30 air-glass surfaces would have a transmittance of only about 20 percent. Thus 80 percent of the light would be lost by reflection losses. This is in itself a serious enough matter, but much of this light may be reflected forward again by preceding surfaces and give a haze of stray light over the image. The resulting severe reduction in contrast is the second serious consequence of using untreated surfaces. The traditional form of construction would have even more air-glass surface and so would be worse in this respect than a rod-lens system.

It is fortunate that postwar technology has produced antireflection coatings with which these reflection losses may be reduced. The simplest technique is that of ordinary "blooming" as used in photographic objectives. A thin film of magnesium fluoride, one quarter of a wavelength thick, is deposited on the glass surface by evaporation in a vacuum. The reduction in the reflection coefficient of such single-layer coatings is shown by the two curves in Figure 23. The significance of light in the different parts of the visible spectrum is indicated in this figure by the relative sensitivity of the human eye. For most practical purposes, the reflection losses may be considered as constant throughout the visible spectrum.

Taking $R = 1.25$ percent as a representative value of the reflection coefficient for a bloomed surface of glass of refractive index $n = 1.52$, the curves of Figure 22 show an increase in transmittance to 69 percent for a system having 30 surfaces. The efficiency of a single-layer coating is greater for glass of higher refractive index, but the dependence on wavelength is also more marked. This is seen by comparing the curves for $n = 1.67$ and $n = 1.52$ in Figure 23. Taking $r = 0.60$ percent as an average for $n = 1.67$, the curves of Figure 22 show an increased transmittance for such a glass to 83 percent for $N = 30$.

Assuming a system of 30 air-glass surfaces composed of some high- and some low-index glass, the mean of the curves for $R = 0.60$ and 1.23 percent gives a transmittance of 76 percent. This improves the transmittance by a factor of 3.80 over the 20 percent transmittance for untreated surfaces.

The reflection coefficient may be still further reduced by the use of multilayer optical coatings. Typical curves are shown in Figure 23. The average reflection coefficient is now reduced to about 0.25 percent for both low- and high-index glasses. As seen from the curve in Figure 22 for $R = 0.25$ percent, the transmittance for 30 surfaces is now 93 percent showing a 1.22-fold improvement over single-layer coatings and a 4.65-fold improvement over untreated surfaces. The accompanying reduction in stray light results in a marked increase in contrast of the image. Moreover, note from the curves of Figure 23 that multilayer coatings can have very uniform efficiency throughout the visible spectrum.

With a rod-lens system the glass is much thicker than in the traditional endoscope. Even for a cystoscope there is a total of some 300 mm of glass, which may increase to around 500 mm for a bronchoscope. Light absorption by glass thus becomes more important, and the glass types used must be selected for low absorption. Fortunately there has also been great improvement in the transmission properties of optical glass.

The curves in Figure 24 show the absorption throughout the range of the visible spectrum of different thicknesses of typical modern flint glass with good transmission properties. The internal transmittance (T_i) of a thickness (D) of glass is the transmittance of a block of this thickness, assuming no reflection losses at the two faces. Note that the absorption increases strongly for the ultraviolet region, i.e., wave-

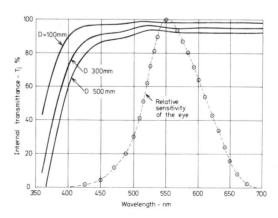

FIG. 24. Internal transmittance for different lengths (D) of an optical glass of good transparency.

lengths shorter than 400 mm. The visible spectrum is the range covered by the relative sensitivity curve of the human eye (Fig. 24). With increasing thickness of glass, the absorption at the blue end of the visible region increases; but for the important part of the visible spectrum (e.g., above 440 mm) the transmittance even for $D = 500$ mm is almost constant. This is of importance in a medical endoscope, where detail is often distinguished by differences in colour. Uniform transmittance throughout the spectrum, which is necessary for the production of good colour, is consequently of particular importance.

DEPTH OF FOCUS

Medical endoscopes are usually made as fixed-focus instruments, since the moving parts of a focusing mechanism would add appreciably to the difficulty of sterilisation. To view objects at different distances, therefore, one relies on there being a sufficient depth of focus. In other than fibreoptic endoscopes the depth of focus in visual use is greatly aided by the power of accommodation of the eye. The normal eye of a young person can focus on distances between infinity and the near point, which is at a distance of 250 mm. The range of exact focus when using an endoscope visually is thus given by the maximum and minimum object distances for which the endoscope produces its image lying within the range from infinity to 250 mm.

To find a formula for this range of focus, consider an endoscope for which the visual magnification for an object distance L_o has the value M_o. If the endoscope is focused so that an object placed at this distance (O_o in Figure 25),

is imaged at a distance $L'_o = 250$ mm from the exit pupil (E'), the visual magnification for this object distance is $M_o = \eta'_o/\eta_o$, where $\eta'_o = L'_o \tan \beta' = 250 \tan \beta'$ and $\eta_o = L_o \tan \beta$. Now the linear magnification between the entrance pupil E and its image, the exit pupil at E', is given by

$$\overline{M} = \frac{n \tan \beta}{\tan \beta'} = \left(\frac{nL'_o}{L_o}\right) \frac{L_o \tan \beta}{L'_o \tan \beta'}$$

where $n' = 1$; or, using the formulae for η_o and η'_o

$$\overline{M} = \frac{250n}{M_o L_o} \tag{30}$$

where L_o is given in millimetres. The quantity $\overline{M}$ is used in the depth of focus formula derived below.

The image of O_o is considered to be at O'_o only in specifying the visual magnification, in accordance with the convention described earlier. In practice an endoscope should be focused such that an object at approximately the greatest distance that occurs (e.g., O_1 at distance L_1 in Figure 25), is imaged at a distance $L' = \infty$. If the object point is now moved from O_1 to O_2, at a shorter distance (L_2), the image moves in from infinity toward the observer. If this image is formed at a distance of 250 mm, the range O_1O_2 gives the range of object distances that can be exactly focused by a normal eye. It follows from the laws of optics that

$$\frac{n}{\overline{M}}\left(\frac{1}{L_2} - \frac{1}{L_1}\right) = n'\overline{M}\left(\frac{1}{L'_2} - \frac{1}{L'_1}\right) \tag{31}$$

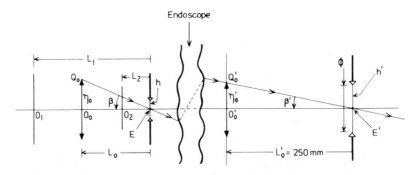

FIG. 25. Calculation of the range of exact focus for an endoscope used visually.

where n is the refractive index of the object space, and $n' = 1$ is the index of the image space. Thus using Eq. (30) for $\overline{M}$, and putting $L'_1 = + \infty$, $L'_2 = 250$ mm, Eq. (31) gives

$$\left(\frac{1}{L_2} - \frac{1}{L_1} \right) = \frac{250n}{(M_o L_o)^2} \qquad (32)$$

from which formula the focal range can be calculated.

Suppose, for example, that a cystoscope has a specification that gives unit magnification (M_o) as 1 for an object distance (L_o) of 30 mm. For water $n = 4/3$, and Eq. (31) gives

$$\frac{1}{L_2} - \frac{1}{L_1} = 0.370 \qquad (33)$$

If the cystoscope has its focus set to give a maximum object distance (L_1) of 40 mm, Eq. (33) gives $L_2 = 2.5$ mm for the nearest object distance that can be exactly focused. This assumes that the observer has the full amplitude of accommodation. If the observer's range of accommodation is between infinity and a near point at any distance L'_2, Eq. (31) gives

$$\frac{1}{L_2} - \frac{1}{L_1} = \frac{250n}{(M_o L_o)^2} \left(\frac{250}{L'_2} \right) \qquad (34)$$

in place of Eq. (32). Thus if $L'_2 = 500$ mm, the range of accommodation, Eq. (33), is halved; and in the example given, the nearest object that can be exactly focused is at $L_2 = 4.8$ mm. This value is more typical of what is expected for older observers.

The above considerations give the range of exact focus made possible by the exercise of accommodation by the observer's eye. The full range of depth of focus is greater at each end of this range by the depth of focus as ordinarily understood. In photography of course there is only this ordinary depth of focus, and for this reason focusing the camera is essential for good results. As in ordinary photography, the smaller the aperture employed, the greater the depth of focus about the position of true focus. It is for this reason that the diameter of the exit pupil of any endoscope should be specified.

In a fibreoptic endoscope the relay systems between the objective and the eyepiece are replaced by a coherent fibre bundle. Such a bun-

dle merely transmits to the proximal end the image formed by the objective on the distal end. If this image is out of focus it is seen out of focus by the observer, and the image seen cannot be refocused by accommodation of the observer's eye. The best that can be done is for the observer to see the proximal end of the fibre bundle in good focus. In this respect fibreoptic endoscopy is more akin to photography. The image detail that can be seen with a fibreoptic endoscope is limited by the finite size of the fibres employed. The resolution of the objective is thus not fully utilised. By contrast, with a well designed and well constructed rod-lens endoscope the resolution of the objective may be fully used. It is for this reason (i.e., the very much better image quality) that a more refined approach to the question of depth of focus is needed, compared with what suffices for a fibreoptic instrument.

Even with a perfectly designed and constructed endoscope (having no aberration and no production errors) the image of a single point of the object is a circular disk of light, the so-called Airy disk, surrounded by alternately dark and light rings. It is the blurring resulting from this diffraction effect that sets a limit to the detail which can be resolved by any optical instrument. The effect of aberration and/or error of focus is to broaden this pattern and thereby increase the size of the smallest detail that may be resolved. The depth of focus, even of a perfect system, thus depends on the size of detail it is desired to resolve.

To deal with this question it is necessary to use the idea of the optical transfer function, also termed the modulation transfer function. A grating-like test object is considered, having an intensity distribution of the form shown in Figure 26 for $C = 1$. The contrast (C) has its maximum value of unity when $C = 1.0$, and $C = 0$ denotes a constant intensity. If p is the peak-to-peak distance of the pattern, the spatial frequency of the pattern is given by

$$N = \frac{1}{p} \qquad (35)$$

and specifies the number of cycles per millimetre if p is given in millimetres. Even for a perfectly focused image the contrast steadily decreases to zero as test objects of increasing spatial frequency (i.e., smaller p) are used. The highest spatial frequency that can be resolved

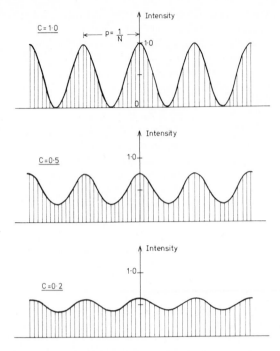

FIG. 26. Intensity variation across gratings of different contrast.

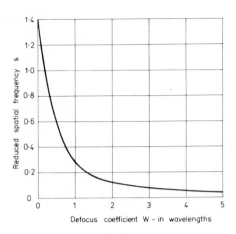

FIG. 27. Maximum reduced spatial frequency *(s)* for which the image contrast *(C)* is not less than 0.20 for a defocused but aberration-free system.

depends on the size of the optical system aperture, the wavelength of the light, and the minimum acceptable contrast in the image.

The curves in Figure 26 show the form of intensity variation for the contrasts $C = 1, 0.5$, and 0.2. A convenient value for the minimum acceptable contrast is the last value $(C = 0.2)$. To estimate the smallest detail whose image has this contrast, it is useful to assume an aberration-free system, using light of the mean wavelength $\lambda = 0.00055$ mm in the visible spectrum, and to calculate the "reduced spatial frequency" *(s)*. The maximum reduced spatial frequency that gives $C = 0.2$ is shown in Figure 27 as a function of the coefficient *(W)* which specifies the focus error.

Let the entrance pupil of the system, E in Figure 28, be of radius h. The semiangle α of the cone of rays accepted from an object point O at a distance L is then given by $\sin \alpha = h/L$. If N is the spatial frequency in the object at O, given in cycles per millimetre, the reduced spatial frequency is defined as

$$s = \left(\frac{\lambda}{n \sin \alpha} \right) N \qquad (36)$$

where the wavelength of the light (λ) is also in millimetres, and n is the refractive index of the object space. Suppose now that the diameter $\varphi = 2h'$ of the exit pupil of the endoscope is known, as indicated in Figure 25. The radius of the entrance pupil is then given by

$$h = \frac{h'}{\overline{M}} = \frac{\varphi/2}{250n(M_oL_o)} = \frac{\varphi(M_oL_o)}{500n} \qquad (37)$$

where $\overline{M}$, given by Eq. (30), is the pupil magnification. Using this value of h to give $\sin \alpha = h/L$, Eq. (36) becomes

$$s = \left(\frac{500\lambda L}{\varphi(M_oL_o)} \right) N$$

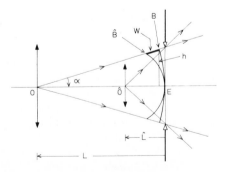

FIG. 28. Specification of the reduced spatial frequency *(s)* and the degree of defocus.

or, with $\lambda = 0.00055$ mm

$$s = \left(\frac{0.275L}{\varphi(M_oL_o)}\right)N$$

$$N = \left(\frac{3.64\varphi(M_oL_o)}{L}\right)s \qquad (38)$$

from which the number of cycles per millimetre in an object (at distance L), which corresponds to any given value of s, may be calculated, and conversely.

For a cystoscope, $n = 1.333$ and a typical value of φ is 2.4 mm. If the visual magnification is $M_o = 1$ for an object distance $L_o = 30$ mm, the value of N for any value s and object distance L is given by

$$s = \frac{LN}{262} \qquad N = \frac{262s}{L} \qquad (39)$$

For a perfectly focused and aberration-free system $s = 1.40$ for an image contrast $C = 0.20$ (Fig. 27). Thus $N = 367/L$ gives the resolution limit, according to the criterion adopted, for any object distance L. For $L = 40$ mm, this gives $N = 9.2$ cycles/mm; or $p = 0.11$ mm is the smallest size of detail. If L decreases to 10 mm, the value of N becomes 36.7 cycles/mm, or $p = 0.027$ mm. It must be stressed that these values are approximate, and they assume a perfect optical system. They nevertheless serve to illustrate how very much finer is the object detail that can be resolved compared with even the best fibreoptic system.

To consider defocused images, it is necessary to specify the appropriate measure of defocus. In Figure 28 O is an object at distance L from the entrance pupil E at the distal end of the endoscope. $\hat{O}$ is a second object at distance $\hat{L}$. The difference in focus between $\hat{O}$ and O is specified by the quantity $W = n(\hat{B}B)$, where $(\hat{B}B)$ is the length shown in the diagram. This is the distance, at the edge of the aperture, between the light wave EB from O and the wave $E\hat{B}$ from $\hat{O}$; as usual n is the refractive index of the object space. For an entrance pupil of radius h, the defocus coefficient W (when measured in wavelengths) is given by

$$W = \left(\frac{1}{2\lambda}\right)nh^2\left(\frac{1}{\hat{L}} - \frac{1}{L}\right) \qquad (40)$$

A positive value of W thus means that $\hat{O}$ is nearer to the endoscope than O, and conversely. Using Eq. (37) for h, with $\lambda = 0.00055$ mm, Eq. (40) gives

$$W = \left(\frac{\varphi(M_oL_o)^2}{275n}\right)\left(\frac{1}{\hat{L}} - \frac{1}{L}\right)$$

$$\left(\frac{1}{\hat{L}} - \frac{1}{L}\right) = \left(\frac{275n}{\varphi^2(M_oL_o)^2}\right)W \qquad (41)$$

where the diameter of the exit pupil (φ), L, and $\hat{L}$ are all expressed in millimetres. For the cystoscope used above, $\varphi = 2.4$ mm, $n = 1.333$, $M_o = 1.0$, and $L_o = 30$ mm; and Eq. (41) gives

$$W = 14.1\left(\frac{1}{\hat{L}} - \frac{1}{L}\right)$$

$$\left(\frac{1}{\hat{L}} - \frac{1}{L}\right) = 0.075W \qquad (42)$$

for the relations between the defocus coefficient W and the difference in the reciprocal distances of $\hat{O}$ and O.

The use of Eq. (38) and (41) in conjunction with the curve in Figure 27 provides a simple procedure for determining the maximum spatial frequency N for which a given focus error has an image contrast C not less than 20 percent. Conversely, given the spatial frequency N, the depth of focus (according to the criterion adopted here) may be found. The advantage of using the spatial frequency and defocus coefficients in the forms s and W is that they enable the single curve of Figure 27 to apply to any endoscope under any conditions of use.

To illustrate the procedure, consider the example of the cystoscope used above, to which Eq. (39) and (42) apply. If the true plane of focus is at a distance (L) of 20 mm and we consider a spatial frequency (N) of 10 cycles/mm in this plane, the reduced spatial frequency (s) is 0.76 by Eq. (39). The curve in Figure 27 shows that for this value of s the permissible defocus (W) is ±0.35. Using this value in Eq. (42) with $L = 20$

$$\frac{1}{\hat{L}} = 0.050 \pm 0.025$$

where $\hat{L}_{max}$ = 40 mm and $\hat{L}_{min}$ = 13.3 mm. For objects lying between these extremes, a detail which seems in the image to be the same size as that for N = 20 for the object at L = 20 has the contrast (C) decreasing to a minimum of 0.20 for the two extreme distances. The number of cycles per millimetre in an object at distance $\hat{L}$ having the same image size at that for N cycles per millimeter at distance L is given by

$$\hat{N} = \left(\frac{L}{\hat{L}}\right)N \qquad (43)$$

since the reduced spatial frequency (s) remains constant for a given size of detail in the image. For the case in question, we have $\hat{N}$ = 5 cycles/mm for $\hat{L}$ = 13.3 mm.

For the case L = 20 mm and N = 5 cycles/mm, the corresponding values of s and W are 0.38 and 0.80, respectively. For this case, then, Eq. (42) gives

$$\frac{1}{\hat{L}} = 0.050 \pm 0.057$$

so that $\hat{L}_{min}$ = 9.3 mm, but $(1/L_{max})$ = −0.007. This negative value merely implies that all object distances to infinity, $(1/L_{max})$ = 0, are within the depth of focus.

The above results indicate that because of the small aperture of an endoscope there is a considerable depth of focus even in photography, where the observer's accommodation cannot aid in maintaining focus. The above method of treating the problem of depth of focus is of course an approximate (but practi-

cal) rule. It gives an estimate of the best performance that may be expected from a high-quality endoscope. Even then the performance of the system at the edge of the field is not usually as good as that at the centre.

The general conclusions to be drawn from these considerations is that even for observers with reduced accommodation a fixed-focus endoscope is usually able to give adequately sharp images over the ranges of object distance that occur in practice. On the other hand, for photography and television cameras, focusing is unquestionably necessary in most cases.

DUAL-VIEWING ATTACHMENTS

A dual-viewing attachment is an optical system that provides a second position for viewing the endoscopic image. Figure 29 shows the essentials of such a system. A beam splitter is used to reflect and transmit equal amounts of light from the endoscope. The endoscopist (E_1) observes the image using the transmitted light, and the reflected light passes through an optical system which forms intermediate images at $I_1, I_2, I_3,$ and I_4, where it is observed by a second observer (E_2). The final lens, which is the eyepiece, is made focusable.

In a fibreoptic system the image formed at I_1 falls on the distal end of a coherent fibre bundle, which conveys the image to the proximal end at position I_4, where it is viewed via the eyepiece. Any focus error of the image at the distal end of the fibre bundle inevitably results in a blurred image, since the eyepiece can focus only on the proximal end of the fibre bundle, which can display only the image it

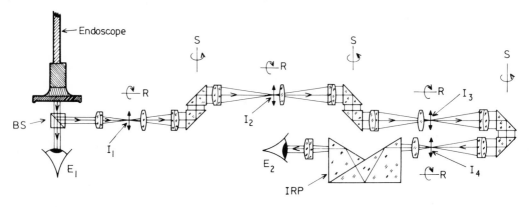

FIG. 29.   Dual-viewing attachment. BS, beam splitter. R, rotation joints. S, swivel joints. IRP, image rotating prism.

receives at the distal end. The depth of focus is thus that which is obtained in photography. This effect, combined with the limited detail resolution resulting from the discrete pattern of dots of light constituting the fibreoptic image, explains the relatively poor image quality obtained with a fibreoptic teaching attachment.

The advantage of a fibreoptic dual-viewing attachment is its great flexibility, thereby causing little inconvenience to the endoscopist. A lesser but still adequate degree of flexibility may be achieved using a lens-type dual-viewing attachment. The type of system in Figure 29, for example, consists of four articulated tubes, each about 20 cm long. The ends of these tubes are linked by means of swivel joints, giving a full 360-degree rotation around the axis of each joint *(S* in Figure 29). The axis of rotation of each swivel joint is the optical axis between the two reflecting prisms. In a recently designed system each of the tubes is made in two parts, joined by a rotation joint *(R* in Figure 29). This provides great flexibility in all directions. With such a system the final image rotates around the optical axis as the whole attachment is flexed. For small degrees of flexure this rotation is not disturbing, but the image orientation may be corrected by rotating the image-rotating prism around the optical axis. A K prism (Fig. 8) is used.

With a lens-type dual-viewing attachment the second observer has the advantage of his accommodation to aid focusing. The eyepiece of the system is also made focusable, with the result that the second observer frequently enjoys a sharper image than that viewed directly by the endoscopist through his fixed-focus instrument.

The image presented by the dual-viewing attachment may be used for photography or television, the camera objective being placed at position E_2. This is advantageous in that photography and filming may be performed without interrupting the work of the endoscopist. Either a fibreoptic or a lens-type attachment may be used. For photographic and television use it is desirable to employ a beam splitter which reflects some 90 percent of the incident light; otherwise there is either too little light for the camera or much too much for the endoscopist. The advantage of the fibreoptic system is its greater flexibility, but this must be weighed in relation to the deterioration in a fibreoptic system with use and the considerably better image quality that is obtained with a well designed lens-type system. The fibreoptic system is also smaller in diameter, but the lens-type systems can be designed with tubes having an outside diameter less than 18 mm, providing a system that is not at all cumbersome.

PHOTOGRAPHY AND TELEVISION

For television and still and ciné photography the endoscopic image may be recorded either by placing the camera directly on the endoscope *(E₁* in Figure 29) or at the second position *(E₂)* if a dual-viewing attachment is employed. In the former case focusing is achieved by the camera objective, whereas with a dual-viewing attachment focus can be set by the focusing eyepiece.

The radius of the image formed in the camera film plane or on the photocathode of a television camera is determined by the angular size of the endoscope image and the focal length (F_c) of the camera objective. As in Eq. (19) and (20), the angular radius of the endoscope image is given by

$$\tan \beta' = \frac{(M_o L_o) \tan \beta}{250} \qquad (44)$$

The radius of the image formed on the film is derived from

$$\eta'_c = F_c \tan \beta' \qquad (45)$$

For an endoscope with a visual magnification (M_o) of 1, when the object distance (L_o) is 30 mm and the semiangle of object field (β) is 35 degrees, Eq. (44) gives $\tan \beta' = 0.084$; and when the camera objective of focal length (F_c) is 75 mm, Eq. (45) gives $\eta'_c = 6.3$ mm for the radius of the image. A focal length of 75 mm is typical of the objectives employed.

The total amount of light leaving the endoscope is distributed over a greater or smaller area depending on the focal length of the objective. Since the area of the image is proportional to the square of its radius, the level of illumination is inversely proportional to F_c^2. That is, if a camera objective is replaced by one having twice the focal length, the level of illumination

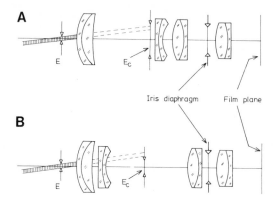

FIG. 30. Zoom camera objective, showing vignetting of an endoscopic image. **A.** Long-focus position. **B.** Short-focus position.

in the image is reduced to one-fourth its original value. For this reason it is usually advisable to employ the shortest focal length consistent with the smallest useful size for the image.

A typical diameter for the exit pupil of an endoscope is $\varphi = 2.4$ mm. Used with a camera objective with a focal length (F_c) of 75 mm, this gives $F/N_o = F_c/\varphi = F/31$. Despite this extremely small aperture, it is nevertheless usually necessary to employ a high-aperture objective if a standard one is employed. This is because of the possibility of vignetting, particularly when a zoom objective is employed. The construction often employed for a zoom lens is seen in Figure 30. The two inner lenses are moved along the axis to vary the focal length of the system. The long-focus position (Fig. 30A) gives a larger image size, and the short-focus position (Fig. 30B) a smaller image size.

The iris diaphragm of a zoom lens is fixed in position; and for a given F/n_o setting it remains constant in size. To pass through the diaphragm itself, any entering beam must appear to fall within the interior of the entrance pupil (E_c), which is the image of the diaphragm as seen through the components preceding it. When the zoom is operated the entrance pupil of the zoom lens moves along the axis; but more importantly it decreases in size as the zoom changes from the long-focus to the short-focus position (Fig. 30). A pencil of light from the edge of an endoscopic image is seen in Figure 30; it emerges from the exit pupil (E) of the endoscope. These rays, when continued, fall outside the camera lens pupil $(E_c$ in Figure 30B) so that light from the edge of the endoscope image does not pass through the zoom lens: it falls outside the aperture of the diaphragm after traversing the first three components of the system. The result is that the outer part of the image is vignetted, and only the central region is imaged onto the film plane.

This effect is present with any standard camera lens. It arises because the exit pupil of the endoscope falls outside the front element of the camera objective, whose own entrance pupil lies to the right and inside the objective. This pupil mismatch is usually more severe for a zoom lens because the entrance pupil tends to fall at a greater distance inside the lens. It is for this reason that vignetting is particularly liable to occur with a zoom camera lens. Quite simple fixed-focus and zoom camera objectives have been specially designed for use with endoscopes, and it is usually preferable to use these rather than standard camera lenses.

2

Physics of the Fibreoptic Endoscope

Harold H. Hopkins

If a beam of light enters one end-face of an ordinary glass rod it is repeatedly reflected at the walls and eventually emerges from the other end-face of the rod. In the ideal case there is perfect "total internal reflection" at the walls; the reflection coefficient is 100 percent, and no light is lost other than by absorption as it travels between reflections through the glass of the rod. It is this trapping of light which forms the basis of the use of fibreoptics in endoscopy. That practically useful fibreoptic endoscopes are possible results from the fact that this property persists in rods with diameters as small as a little less than 8μ, when the glass rod becomes flexible and is then more properly termed a fibre.

The light entering any such fibre is trapped; and after a great number of reflections at the walls it emerges uniformly distributed over the other end-face of the fibre. It is this fact which sets a limit to the smallest size of detail that may be resolved by a fibreoptic endoscope.

In practical fibreoptic gastroscopes, colonoscopes, and the like, the fibres employed have diameters of about 10μ. It is not the increased difficulty of working with fibres of smaller diameter that prevents their use in endoscopes but rather that there is a fundamental physical limitation. In elementary optics light emerging from a source is pictured as travelling along rays, which are refracted or reflected at any surface they meet and then continue as rays. This concept adequately explains many aspects of the propagation of light and of the action of lens systems, but it fails to explain other phenomena such as interference and diffraction. Here it is necessary to regard light as a propagating wave, in terms of which theory the ideas of ray optics appear as a first approximation.

The wave theory of light serves to explain why total internal reflection occurs and why light is no longer trapped in a fibre when the radius of the fibre is smaller than several times the wavelength of the light in question. The visible spectrum includes light waves whose wavelengths are 0.4 to 0.7 μ; for such wavelengths ray optics fails for fibres having a diameter smaller than about 8 μ. When the fibres have a smaller diameter, each fibre behaves as a wave guide and only certain "modes" are transmitted along it without loss. Any general form of light wave entering the fibre contains both these "permitted" modes and modes which are forbidden. Energy from the forbidden modes is lost through the walls of the fibre, constituting the "diffraction losses." As the fibre diameter is increased the number of permitted modes increases very rapidly, with the result that fibres of 10 μ diameter transmit any form of entering wave without significant loss over lengths of 1 metre or more. It is in these circumstances also that we expect ray optics to be valid, and fortunately this is the case. For this reason it is possible to explain the properties of practical fibreoptic endoscopes using the simple methods of ray optics. Were this not so, it would be impossible to treat adequately the physics of these systems without the use of appreciably more advanced mathematics.

For the present purposes, however, the important fact is that we cannot reasonably hope for long endoscopes using fibres with a diameter smaller than about 10 μ, since it is essential that light falling on any one fibre is trapped and transmitted to the exit-face of that fibre without leakage of light through the walls. Some improvements in the technology of producing fibreoptic endoscopes will doubtless occur, but no fundamental improvement in the resolution of finer detail can be expected.

There are two uses of fibreoptic bundles in endoscopy: illumination and transportation of images. For conveying light from an external lamp to the distal end of an endoscope, fibres with a diameter of about 25 μ are generally used; there is no need to have any precise order in the bundle (*incoherent bundles*). For transporting an image from the distal to the proximal end of an endoscope, fibres of smaller diameter, typically 10 μ, are used and the ordering of the fibres over the proximal end of the bundle must coincide with the ordering of the same fibres over the distal end. Such ordered bundles of fibres are termed *coherent bundles*.

To appreciate the role of a coherent bundle in a fibreoptic instrument, it is useful to consider the construction of a typical endoscope using lenses. This is illustrated in Figure 1, where light from an object $P_1O_1Q_1$ passes through the endoscope and enters an observer's eye (E). The front group of lenses constitutes the *objective*, which forms a reduced image of $P_1O_1Q_1$ at $P'_1O'_1Q'_1$ in the tube of the endoscope. The paths of a cone of rays from the object point Q_1 is shown, forming the image of this point at Q'_1. This light proceeds beyond Q'_1 and is refocused by a *relay system* to form a second image of Q_1 at Q'_2. Thus $Q'_1 = Q_2$ acts as the object point for the relay system. In a similar way $Q'_2 = Q_3$ acts as the object point

for the *eyepiece*, which then forms an enlarged image of the final relayed image $(P'_2O'_2Q'_2)$ at a convenient distance from the *exit-pupil* at E so that it may be seen by the observer. In a practical endoscope there is of course more than one relay system between the image produced at O'_1 by the objective and that at O'_2, which is magnified by the eyepiece. In the simple case shown, the image at O'_1 is inverted; and since each relay system gives an inverted image of the object presented to it, the final image at O'_2 is corrected, in that the lower point Q_1 is imaged as the lower point Q'_2. The observer then sees a correctly oriented image, and this remains true provided an odd number of relay stages is employed.

In a fibreoptic endoscope the relay stages are replaced by a coherent fibre bundle (Fig. 2). An objective is used, as in the lens-type endoscope, to form an image on the distal end of the fibre bundle. Thus light from the object point Q_1 is focused at the image point Q'_1, and this light travels along the shaded fibre of the coherent bundle and emerges at Q'_2. This point in turn acts as the object point for the eyepiece, which produces a magnified image of the proximal end-face of the fibre bundle at a convenient viewing distance from the exit-pupil at E, where the observer's eye is placed. With each fibre of the bundle acting in this way, an image of the object is seen, this image consisting of a raster of small light spots whose colour and level of illumination are determined by the total amounts of light of the different wavelengths received by the distal ends of the corresponding fibres of the bundle.

The image of the lower point Q_1 of the object (Fig. 2) is formed in the upper half of the fibre

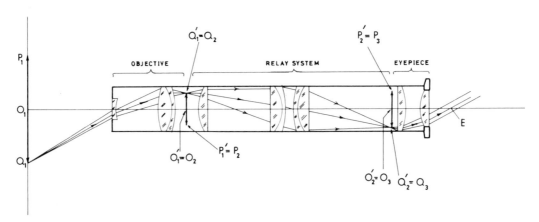

FIG. 1. Conventional endoscope.

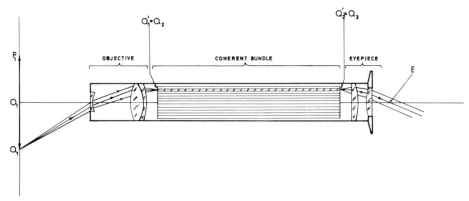

FIG. 2.   Fibreoptics endoscope.

bundle and emerges to give a final image point also in the upper part of this image. This inversion of the image may be corrected by arranging for the coherent fibre bundle to be twisted through 180 degrees between its distal and proximal ends.

If the central ray of each pencil of light falls normally on the distal face of the coherent bundle (Fig. 2) the pencils of light emerging from the different fibres at the proximal end also have their central rays parallel to the axis. This is an important condition, since the pencils entering the observer's eye then all intersect to form an exit-pupil at E exactly as for a lens-type endoscope. Unfortunately this is not always appreciated by the manufacturers of fibreoptic endoscopes.

TOTAL INTERNAL REFLECTION: USE OF CLAD FIBRES

A block of glass is shown in Figure 3 (top), with light incident from air on the face AA, giving "external" reflection, and light incident from the glass on the face BB, termed "internal" reflection. At near normal incidence—i.e., with the angle of incidence (I) small as in the cases of the upper rays shown—approximately 5 percent of the incident light is reflected in both cases, the remainder being transmitted. As the angle of incidence increases, the percentage of light reflected increases, but there is a marked difference for the two cases. For external reflection the coefficient of reflection increases with the angle of incidence, as shown by the curve R_A in the lower part of Figure 3. The reflection coefficient increases slowly, and

only attains 100 percent for grazing incidence $(I = 90$ degrees). By contrast, for internal reflection there is a rapid increase in the reflection coefficient as the angle of incidence approaches the so-called critical angle $I = I_c$, where I_c has a value of 36 to 42 degrees for most types of glass. For angles of incidence greater than the critical angle there is no transmitted light, as shown for the lower ray at

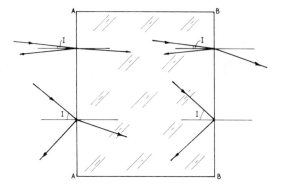

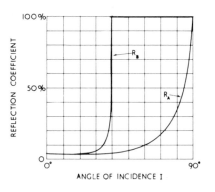

FIG. 3.   Reflection of light at an air-glass interface.

the face *BB* (Fig. 3), and the reflection coefficient is 100 percent for all such rays. This is the phenomenon of *total internal reflection.* It forms the essential basis of fibre optics.

Rays reflected along a 10 μ diameter fibre 1 metre long may experience as many as 10,000 reflections at the walls. Consequently it is essential to ensure that there is perfect total reflection. If there is any mechanical damage or contamination of the glass surface at the point of reflection, the reflection coefficient is less than 100 percent, and some light escapes. It is for this reason that "clad" fibres are used.

A clad (sheathed) fibre consists of a core fibre with a high refractive index and a cladding of glass that has a lower index. The thickness of the cladding is typically about 1 μ for the fibres used in coherent bundles. The composite fibre is produced in such a manner that the cladding is optically fused to the core.

The use of clad fibres is possible because total internal reflection always occurs on reflection at the interface of two transparent media such as glass, provided the light is incident in the "denser" medium (i.e., the medium with the higher refractive index) and the angle of incidence is greater than the critical angle for the particular case. If n is the refractive index of the denser medium in which the reflection occurs, and n' is that of the external medium of lower refractive index, the critical angle I_c is

$$\sin I_c = \frac{n'}{n} \qquad (1)$$

The dependence of I_c on the ratio of the two refractive indices is shown in Figure 4. The critical angle for a glass of index n with air as the external medium is given by Eq. (1) with $n' = 1.0$.

For the nominal values $n = 1.60$ and $n' = 1.50$, the critical angle is $I_c = 69.5°$. A ray reflected down a clad fibre is illustrated in Figure 5. All rays for which $I \geqslant I_c$ suffer total internal reflection at the walls. The angle of the ray to the fibre axis is $\alpha = 90° - I_c$, so that all rays for which $\alpha \leqslant (90° - 69.5°) = 20.5°$ are trapped in the fibre. This is already a large cone of rays compared with what is common: It corresponds to an effective F number of $F/0.8$, or to a numerical aperture *(N.A.)* of 0.56. This size of aperture is appreciably higher

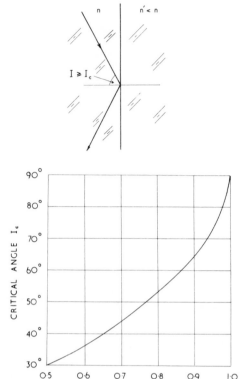

FIG. 4. Critical angle for reflection at a glass-glass interface.

than that normally required for an image-transmitting bundle but is not as high as the aperture angle often required for illumination. High-aperture fibres can be made using indices of the order of $n = 1.70$ and $n' = 1.52$, giving $F/0.62$ (i.e., N.A. = 0.80), and values of $n = 1.79$ for the core glass have been reported. Fibres of this type are useful when it is necessary to provide a wide-angle cone of light for illumination for endoscopy.

PROPAGATION OF LIGHT ALONG A STRAIGHT FIBRE

In Figure 5 a ray of light, making an angle (α_o) with the axis, enters one end of a clad fibre. This ray is refracted at O and makes a smaller angle (α) with the fibre axis. By the law of refraction, the angle α is

$$\sin \alpha = \frac{\sin \alpha_o}{n} \qquad (2)$$

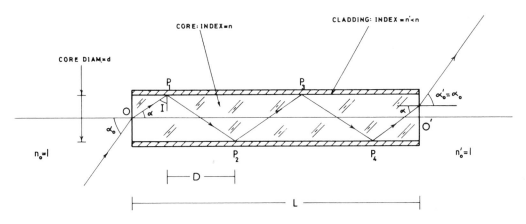

FIG. 5. Path of a ray in a straight fibre.

where n is the refractive index of the core glass. The ray inside the fibre is successively reflected at the points P_1, P_2, P_3, and P_4, finally emerging from point O' on the exit-face of the fibre.

The angle of incidence at P_1 on the fibre wall is given by $I = 90° - \alpha$, and total internal reflection occurs provided $I > I_c$ (i.e., when $\alpha < 90° - I_c$). Since the angles of incidence and reflection are equal, and the wall of the fibre is a cylinder, the angles of incidence at P_1, P_2, P_3, and P_4 are all equal. Consequently each segment of the multiply-reflected ray makes the same angle (α) with the fibre axis, and the angle of incidence of the ray at O' on the exit face is also equal to α. The law of refraction gives for the angle α'_o between the emergent ray and the normal to the exit-face the equation

$$\sin \alpha'_o = n \sin \alpha \qquad (3)$$

so that, in view of Eq. (2), $\alpha'_o = \alpha_o$. Thus if a cone of light of semiangle α_o is focused on the entry-face of a fibre, it emerges from the exit-face as a cone of precisely the same semiangle. This assumes that the central ray of the incident cone is normal to the entry-face and that the light emerges from the fibre into air.

The above is an extremely important result and explains why in the fibreoptic endoscope of Figure 2, for example, the light cone emerges from the image point O'_2 as shown and can enter the observer's eye at E. If the emergent light cone were of much larger angle than the entering cone, only a small fraction of it would be received by the observer's eye, with a conse-quent serious reduction in the level of illumination in the image.

It is important to know the number of reflections suffered by any given ray in travers-ing a fibre. From Figure 5, if d is the diameter of the fibre, the axial distance between succes-sive reflections is given by

$$D = \frac{d}{\tan \alpha} \qquad (4)$$

For an endoscopic image bundle a typical value would be $d = 10 \ \mu$; and if $\tan \alpha = 0.1$, the successive reflections occur at distances along the fibre separated by only $100 \ \mu = 0.1$ mm. For this ray, then, there would be 100 reflec-tions per centimetre, i.e., 10,000 per metre. It is because of this very large number of reflections that clad fibres must be used to en-sure that total reflection is not frustrated by damage or contamination of the surfaces of the fibres.

Another source of light loss is by absorption as the ray propagates through the glass of the core. This absorption depends on the total length of the ray in the material. In Figure 5 the length of the segment $(P_1 P_2)$ of the ray is given by $D/\cos \alpha$, and similarly for all other segments of the ray. The length of path (P) of the ray is thus given by

$$P = \frac{L}{\cos \alpha}$$

where L is the length of the fibre. For $\tan \alpha = 0.1$, the value of $1/\cos \alpha$ is equal to 1.005.

Hence in this case the length along the ray differs from the fibre length by about 0.5 percent; and the absorption is thus sensibly the same as for direct transmission of a ray through a thickness (L) of the core glass.

If in Figure 6 we consider a cone of rays entering the fibre at point O of the entry-face, the rays of the emergent beam fill the exit-face PQ, as shown in the upper diagram; but, as seen earlier, the extreme rays of the emergent beam always make the same angle with the fibre axis as those of the entering pencil. Why the emergent light fills the whole exit-face is illustrated in the lower diagram of Figure 6, where two rays entering at O emerge from two different points $(O'_1$ and $O'_2)$ of the exit-face. In practice of course there are a great number of reflections, resulting in there being uniform illumination of the exit-face no matter how the entering light is distributed over the entry-face.

A single fibre thus transmits the light to give a uniform patch of light at the exit-face, whose brightness is determined by the total amount of light falling on the entry-face. The detailed light distribution over this face is completely blurred on transmission down the fibre.

If the small losses due to imperfect total reflection and absorption are neglected, the amount of light that is accepted and transmitted by a fibre of given diameter is determined by its *numerical aperture*. In Figure 5 the maximum cone angle (α_o) accepted by the fibre occurs when the angle of incidence at the wall is equal to the critical angle (I_c). Rays incident at

O at greater angles to the axis have only a small amount of light reflected back into the fibre, the remainder passing out through the wall and cladding. In a fibre bundle this light is finally absorbed at the containing sheath.

Using Eq. (1) and some simple geometry, the maximum value of α_o occurs when

$$\sin \alpha_o = (n^2 - n'^2)^{1/2} \qquad (5)$$

or if the external medium has refractive index n_o the left-hand side must be replaced by $n_o \sin \alpha_o$. This is the numerical aperture, so that

$$N.A. = n_o \sin \alpha_o = (n^2 - n'^2)^{1/2} \qquad (6)$$

which reduces to Eq. (5) when the external medium is air, having $n_o = 1.0$.

If light emerges from the exit-face into a medium such as water, for which $n'_o = 1.333 > 1.0$, a ray such as that entering in air at O in Figure 7 suffers only a slight refraction on emerging from the fibre at O'. By the law of refraction, we have at O'

$$\sin \alpha'_o = \frac{n \sin \alpha}{n'_o}$$

or by Eq. (2)

$$\sin \alpha'_o = \frac{\sin \alpha_o}{n'_o} \qquad (7)$$

so the emergent cone is of a smaller angle than

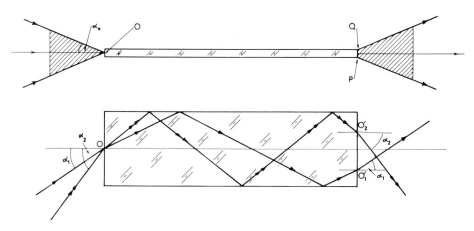

FIG. 6.   Light beam emerging from a fibre.

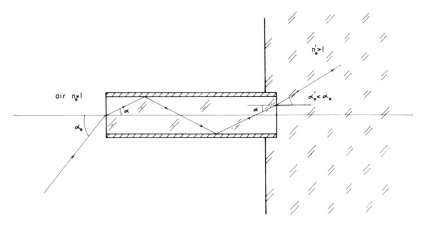

FIG. 7. Light emerging into a medium such as water: $\eta'_o > 1$.

the incident cone of light. For water the angle α'_o is given approximately by $\frac{3}{4}\alpha_o$. This is an important factor when as in cystoscopy illumination of a wide angle of field is desired with water as the medium.

PROPAGATION OF LIGHT ALONG A CURVED FIBRE: INFLUENCE OF FIBRE CONSTRICTION

The two decisive advantages of fibre optics in endoscopy are: (1) the high numerical aperture, which permits high levels of illumination from an external lamp; and (2) the great flexibility of both light guides for illumination and coherent bundles in those endoscopic procedures not possible with a rigid endoscope.

With a straight fibre a pencil of light entering with its central ray perpendicular to the entry-face emerges as a cone of rays (of the same angle as the incident cone) with its central ray perpendicular to the exit-face. The fundamental importance of this fact was noted above. It is fortunate that this result also holds for a curved fibre. Were this not so, the light cone emerging from the distal end of a flexible light guide used for illumination would swing about and illuminate a different part of the object being observed each time the light guide was moved. The same difficulty would be experienced in observing the image formed by a flexible fibreoptic endoscope. In Figure 5, for example, the light cone emerging from the image point O'_2 at the proximal end of the coherent bundle would not remain normal to the

exit-face and consequently would then pass only partly or not at all to the observer's eye at E. The usefulness of the flexibility of a fibreoptic endoscope thus rests on the fact that a curved fibre has substantially the same properties as a straight fibre.

The reason for this at first surprising result may be understood by reference to Figure 8. An entering ray is reflected at P_1, P_2, and P_3 in a straight portion of fibre. It then enters a curved portion of fibre, where it is reflected at P_4, P_5, and P_6; this length of fibre is a circular arc with its centre at C and of bending radius R. On leaving the curved part of the fibre the ray is reflected at P_7 and P_8 in a second straight portion of fibre and emerges at O'.

The angles of incidence at P_1, P_2, and P_3 are all equal; thus at P_3 the angle of incidence is $I_3 = I$, where I is the angle of incidence in the straight length of fibre. The angle of reflection at P_3 (i.e., $\angle CP_3P_4$) is also equal to I. If I_4 and I_5 are the angles of incidence (equal to the angles of reflection) at points P_4 and P_5, the sine rule applied to the triangles P_3CP_4 and P_4CP_5 gives

$$\frac{\sin I_4}{\sin I_3} = \frac{CP_3}{CP_4} \tag{8}$$

$$\frac{\sin I_5}{\sin I_4} = \frac{CP_4}{CP_5} \tag{9}$$

The radius of bending of the fibre is R; so that if r is the radius of the fibre, $CP_3 = R + r$, $CP_4 = R - r$, and $CP_5 = R + r$. Using these values in Eq. (8) and (9) and noting that $I_3 = I$

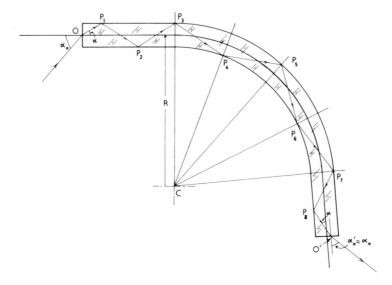

FIG. 8. Path of a ray in a curved fibre.

$$\sin I_4 = \left(\frac{R + r}{R + r}\right) \sin I$$

$$\sin I_5 = \left(\frac{R - r}{R + r}\right) \sin I_4$$

$$= \left(\frac{R - r}{R + r}\right)\left(\frac{R + r}{R - r}\right) \sin I$$

hence

$$\sin I_4 = \left(\frac{1 + r/R}{1 - r/R}\right) \sin I \qquad (10)$$

$$\sin I_5 = \sin I$$

so that $I_5 = I$.

In a similar manner it is found that after any number of reflections in a curved part of the fibre the angle of incidence at the outer edge of fibre is always equal to I. For the case shown in Figure 8, therefore, the angles of incidence and reflection at P_7 are both equal to I. It follows that the angles of incidence (e.g., at P_7 and P_8) in the final straight portion of fibre are also equal to I; consequently these ray segments all make the same angle (α) with the fibre axis as in the first straight portion of fibre. Thus if the ray enters the fibre at O making an angle (α_o)

with the fibre axis, it emerge from O' making the same angle ($\alpha'_o = \alpha_o$) with the direction of the axis of the fibre at the exit-face.

The angles of incidence at the inner edge of the fibre (e.g., those at P_4 and P_6) are also all equal to I_4. For fibres of diameters as large as 50 μ, with a radius *(r)* of 0.025 mm, and a very short bending radius *(R* = 10 mm)*, the angle I_4 is given by $\sin I_4 = 1.0050 \sin I$. Hence the angles of incidence in the curved part of the fibre never differ from those in the straight portion by more than 0.5 percent, even in the extreme case considered. Therefore in Figure 8 if the ray had entered the final straight portion of the fibre after a reflection at the inner edge of the curved part of the fibre, the direction of the emergent ray would not have been sensibly different.

In practice a fibre bundle is prevented from flexure into too short a bending radius by means of the containing sheath. This is to minimise the danger of fibre breakage; a short bending radius *(R)*, typically in excess of 50 mm, is usually imposed. The propagation of light in the fibres of such a flexible endoscope does not differ essentially from its propagation in a straight fibre.

Careful control is exercised in the production of optical fibres to maintain a constant diameter. There is nevertheless always some residual variation in diameter, leaving constrictions (Fig. 9). The reflections at P_2 and P_3 take place

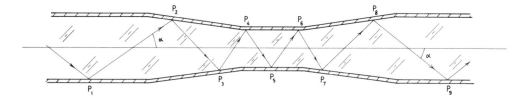

FIG. 9.   Path of a ray along a constricted fibre.

at the walls of a tapered portion of the fibre. The angle of incidence at P_2 is less than that at P_1, by an amount equal to the angle Θ that the tapering wall makes with the fibre axis. If α is the angle between the axis and the ray segment P_1P_3 after reflection at P_1, the inclination of the ray segment P_2P_3 to the axis is $\alpha + 2\Theta$; and this angle increases by 2Θ after each reflection. The result is that on entering the narrower length of fibre between P_4 and P_6 the inclination of the ray segments to the axis is greater than α and the angles of incidence at P_4, P_5, and P_6 are correspondingly smaller than at P_1. Consequently if the rays shown were at the full numerical aperture permitted by the given fibre, the angles of incidence at P_4, P_5, and P_6 would be less than the critical angle, and light would leak out of the fibre.

In practice loss of light from this cause is avoided in the case of coherent bundles because the numerical aperture of the light beams to be transmitted by the fibres of the bundle is appreciably less than the full aperture that the fibres would accept. It is the need for depth of focus in an endoscope that usually entails the use of numerical apertures some five times smaller than the maximum permitted by the fibres used. In these circumstances the reduced angles of incidence following reflections at a converging tapered portion of fibre can remain greater than the critical angle so that the light remains trapped.

Following the narrowed length of fibre in Figure 9, the light enters a diverging taper in which the reflections at P_7 and P_8 restore the original value of α, the inclination of the ray to the fibre axis. Thereafter the ray proceeds to be reflected at P_9 and so along the part of the fibre beyond the constriction. For small angles of aperture no light is lost at the constriction, and the fibre behaves as if the diameter had remained constant. In the case of an illuminating bundle used at its full numerical aperture, the effect of a constriction is to reduce the light

transmitted to that of a fibre of diameter equal to the smallest diameter at the constricted part of the fibre. Thus for light guides the effect of constrictions is to reduce the total amount of light transmitted. For an image-transmitting bundle, if used with the full permitted aperture, there would be deleterious effects on the image in that fibres with different constrictions would show different light losses and so fail to reproduce faithfully the image received at the distal end of the bundle.

ILLUMINATION SYSTEMS: FACTORS AFFECTING BRIGHTNESS AND COLOUR

A typical illuminating system for an endoscope is illustrated in Figure 10. Light from the lamp passes through a heat filter and then high-aperture condensor lenses, which form an image of the light source on the entry-face of the flexible light guide. This comprises an incoherent flexible fibre bundle and is commonly up to 2 metres in length. The light guide is coupled to the endoscope to place the exit-face of the flexible light guide substantially in contact with a corresponding light guide, also an incoherent bundle, which lies inside the endoscope; a cone of light emerges from the distal end of the light guide to illuminate the area being viewed.

The two important properties of such an illuminating system are the total light transmitted and the angle of field illuminated by the light cone emerging from the distal end of the light guide in the endoscope. In Figure 10 α' is the angle of the edge ray of the cone of light focused on the entry-face of the flexible light guide. The light emerging from the exit-face is a cone with a semiangle equal to α'. This is also the angle of the extreme rays entering the light guide in the endoscope, which accordingly gives an emergent cone with $\alpha'' = \alpha'$ when it

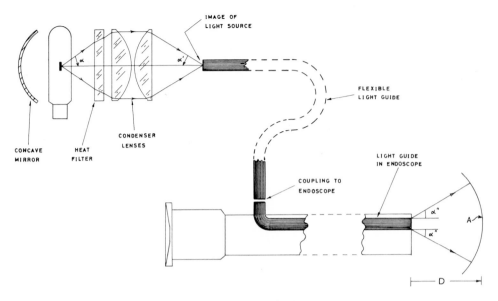

FIG. 10. Endoscope illuminating system.

emerges into air. A typical condensor system gives cones for which sin α' is not greater than about 0.50, so that $\alpha' \leq 30°$. Therefore when the endoscope is used in an air-filled cavity, for example, the total angle of field is $2\alpha' \leq 60°$.

If, as in cystoscopy, the illuminating cone emerges into water (whose refractive index is 1.333) the value of α'' is given, using Eq. (7), by sin $\alpha'' = 0.3751$ so that $\alpha'' = 22°$ and the total angle of field is only $2\alpha'' = 44°$. In practice the total angle of field used by a cystoscope may be as large as 70 degrees, so the illumination must provide a cone of at least this angle. This may be achieved in part by dividing the illuminating bundle in the endoscope into two or more smaller bundles at the distal end, which are then suitably "angled." Alternatively the light guide in the endoscope may use fibres of higher numerical aperture. For *N.A.* = 0.80, the angle α'' is given by sin $\alpha'' = 0.80/1.333 = 0.60$, from which $\alpha'' = 37°$ and the total field angle is $2\alpha'' = 74°$. To achieve this of course the light cone entering the proximal end of the light guide in the endoscope must also have a numerical aperture of 0.80. This can be obtained by using a fibre cone to feed light from the coupling to this light guide, when the angles of rays to the axis are increased after each reflection at the walls, as with the effect of constriction in a fibre.

The problem of illumination in the case of a wide-angle endoscope working in water is far from trivial. In the case of endoscopy of the digestive tract, however, providing illumination of the desired angle of field is well within the performance capability of ordinary light guides.

We come now to the questions of the overall transmittance of light by an endoscope illuminating system and the level of illumination received at any distance *(D)* from the distal end of the endoscope. These are affected by the following factors, some of which are interdependent:

1. Total light accepted by the condensor from the lamp
2. Reflection losses at air-glass surfaces
3. Transmittances of the two light guides
4. Losses at the coupling of the two light guides
5. Angle (α'') of the final illuminating cone
6. Distance *(D)* of the object from the distal end of the endoscope

If the source itself (e.g., a filament) presents an area *S*, the total light accepted from it by a condensor of aperture angle α (Fig. 10) is given by the formula

$$F = \pi BS \sin^2 \alpha \qquad (11)$$

The quantity *B* is a measure of the intrinsic luminosity of the source. If the source consists of an open filament, its effective area can be increased with a concave mirror (Fig. 10), which can re-image light travelling backward from the filament into the spaces between the coils of the filament itself. In favourable cases this can increase the effective value of the source area (S) by about 50 percent. It is assumed that this increase in effective area is included in S in Eq. (11).

The source (S) is imaged by the condensor lenses on the entry-face of the flexible light guide, where the aperture angle is α'. The linear magnification between this image and the source is given by

$$M = \frac{\sin \alpha}{\sin \alpha'} \qquad (12)$$

so that the magnification for areas is

$$\frac{S'}{S} = M^2 = \left(\frac{\sin \alpha}{\sin \alpha'}\right)^2 \qquad (13)$$

where S' is the area of the image of the source. Using Eq. (13) the total light flux (F) given by Eq. (11) may be written alternatively as

$$F = \pi B S' \sin^2 \alpha' \qquad (14)$$

The maximum value of S' exists when the source image just fills the entry-face of the light guide and $\sin \alpha'$ has its maximum value corresponding to the numerical aperture accepted by the fibres of the guide.

The total light flux falling on the entry-face of the light guide is thus determined by the luminance of the source and the product of the area and the square of the numerical aperture of the guide. It must be strongly emphasised that this is the maximum useful light that can be taken from the source. A great deal of fruitless effort has been expended in the hope of defeating this fundamental law of the photometry of optical systems. Provided the image of the light source completely fills the entry face, and the cones of light forming this image have $\sin \alpha'$ equal to the N.A. of the fibres, no increase in the amount of usable light from the source is possible.

Equations (11) and (12) give the light flux arriving at the entry face of the flexible light guide on the assumption that no light is lost by reflections at the air-glass surfaces of the heat filter and condensor lenses, or by absorption in the glass of those components. To find the ef-

fects of such light losses, it is necessary to find the transmittance (always expressed as a fraction) of each surface and of the given thicknesses of glass. The overall transmittance is then given by the product of the separate transmittances.

When there is loss by surface reflections, R denotes the fraction of light reflected. The fraction of light transmitted by a single surface is then equal to $(1 - R)$, and the transmittance of N surfaces is given by

$$T = (1 - R)^N \qquad (15)$$

The percentage transmittance is obtained by multiplying this value of T by 100. The curves of Figure (11) show this percentage transmittance for N values up to 20, for untreated air-glass surfaces when the refractive index of the glass is either 1.55 or 1.65. For these cases the reflection losses for a single surface are 4.65 and 6.02 percent, respectively, so that R is 0.0465 and 0.0602, respectively. The higher the refractive index of the glass, the greater the reflection losses. Curve A shows the improvement expected from ordinary blooming of the surfaces, which reduces the reflection loss per surface to about 1.5 percent. The above reflection losses do not differ greatly in the different parts of the visible spectrum, i.e., for wavelengths between 0.4 and 0.7 μ. Using multilayer antireflection coatings the reflection loss per surface can be reduced to less than 0.5 percent throughout the visible region.

For the heat filter and condensor lenses in

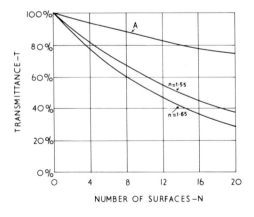

FIG. 11. Transmittance through N air-glass surfaces. Curve A, Single-layer antireflection coated surfaces.

Figure 10, there are six air-glass surfaces, for which the transmittance *(T)* is 0.68 to 0.75 for refractive indices (λ) of 1.65 to 1.55. On this account alone, therefore, the light loss can amount to between 32 and 25 percent. Even with ordinary blooming this loss is reduced to less than 10 percent.

The curves in Figure 11 show that the improvement resulting from the use of antireflection coatings rapidly becomes greater as the number of air-glass surfaces increase. In this connection the light in the illuminating system of Figure 10 encounters a total of 10 air-glass surfaces. For $N = 10$, the curves in Figure 11 show that the reflection losses are 40 to 45 percent for untreated surfaces; with ordinary blooming the loss is reduced to 15 percent, and to less that 5 percent for multilayer anti-reflection coatings. These results make clear the importance of keeping the number of air-glass surfaces in the light path to a minimum, and of using good antireflection coatings on those surfaces which are unavoidable.

When light traverses a plate of glass or a lens, there is absorption in the glass in addition to reflection losses at the two surfaces. *Internal transmittance* is the ratio of the light reaching the exit-face to that which came in at the entry-face; this definition assumes perfect antireflection coatings on the two surfaces. The *overall transmittance* of a given component is then equal to the product of the internal transmittance and the separate transmittances of the two bounding surfaces.

The absorption of glass is specified by giving the value of the internal transmittance (T_o) for a standard length (L_o). For any other length *(L)* the internal transmittance is given by the formula

$$T = T_o^{(L/L_o)} \qquad (16)$$

For ordinary optical glass the value of T_o usually refers to a length (L_o) of 25 mm. The internal transmittance for a length *(L)* of 1 metre, for example, is then given by $T = T_o^{40}$; for a length *(L)* of 100 mm the internal transmittance would be $T = T_o^4$. Curves showing the variation of T with wavelength for these two *L* values are shown in Figure 12 for a good quality ordinary optical flint glass having a refractive index (λ) of 1.62 for the green wavelength in the middle of the visible spectrum.

The total thickness of glass of the two con-

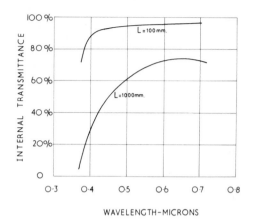

FIG. 12. Internal transmittance of an ordinary optical flint glass; $n = 1.62$.

densor lenses shown in Figure 10 would not exceed 40 mm, so that their loss by glass absorption would be only 1 to 2 percent throughout the entire visible spectrum. For greater thicknesses the fact that there is greater absorption in the blue end of the spectrum (i.e., shorter wavelengths) becomes significant. The longer the length of glass traversed, the greater the relative depletion of blue in the transmitted light.

In most glasses the transmittance becomes zero at wavelengths just below 0.4 μ, and they are therefore opaque for almost the entire ultraviolet region of the spectrum. However, even the absorption at 0.4 μ is of little account visually, because the eye responds only to light with wavelengths in the region 0.4 to 0.7 μ, with a relative efficiency of the form shown in Figure 13. This curve does not apply in the

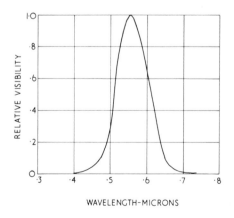

FIG. 13. Relative efficiency of the eye at different wavelengths.

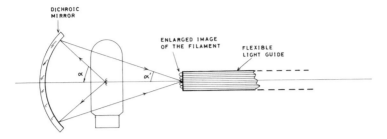

FIG. 14. Use of dichroic mirror for an illuminating system.

case of extremely weak illumination, when it is the rods of the retina rather than the cones that detect light. In this case the maximum visibility is for light of a wavelength equal to 0.50 μ, i.e., about 0.05 μ nearer the blue end of the spectrum than is the case for ordinary vision, which is that shown in Figure 13.

For the system illustrated in Figure 10 approximately 30 percent of the useful light leaving the source may be lost by reflections at the air-glass surfaces before it reaches the entry-face of the flexible light guide. Only a certain fraction of this light is transmitted.

An alternative to the use of a heat filter and condensor lenses is shown in Figure 14. The concave mirror is a dichroic reflector, being transparent to infrared radiation but having high reflectivity for visible light. After reflection at the dichroic mirror an enlarged image of the filament is formed on the entry-face of the flexible light guide. This mirror acts as both a heat filter and a condensor. The reflection coefficient can be made greater than 95 percent for the entire visible region of the spectrum—from 0.4 to 0.7 μ—while the reflection coefficient for the infrared region can be made as low as 20 percent or smaller. Thus 80 percent of the heat is removed from the beam. Nevertheless with high-intensity lamps sufficient heat to damage the fibres at the entry-face of the flexible light guide may remain.

The image of the filament in this case is also free from the colour effects arising from the chromatic aberration that is present when a lens system is used for the condensor. The mirror system thus has a number of advantages; but since most of the light must pass again through the lamp, it encounters four additional air-glass surfaces, the reflection losses which cannot be avoided by using antireflection coatings. Moreover, the acceptance angle (α) must be larger than the desired value of α', in

accordance with the magnification law stated in Eq. (12).

We now consider what fraction of the light is transmitted by the light guides of the endoscope. The fibres of any light guide are, as usual, clad with a glass of low refractive index, and the separate fibres are bonded together at each end of the light guide. Bonding is effected either with an epoxy cement or by fusing the glass claddings. The latter method is often preferred because heat from the lamp, not all of which is removed by the heat filter, can affect the epoxy cement. In either case it is only the core glass of each fibre that traps entering light and transmits it along the guide. Light falling on the cladding or the cement is not trapped and is eventually lost by absorption at the walls of the containing sheath.

A typical arrangement of the fibres in a bundle is illustrated in Figure 15. The ratio of the total area occupied by the fibre cores (hatched areas, Fig. 15) to the whole area of the bundle defines the *core packing fraction (G)*. The value of this packing fraction is customarily about 0.70, so that only 70 percent of the area of the bundle is active. In addition to this factor there are reflection losses at the two air-glass surfaces at the ends of the fibre cores. These use

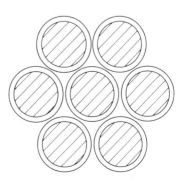

FIG. 15. Packing fraction *G*.

glass of high refractive index, so that the reflection loss may amount to 6 percent per surface. If R (equal to 0.06 in this case) is the fraction of light reflected at each face, the transmittance of the light guide is given by

$$T = G(1 - R)^2 \qquad (17)$$

assuming no losses by absorption or by imperfect total reflection. For $G = 0.70$ and $R = 0.06$, the transmittance is 0.62, i.e., 62 percent.

The effects of both absorption and imperfect total reflection may be taken into account by defining an *internal transmittance* for a fibre of specified length. Thus if T_o is the internal transmittance for a length (L_o) of fibre, the overall transmittance of a light guide of length L, using Eq. (17), is

$$T = G(1 - R)^2 T_o{}^{(L/L_o)} \qquad (18)$$

Reported values for the overall transmittance of good quality light guides for white light are typically about 50 percent for lengths of 1 metre. If T_o in Eq. (18) is taken to refer to $L_o = 1$ metre, Eq. (18), for the overall transmittance, gives for $L = 1$ metre

$$T = G(1 - R)^2 T_o$$

or, since $G(1 - R)^2 = 0.62$ as found above, the reported transmittance (T) of 0.50 for a 1-metre light guide implies a T_o value of 0.80. Thus if the length of guide L is given in metres, Eq. (18) for the overall transmittance of the guide may be written

$$T = G(1 - R)^2 T_o{}^L \qquad (19)$$

where the internal transmittance (T_o) has a value of about 0.80. For a 2-metre guide, using $G(1 - R)^2 = 0.62$ and $T_o = 0.80$, Eq. (18) gives $T = 0.40$. This value of 40 percent is again typical of the overall transmittance of white light reported for good quality 2-metre light guides.

In Eq. (19) the quantity G is independent of the wavelength of the light, as is R. The final factor T_o is determined predominantly by absorption in glass, and this can vary appreciably with the wavelength. Because of the greater absorption for shorter wavelengths, the longer the length of the guide, the greater the relative depletion of blue in the transmitted light.

This consideration is of particular importance in medical endoscopy where detecting detail often depends on perceiving differences in colour.

The dependence on wavelength of the overall transmittance of a light guide may be usefully specified in the following manner. Let $T_o(\lambda)$ be the internal transmittance for light of wavelength λ of a 1-metre fibre. The overall transmittance for light of this wavelength is then given by

$$T(\lambda) = G(1 - R)^2 \{T_o(\lambda)\}^L \qquad (20)$$

as in Eq. (19) for white light. If

$$W_\lambda = \frac{T_o(\lambda)}{T_o} \qquad (21)$$

is used to denote the ratio of the internal transmittance for light of wavelength λ to the internal transmittance for white light, both being for a 1-metre fibre, combining Eq. (19) and (20) gives

$$T(\lambda) = T W_\lambda{}^L \qquad (22)$$

This formula expresses the overall transmittance for light of wavelength λ in terms of the overall transmittance for white light and the weighting factor W_λ.

If the internal transmittance $T_o(\lambda)$ for a given type of fibre is known for a set of N equally spaced wavelengths, the weighting factors W_λ may be found using Eq. (22) together with the formula

$$T_o = \left[\frac{1}{N-1}\right]\left[\frac{1}{2}T_o(\lambda) + T_o(\lambda_2)\right.$$
$$\left. + \ldots + T_o(\lambda_{N-1}) + \frac{1}{2}T_o(\lambda_N)\right] \qquad (23)$$

used to give the internal transmittance for white light. Equation (23) assumes "white" to mean light having constant energy throughout the entire visible spectrum.

An example is given in Figure 16. Using the four values of $T_o(\lambda)$ at wavelengths (λ) of 0.4, 0.5, 0.6, and 0.7 μ, Eq. (23) gives $T_o = 0.75$. This is rather less than the value $T_o = 0.80$ deduced above on the assumption of a meas-

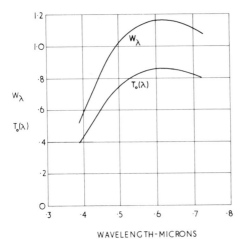

WAVELENGTH-MICRONS

FIG. 16. The internal transmittance $T_o(\lambda)$ and the wavelength weighting factor W_λ for a 1-metre fibre.

ured overall white light transmittance *(T)* of 0.50 for a good light 1-metre guide. This could be due to the "white" light used in these measurements having less blue than that of the equienergy spectrum used above to specify what is meant by "white" light. The values of W_λ given by Eq. (21) and (23) are also shown in Figure 16.

By Eq. (22) the quantity $W_\lambda{}^L$ is equal to the ratio of the overall transmittance (for light of wavelength λ) of a light guide L metres long to the overall transmittance of the same guide for white light. This ratio is shown as a function of wavelength in Figure 17 for light guides 1, 2, 3, and 4 metres long *(L)*. These curves show how serious the depletion of light in the blue region of the spectrum can be. A fibreoptic colonoscope, used with a flexible 2-metre light guide would have an overall length *(L)* at least equal to 4 metres. In this case if the source does not have a high colour temperature, the images seen inevitably are markedly yellow. In fact the transmittance is a maximum for the wavelength 0.6 μ (Fig. 17); this is yellow light, the colour of a sodium lamp.

Losses occur at the coupling of two light guides, e.g., at the junction of the flexible light guide in Figure 10 and the light guide in the endoscope. Unless the exit-face of the first bundle is placed in close contact with the entry-face of the second bundle, light is lost (Fig. 18A). For the large separation shown in Figure 18A, some light is lost even from the cones emerging from the central fibres of the bundle.

The peripheral parts of the cone of light emerging from O'_1, for example, fall outside the entry-face of the second bundle, and light in the shaded region is lost. For a fibre at the edge of the first bundle (e.g., that at O'_2) half of the emergent light beam falls outside the second bundle. This source of loss is of course easily avoided by ensuring close contact between the abutting ends of the two bundles.

An unavoidable source of loss is that arising from a *mismatch* between the individual fibres of the two bundles. If each fibre of the first bundle were exactly opposite a corresponding fibre of the second bundle, there would be no light loss apart from that from the two air-glass surface reflections. In practice there is a greater or less degree of mismatch, the worst case of which is illustrated in Figure 18B. Light emerging from the core of the fibre of the first bundle and falling on the claddings or in the interspaces between fibres of the second bundle is not trapped and is not transmitted. For the case shown, only light from the hatched region of the fibre of the first bundle in

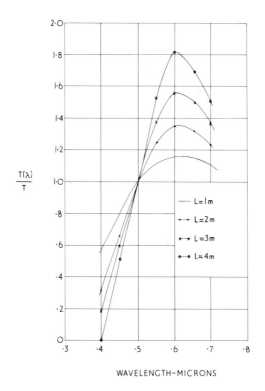

WAVELENGTH-MICRONS

FIG. 17. Ratio of the overall transmittance of a fibre bundle for different wavelengths to the overall transmittance for white light.

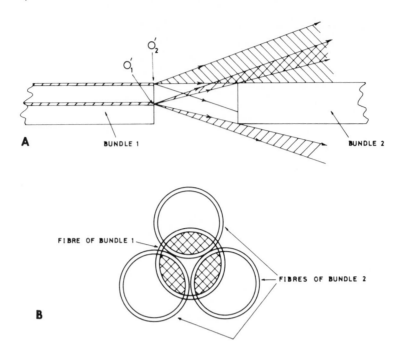

FIG. 18. Light losses on coupling two light guides. **A.** Separation effect. **B.** Mismatch.

Figure 18 is transmitted along the fibres of the second bundle.

The area of overlap of the core regions of fibres in the two bundles varies from complete overlap of two corresponding fibres to that seen in Figure 18B. The *mismatch factor (M)* is defined as the ratio of the total area of overlap of all the fibres of the two bundles to the total active area (i.e., of the cones) of the first bundle. An estimated value to be expected for M is 0.80; i.e., 20 percent of the light may be lost from this cause alone.

The overall transmittance of a second bundle L metres long, when fed by light from a preceding bundle, is given by

$$T = M (1 - R)^2 T_o^L \qquad (24)$$

the factor $(1 - R)^2$ taking into account the two surface reflection losses. Equation (24) is simply Eq. (19) with the core packing fraction G replaced by the mismatch factor M.

If there are two light guides in tandem (of lengths L_1 and L_2) the transmittance of the whole guide is given, combining Eq. (19) and (20), by

$$T = G(1 - R)^2 T_o^{L_1} M (1 - R)^2 T_o^{L_2}$$

This formula may be written

$$T = G(1 - R)^2 T_o^{(L_1 + L_2)} \left[M(1 - R)^2 \right] \quad (25)$$

which is equal to the overall transmittance of a single guide of length $(L_1 + L_2)$ multiplied by the factor $M(1 - R)^2$, which is the transmittance of the coupling. With $M = 0.80$ and $R = 0.06$, this coupling transmittance has the value $M(1 - R)^2 = 0.71$; i.e., the coupling reduces the transmittance by 29 percent. It is for this reason that, to obtain a higher level of illumination, the light cable is frequently made integral with the light guide of the endoscope.

The effect of replacing a coupling by an integral guide is to increase the light transmittance by the factor $1/0.71 = 1.41$; i.e., elimination of the coupling can increase the light by 41 percent of that obtained using a coupling. It is not always feasible to do this in practice, particularly where a large angle of field in a medium such as water must be illuminated. In such cases a coupling consisting of a conical fibre bundle may be employed, in order to increase the numerical aperture of the light entering the light guide in the endoscope. Couplings of this kind are described later.

A typical flexible light guide is approximately 2 metres long and has a diameter of 3 to 4 mm; it provides an illuminating cone in air of half-angle equal to about 35 degrees. The numerical aperture is thus $N.A. = \sin 35° = 0.57$. A numerical aperture of this size may be obtained using glasses of refractive index equal to around 1.60 for the core and 1.50 for the cladding glass. Even with such a relatively low index for the core glass, special precautions are necessary to obtain glass of lower absorption in the blue end of the spectrum than that customarily found even with good-quality optical glass. To obtain a larger numerical aperture the core must have glass of higher refractive index, and this carries with it greater absorption for the shorter wavelengths in the visible spectrum. It is for this reason that it is desirable to use as short a high-aperture light guide as possible in any system.

The angles of field usually employed in fibre-optics endoscopes for the digestive tract may be illuminated using relatively low-aperture bundles. In other cases, notably in wide-angle cystoscopes, the light guide in the endoscope demands a higher numerical aperture. For example, with a total angle of field of 70 degrees in water, the necessary numerical aperture is given by $1.333 \times \sin 35° = 0.76$. In such cases a low-aperture flexible light guide from the lamp may be coupled to a high-aperture guide in the endoscope by means of a conical fibre bundle.

The arrangement is shown in Figure 19, where pencils of light of a smaller aperture (α_I) enter bundle 1. After traversing the fibre cone this light enters the fibres of bundle 2 to emerge as pencils of larger aperture (α'_2). The action of the converging fibres in the fibre cone is as was depicted in Figure 9. Each fibre of the cone tapers to a smaller diameter, the reduction ratio (K) being equal to the ratio of the larger to the smaller diameter of the whole fibre cone. In the air space between bundle 1

and the fibre cone, the aperture angle of the light pencils is $\alpha'_I = \alpha_I$. On emerging from the fibre cone the aperture angle in the following air space is given by

$$\sin \alpha_2 = K \sin \alpha_I \qquad (26)$$

and this light emerges from bundle 2 with the increased aperture angle $\alpha'_2 = \alpha_2$. If the medium at the distal end of bundle 2 were of refractive index n'_2, the aperture angle would be given by

$$\sin \alpha'_2 = \frac{\sin \alpha_2}{n'_2}$$

or, using Eq. (26),

$$\sin \alpha'_2 = \left(\frac{K}{n'_2}\right) \sin \alpha_I \qquad (27)$$

The action of the fibre cone is simply to increase the aperture by the factor K while reciprocally reducing the diameter of the illumination area by the same factor.

The fibres of the cone must have the higher aperture $(\sin \alpha_2)$. Because of the taper of each fibre, if light of an aperture greater than $\sin \alpha_2/K$ enters the cone, the outer rays are not trapped and are lost. Fortunately all entering rays of aperture $\leq \sin \alpha_2/K$ are transmitted, provided the fibres transmit the larger aperture of the finally emergent light.

To find the transmittance factor for such a fibre cone coupling, it has simply to be noted that there is a mismatch at both the entry- and exit-faces of the fibre cone, and four reflection losses at air-glass surfaces. The transmittance of a fibre cone coupling is thus given by

$$T = M^2(1 - R)^4 \qquad (28)$$

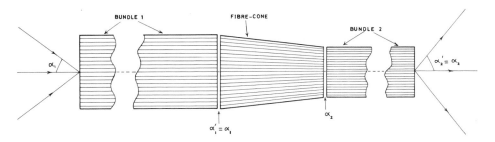

FIG. 19. Use of a conical fibre bundle to couple two light guides.

For $M = 0.8$ and $R = 0.06$, $T = 0.50$; thus 50 percent of the light may be lost at such a coupling, compared with 29 percent at a simple coupling. The advantage of a fibre cone coupling is that it permits a low-aperture bundle for the flexible light guide, thereby keeping to a minimum the length of the high-aperture guide. The transmittance may be increased if the fibre cone is cemented to the endoscope light guide, thereby eliminating two of the surface reflections.

The total light flux emerging from the distal end of the illuminating light guide of an endoscope is given by the flux (F) accepted from the lamp multiplied by the product of the transmittance factors $(T_1, T_2, \ldots, T_k)$ of the condensor system, light guides, and couplings. The intensity of illumination of the object depends on the area (A) of the object over which this total light flux is distributed and is given by

$$I = \frac{F(T_1, T_2 \ldots T_k)}{A} \qquad (29)$$

For the special case shown in Eq. (11), where the surface of the object is assumed to be a sphere of radius D, the area (A) is given by

$$A = 2\pi D^2 \, (1 - \cos \alpha'')$$

provided the size of the exit-face of the light guide is assumed to be small compared with the distance (D) of the object. Even for angles as large as 35 degrees the approximation $2(1 - \cos \alpha'') = \sin^2 \alpha''$ has an error of less than 10 percent, which reduces to about 3 percent for $\alpha'' = 20°$. The area illuminated may thus be written

$$A = \pi D^2 \sin^2 \alpha'' \qquad (30)$$

and since this increases with the square of the distance (D) the intensity of illumination at any surface varies inversely as the square of its distance from the distal end of the light guide. Consequently in endoscopic photography, for example, the greater the distance of the object from the endoscope, the longer the exposure times must be.

The dependence of the area illuminated on the value of $\sin^2 \alpha''$ does not affect the level of illumination, since obtaining an increased value of $\sin \alpha''$ demands a proportionately larger value of $\sin \alpha$ at the source. Consequently the total light flux $(F = \pi BS \sin^2 \alpha)$ accepted from the source is increased by precisely the same factor as the illuminated area $(A = \pi D^2 \sin^2 \alpha'')$.

To find the necessary accepted aperture $(\sin \alpha)$ at the source, let the light fall on the entry-face of the first light guide, with aperture $\sin \alpha'$. If S is the area of the source imaged to fill the area S' of this entry-face, then

$$S \, \sin^2 \alpha = S' \, \sin^2 \alpha' \qquad (31)$$

Suppose now that the first light guide is coupled by means of a fibre cone to a second light guide of area S''. As seen earlier the numerical aperture of the emergent pencils of light is then given by $\sin \alpha'' = K \sin \alpha'$, and the area of the exit-face of the cone is $S'' = S'/K^2$, where K is the ratio of the larger to the smaller diameter of the cone. Thus

$$S'' \, \sin^2 \alpha'' = (K^2 \, \sin^2 \alpha) \frac{S'}{K^2}$$

$$= S' \, \sin^2 \alpha'$$

and using Eq. (31) the angle (α'') of the pencils emerging from the second light guide is seen to be such that

$$S'' \, \sin^2 \alpha'' = S \, \sin^2 \alpha \qquad (32)$$

This equation provides the necessary acceptance aperture (α) of the condensor system, which must also image the source area (S) to fill the entry-face of the first light guide.

Using the relations $F = \pi BS \sin^2 \alpha$ and $A = \pi D^2 \sin^2 \alpha''$, the intensity of illumination given by Eq. (29) becomes

$$I = \frac{BS}{D^2} \left(\frac{\sin \alpha}{\sin \alpha''} \right)^2 (T_1, T_2 \ldots T_k) \qquad (33)$$

or, using Eq. (32) for the value of $S \sin^2 \alpha$

$$I = \frac{BS''}{D^2} (T_1, T_2 \ldots T_k) \qquad (34)$$

From this equation it is seen that for a given distance (D) the level of illumination depends only on the luminance (B) of the source, the total area of the distal end of the second light guide, and the product of the transmittance factors $(T_1, T_2 \ldots T_k)$. This important result assumes only that the source image completely fills the entry-face of the first light guide. If the angle (α) of the light accepted from the source is too small, it reduces the angle of field illuminated but not the level of illumination. The colour of the illumination depends on the colour temperature of the source and the variation with wavelength of the internal transmittances of the fibres used in the light guides.

If the light guide terminates in a medium of refractive index n'', the angle α'' is smaller than when emerging into air. As seen earlier $\sin \alpha''$ must then be replaced by $\sin \alpha''/n''$ in Eq. (32) and (33). Eq. (34) for the intensity of illumination must also be multiplied by the square of n''.

IMAGE-TRANSMITTING BUNDLES: FACTORS AFFECTING IMAGE BRIGHTNESS AND QUALITY

The intensity of illumination provided by a light guide is inversely proportional to the square of the distance of the surface being illuminated. The images of more distant parts of an object are thus less brightly illuminated than closer parts of the same object. There are, however, several other factors which play a significant role in determining the brightness of different regions of the image of an object when viewed endoscopically. In discussing these factors it is assumed that the fibre bundle radiates light uniformly in all directions within the cone of illumination it provides.

The object surface was assumed earlier to be a sphere with its centre at the distal tip of the endoscope. In these circumstances all parts of the object surface are at the same distance, giving uniform illumination; also the illumination falls everywhere normal to the surface and so gives the maximum amount of light reflected back to the objective lens of the endoscope. Figure 20 shows a different situation, where the object is a plane surface perpendicular to the axis of the endoscope. This case shows how the brightness of the endoscopic image depends on the axial object distance $(EO) = D_o$ and the field angle β.

It is assumed that the object distance is large compared with the separation between the light guide and the objective. To include explicitly the dependence of the illumination on the distance of any part of the object surface, it is convenient to let I in Eq. (34) refer to the illumination at a unit distance of 1 cm from the light guide, i.e., with $D = 1$ in Eq. (34)

$$T = BS''(T_1, T_2 \ldots T_k) \qquad (35)$$

and the illumination at any other distance (D), expressed in centimeters, is then given by

$$I(D) = \frac{I}{D^2} \qquad (36)$$

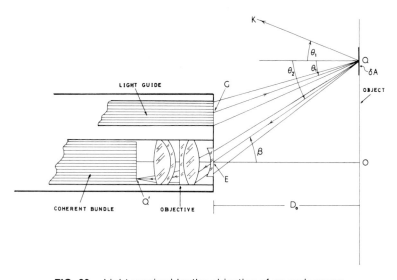

FIG. 20. Light received by the objective of an endoscope.

The intensity of illumination $I(D)$ is the amount of light per unit area falling on an element of surface perpendicular to the illuminating cone. For the obliquely illuminated element of area δA at Q in Figure 20 the light received from the light guide is given by $I(D)$ $\delta A \cos \Theta_1$, where D is the distance (GQ) and Θ_1 is the angle of incidence of the cone of light at Q. If the separation (EG) is small compared with the axial object distance $(EO) = D_o$, the angle Θ_1 is not significantly different from the field angle β. The total light falling on δA at Q is then given by $I(D)\delta A \cos \beta$.

The light falling at Q would all be reflected along the direction QK if the object at Q were a perfect mirror; this is the case of specular reflection from a perfectly smooth surface. For a completely rough surface the light falling at Q would be scattered almost uniformly in all directions, no matter what the direction of the incident cone of light; this is the case of completely diffuse reflection. The surfaces encountered in endoscopy have reflection properties lying between these two extremes. In Figure 20 the angle under which the light reflected from Q is observed is denoted by Θ_2. Again assuming that the separation (EG) is small compared with D_o, the angle Θ_2 is not greatly different from Θ_1. We thus need to consider the fraction of light falling on a surface at any angle of incidence Θ that is reflected back along approximately the same direction. This directional coefficient of reflection is denoted by $R(\Theta)$. It has its maximum value when $\Theta = 0$, (i.e., at normal incidence), and it decreases with increasing Θ, except for a perfect diffuser, for which this reflection coefficient is small but nearly constant for all values of Θ. With the approximation $\Theta_1 = \Theta_2 = \beta$, the part of the light $I(D)\delta A \cos \beta$ falling on the area δA at Q which is reflected back is given by $I(D)\delta A \cos \beta R(\beta)$.

Of this reflected light the amount accepted by the endoscope is determined by the solid angle that the objective, or more precisely the entrance pupil, subtends at Q. If P_o denotes the area of the aperture, this solid angle is given by $P_o \cos \beta / D^2$, and the total light flux accepted by the objective is thus given by

$$E = I(D)(\delta A \cos \beta)R(\beta) \frac{P_o \cos \beta}{D^2} \qquad (37)$$

where D is again the distance (EQ). From Figure 20, $(EQ) = (EO)/\cos \beta$—i.e., $D = D_o/\cos \beta$

where $D_o = (EO)$ is the axial object distance. Using this value for D and Eq. (36) for $I(D)$, Eq. (37) becomes

$$E = \left(\frac{IP_o}{D_o^4}\right) R(\beta) \cos^6 \beta \, \delta A \qquad (38)$$

This is the total light flux from the element δA at Q accepted by the objective to form the image δA at Q'.

The intensity of light found in the image formed on the distal face of the coherent fibre bundle (i.e., the light flux per unit area) is given by

$$I(\beta) = \frac{E}{\delta A'}$$

$$= \left(\frac{IP_o}{D_o^4}\right) R(\beta) \cos^6 \beta \left(\frac{\delta A}{\delta A'}\right) \qquad (39)$$

where $\delta A'$ is the area of the image of the element of area δA of the object; reflection losses at the surfaces of the objective are ignored. If the usual sign conventions of geometric optics are disregarded and all quantities are taken to be positive, the linear magnification between the object O and the image O' is given for the case of a simple lens by

$$M_o = \frac{F_o}{D_o - F_o}$$

where F_o is the focal length of the lens. For an objective of the kind shown in Figure 20, where the central ray of the pencil from Q falls perpendicularly on the entry face of the coherent bundle, point E is very close to the front focal point of the objective. When the distance $(EO) = D_o$ is measured from the front focal point, the linear magnification is given by

$$M_o = \frac{F_o}{D_o}$$

where F_o is now the equivalent focal length of the compound objective. The magnification for areas is then given by

$$\frac{\delta A'}{\delta A} = M^2 = \frac{F_o^2}{D_o^2} \qquad (40)$$

Using the reciprocal of this in Eq. 39 gives

$$I'(\beta) = \left(\frac{IP_o}{F_o{}^2D_o{}^2}\right) R(\beta) \cos^6 \beta \qquad (41)$$

for the intensity in the image, with I given by Eq. (35).

The intensity of the image produced at the distal end of the coherent bundle of the endoscope is thus inversely proportional to the square of the distance D_o of the object and to the sixth power of the cosine of the field angle (β). The variation of intensity from the centre of the image to the outer parts is given by

$$\frac{I'(\beta)}{I'(o)} = \frac{R(\beta)}{R(o)} \cos^6 \beta \qquad (42)$$

or for a perfectly diffusing object

$$\frac{I'(\beta)}{I'(o)} = \cos^6 \beta \qquad (43)$$

This variation is shown by curve I in Figure 21. In endoscopes for the digestive tract the total angle of field may equal 40 degrees so that $\beta = 20°$. For this size of field the variation of intensity across the image is significant but not of the importance sometimes found in cystoscopy, where β can have values up to 35 degrees.

Fortunately in the latter case the object surface (i.e., the urinary bladder) can more closely approximate the curved form of object surface assumed in Figure 10, for which the intensity of illumination is more nearly constant and the

reflection coefficient always has its maximum value $R(o)$, since the illumination falls everywhere at very near normal incidence. In this case the intensity at points in the image on the distal face of the coherent bundle is given by

$$I'(\beta) = \left(\frac{IP_o}{F^2D_o{}^2}\right) R(o) \cos^4 \beta \qquad (44)$$

and the variation of illumination over this image has the form

$$\frac{I'(\beta)}{I'(o)} = \cos^4 \beta \qquad (45)$$

in place of Eq. (43). One factor, $\cos \beta$, occurs in Eq. (44) and (45) because the projection of the area of the objective lens as seen by the object surface is $P_o \cos \beta$, and the further factor $\cos^3 \beta$ arises from the magnification properties between a curved object and a flat image surface. The form of Eq. (45) is shown by curve II in Figure 21.

Both curves in Figure 21 assume that the distal end of the fibre bundle radiates light uniformly in all directions within the cone of illumination. In practice it is more likely for the emitted light intensity to be maximal in the forward direction and to decrease in directions away from this. This effect could easily bring another factor, $\cos \beta$, into Eq. (43) and (45). Moreover, curve I assumes completely diffuse reflection at the illuminated surface, when the reflection coefficient $R(\beta)$ is constant. Again in practice $R(\beta)$ decreases with increasing field angle β. The curves in Figure 21 for the nonuniformity of intensity across the image are therefore optimistic.

Equation (44) for the intensity of the image formed at the distal end of the endoscope also ignores reflection losses at the air-glass surfaces of the objective. These give an additional transmittance factor, $T = (1-R)^N$, where N is the number of surfaces, as seen earlier for the condensor system.

The image received at the distal end of the coherent bundle is transmitted to the proximal end (O'' in Figure 22), where it is viewed by the eyepiece, the role of which is to produce a magnified virtual image of the exit-face of the bundle at a convenient distance from the observer's eye. The position of this enlarged image is shown at O'''. It is assumed here that

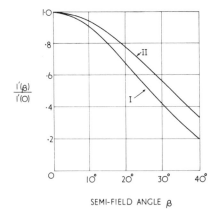

SEMI-FIELD ANGLE β

FIG. 21. Variation of image intensity with field angle. I, Flat perfect diffuser as object. II, Spherical object surface.

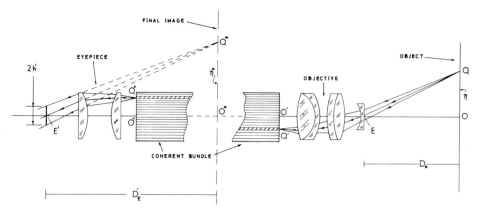

FIG. 22.   Successive images formed by a fibreoptics endoscope.

the coherent bundle has been twisted through half a turn, so that the fibre (shaded) receives the light from the image point *(Q)*, which is formed below the axis, and transmits this light to emerge at the proximal end of the bundle at the second image point *(Q″)* above the axis. The final image *(O‴Q‴)* of the object *OQ* is then seen correctly oriented and not inverted.

So far as the intensity and colour of the proximal image at *O″* are concerned, the transmittance of the coherent bundle is treated exactly as in the case of the illuminating light guide. That is, there are reflection losses at the two end-faces of the coherent bundle, reduced transmittance because of the core-packing fraction of this bundle, and a wavelength-dependent internal transmittance for the fibres. The proximal image at *O″* is thus less bright than the distal image at *O′*, and it is further depleted in intensity in the blue end of the visible spectrum.

With the type of objective in Figure 22 the central rays of the light cones forming the distal image at *O′Q′* all fall normally on the entry-face of the coherent bundle. This is shown for the pencil of light forming the image at *Q′* of the object point *Q*. This arrangement is termed a *telecentric objective*. The importance of using such an objective for a fibreoptics endoscope lies in the fact that the central rays of the pencil emerging from the proximal end of the coherent bundle are then also perpendicular to the end-face of the bundle (Fig. 22) for the cone of light emerging from the fibre at *Q″*. The central rays of all such emerging pencils of light are thus parallel to the axis, and they all therefore pass through the back focal point *(E′)* of the eyepiece. Furthermore all of the other rays of each bundle pass through a circle at *E′* of definite radius ρ' (Fig. 22). This circle at *E′* is the *exit-pupil* of the system, and an observer's eye placed with its own pupil at *E′* receives all the light from all points of the proximal image.

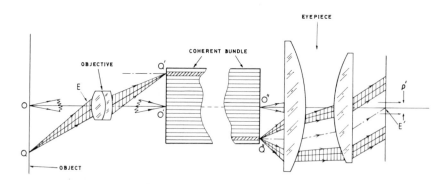

FIG. 23.   Annular pupil for extraaxial object points when using a nontelecentric objective.

If an ordinary (i.e., a nontelecentric) objective is used for a fibreoptics endoscope, the rays from any extraaxial object point emerge from the eyepiece as an annular tube of rays. The effect is shown in Figure 23. Light from point Q travels from the left and falls on the distal face of the coherent bundle at Q'. The cone of rays from the objective falls obliquely on this end-face; consequently a hollow cone of rays emerges from the proximal end of the fibre at Q''. These rays then give an annulus of rays falling on the observer's pupil at E'. By contrast, the rays from the axial object point O give a cone of rays focusing at O' on the coherent bundle. The central ray of this cone is along the axis and so falls normally on the bundle face. As a result these rays emerge from the fibre at O'' to give a narrow pencil of rays at E'.

The reason for the effect shown in Figure 23 is illustrated in Figure 24. A cone of rays falls obliquely on the end-face Q' of a fibre. The rays emerging from the other end of the fibre at Q'' form the same angles with the fibre axis, shown by the broken line in the diagram, as the entering rays. If the paths of all rays of an oblique cone enter the fibre at all points of its end face, the exit-face of the fibre is uniformly illuminated and the rays leaving it form a hollow cone (Fig. 24). If the axis of the entering cone of rays makes an angle α_o with the fibre

axis and α is the semiangle of this cone, the emergent rays lie in a hollow cone whose inner and outer rays make angles $(\alpha_o - \alpha)$ and $(\alpha_o + \alpha)$, respectively, with the fibre axis at the emergent end.

If a telecentric objective is not used for a fibreoptics endoscope, no clearly defined exit pupil is formed at E'. In practice some of the light may therefore not enter the observer's eye; but of potentially greater importance is the fact that light from points such at Q'' passes only through the outer parts of the observer's pupil, where the aberrations of the human eye degrade the image quality. Unfortunately, as examination of a number of fibreoptics endoscopes has shown, nontelecentric objectives are used not infrequently.

Consider the influence of the eyepiece on the intensity of illumination of the final image at O''' (Fig. 22). There are reflection losses at each of the N air-glass surfaces of the eyepiece, giving again a transmittance $T = (1-R)^N$, but the absorption losses in the glass of the lenses are very small, exactly as for the condensor and objective lenses. The remaining effect is that of the eyepiece magnification.

The formation of the magnified image by an eyepiece is illustrated in Figure 22, where rays from Q'' emerge from the eyepiece and appear to come from point Q'''. The eyepiece image is thus a virtual image. The exit pupil E' in the

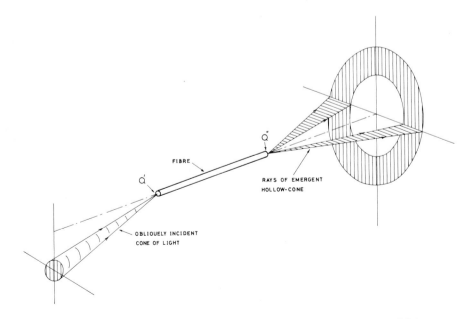

FIG. 24. Hollow cone effect produced by an obliquely incident cone of light.

case shown is at the back focal point of the eyepiece. If the eyepiece is focused to form the image $O'''Q'''$ at a distance D'_E from E', the linear magnification for the eyepiece is given by

$$M_E = \frac{F_E}{D'_E} \qquad (46)$$

where F_E is the equivalent focal length of the whole eyepiece. The area magnification between O'' and O''' is thus given by

$$\frac{\delta A'''}{\delta A''} = M_E^2 = \left(\frac{F_E}{D'_E}\right)^2 \qquad (47)$$

where $\delta A'''$ is the area of the image of an element of area $\delta A''$ at the proximal face of the endoscope bundle. For an area at the centre of the field of view, the intensity at the proximal end of the endoscope bundle is given by

$$I''(O) = \left(\frac{IP_o}{F_o{}^2 D_o{}^2}\right) R(O) \left(T'_1 T'_2\right) \qquad (48)$$

Where T'_1 and T'_2 are the overall transmittances of the objective and of the coherent bundle, and the remaining factor is $I'(O)$ of Eq. (41)—i.e., the intensity of the distal image when $\beta = 0$. The total light received by the area $\delta A''$ is given by $I''(O)\delta A''$, and the fraction of this light transmitted by the eyepiece is spread over the area $\delta A'''$ in the final image. The intensity at the axial point of this image (i.e., the light per unit area) is thus given by

$$I'''(O) = \frac{I''(O)\delta A'' T'_3}{\delta A'''}$$

where T'_3 is the transmittance factor of the eyepiece, which depends on the reflection losses. Thus using Eq. (47) and (48)

$$I'''(O) = \left(\frac{IP_o}{F_o{}^2 D_o{}^2}\right) \frac{R(O)}{M_E^2} \left(T'_1 T'_2 T'_3\right) \qquad (49)$$

gives the intensity for the axial point of the final image. The variation of this intensity with the field angle β is given by Eq. (42) or (45) for the two cases considered there.

If the value of I from Eq. (35) is inserted in Eq. (49) the equation for the final image intensity becomes

$$I'''(O) = BS''\left(T_1, T_2 \ldots T_k\right) R(O)$$

$$\frac{P_o}{F_o{}^2 D_o{}^2 M_E^2} \left(T'_1 T'_2 T'_3\right) \qquad (50)$$

in which the successive factors are B, the luminance of the source; S'', the area of the distal end of the illuminating light guide; $T_1, T_2 \ldots T_k$, the product of the transmittance factors between the source and the object; $R(O)$, the reflection coefficient of the object; $P_o/F_o{}^2$, the ratio of the area of the entrance pupil to the square of the focal length of the objective; $D_o{}^2$, the square of the object distance; M_E^2, the square of the eyepiece magnification; and T'_1, T'_2, T'_3, the product of the transmittance factors between the object and the observer.

The importance of Eq. (50) is in showing explicitly all the factors that determine the level of illumination of the image. Consequently it shows those factors to which attention must be given if it is necessary to have more light. This is particularly important in still or cinephotography, where M_E has merely to be replaced by the overall magnification between the proximal end of the bundle and the final image formed on the film, and the eyepiece transmittance factor T'_3 also includes the transmittance of the elements in the photographic system employed.

For example, consider an endoscope employing the illuminating system of Figure 10 together with a fibre cone coupling and a telescope of the form represented in Eq. (37). There are then 12 air-glass surfaces in the illuminating system and 12 in the telescope. The product of the average transmittances for two such systems with untreated surfaces is then given from Figure 11, by $(0.5)^2 = 0.25$, i.e., only 25 percent. Using only ordinary blooming for each of these surfaces would increase the figure to $(0.83)^2 = 0.69$, i.e., 69 percent. This represents a 2.8-fold increase in the intensity of the image. It is thus of great importance that as many air-glass surfaces as possible be given antireflection coatings.

Equation (50) for white light has the same form for monochromatic light of any wavelength (λ), provided the white light values of wavelength-dependent factors are replaced by their values for the wavelength in question. These factors are the source luminance, $B(\lambda)$, for the given wavelength, the reflectance of the object at that wavelength, and the internal transmittances of the fibre bundles. The other factors do not normally vary appreciably with the wavelength of the light. It is thus predominantly the colour temperature of the source and absorption in the fibre bundles that affect colour rendering.

The remaining aspects of image quality are contrast and resolution of detail. The contrast of an image can be seriously affected by stray light in the telescope, which derives principally from light scattered and reflected at the edges of lenses, the internal surfaces of the containing tubes, and reflections from untreated air-glass surfaces. Good optical practice can reduce this stray light to an acceptable level provided efficient antireflection coatings are used for the air-glass surfaces. Part of the light reflected at an untreated surface is liable to be reflected forward again, which produces a general haze over the image. With a large number of air-glass surfaces this effect can result in very poor contrast in the image, and the improvement obtained with good antireflection coatings is thus not only an increase in the overall transmittance but also improved contrast.

There is also the possibility of reduced contrast with a fibreoptic telescope arising from leakage of light into adjacent fibres. With good quality bundles this effect seems to be very small, possibly because very little of any light that does leak out of a fibre is retrapped and conducted to the exit-face of the fibre bundle.

The two most important factors which determine the smallest detail that may be resolved by a fibreoptic endoscope are the finite size and spacing of the fibres in the coherent fibre bundle and the depth of focus of the objective. The objective and eyepiece also each have a resolution limit determined by the size of aperture employed and the residual aberrations of these systems. These must both be of high quality; but, given this, in most practical systems these components of the system do not ultimately limit the optical performance.

The limit of resolution of a fibreoptic endoscope is usually set by the discrete structure of the coherent fibre bundle. All of the light falling at points at the distal end of any given fibre appears uniformly spread over that fibre at the proximal end. Any detail smaller than the fibre diameter is therefore lost. The proximal image consists of a lattice of small spots of light, each with uniform intensity and colour corresponding, apart from transmittance losses, to the average intensity and colour of the total amount of light falling on the particular fibre. A useful general assessment of the image quality that may be expected from a fibreoptic system is thus to compare it with a television picture, which is similarly composed of discrete picture elements. A typical coherent bundle has fibres of 10 μ diameter and may have a cross section of 4×4 mm. There are then 400 picture elements across the width or height of the image, corresponding roughly to the picture quality given by a 400-line television system.

A more precise method of characterising the ability of an optical system to reveal fine detail is the limit of resolution. Suppose, for example, that the object consists of two adjacent striae or bars, as suggested in Figure 25A, where the hatched areas represent the light in two separated lines that are imaged on the distal face of a coherent fibre bundle. The light falling on the fibres of rows 1, 3, and 5 all appear at the proximal ends of these fibres (Fig. 25B). However, the two strips of light fall astride two adjacent fibres in rows 2 and 4, and consequently light appears in four fibres of each of these rows at the proximal end of the bundle. For two lines closer than the separation shown there would be no fibre between them in any row that did not receive light. The case shown therefore represents a limit of resolution. The centre-to-centre spacing of the lines shown is $p = 2d$, where d is the centre-to-centre spacing of the fibres. The limit of resolution in lines per millimetre is thus given by

$$N = \frac{1}{2d} \qquad (51)$$

and the smallest resolvable separation is given by

$$p' = 2d \qquad (52)$$

The case in Figure 25 is optimal, the fibres being perfectly aligned with their centres in a triangular pattern. Moreover, if d is the fibre diameter, the centre-to-centre spacing of the

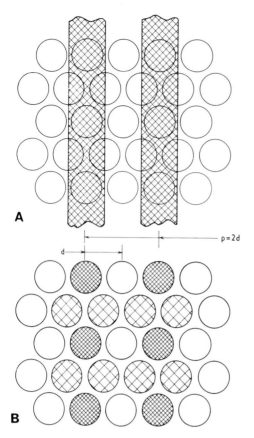

A

$p = 2d$

d

B

FIG. 25. Image of two bars as transmitted.

fibres are rather greater than d. Taking these factors into account and noting that the bars in Figure 25 would not appear perfectly resolved, a more realistic value for the least resolvable separation is taken to be

$$p' = 2.5d \qquad (53)$$

with the resolution limit of

$$N' = \frac{1}{2.5d} \qquad (54)$$

where d is the fibre diameter in millimetres, and N' is the number of lines per millimetre. Equations (53) and (54) constitute only a rule of thumb of course, but they have the advantage of not overestimating the detail to be expected in a fibreoptic image.

For 10 μ diameter fibres $d = 0.010$ mm, and Eq. (53) gives the smallest resolvable separation to be $p' = 25\ \mu$ when measured on the

distal face of the coherent bundle. By Eq. (54) this corresponds to 40 lines/mm, again as seen at the fibre bundle. If M_o is the magnification between the object and the distal end of the bundle, where M_o is less than unity the smallest resolvable separation in the object is $25/M_o\ \mu$; expressed as a number of lines per millimetre, this is 40 M_o. Since the proximal image formed by the fibre bundle is the same size as the distal image formed on it by the objective, the smallest resolvable separation in the visual image is given by $25M_E\ \mu$, or $(40/M_E)$ lines/mm, where M_E is the eyepiece magnification. For photography M_E must be replaced by the magnification between the proximal end of the fibre bundle and the final film plane. We thus need to consider equations for these magnifications.

Figure 26 shows pencils of light from points O and Q of an object at a distance D_o from the entrance pupil (E_o) of a compound objective, represented by its "principal planes" at H and H'. If E_o is at the front focal point of the objective, the size of the image $(O'Q') = \eta'$ is given by

$$\eta' = F_o \tan \beta \qquad (55)$$

where β is the semiangle of field. In the form

$$F_o = \frac{\eta'}{\tan \beta} \qquad (56)$$

Eq. (55) is used to find the necessary equivalent focal length of the objective if a field angle 2β is to be imaged at the edges of a bundle of width $2\eta'$. In a typical example of a narrow-field endoscope $2\beta = 37°$ and $2\eta' = 4$ mm, giving an equivalent focal length $F_o = 6$ mm for the objective. For a wider-field system (e.g., $2\beta = 65°$) the focal length is $F_o = 3.1$ mm, with η' again equal to 2 mm.

Given the focal length (F_o) of the objective, the linear size of object $(OQ) = \eta$ seen at a distance D_o is given by

$$\eta = D_o \tan \beta \qquad (57)$$

and then, using Eq. (55), the magnification for the objective is given by

$$M_o = \frac{\eta'}{\eta} = \frac{F_o}{D_o} \qquad (58)$$

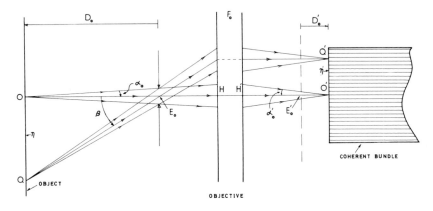

FIG. 26. Object and image for the objective of an endoscope.

The smallest resolvable detail in the object is thus given by

$$p_o = \frac{p'}{M_o} = \left(\frac{D_o}{F_o}\right)p' \qquad (59)$$

In the example quoted above, $p' = 25\,\mu$ when measured at the fibre bundle. When F_o is 6 mm and the object distance (D_o) is 36 mm, the magnification is equal to $M_o = 1/6$, so that the smallest resolvable detail in an object at this distance is $p_o = 150\,\mu$ (0.15 mm). This size clearly increases proportional to the object distance (D_o). For the wide-field system having F_o = 3.1 mm, the magnification $M_o = 1/6$ occurs for the smaller object distance $(D_o = 18.6$ mm). In this case the resolution limit of the bundle would correspond, for $D_o = 36$ mm, to a size $p_o = 290\,\mu$ (0.29 mm). The above considerations refer to the image of an object for which the objective is perfectly focused. The important question of depth of focus is treated later.

Equations similar to the above apply to the eyepiece of an endoscope (Fig. 27). With a correctly designed objective the rays from points such as O and Q at the proximal end of the fibre bundle emerge with the central rays of each pencil parallel to the axis. These pencils of light then leave the eyepiece to intersect as

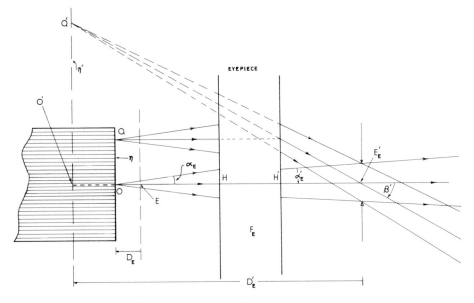

FIG. 27. Object and image for the eyepiece of an endoscope.

shown, forming a clearly defined exit pupil at the rear focal point (E'_E) of the eyepiece. If the central ray from Q on leaving the eyepiece makes an angle β' with the axis, the object and image sizes, $(OQ) = \eta$ and $(O'Q') = \eta'$, are given by

$$\eta = F_E \tan \beta'$$

$$\eta' = D'_E \tan \beta' \tag{60}$$

so that the linear magnification produced by the eyepiece is given by

$$M_E = \frac{\eta'}{\eta} = \frac{D'_E}{F_E} \tag{61}$$

and it depends on the distance D'_E from E'_E at which the eyepiece is focused by the observer to form the image $O'Q'$.

Thus the image distance (D'_E) changes when the eyepiece is focused to suit different observers; consequently the linear size (η') of the image changes. However, the angular size of the image (β') does not change, and for this reason the apparent size of the image seen by the observer remains constant. To take account of this fact the *visual magnification* of an eyepiece is conventionally defined to be the linear magnification when the image is formed at the normal least distance of distinct vision, i.e., when $D'_E = 250$ mm. Equation (61) then gives

$$M_E = \frac{250}{F_E} \tag{62}$$

where F_E is the equivalent focal length of the eyepiece expressed in millimetres. The practical effect of this is that the visual magnification expresses the increase in apparent size for an observer viewing the object magnified M_E times and placed a distance of 250 mm when compared with the object itself viewed from the same distance. The visual magnification of the whole endoscope is similarly expressed and is given by

$$M = M_o M_E \tag{63}$$

i.e., by the product of the linear magnification of the objective and the visual magnification of the eyepiece.

A typical value for the eyepiece magnification is $M_E = 10$, corresponding to a focal length (F_E) of 25 mm, by Eq. (62). The smallest

resolvable detail referred to the eyepiece image at a distance $D'_E = 250$ mm is thus given by $p'_E = M_E p'$, or $p'_E = 10 \times 25 = 250\ \mu$ (0.25 mm). The same considerations apply in photography provided M_E is replaced by the overall linear magnification M_{EC}, between the proximal end of the fibre bundle and the camera film plane. To calculate this magnification, we assume the eyepiece to be focused to give an image at infinity. The required linear magnification between the proximal end of the bundle and the film plane of the camera is then given by

$$M_{EC} = \frac{F_c}{F_E} \tag{64}$$

where F_c is the focal length of the camera objective. Using Eq. (61) with $D'_E = 250$ mm for F_E, this gives

$$M_{EC} = \left(\frac{F_c}{250}\right) M_E \tag{65}$$

where F_c is expressed in millimetres. Thus for an eyepiece magnification $M_E = 10$ and a camera lens of focal length $F_c = 76$ mm, the magnification is given by $M_{EC} = 3$. The image of a 4×4 mm bundle would then be 12×12 mm on the film plane.

Depth of focus is an important consideration. Figure 28 shows the objective and the distal end of the coherent bundle of an endoscope. The objective is set for focus on the object plane at O_o, giving a sharply focused image of this plane at O'_o. A second object point at O_1 then produces an image point at O'_1, and this light thus gives an out-of-focus patch of light on the coherent bundle. With a lens relay system the out-of-focus image point O'_1 would be transferred to the object space of the eyepiece as an out-of-focus image point, which could be seen in sharp focus either by exercising visual accommodation on the part of the observer or by adjusting the focus of the eyepiece. This is not possible with a fibre bundle since whatever light pattern falls on the distal end of the bundle is merely reproduced at the proximal end so that light from the object point O_1, for example, falls on several fibres which transmit this light to their proximal ends; no refocusing of the eyepiece can make this light appear to emerge from a single fibre. Thus any loss of image quality at the distal end of the bundle due to

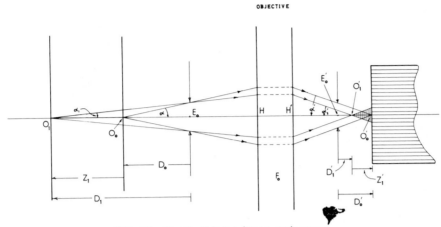

FIG. 28. Depth of focus for an endoscope.

focus error is an irretrievable loss. Therefore in respect to depth of focus, a fibreoptic endoscope is at some disadvantage compared with a lens relay system.

The simplest manner by which to estimate the effect of focus error is to consider the out-of-focus patch of light using the methods of geometric optics. In Figure 28, for example, if the objective is assumed to be accurately focused for the object O_o at distance D_o, the image of point O_I is formed at O'_I, which is at a distance $Z_I = (O'_I O'_o)$ short of the face of the coherent bundle. The radius of the circular patch of light formed on the coherent bundle is then given by

$$\rho' = Z_I \tan \alpha'_I \qquad (67)$$

where α'_I is the angle of the edge ray from O_I which passes through O'_I. With the aperture stop (i.e., the entrance pupil E_o) at the front focus of the objective the angle α' is the same for the edge ray coming from any object point. The easiest way to see this is to note that any rays coming from a point in the front focal plane of the objective are parallel in the image space. Alternatively, we may note that the magnification between O_I and O'_I is given by

$$M_o = \frac{\sin \alpha_I}{\sin \alpha'_2}$$

or, using Eq. (58) for M_o

$$\sin \alpha'_I = \sin \alpha_2 \left(\frac{D_o}{F_o} \right)$$

Now $D_o \sin \alpha_I = h$, the radius of aperture at E_o, so that

$$\sin \alpha'_I = \frac{h}{F_o} \qquad (68)$$

which is independent of the object distance $D_I = (O_I E_o)$. Hence $\alpha'_I = \alpha'_o$, the aperture angle of the edge ray from O_o, which focuses at O'_o on the face of the bundle. Equations (67) and (68) may thus be written

$$\rho' = Z'_I \tan \alpha'_o$$
$$\qquad (69)$$
$$\sin \alpha'_o = \frac{h}{F_o}$$

For the small angles in question $\tan \alpha'_o \approx \sin \alpha'_o$, so that from Eq. (69)

$$\rho' = \frac{h Z'_I}{F_o} \qquad (70)$$

gives the radius of the out-of-focus patch of light.

From Figure 28, $Z'_I = D'_o - D'_I$; also, using Newton's form of the lens equation, we have $D'_o = F_o^2/D_o$ and $D'_I = F_o^2/D_I$. Thus

$$Z'_I = F_o^2 \left(\frac{1}{D_o} - \frac{1}{D_I} \right)$$

and this used in Eq. (70) gives

$$\frac{1}{D_{max}} = \frac{1}{D_o} - \frac{\rho'}{h F_o} \qquad (71)$$

This equation gives the largest object distance $(D_1 = D_{max})$ for which the out-of-focus patch on the fibre bundle has a radius $\leqslant \rho'$. In a similar manner it is found that

$$\frac{1}{D_{min}} = \frac{1}{D_o} + \frac{\rho'}{hF_o} \qquad (72)$$

gives the nearest object distance (D_{min}) for which the radius of the out-of-focus patch is $\leqslant \rho'$. If the largest permissible value of ρ' is stipulated, Eq. (71) and (72) serve to find the depth of focus.

From the latter two equations it is seen that the difference between D_{max} and D_{min} (i.e., the depth of focus range) becomes larger as the value of the quantity ρ'/F_o increases. If the criterion for permissible focus error is taken to be that the diameter of the out-of-focus patch just covers two fibres (i.e., $2\rho' = 2d$), ρ' must be replaced by the fibre diameter (d). For the narrow-field endoscope $F_o = 6.0$ mm; and using $\rho' = d = 10\ \mu$, with $h = 0.50$ mm, corresponding to an entrance pupil of diameter 1.0 mm, the depth of focus extends from $D_{max} = 40.9$ mm to $D_{min} = 32.1$ mm. For the wide-field endoscope, using $F_o = 3.1$ mm, $\rho' = d = 10\ \mu$, $h = 0.4$ mm, and $D_o = 18.6$ mm, the depth of focus range is found to be from $D_{max} = 21.9$ mm to $D_{min} = 16.2$ mm.

The larger the value of the distance D_o for which the objective is exactly focused, the greater the range of focal depth $(D_{max} - D_{min})$; but of course the value of D_{min} is then also larger. Nevertheless, a useful indication of the available depth of focus is the value of D_{min} obtained when D_o is chosen to make $D_{max} = \infty$. From Eq. (71) the value of D_o is then given by

$$D_o = \left(\frac{hF_o}{\rho'}\right) \qquad (73)$$

and from Eq. (70) the minimum object distance is then

$$D_{min} = \frac{1}{2}\left(\frac{hF_o}{\rho'}\right) \qquad (74)$$

Thus for the narrow-field endoscope, using $h = 0.5$ mm, $F_o = 6.0$ mm, and $\rho' = d = 10\ \mu$, the value $D_{min} = 150$ mm. For the wide-field system, using $h = 0.4$ mm, $F_o = 3.1$ mm, and

$\rho' = d = 10\ \mu$, the corresponding value is $D_{min} = 62$ mm. It follows that the wide-field system has the greater inherent depth of focus.

An alternative to the above is to take the difference between Eq. (72) and (73), giving

$$\frac{1}{D_{min}} - \frac{1}{D_{max}} = \frac{2\rho'}{hF_o} \qquad (75)$$

which specifies the focal depth range in terms of reciprocal distances. The range is thus greater as the values of h and F_o become smaller and the permissible radius ρ' of the out-of-focus patch of light becomes larger.

The above examples illustrate the severity of the problem of depth of focus in fibreoptics endoscopes. The focal length of the objective F_o is fixed, in accordance with Eq. (56), once the width of the bundle $2\eta'$ and the total field angle 2β are decided. For any permissible value of the radius of the out-of-focus patch (ρ') the only way to increase the depth of focus is thus to reduce the radius of aperture h. However, the area of the pupil is given by $P = \pi h^2$, so that if the aperture is reduced to one-half its size, for example, the depth of focus is doubled, but the value of P and therefore the brightness of the image is reduced by a factor of four.

In some fibreoptics endoscopes the focus is made adjustable by arranging for one lens of the objective assembly to slide within the endoscope under the control of a focusing knob. For medical endoscopes a fixed focus is often preferred, carrying with it a very limited range of object distances within which the image quality is really comparable with that obtained for an object at the distance for which the exact focus is set. A consequence of this is that the ranges of focal depth quoted for commercial instruments often imply that a markedly reduced image quality may be tolerated. For example, a system giving a field angle $2\beta = 60°$ with a coherent bundle 4×4 mm has an objective of focal length given by Eq. (55) to be $F_o = 2/\tan 30° = 3.464$ mm. The relative aperture is stated to be $F/4$, i.e., $2h = F_o/4 = 0.866$ mm, or $h = 0.433$ mm. The range of focal depth is given as $D_{max} = 100$ mm to $D_{min} = 10$ mm, which requires that the objective be focused for a distance D_o, given by

$$\frac{1}{D_o} = \frac{1}{2}\left(\frac{1}{D_{max}} + \frac{1}{D_{min}}\right) = 0.0550$$

or $D_o = 18.18$ mm. Using the above values in either Eq. (71) or (72) gives $\rho' = 0.068$ mm (68 μ). The diameter of the out-of-focus patch for the two extremes of the quoted focal depth range is thus 136 μ, or $2\rho' = 13.6d$, with the fibre diameter assumed to be $d = 10$ μ. To allow $\rho' = 6.8d$ of course represents a serious degradation in image quality.

To appreciate how serious these effects can be for the detail perceived in the final image it is necessary to introduce some aspects of the wave theory of image formation and also the concept of the optical transfer function (OTF). This latter is often termed the modulation transfer function (MTF). By means of the MTF it is possible to assess in a simple manner the loss of image detail resulting from the limited depth of focus of an endoscope.

Figure 29 shows rays diverging from a point object at O, focused by the lens to pass through the image point at O'. If the lens has no aberration, all of these rays pass exactly through the image point at O'; elementary ray optics then suggests that all of the light from O passes through a single point at O'. In practice, however, it is found that the image of a point object consists of a disk of light surrounded by a dark and bright ring (Fig. 29, at right). The curve drawn at O' shows the variation of intensity across the diameter of this diffraction pattern. The central disk and the whole pattern are termed the *Airy disk* and Airy diffraction pattern, respectively, after Airy, who appears to have been the first to explain this effect. For this explanation it is necessary to invoke the wave theory of light, in terms of which light diverges from O in the form of spherical waves. These waves travel more slowly in glass than in air, and the action of

the lens is thus to retard the centre relative to the outer parts of each wave. Consequently a converging wave with its centre at O' leaves the lens. Away from the region of focus at O' the elements of the wavefront may be considered to travel along the rays, and elementary ray optics is then applicable. This is not so at or near the focus O'. The effects produced at the focus of a wave are an example of *diffraction.*

Diffraction theory shows that the radius of the Airy disk is given by

$$\xi'_o = \frac{0.61\lambda}{n' \sin \alpha'} \tag{76}$$

where λ is the wavelength of the light, n' is the refractive index of the image space, and α' is the aperture angle. By Eq. (69) the value of $\sin \alpha'$ for the objective of an endoscope is given by the reciprocal of twice the F number, which is the value of $(F_o/2h)$; $n' = 1$ in the present case since the image is formed in air. A typical aperture ratio is $F/4.5$, giving $\sin \alpha' = 1/9$. For the middle of the visible spectrum $\lambda = 0.55$ μ, and Eq. (76) then gives $\xi'_o = 3$ μ for the radius of the Airy disk. The focused image of each point of the object thus consists of a central disk of light of diameter $2\xi'_o = 6$ μ, surrounded by a weak diffraction ring. This result assumes not only perfect focusing but also that the lens is perfectly corrected for aberration. The effect of focus error and/or aberration is to modify the diffraction pattern, causing a loss of intensity from the centre and a general spreading of the light over a larger area.

One consequence of the above result is seen immediately in connection with Figure 25. The two bars of light falling on a coherent bundle

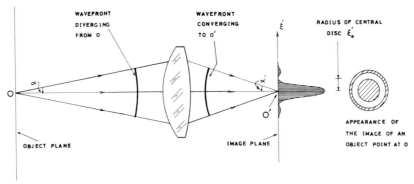

FIG. 29. Diffraction image of a point source.

were assumed in Figure 25 to be produced by an object placed in contact with the bundle. If these bars are produced as images using a lens of aperture $F/4.5$, each point along the edges of the bars is imaged as an Airy disk, so that the images spread about 3 μ outside the edges of the bars as given by elementary geometric optics. Thus some light also falls on the central fibres of rows 1, 3, and 5, further degrading the images seen at the proximal end of the bundle. This spreading of light in the image would be increased by the presence of focus error and/or aberration.

It proves not practicable to treat the influence of the spreading light by diffraction, focus error, and aberration on the images of extended objects by summing explicitly their effects on the images of the individual points of such objects. Fortunately this problem is easily handled by means of the modulation transfer function (MTF), which is, simply, as follows. A typical object is a line grating, or grid, consisting of alternately bright and dark lines, with a variation of intensity of the form

$$I(\xi') = A + B \cos (2\pi N'\xi') \qquad (77)$$

when referred to the image plane. That is, $I(\xi')$ gives the form of intensity variation over the object but scaled in size according to the magnification between the object and image. This is termed a *cosine wave grating* by analogy with the terminology used in electronics. The quantity ξ' is a coordinate distance in the image plane. As ξ' varies the form of $I(\xi')$ is as shown by the curves in Figure 30. The contrast in this *cosine wave grating* is defined to be

$$C = \frac{B}{A} \qquad (78)$$

in which $\pm B$ is the amplitude of modulation above and below the mean intensity A. For the case $B = A$, the contrast is $C = 1$ and the intensity varies between maxima equal to $2A$ and zero.

It may be shown that the image of a cosine wave grating is also a cosine wave grating, but of reduced contrast. The image of the object $I(\xi')$ is thus of the form

$$I'(\xi') = A' + B' \cos (2\pi N'\xi') \qquad (79)$$

which is of contrast

$$C' = \frac{B'}{A'} \qquad (80)$$

where $C' < C$. The quantity N' in the above equation is the *spatial frequency* of the grating; that is, if p'_o is the centre-to-centre spacing of the bright lines in the image of the grating

$$N' = \frac{1}{p'_o} \qquad (81)$$

gives the number of lines per millimetre, in the case where p'_o is specified in millimetres.

The MTF for a grating of spatial frequency N' is defined as

$$T(N') = \frac{C'}{C} = \frac{\text{image contrast}}{\text{object contrast}} \qquad (82)$$

and it represents the attenuation in contrast

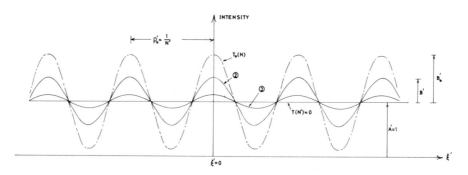

FIG. 30.   Images of cosine wave gratings.

resulting from the process of forming the image. If the object is of the form

$$I(\xi') = 1 + \cos (2\pi N'\xi') \tag{83}$$

which has contrast $C = 1$, the intensity in the image is given by

$$I'(\xi') = 1 + T(N') \cos (2\pi N'\xi') \tag{84}$$

with contrast $C' = T(N')$, where $T(N') < 1$, this contrast attenuation becoming greater the larger the spatial frequency N' (i.e., the finer the grating).

The loss of contrast in the image arises simply because of the spread of light in the image of each point of the object. The brighter parts of the object lose more light to the darker parts than they gain back from them. The loss of contrast thus becomes increasingly serious as the grating period $p'_o = 1/N'$ becomes smaller than the spread of light in the image of a single point. The radius of the Airy disk, ξ'_o in Eq. (77), is larger for longer wavelengths (λ) and for small-aperture angles (α'). For this reason it often proves useful to introduce a *reduced spatial frequency*, defined by

$$s = \left(\frac{\lambda}{n' \sin \alpha'}\right)N' \tag{85}$$

where N' is the spatial frequency, expressed as lines per millimetre when the wavelength of the light (λ) is given in millimetres. The absolute limit of resolution for any optical system occurs for the reduced spatial frequency $s = 2.0$. For a typical fibreoptic endoscope using an objective of aperture $F/4.5$ with a coherent bundle having fibres of diameter $d = 10 \mu$, the spatial frequency at the limit of resolution of the bundle is $N' = 1/2.5d = 40$ lines/mm. The angle of aperture (α') is such that $\sin \alpha' = 1/9$, so that this as a reduced spatial frequency is $s = 0.20$, which is one-tenth of the theoretical limit $s = 2.0$, for the objective. This fact has two important consequences.

The spread of light due to diffraction alone (i.e., for a perfectly focused aberration-free objective) gives a transfer function of the form denoted by $T_o(N')$ in Figure 31. For $s = 0.2$ the MTF has fallen only to 0.87, so that diffraction alone does not seriously reduce the image con-

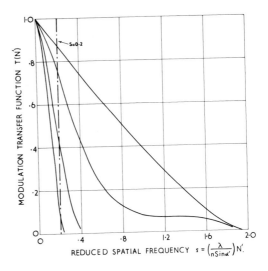

FIG. 31. Influence of focus error on the modulation transfer function of an aberration-free system.

trast for spatial frequencies up to the limit of resolution of the fibre bundle. The intensity variation across the image of an object grating of contrast $C = 1$ for this case of a perfectly focused image is shown by the chain curve in Figure 30. The curves numbered 1, 2, and 3 in Figure 30 show the effect on the MTF of progressively larger focus errors, such that the out-of-focus ray patch is of radius

$$(1) \qquad \rho' = \frac{\lambda}{\sin \alpha'_o}$$

$$(2) \qquad \rho' = \frac{2\lambda}{\sin \alpha'_o}$$

$$(3) \qquad \rho' = \frac{3\lambda}{\sin \alpha'_o}$$

respectively. For $\lambda = 0.55 \mu$ and an $F/4.5$ objective, having $\sin \alpha_o = 1/9$, these correspond to $\rho' = 4.95, 9.90$ and 14.85μ, respectively. The image intensity curves for $\rho' = 9.90$ and 14.86μ are shown as (2) and (3) in Figure 30. For a focus error specified by $\rho' = 15 \mu$ the MTF has the value $T(N') = 0$ for $s = 0.2$; the image then shows no contrast (Fig. 30).

For the lower spatial frequencies (in the range $s \leqslant 0.2$) it is possible to find the MTF for a perfectly focused image using the approximate formula

$$T_o(N') = \left(\frac{0.64\lambda}{n' \sin \alpha'} \right) N' \qquad (86)$$

Also for $s \leq 0.2$, the relative MTF defined by

$$M(N') = \frac{T(N')}{T_o(N')} \qquad (87)$$

is given for a defocused but aberration-free objective by the curve shown in Figure 32. This curve shows that $M(N')$, and therefore $T(N')$, falls to zero for $(2\pi\rho')N' = 3.83$; i.e., when

$$N' = \frac{0.61}{\rho'} \qquad (88)$$

This serves to give the resolution limit for a defocused objective, it being assumed that the objective is highly corrected for aberration.

It is instructive to apply Eq. (88) to the focal depth range from $D_{max} = 100$ mm to $D_{min} = 10$ mm claimed for a commercial endoscope. At the extremes of this range, the radius of the out-of-focus ray patch on the coherent bundle is $\rho' = 0.068$ mm (*vide supra*). Hence the limit of resolution on the fibre bundle for objects at either $D_{max} = 100$ mm or $D_{min} = 10$ mm would be given by Eq. (88) as $N' = 0.61/0.068 = 8$ lines/mm, compared with the limit $N' = 40$

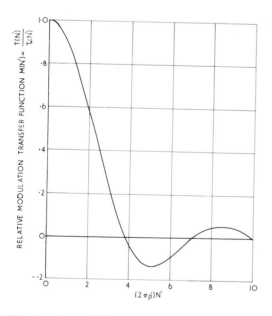

FIG. 32.   Form of $M(N')$ for low spatial frequencies.

lines/mm imposed by the bundle, which is detail of a size easily resolved in the focused image of the object.

For a defocused image the spatial frequencies beyond $(2\pi\rho')N' = 3.83$ up to $(2\pi\rho')N' = 7.01$, i.e., from $N' = 0.61/\rho$ to $N' = 1.12/\rho$ have negative values of $M(N')$. Therefore for this range of spatial frequencies the image has spurious resolution, with the image having reversed contrast.

The second consequence of the fact that the limit of resolution of a typical fibre bundle corresponds to a value of $s = 0.2$ for the reduced spatial frequency relates to the degree of aberration correction and the precision of manufacture demanded of the objective. The MTF curves of Figure 31 refer to an aberration-free objective. The effect of aberration, even at the best focus, is to give curves qualitatively similar to the out-of-focus curves, which are numbered in the figure. If we impose the criterion that the aberration should not reduce the image contrast to less than 80 percent of its value for a perfectly focused aberration-free system—i.e., $M(N') \geq 0.80$—for values of N' corresponding to $s \geq 0.2$ the system must have a degree of aberration correction and a precision of manufacture comparable with those obtaining for a good-quality microscope objective. This is a surprising result since $s = 0.2$ denotes a spatial frequency only one-tenth of the theoretical resolution limit $s = 2.0$. It is nevertheless a well-founded conclusion.

If the cone of rays entering the distal end of the coherent bundle of an endoscope has an aperture angle α_o (Fig. 26), the cone of rays emerging from the proximal end of the bundle (Fig. 27) has the same aperture angle $\alpha_E = \alpha_o'$. It follows from this that the F/N_o of the eyepiece is exactly the same as that of the objective. The aberration correction and production standards demanded by the eyepiece are consequently also high, even though the eyepiece is required only to focus on the proximal face of the bundle, so that depth of focus considerations do not arise.

The final component of the overall endoscopic system is either the human eye or a camera. To consider the functioning of either it is necessary to know the diameter ($2h'$) of the exit pupil of the endoscope. Now the F/N_o of the eyepiece is defined by $F_E/2h'$; and since this is equal to the F/N_o of the objective, the exit pupil diameter is given by

$$(2h') = \frac{F_E}{(F/N_o)_o}$$

For a magnification M_E the focal length of the eyepiece is given by Eq. (62), so that the diameter of the exit pupil for such an eyepiece is given by

$$(2h') = \frac{250}{M_E(F/N_o)_o} \qquad (89)$$

where M_E is the eyepiece magnification and $2h'$ is expressed in millimetres. Thus for a typical case the objective has a relative aperture $F/4.5$ and the eyepiece magnification is $M_E = 10$; using Eq. (89) these values give $2h' = 5.6$ mm. This is the diameter of the circular region at the exit pupil through which all the beams originating at different points of the original object pass. It is accordingly the necessary diameter of the pupil of the eye or of the aperture of a camera lens placed following the eyepiece in order to photograph the image.

Under ordinary conditions of ambient lighting the pupil of the human eye has a diameter of 4 to 6 mm, the value being smaller when exposed to relatively bright light. In dimmer light the larger diameter (6 mm) is attained, but even then the pupil of the eye is only just large enough to accept all of the light from a typical fibreoptic endoscope with an exit pupil of diameter $(2h') = 6.5$ mm. Note also that if a nontelecentric objective is used, producing hollow tubes of rays for off-axis image points (Fig. 23), some of these rays can easily pass outside the pupil of the observer's eye even when the effect is not as severe as in the case depicted in Figure 23.

If the endoscopic image is to be photographed with a camera placed at the proximal end of the endoscope, the passage of rays through the camera lens to the film plane is as illustrated in Figure 33. Provided a telecentric objective is used for the endoscope, the image-forming pencils of rays all emerge to pass through the exit pupil, of diameter $(2h')$, located at E'_E. The unshaded pencil of rays, forming the axial image at O'_c, passes centrally through the iris diaphragm of the camera lens. The necessary F/N_o of the camera to accommodate this pencil is thus $F_c/2h'$, where F_c is the focal length of the camera lens. Typical values of these quantities are $2h' = 5.6$ mm and $F_c = 75$ mm, giving an aperture ratio of $F/13.4$. Therefore so far as the axial image is concerned the camera lens could be stopped down with no effect on the image.

The situation is different for the pencil of rays forming the extraaxial image point at Q'_c (Fig. 33, shaded area). Because the exit pupil of the endoscope (E'_E) is situated in front of the camera lens, this pencil of rays passes eccentrically through the iris diaphragm of the camera lens and would not pass the diaphragm if this were stopped down to the size of the axial pencil. This tendency to vignette the outer parts of the image is particularly marked in the case of zoom objectives when used at the shorter focal length end of the zoom. Moreover it is for this reason that the camera lens usually needs to be used at full aperture, even though the F/N_o of the pencils of light forming the image may be much smaller than the rated F/N_o of the camera objective.

To find the F/N_o at which the camera lens works, it is merely necessary to scale the F/N_o of the endoscope eyepiece by the ratio of the

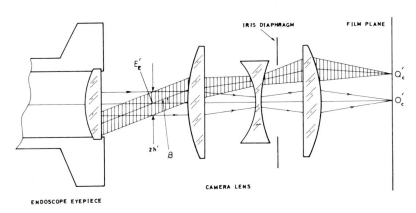

FIG. 33. Ray paths in endoscopic photography.

focal lengths (F_c/F_E). Thus since the F/N_o of the eyepiece is the same as that of the endoscope objective, the camera lens works at an aperture

$$(F/N_o)_c = \left(\frac{F_c}{F_E}\right)(F/N_o)_o$$

or since $F_E = 250/M_E$, where M_E is the magnification of the endoscope eyepiece

$$(F/N_o)_c = \left(\frac{M_E F_c}{250}\right)(F/N_o)_o \qquad (90)$$

with the camera lens focal length (F_c) expressed in millimetres. The values $M_E = 10$, $F_c = 75$, and $(F/N_o)_o = 4.5$ in Eq. (90) give $(F/N_o)_c = 13.5$ for the camera lens, agreeing to the accuracy used there with the value $F/13.4$ found above.

The angle of field required of the camera lens $(2\beta')$ is given by Eq. (60) for the field angle (β') of the eyepiece, i.e.,

$$\tan \beta' = \frac{\eta}{F_E}$$

where (2η) is the width of the coherent fibre bundle. Using $F_E = 250/M_E$ gives

$$\tan \beta' = \frac{M_E \eta}{250} \qquad (91)$$

where η is given in millimetres. With $M_E = 10$ and $2\eta = 4$ mm, the above formula gives $\tan \beta' = 0.08$, from which the total field angle for the camera lens is found to be $2\beta' = 9°$.

It remains to consider the influence of the mosaic structure of the coherent fibre bundle on the visual appearance of the image, as well as the role this structure plays in the images seen using a fibre optic teaching attachment. With regard to the first question, it has only to be said that a single fibre of diameter d appears to the observer as a spot of light of diameter $M_E d$ seen at a distance of 250 mm. For the typical values $d = 10 \ \mu$ and $M_E = 10$, this diameter is $100 \ \mu$ (0.10 mm). Two adjacent fibres appear as two spots of light whose centre-to-centre separation is equal to the magnified fibre diameter plus the thickness of the small interspace between them. Therefore

in the example given, the separation between the images of adjacent fibres are also about 0.10 mm. An eye with good visual acuity can resolve two points of light, such as a double star, provided they subtend an angle of not less than 1 minute of arc at the observer's eye. Good visual acuity therefore is able to resolve a separation of 0.09 mm at a distance of 250 mm. Fibres of $10 \ \mu$ diameter observed with an eyepiece magnification of $\times 10$ are thus on the limit of visual acuity. With larger eyepiece magnification the mosaic structure of the fibre bundle is expected to be observable.

The discrete structure of fibre bundles plays a further role when a fibreoptic teaching attachment is used in conjunction with a fibre-optic endoscope. The system used is shown in Figure 34, in which the path of light from one fibre is indicated. The cap of the teaching attachment carries a beam splitter and objective. In the form of beam splitter shown, the diagonal face of the cube is metallised to make it partially reflecting. It thus reflects part of the light and transmits the remainder, apart from absorption in the metal film. For an equally reflecting and transmitting film there can be as much as 30 percent loss by absorption, leaving 35 percent for the reflection coefficient and 35 percent for the transmission coefficient of the beam splitter. The endoscopist views the image directly through the beam splitter, while the objective of the teaching eyepiece forms an image on the distal end-face of its own coherent fibre bundle. This image is transmitted to the proximal end of the flexible coherent bundle, where it is viewed through an eyepiece by a second observer or a camera.

What was discussed above concerning light losses, image quality, and the need for good-quality lens systems applies equally to the components of a teaching attachment. There are, however, two further factors which influence the image quality seen by the second observer. The first of these is the need for the focus settings of the endoscope eyepiece and of the teaching attachment objective to be compatible in the sense that the proximal end of the endoscope bundle is sharply focused on the distal end of the bundle of the teaching attachment. This is of course easy to arrange provided there is focusing for both the endoscope eyepiece and the objective of the teaching attachment. The endoscopist sets the focus of the endoscope eyepiece to suit his own

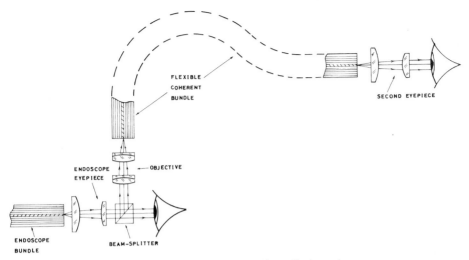

FIG. 34. Fibreoptics teaching attachment.

eyesight, but this does not usually guarantee that the light emerging from the endoscope is sharply focused by a fixed-focus objective on the bundle of the teaching attachment. Therefore the image formed on the bundle of the teaching attachment may easily be greatly inferior to that seen by the endoscopist. Focusing of the eyepiece of the teaching attachment is of course necessary to suit the eyesight of the second observer, but focusing of the eyepiece alone cannot compensate for poor focus at the distal end of the bundle.

The second factor affecting the image quality observed through a fibreoptics teaching attachment is that of mismatch between the fibres of the two bundles. If each fibre of the endoscope bundle were imaged exactly on a corresponding fibre of the bundle of the teaching attachment, there would be no loss of image quality apart from a small reduction in contrast resulting from the modulation transfer function of the combination of the endoscope eyepiece and the objective of the teaching attachment. In practice there is never exact matching between the images of the fibres of one bundle and the positions of the fibres in the other. There is consequently an unavoidable loss of resolution whenever two coherent fibre bundles are used in tandem, as with a fibreoptics endoscope and teaching attachment. It has been estimated theoretically that the limit of resolution is impaired by a factor of $\sqrt{2}$; i.e., an endoscope with a coherent bundle giving a resolution of $N' = 40$ lines/mm has its resolution reduced to $40/\sqrt{2} = 28.4$ lines/mm. This effect, together with the residual focus error between the endoscope eyepiece and the objective of the teaching attachment, can result in an extremely poor quality of image seen by the second observer.

3

Light Sources

Valerie Olson

Early illumination schemes which employed distally located light sources were cumbersome, produced marginal intensity, and proved in general to be highly unsatisfactory. There are several principal considerations in the design of a suitable illumination system.

LIGHT TRANSMISSION

Incoherent Fiber Bundles

With the introduction of incoherent, flexible fiber optics, a tremendous advance was made in the field of endoscopic illumination. These light fibers, when packaged into bundles, allow light to be transferred from a fairly intense light source, located outside the sterile operating field, to the telescope. However advantageous flexible fiber optics appears, it has serious inherent physical limitations. Some can be minimized, but all must be carefully considered when designing optical systems that interface with fiber optic assemblies.

The maximum entrance and exit angles (or field of view) of a given fiber are equal and uniquely determined by the indices of refraction of its core and cladding glasses. Therefore it is useless to attempt interfacing fiber optics with optical systems having greater fields of view.

Several unavoidable phenomena contribute to significant light transmission losses. A characteristic loss for a 6-foot bundle is about 65 percent. Absorption that arises from bulk absorption mechanisms in the glass itself, as well as during the thousands of reflections from the core-clad interface, contribute an unfortunate 5 to 8 percent transmission loss for every foot of glass. Thus it becomes very important to select a low-loss combination to minimize this effect. A second, large-loss mechanism is the packing fraction loss and can be somewhat minimized by selecting only carefully constructed bundles. Packing fraction losses are approximately 25 to 30 percent. Simple Fresnel losses due to reflection at the two air-glass surfaces are responsible for another 10 to 12 percent loss. This loss may be reduced by antireflection material coating the fiber ends,

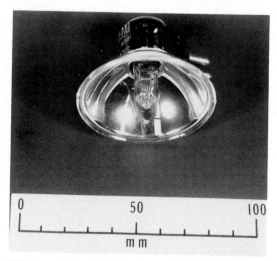

FIG. 1. This 150 tungsten lamp was originally designed for projectors. The paraboloidal mirror is not designed to match the active entrance angle of commonly used fiberoptic bundles. Heat production is significant. The majority of examining light sources employs this or similar globes.

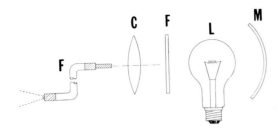

FIG. 2. An examining light source: the spot size (filament) of the lamp (L) should be matched with the active area of the fiber bundle. If reflecting mirrors (M) are used they should be designed especially for this application. Appropriate filters (F, at center) for ultraviolet and infrared should be employed. Incorporating a condenser lens (C) increases the density but also the heat production. Appropriate lamp and mirror design can eliminate the condenser. F (at left), fiber cable.

but coating fibers is a somewhat sophisticated undertaking and is not generally considered cost effective.

In addition to the inherent transmission losses, broken fibers can contribute significantly to transmission loss. In this case bundle selection again becomes extremely important.

Still another area where selection plays a large role is color purity. Fibers must be chosen that transmit equally over the entire visible spectrum in order to maintain correct color perspective of the tissue and organs being viewed. It is especially important to get true color rendition of the red region of the visible spectrum.

A further consideration is the requirement that fiber ends be cemented with high-temperature epoxy to protect them against heat damage, which is likely to occur when using very-high-intensity or pulsed light sources.

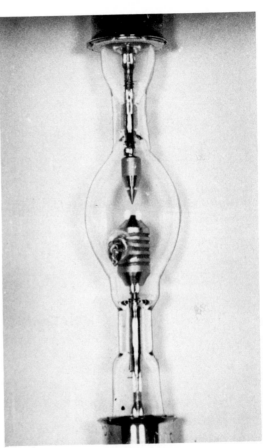

FIG. 4. Quartz glass high-pressure xenon arc (point source) globe (350 watts). Lifetime is 1000 hours. Color purity for endoscopy is excellent. The optical system can be designed to match both reflective and refractive aspects and to match the field of view of the matching fiberoptic cables. The ultraviolet and infrared outputs are high and must be carefully filtered. The necessary igniting and power units are large, cumbersome, and costly. These types of xenon lamps are dangerous as they can explode and so must be encased in heavy armor-plated housing. The X-Y alignment is critical.

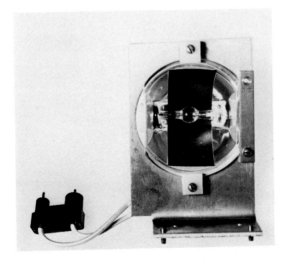

FIG. 3. General Electric Marc-300 lamp. (The mirror is blacked out to avoid reflection for this photograph.) This is a mercury high-pressure globe developed for movie projectors. The color temperature is higher than that of a tungsten globe. The large heat production is objectionable. Both intensity and color purity degrade continuously during a short 25-hour lifetime.

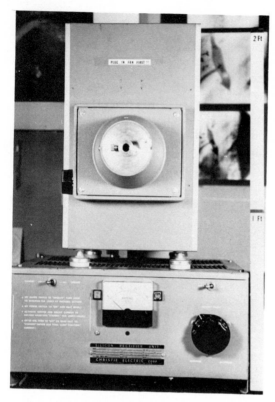

FIG. 5. Same xenon globe as shown in Figure 4, but with the housing and power supply.

LOW-INTENSITY (EXAMINATION) LIGHT SOURCES

Requirements

A light source used for viewing only should incorporate the following features:

1. Sufficient illumination should be provided over the required field of view, with good color purity, to permit thorough, detailed endoscopic examinations.
2. Infrared radiation, which might produce contact burns, as well as result in radiative heat transfer to body cavities, must be minimized.
3. Electrical components such as transformers must be isolated and present no hazard to operating-room personnel.
4. Fans used for heat removal should not move such large volumes of air that it causes excessive turbulence and noise.
5. It is desirable that the unit be rugged and easy to operate.

History

Tungsten projection lamps (Fig. 1) have been employed as endoscopic light sources. While tungsten lamps work reasonably well, they have not been specially designed for endoscopy and therefore do not result in the most efficient configuration possible for endoscopy. Some of the light output is lost because the output spot size of the lamp is not optically matched to the active area of common fiber optic bundles. Moreover, the characteristic "yellow" of tungsten bulbs tends to affect tissue color appearance, which can affect the actual appearance of inflammation. This is commonly called a low "color temperature." Color temperature refers

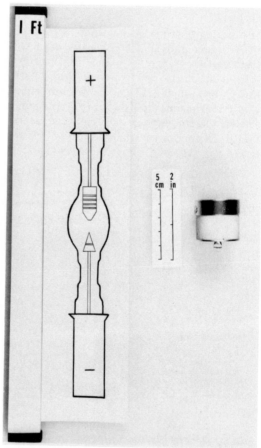

FIG. 6. New type of xenon arc globe. Note the difference in size compared with the 350-watt quartz glass xenon globe in Figure 4. The output of this "miniature" xenon globe is compatible with the standard large ones. This small and compact light source can be made to match the 70-degree field of view of most fiber optics.

to how closely a given source approximates a true blackbody radiation at a certain temperature. Color temperatures of tungsten sources range between 2800 and 3500° K. The higher the color temperature, the closer the color approximates what is seen in daylight. Last, very little attempt has been made to reduce infrared output beyond the routine heat rejection coatings found on projection lamps.

Some recently available examining sources satisfy most of the requirements discussed previously. Operation with a hotter filament results in higher visible output with a more desirable color temperature. Condensing optics ensures that minimum energy is lost and that the fields of view of lamp and fibers match. Sophisticated heat rejection filters reduce infrared radiation (Fig. 2).

HIGH-INTENSITY LIGHT SOURCES

In addition to the requirement for examination sources, there is a smaller but rapidly growing demand for high-intensity light sources. These devices are required for: (1) procedures utilizing extremely long, flexible fiberoptic endoscopes; (2) procedures employing flexible, fiberoptic teaching attachment; and (3) documentation, which may be in the form of cinematography or television.

Requirements

The requirements for high-intensity sources are similar to those outlined for low-intensity sources. However, the visible intensity requirement increases approximately 10-fold. For documentation this increase is necessitated by two factors; additional light is needed to film, and there are two simultaneous activities ongoing. These two activities are the examination itself and filming (or television). Therefore some fraction of the light coming through the telescope must be used for one and the remainder, which has been somehow separated out, for the other. This separation or splitting is accomplished by an optical beam splitter. Beam splitters may be flat plates or cubes, depending on the particular application.

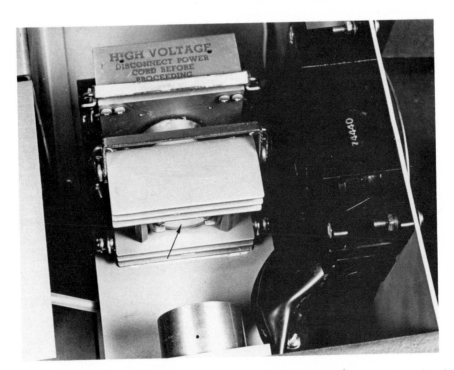

FIG. 7. Same small, compact xenon lamp seen in Figure 6, encased in a housing (view from above). Special filters placed in front of the globe (arrow) reject both infrared and ultraviolet radiation. The entire lamphouse or lamp itself can be interchanged with ease, without the necessity of wearing protective helmets.

Specifications concerning heat production are much more difficult to meet with high-intensity sources. This is because invariably no matter how efficient the heat rejection schemes employed some of the visible light is converted to infrared through absorption phenomena. Design of such systems then becomes a detailed trade-off study of visible light versus heat; i.e., the more heat that must be rejected, the less visible light there is available.

As with the examining sources no effort has been made to design a unit specifically for endoscopic purposes. Rather, most units are assembled from components designed for different purposes. As a result most currently available sources are unsatisfactory with regard to one or more of the desired features.

The most widely used high-intensity source employs a General Electric (GE) MARC-300 lamp (Fig. 3). This is a mercury, high-pressure globe that produces adequate light for most procedures. Its apparent color temperature is higher than that of tungsten. It is not correct to speak of color temperature with line sources. For these sources it is more accurate to refer to color purity or the psychophysical effects on the viewer; i.e., the color looks the same as it does in daylight. However, the large heat produced along with the visible output is objectionable. Both intensity and color purity degrade continually during the short 25-hour lifetime of the GE MARC-300 globe. This unit is also heavy and cumbersome.

Point source xenon lamps have also been used. They have much longer lifetimes (on the order of 1000 hours) and good color purity. Because special optical systems (both reflective and refractive) have been used, these units match the fields of view of the mating fibers more closely than the MARC-300. However, both ultraviolet and infrared outputs are still objectionably high, and the units tend to be large, heavy, cumbersome, and costly. Xenon lamps are notoriously erratic and have been known to explode for no apparent reason. Therefore explosionproof mechanical housings are required (Figs. 4 and 5).

Recent Developments

There is now available a unit which meets all the requirements outlined above (Fig. 6). This unit employs refractive condensing optics to match the 70-degree field of view of most fiber optics. Special filtering rejects both infrared and ultraviolet. The small, compact xenon lamp is encased in a housing (Fig. 7), and the total system, weighing 42 pounds, is contained in a cabinet no larger than a conventional xenon power supply (see Chap. 18).

4

Teaching Attachments

Valerie Olson
George Berci

The current widespread use of endoscopy for examining, manipulating, operating, and treating various conditions brings to light several pressing requirements. One of these is the need for auxiliary personnel capable of assisting during different procedures. In order to assist properly the doctor or nurse must be permitted a simultaneous view of the operative field with the examiner. The ability to view simultaneously is also immensely important in teaching institutions. It is obvious that as endoscopy grows, so does the necessity of training skilled endoscopists. The reasons for having a simultaneous viewing device are then twofold: assisting and teaching.

Simple devices of this nature are commonly called teaching attachments. In principle they consist of: (1) a beam splitter, which divides the light-exiting image from the eyepiece of the endoscope to the examiner and to the observer; (2) an optical relay system, which transmits the image from the beam splitter to the eyepiece of the observer; and (3) the ocular of the observer end (Fig. 1).

REQUIREMENTS

Proper functioning of the teaching attachment necessitates fulfilling the following optical requirements:

1. The examiner and assistant must be able to view the operative field simultaneously.
2. The fields of view at both viewing positions must be identical.
3. Contrast and resolution at both the examiner's and the assistant's ends must not be degraded.
4. There should be no evidence of vignetting.
5. Sufficient light must reach the examiner's and the assistant's viewing positions to present a

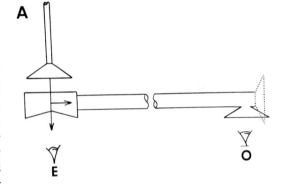

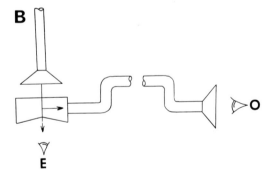

FIG. 1. Rigid (**A**) and flexible (**B**) teaching attachments. The image from the endoscope is split via a beam splitter to the examiner (E) and transmitted through (**A**) a rigid optical relay system or (**B**) a flexible coherent fiber bundle to the observer (O).

bright, clear image without having to employ high-intensity light sources.
6. The interposed teaching attachment should not interfere with the routine of the examination.

It is also desirable that this unit be fairly rugged. It should be capable of being sterilized in gas and of being attached and released quickly and smoothly from the endoscope.

HISTORY

The teaching attachments available in the past generally fall into three catagories: rigid, flexible (Fig. 2), and articulated optical arms (see Chap. 19).

FLEXIBLE TEACHING ATTACHMENTS

Flexible teaching attachments are fairly straightforward devices utilizing a beam splitter (to direct the light in two different paths) and a flexible coherent fiberoptic cable. Unfortunately these instruments, by definition, must suffer from all the problems inherent with coherent flexible fiber optics, i.e., large transmission losses (up to 15 percent per foot), a disturbing mosaic pattern, and severe resolution loss. In addition, they are quite fragile. This fragility can be attributed to unavoidable broken fibers, which tend to cause other broken fibers (cascading). With this effect it is possible for instruments to become inoperative in a comparatively short period of time. Further, when flexible teaching attachments are coupled to flexible endoscopes, the mosaic pattern tends to overlap and cause an even greater reduction in resolution (Fig. 3). This effect is detailed in Chapter 2. Finally, flexible teaching attachments are relatively costly.

However, there are situations in which the flexible teaching attachment must be applied because, due to space and movement limita-

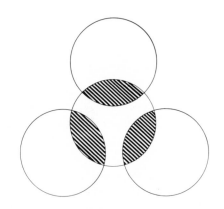

FIG. 3. Mismatch phenomenon. If coherent (size approximately 10 to 15 μ) fiber threads are coupled mechanically but not optically, the continuity of image transmission of the individual fibers is interrupted or partially transmitted. This results in loss of resolution or in a disturbing pattern.

tions of the endoscope, the manipulation cannot be performed with ease using a rigid attachment, e.g., cystoscopy. In these particular applications optical requirements must be compromised.

RIGID TEACHING ATTACHMENTS

Rigid teaching attachments also use a beam splitter to separate light into two paths. However, they employ more conventional (rigid) optical systems to relay the image to the assistant's viewing port. All of the rigid teaching attachments available until quite recently exhibited one or more of the following objectionable characteristics: (1) incorrect eye relief; (2) field of view mismatch; (3) severe vignetting; or (4) insufficient light intensity at the examiner's or the assistant's end. Because of these problems they have not been widely used or accepted.

NEW ADVANCES

Recently a rigid teaching attachment was made available that meets all of the requirements outlined earlier. It allows simultaneous viewing of the exact same field with crisp, clear, well-illuminated, nonvignetted images.

The unit is rugged and capable of being gas-sterilized or soaked in sterilizing solution. In addition it is economical and well within the

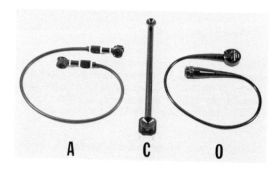

A   C   O

FIG. 2. Flexible and rigid teaching attachments. A, ACMI flexible coherent fiber teaching attachment. C, Storz rigid teaching attachment. O, Olympus flexible coherent teaching attachment.

means of the smaller teaching institution or hospital.

The optical system of this unit was carefully designed to match the telescopic field of view and uses the most advanced optical engineering techniques. Transmission losses were minimized by means of sophisticated antireflection coatings on all optical interfaces. Maximum absorption of the relay system is 6 percent. The beam splitter was also specially designed and fabricated to give optimal illumination in both paths.

Two variations of this device are available. One of these permits the examiner and assistant to stand side by side—they are perpendicular to one another in the standard configuration (Fig. 4A). Additional rotation

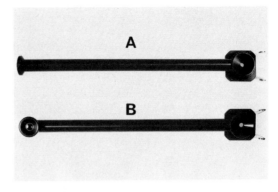

FIG. 4. Teaching attachments with (**A**) a quick adapter and straight perpendicular view; and (**B**) a quick adapter but viewing conditions identical to those of the operator. (Courtesy Storz Co.)

FIG. 5. A. Articulated optical arm. The outcoming image from the endoscope is split. One part is transmitted through the beam splitter to the examiner (E) whereby the rest of the image (90 percent) is transmitted through several rigid optical relay systems interconnected with rotating optical joints (prisms or mirrors) to the camera (C) or second observer (O). (For details see Figure 29 in Chapter 1.) **B.** Articulated optical arm attached at the viewing end to cystoscope and the other end to a (16-mm movie) camera. (Courtesy of Professor Hopkins).

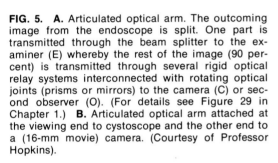

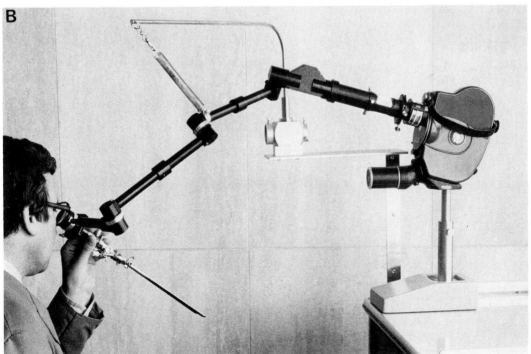

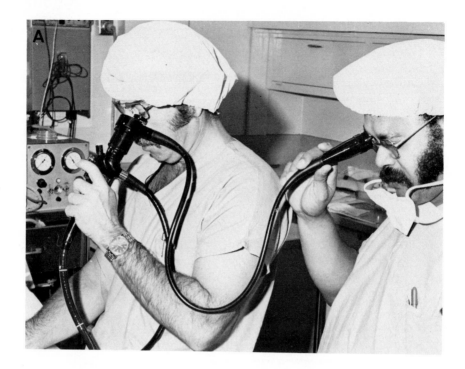

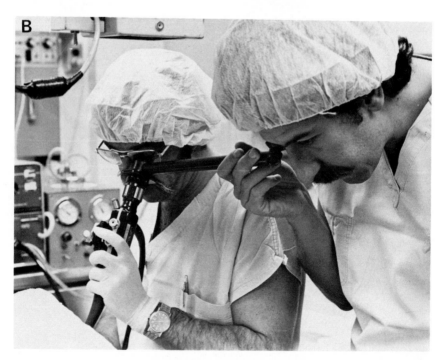

FIG. 6. **A.** Flexible (colon) fiberscope with flexible teaching attachment. **B.** Same flexible fiberscope but coupled to the rigid teaching attachment. The transmitted image to both examiner and observer is brighter. The image quality at the examiner's viewing end is the same as at the observer's eyepiece. (Courtesy Gastrointest Endo 22:30, 1975)

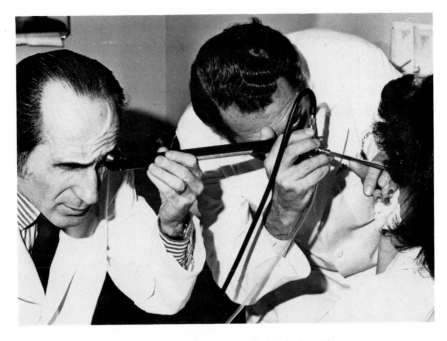

FIG. 7. Rigid teaching attachment coupled to indirect laryngoscope.

around the eyepiece anticipates movements required for following various positions, e.g., during laparoscopy. The second version (Fig. 4B) gives the same relative viewing position to the assistant as to the operator.

ARTICULATED OPTICAL ARM

The articulated optical arm consists of several rigid relay systems connected by joints. The joints consist of mirrors or prisms that can rotate (Fig. 5). Again a beam splitter is employed to permit an unobstructed view for the examiner and simultaneously allow the other end to be coupled to a recording (television or movie) camera (Chap. 19). The total absorption of the various rigid relay components is approximately 20 percent. An additional 10 percent of the light is directed to the operator, resulting in a total light loss of approximately 30 percent. The articulated optical arm transmits a higher resolution image than does a coherent fiber bundle. It is well designed, and the quality of the displayed image at the camera end is excellent. Its construction is delicate and expensive, and only prototypes are currently available. The articulated joints permit movement of the telescope without the burden of having a heavy recording apparatus attached.

CONCLUSION

Increasingly sophisticated endoscopic procedures, proceeding from simple examination to manipulation, operation, or treatment, require the help of an assistant. Teaching a complex procedure requires that the student see the technique (Figs. 6 and 7). Progress in endoscopy necessitated the development of a teaching attachment to serve the purpose.

It is hoped that the flexible teaching attachment can be improved with respect to better transmission parameters and elimination of the disturbing mosaic pattern. It should be carefully noted, however, that because of physical limitations resolution of flexible fiber optics can never be made comparable to that of rigid optical systems.

5

Instrumentation I: Rigid Endoscopes

George Berci

Progress in diagnostic and therapeutic medicine was mainly achieved with the help of new technologic ideas. There are few areas in medicine where we are so dependent on instruments and their performance as in the field of endoscopy. We could not dream of examining the urinary bladder without a cystoscope, performing a tubal sterilization or aimed target biopsy of abdominal organs without a laparoscope, assessing a gastric or duodenal ulcer (or doing a noninvasive colonic polypectomy) without a flexible fiberscope, and so on. The list is almost endless.

The physiologic and pathologic aspects are of course the dominant ones, but it seems to me that the instrument itself does not receive the attention it deserves because the members of our profession are predominantly trained and interested in the clinical part. Well-organized research activities are found in many institutions in a number of areas—cardiology, nephrology, radiology, etc.—but laboratories dealing with the basic parameters or research possibilities to help to develop endoscopy per se are practically silent. There is little to be found in the literature, and where reports do appear they deal with a particular endoscopic subspecialty, emphasizing mainly the diagnostic or therapeutic application.

Approximately 10 million endoscopic examinations are performed each year in the United States alone. The time has come to recognize the importance of these facts and figures and the need for well-organized laboratory and clinical research projects in this neglected area.

GENERAL ASPECTS

Amnio-, arthro-, broncho-, choledocho-, culdo-, cysto-, esophago-, hystero-, laparo-, laryngo-, mediastino-, procto-, rhino-, recto-, stereo-, encephalo-, thoraco-, and transconioscopy are procedures to be considered as forms of endoscopy. A set of instruments for endoscopic techniques consists in general of four major components: (1) outer sheath; (2) illuminator; (3) optics; and (4) accessories (Fig. 1).

Outer Sheath

The outer sheath allows exploration of the organ and keeps it in a distended position to facilitate vision and manipulation by means of a straight (optical) access. The design and manufacturing process of metal sheaths (e.g., a laryngoscope or bronchoscope) is at least 40 to 50 years old. Brass was used, resulting in a relatively thick wall; this decreased the lumen size as well as the viewing area. Modern metallurgy produced various alloys which permit a thinner wall, with the same stress or durability but a larger lumen for better observation (Fig. 2).

Illumination

Distal. In older instruments a small electric globe was inserted in a bulb carrier that was introduced to the working end of the

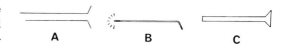

D− ACCESSORIES

FIG. 1. Main components of a rigid endoscope. **A.** Outer sheath. **B.** Illumination. **C.** Optics. **D.** Accessories.

FIG. 2. A. Standard (adult) bronchoscope examining sheath. Outside diameter 12.5 mm; inside diameter (lumen) 8.0 mm. **B.** Modern (adult) bronchoscope (aluminum alloy) sheath. Outside diameter 11.3 mm; inside diameter (lumen) 10.0 mm. Despite the smaller outside diameter this sheath provides a larger lumen. **C.** A small electric globe inserted in a bulb carrier. It was most disconcerting if the bulb burned out during the examination. This type of illumination is today replaced by fiber optics.

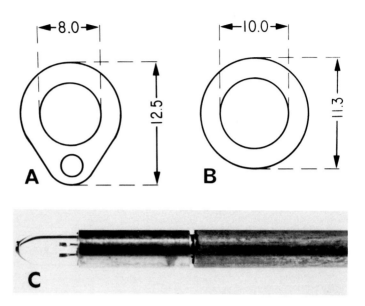

endoscope. It was very disconcerting if during an examination the bulb burned out and the procedure had to be interrupted. This type of illumination is today obsolete, replaced by the proximal ones described below (Fig. 2C).

Proximal. Light is reflected by means of a mirror from an outside light source. Since the light source is placed externally, its intensity can be increased. The larger globe poses heat and space problems, however. In a more modern version the light is conducted via a flexible (incoherent) bundle from an external light source to a prismatic light deflector, which is inserted into the sheath (Fig. 3).

Advantages. Light intensity is greater with a proximal light source than with a distal one. Some types can be withdrawn into the sheath (Fig. 4) and a telescope introduced with its built-in illumination. This provides the examiner with a "double" lighting system. If the telescope becomes dirty (blood, secretion, etc.) and is withdrawn, the prismatic light deflector is pushed back into the sheath within seconds and the examiner is never left in the dark. In a case of bleeding or manipulation, suction can be instituted immediately. Proximal illumination is advantageous during rectoscopy (a better term for sigmoidoscopy), laryngoscopy (direct), adult and pediatric bronchoesophagoscopy, and proctoscopy because it is located a safe distance from the working end and it avoids the obliteration of light by secretions. It can be employed only in those systems where a short, open tube suffices. In applications where the outer (explorative) sheath is long and/or has a small diameter, proximal illumination cannot be used because of the small "keyhole" or tunnel vision effect. For instance, in such procedures as adult bronchoscopy, pediatric and adult urologic examinations, arthroscopy, etc., a telescope must be introduced.

Disadvantages. The protruding part (prismatic deflector) is sometimes in the way during manipulations. Moreover, minor but disturbing reflections from the inside wall of the sheath are sometimes observed.

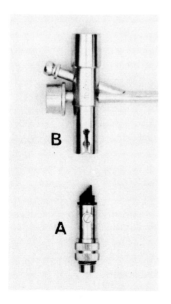

FIG. 3. A prismatic light deflector (**A**) to be inserted into a sheath (**B**).

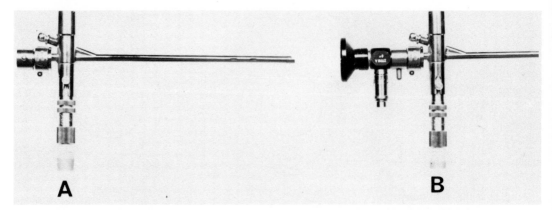

FIG. 4. If a telescope with fiber illumination is introduced, the prismatic light deflector (**A**) is pulled back into the sheath (**B**). If the telescope is removed, the deflector is pushed back within seconds (**A**) and illumination is provided (double lighting system). Applications: pediatrics, direct laryngoscopy, and procto-, recto-, sigmoido-, and mediastinoscopy.

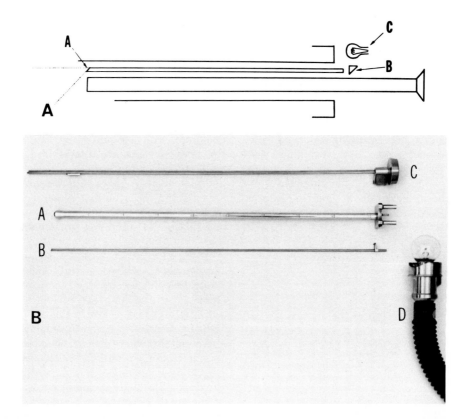

FIG. 5. **A.** Quartz rod illumination. A quartz rod is inserted into the sheath (A) between the telescope and the wall of the sheath. It is connected via a small prism (B) to a projector globe (C). **B.** Bronchoscope with quartz rod light transmission. A, sheath. B, quartz rod. C, telescope. D, projector globe. Lamphouse with condensor, deviating prism, and cooling system is removed. Lamp has a 16-volt tungsten filament. Quartz rods are excellent light-conducting media; they are more efficient than fiber incoherent light transmitters.

Quartz Rod Light Transmission.
Quartz rod lighting is a proximal illumination system. A small projector globe is attached in a housing to the viewing end of the endoscope. A small quartz rod is inserted below the telescope (Fig. 5). It was introduced by Fourestier et al. in 1952.[9] Quartz rods are excellent light-conducting media; 95 percent of visible light is transmitted with excellent color temperature. This was the first device that made cinematography or still picture documentation easier (Fig. 5B).

Disadvantages. It is clumsy to hold a projector globe with housing and a cooling system in your hand, and the quartz is very fragile and expensive. Furthermore, using continuous illumination the "ring effect" of the quartz rod is visible at longer object distances.

We must give credit to this illumination design, however, because it was the first that produced bright light and opened the field to documentation for rigid endoscopes of normal sizes.

Fiber (Incoherent) Illumination. A small fiber rod is inserted into the bottom part of the sheath and connected via a fiber cable to an external light source (Fig. 6). In longer tubes the viewing field cannot be illuminated properly with a proximal deflecting lighting system. The working end of the fiber rod is slightly recessed into the tube to avoid frequent withdrawal due to blocking of the illumination with blood or secretion (Fig. 6B).

If telescopes are employed the image-transmitting part (lenses) are assembled together with fibers carrying light for illumination. There are other ways and means to "package" light-transmitting fibers in a rigid sheath, e.g., building it together with the wall in a semicircular or other shape. This design depends on the allotted space, application, etc. The quick interchangeability of any light-transmitting system is preferable to one that is built in. Occasionally there is excessive secretion or bleeding, and when this occurs it is very helpful to be able to withdraw the fiber light

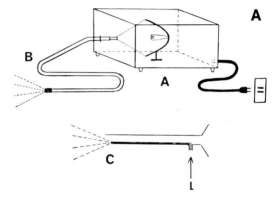

FIG. 6. A. Proximal, flexible fiber illumination. An external light source (A) is connected through a 6-foot flexible fiber bundle (B) to the light input (L) of an endoscope sheath to a fiber light carrier (C). **B.** If a fiber rod (B) is recessed (at bottom) —e.g., in the adult bronchoscope sheath (**A**)— frequent withdrawal to clear blood or secretion can be avoided. It can still be withdrawn, cleaned, and reinserted if required, keeping the sheath in position. **A.** Sheath. **B.** Fiber rod connected to external light source.

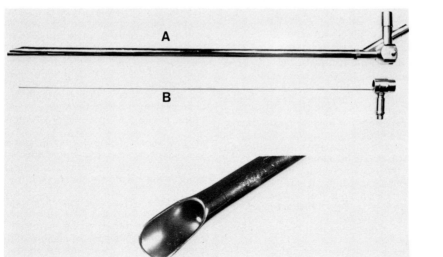

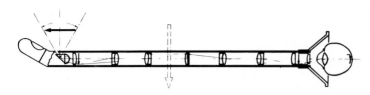

FIG. 7. Standard lens system, first described by Nitze. Small lenses are placed in a certain air intervals with an objective lens and prism on the working end, the ocular, and the eyepiece. This design—the cystoscope—served for decades as the most important diagnostic tool in urology.

system and clean and reinsert it without removing the sheath. Fiber light illumination can be also classified as proximal because of the location of the light source.

Disadvantages. The system is fragile and needs careful handling. There is also significant light absorption and a yellowish tint.

Optics

Since the invention of the medical telescope by Nitze[24] in 1879 the principle of optics has remained generally the same. Small lenses were placed in certain air intervals with the help of spacers (Fig. 7). An objective lens with an optical deviating system determines the direction of view in the case of any optical axis or direction of view other than 0 degrees. The ocular system with the eyepiece completed the design. This system underwent improvement but served for 75 years in various applications, e.g., urology, bronchology.

There were several disadvantages encountered. The small-diameter (high-aperture) air interspace, optical alignment problems, difficulties in producing quality lenses in this small diameter all contributed to a high degree of light absorption and narrow viewing angle. If this system was miniaturized (lens diameter decreased) further light absorption resulted in an extremely dim image. (Flexible fiber optics are dealt with in a separate chapter.)

To enable us to communicate better, let us briefly review terminology:

Resolution. This may be measured by the smallest distance between two objects that an endoscope can register by displaying two separate images. Very often we are misinterpreting two physical concepts: *resolution* and *magnification*. Resolution has nothing to do with magnification; they are two different entities. An indistinct image remains indistinct no matter how many times it is magnified. The only effect of magnification is that a small indistinct image is produced as a large indistinct image. For example, if an image is painted on a sheet of rubber, stretching this sheet reveals no more detail.

Definition. This is the sharpness of the image.

Ideally the edges of the image are reproduced without optical distortion and the continuity of the image is not interrupted, e.g., in the case of flexible fiber endoscopes through breakage of individual fiber threads.

Aberration. The quality of the image seen depends primarily on the quality of the real image formed as an end result. Any imperfections in this image are magnified if it is viewed through the ocular eyepiece from a close distance. The aberration of a telescope should therefore be reduced to the smallest practicable values. Spherical aberration produces a hazy image, whereas chromatic aberration produces color fringes at the boundaries of the object and reduces the contrast of the image.

Contrast. This is the observer's subjective impression created by the differences between the darkest and the lightest part of the field of view. It can be measured by applying special optical tests. This factor plays a role in color reproduction and interpretation.

Direction of view. This term is often confused with the viewing angle. The direction of view or viewing direction of the optical system represents the relation of the optical system to the horizontal axis of the telescope, which is expressed in degrees (Fig. 8). The direction of view corresponds also with the middle of the viewing angle (Fig. 9).

Viewing angle. This is the angle formed by the two outer visual limits determining the diameter of the field of view and represents the size of objects seen (Fig. 9). If the viewing angle is narrow the magnification can be greater, or vice versa. In telescopes with a wide viewing angle but low magnification, this can be compensated for by advancing the optic, thereby enlarging the object. The size of the viewing angle of a telescope or fiber endoscope determines an important feature. If it affords a wide-angled view but still provides sufficient information, orientation becomes much easier because a larger part of the organ can be seen in a single viewing field.

Magnification. The object seen and magnified is dependent on the design of the optical components where the viewing angle, ocular enlargements, and object distance are significant factors.

Virtual field. This is the total diameter of the actual image as seen through the ocular of the endoscope. This is constant for any one instrument and is independent of the distance of the lens to the object. Its precise diameter cannot be accurately determined,

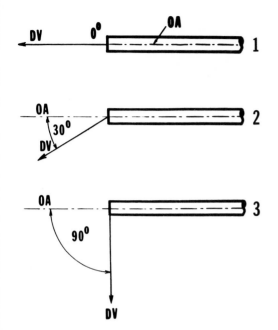

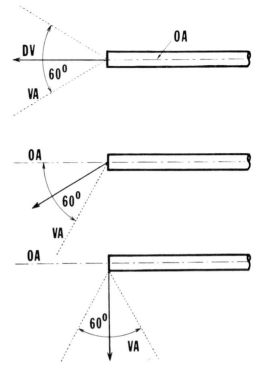

FIG. 8. Direction of view (arrow). 1, If the optical axis (OA) of the telescope is extended, it produces a straightforward view (0 degrees). The deviation or direction of view (DV) from the horizontal optical axis is expressed in degrees. 2, Forward-oblique view (30 degrees). 3, Lateral view (90 degrees).

but for comparative purposes it can be assessed as follows: One eye is applied to the endoscope, and circular test objects of various diameters are placed at the optimum viewing distance for the other eye. When the size of the test object matches that of the field of view of the endoscope, the virtual field can be compared to the test object diameter.[19]

Light transmission. The light absorption of an endoscope is relatively high, and the problems of light absorption continue to limit the efficiency of our instruments. It can be measured accurately by optical means. With the development of modern, more powerful light sources, this can be compensated for somewhat by transmitting more light into the cavity. The complex design of high-intensity light sources have accompanying problems—e.g., heat production, wavelengths dangerous to tissues (ultraviolet and infrared)—that at this stage limit their use. Further optical improvements are required to increase the light or image transmission through our currently available systems. This applies to both rigid and flexible endoscopes.

Depth of field. This is the shortest and longest object distance seen in a single viewing field. In the field of endoscopy the depth of field is dependent on many parameters of the optical design and illumination.

It is very important to see with enough detail well-defined lesions located near the objective

FIG. 9. Viewing angle (VA) is shown with dotted lines. This angle (60 degrees) is formed by two outer visual limits determining the diameter of the field of view or the size of the object. The direction of view corresponds also with the middle (arrow) of the viewing angle (dotted lines). Various directions of view with a 60-degree viewing angle are displayed.

(distal end of scope) as well as those at a distance (e.g., the mucosal lining) *without moving the instrument.* It is a complex problem in physics and medicine. How far and how near must we be able to see sharply? We require depth perception with adequate resolution, and this is determined separately for each endoscopic application according to the anatomy and diagnostic need (Fig. 10).

The invention by Hopkins* of his rod-lens system[4] created a breakthrough in image transmission of rigid telescopes† with the following features:

1. Significantly less light absorption (compared with a standard lens system). The image is therefore brighter, and there is faster perception.

*Patents: Great Britain 954629, United States 3257902.
†Manufacturer: K. Storz Endoscopy Co., Tuttlingen, West Germany. Distributor: K. Storz Endoscopy America Inc., 658 So. San Vicente Boulevard, Los Angeles, California 90048.

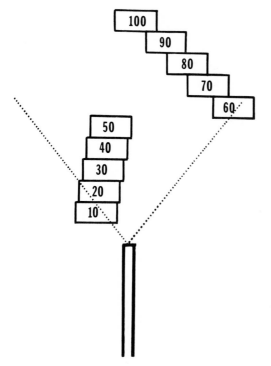

FIG. 10. Depths of field. The shortest and longest object distance seen clearly in a single viewing field. This diagram displays the relation of various object distances (0 to 100 mm) seen through an endoscope without moving the instrument itself.

2. Wide viewing angle. A large part of the organ can be seen in a single viewing field. Orientation therefore is easy and the examination fast.
3. Excellent image quality (resolution, contrast, and color reproduction).
4. Facilitates documentation (permanent film records or television) because of aspects mentioned in items 1 through 3.
5. Miniaturization. The above parameters made it possible to decrease the diameter. This in turn permitted the production of smaller instruments, and so there is safer introduction and easier manipulation.
6. New applications. It opened new vistas in pediatric endoscopic procedures[12] or areas where the size is important, e.g., arthroscopy, encephaloscopy, and pediatrics in general. Even through these "miniscopes" (rod-lens diameter 1.8 mm) sufficient light and image quality is transmitted to expose a 16-mm movie film.

The rod-lens system opened a new chapter in rigid endoscopy (Fig. 11). A similar approach is the Microlens* in which the air interspace is also largely replaced with glass.

*American Cystoscope Makers, Inc., 8 Pelham Parkway, Pelham Manor, New York 10803.

The Selfoc* system is a new development, which is a single image-transmitting fiber thread. It is manufactured in such a way that the refractive index of this fiber is improved by chemical methods. The single-fiber thread can be as small as 0.5 to 1 mm in diameter, and with a minimum of light transmitting fibers surrounding it the entire image and light-transmitting system can be decreased to 1.7 mm total outside diameter (Fig. 12). It is an intriguing idea but in our opinion is still in the experimental stage. This Needlescope is advocated for arthroscopy but suffers from limitation in image quality compared with the rod-lens system (Fig. 12B). Another disadvantage is that a large magnifying lupe system must be employed at the other end of this single-fiber transmitting part for convenient viewing, which makes the instrument clumsy. It does have potential, however, if the optical quality can be further improved.

Accessories

If the telescope is introduced in a body cavity where the temperature is higher (e.g., in the larynx, bronchial tree, esophagus, rectum) the lens can become fogged, which is disturbing. This can be overcome by: (1) prewarming the lens in (sterile) warm water; (2) preheating with a hairdryer[16] or a thermoelement; or (3) using a very thin outer sheath or tube connected to an external, small (aquarium) pump which blows room air in the front of the lens to keep it clean—a "window wiper" (Fig. 13). This small positive-pressure system compared with techniques mentioned under (1) and (2) has the advantage of keeping secretions, blood, or products of forced expiration (cough) out of the way of the working end (objective) better than any sort of lens cleaners, mainly in the respiratory or alimentary tract.

We have problems in manufacturing precision hand instruments. These microsurgical tools can be mass produced only with difficulty, and so usually they are handmade individually. As a good example, some of our greatest problems in instrumentation are the small biopsy forceps (Fig. 14) and the microsurgical instruments required for laryngeal surgery, such as small, fine scissors or variously shaped

*Manufacturer: Nippon Glass Company, Tokyo, Japan. Distributor: Dyonics Company, 1450 Brooks Road, Memphis, Tennessee 38116.

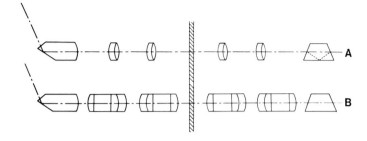

FIG. 11. Hopkins rod-lens system. **A.** Standard lens system. **B.** Rod-lens system. The air interspace is largely replaced by glass rods with appropriate optics on both ends. This system created a breakthrough in rigid endoscopes. The parameter and advantages are listed in the text.

cup forceps on a long handle (Fig. 15). There is a definite shortage in skilled manpower among our younger, well-trained instrument makers. The situation has deteriorated in recent years and deserves serious consideration from the medical profession, health authorities, and the industry itself. The demand is much greater than the availability of these much-needed and delicate instruments. Rigid endoscopic instruments are still used more frequently than flexible fiberscopes (approximate ratio 4:1).

RIGID ENDOSCOPES

Aspects to be considered when using the tools which play a crucial role in the final outcome of an endoscopic examination include their diagnostic accuracy, effectiveness of treatment, and risk to the patient. *The endoscopes described here were chosen on the basis of the author's personal experience. Hence it is not meant to be implied that other types of instruments are not useful.*

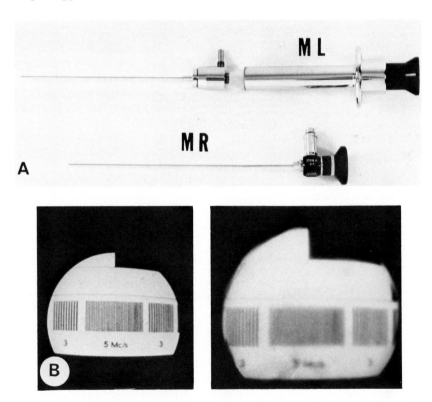

FIG. 12.   A. Selfoc system (Needlescope), consisting of a single small fiber thread where the refractive index of the fiber is created by chemical methods. A small number of fibers are surrounding the image-transmitting part to provide illumination (OD 1.7 mm). A large magnifying lupe (ML) must be employed on the other end. A miniature rod-lens system (MR) including fiber illumination (OD 2.7 mm) is shown for comparison.   **B.** Resolution test pattern through the miniature Hopkins rod-lens telescope (left) and the Needlescope or Selfoc system (right). (Photographs were taken under identical conditions.)

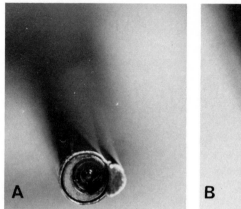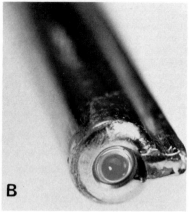

FIG. 13.   Antifog system.   **A.** A thin outer sheath is pulled over the telescope and connected to a small air pump to create positive pressure at the front of the lens to act as a "window wiper."   **B.** Another approach is to attach a small needle to the telescope and blow air in front of the objective to keep it clean.

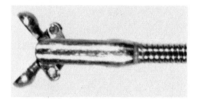

Amnioscope

Amnioscopy is performed through the vagina. A cone-shaped exploratory tube is required with a proximal fiber light to examine the color of the transparent fluid seen through the cervical os. (Preferred instruments are described in Chapter 35.) A telescope can also be inserted.

FIG. 14. A major problem in tissue sampling through small endoscopes is designing and manufacturing a delicate but powerful biopsy forceps with sharp cutting edges (cutting and not tearing).

The other approach is to investigate prenatal

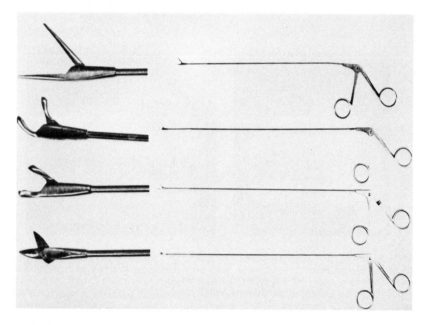

FIG. 15.   Examples of handmade precision microsurgical instruments used for laryngeal surgery.

or fetal physiology through the transabdominal, transuterine routes by inserting a small rigid or flexible endoscope within the womb. Fetoscopy is still in an early experimental stage (see Chap. 37).

Arthroscope

Because of the small size and required excellent image quality and manipulation, rigid instruments are used for arthroscopy. A cannula with sharp and blunt stylets (trocar) is employed. The sharp stylet is inserted first and then after the trocar is in position the blunt stylet replaces the sharp stylet to ensure further safe advancement. As soon as it is in the joint cavity a telescope is introduced under visual control, replacing the blunt stylet. Irrigation is applied to distend the knee or other joints. Additional accessories include small curved hooks, which can be advanced from a separate incision; and a biopsy forceps, which can be introduced through the trocar with the telescope. The maximum diameter of the trocar is 3 to 4 mm. For further details see Chapter 55.

Bronchoscope (Adult)

The instruments for bronchoscopy have now become smaller. We can now perform adult examinations with a sheath of 6.5, 7.5, or 8 mm. The old open brass tubes provide a much smaller view through the lumen. The numbers engraved on these sheaths are arbitrary, and if the inside (ID) or outside diameter (OD) is measured there is a slight discrepancy between these figures and the actual measurements

(Table 1). This must be kept in mind. Perhaps a more accurate indication (e.g., ID/OD) would give the examiner a better idea about the actual size.

Bronchoscopy is one of the oldest endoscopic procedures. It is amazing how many difficulties we had to overcome before feeling that we could recommend the use of already existing telescopes. If a test pattern is placed at a distance of 10 mm from an open 43-cm tube and is looked at with the naked eye, and then a telescope is introduced, the vastly improved visual acuity becomes evident (Fig. 16). Various directions of view facilitate observation of the different locations of the orifices and anatomy (Fig. 17). The superiority of observation is even more obvious when small lesions have to be identified or when the instrument must be of pediatric size (Fig. 18).

The greater detail of perception is obvious, but despite these facts it will take time to convince the experienced bronchoscopist—whose vision is trained for a tunnel view—to change his approach to the telescopic inspection. It is easier for the trainee, who starts with this technique. Even a small magnifier lupe on a hinge that can be easily flipped in position (Fig. 19) improves observation and detection of small lesions.

Biopsy. Often a biopsy is performed after locating the lesion with the naked eye through the open tube. The biopsy forceps is then introduced, obscuring the view. Thus the actual biopsy specimen is obtained by aiming at the lesion, i.e., the procedure is done semiblindly (Fig. 20). With optical biopsy forceps (Fig. 21) the aim is accurate and the actual bite is taken under good visual control; this is referred to as a *target biopsy*. It is astonishing how many biopsies are performed with an outdated, inadequate technique despite the fact that a safer, more accurate method is now available. We do not have figures or controlled studies, but it is encouraging to see Figures 20 and 21. Similar optical forceps but with alligator jaws are available for foreign body removal under precise visual control (Fig. 22).

Second Observer. Teaching bronchoscopy without extending the examining time or increasing the risk to the patient with unnecessary movements can be accomplished by using a telescope and the newly developed teaching attachment (Fig. 23). Today this should be the method of choice in every institution where bronchoscopy is taught (see Chap. 4).

TABLE 1. Adult Broncoscope

Type and Arbitrary Size*	Length (mm)	Sheath	
		Outside Diameter	Inside Diameter
Pilling			
7	395	11.6 × 8	7
8	465	12.5 × 9	8
Storz			
7.5	435	11.5	9
8.5	435	12.5	10

*It would be worthwhile to consider a common nomenclature or actual figures instead of employing arbitrary sizes or designations, e.g., OD/ID.

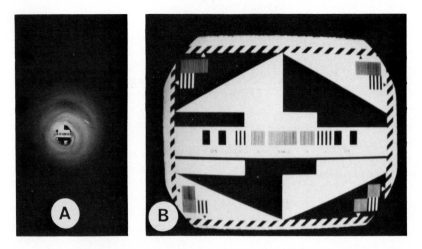

FIG. 16. Open tube (adult) bronchoscope. Resolution test pattern is placed 10 mm from the working end. **A.** View obtained with the naked eye. Reflection is disturbing. **B.** Same view but seen through a telescope.

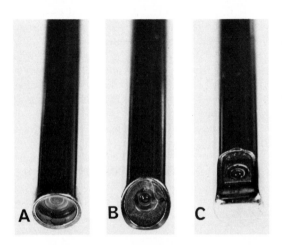

FIG. 17. Bronchotelescopes (adult) with directions of view: 0 degrees (**A**); 30 degrees (**B**); and 90 degrees (**C**). Light-transmitting fibers surround the optic lens (**A** and **B**) or are placed beside the objective lens (**C**).

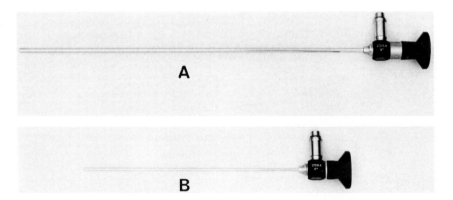

FIG. 18. Pediatric bronchotelescopes. **A.** Intermediate size (OD 4 mm). **B.** Newborn size (OD 2.7 mm).

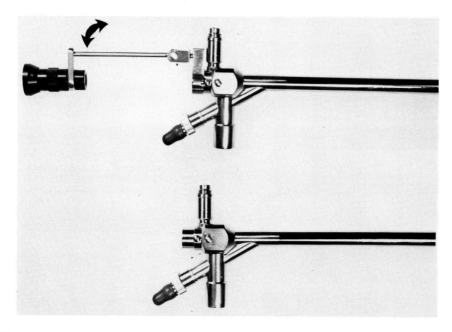

FIG. 19. Bronchoscope with a lupe magnifier that can be easily flipped in position to provide a ×2 or ×4 magnification. An intermediate solution is used to improve vision between a naked eye observation and a telescopic view.

FIG. 20. Bronchoscopic biopsy. **A.** Optical biopsy forceps. **B.** Using an open-tube system, the forceps is introduced. The instrument is aimed, but the actual bite is performed semiblindly.

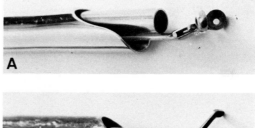

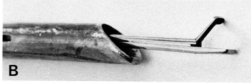

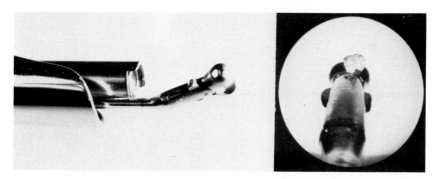

FIG. 21. Using the optical biopsy forceps the positioning and movements of the jaws can be seen without obstruction. The photograph at right was taken through the telescope.

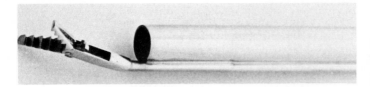

FIG. 22. Optical foreign body forceps with alligator jaws for foreign body removal (telescope is not inserted).

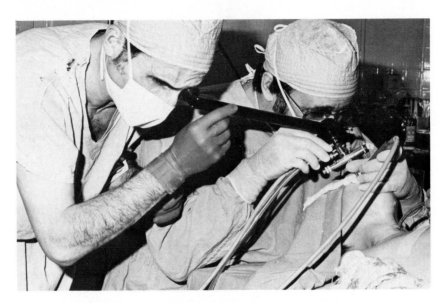

FIG. 23. Teaching bronchoscopy without extending the examination time can be achieved by having the procedure observed simultaneously by the operator and a second observer employing a newly designed teaching attachment. (For details see Chap. 4.)

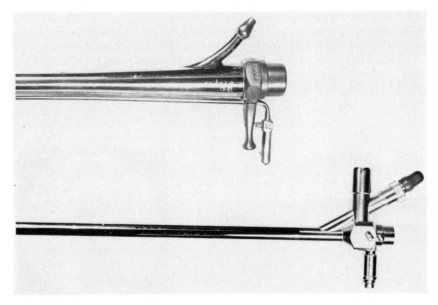

FIG. 24. Adult bronchoscope with a large-bore ventilation outlet for attaching to a respirator or anesthesia machine (bottom). Top, Ventilation outlet of standard bronchoscope.

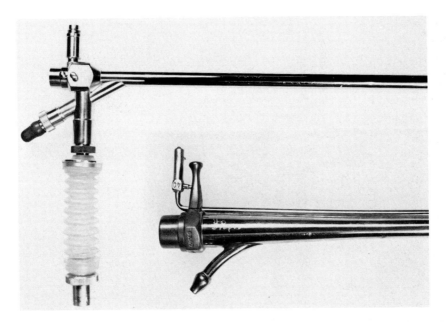

FIG. 25. Bottom, Standard bronchoscope. Top, Flexible connection to facilitate the link between the bronchoscope and the respirator.

Ventilation. Optimal patient ventilation or assisted respiration in a closed system is of paramount importance in every bronchoscopic examination whether it is done under local or general anesthesia. The new bronchoscope with a large-bore outlet attached to a respirator or anesthesia machine (Fig. 24) with which controlled oxygenation and air exchange can be maintained is preferable. A flexible connection (Fig. 25) provides the link between bronchoscope and respirator. An instrument channel (Fig. 26) can also be utilized by being connected to an assisted positive-pressure respiration apparatus[27] or other similar systems.[7·33]

Manipulation. An additional instrument channel can be helpful if the telescope is in position. A small biopsy instrument, foreign body forceps, or flexible suction tube can be advanced beyond the working end of the telescope if required (Fig. 26). Tissue secretion or tissue samples for cytology can be obtained under visual control.

Upper Lobe. The upper lobe represents a problem because of the anatomy in angulation of the bronchial tree. Looking "around corners" was never an easy proposition. However, with a wide-angle system and a good depth of field, the results are quite satisfactory with rigid endoscopic systems (Chap. 43). A deflector (Fig. 27) facilitates advancement of the biopsy forceps in a bent position (upper lobe) toward a peripheral lesion that can be still seen through the lateral telescope. Of course the biopsy cup is smaller than in the case of the rigid, straightforward one, but the obtained tissue sample is larger than one obtained by suction cytology.

The same deflector mechanism (Fig. 28) can be used for directing a radiopaque catheter into the orifice and advancing it toward the peripheral lesion that is out of the visual range but which can be located under fluoroscopic control. A bronchocatheter with remote-controlled tip*—similar to those employed in angiography (Fig. 29)—is available for this purpose. This catheter, because of its small size (Fr. 7), can be advanced far into the periphery of the bronchial tree. Some investigators claim high diagnostic accuracy using small catheters.[11]

Bronchoscope, Pediatrics

The aspects discussed for adult bronchoscopy are even more important for pediatric usage.

Manufacturer: Medi-Tech, Inc., 407 Belmont Street, Belmont, Massachusetts 02178.

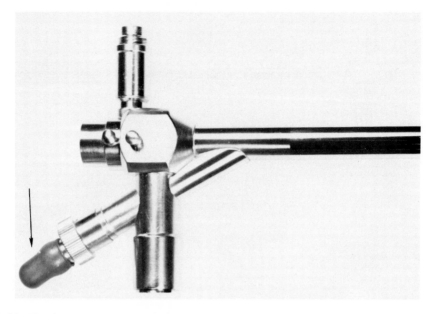

FIG. 26. The instrument channel (arrow) can also be connected to a positive-pressure respiration system.

In some centers highly skilled and experienced endoscopists are available and they have a special aptitude and remarkable ability to be able to see so much through those tiny open tubes under trying circumstances. But even in their hands, and more often in less talented hands, serious errors have been made, and procedures in critically ill infants have been unduly prolonged or even abandoned, and often repeated. Moreover, the difficulties in teaching endoscopy under these conditions are overwhelming. Training in this art is hard to come by leaving this critical ability as the possession of a few experts.[12]

Miniaturized tubes (2.5, 3.0, and 3.5 mm) are made with remarkable craftmanship. The lumen of the smallest bronchoscope sheath (2.5) is only 3 mm. The total length of the newborn tubes is 20 cm. Despite this small diameter the telescope can be introduced, and vastly improved inspection (magnified view) can be obtained with controlled respiration. It is extremely difficult and requires outstanding skill and adaptive ability to detect pathologic changes through a tube 20 cm long with a 3- to 4-mm "keyhole" lumen (Fig. 30).

Foreign Body Removal. Foreign body removal under telescopic control is of great importance. Many complications can be avoided by accurate and fast manipulations (see Chap. 24).

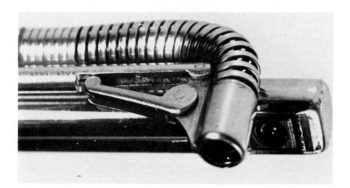

FIG. 27. Remote-controlled deflector to facilitate the advancement of a biopsy forceps in a bent position toward a peripheral or upper lobe lesion that can still be seen through the lateral telescope.

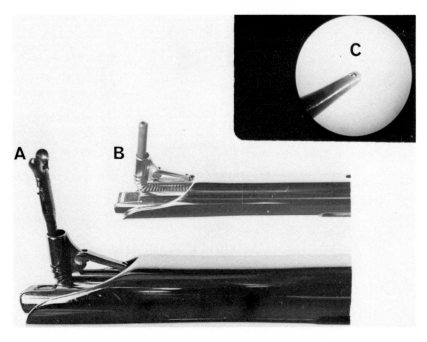

FIG. 28. Same deflector mechanism as shown in Figure 27 used to manipulate a radiopaque catheter into the orifice and advance it further toward the periphery under fluoroscopic control. **A.** Flexible biopsy forceps. **B.** Radiopaque catheter. **C.** Catheter as seen through the telescope.

Cystoscope

There is no subspecialty where instrumentation is of such dominant importance as in the field of urology. This was the first endoscopic examination using the Hopkins rod-lens system, and its introduction paid great dividends. After years of diligent research and redesigning, we produced our first clinical results 7 years ago.[4]

In adult cystoscopy the major advantage of using a telescope with a 4.0 mm diameter, a

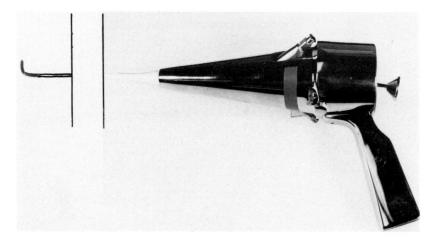

FIG. 29. Remote-controlled radiopaque bronchocatheter directed by a "joy stick" similar to the angiocatheter technique used in radiology.

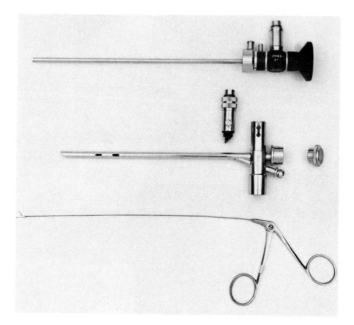

FIG. 30. A newborn broncho- scope set is available in three sizes: 2.5, 3.0, and 3.5 mm. The outside diameter of the 3.5-mm in- strument is 5.6 mm, and the lumen diameter is 4.5 mm. Length of the newborn set is 20 cm. Top, Tele- scope with antifog sheath. Middle, Sheath with prismatic reflector and glass window. Bottom, Minia- ture alligator foreign body forceps.

wide viewing angle, and more light transmis- sion made it possible to decrease the smallest adult examining sheath to Fr. 15.5. Two tele- scopes (a forward-oblique and a lateral direc- tion of view) are needed for examination, instrumentation, and transurethral resection (Fig. 31). With the additional resectoscope sheaths (24 and 27 Fr.) and one working ele- ment the entire uro-set is complete. The ver- satility of these telescopes has proved very use-

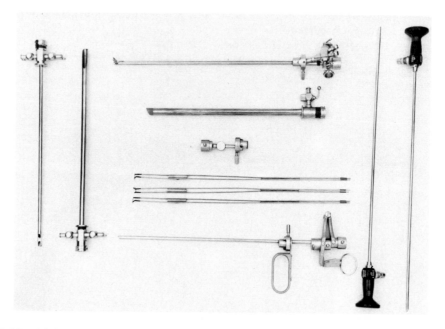

FIG. 31. Adult uro-set, permitting the use of two telescopes only (forward-oblique and lateral). The smallest size of adult examining sheath is 15.5 Fr., and the largest 23 Fr. The same telescopes can be utilized for resectoscope sheaths (24 and 27 Fr.).

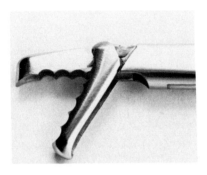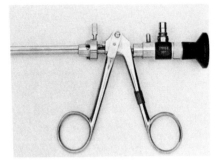

FIG. 32. Telescope with stone-crushing forceps, to be introduced through a sheath (23 Fr.).

ful in combination with examination, orifice catheterization, the use of a stone-crushing forceps (Fig. 32), the lithotrite (Fig. 33), biopsy forceps (Fig. 34), and transurethral resection.

During transurethral surgery if the 24 or 27 Fr. sheath is in position the forward-oblique telescope can be changed with ease to a lateral one, the ureter-catheter deflector can be inserted, or the trigonum can be inspected without interchanging the sheath.

Using a straightforward 0-degree telescope to resect a prostate is another aspect which has merits and needs further evaluation. Why do we use an oblique view during transurethral resections if the direction of manipulation (urethra) is straight ahead?[18] The irrigation

resectoscope reduces the operating time since continuous withdrawal of the telescope for forced rinsing during transurethral surgery is avoided because of continuous increased volume of water exchange.[17]

Pediatric Cystoscopy. A large number of congenital and acquired lesions of the urinary system and the great frequency of their occurrence makes endoscopic examination of the urinary tract in the newborn or infant a necessary routine. In the past many efforts were made to miniaturize adult instruments for use in pediatrics, but they fell far short of being satisfactory. The major drawback was the telescope itself because when the standard lens system was decreased in diameter light

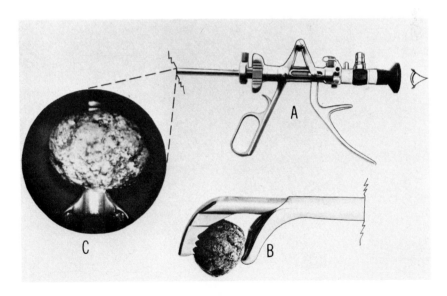

FIG. 33. Telescope with a lithotrite for disintegrating larger stones under visual control (24 Fr.). **A.** Instrument. **B.** Grasped stone. **C.** Stone seen through the telescope.

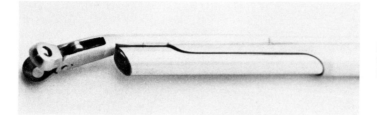

FIG. 34. Biopsy forceps with a forward-oblique telescope can be introduced in the sheath (19 Fr.).

absorption became so high, the image so dim, and the viewing field so small that orientation and observation were difficult.

Newborn Cystoscope. There is now an instrument for use in the newborn where the total outside diameter of the telescope, including fiberoptic light transmission, is 1.8 mm (Fr. 5.4). To the best of our knowledge this is the smallest reported examining cystoscope; it has a 2.7-mm sheath (Fr. 8) and a removable telescope for irrigation (Fig. 35). The direction of view is 30 degrees.[12]

Cystoscope for Children. A set is also available (Fr. 10, 11, 13, and 14) for larger infants. Each can be used with two miniature telescopes. The directions of view are 0 and 30 degrees. According to the size and space available, one or two (ureteral) catheters can be in-

serted. A slightly curved tip facilitates passage of the instrument or manipulation in the posterior urethra. Urethroscopy and visualization of the bladder neck may be carried out in one examination through the same sheath (Fig. 36). A Fr. 10 or 11 cystoscope can also be used with a small (Fr. 3) electrode to destroy (coagulate) urethral valves.[14]

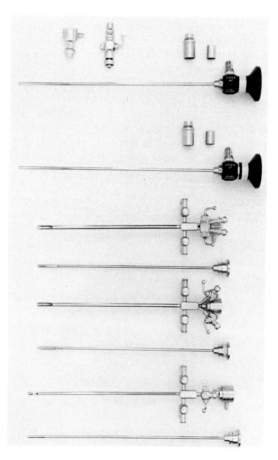

FIG. 35. Newborn cystoscope. Outside diameter of sheath is 8 Fr., incorporating a removable telescope with fiber light. Even in this miniature size the telescope can be removed for irrigation purposes.

FIG. 36. Cystoscope set for infants (Fr. 10 to 14). A miniature manipulator (not shown) can be introduced to direct the ureter catheters. Two telescopes are available: 0 and 30 degrees.

Pediatric Resectoscope

A miniature telescope (OD 2.7 mm, including fiberoptic light transmission) can be introduced in the Fr. 13 and recently the Fr. 10 and 11 resectosheath (which has a working element) and a miniature cutting or coagulating loop incorporated. This is of great value for resecting bladder neck obstructions, valves, etc., and has already proved its clinical usefulness (see Chap. 57).

Choledochoscope

The obvious way of decreasing the frequency of reoperations for stones in the extrahepatic biliary system is to increase the accuracy of the intraoperative diagnostic methods.[31] For clinical details see Chapter 20.

Direct observation of the intraluminal appearance of the extra- and intrahepatic duct system was obvious since Bakes in 1923 conceived the idea of direct visualization of the papilla of Vater. In 1941 McIver[21] designed a right-angle endoscope with standard lenses and a small distal bulb. It is true that his design of the right-angle shape was more suitable to the need, but the poor image due to the small size and insufficient illumination using a distal electric bulb were the main obstacles for a wider acceptance (Fig. 37).

In 1953 Wildegans[38] reported the first series of patients who underwent choledochoscopy. He used an instrument which had a horizontal limb that was 8×4 mm in diameter and 60 mm long, and a 260-mm vertical limb placed at a 60-degree angle. The instrument contained standard lenses and a distal electric bulb (Fig.

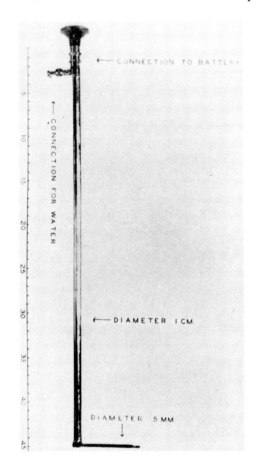

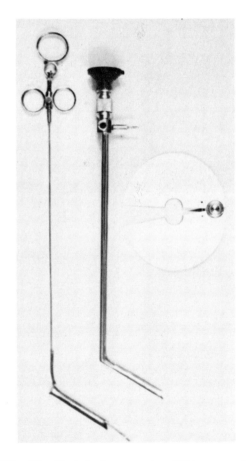

FIG. 37. McIver's right-angle choledochoscope, employing a standard lens system and a distal electric bulb. (From McIver: Surgery 9:112, 1941)

FIG. 38. Choledochoscope by Wildegans with standard lenses and a distal light bulb. Diameter of horizontal limb is 8 × 4 mm. (Courtesy Med J Australia 2:653, 1962)

38) with an irrigation system. I advocated the use of this endoscope 14 years ago,[2] but because of the 60-degree angulation and large size, we had difficulty introducing it into the reexplored patient. In these cases the dissected common bile duct and the duodenum-liver distance are short. Using a 60-degree angulation and a 60-mm limb we encountered problems when placing it in the distal part of the common bile duct to visualize the sphincter because of the nearby rib cage.

Shore and Lippman[30] introduced the flexible fiber choledochoscope to overcome the disadvantages of a rigid system. Using a coherent fiber image transmitter the following shortcomings were encountered: (1) inferior image quality compared to lens system; (2) a need for continuous focusing and therefore limited depth of field; and (3) difficulties in maneuvering the floating tip in the hepatic part.

It was felt that additions such as a remote-controlled tip and a fixed focus would probably eliminate the deficiencies.[23] It resulted in a larger outside diameter, incorporating light, irrigation, and a control mechanism for the movements of the tip with a fixed focus. The diameter of the image-transmitting bundle had to be decreased—compared with the Shore-Lippmann design—resulting in significant deterioration of the image quality. Figure 39 demonstrates comparative tests between the Storz-Hopkins rigid and the flexible fiber choledochoscope.

It is simpler during choledochoscopy to use a small, rigid instrument with a better image quality than the fiber one, with fixed focus but excellent resolution and superior depth of field. Maneuvering is easier than with an instrument that is complicated and needs more coordination. We are dealing with general surgeons and not specially trained endoscopists. The problems involved in the durability of fiberoptic instruments (breakage of coherent fibers) and continuous gas sterilization (water condensation) must be also taken into account. The capital outlay for a fiber choledochoscope is approximately four or five times greater than for a rigid one.

The Hopkins-Storz system[5] facilitated the design of a choledochoscope with a diameter of only 5×3 mm, including irrigation, fiber illumination, and optics (Fig. 40). The right-angle version is more suitable for the purpose. This "mini" size can be used in patients with a small duct or for reexploration in the presence of difficult anatomy. The horizontal limb is 40 mm, and the vertical one 300 mm. The viewing angle is 90 degrees; there are extreme depths of field with fixed focus and excellent resolution (Fig. 39). Any standard external light source with a fiberoptic light and cord can be employed.[32] The instrument is sterilized in gas.

For stone removal an additional instrument channel can be clipped on the choledochoscope, increasing the diameter to only 4.5×8 mm. The duct is dilated in the majority of these cases of choledocholithiasis. A flexible forceps with alligator jaws can be introduced to retrieve stones under visual control; the diameter of the alligator forceps is 2.2 mm (Fig. 41). A Fogarty catheter can also be advanced through the same channel. Bypassing the stone, the balloon is inflated and withdrawn, with the instrument recovering the stone from its deep location.

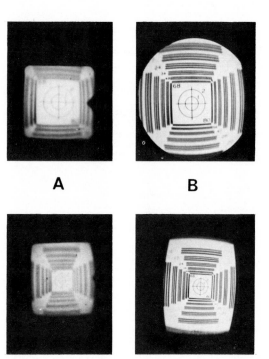

A   **B**

FIG. 39. Comparative resolution test (object distance 10 and 20 mm). **A.** Flexible fiber choledochoscope with remote-controlled tip by Nishimura (manufactured by Olympus). **B.** Rigid choledochoscope (manufactured by Storz). The image quality in a rigid system is superior to the flexible one. In this application a small, rigid scope is easier and simpler to manipulate.

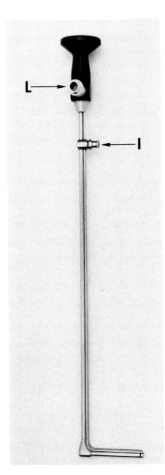

FIG. 40. Choledochoscope with Hopkins rod-lens system (manufactured by Storz) designed by one of the authors (G.B.). Outside diameter is only 5 × 3 mm, including irrigation, fiber illumination, and optics. Horizontal limb is 40 mm and the vertical limb 300 mm long. The larger version (nephroscope) is identical except that the horizontal limb is longer (60 mm). The viewing angle is 90 degrees with extreme depths of field, fixed focus, and excellent resolution (Fig. 39). L, fiber light. I, irrigation.

The design of an ideal choledochoscope was our greatest test in respect to simplicity and acceptance by the surgeons. In our experience with other type of choledochoscopes we found that if an instrument needs "a driver's license" or special training in how to use it it will not be accepted by the general surgeon. This new choledochoscope is employed in several institutions today and has become the additional but essential "visual probe" on the tray of biliary stone retrievers.

Nephroscope

The nephroscope is the same as the choledochoscope in size and shape, except that the horizontal limb is 60 mm long. Recurring stones constitute one of the main indications for reexploration of the kidney; since the renal pelvis is enlarged in these patients, the longer horizontal limb in the nephroscope would be more useful.[35] Of course the shorter choledochoscope can be used for the same approach, and the accessories are identical in both scopes. Hertel[15] designed a special round forceps to facilitate retrieval of smaller or floating stones.

Various parts of the caliceal system and the renal papillae can be well observed. The tech-

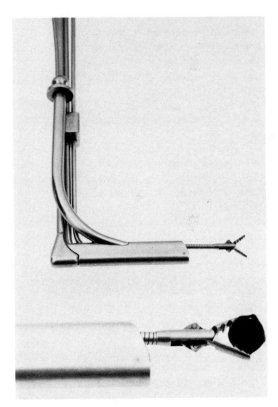

FIG. 41. Accessory instrument channel, which slightly increases the overall diameter of the horizontal limb (Fig. 40) to 4.5 × 8 mm. In dilated ducts there is no difficulty in introducing the instrument with this guide channel. A flexible stone forceps with alligator jaws is directed into the visual (optical) axis. If the location of the stone or other technical difficulties prohibit the use of the flexible stone forceps, a Fogarty balloon catheter or Dormie basket can be introduced through the same channel.

nique is also useful in patients with hematuria due to small lesions, helping the surgeon decide on whether to perform a partial or total nephrectomy.[13]

The choledochoscope-nephroscope is a simple instrument that can be assembled with ease by a nurse in the operating room. By extending the operating time only a few minutes, retained stones can be observed or valuable information gained that was impossible to obtain when working "blindly."

Culdoscope

Culdoscopy has lost its wide application since the introduction of laparoscopy. There are still conditions (e.g., obesity), however, where the examination should be performed. The instrument consists of a telescope with fiberoptic light and a cannula. The trocar is introduced in the appropriate location through the vaginal wall. The sharp stylet is withdrawn and the telescope introduced with a forward-oblique or lateral direction of view.

Esophagoscope

Adult Size. There are certain situations where a rigid esophagoscope is still the method of choice in esophagoscopy, although its use requires more skill and know-how than a flexible scope. For safer introduction a thin outer plastic tube 30 cm (12 inches) long with a flexible rubber mercury bougie is inserted first into the esophagus. The plastic tube is left in position and the mercury bougie withdrawn. The metal sheath is now advanced through this plastic guide (tube) into the esophagus. The metal esophagoscope provides better exploration than the flexible ones. More effective suction is achieved partially because of the wider exploration and partially because a larger (lumen) suction tube or built-in suction in the wall of the sheath is used. If a telescope is employed in adult esophagoscopy, accurate and large tissue samples can be taken or a larger foreign body removed.

It is not the aim of this chapter to debate the desirability of using rigid versus flexible instruments, but note that it is still too early to discard the rigid ones. For the patient it is just as distasteful to have a 13-mm flexible tube in his gullet causing unpleasant reflexes or the sensation of choking as it is to have the same

feeling triggered by a similar diameter but metal tube. Figure 42 displays one type of modern rigid esophagoscope.

Pediatric Size. There is no doubt at this stage that a rigid scope is the instrument of choice in infants. Miniaturization of the coherent (image) fibers causes deterioration of the image quality, and the operating or manipulating instrument channel is extremely small. The rigid scope is the instrument of choice for foreign body removal.

The pediatric esophagoscope is available in two sizes: The newborn has sheaths 3.5 and 4 mm in diameter and 20 cm in length, with a prismatic light deflector, instrument channel, and telescope (Fig. 43). The intermediate pediatric esophagoscope consists of 4-, 5-, and 6-mm sheaths and is 300 mm long. The accessories are the same as in the newborn instrument but are proportionally larger. A longer telescope with an antifog tube is employed in this set. A miniature alligator forceps (Fig. 44) can be introduced through the instrument channel beside the telescope in both sets, and foreign body removal is performed under accurate visual control.

Hysteroscope

The clinical and some of the technical details pertinent to hysteroscopy are described in Chapter 38. This examination was advocated by Menken[22] as an office procedure; he used a miniature telescope (2.7 mm) with a sheath that was introduced without dilating the cervical canal. He injected a highly viscous material* through the instrument channel to dilate the uterus; it did not spill into the abdomen, and it allowed good visibility. Lindemann employs a suction cap and a larger telescope (diameter 4 mm). As a distending medium carbon dioxide is insufflated under high pressure but low flow, limiting the time of the examination.[20] Other investigators prefer high-molecular-weight dextran for dilatation.[8]

The sheath incorporates an instrument channel through which a biopsy forceps or a coagulation probe can be introduced under visual control. The probe is advanced into the ostium to coagulate or destroy the lining of the tube for sterilization purposes.[29]

The larger instruments require dilatation of

---

*Luviskol-K; not available in the United States.

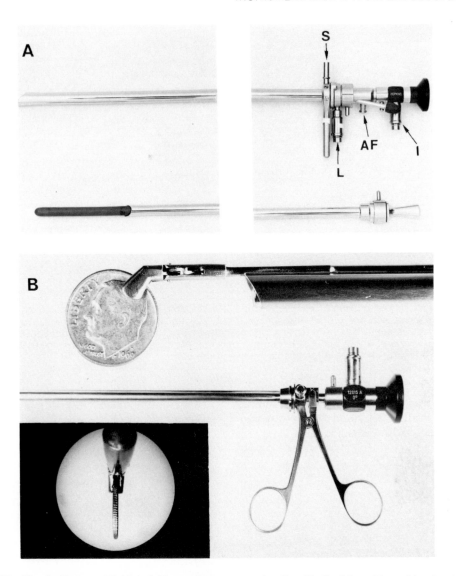

FIG. 42. A. Bottom, Rigid (adult) esophagoscope sheath with flexible rubber obturator to facilitate introduction. Top, Esophagoscope assembled. The sheath has a built-in suction channel (S) and a separate fiber light guide (L) for open-tube introduction. The telescope with fiberoptic light (I) is inserted into the tube. An antifog (AF) outlet is connected to a small air pump to provide positive pressure in front of telescope. **B.** Optical foreign body forceps, which can be introduced through the esophagoscope sheath. Top, Enlarged side view from the working end. Middle, Forceps with telescope. Bottom, Grasped object as seen through the telescope. The optical forceps allow accurate and precise manipulations.

the cervical canal. Various methods were employed for intratubal sterilization, including unipolar, bipolar, and direct-contact heat. The introduction of foreign bodies to block the tube, which could be removed at a later stage, were reported.[1,25] Instillation of chemicals to achieve the same effect as coagulation were also mentioned. It is too early to make any definite statement about the proper instrumentation, as I am sure there will be changes according to clinical results during the follow-up period.

Laparoscope

Despite their wide experience earlier investigators in the United States[26,39] did not gain

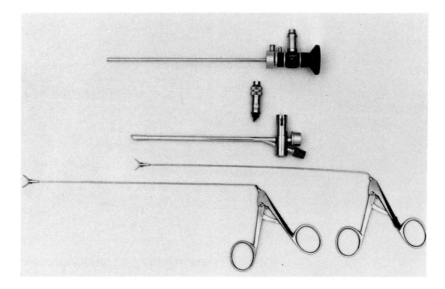

FIG. 43. Newborn pediatric esophagoscope. It is available in two sizes—3.0 and 3.5 mm, each 20 cm long—and has a built-in prismatic light deflector and instrument channel. The same telescope is applied as used in newborn bronchoscopy. The intermediate esophagoscope is similar to the newborn one just larger in proportion (4-, 5-, and 6-mm sheaths, each 300 mm long). Alligator and peanut forceps are shown at the bottom.

many followers. The inadequacy of existing instruments was probably responsible. Visualization through the older standard telescopes was poor compared with those available today. The invention of the rod-lens system made it possible to produce examining trocars not exceeding 7 to 8 mm in diameter (Fig. 45). Moreover, the larger diameter of the trocar, the greater the danger of visceral injury during abdominal wall penetration (Fig. 46). The smaller size

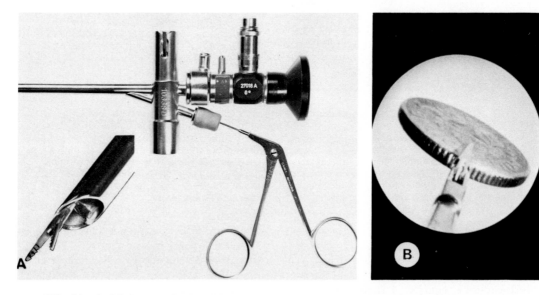

FIG. 44. **A.** Miniature alligator forceps introduced through the instrument channel in the newborn and intermediate broncho- or esophagoscope beside the telescope. Accurate visual control is secured during foreign body removal. **B.** View through the pediatric (newborn) telescope grasping a coin (dime).

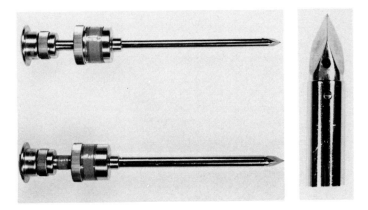

FIG. 45. The most dangerous tool for laparoscopy is the examining trocar. Two diameter sizes are shown: 4 mm (top) and 7 mm (bottom). At right, Enlarged view of cannula and stylet with a side hole.

facilitates safer penetration of the abdominal wall. The increased light transmission, brighter image, improved resolution, wide viewing angle and therefore easier orientation, greater depths of field without focusing, and incorporation of fiberoptic light transmission facilitate prompt endoscopic orientation, examination, and manipulation. The excellent image quality contributes significantly to an improved overall diagnostic accuracy.[6]

The prewarmed (sterile, hot saline) telescope is introduced through the examining trocar. The trocar itself has a "no-escape" valve which closes automatically as soon as the telescope is withdrawn to avoid desufflation of the pneumoperitoneum. The viewing angle of the telescope is 70 degrees; the relationship of object distance versus size of object is shown in Figure 47. The resolution is displayed in Figure 48. Even at 15 mm object distance, 37.5 μ can

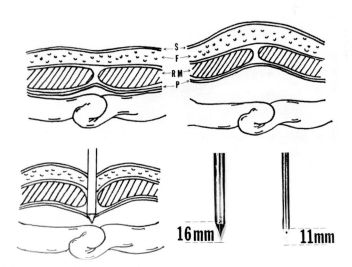

FIG. 46. In a large-diameter trocar the length of the sharp tip of the stylet is increased. Even a 4- or 5-mm difference in the length can contribute to a higher incidence of injuries. If pneumoperitoneum is achieved with the drilling-pressing action, the distance of parietal peritoneum and abdominal viscera is decreased; therefore if a sharp trocar tip is shorter it is safer. The tip of a 10-mm trocar is 16 mm and that of a 7-mm trocar 11 mm. S, skin. F, subcutaneous fat. RM, rectus muscle. P, peritoneum. (Courtesy J Reprod Med 10:276, 1973)

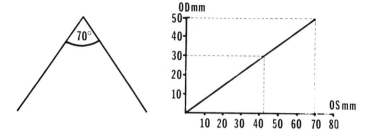

FIG. 47. The wide-angled view of the laparoscope telescope is 70 degrees, facilitating fast observation. The relation of object distance (OD) to size of the object (OS) is displayed. At 30 mm object distance, 42 mm can be seen, and at 50 mm object distance, 70 mm can be seen.

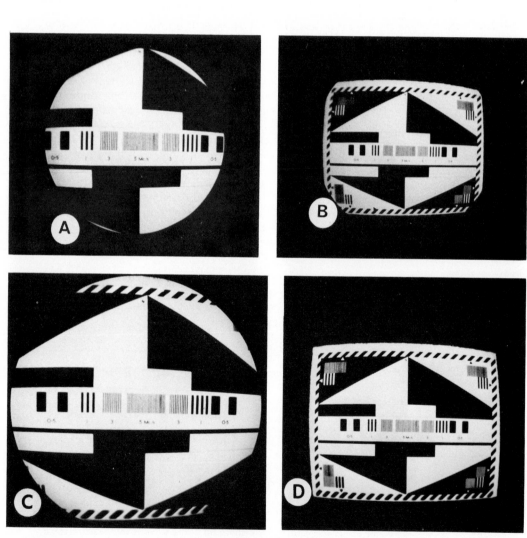

FIG. 48. **A** and **B.** Hopkins-Storz standard laparoscope telescope. Object distances are 10 mm (**A**) and 20 mm (**B**). **C** and **D.** *Hopkins-Storz enlarging laparoscope. Object distances are 10 mm (**C**) and 20 mm (**D**). The viewing angle for all four is 70 degrees. Both telescopes can be introduced through the standard (7 mm) examining trocar.* Note the crisp, bright, enlarged image covering a large area with excellent resolution. Displayed image is also enlarged on film. The second generation Hopkins system is a great improvement.

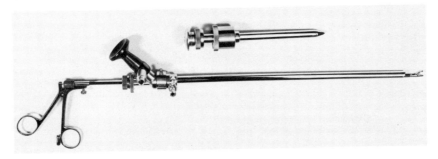

FIG. 49. Single-puncture laparoscope. A much larger trocar (11 mm) must be employed to incorporate the telescope and the operating instrument in a common channel.

still be defined. Maintaining a wide-angled view (70 degrees) and this high resolution, it is more than sufficient for visual scrutiny and the discovery of minute lesions.

The manipulating or operating instruments are introduced under visual control. The smaller accessory trocar is introduced via a separate incision.

Single-Puncture Approach. The design of the eyepiece of the telescope in an angle to facilitate manipulations through the same instrument in order to avoid insertion of a second accessory trocar, but increasing the total diameter of the trocar (10 to 11 mm), has been known for many years (Fig. 49). The trocar must be enlarged in order to insert a telescope and an operating instrument through a common cannula. Despite the larger trocar, the telescope diameter had to be reduced, resulting in a less efficient optical performance. In the single-puncture approach the direction of view of the telescope is 0 degrees (straight forward).

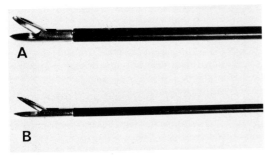

FIG. 50. A. Biopsy forceps employed through a second accessory trocar (5.5 mm in diameter). **B.** Size of biopsy forceps introduced through the single-puncture laparoscope.

It is much more cumbersome to use it for observation and manipulation than the 30-degree forward-oblique ones.[6,10,34] Using the single-puncture laparoscope it is more difficult to deal with complications such as bleeding or oozing surfaces, where fast and accurate suction-coagulation is important. The operating instruments are smaller (Fig. 50) and therefore less efficient.

Working through a second, smaller accessory trocar we have complete freedom of movement and are able to change instruments without moving the telescope and thereby losing the visual field, because we do not have to perform manipulations through the same common (operating and visual) cannula. Employing the two-puncture technique and working through a second trocar, the viewing field remains the same throughout the procedure.

Pneumoperitoneum. Pneumoneedle. A special pneumoperitoneum needle (Fig. 51) described by Veress[36] is recommended. It consists of the needle proper and a spring-loaded, blunt stylet, which is retracted during penetration of the abdominal wall. If the last layer, the parietal peritoneum, is penetrated the spring pushes the blunt stylet into the abdominal cavity to prevent visceral injury.

Insufflator. For years pneumoperitoneum was accomplished by room air insufflation using a syringe with an air filter. The trend today is to use gas: carbon dioxide or nitrous oxide (see Chap. 29).

The sophisticated insufflator by Semm[28] (Fig. 52) measures intraabdominal pressure by means of a gauge. This is helpful in determining the position of the pneumoneedle. Monitoring the volume is time-consuming and unnecessary. There are large individual variations from patient to patient, and pressure losses due

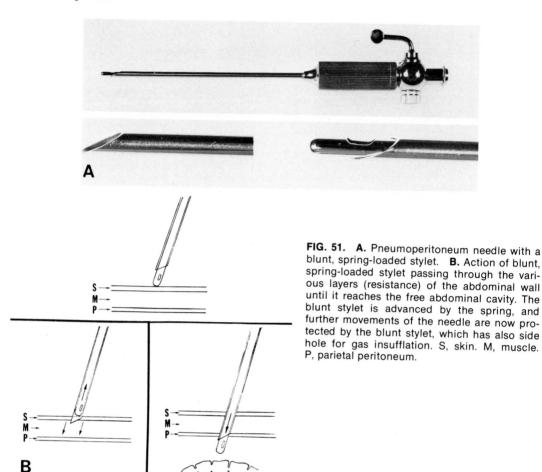

FIG. 51. A. Pneumoperitoneum needle with a blunt, spring-loaded stylet. **B.** Action of blunt, spring-loaded stylet passing through the various layers (resistance) of the abdominal wall until it reaches the free abdominal cavity. The blunt stylet is advanced by the spring, and further movements of the needle are now protected by the blunt stylet, which has also side hole for gas insufflation. S, skin. M, muscle. P, parietal peritoneum.

to leakage can occur at any time. The clinical impression, palpation of the abdominal wall, symmetrical tympanic percussion, and the required optimal intraabdominal pressure (which is in the vicinity of 20 mm Hg) are important indicators. We felt that a wide range is very efficient and found that an insufflator* in which the pressure and flow can be adjusted and regulated from 0 to 50 mm Hg (Fig. 53) is practical. It incorporates an automatic shut-off system. Wherever the dial is set (0 to 50 mm Hg), if the intraabdominal pressure should drop the device refills to the preset pressure. This can be adjusted according to the need; it may be high in cases of leakage because of insufficient gas cushion or low in pediatric or high-risk patients.

Automated Medical Devices Corp., Suite 365, Avenue of the Stars, Los Angeles, California 90067.

Trocar. This can be a very dangerous tool. Since a large percentage of intestinal or other organ injuries have been caused by this cannula, the smallest possible examining trocar should be used. If a large cannula is employed the tip of the sharp stylet is longer (Fig. 46). The protective gas cushion or the distance between the abdominal wall and the organs lying beneath is decreased during the penetrating maneuver of this instrument. The smallest trocar with the shortest tip is preferable. Even a few millimeters difference in the length of the sharp stylet can be significant in the morbidity statistics of laparoscopy.

Accessory (Operating) Trocar. The second trocar diameter can vary from 4 to 5.5 mm. When employing (unipolar) electrosurgery insulated cannulas are recommended to avoid skin burns. Operating instruments (Fig. 54) for tubal sterilization, adhesiolysis, biopsy, or other maneuvers can be introduced. The pene-

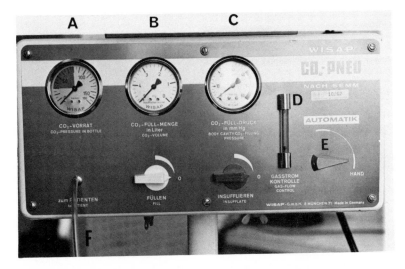

FIG. 52. Pneumoinsufflator by Semm. **A.** Cylinder pressure. **B.** Volume of gas used (which is not identical with the actual consumed volume because of the large variety of leakage possibilities). See Chapter 29 for further discussion. **C.** Intraabdominal pressure gauge. **D.** Flowmeter. **E.** Switch "hand" or "automatic" (for details see Chap. 29). **F.** Outlet to patient.

tration of this trocar is safer because the site of insertion can be carefully selected and the actual introduction observed under visual control.

Biopsy and Hemostasis. There is a variety of forceps available that can be operated through the second accessory or instrument trocar. I did not find it advantageous to have the biopsy forceps insulated. After the forceps is closed in liver or parenchymal biopsies the surrounding tissue can be coagulated to arrest oozing or bleeding. Despite the fact

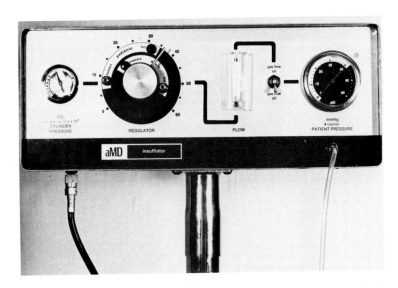

FIG. 53. Another type of automatic insufflator. Pressure can be adjusted stepwise from 0 to 50 mm Hg with incorporated automatic shutoff system. If the dial is set and the intraabdominal pressure exceeds the preset value, the gas inflow is interrupted. If the intraabdominal pressure drops below the preset value it refills automatically. This instrument gives a larger range of preset values, which is important in high-risk or pediatric patients.

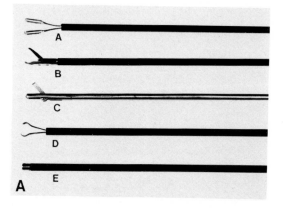

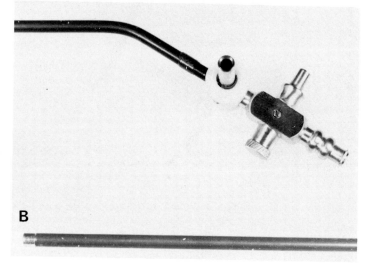

FIG. 54. **A.** A few important operating instruments: A, ATR: atraumatic grasper. B, Biopsy forceps. C, Punch forceps. D, Gynecologic grasping forceps. E, Coagulation-suction probe. A, B, D, and E are insulated. **B.** One important instrument to arrest bleeders is the suction-coagulation cannula with a trumpet valve and insulation for immediate hemostasis without desufflating the pneumoperitoneum. (See Chap. 29 for further discussion.)

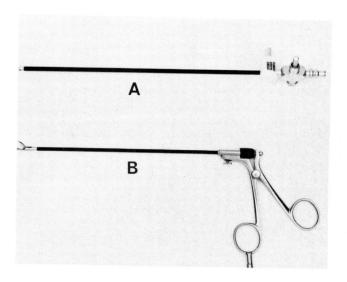

FIG. 55. Accessory (operating) instruments for pediatrics. These are introduced through a trocar whose outside diameter is 4 mm. **A.** Insulated coagulation-suction probe. **B.** Biopsy forceps.

that tissue in the forceps could remain undamaged during coagulation—which is questionable—appropriate hemostasis was not achieved in my experience. For these purposes the coagulation-suction probe is of much greater help and should be applied (Fig. 54B). Bipolar coagulation and hemostasis is a new approach that can decrease coagulation or skin injuries.

Any biopsy forceps cup should be kept extremely sharp and be resharpened from time to time to avoid squashing or tearing the tissue. A slightly sharp tip facilitates introduction into hard lumps or solid lesions. Tangential tissue samplings from the parietal peritoneum or other areas are perhaps better achieved with a punch forceps. The punch system is also preferable for tubal division if representative samples are required in previously destroyed (coagulated) tissue.

Miniaturization of biopsy forceps decreases the closing power of the jaws and the amount of tissue obtained. For pediatrics, however, microsurgery requires the use of smaller sizes and more delicate instruments (Fig. 55). Biopsy forceps production is one of the great problems in rigid instrument manufacturing.

A large variety of punch-coagulation forceps is available; a sample of a small punch forceps recommended by Frangenheim is shown in Figure 56. The configuration of this forceps allows the tube or round object to be gently grasped without cutting through, just holding it, but providing contact for coagulation. By closing the jaws a small tissue sample remains in the lower jaw (punch action).

We have no experience with the Palmer-Cohen-Eder punch biopsy forceps.

For pediatric laparoscopy instruments, see Chapter 31.

Laryngoscope

Indirect Laryngoscopy. This is a simple and useful procedure that became widely accepted in outpatient clinics and is used as an office procedure. The mirror served us well for more than a century.

The average distance from the vocal cords—which are approximately 275 mm (11 inches)—to the visualizing instrument creates very difficult viewing circumstances when trying to inspect and illuminate the object with a head mirror. The anatomy is reversed using a mirror image, and so we are faced now with the problem of adapting ourselves to viewing the vocal cords "right side up" rather than "upside down" as they are seen using the conventional technique. Using an optical system, the area inspected is larger than a mirror. In one viewing field the adjacent area of the vocal cords and/or lesion can be better seen and enlarged with much more detail than with the old, outdated mirror[3]. The appearance of a simulated vocal cord and the observation under identical conditions using a mirror and a telescope are seen in Figure 57.

The Hopkins-Storz system provided a milestone in the examination of the larynx (Fig. 58). The instrument consists of a 90-degree telescope with a 50-degree viewing angle,

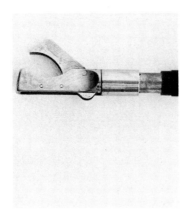 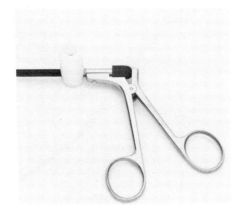

FIG. 56. Punch forceps (by Frangenheim) has a curved beak. Used for simultaneous grasping, coagulation, and transection of tubes. A small section of the tissue remains in the punched-out jaws.

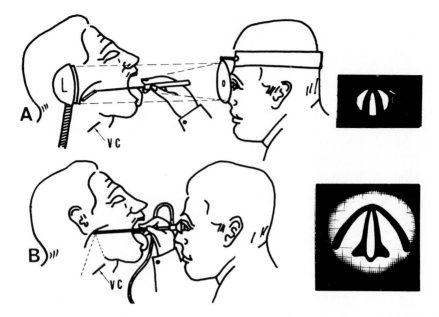

FIG. 57. Indirect laryngoscopy. Diagram of the vocal cord as seen through a laryngeal mirror **(A)** or observed through the telescope **(B)**. VC, vocal cords. L, light.

which means that we can see an area of 43 mm from a 50 mm object distance (Fig. 59). The illumination is aligned with the viewing angle and moves with the telescope. Therefore the difficulties we had with a reflecting head and laryngeal mirror alignments caused by movements of a patient's head or the head mirror, or difficult anatomy, are not encountered with the Hopkins-Storz system.

Figure 60 shows the telescope, which is conveniently held in the examiner's hand. An external light source is employed to couple a flexible fiberoptic light carrier to the incoherent fibers of the telescope. The continuous, disturbing fogging of the mirror, which requires pre- and rewarming, is eliminated by incorporating an antifog system, by blowing a small amount of air in the front of the lens, providing

positive pressure, and avoiding temperature differences or moisture formation by cough or forced phonation.

In our opinion telescopic examination will eventually replace the mirror examination.[37] The simplicity, greater detail, and easier perception due to the brighter image and magnification are the main supporting factors for this significantly improved examination technique of laryngeal pathology.

Direct Laryngoscopy. It is difficult if not impossible to employ telescopes for mag-

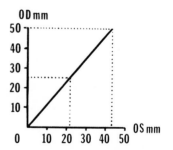

FIG. 59. Relation of size of object (OS) and object distances (OD) observed through the 90-degree indirect laryngoscope with a 55-degree viewing angle (Hopkins rod-lens system). From 25 mm object distance a 22-mm object can be seen, and from 50 mm, a 43-mm area can be observed. Orientation, good overall view with sufficient detail, and magnification are of great importance.

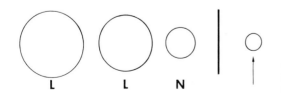

FIG. 58. Various sizes of mirrors employed compared with the diameter of a telescope (arrow). L, laryngeal mirrors. N, nasopharyngeal mirror.

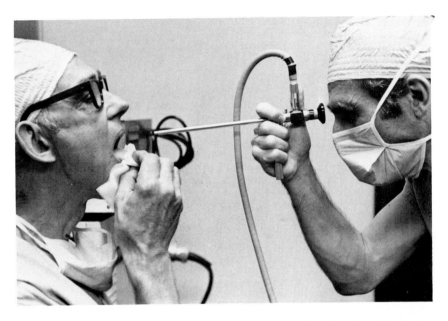

FIG. 60. The indirect laryngoscope can be conveniently introduced and held in the hand of the examiner. Illumination and vision is properly aligned and always maintained.

nification because in the majority of indications (e.g., stripping of the cords, biopsy, removal of polyps), or when other sophisticated procedures are involved, the telescope would interfere with manipulations through the laryngoscope.

There are several types of open-tube laryngoscopes available. The one most commonly preferred is the Holinger type because of its shape and small size, which facilitate exploration and operation. The obsolete distal light globe is replaced with brighter fiber light transmission, providing much better illumination.

Kleinsasser, the pioneer of microlaryngeal surgery, introduced his larger laryngoscope in conjunction with the binocular operating microscope. It is hoped that further improvement of this optical system (i.e., an increased depth of field) will eliminate the present necessity of continuous refocusing if the object distance is only slightly changed.

The above-mentioned laryngoscopes (blades or spatulas) are kept in a fixed position by an attached chest support, allowing the examiner to use both hands. Further details are described in Chapter 46.

Posterior Rhinoscopy. Inspection of the nasopharynx is more difficult than of the larynx, using smaller mirrors. The instrument is the same as described for indirect laryngos-

copy *(vide supra)*. After examining the larynx the 90-degree telescope is turned around 180 degrees—or introduced immediately in this position—to see the posterior nasopharynx. Because of the wide-angled view the septum and

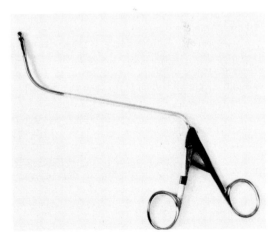

FIG. 61. S-shaped biopsy forceps. When the indirect laryngoscope is turned 180 degrees the nasopharyngeal area comes into full view. Biopsy of the posterior nasopharyngeal area is one of the most difficult procedures. This forceps can be introduced beside the telescope, and an aimed target tissue sampling can be obtained under visual control.

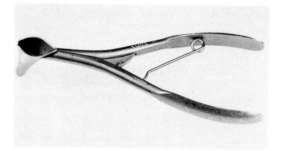

FIG. 62. Anterior rhinoscopy was performed for decades with this dilating speculum and a head mirror that reflects light into the front part of the nostrils only. This exploring technique has been replaced with the telescope. (For details see Chap. 51).

conchae are very well seen, as is the opening of the Eustachian tubes and the recess of Rosenmüller.

Tissue sampling in these areas is extremely difficult. Various techniques have been described—some performed blindly and some done via a mirror. The operator has only one opportunity to obtain a biopsy—at the first bite because the consequent oozing or bleeding interferes with further attempts. An excellent view is obtained using the 90-degree telescope; and by introducing an S-shaped biopsy forceps (Fig. 61), which is available in two sizes, an aimed target biopsy can be obtained under accurate visual control.

Anterior Rhinoscopy. This examination has been known for decades and is performed with a dilating speculum (Fig. 62) and a head mirror to reflect light into the front part of the nostrils.

The new approach is a forward-oblique or straightforward telescope as detailed in Chapter 51. It gives a much better view of the hidden areas and small lesions on the surface of the mucosa; furthermore, it can be advanced far back to see the posterior part of the nostrils, which are impossible to observe with the standard speculum.

Mediastinoscope

Mediastinoscopy is performed with an exploring speculum that has a built-in fiber light and a side slit (Fig. 63). The latter is used to introduce various accessories that enable us to dissect the paratracheal area and to obtain tissue samples from the lymph nodes for his-

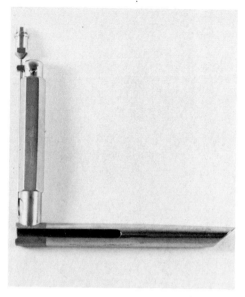

FIG. 63. This mediastinoscope is an oval speculum with a slit on the side for easy introduction of manipulating instruments. The handle has a built-in light carrier (fiber).

tologic examination. A telescope can be used for an enlargement technique, or the operation microscope can be utilized; but the positioning of the speculum and the fixation in this critical area must exclude unnecessary movements so as to avoid injury. Before this procedure is used for staging primary and secondary lesions from the lung or as a differential diagnostic tool, it must first gain far wider acceptance among thoracic surgeons than it now enjoys.

Proctoscope

We need an exploring tube with proximal illumination for proctoscopy. Proximal lighting is more suitable than distal lighting for this purpose; it also permits easier cleaning and suction to keep the viewing area unobstructed. A handle on the tube facilitates positioning (Fig. 64). It should be available in various sizes, according to the anatomy, age of the patient, and situation.

If the instrument is employed for treatment (e.g., coagulation) it is advisable to use large tubes and/or insulated surfaces to avoid an electrical shorting of the unipolar electrosurgical system (Fig. 65). We hope that further developments of the bipolar systems will improve this application of electrotherapy.

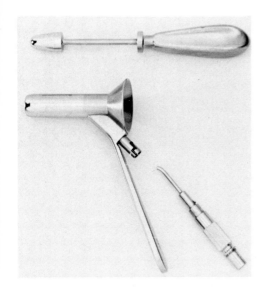

FIG. 64. Proctoscope for examination of the anus and the first part of the rectum. It consists of an exploring outside sheath with a handle and proximal fiber light. It is available in various sizes and shapes.

Sigmoidoscope (Rectoscope)

The term "rectoscope" is perhaps more realistic than "sigmoidoscope." It is sometimes difficult and painful to introduce a 20- to 30-cm tube into the sigmoid colon.

The general principle comparing an open-tube system 30 cm (12 inches) or 25 cm (10 inches) in length with a telescopic view is similar to that mentioned under bronchoscopy. Although these tubes are rather wide (12 to 20 mm in diameter), it is still a great help to use some sort of magnification. The instrumentation consists of the exploring outer sheath with an obturator (Fig. 66), and a plain glass window to seal the tube and facilitate distention by a small amount of air insufflation through a hand bulb. The small, distal light bulb with a carrier is already outdated. It is most disconcerting if this bulb burns out; moreover, when there is secretion (e.g., ulcerative colitis) or bleeding the viewing area suddenly becomes dark.

The rectoscope can also be used with a lupe magnifier (Fig. 66) similar to that of the bronchoscope, mounted on a hinge that can be flipped over the window.* The tubular vision is decreased and the object enlarged.

Recently available in a rectangular form facilitating free manipulations.

For biopsy purposes the rectosigmoidoscope as a closed system is interrupted by removing the window to introduce a biopsy forceps. In this case the view is partially or totally obscured by the forceps and provides an aimed but semiblind procedure. Another problem sometimes occurs when the lesion can be located or well displayed only by slight insufflation; then as soon as the small air inflow (distention) is interrupted, the lesion bulges into the tube or changes position. Using a "sealed" optical biopsy system, superior vision target biopsies and optimal explorative conditions are maintained (Fig. 66B).* A telescope is very helpful in locating small lesions, in seeing the pathology in greater detail, and in documenting the findings.

Suction and/or coagulation in cases of oozing or after a biopsy can sometimes be difficult. In general if a simple metal suction device is employed and the vacuum is too high, the friable mucosa can be "sucked in" and start to bleed. It is helpful to use a suction apparatus that holds the mucosa away in order to avoid close contact or to block suction. The same instrument can be connected to an electrosurgical unit, employing coagulation current and suction simultaneously.

Various insulated snares are available for transection of polyps.

Stereotactic Encephaloscope

Stereotactic encephaloscopy, a new examination technique, is discussed in Chapter 59.

Thoracoscope

Thoracoscopy is very useful in assessing various types of pathology (see Chap. 52). There are two types of instruments available.

Operating Thoracoscope. This is the larger of the two instruments. It consists of a trocar and cannula with an outside diameter of 9 mm through which another sheath incorporating a telescope and instrument channels can be advanced (Fig. 67). For biopsies the forward-oblique telescope with a rigid biopsy forceps permits relatively accurate tissue sampling.

Examining Thoracoscope. The same procedure can be performed with a smaller instrument but two punctures. A 7-mm examin-

Manufacturer: Storz Endoscopy Co., Tuttlingen, West Germany.

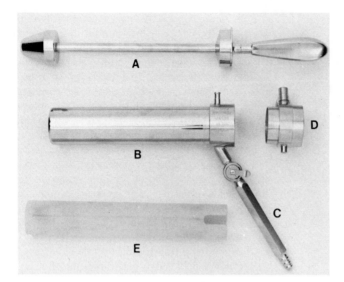

FIG. 65. Operating proctoscope. It is large in diameter (OD 20 to 30 mm) and is 15 to 20 cm long. Because of its frequent use in electrosurgery it is advisable to employ an insulated inlet to avoid shorting or skin burns by touching the metal sheath with the probe during coagulation. a, Obturator. b, Sheath with build-in suction. c, Handle with stopcock for suction. d, Window with proximal light (window cover can be removed). e, Insulated inlet.

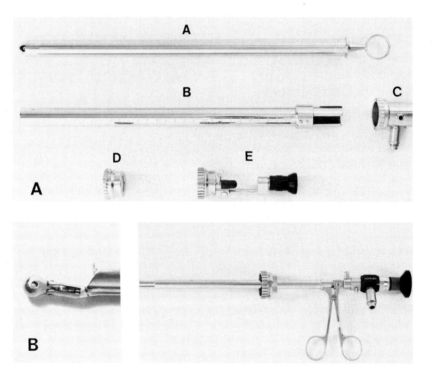

FIG. 66. **A.** Rectoscope or sigmoidoscope. Independent of the brand or type of instrument, it consists of the following main parts. A, Obturator. B, Exploring sheath. C, Proximal illuminator with air inlet for insufflation. D, Glass window. E, Another type of window but with attached lupe magnifier to decrease the tubular vision and enlarge the object. **B.** When a lesion is sited using the standard sigmoidoscope and a biopsy is deemed necessary, the glass window is removed and the air pressure lost. It is not uncommon therefore that the lesion changes its position, disappears from view, or bulges completely into the tube. Using this optical biopsy forceps the closed or sealed situation can be maintained. A slight distention is sometimes required; employing a telescope (magnification with the optical biopsy forceps) the lesion is not obscured by the forceps and the bite can be taken with much more precision and control. Left, Close-up from forceps with telescope. Right, Forceps with telescope assembled.

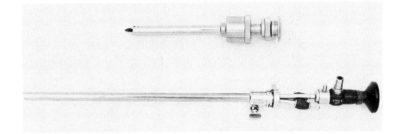

FIG. 67. Operating thoracoscope. Outside diameter of the trocar is 9 mm. The instrument consists of a trocar, an insert with two instrument channels, and a telescope. Biopsy, coagulation, and suction can be performed under visual control.

ing trocar penetrates the chest wall in the appropriate anatomic location and carries only the observing telescope. If a lesion is located, the operating instrument (suction, coagulation, biopsy forceps) can be advanced through a second, smaller (4 mm) trocar. Working with two trocars needs more coordination; but on the other hand, it requires smaller incisions.

Transconioscope

The transconioscope is a 5-mm trocar with various telescopes (forward-oblique, lateral, and straightforward views). For details see Chapter 53.

COMMENTS

Introduction of the rod-lens system in rigid endoscopy instituted an epoch of improved image transmission. The smaller size allowed the redesign of our traditional "hardware" to more effective and physiologically sound instruments. It opened a variety of new diagnostic modalities in pediatrics and rigid endoscopy in general, and prompted much wider acceptance of procedures that were previously abandoned because of the poor performance of the instruments.

The previous "monopoly" of viewing the procedure by the examiner only has been changed with the development of teaching attachments, allowing observation by a second person—assistant or student—and allowing him to help or observe without interfering with the examiner.

Documentation, which is very important as an objective record of our visual examination, became a feasible proposition (see Chap. 18). It stimulated many new developments and triggered the endoscope manufacturers to step out from the "sleeping beauty" stage to a progressive phase.

REFERENCES

1. Alvarado A, cited in Sciarra et al: Hysteroscopic sterilization. Symposium. Intercontinental Medical Book Corp, New York, 1974, pp 85–94
2. Berci G: Choledochoscopy. Med J Aust 2:860, 1961
3. Berci G, Calcaterra T, Ward P: Advances in endoscopic techniques for the examination of the larynx and nasopharynx. Can J Otolarygol. In press, 1976
4. Berci G, Kont LA: A new optical system in endoscopy with special reference to cystoscopy. Br J Urol 41:564, 1969
5. Berci G, Shore JM: Advances in cholangioscopy. Endoscopy 4:29, 1972
6. Berci G, Shore JM, Panish J, et al: The evaluation of a new peritoneoscope as a diagnostic aid to the surgeon. Ann Surg 178:37, 1973
7. Carden E, Trapp WG, Oulton J: A new and simple method for ventilating patients undergoing bronchoscopy. Anesthesiology 33:454, 1970
8. Edstrom K, Fernstrom I: The diagnostic possibilities of a modified hysteroscopic technique. Acta Obstet Gynecol Scand 49:327, 1970
9. Fourestier M, Gladu A, Vulmiere J: Perfectionnements a la endoscopie medicale. Presse Med 60:1291, 1952
10. Frangenheim H: Laparoskopie und Culdoskopie. Thieme, Stuttgart, 1972
11. Friedel H: Die Katheterbiopsie des peripheren Lungenherdes. Barth, Leipzig, 1961
12. Gans St L, Berci G: Advances in endoscopy of infants and children. J Pediatr Surg 6(Suppl): 199, 1971
13. Gittes RF, Elliott ML: Renal cortical rest and chronic hematuria. J Urol 109:14, 1973
14. Hendren WH: Posterior urethral valves in boys. J Urol 106:298, 1971
15. Hertel E: Entwicklung der operativen Pyeloskopie. Urologe [A] 12:116, 1973

16. Holinger P: Personal communication, 1971
17. Iglesias JJ: Personal communication, 1974
18. Kaufman JJ: Personal communication, 1974
19. Kont LA, Berci G: A comparative assessment of optical and fiber gastroscopes. Med Biol Ill 17:181, 1967
20. Lindemann JH: Eine neue Untersuchungsmethode für die Hysteroskopie. Endoscopy 3:194, 1971
21. McIver MA: An instrument for visualizing the interior of the common bile duct during operation. Surgery 9:112, 1941
22. Menken FC: Ein neues Verfahren mit Vorrichtung zur Hysteroskopie. Endoskopie 3:2–0, 1971
23. Nishimura A, Norikatsu D, Hiroshi S, et al: Exfoliative cytology of the biliary tract with the use of saline irrigation under choledochoscopic control. Ann Surg 178:594, 1973
24. Nitze M: Eine neue Beobachtung und Untersuchungsmethode d. Harnblase. Wien Med Wochenschr 24:649, 1879
25. Quinones R et al, cited in Sciarra et al: Hysteroscopic sterilization. Symposium. Intercontinental Medical Book Corp, New York, 1974
26. Ruddock JC: Peritoneoscopy. Surg Gynecol Obstet 65:623, 1937
27. Sanders DR: Two ventilating attachments for bronchoscopy. Del Med J 39:170, 1967
28. Semm K: Die Laparoskopie in der Gynekologie.

Geburtshilfe Frauenheilkd 27:1029, 1967
29. Sciarra JJ, Butler JC, Speidel JJ: Hysteroscopic sterilization. Symposium. Intercontinental Medical Book Corp, New York, 1974
30. Shore MJ, Lippman HL: A flexible choledochoscope. Lancet 1:1200, 1965
31. Shore MJ, Berci G: The clinical importance of cholangioscopy. J Endoscopy 2:117, 1970
32. Shore JM, Morgenstern L, Berci G: An improved rigid choledochoscope. Am J Surg 122:567, 1971
33. Spoerel WE, Grant PA: Ventilation during bronchoscopy. Can Anaesth Soc J 18:178, 1971
34. Steptoe P: Laparoscopy in Gynecology. Livingstone, Edinburgh, 1967
35. Vatz A, Berci G, Shore JM, et al: Operative nephroscopy. J Urol 107:355, 1972
36. Veress J: Neues Instrument zur Ausführung von Brust oder Bauchpunktionen und Pneumothoraxbehandlung. Dtsch Med Wochenschr 64:1480, 1938
37. Ward P, Berci G, Calcattera T: Advances in endoscopic examination of the respiratory system. Ann Otolaryngol 83:754, 1974
38. Wildengans H: Grenzen der Cholangiography und Aussichten der Cholangioscopie der tiefen Gallenwege. Med Klin 48:1270, 1953
39. Zoeckler SJ: Peritoneoscopy. Gastroenterology 34:969, 1958

6

Instrumentation II:
Flexible Fiber Endoscopes

George Berci

Transmitting an image or light through a flexed transmitting media has intrigued physicians for more than half a century. Rudolph Schindler had the idea to incorporate prisms or lenses in a flexible tube that tolerates a 30-degree bending radius in one or the other direction. The semiflexible gastroscope[8] opened the field of gastroscopy but suffered from inherent limitations: The light absorption was significant, the image was "cut" like a half-moon if the scope was flexed, the bending radius was limited, and several (blind) spots were not visualized.

In 1930 Lamm[7] demonstrated that if fine glass-fiber threads are pulled and put together in a bundle, this bundle can be flexed in the form of a loop and an image and/or light is transmitted even in a bent position. It is still unknown why this ingenious idea did not gain more attention among physicians or physicists, and why we had to wait several decades to see the clinical results.

The peculiar shape of some organs (e.g., the stomach, the gastrointestinal tract) made it necessary to devise a system other than the rigid endoscope with its limitation. Another system, although perhaps from the point of image transmission is not ideal in respect to image quality, does enable us to gain access to corners we were unable to see with rigid or semirigid endoscopes or with the naked eye.

There are other methods (e.g., radiologic techniques) by which we can see the outline of the interior of these organs with a radiopaque material (indirect technique), but they do not enable us to look directly into the organ itself. In 1954 Heel[4] reported a flexible image-transmitting system. That same year Hopkins and Kapany[6] described the first prototype of coherent fiber threads and pointed out the potential for their application as a flexible instrument for investigating the stomach. Hirschowitz with his coworkers[5] in 1958 made history with the first flexible gastroduodenoscope.

Less light is absorbed during passage through a fiber bundle than through an equal length and diameter of any existing endoscopic lens system. If the individual fiber glass threads (10 to 20 μ) are assorted precisely on both ends an image can be transmitted, even if it is in a bent position. This type of bundle is called a *coherent bundle*. If the individual fiber threads are held together but are nonassorted, it is called an *incoherent bundle*. Each individual fiber conducts light, but no image can be compiled (see Chapter 2).

The incoherent fiber threads as a flexible medium for light transmission are used extensively for piping illumination from an external light source to the deeply located viscera. Separating the light source from the instrument is advantageous, despite the fact that the losses through a fiber light pipe (bundle) are significant and larger light sources must be used because more than half of the light is absorbed during a 6-foot transmission. However, more light can be pumped into the cavity of the organ with more illumination than the previously used distal tungsten filament globes. The currently available incoherent bundles account for an absorption in the vicinity of 10 to 15 percent per foot. This is the reason we require a many times higher output light source than

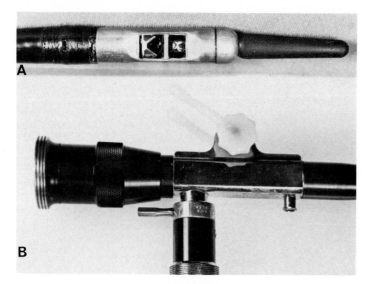

FIG. 1. First model of the Hirschowitz flexible fiber gastro-duodenoscope, with a floating working end. **A,** Electric globe. **B,** focusing device.

we would need if our incoherent bundles had better light-transmitting qualities. The yellowish tint is sometimes disturbing and can cause compression in the lighter part of the spectrum. During endoscopic procedures we are dealing mainly with colors *within* the red spectrum. This compression is extremely visible on still photographs taken with fiber light when compared, for example, with quartz rod light transmission. The advantages outweigh the disadvantages, however. It is true that we are far from the ideal or a final developmental stage, but we have shown progress by employing flexible incoherent fiber bundles rather than minielectric globes.

FLEXIBLE FIBER GASTROSCOPE

The appearance of the first flexible gastroscope by Hirschowitz et al.[5] was a breakthrough in the examination of the stomach, duodenal bulb, and esophagus. The first instrument* was produced as a lateral-view gastroscope with a distal electric bulb (Fig. 1). The tip of the instrument was "loose" and acted as a "floating working end" in the stomach. The first intragastric movie films were made with this instrument. Despite the fact that the light absorption factors of fiber glass are better than a lens system of similar length and diameter, a large amount of illumination was required to

ACMI, 8 Pelham Parkway, Pelham Manor, New York 10803.

expose a 16-mm ciné film. These distal electric bulbs were overburned to "squeeze out more energy," which resulted in excessive heat production and occasionally burn injuries to the stomach wall.[1] Colcher and Katz[3] synchronized the overburned distal globe with the movie camera shutter to avoid continuous heat accumulation.

Within a short time the distal electric bulb was replaced with the incoherent light fiber bundle, which was directly guided from the working end (objective) of the fiber endoscope right into the output or focal plane of the illuminating light source, called an integral (without interruption) light-conducting bundle. This decreased the complication of excessive heat production but triggered other problems. For instance, these incoherent light bundles are small—2 to 3 mm in diameter (or in smaller instruments it is further decreased significantly)—and 270 to 370 cm long, and the significant light absorption (10 to 15 percent per foot or per 30 cm) became even more plausible. To win this "game," larger, more powerful (and expensive) light units were built to overcome the loss and to provide a better illuminated area.

It was obvious that the free-floating tip will not be the final design, and it would be advantageous to have a flexible fiber image-transmitting system that incorporates illumination and a *remote-controlled movable tip.* After diligent research a scope was devised where during the first phase of development the tip was flexed in one way or the other (one

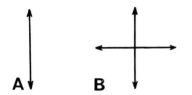

FIG. 2. It became evident that a remote-controlled tip is essential. The first models appeared with tip movements (up and down) in one plane only (**A**), but during the following years four-way or biplane (**B**) movements were incorporated in every upper GI scope used for adults.

plane) and was operated below the eye piece. Years later the same system was developed to a four-way (biplane) control (Fig. 2).

The main target was first the upper gastrointestinal tract, which was followed with many other partially successful, partially abortive experiences in other areas that needed smaller or miniature instruments. Currently a major diagnostic and therapeutic breakthrough has been achieved for exploring the upper gastrointestinal tract and colon. Without further discussion of the evolution of instruments let us start in *medias res*.

It became obvious that using separate instruments for examination of the esophagus, stomach, and duodenal bulb would be difficult, as well as inconvenient for the patient. For routine gastroscopy it is important during passage of the instrument to inspect the esophagus, esophageal cardiac junction, stomach, and duodenal bulb *in one session with one instrument*. There are many pathologic entities located in various parts of the above-mentioned anatomic region which are related and must be observed during the same examination without changing instruments. We started with a lateral view (90 degree) scope, changed to a forward-oblique, and ended up with a 0-degree straightforward one.

ESOPHAGOGASTRODUODENOSCOPE

In recent years we have used a flexible scope with a four-way tip control, air and water insufflation, a suction channel that is also employed as a biopsy channel, and a straightforward (0 degree) view. We use a scope with a lateral view only for the small number of cases in which extreme difficulties are encountered (e.g., a small, enlongated stomach) in order to see, for example, the angulus or parts of the

cardia. The lateral scope is therefore seldom employed, but it is essential to have one on hand for inspecting any blind areas that cannot be seen satisfactorily with the 0-degree scope. The ideal solution for investigating the esophagus, stomach, duodenal bulb, and first portion of the duodenum would be a scope *with both directions of view:* 0 and 90 degrees. This idea was incorporated in some designs (Eder and Machida Co.). It is a difficult mechanical and optical task to divert the viewing direction. Problems are also involved in providing similar manipulation possibilities for the biopsy forceps. A guide mechanism with an optical deflection for both directions is not simple. It will take time and new concepts in design to perfect a "universal" scope.

Table 1 gives some figures for two scopes available to us. The useful length is 1,000 to 1,095 mm. If the outside diameter exceeds 13 mm, it can cause difficulties or complications during introduction of the instrument. The flexibility and length at the working end is of great importance in maneuvering and performing the J curve (inversion) for inspecting the cardia or fundus. The length of the flexible tip is 115 to 125 mm. The turning radius of the tip is shown in Figure 3. If the flexion is not small or sharp, we need additional "tricks" (e.g., using the wall of the curvature as a further "assisting deflector" during advancement, enabling us to see the cardia).

Introduction of the biopsy forceps is still a problem. If the scope is in the maximally flexed position and bent simultaneously in both planes, the biopsy forceps in many instances

TABLE 1. Physical Characteristics of Two Upper Gastrointestinal Scopes

Parameter	Olympus GIF-D2	ACMI F8
Useful length (mm)	1,045	1,000
Flexible tip (mm)	125	115
Tip diameter (mm)	15	12.6
Smallest diameter (mm)	12.5	12.4
Pupil (mm)	9	14.5
Biopsy channel (mm)	2.8	3.3
Light-carrying fiber bundle (mm)	2,770	2,730
Control	Double reel	Joy-stick
H_2O/air	Separate	Common
H_2O	In handle	Separate

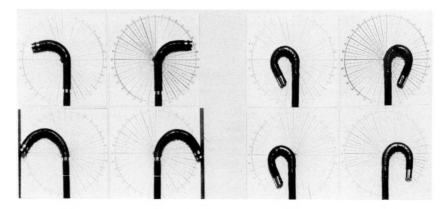

FIG. 3. Turning radius of the ACMI FO-7089P (right) and Olympus GIF-D2 (left) upper GI gastroscopes. If the tip is in a maximum flexed position in both planes, it is difficult to advance the biopsy forceps.

just do not pass through. In the stomach this can be overcome by straightening the scope, advancing the forceps, and locating the lesion again; but in the colon (see below) this creates significant difficulties.

Viewing Angle

We started with smaller viewing angles (30 to 40 degrees) but found out very quickly that orientation is then difficult and the examination time extended. With improved technology this angle became larger and the orientation easier (Fig. 4).

Depth of Field

When focusing devices were incorporated the object was sharp, but the areas in front and behind were not seen well (shallow depth of field). Continuous refocusing was necessary during movements and was time-consuming. We require a relative sharp picture in the stomach from a 10 to 150 mm object distance

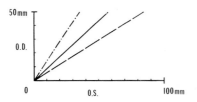

FIG. 4. Viewing angles of various scopes (relation of object distance versus size of object), which is an important aspect for orientation. The trend to increase the viewing angle becomes obvious. Interrupted line, 40°. Straight line, 60°. Dotted line, 80°.

without the need of refocusing. If the objective is supplied with a smaller iris the depth of field can be improved but also requires much more light because our working "pupil" is then smaller. We made a simple test to obtain some information about this parameter. Figure 5 shows the test arrangement and Figure 6 the comparative tests of two scopes. An optimal design of optical and fiber components is important because some improvements in this performance are still required.

Resolution

The amount of detail we can see is dependent on many factors: among others, the optical design and the quality of fibers (coherent bundle), e.g., the quality of assorting and packaging the fiber threads. The interspace between the individual fibers is a dead space for image transmission. It can be kept fairly symmetrical (square packaging); or if the fibers are smaller, assorted more closely, it ends up in a circular shape (Fig. 7). The resolutions of both scopes are shown in Figure 8.

The contrast, detail, illumination of the object, and magnification at the eyepiece all contribute to the appearance of the object. Three major components play a role in the displayed image quality: (1) the quality of the coherent bundle and its arrangements; (2) design of the optics on both ends; and (3) illumination.

The question is how much resolution we need. At this stage we can resolve an object 1 to 2 mm in diameter at a distance of 50 mm (2 inches). When examining patterns we are deal-

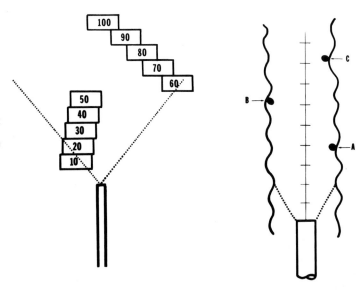

FIG. 5. Left, Simple test arrangement to assess the depths of field of the scope to be seen in a single viewing field without moving the instrument. Small test patterns are placed from 10 to 100 mm OD. Right, Lesions (**A**, **B**, and **C**) in the colon should be seen sharply without moving the scope.

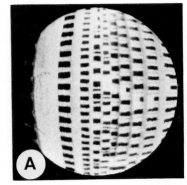
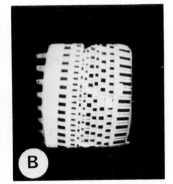

FIG. 6. Comparative test of depth of field. A, ACMI. B, Olympus gastroscope. Each 10 mm wide strip with black and white lines is placed at 10-mm intervals (cf. Fig. 5, left) and is photographed through the eyepiece.

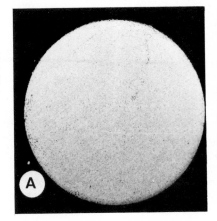
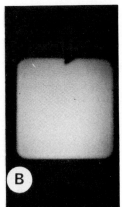

FIG. 7. Arrangement of the coherent individual fiber threads in two instruments. **a**, Round, circular packaging (ACMI). **b**, Square packaging (Olympus).

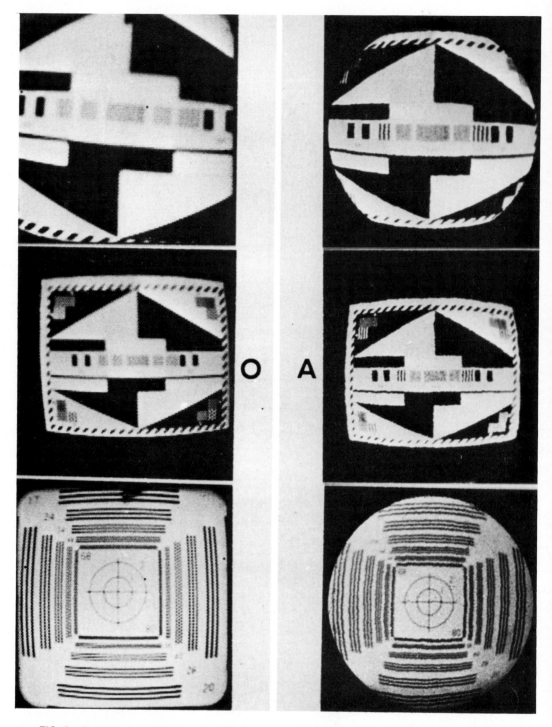

FIG. 8. Resolution test as it appears looking through both scopes under identical conditions. A, ACMI. O, Olympus. Object distance: 10 mm (top), 20 mm (middle), and 50 mm (bottom).

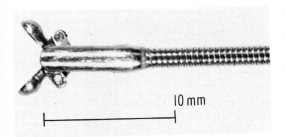

10 mm

FIG. 9. Flexible biopsy forceps. Unfortunately the narrow biopsy channel determines the diameter and the length of jaw of the small biopsy forceps. The rigid part also plays a role in the advancement if the scope is flexed. Because of the superficial bite, several tissue samples are required to decrease the existing risk of a false-negative result. It is recommended that in doubtful attempts biopsies be combined with brush or wash cytology.

ing with ideal conditions: straight lines with peak contrast differences (black and white). In the esophagus or stomach nothing is straight with sharp edges, or black and white lines, as these patterns are. The fact is that we can see (directly) a small lesion 2 mm in diameter, compared with an x-ray film where the shape the contrast material assumed determines our findings. A 2-mm lesion is difficult to interpret via x-ray, and so fiber endoscopy has contributed to an improvement in our findings. I have no intention of comparing the diagnostic accuracy of gastroscopy with a barium meal. Both examinations should be carried out with appropriate indications because the two proce-

dures are complementary. We should not give up the hope, however, of finding a better optical technique to improve on our present limiting factors, e.g., resolution, depth of field, contrast, and mechanical design.

Tissue Sampling

Obtaining a target biopsy or aimed (jet) washings for cytologic study helped greatly to increase our diagnostic capabilities by providing us with histologic proof. The biopsy forceps are unfortunately somewhat small (Fig. 9) owing to the space available in the design of the instrument and diameter of the biopsy channel. False-negative results are possible, but with increased experience and combined technique (biopsy and cytology) the incidence can be decreased. The problems arise mainly with large carcinomas (where the edges contain more necrotic tissue than typical malignant cells) and lymphomas, or when malignancy is combined with inflammatory components. The experienced endoscopist is alarmed by the appearance, color changes on edges of the lesion, etc. The response of distention and other visible indirect signs are also helpful.

The development of better biopsy forceps needs more manufacturing "homework." We require a deeper and sharper bite, more flexibility, and greater power on the small jaws. These are difficult problems to be solved. The protuberating needle in the middle is claimed to be helpful in "fixing" the position of

FIG. 10. These forceps are very vulnerable. If the tip of the scope is flexed the outer spiral breaks very easily when force is needed to push it through. The forceps exits the channel on one side (unilateral), making it difficult to attack a lesion on the opposite side immediately behind or in a curvature. The biopsy forceps is one of the most common and frequently replaced items. The situation in which the lesion is in an area where access is difficult (e.g., hepatic flexure or ascending colon) and the forceps cannot be advanced in the last stage is extremely difficult and frustrating.

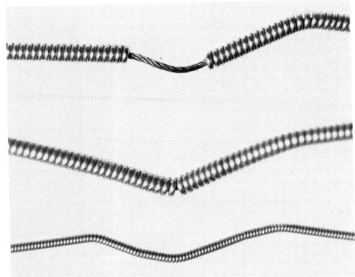

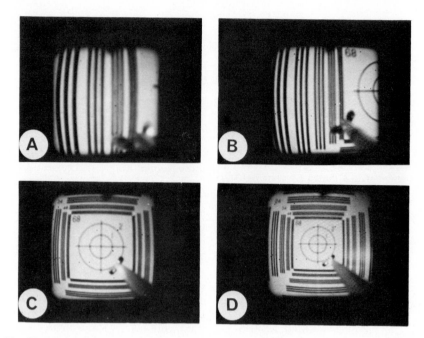

FIG. 11. Biopsy forceps advanced 10 mm (**A**), 20 mm (**B**), 30 mm (**C**), and 40 mm (**D**) object distance. The problem in accurate visibility and limitation of depths of field are plausible (Olympus).

tissue before the jaws are closed. These forceps are very vulnerable, and the spiral breaks easily when we have to apply force to push it through a bend (Fig. 10). Meticulous maintenance (cleaning and lubrication) and the dexterity of the operator helps to prolong the "survival time" of these not inexpensive accessories. A lever on the outlet of the biopsy channel (as in some colonoscope models) can help in directing the forceps. The forceps exits the channel on one side. If the lesion is located on the opposite wall from the exit of the forceps, the entire working end of the scope must be bent in order to help in directing the forceps. The visibility of a biopsy forceps versus object distance is shown in Figure 11. The limitation of visibility for a 30 mm object distance is obvious. In general improvements are needed in the biopsy forceps per se, its maneuverability, and the provision of better vision if the object distance is longer than 20 mm.

Air–Water–Suction Channels

A common air–water channel is not the best solution because after irrigation followed by air insufflation the rest of the water is always retained in the long tube of the front lens until it

is completely emptied. With separate channels this is avoided and expedites examinations —but this requires more space. The common suction-biopsy channel diameter is given by the diameter of the scope. A larger size would ease the passage of biopsy forceps when the

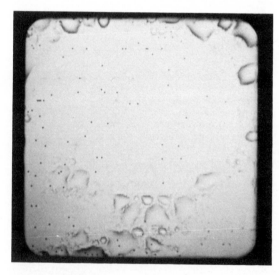

FIG. 12. Another known repair problem: water behind the front cover lens due to a damaged cover sheath, seal, or leakage.

scope is flexed. This channel is a plastic tube that can be easily kinked in a flexed position. Its connection to a small metal tube at the working end (biopsy or air–water channel) can come loose, and moisture or water infiltrates the front between the objective lens and the cover (Fig. 12). Appropriate cleaning and drying of these delicate channels is greatly important. Mixing the rinse water with an antifoam agent (Mylicon*) can be helpful.

Operation of Scope

The water–air system of suction is now operationally uniform, using a trumpet, electric, or mechanical contact valve system. Handling one valve for two functions (air and water) sometimes complicates the procedure because the examiner is concentrating on many other facets of the examination. The use of three valves instead of two is perhaps easier; and placing these valves at different heights would also be helpful, enabling the operator to determine immediately which is the right one by feeling it instead of losing the visual field by mistakenly pushing the suction instead of the air valve. A separate water injection apparatus (syringe) operated by the assistant is time-consuming and interferes with the routine. Another possibility is a footswitch control for the two actions (suction and water) leaving only one valve function in the already crowded handle.

Vacuum and Air Pressure

Suction is not always adequate. When a central wall vacuum system is used during busy hospital hours (if several rooms are in use simultaneously) the vacuum can drop significantly. The long connecting tubes not coupled with care may result in reduced suction. The resistance of the small tube or channel in the scope is high. To exclude as many factors that can go wrong as possible, it is advisable here to use a separate suction machine located near the scope which provides a maximum of 700 mm Hg vacuum—adjustable according to the length of the instrument and the requirements.

The air inflow should be also adjustable. Gauges on a simple suction-air inflow ap-

paratus should indicate the vacuum/air pressure so as to adjust the two safely but adequately (Fig. 13).

For illumination and documentation see Chapters 3 and 18).

Discussion

Since 1958 upper gastrointestinal endoscopy has undergone significant changes and improvements in instrumentation. The better visualization and maneuverability have improved tissue sampling possibilities, which in turn have greatly contributed to higher diagnostic accuracy, which in turn has resulted in wide acceptance of this important diagnostic tool. The introduction of a single scope for examining the esophagus, stomach, duodenal bulb, and sometimes the first part of the duodenum was a great step forward. This instrument, the 0-degree viewing fiberscope, had flexibility and wide viewing angle, relatively good depth of field and resolution, and sufficient length.

An objective evaluation should be carried out to determine whether the 0- or the 30-degree forward-oblique view is more suitable for visualizing certain areas (e.g., the duodenal bulb) that are difficult to observe. A 90-degree (lat-

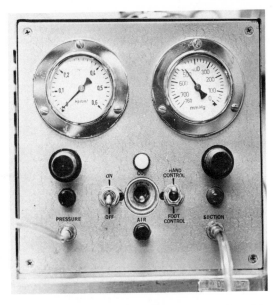

FIG. 13. "Home made" unit providing adjustable air (or CO_2) inflow (left) and vacuum (right). Suction requirements must be adjustable up to 700 mm Hg and are needed for longer instruments (e.g., for colon polypectomy).

Manufacturer: Stuart Pharmaceuticals, Division of ICI America Inc., Wilmington, Delaware 19899.

eral) scope must be available for visualizing those anatomic areas that are difficult to see or impossible to obtain a biopsy from with the 0-degree (straightforward view) scope. Combining both of these viewing angles in one scope at this stage is too difficult from the mechanical and optical points of view.

Good maintenance by a skilled nurse and adequate training of the endoscopist help significantly to extend the "lifetime" of scopes, an aspect that must be recognized before the tool is purchased. Spiraling costs make it mandatory for manufacturers not to release obvious instrument improvements only on a year by year basis. An instrument that costs $4,000 today should be good enough for a minimum of two years on the average.

COLONOSCOPE

In recent years the colonoscope opened a new chapter in the detection and evaluation of colonic pathology. Its use does not replace the barium enema, but it has already become a valuable diagnostic adjunctive device for examining this organ. If a part of the colon can be seen well, the image quality and detail are greater than those seen on x-ray. Smaller lesions (less than 5 mm) can be detected more precisely with the colonoscope. The misleading x-ray findings of fecal matter and protuberating mucosa simulating lesions or polyps can be identified readily through the scope. The possibility of obtaining tissue samples has immense value, and the removal of polyps is associated with decreased morbidity and mortality compared with open surgery (see Chap. 21).

The instrument is still in a "redesigning" stage, needing further refinements. There are many aspects in instrumentation where changes can make this examination easier and safer. Despite some shortcomings this examination has made and its undisputable value as a new tool for examining colonic pathology and discovering disease in early stages, there are still many unsuccessful examinations and complications. Among the factors responsible for this are the inability to clean the bowel, anatomic or pathologic changes of the colon, the competence of the examiner, and finally problems caused by instrumentation.

Image Quality

Details of the object within a given distance should be seen under optimal conditions and therefore well observed. We are still far from the ideal if the lesion is at a long object distance.

Depth of Field

The depth of field should be improved (Fig. 14).

Viewing Angle

Do we need the present viewing angle (approximately 70 degrees) in a tube-shaped organ? Would a smaller angle be sufficient? Greater depth of field and a larger magnification can be provided with less light absorption.

We experience occasional difficulties in visualizing radiologically manifest lesions on crit-

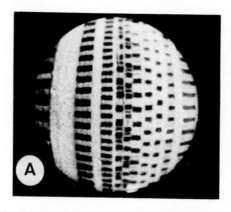 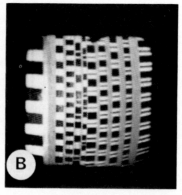

FIG. 14.   Depths of field as seen through the colonoscopes. Left, ACMI. Right, Olympus. (See also Fig. 4.)

ical locations, near a flexure or in a sharp curve. Those who perform colonoscopy know how frustrating it can be if we must waste time going backward and forward several times around suspected areas if the lesion is visible only for a short period of time or is partially covered. If the scope is withdrawn 0.5 inch or so, the flexure suddenly "swallows" the view or the peristaltic wave obscures it and we must start all over again. I wonder if it would not be worthwhile to test, instead of the straightforward (0-degree) view, a forward-oblique 30-degree view to determine if we might see around corners better.

Dimensions

Generally two lengths are available: a short and a long one. The parameters of various scopes are shown on Table 2.

Bending Mechanism of Scope

The four-way movements of the tip are essential, and the flexible tip should be as short as possible. On numerous occasions the maximum flexion in both planes provides only a "half-moon" appearance of the lumen or the edge of the lesion, despite the fact that both controls are in the extreme position. When it cannot go further, the "third hand"—that of

the assistant or the examiner—sometimes must be used. The instrument is twisted (torque) around its axis to force a better position of the tip. This stress is very harmful to the instrument but cannot be avoided at this stage of instrument design. The additional stress can add significantly to earlier impairment of the coherent bundle, flexible channels, and function of the instrument.

Flexibility Versus Rigidity

We need as much flexibility as possible. In my experience the "softer" scope in those cases where we are dealing with a short mesocolon, patients after pelvic surgery, or diverticula is somehow safer than a rigid one. We also sometimes require a stiff instrument. Perhaps the flexibility of the scope might vary within the instrument (e.g., the first third soft and the following parts somewhat stiffer); or we might incorporate a mechanism whereby we could change the flexibility of the scope at will.[2] The currently used outer stiffening sheath straightens or splints only the sigmoid colon if introduced.

Problems with Biopsy

If the tip of the scope is bent in a sharper angle, it is impossible to pass the biopsy forceps through it. It is most frustrating when a large sessile lesion is located in the transverse or ascending colon, and it is dangerous or difficult to snare and impossible to obtain tissue samples.

During advancement of forceps in these cases the resistance to the biopsy forceps is increased. The examiner often tries to overcome it by exerting more pressure to pass the forceps through. This manipulation may cause a sharp, irreparable bend or break in the outer spring coil, with the result that the forceps must be replaced.

How might we overcome difficult introduction of biopsy forceps?

1. The diameter of the biopsy channel could be increased.
2. The length of the rigid part of the biopsy forceps could be decreased to allow sharper turns.
3. The spring coil outer sheath could be replaced with a Teflon tube, into which is inserted only the jaws of the biopsy forceps, with one wire operating the movements.
4. The wall of the biopsy channel tube could be thickened, since if it is too thin it can be kinked

TABLE 2. Physical Characteristics of Colonoscopes

Parameter	Olympus Long	Olympus Short	ACMI
Useful length (mm)	1,780	1,040	1,600
Flexible tip (mm)	100	100	124
Tip (mm)	18	18	18.2
Smallest diameter (mm)	13.9	13.9	15.4
Pupil (mm)	6.5	6.5	14
Biopsy channel (mm)	3.5	3.5	4
Light-carrying fiber bundle (mm)	1,580	1,560	2,500
Control	Double reel	Double reel	Joy-stick
H_2O/air	Common	Common	Common
H_2O	In handle	In handle	Separate

when the scope is in a bent position, obstructing further advancement.

The solution has yet to be found, but something must be done to solve the problem of advancing the biopsy forceps when the scope is in a critical position.

Biopsy-Suction Channel

Using the same (common) channel for suction and biopsy results in a dirty working end if the forceps is introduced, as feces particles are pushed back in front of the lens. Time must be taken to clean it with repeated washings and air inflow. If the forceps or snare is introduced, it may interfere with the suction (which sometimes is required) because of the space-occupying instrument in this common suction channel. Two separate channels would be helpful in solving this problem, but this increases the outside diameter of the instrument, and the flexibility is then changed (stiffer scope).

Polypectomy Snares and Electrosurgery

There are various types of snares available: (1) a single, thin wire, which opens symmetrically; (2) a braided wire loop, which opens

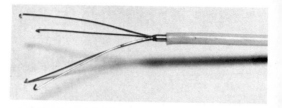

FIG. 16. Four-prong grasping forceps which can be introduced through the biopsy channel to fix the transected polyp for recovery, or in the case of a double-channel instrument to pull it through the open loop for easier snaring. (Manufacturer: Medi-Tech Co., Boston.)

asymmetrically; and (3) the coiled spring, which opens symmetrically (Fig. 15). The snare of choice is probably simply the examiner's preference. The main object is to place the loop in the proper position.

There are grasping instruments available (Fig. 16). In case of a double-channel scope, if the polyp is "lassoed" and the examiner is not satisfied with the position of the snare, the grasper can be forwarded through the second channel and the head of the polyp grasped and pulled into the open snare. A double-channel scope is needed for this maneuver.

If the snare is closed around the polyp, only pure coagulation current should be used. There are large variations from patient to patient regarding the strength of current required. The polyp is desiccated and transected by mechanically increasing closure or by moving the closed snare. In other instances a longer time is required to achieve the same changes that are seen through the scope: the whitish color, demarcation, smoke, bubbling, etc. Many physiologic factors are causing these variations that require different times and currents for adequate coagulation.

Using a unipolar electrosurgical system, it is essential to check the elementary prerequisites (contacts) before the system is applied to the patient. The plate should have a large surface contact, and all wires and contacts (including the snare) should be tested before the patient is put on the table.

The interposed tissue resistance between the patient's plate and the active lead (snare loop) varies according to interposed tissue resistance. Using a unipolar electrosurgical unit, if the opposite wall of the colon is touched by the snared polyp during the coagulation for a period of time, a necrotic (burned) lesion can develop. It is therefore advisable to move the

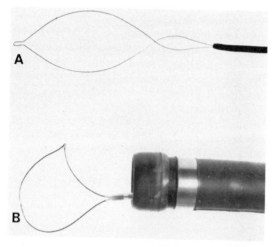

FIG. 15. A. Deyhle polypectomy snare (manufacturer: Storz Co.), which is a single wire and opens symmetrically. It is inserted in a Teflon tube with an insulated handle. **B.** Another approach is the braided wire loop which opens and closes asymmetrically (ACMI-Olympus Co.). Both loops have advantages and disadvantages, so generally the loop used is simply a matter of the operator's preference.

polyp during coagulation if the wall is near. Coagulation is not performed if vision is impaired or the position is not satisfactory. *Special attention should be paid to patients with a pacemaker.*

A new approach would be a bipolar snare that needs much less current and has better efficiency. No patient's plate would be required, with the current flowing from one pole to the other—i.e., from one side of the wire loop to the other without needing to overcome the resistance of a large, interposed tissue complex between the patient's plate and the active electrode (patent pending).

Every snare should be checked before and after each polypectomy. Heat production during coagulation can affect the elasticity and the full opening of the loop.

Recovery of Transected Polyp

Recovery must be attempted if the polyp is transected. In the majority of cases this is achieved by removing the snare, approaching the transected polyp with the front end of the scope, and applying sudden suction. (A minimum of 700 mm Hg vacuum is required for a long colonoscope.) High suction is important as polyps can be lost during the withdrawal if the vacuum is incomplete. The development of a grasper (Fig. 16) has made it easier. This instrument is inserted through the suction-biopsy channel; it is then held in position (or pulled into the opening of the biopsy channel) while suction is applied.

If a larger biopsy channel is provided (e.g., on the double-channel scopes), the same suction (700 mm Hg) is more effective because of the larger diameter. We apply high suction only if the polyp sits properly in position. High suction should not be used with larger channels during normal examination. The sudden and vehement aspiration can cause mucosal bleeding. The vacuum should be adjustable, the experienced examiner easily assessing the amount required.

Air–Water Channels

Rinsing and air (CO_2) insufflation is provided by means of a small channel. (It is advisable to have these channels separated.) If the same channel is used for air and water in long instruments after discontinuing the water rinse

and proceeding with air insufflation there is a short period of time when water bubbles in front of the lens disturb the view, thereby extending the examination time (thus the advantage of separate channels). Instead of combined trumpet valve action for air and water administration, separate valves would make the procedure easier.

Testing Instrument Functions

The ocular should be adjusted to fit the examiner's vision, and the instrument should be so constructed that it can be fixed in this position. During examination or manipulation this ocular position can be changed inadvertently with the view becoming hazy. Before inserting a scope and starting the examination the following should be tested: vision (clear view), proper adjustment of the ocular (seeing the sharp, distinct fiber structure), light source, operation of valves and their functions (suction

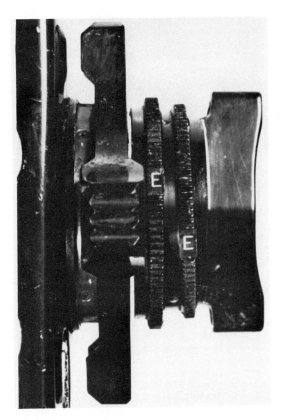

FIG. 17. The locking mechanism of the remote-controlled tip can be disturbing if both fixing reels (E) are placed beside each other instead of being apart (already improved in recent models).

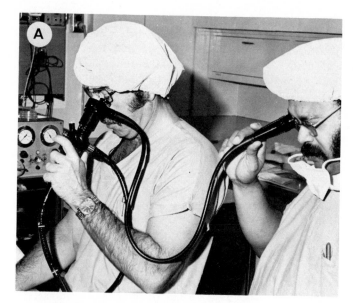

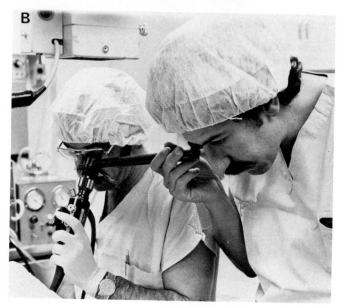

FIG. 18. A. Use of the colonoscope with its flexible teaching attachment. **B.** Same instrument except that a rigid teaching attachment is coupled to it. The performance and image quality of the rigid teaching arm is superior to the flexible ones. For detail see Chap. 4.

and air), bending mechanism, biopsy forceps, snare and electric wire contacts, and patient's plate.

Locking Mechanism

There are certain positions where we need to lock the flexed tip in one way or the other in a bent position. It is advisable that these locking devices not be hidden (Fig. 17) but be designed to operate with ease.

Teaching Attachment

The assistant is of great importance on many occasions, and so the attachment with which he can visualize the field simultaneously with the operator is essential here as well as for teaching (Fig. 18). This (teaching) attachment (see Chap. 4) is a beam splitter which divides the image that comes through the eyepiece and conveys it to the second observer as well as the examiners. Using a flexible fiber coherent

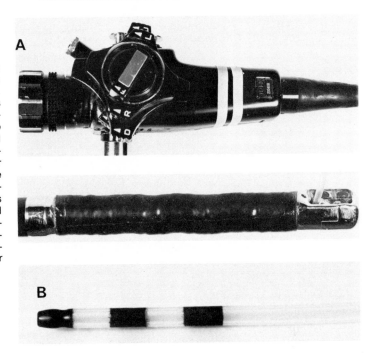

FIG. 19. **A.** Duodenoscope with lateral view for cannulating the papilla of Vater (JF-B2, Olympus). It has a built-in lever that bends the introduced cannula into position. **B.** Plastic cannula (close-up view). OD, 1.7 mm. ID, 1.0 mm, and in the tapered end 0.7 mm. Because of the small inside diameter it is very difficult if not impossible to collect or aspirate pure pancreatic secretion. It also causes problems if highly concentrated (50 to 60 percent) contrast material is injected (e.g., pancreatography) because of the large resistance due to the small catheter lumen.

teaching attachment we found a significant light loss. The image viewed through the beam splitter by the examiner became extremely dim, and we therefore had to employ larger and more expensive high-intensity light sources. The eyepiece also became larger and more clumsy. There is another aspect that must be emphasized. If two coherent bundles, which according to their characteristics are precisely assorted, are coupled *mechanically only* (not optically)—as in the case of a flexible teaching attachment—this results in a loss of resolution: "mismatch phenomenon." It is interesting to note how this was overlooked by our profession. If each individual coherent fiber thread is not aligned with its exact counterpart, there is no assurance that the image will be properly transmitted. Those that are misaligned cut the image and transmit half (which half depends on the position). Significant information is lost when our present mechanical adaptor is used (see Chaps. 2 and 4).

The colonoscope has been improved during recent years, but there are still areas in optics and mechanics that need further refinement. This instrument, however, has become one of the most important tools in the investigation of colonic pathology. A short (approximately 60 cm) colonoscope for examination and biopsy of the first part of the sigmoid colon would be a valuable extension of the rigid rectosigmoidoscope.

DUODENOSCOPE FOR ENDOSCOPIC RETROGRADE CANNULATION OF PAPILLA (ERCP)

We use the Olympus JF-B2 duodenoscope with a lateral (90 degree) view for duodenoscopy. This scope was designed for cannulating the papilla of Vater (Fig. 19A). It has a built-in lever that can bend the cannula into position if the papilla is in vision. The scope parameters are shown in Table 3.

This scope is always used with fluoroscopy and radiography. Radiation affects the bundles by increasing the yellowish tint; it also affects light absorption. In our experience it has to be replaced after approximately 100 procedures.

The small-lumen catheter (cannula)—outside diameter 1.7 mm, lumen diameter 0.7 to 1.0 mm—does not allow aspiration (Fig. 19B). When a high-concentration (50 percent) contrast medium is injected the small lumen presents a high resistance, requiring that the operator exert more pressure during injection. This can eliminate the "feeling" of what the

**TABLE 3. Parameters of
the JF-B2 Duodenoscope**

Parameter	Olympus JF-B2
Useful length (mm)	1,305
Flexible tip (mm)	87
Tip diameter (mm)	10.8
Smallest diameter (mm)	10
Pupil (mm)	6.5
Biopsy channel (mm)	2.5
Light-carrying fiber bundle (mm)	1,560
Control	Double reel
H_2O/air	Common
H_2O	In handle

actual resistance of the pancreatic duct system is during injection and can play a role in some of the complications due to high pressure and consequences of tissue destruction in the pancreatic parenchyma. The examiner is guided only by the television-fluoroscopic image, which does not always display the details required for this purpose (see Chapter 17). The instrumentation for cannulation is still in a developmental stage.

The biopsy forceps is smaller because the instrument channel is narrower. Only a small bite is therefore possible, although it is still useful for examining lesions of the papilla.

The duodenoscope is useful for examining the duodenal bulb because of its optical ability to visualize objects from a short distance with a lateral view.

PEDIATRIC FLEXIBLE FIBER ENDOSCOPES

On a few occasions we tested a scope (OD 8.5 mm) with a two-way and a four-way control. All the compartments (image transmission, light transmission, etc.) are decreased or miniaturized. The era of using scopes in infants and children for examining the upper or lower gastrointestinal tract has just begun, and time and experience will show the clinical value and the changes required in the instruments. The smaller scopes have been tried in adults, but we do not have enough experience to provide a clinical evaluation.

A few prototype experimental scopes of small diameter size but longer are used with a mer-

cury bag attached to the end similar to the Miller-Abbot tube, but providing visibility. The weight-bearing portion guides the tube into deeper sections of the small intestine. Evaluation of the clinical merits of visualizing the entire gastrointestinal tract needs more time and more convincing data.

FLEXIBLE BRONCHOSCOPE

The desire to make bronchoscopy somewhat more pleasant than what is experienced with the rigid instrument and to advance it further to the periphery caused the flexible fiber bronchoscope to be created. The physical sizes and diameters of the ACMI and Olympus bronchoscopes are shown in Table 4. The best image is seen at approximately 10 mm object distance.

The use of fiber bronchoscopy is indicated in patients with peripheral malignant lesions, as well as in other situations, e.g., in intensive care units, for acute respiratory distress, at the bedside. Sterilization can create a problem in the latter application. If cold sterilization (soaking) is applied it can be harmful for the scope, and bacteriologically its effect is debatable (see Chap. 8). If gas sterilization is used we found that ethylene oxide "stiffened" the scope somewhat after repeated applications. This in-

**TABLE 4. Parameters of Olympus
BF 582 and ACMI FO
8800 Fiber Bronchoscopes**

Parameter	Olympus BF 582	ACMI FO 8800
Useful length (mm)	550	494
Flexible tip (mm)	70	34
Tip diameter (mm)	5.2	6.5
Smallest diameter (mm)	5.2	6.3
Pupil (mm)	6.5	13.5
Biopsy channel (mm)	2	2
Light-carrying fiber bundle (mm)	1,560	2,300
Control	Lever	Reel
H_2O/air	Air only	Air only
H_2O	—	—

Both instruments move the tip in only one plane. Flexible fiber endoscopes in these small sizes are extremely difficult to manufacture, are very vulnerable, and need delicate care. Because of the small diameter of the light and image bundle, the performance of image quality and illumination is limited.

strument requires extreme care and maintenance because of its delicate nature. The clinical aspects of fiber-bronchoscopy are discussed in Chapter 44.

"MINI" SCOPES

When the total outside diameter of a flexible fiberscope is less than 4 mm, including image and light transmission as well as a bending mechanism, the smaller size of the bundle contributes to deterioration of the image quality. Are the inferior resolution, poor contrast, and limited information so derived sufficient for the purpose? If we are introducing it in areas which are not clean, can we be satisfied with the lack of our water-air channel to "wipe" or clean the front of the lens and thereby avoid unnecessary reintroduction? Can we omit the possibility of obtaining tissue samples?

Miniscopes are extremely vulnerable regarding breakage of the bundles and impairment of mechanisms. The ratio of the individual fiber thread size to the total outside diameter of the bundle here is larger, so each fiber thread breakage is more visible as a larger black dot.

ILLUMINATION

The situation concerning light sources for flexible scopes is chaotic at the moment. The majority of manufacturers are using the same globe, but the different fittings made it impossible to use various types of scopes with the same light. In larger hospitals, where rigid and flexible fiber endoscopes of different brands are used, it is economically important to use light sources that are interchangeable.

It is very helpful if adaptors are available that optimally align the light beam with the light fiber bundle. A 150-watt halogen lamp with a dichroic mirror is sufficient for a routine examination with a short fiber scope. The ultraviolet (UV) and infrared (IR) range should be filtered and only the visible spectrum transmitted. This also decreases heat production in the focal plane and at the working end of the fiber. This light source is not strong enough when flexible fiber (coherent) teaching attachments or long scopes are used. It is also inadequate for still photography.

The features of incoherent bundles are detailed in Chapter 2. The light-transmitting fiber bundles are integral. This means that the bundles are pulled in, in one piece, from the working end of the scope up to the light source. Every connection increases the light loss. These integral bundles are very small in diameter and contribute further to the light loss. The characteristic yellowish tint of the light-transmitting bundle and a tungsten filament globe spectrum contribute to a more yellowish illumination compressing the red spectrum of the object. The color of the visceral linings is within the red spectrum. A light source with a higher color (Kelvin) temperature than the tungsten filament globe—as in the case of fiber light transmission—is advantageous. The General Electric Marc 300 quartz iodine globe has a better color temperature than a tungsten globe but as a light source is not the most efficient. Its lifetime is limited (25 to 30 hours), and the output decreases gradually. We installed a timer in the commercially available light units to indicate the exchange of globes in time. The beam of the Marc 300 and its angle are much wider than required, and we are "shooting beside" a large amount of light, which is wasted; the heat production is significant.

A well designed high-intensity light source with a long lifetime and little heat production is desirable. It should be made with better interchangeable attachments to fit every available endoscope light-transmitting bundle (see Chapter 3).

CONCLUSION

Light Transmission

The introduction of flexible fiber incoherent light transmission opened new avenues for more convenient and efficient illumination systems in endoscopy. These fibers are packed around rigid telescopes connected to a flexible fiber bundle and an external light source (Fig. 20).

The same incoherent fibers are employed in flexible fiber endoscopes as an integral light-transmitting medium (Fig. 21). The light-transmitting quality and other characteristics of the existing bundles are not optimal. The absorption is too high, and the dominant yellowish tint is sometimes disturbing, especially when distinct color differentiation is important.

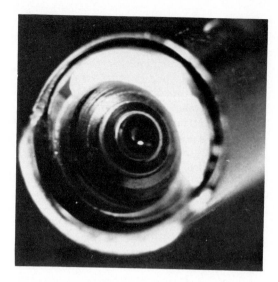

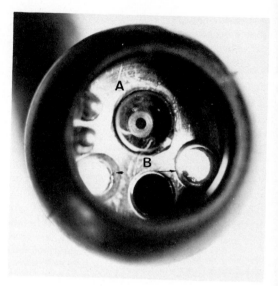

FIG. 20. Small amount of incoherent fibers is packed around the 0-degree rigid telescope. It is connected to the external light source via a 6-foot flexible glass fiber cable.

FIG. 21. The same incoherent fibers as seen in Figure 20, but this time integral, are guided from the light source without interruption to the working end of the flexible fiberscope. In this instrument (Olympus) a 4-mm bundle is divided in two smaller parts (**B**) and placed below the objective (**A**) of the image (coherent) bundle.

Flexible Fiber Endoscopes

The introduction of flexible fiber endoscopes in the upper and lower gastrointestinal tract revolutionized direct examination of the esophagus, stomach, duodenal bulb, first part of the duodenum, and recently the colon. It took us 15 years to devise a controlled tip with maneuverability and to perform procedures under visual control: biopsy, cytology, polypectomy, hemostasis, cannulation, etc. The sudden increase in number of examinations performed today compared with the prefiber era speaks for itself. Clinical results support the wide indications noted for these examinations.

However, there are still some areas left for improvement: the mechanism, durability, design of accessories (mainly biopsy forceps), and the image- and light-transmitting qualities of the coherent and incoherent bundles. Despite their shortcomings, these instruments have become some of the most important tools for diagnosing gastrointestinal lesions; they are also valuable adjuncts to other diagnostic examinations.

By coupling a beam splitter (teaching attachment) to the eyepiece, the examination or procedure could be viewed and/or assisted simultaneously. This then extended the one-man procedure to a team effort and provided a basis from which more complex examination and procedures can be developed.

There would be a significant impact on the future of these promising diagnostic modalities if basic and clinical research projects could be initiated dealing with one of the most important factors of our diagnostic procedure: *the instrument itself*. Coordination of the varied opinions of endoscopists and improved communication with the manufacturers would result in a higher diagnostic accuracy due to better or new instruments. As an example: assessing the durability of the instruments could lead to an extended lifetime of these expensive items; and better and faster repair services would eliminate the present aggravations and interuptions in the continuity of patient care. It would be advisable to concentrate on further refinement and improvements designed to explore the upper and lower gastrointestinal tract, which is where the overwhelming majority of these examinations are performed and where the clinical value of endoscopy is already established.

Small scopes are fragile and difficult to

handle, so the lifetime is significantly shorter than that of the large scope, creating economic problems because of replacement expenses. The image quality, as mentioned before, deteriorates as soon as the diameter of the coherent bundle is decreased. The production of small fiber threads (less than 10 μ) poses significant technologic problems and adds further chances of increased breakage of these fragile fibers. Below a certain diameter (7 μ), physicists reported the "wave guide phenomenon," which interferes with image transmission. This problem—if it can be solved at all—needs further study before miniaturization is attempted.

In summary, flexible fiber endoscopes contributed to a significant improvement in diagnostic accuracy of lesions in the gastrointestinal tract and bronchial tree. It furthermore produced new treatment modalities whereby

surgery could be replaced with noninvasive techniques.

REFERENCES

1. Beck TE, Lacerte M, Rona G: Thermal injury of the stomach following intragastric colour cinematography. Can Med J 89:216, 1963
2. Berci G, Panish JF: Suggestions for a better colonoscope. Gastrointest Endosc 19:38, 1972
3. Colcher H, Katz GM: Cinegastroscopy. Am J Gastroenterol 35:518, 1961
4. Heel ACS: A new method of transporting optical images without aberrations. Nature (Lond) 173:39, 1954
5. Hirschowitz BI, Curtis LE, Peters CW, et al: The fiberscope. Gastroenterology 35:50, 1958
6. Hopkins HH, Kapany NS: A flexible fiberscope. Nature (Lond) 173:39, 1954
7. Lamm H: Biegsame optische Geraete. Z Instr 50:579, 1930
8. Schindler R: Gastroscopy with a flexible gastroscope. Am J Dig Dis 2:656, 1936

EDITORIAL COMMENT

At a recent (1975) meeting on endoscopy a prominent manufacturer of flexible fiberscopes offered eight different models with various functional parameters for examination of the esophagus, stomach, and duodenum. This seemed to be one extreme, and the "unimodel" another.

The working head of the "unimodel" is designed to provide a straightforward (0-degree) view but only a 40-degree viewing angle. This straight direction of view can be moved into a lateral position, converting two scopes into one instrument. In addition, the optical head can be rotated (panning). It is a fascinating idea to have a universal instrument. Of course the diameter had to be increased (14 mm), which in my opinion is the upper limit for safety and convenient introduction of an upper gastrointestinal endoscope. The "panviewscope" idea is not new, but I am leery of the overcomplicated mechanism and the increase in repair problems. Six separate knobs are available to control the various functions.

With soaring instrument prices we have to make decisions, based on sound protocols, somewhere between these two extremes. For instance, would a 0-degree instrument with a small diameter and short turning radius be just as good as the rediscovered 30-degree forward-oblique one? We should note certain facts about the diagnostic accuracy in the duodenal bulb before we trade in our scopes.

Single- or Double-Channel System.

Upper Gastrointestinal Scope. The outside diameter is limited by the anatomy. If a second channel is inserted it must be done by reducing other vital structures (e.g., smaller images bundles; or instead of one or two large light bundles, one smaller one). The instrument will be less flexible because more internal components (channels) are inserted.

We must have convincing clinical data (e.g., in the diagnosing or treatment of bleeders or polyps) to sacrifice some of our image light and other factors influencing performance.

Colonoscope. The outside diameter here is not so critical but still plays a role. The possibility of grasping and pulling a pedunculated polyp through an open snare is very impressive as described in the advertisements, but it is somewhat more difficult in practice.

Conclusion

We need more coordination in our assessments with a realistic input toward necessary alterations before a new scope is released. Furthermore, how many scopes do we need to examine successfully the upper and lower gastrointestinal tract?

THE EDITOR

7

Instrumentation III: Cleaning, Storage, and Maintenance and Supervision

Gabriella Nemethy

CLEANING ENDOSCOPIC EQUIPMENT

The cleaning procedure is one of the most important aspects of upkeep, maintenance, and performance of instruments. It must be clearly understood by operating room (OR) supervisors, nurses, doctors, and hospital administrators that if appropriate endoscopic service is to be provided merely generating capital investment to purchase expensive instruments is not enough: The equipment must be cleaned properly, or its function will not be good enough to achieve the expected diagnostic accuracy. Furthermore, if these aspects are not considered, patient care suffers.

Endoscopic equipment is expensive, delicate, and extremely vulnerable; and some of the miniaturized pediatric scopes with their thin walls need even further care. Some of the adult scopes occupy space because of the peculiar configuration or extreme length (e.g., fiberscopes). As with any other expensive diagnostic equipment (e.g., radiologic) it is not only the instruments that are purchased but also their serviceability. In this particular application the operator must be able to see in order to provide the best service available.

For achieving appropriate cleaning we need the following: (1) working (bench) space; (2) facilities for sufficient cleaning; and (3) enough time to perform an adequate job.

Working (Bench) Space

1. The space alloted should be located if possible in the endoscopy room or adjacent to it so that the nurse does not waste valuable time running back and forth with dirty or clean instruments.
2. The actual working area (bench) should be large enough to place dirty and clean instruments on it without being forced to place one instrument on another. The area should be deep enough (20 to 24 inches) and long enough (50 to 60 inches) to permit easy and fast operation.
3. The dirty area should be separated from the clean one, and each should be large enough. The logical arrangement is to place the actual washing facilities (water outlets and double sink) between the clean and dirty areas.
4. The bench space should be covered with a material that is easy to clean (e.g., commercially available plastics) in a color that contrasts with the instruments so that if a small accessory disappears it is easily discovered against this contrasting background. These materials are readily available from bench manufacturers.

All four of these items are important from the logistic point of view. They save time, which here also means saving dollars.

Facilities

Cold and hot water with a mixing tap and swivel arm outlet are needed (Fig. 1). A double sink is required, one with a normal depth and one with an increased depth for the longer (fiber) scopes. A holder for the fiberscopes dur-

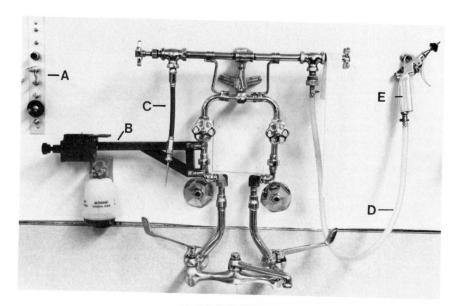

FIG. 1. Cleaning assembly. Hot and cold water with the mixing tap and cleaning pistol, assembled above a double sink. **A.** Several types of nozzles can be attached to the (rinsing) pistol according to the openings of the instruments. **B.** Plastic holder on a hinge to support various types of long, flexible scopes. It facilitates manipulation and cleaning of these scopes. **C.** Previously available endoscope cleaners consisted of a rubber tube and a cone-shaped metal tube on the end. This system is outdated. **D.** Hose connected by the hospital plumber to the existing cold water outlet. **E.** Cleaning pistol. The rinsing pressure can be adjusted using various nozzles (**A**), which can be attached according to the configuration of the instrument. The hose provides flexibility and easy cleaning. We rinse every rigid endoscope inside and out. It decreases the cleaning time and is more thorough. The biopsy channel of the flexible scope cannot be rinsed with pressure because of its delicate nature. It does not stand pressure in general and we therefore simply aspirated it, using only the pressure produced by the water channel. However, even with this procedure we had so many repair problems we gave up even the low-pressure rinsing of flexible scopes.

ing cleaning facilitates easier manipulation because these are extremely long instruments (Fig. 2). The double sinks should be placed between the dirty and clean areas of the working benches. The wall around the working area should be covered with a waterproof material (wall).

Rinsing small tubes or channels is difficult. One of the older designs had rubber outlets with a cone-shaped tube, which proved to be short and cumbersome. A very simple solution is a water pistol (Fig. 1); this can be installed by a hospital plumber to the normal water outlet and has a number of different attachable nozzles which fit in the various diameter holes. It is a very efficient and rapid rinsing system. Every tube, channel, or accessory can be approached with ease without making a mess or splashing water around. It is very important to have proper rinsing and a deep sink available where the instruments can be held conve-

niently. To accomodate the various instruments in their entire lengths, the sink should also be large enough to accomodate a large pan or container.

The usual paraphernalia for cleaning—a variety of brushes, cleaning solutions (Betadine*), soft tissues, Q-tips, a cotton wool ball on a long carrier, Kleenex tissue, towels, etc.—should be available under the bench in drawers.

For rigid endoscopes (e.g., for use in bronchoscopic and urologic examinations), with small, long channels or tubes, it is of paramount importance that there are directed water streams (rinsing) with required pressure to remove lubricating jellies, dried secretion, or blood clots. This is much easier to achieve with a water pistol than taking the chance of

Manufacturer: Purdue Frederick Co., 50 Washington Street, Norwalk, Connecticut 06856.

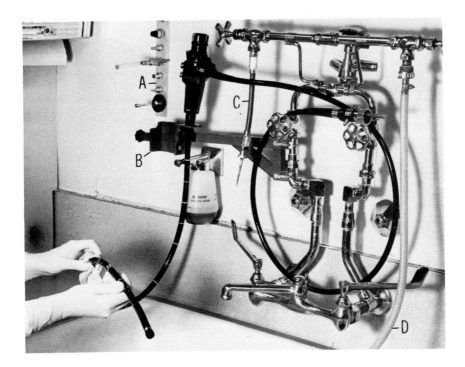

FIG. 2. Fiberscope. Thorough cleaning of a long scope is facilitated by suspending it above the sink; this frees the nurse's hands and at the same time secures the scope into position. The outside can then be wiped or rinsed carefully. **A.** Nozzles of the water rinsing pistol (pistol not seen). **B.** Scope holder; made locally. **C.** Old type of flexible endoscope cleaner with a cone-shaped metal tube on the end that has proved to be outdated for modern endoscopes. **D.** Hose of water pistol connected to water outlet.

scratching the surface with rough brushes or wasting time pushing through loose cotton wool balls, which does not help very much anyway. (Moreover, if the ball fits too tightly it sticks in the middle of the tube.) Small channels must be cleaned meticulously. The pistol has another advantage with its long hose connection in that it can easily be brought into any suitable position. When not in use, it can be kept on a wall hook. It is advisable to soak some instruments (e.g., a laparoscopy set or accessories that cannot be dismantled completely) in a pan in a specific solution such as Betadine before rinsing.

Fiberscopes

Flexible upper and lower gastrointestinal scopes need extremely careful handling because they are very vulnerable. Furthermore, special attention should be paid to the small-diameter scopes, which are even more vulnerable, e.g., the bronchoscope. The scope is placed in a holder (Fig. 2) and its outer surface rinsed

to remove debris, blood clots, or feces particles (Fig. 3) *(Note: If a biopsy is performed and suction used, the suction bottle content should be strained to remove further tissue samples for histologic examination.)* The fiberscope unfortunately cannot tolerate forced rinsing; therefore we must be satisfied here using suction only, applying solutions (Betadine) or clear fluid through the suction-biopsy channel and rinsing water through the water-air channel (Figs. 4, 5). It is advisable before aspirating through the biopsy–suction channel that an available brush be advanced through the biopsy channel to remove debris from the wall of the channel; then the already pushed through dirty brush should be cleaned before it is withdrawn. Fluid is then aspirated until clean water enters the suction container. After the biopsy-suction channel is properly cleaned by suction, or the water channel by rinsing, the same two channels are dried by simply aspirating air or pushing it through the water channel and cleaning the cover glass with a wet Q-tip (Fig. 6).

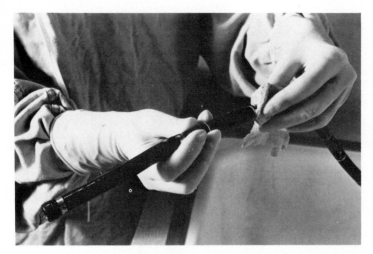

FIG. 3. Flexible fiberscope, for upper and lower gastrointestinal tract. After the procedure is completed and a biopsy is taken or polypectomy performed, the first step is to strain the content of the (suction) bottle to preserve aspirated tissue samples for histologic study. Small polyps are easily aspirated through a large biopsy channel. After the bottle is emptied it is replaced and the outside sheath cleaned using a wet (4 × 4) gauze soaked in water or Betadine solution.

Drying

After rinsing the outside or inside of an instrument and accessories, the wet areas are dried. This step is complicated in rigid instruments because of the larger number of accessories and the small channels. If these instruments are not properly rinsed or dried, a crust of unremoved debris or blood clot forms. We found the same type of pistol mentioned before very useful; connecting it to the compressed air outlet on the wall with the various attachments enabled us to dry the outsides and insides of the various instruments in a very short period of time much more efficiently than with any other drying technique available (Fig. 7). Every small hole and channel is accessible, and the job is performed rapidly and better (Figs. 8, 9). If central compressed air is used it sometimes produces too much condensed water; therefore an inexpensive filter (Figs. 3 and 4) is interposed by the hospital plumber that provides dry air. There are many hospitals where compressed air is not available, especially in the endoscopy room. A very reasonable solution is to order a compressed air cylinder that can

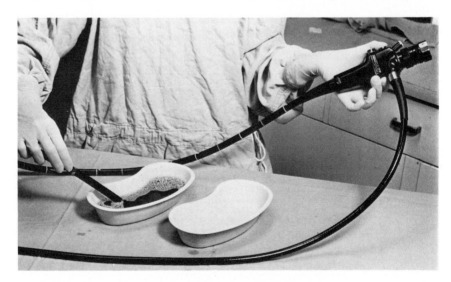

FIG. 4. Fiberscope. If the outer skin is clean, continued suction is applied using first Betadine solution and later clean water. In "dirty" cases (e.g., the colon) it is advisable to advance a brush through the biopsy channel to remove hard debris. After sufficient suction has been applied and clean water appears in the collection bottle, air is aspirated through the suction channel to dry it or to remove fluid particles.

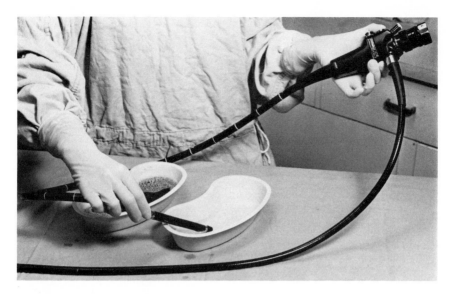

FIG. 5. After the suction channel is completed, the water-air channel is next cleaned by immersing the tip and aspirating water from a container and then air.

be kept in the corner of the room with a reduction valve and to which the cleaning pistol can be attached. One cylinder lasts for several months, and the cost of a new one is very little. This is a very important aspect of the cleaning procedure as it saves the nurse a tremendous amount of time and improves the quality of the work.

The cleaning and checking of the image-transmitting and illumination parts must be emphasized (Figs. 10–13). The objectives are protected with a cover glass and can be rinsed with the pistol (Fig. 10) or a wet Q-tip (Fig. 6). Drying the objective with compressed air is safe. The strength of the compressed air can be adjusted on the second stage of the reduction valve or directly on the pistol itself. It does not have to be very strong, and the nurse can check it with ease. The best drying technique for an objective cover glass or illumination (fiber) outlet after proper rinsing or cleaning is air. Any small water drops that are left do not evaporate properly if left to dry themselves and so show up later in the form of a gray spot. For specific cleaning aspects, see Figures 14–18.

Appropriate Time for Cleaning

The best time to clean the instrument is immediately after the procedure. It must not be stored in a dirty condition. Although it is more lucrative to book one case immediately after another, it does not allow the time needed for appropriately cleaning the instruments. It is much more difficult to clean endoscopes after they have been left for several hours, than immediately after a procedure. If several endoscopic procedures are performed on the same floor, they can be done by the same personnel after the main schedule for the day is completed, but arrangements must be made concerning which parts of the dirty instruments can be stored and which should be rinsed immediately.

The entire endoscopy organization must be tailored to the turnover of the individual department. It also must be understood that a properly functioning endoscopy unit requires appropriately cleaned equipment, which is an impossible goal without adequate space, proper facilities, and allotted time. We spend tremendous amounts of money on the capital outlay and so should not omit from our priority list those items and factors which are of equal importance to the proper operation of this expensive equipment.

INSTRUMENT STORAGE

Whenever a new rigid or flexible instrument is received, the enclosed packaging (shipping) document is checked to verify that it meets the specifications on the order. The serial number

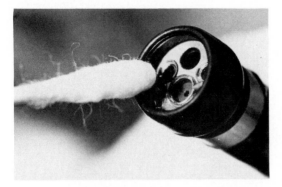

FIG. 6. Fiberscope. After cleaning the outer sheath and aspirating the channels, the working end (which was previously immersed in clean water) is now cleaned separately with a wet and dry Q-Tips. Special attention is paid to the objective lens and the illumination outlet. The cleanliness of the image and light-transmitting section are checked by looking through the eyepiece, observing the clean, sharp structure of the fiber bundle with its round, sharp, black dots (broken fibers). The eyepiece sometimes contains fingerprints, so the cover glass of the ocular should be similarly cleaned before placing it in the storage cabinet. The operating function of the tip's movement should also be tested. It is advisable that the trumpet valve of this type of scope (Olympus) be lubricated. The upper valve at the inlet of the biopsy channel can be removed and cleaned occasionally (twice weekly).

(on flexible scopes) or the type number is noted immediately in the inventory. The serial number is a good mark for future reference should the instrument ever need to be repaired. The next step is to check the instrument functions before storing it. The image bundle is observed for optics and for broken fibers in flexible scopes (Fig. 19). To check the light transmission of the illuminating fiber bundle, the end that is inserted into the light source is held up to a dim light (or daylight), and the working end of the incoherent light optic bundle observed (Fig. 20). The number of broken fibers can be easily seen as a dark, round dot(s). At this stage there are no standards as to how many broken fibers (percent) are acceptable, but if there are more than expected the physician in charge of the endoscopy unit is consulted.

All the functions of the instrument are now simulated. In flexible fiberscopes the various movements of the tip, as well as the suction, water, and air channels are tested. The maximum movements of the instrument are described (in degrees) in the specifications pro-

vided by the manufacturer; this provides a base line against which to test the instrument.

If the instrument is unfamiliar, it *must not be tested* before the instruction manual is read carefully (or if this is not available the representative of the company is called in to demonstrate the function and care of these delicate and expensive instruments). It is advantageous to arrange systematic visits from the salesmen of the various endoscopic companies to discuss any questions that might arise. Communication with companies, including early feedback of problems, are important factors in helping the manufacturer to over-

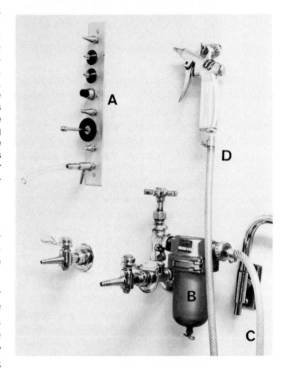

FIG. 7. The same type of pistol used for water rinsing is employed for drying with compressed air, the screw under the trigger adjusting the air pressure. Small channels, holes with difficult configurations, cannot be dried using conventional techniques. It is of utmost importance that small channels or delicate mechanisms be appropriately rinsed and dried before they are (gas) autoclaved, soaked, or reused. **A.** Series of nozzles that can be attached to the pistol to fit various holes, etc. **B.** In case of centrally supplied compressed air, a water filter should be inserted into the compressed air line. **C.** Flexible hose. **D.** Pistol with convenient grip. If central compressed air is not installed, a commercially available compressed air cylinder with a reduction valve will last for months and can be replaced inexpensively. The hose is easily connected to the outlet of the cylinder.

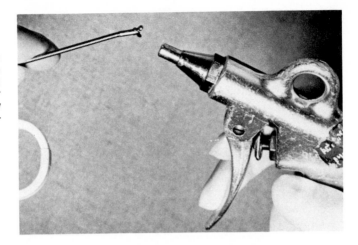

FIG. 8. The biopsy forceps (flexible) can easily be put out of service if the delicate jaw is not rinsed and cleaned properly. The moving jaws and their mechanism must be dried completely with compressed air, an easy procedure.

come shortcomings in instrument design or function.

Storage

The instrument should be stored in a safe manner, with easy access, good visibility, and under lock and key. An identification tag is attached to flexible scopes and on the trays of rigid scopes.

Flexible Fiberscopes. The flexible scope can be kept in its carrying case after cleaning, but if it is used at a single location it is more convenient to store it in a separate (locked) area (Fig. 21). The storage of accessories (biopsy forceps, polypectomy snares, etc.) can be kept beside the corresponding instru-

ment. This allows fast handling and avoids wasting time to find out, for example, which biopsy forceps belong to which scope. If there are instruments other than the scope in the storage area, they can all be color-coded for easier recognition.

Rigid Endoscopes. We found that separate storage and sterilizing trays are a burden to the nurse, who must remove the instruments from one tray and place them in another. We devised trays (aluminum) with holes on the bottom in which plastic holders are fixed to keep the individual instrument and its parts or accessories in position. The tray has spacers to hold a perforated plastic lid. The same tray is used for holding and sterilizing. All trays are grouped according to the proce-

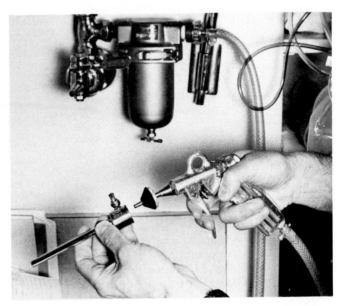

FIG. 9. Drying a wet laparoscopy trocar sleeve. This attached Luer nozzle with rubber protection can be easily and well fitted to the female outlet on the trocar stopcock in order to flush this area. The wall outlets of compressed air used in some hospitals generally contain water and have an inexpensive filter in the line attached to the wall (easily inserted by the hospital engineer); this can be drained bimonthly (at top). If separate compressed air cylinders are used, water condensation is less common.

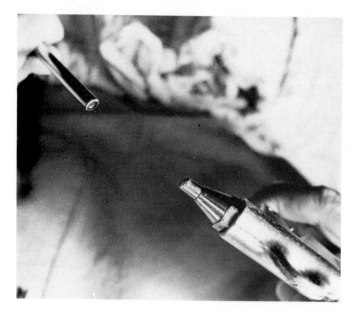

FIG. 10. Rigid telescope. After a short period of soaking and rinsing the outside is totally cleaned with a soft, wet cloth, and then the objective is dried; drying is critical. It is very easy to scratch the cover glass. If compressed air is unavailable, a soft, wet tissue may be used followed by drying with a soft material. However, compressed air is by far the best and safest method of drying lenses.

dure, e.g., adult cysto- resecto-, laparoscopy sets. After cleaning, the sets are wrapped and placed in the gas autoclave. This type of storage system (Fig. 22) allows easy orientation because each instrument or part has its own place. When sets consist of 10 to 20 parts it is difficult to determine immediately what instrument or part has gone astray, especially if there is a busy schedule. In our system the empty place immediately indicates the missing part.

The telescopes need special attention. The tip can be damaged, even with plastic holders, if it is loose in the tray. A loosely fitting rubber tip with open ends or a plastic tube placed loosely above the end of the telescope protects it from unwarranted damage. The telescope is kept in the sterile tray on the instrument table and after use is not mixed with heavy metal instruments. It is always replaced in its own area of the tray (Fig. 23).

We found that using a separate tray for storing each rigid endoscope is very efficient and protects against damage during handling. If there are several sets for the same procedure, color-coding with autoclavable tapes (each instrument, accessories, and tray) expedites handling the sets by the nurses. Spare parts are stored with the full sets (Fig. 24).

The rigid endoscopes are soaked or gas-sterilized, and so the compartmentalized tray (one per endoscope set) proved to be the method of choice.

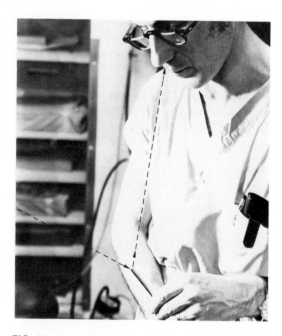

FIG. 11. If a dirty spot is discovered, the telescope is grasped and held at an angle toward room light. If in the reflected light the flat cover glass can be observed at a certain angle, the areas that are damaged or not appropriately cleaned can be seen immediately.

There are other ways and means to store these delicate and expensive items, and methods can be tailored to the local circumstances. Whatever procedure is chosen, however, it must be borne in mind that appropriate storage

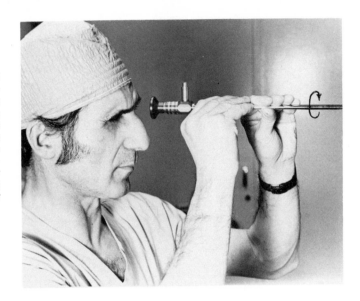

FIG. 12. After cleaning and drying, the telescope is examined against room light; it is rotated during inspection because even a small dirty area or a localized optical transmission problem can be recognized in this manner. (The spots can be seen to move with the rotation of the telescope.) If it is "foggy," check cleanness of objective (working end) or eyepiece (ocular); if the image is "cut" like a half-moon shape, look for a dent on the telescope sheath.

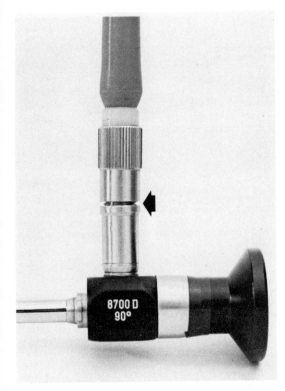

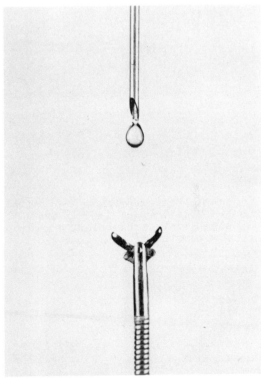

FIG. 13. If the rigid telescope is assembled or connected to the fiber cord, the thread or clip connection must be properly attached lest light be lost. If the telescope is disconnected, the fiber ends or surfaces in the telescope and the fiber surface of the fiber cord are cleaned with a wet Q-tip and dried with compressed air.

FIG. 14. After rinsing and cleaning the jaws and outside, and drying with compressed air, the jaws are lubricated separately, opening and closing them during lubrication. The outside is also lubricated. The operation (jaw movement) is always checked and the outside lubricated before insertion into the biopsy channel. Oil is dropped into the open jaws.

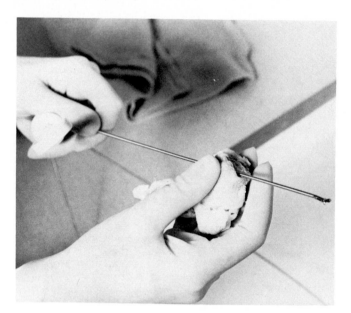

FIG. 15. Fiberscope biopsy forceps. This is cleaned first externally with a wet gauze soaked with Betadine solution or soapy water. Special attention is paid to the working end of the jaws, where debris, secretion, blood clots, or feces can be hidden; it is rinsed with the water pistol (Fig. 1). It is advisable to put a few drops of mineral oil in the jaws.

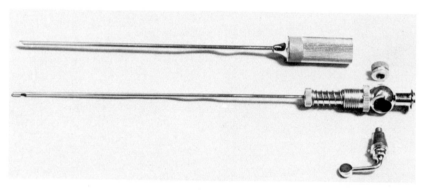

FIG. 16. Disassembled laparoscopy pneumoperitoneum needle. Top, Outside of needle. Bottom, Blunt stylet with side hole. Stopcock is removed. If the various small areas are not properly handled or cleaned (of the usual blood clots) and not dried, they start to stick within a short period of time.

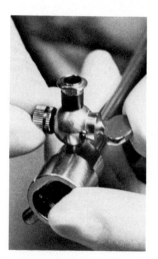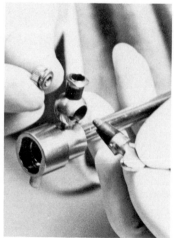

FIG. 17. Left, Disassembling a stopcock should always be done over a bench space on which a towel is placed first in case some of the small screws are dropped. A stopcock must be removed and disassembled (right) after each use. The cone-shaped part, as well as the female part, should be cleaned, dried, and relubricated after each use. The stopcock does not operate properly if it is not maintained systematically and cleaned after each use.

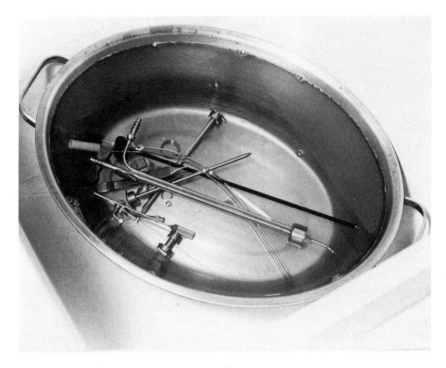

FIG. 18. A laparoscopy set should never be thrown in the soaking pan after use, as is shown here. The uterine suction cannula should be rinsed first—separately because it is always heavily contaminated with vaginal mucus and blood—before placing it with other instruments. The individual instruments should be disassembled and placed in a pan beside each other.

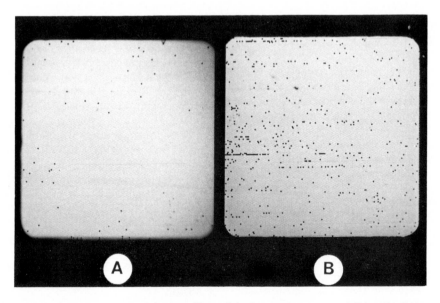

FIG. 19. The small number of broken fibers (black spots) are very visible (**A**). If they are excessive (**B**) in a new instrument the bundle should be rejected since broken fibers do not transmit an image. With a used instrument, keeping a log helps to determine the deterioration of the bundle after a certain number of procedures.

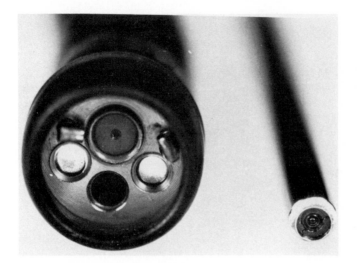

FIG. 20. The (incoherent) fiber end of the bundle (which should be inserted into the light unit) is held up to a dim light (e.g., x-ray viewer) and the other (working) end of the light transmitting bundle observed. Left, Flexible scope. Right, Rigid scope.

and handling extend the lifetime of these costly instruments and makes life easier for both the nurses and doctors by averting those well known episodes wherein there is a search for missing parts after the instrument is already inserted in the patient. Certainly, any group who has spent several thousand dollars for a set of instruments must be willing to set aside $100 to $150 more per set to avoid the frustration of increased repair costs by providing safe handling and proper storage.

MAINTENANCE AND SUPERVISION

All parts, instruments, and functions should be checked. The rigid endoscopes should be checked: (1) before they are inserted into the tray for sterilizing; (2) after the instruments are removed (sterile) from the sterilizing tray by the scrub nurse and before being handed over to the doctor (parts and function); and (3) immediately after use to discover any damage or malfunction. Flexible fiberscopes should be checked: (1) immediately before use; and (2) after cleaning but before being stored.

Records

The following records are of great help in evaluating care and lifetime of instruments.

Repair Log.   To assess the running cost and the depreciation of instruments, it is recommended that a log be kept in which the specific breakdown of each instrument is inserted. The date of sending and return from repair and its cost should be noted, and for fiber endoscopes the serial number should be included. It is also worthwhile to mention whether the returned instrument functioned as expected or had to be repaired again.

The existence and upkeep of a repair log gives information concerning how the medical and nursing personnel are handling the equipment. Certain types of repairs (damages) are characteristic of the staff's lack of knowledge on handling and maintaining the scope. These aspects can be overcome by in-house education in the form of seminars, etc. On the other hand, if the instrument design is inadequate for the purpose, it is demonstrated by the same repeated malfunction requiring service calls. The "lifetime" or depreciation of an instrument can also be calculated from the log's entries.

Endoscopy Log.   The endoscopy log is another important document that should contain the following data: the entry number, date, patient's name and hospital number, the procedure performed, if a biopsy is included, name of the operator and assistant(s), and any appropriate remarks. Flexible fiberscope examinations can be given a separate consecutive number in the "remarks" column—e.g., colon (23),* colon (24), ERCP (88)—which can be transferred to the repair log. In this way it can be determined that, for instance, a particular endoscope failed after a certain number of procedures.

Consecutive case number of this particular procedure.

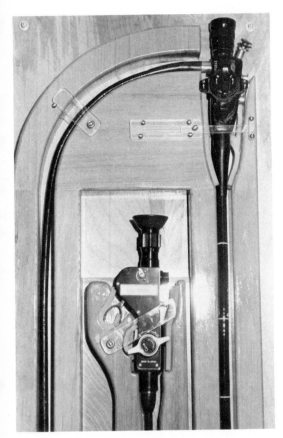

FIG. 21. There are many ways to store flexible scopes. We use a fixed, wooden storage space mounted on the wall. Several instruments can be kept beside each other, and there is easy access and good visibility. The storage area should be locked. (Courtesy of the Department of Gastroenterology, UCLA.)

importance for rigid endoscopy procedures, where telescopes and certain other parts are extremely delicate (e.g., in pediatric instruments).

Improved nursing education is tremendously helpful when we know what should be done. The majority of endoscopists are aware of the extremely gentle care and handling of equipment, but in teaching institutions the yearly turnover of residents, interns, and trainee nurses requires that appropriate instructions be given periodically. It is up to the individual medical or surgical department heads and the nursing department to make it clear to the fellows, trainees, and nurses that because they are knowledgeable about the diagnostic or treatment aspects does not necessarily mean that they are specialists in handling new equipment—especially if they have a minimum of experience. When the principles of proper communication and mutual respect between well-trained endoscopy nurses and doctors is appreciated and followed through, it decreases the problems in maintenance and early replacement of instruments.

The endoscopy log can be useful for collecting medical data for the departments in establishing a cross index based on this book. Reports issued from time to time can be useful in indicating the type of procedure, frequency, and other figures which reflect the operation of the unit. The same report can carry (e.g., on a monthly basis) the cost-effectiveness and balance indicating the economical aspect of this unit.

Flexible Fiber Endoscopes

We check the image-carrying bundle after each repair (or after 50 or 100 procedures) by photographing a simple test pattern (black and white) with the scope. With the dates and data from the endoscopy log we know exactly the rate of deterioration of the image bundle and the rate of other repair problems according to the number of patients examined with the scope.

The questions which then arise are: What is the cause? Is it due to lack of appropriate handling or maintenance, or is it the manufacturer's fault? The cause can be traced only if the data are available for analysis. Although we are anxious to avoid additional administrative burden, the endoscopy and repair logs are essential for evaluating the effectiveness of instruments, repair, and nursing service.

This record-keeping system is of importance first in cases of flexible fiberscopes where the fragility, lack of durability, and variety of deficiencies or damages manifest more frequently. The steadily rising repair cost (which is not negligible) can sometimes be lessened by knowing exactly what the problems are and how they should be overcome. It is also of

The image bundle should be checked after cleaning—before it is stored and before actual use. If the image is "foggy" it must be ascertained that the objective lens is not dirty and that the eyepiece is clear. The ocular is adjusted to maximum sharpness (to see the individual fiber structure and broken fibers as

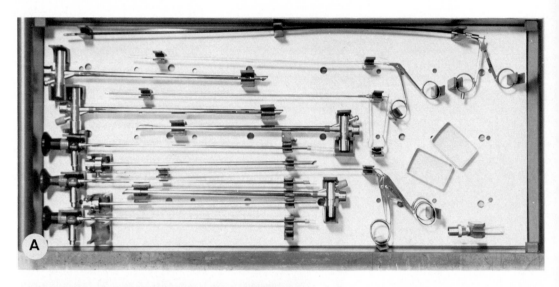

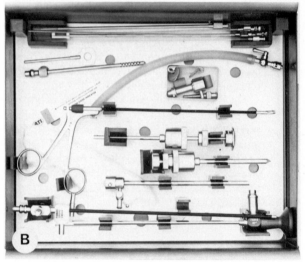

FIG. 22. A. Holding (aluminum) tray for adult instruments. Small plastic blocks are milled to the shape of the holding telescope, the instruments, or its parts to keep them in position. The tip of the telescope is also protected with a loose rubber tube (removed). The bottom and the lid are perforated. The same tray is used for holding and for (gas) sterilization. Between cases the instruments are soaked and cleaned and then replaced in their individual spots in the tray. When there are many accessories this system provides the nurse with a quick reference for what is missing, as well as protecting the valuable instruments from damage. If several sets are available for the same procedure (e.g., cysto- or laparoscopy) each part and the tray are color-coded with autoclavable tape. **B.** Same system as shown for adult instruments, but this time a smaller tray was made for holding smaller (miniature) or pediatric sets.

clear, sharp, black dots). With reflected light at the working end we can easily discover dirt or cracks on the cover glass (Fig. 25). If a small crack is visible an inexpensive magnifier is used to inspect the cover glass (image- and light-carrying bundles). At the same time the position of the small water and air nozzles are checked for damage. In the case of a mechanical (trumpet or other type) valve the air-water and suction operations are checked after the procedure is completed and the apparatus cleaned before use in a patient. Small, wet Q-tips are used for cleaning the cover glass. Other types of valves (electromagnetic) are checked in a similar manner. If plastic tube connections from the "umbilical cord" (com-

bined cord of the fiberscope incorporating light, suction, and water) are loosened, they are replaced before use, not taking a chance of their becoming disconnected in the patient.

The outer skin of the working end of the fiberscope is lubricated, making certain that the jelly is not smeared into the actual viewing-illuminating end of the scope, obscuring vision and light or plugging water-air channels; only the outside of the cover (black plastic) sheath is lubricated. The continuity or the intact outside of this cover sheath is checked. The moving distal (working) end of the scope is covered with a thin, black, rubber sheath that is especially vulnerable. A small hole here can cause water to enter the most

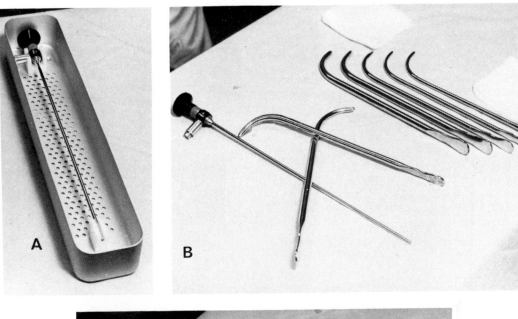

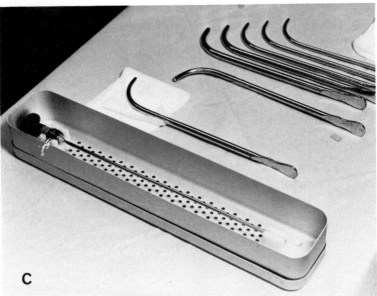

FIG. 23. A. An alternative approach for keeping the telescope separately is a small autoclavable holder (lid removed) even on the sterile instrument table. Instead of placing it back among other instruments after use, it is put in the protective holder, thereby ensuring that this telescope "survives" longer. **B.** Urologic procedures are notorious for damaging expensive telescopes. It is easy to make a dent on these sheaths with other metal instruments. **C.** With minimal effort the optics can be replaced into a separate protective holder, which is also sterilized with the telescope and perforated lid.

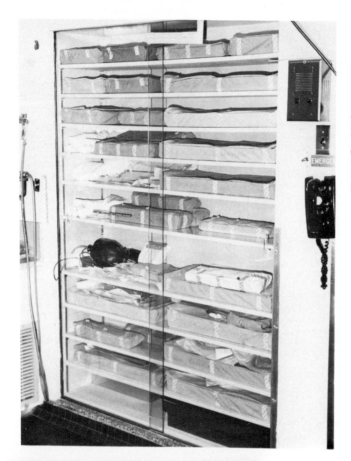

FIG. 24. Presterilized and marked trays (set of instruments per procedure). Spare parts to replace those that are sometimes dropped or damaged during procedures are sterilized separately and kept in a glass cabinet. This layout makes the instruments easy to find, and it is also easy to determine what if anything (e.g., a tray) is missing. The cabinet should always be strictly kept under lock and key.

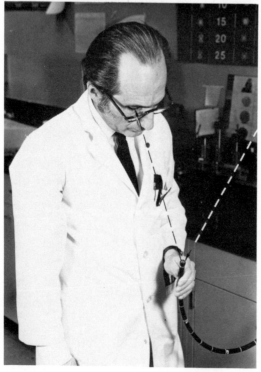

FIG. 25. The working end of the scope is held toward the ceiling light and tilted at a certain angle, which is a means of detecting minute cracks or dirt dried on the cover glass of the objective (which should be a shiny, smooth surface). An inexpensive magnifier is handy for inspecting it further if some changes are discovered.

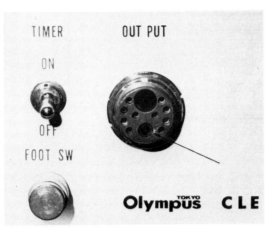

FIG. 26. Female plug of the Olympus light unit. The lower hole (arrow) holds a plastic tube to improve the seal during connection with the male part of the scope (water-air). Force is avoided during insertion as the plastic or rubber tube can be easily damaged and the water-air tight connection disrupted. The tightening outer ring on the male (umbilical cord) part should be fixed to secure the connection. It should also be noted if the light-transmitting bundle, which is inserted here, is chipped, damaged, or contains too many broken fibers.

delicate compartment, resulting in condensation between the cover glass and the objective lens. After a number of examinations this part becomes "floppy" and soft, and it should be replaced before a major repair is required.

The major movements or controls of the tip are checked, making sure that the "breaks" of the tip movements are open. Breakage of some wires interfere with certain (plane) movements.

Light Unit

Before starting the examination the light source, light output, and air pump-suction (vacuum) connection are checked. The Olympus female plug in the light unit has a plastic tube that provides a seal for the male part in the umbilical cord (Fig. 26). This connection provides transport for air and water. Because of continuous movements (connections-disconnections) this part is notorious for being damaged. With other types of light units, the unit is not switched on if the patient is already on the table; it must be done beforehand. The globe is checked weekly. If the globe becomes "charred" or blackish it is exchanged, not waiting until it burns out during an examination.

Spare globes are always kept with the units. Some light units employ fuses; with these, spare fuses are kept in the vicinity of the spare globes in a box marked with the name or type of unit it is to be used with.

Some light units have a built-in spare globe that can be switched on with ease during the examination if the other burns out. In this situation the expired globe is exchanged after the procedure. If there are faulty wires or plugs, the hospital electrician is called immediately. Some light units have a limited life span (e.g., ACMI 1000 with GE Marc 300 globe = 25 hours). In such cases the unit is exchanged prior to expiration of its lifetime. Although it can function longer, the results (output) will deteriorate. It must be ascertained that any newly purchased light unit is built according to an accepted safety code.

Accessories for Flexible Scopes

The items most frequently damaged or exchanged are accessories to the flexible scopes. Many anxious moments can be avoided if the biopsy forceps are checked ahead of time to determine that they open properly. These instruments are far from ideal because of their small size and the force that is applied. The jaw movements are checked in a bent position after careful cleaning. A few drops of mineral oil are placed in the jaws (Fig. 14) and allowed to run into the inside of the spiral cover. After the outside of the spiral is cleaned and dried, it is lubricated with oil. The forceps is stored without stress, hanging down (Fig. 27). Before use the action and power of the jaws are checked again, and the jaws are lubricated outside with mineral oil (or whatever lubricant the hospital provides) just prior to starting the procedure. *A procedure is never started without having one spare functioning biopsy forceps or other spare accessories on standby.* It is unfair to the patient to jeopardize a difficult, sometimes risky (and costly) procedure because the only available biopsy forceps may break, requiring that the examination be repeated at another time.

Polypectomy Snare

There are various types of polypectomy snare available (see Chap. 6). The snare must be dismantled, cleaned, and reassembled after each use. With repeated opening and closing the maximal opening may be visualized; this

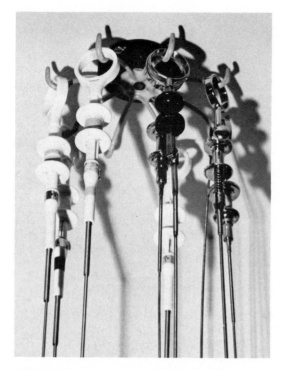

FIG. 27. Forceps are stored without stress or sharp bending. We found the hanging system satisfactory. If there are different types they may be kept supported beside the scope or color-coded with autoclavable tape.

can be decreased after repeated use by heating. If it is bent or overheated, however, it does not form the same large required loop and should therefore be replaced. The major malfunctions are at the electrical contact points. A small piece of meat placed on the patient's plate, with a low coagulation current, can be used to determine if the electric circuit is complete and functioning well; the sparks can be observed. If the snare just touches the patient's plate without the piece of meat (resistance) and the output of the electrosurgical unit is not low, the tip of the loop burns (melts). The snare should be checked after each cleaning, both mechanically (opening, closing, and spring action) and electrically. Polypectomy is never begun without making sure that all these aspects are in good operating condition and that minimally one or two spare snares are ready for use.

Miniature Brush

A brush on a flexible (spiral) stem is available for thorough cleaning of the biopsy channels of large flexible scopes. This is a useful instrument for removing blood clots or (feces) debris from the biopsy channel, even during the procedure if required. It is also useful for cleaning the biopsy channel systematically during the routine cleaning, followed by aspirating fluid through the channel. The brush helps to remove small debris.

Suction Unit

In general variable vacuum must be available, its use depending on the procedure length and the diameter of the instrument's suction channel. The maximum vacuum required is 700 mm Hg. If wall (central) suction is employed it must be ensured that during the peak time (8 to 12 AM) the suction does not decrease significantly. Moreover, with central suction outlets it also must be ascertained that the connections are tight lest vacuum is lost. The most handy system for the nurse is to have a separate (small pump) suction with a collection bottle and a small air pump built together so that there are few if any tubes on the floor (which can disturb traffic in the endoscopy room). If the collection bottle is emptied, important tissue samples for histologic examination must not be thrown down the drain. In those cases where biopsy and suction are applied, it is advisable to strain the collected material. The suction unit is checked daily according to the instruction manual.

Electrosurgical Unit

The electrosurgical unit is described in Chapter 16. It is recommended that the same type of units be used in a given hospital in order to facilitate interchangeability and maintenance. The patient's plate position should be carefully checked to obtain maximum surface contact. In our applications (e.g., polypectomy) patients are positioned on their side. Inadequate contact can result in skin burns or inadequate performance. The hospital should arrange systematic monthly service with a company or biomedical engineering department. These units must be kept under constant control. For polypectomy (colon or stomach) only pure coagulation current should be used. The proper position of the "mixing" (blend) switch is monitored. It is handy to have these units wall-mounted in the endoscopy and cystoscopy rooms. The space in these rooms is usually restricted, and so any unnecessary floor-occupying equipment is eliminated.

The electric cables can be broken or damaged anytime. Again, monthly control by a serviceman is important. The bipolar system is introduced during laparoscopy. This "new-old" idea requires that nursing and medical personnel be retrained. The majority of modern solid state electrosurgical equipment works with both modes. Electrosurgery is one of the most important instruments in cystoscopy rooms; therefore a daily check of proper equipment function by the nurse or nurse-technician is mandatory. The patient's plate, the cable condition, the condition of the resectosnares, and contact in the working element are items of possible electrical faults, which in the majority of cases can be overcome if the personnel is well trained and aware of potential problems. A procedure is never started when electrosurgery is involved without having on hand a standby spare patient's plate, or (autoclaved) active electrodes with connectors. The external wiring system can be broken or disrupted at any time, so spares should be available. Electrosurgical units should be built according to the hospital safety code and tested by laboratories earmarked for this job. Nursing education departments should make a special effort in their training program to include a minimum requirement for trainees to ascertain that the personnel in the operating room know how to handle electrosurgical equipment.

Rigid Endoscopes

As mentioned in the storage section, rigid endoscopes (including accessories) are kept in trays labeled according to the procedure for which they are used.

Fiberoptic Cables

Despite their flexibility fiberoptic cables are vulnerable to a short turning radius. If this precaution is not kept in mind the operator will notice an increased number of black dots (broken fibers). The best precaution is to keep the cables together in a slightly curved fashion in the tray. If kept separately, they should not be wrapped loosely in only a towel because the weight of other instruments in the autoclave can damage them (Fig. 28). If they have to be

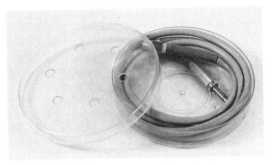

FIG. 28. If the fiberoptic light cables are stored separately—it is advisable to have a few presterilized—they are kept in a proper container. Here an inexpensive, round plastic container with holes is used. A short radius or too much curving can damage the bundle.

soaked (as during consecutive urologic cases) a narrow soaking pan should not be used as it would require jamming the cable to make it fit.

Both ends are wiped dry after rinsing—a wet end must not be inserted into the hot light source. The light transmission is checked by observing the ends on a weekly basis. A bundle is never disconnected from the light source by

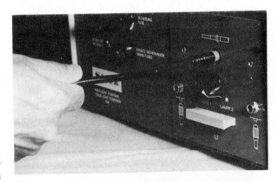

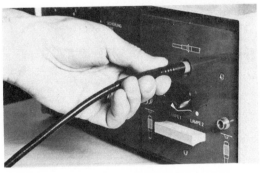

FIG. 29. The cable must not be removed from the light unit by pulling on the cable (top); the strain must be placed only on the solid part (bottom).

holding onto the cable (Fig. 29); the metal or plastic strain-relief part is held. Sometimes the epoxy cement at the end (toward the light unit) melts and darkens. When this occurs it is returned to the manufacturer for repair; it can be polished and reused.

Telescopes

The telescope is checked very carefully for optical image transmission quality before being sterilized and again immediately before use. After return from the operating room it is rinsed very carefully and wiped with a soft cloth (only). The objective (working end) should be dried with compressed air only, if possible. If not available, a soft, wet tissue is used first and then it is dried. The telescope is rotated slowly around the optical (eye axis) while looking through it against room illumination (Fig. 12). This maneuver reveals small (dirt) spots on the objective. The objective is inspected at an angle to reflected light (Fig. 25) or using an inexpensive magnifier. If dirt (dried secretion or blood) is on the cover glass it can be removed carefully with wet and dry soft cloths. The light inlet of the illuminating fibers is noted and cleaned with a Q-tip. The cover glass of the eyepiece, which very often has fingerprints on it, is inspected and cleaned.

Optics. If, when looking through the telescope toward a room light, the picture looks hazy, the following should be checked: (1) Is the objective (working end) clear? (2) Is the ocular (eyepiece) clear? (3) Does the telescope sheath have a dent on the outside? This can be seen or felt by palpating the sheath. Sometimes the image is clear but cut like a half- or quarter-moon. If there are doubts about the optical performance and two identical telescopes are available, the one in question can be compared with the other.

If a telescope is sent to be repaired accurate notes must be made. Dispatch and return dates, reason of damage, repair cost, etc. should be noted in the repair log. The telescope should never be kept loose or put into the autoclave in a cellophane cover with only a cardboard support. A telescope is very expensive and should be handled with extreme care. We keep them on the holding-sterilizing trays. There are also small, separate perforated metal trays with lids available in which the telescope can be kept sterilized and put on the instrument table. The telescope is never put with heavy hardware on the table but is replaced in the tray or telescope holder.

Telescopes have an extremely thin outer metal cover, and their repair is time-consuming and costly. With minimal understanding and careful handling, the life of these telescopes can be extended. For instance, when they are grasped and transferred from the soaking fluid (sterilization) to the sterile table,

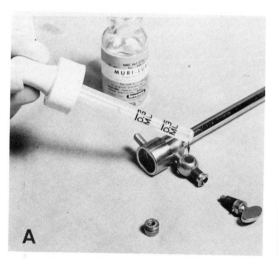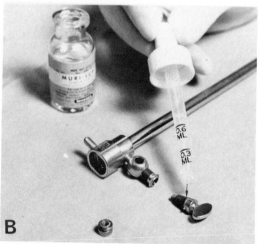

FIG. 30. If instruments have not been used for while, they should be dismantled, so that the female (**A**) and the male (**B**) stopcock parts can be cleaned thoroughly. A drop of lubricating oil should be put on the (male) thread of the stopcock-holder screw to make its movements smoother.

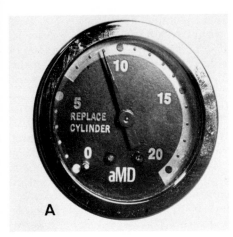

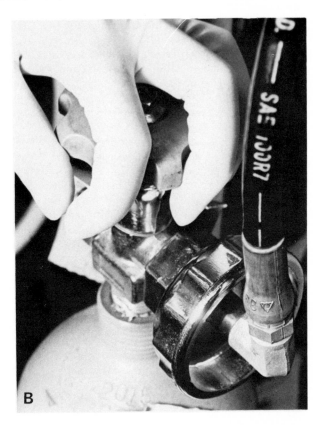

FIG. 31. Gas-cylinder replacement in laparoscopy. **A.** Every type of insufflator has a built-in cylinder pressure gauge. When the handle indicates that the cylinder is nearly empty of gas, a replacement should be made. **B.** The cylinders are filled under high pressure. The valve on the cylinder should be closed tightly before the connecting hose is released.

conventional metal instrument holders are not used. Inexpensive telescope holder forceps with serrated rubber inlets (similar to a surgical swab holder but with rubber inlets) are available that provide safer handling of these instruments.

Accessories

There are hundreds of small gadgets, bridges, gaskets, washers, etc. used during endoscopy, and a systematic approach is needed for their storage and maintenance in order to find the item in time and to make sure that it is still in working order. A few examples for proper maintenance and supervision are shown in Figures 30–32. A time should be set aside on a daily, weekly, or monthly basis according to the need of the individual instrument when someone is responsible for systematically checking the performance, appearance, lubrication, etc. of each item. Appropriate maintenance and prevention is much less expensive than the time spent on administrative paper work to fill out repair or purchase orders to

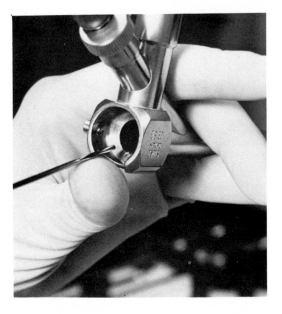

FIG. 32. Small fiber light carriers must be carefully removed and cleaned and slowly and accurately replaced. They are used in rigid bronchoscopes, esophagoscopes, etc. If not handled with care, they can break with ease.

replace expensive items. This principle must be accepted by supervisors and collaborating doctors. There is no more aggravating aspect in endoscopy than discovering, after the examination has began, that the optic is dirty, the biopsy forceps do not open, the light bulb in the unit is burned out and no one knows where the spares are, etc.

A small set of tools to release a screw, open a valve, etc. is kept nearby. Long wires of various gauges (for surgical skin closure) are helpful in cleaning or unplugging channels. The nearest endoscope repair serviceman should be familiar to the endoscopy team. With experience, the endoscopy technicians come to know which parts become damaged most frequently and so keep spares for these items in stock.

Before a new nurse starts her/his duty, she/he should be aware of the schedule, instruments, maintenance plan, and the doctors' working habits. This work requires devotion and endless care in order to be able to account for and keep in good operating condition the expensive (optical), small, innumerable accessories.

The well-trained endoscopy nurse or technician is an important team member. Without her/his close collaboration the procedure cannot be completed properly or on time. The time spent on teaching such personnel to understand the need and necessity of good maintenance and supervision is worthwhile. It is also rewarding to be a member of a team providing excellent patient care.

8

Microbiology and Sterilization of Endoscopes

Irving J. Slotnick

The problems of infection and its control confronting the endoscopist and the entire medical profession today are as great as ever before, and in some respects even greater than during the preantibiotic era.[24] They relate to the changing incidence and patterns of infection in the hospital community; the dilemma of drug-resistant strains of microorganisms, with the relatively recent recognition of infectious drug-resistance transfer (i.e., resistance not to merely a single drug but to multiple agents arising by genetic exchange);[4] the current nature of infection and disease in hospitalized patients;[3,7,24] the specter of contamination of blood and blood components with viruses of hepatitis and cytomegalic inclusion disease; the disruption of homestatic mechanisms by antibiosis leading to changes in microbial flora and superinfection; and the use and continued development of surgical equipment that cannot be heat-sterilized.

Although the impact of infection falls heavily on the surgical units, these personnel should in no way consider themselves unique in the hospital milieu, as the entire staff and all hospital personnel face similar interdigitated and complex infectious disease challenges. Because of the multiple, linked factors that account for surgery-associated and intramural cross-infection, it is requisite that today's and tomorrow's surgeon be familiar with all aspects and causes of infection. In this respect the surgeon at every operation must also act as a practicing microbiologist and epidemiologist.

Endoscopy is confronted with two facets of infection of special interest. First is the current use of skillfully designed, rigid and fiberoptic endoscopes that cannot be autoclaved or heat-sterilized without damage, and which also must be protected from certain kinds of chemical trauma. Conventional methods of cold sterilization[41,43] may have to be altered or new systems discovered to sterilize this type of instrument effectively, not only to protect the patient from virulent organisms but to keep the endoscopist and assisting personnel from being infected as well. Second is the threat of attendant bacteremia and sepsis following instrumental manipulation of tissues that contain a microbial flora.[37] Bacteremia occurs not uncommonly following oral surgery, dental extraction, and gum manipulations, tonsillectomy, bronchoscopy, sigmoidoscopy, instrumentation of the genitourinary tract,[21] and surgery on the lower intestinal tract.[23]

Although a preliminary study of blood cultures on 40 patients following endoscopy of the esophagus and stomach yielded no growth, a larger series of this kind and one that includes mycoplasma, L-forms, and viruses is needed to shed more light on this matter.[34] The entire issue of the nature and occurrence of oncogenic viruses in man awaits resolution, but if we extrapolate from documented situations of animal oncogenic viruses of aerosol transmission, excretion in urine and feces, and the detection of antibodies of laboratory staff, the laboratory ecology of at least some oncogenic viruses is the same as that of other types of infective agent.[19] If viral oncogenesis ultimately should be the case in man, it is evident that the endoscope could be one of the critical factors in the epidemiology of such an infectious process.

INCIDENCE AND PATTERNS OF HOSPITAL INFECTIONS

The exact incidence and frequency of postoperative as well as overall hospital infections is still not precisely determined. Lack of defined criteria for differentiation of operative from preoperative infection coupled with the well known reluctance by the surgeon to document these scrupulously invalidates many published reports or makes them impossible to interpret. However, the introduction of the infection prevalence survey in 1964 for the evaluation of hospital-acquired infection and the establishment of the National Nosocomial Infections Study (NNIS) as a nationwide cooperative hospital surveillance network for hospital infections in 1969 by the Center for Disease Control (CDC) currently provide a useful means of estimating these data and the character of nosocomial infections in any local situation as well as on a nationwide basis.[22,31]

The results of such surveys and any number of case histories testify that a patient entering the hospital today faces many risks for a variety of iatrogenic infections. These can be extremely serious and are often life-destroying. A routine appendectomy leads to complicating *Bacteroides* peritonitis;[7] urinary catheterization becomes responsible for *Proteus* septicemia;[35] inhalation therapy medications produce a *Serratia marcescens* outbreak;[46] a life-saving set of blood transfusions produces a case of viral hepatitis; an *Enterobacter agglomerans* abscess occurs under a plaster cast for a fractured ankle;[49] and five eyes are lost due to endopthalmitis during a single morning in surgery because of *Pseudomonas aeruginosa* contamination of the benzalkonium skin preparation.[40]

Recent infection rates compiled according to hospital type show an average of five infections per 100 discharged patients, varying from a low of 1.7 in the community hospital with less than 300 beds to a high of 11.4 in chronic disease hospitals.[8] Multiple infections are reported for 7.4 percent of all patients. Services with the highest frequencies, in descending order, are surgery, gynecology, pediatrics, obstetrics, and the nursery. High on everyone's list of direct causes of invasive infection is the frequent use of several diagnostic and supportive instrumentations which penetrate internal portions of the body, i.e., arteriography, continuous intravenous therapy, repeated urinary tract catheterizations, endotracheal respiratory assists, central venous pressure systems. As expected, figures comparing postoperative infection rates reveal marked differences between "clean" versus "contaminated" types of operations (Table 1). Notwithstanding the ever-increasing body of infection surveillance data, a working index is not yet available that allows us to predict where or when a specific infection problem will take place in any individual case. However, it is clear that any lack

TABLE 1.   Estimated Incidence of Infection Rate for Different Operations

Operation	No. of Cases	Estimated Incidence of Postoperative Infection	
		No.	%
Appendectomy	186,662	21,279	11.4
Inguinal hernioplasty	143,742	2,731	1.9
Hysterectomy	129,124	7,877	6.1
Gastrectomy	114,676	11,582	10.1
Salpingectomy	84,777	3,137	3.7
Prostatectomy	64,176	7,316	11.4
Open reduction fractures	39,640	1,665	4.2
Colectomy and abdomino-perineal resection	30,665	3,404	11.1
Total	793,462	58,991	7.4

From Altmeier: Proceedings, International Conference on Nosocomial Infections. Atlanta, CDC, 1970, p 82.
Data obtained from 1,118 hospitals.

**TABLE 2. Incidence and Relative Frequency of Selected
Isolates by Sites**

Isolate	Urinary Tract	Surgical Wound	Respiratory	Cutaneous	Primary Bacteremia
Coagulase-positive staphylococcus	* (*)	17.6 (16)	6.9 (11)	5.0 (25)	1.3 (12)
Enterococcus	21.0 (12)	8.2 (8)	* (*)	* (*)	0.7 (6)
Escherichia coli	53.4 (31)	19.0 (18)	5.9 (9)	1.4 (7)	2.0 (18)
Klebsiella	17.0 (10)	6.7 (6)	7.6 (12)	1.0 (5)	0.9 (5)
Proteus	24.4 (14)	10.6 (10)	3.4 (5)	2.5 (13)	0.5 (5)
Pseudomonas	14.5 (8)	7.6 (7)	6.3 (10)	1.9 (10)	0.9 (8)
Other	42.7 (25)	40.1 (36)	35.9 (53)	8.3 (40)	4.6 (42)
Total	172.4 (100)	107.1 (100)	63.7 (100)	20.0 (100)	10.9 (100)

*Figures give the number of isolates per 10,000 patients discharged. Figures in parentheses are
percentage of all isolates from each site.*
Incidence and relative frequency are very small compared to other pathogens at that site.
*From Center for Disease Control: National Nosocomial Infections Study Quarterly Report, Second
Quarter 1972, issued May 1973.*

of strict adherence to known principles of asepsis during operative techniques and procedures regularly proves to be disastrous.

Profiles of the incidence and relative frequency of specific pathogens isolated from infections when listed by specimen or site (Table 2, Fig. 1) and from medical centers around the world depict that striking changes have taken place since the introduction and widespread use of penicillin and other broad-spectrum antibiotics. Most noteworthy of these changes are: (1) the marked increase in gram-negative bacilli infections, especially the enteric bacilli,

Pseudomonas strains, and members of the anaerobic non-spore-forming *Bacteroides* group; and (2) a significantly greater number of infections caused by several groups of bacteria, fungi, protozoa, and some viruses heretofore considered quite harmless or presumed to be nonpathogenic (Table 3), commonly referred to as opportunists. Characteristically, most of the opportunists are found in the endogenous microbial flora of man. Most reside regularly in the gastrointestinal, genitourinary, and respiratory tracts, and on the skin. Others are inhabitants of soil and water, and contaminants

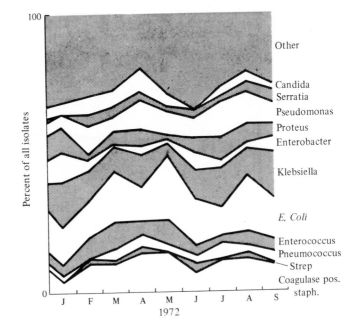

FIG. 1. Relative frequency of isolation of selected pathogens, primary bacteremia, January through September 1972. (From Center for Disease Control: National Nosocomial Infection Study Quarterly Report, Second quarter 1972, issued May 1973)

TABLE 3.   Some Outstanding "Opportunists"

Bacteria
  Acinetobacter and *Achromobacter* spp. (Mimae-
    Herellea-Moraxella group)
  Aeromonas hydrophila
  Bacillus subtilis, B. cereus
  Bacteroides spp.
  Cardiobacterium hominis
  Corynebacterium spp., diphtheroids
  Enterobacter agglomerans (Erwinia spp.)
  "Enterics"
   Escherichia coli
   Klebsiella spp.
   Enterobacter spp.
   Serratia spp.
   Proteus spp.
  Flavobacterium spp.
  Neisseria spp.
  Pseudomonas aeruginosa, Pseudomonas spp.

Fungi
  Mucor spp.
  Aspergillus spp.
  Penicillium spp.
  Phizopus spp.
  Candida albicans
  Torulopsia glabrata

Viruses
  Herpes
  Rubella
  Vaccinia
  Cytomegalovirus

Protozoa
  Pneumocystis carinii
  Toxoplasma gondii

This list is not complete. The numbers of unusual or rare isolates reported is legion.

of the many environmental surfaces in hospital areas.

Despite a heightened awareness of the increased occurrence and importance of this "commensal" or "saprophytic" type of infection, there is a singular lack of long or thorough case experience with these pathogens on the part of most clinicians.[49] Many isolates are notoriously resistant to currently available chemotherapeutic regimens, thus posing a difficult and unsatisfactory treatment problem. Since so many are part of the patient's own flora, epidemiologic analysis and isolation techniques are difficult. Traditional concepts of protective and preventive isolation techniques and procedures to control cross infection by typical "opportunists" are proving to be inadequate or limited.[28]

The epidemic potential of opportunistic infections in the nursery, intensive care units, cardiac care units, and pediatric wards has singled out the need for more stringent hospital environmental microbial surveillance programs as well as improved epidemiologic monitoring. The complexity of determining specific cause and etiology of many nosocomial infections has increased the legal suit vulnerability of the hospital considerably. A sometimes scanty, or simply controversial literature has resulted in insufficient laboratory agreement or documentation of their taxonomy and classification. In some instances it is not possible to distinguish the agent as a contaminant or causal organism. The researcher, handicapped by the lack of appropriate experimental biologic systems to study these and reluctant to pursue unrewarding projects, has provided only fragmentary evidence regarding the immunology and pathogenesis of most of the opportunistic microorganisms. Projected morbidity and mortality figures strengthen the conviction that the trend of infection by opportunists will not be readily reversed in modern medical practices but will dominate infectious disease experience for some time to come.

INFECTION AND THE HOSPITALIZED PATIENT

Infectious disease in any hospital patient is determined not only by the fact of mere parasitism—whether it be by an extremely invasive pathogen such as the streptococcus or staphylococcus or by some opportunist with little intrinsic virulence—but is importantly equated to the patient's ability to neutralize or eliminate the offending microbe. This is accomplished by the sum total of the mechanical and physiologic barriers, as well as the natural and acquired mechanisms of humoral and cellular host resistance. At this point the hospital patient is no different from the normal person in the community, but here the resemblance ends. Once admitted to the hospital, a patient is subjected to one or more stress factors that operate to predispose to infection:

1. Drug therapy (antibiotics, antimetabolites, steroids, and other cytotoxic agents)
2. Catheterization and intubation (urologic and vascular—all types)
3. Radiation (radioisotopic and x-ray)

4. Inhalation therapy (nebulization and endotracheal devices)
5. Blood transfusion
6. Organ transplant, renal and peritoneal dialysis
7. Prosthetic implantation
8. Immunosuppressant therapy
9. Surgery
10. Biopsy
11. Bone marrow aspiration
12. Hyperalimentation
13. Hypothermia
14. Endoscopy

A point often overlooked is that in any given patient multiple determinants favoring increased susceptibility to infection usually are operative. In some sense patients undergoing surgery and anesthesia are typical. They are subject to the special risks of surgical infection plus all the rest of the risks common to all hospitalized patients.

The deep concern of the surgeon over postoperative wound infection may also not take into account that today the principal life-threatening infections during this period are usually much the same as those seen in medical patients. Patient status becomes critical in the outcome of the initiation and course of an infection whether it occurs with or without surgical intervention. The following conditions may predispose him to infection:

1. Diabetes
2. Malignancy (including leukemia, lymphoma)
3. Surgery
4. Aplastic anemia
5. Cushing's disease
6. Collagen disease
7. Alveolar proteinosis
8. Lipid histiocytosis
9. Fibrocystic disease
10. Low birth weight (infants)
11. Agammaglobulinemia
12. Burns
13. Malnutrition

Individuals falling into any of the categories are extremely susceptible to infection because of faulty or missing cellular and humoral lines of defense. Whether the stress in a patient is due to a necessary clinical procedure or is a result of the patient's intrinsic status, such a host is "compromised" and it is in such patients that opportunistic infection flourishes.

There are special situations in which sepsis in surgical patients attributable to surgical and anesthetic stress per se differ from that in other hospitalized patients. These concern a group of factors favoring development of wound infection:

1. Presence of devitalized or dead tissue (inadequate wound debridement, necrosis)
2. Retained foreign body
3. Nature of surgical procedure (clean versus contaminated; duration; type)
4. Anatomic site of wound (neck or face versus other sites; extent of tissue damage)
5. Hemostasis
6. Impaired wound drainage
7. Age of patient (high in newborns and the elderly; lowest at age 15 to 24)
8. Alteration in microbial flora (prophylactic chemotherapy; prolonged preoperative hospitalization)
9. Extent of wound
10. Obesity

The operative stress may be active systemically or just in the local area of dissection, but both act to reduce host resistance. In either case the extent to which the amount and length of time this period can be minimized or excluded can aid in the prevention of wound sepsis.[12]

Final arguments have yet to be heard whether airborne sources of microbial contamination are more important than surgical or person-to-person contact or whether the patient's indigenous parasites contribute more critically to surgical sepsis than the gamut of exogenous environmental microorganisms.[9,17,42,47] The role of human microflora in hospital infection—its composition and changes—has taken on added significance in the face of much evidence that endogenous host organisms constitute the bulk of offending hospital-acquired infectious agents. Analysis of the organisms involved in hospital cross-infection (Table 3, Fig. 1)—those making up the resident flora of the skin, upper respiratory tract, intestinal tract, and genitourinary tract of healthy individuals—reveals that categorization of flora as "normal" and "pathogenic" is meaningless. Most laboratories have abandoned these terms in reporting culture results. Coagulase-negative staphylococci, long regarded as nonpathogenic commensal organisms found regularly on skin and mucous membranes, may be responsible for endocarditis, wound infections, and septicemia. Diphtheroids and other *Corynebacteria* spp., traditionally considered nonpathogenic, have been reported as a cause of serious disease in man.[5,29]

A partial answer for this state of the art lies

in more quantitative assessment of organisms isolated from clinical specimens, as is the case in urinary culture counts[30,48] and as has been suggested for sputum cultures.[44] However, quantitation does not help in the case of the carrier state and its effect on flora; in many cases personnel harbor virulent *Staphylococcus aureus* in the nose or throat. Respiratory carriage is prevalent for *Corynebacterium diphtheriae meningitidis, Streptococcus pyogenes,* and *Pseudomonas aeruginosa,* among others. The intestinal tract is a jungle of potentially dangerous microorganisms. Less appreciated is the phenomenon of "microbial persistence,"[38] which has often been demonstrated in vivo and in the laboratory. These are descendant organisms isolated after a chemotherapeutic failure. Interestingly the descendant organisms are no more resistant than the original population to the chemotherapeutic agent. It is assumed that the persistent organisms arise in cells that, for reasons still unknown, are metabolically blocked at the point at which a bactericidal response would result; and that the block is overcome when the agent is not present and conditions are favorable for the cells' growth.

Another facet concerning host flora, certainly relevant to possible sepsis, is that involving "latency." Here the microbe remains within the cell in a potentially active state but produces no obvious effect on the cell's function. Adenoviruses have a marked tendency toward latent infection in tonsils and adenoids. Recurrent *Herpes simplex* vesicles at mucocutaneous junctions reflect this phenomenon. Other organisms often associated with latent infection are the varicella-zoster viruses, cytomegaloviruses, and the rickettsial agent of Brill's disease. The relationship between latency and opportunistic infection is a very close one since the same factors that tend to activate latent infections predispose toward opportunism.[39,52]

The resident microflora of an individual host are profoundly altered following prophylactic or therapeutic administration of most antibiotics and a variety of antimicrobials. Although a causative infectious organism is depressed or eliminated, a serious and frequent complication of the therapy is superinfection or secondary infection by organisms that are resistant not only to the drug being used but to many other available antibiotics. The secondary organisms most commonly involved are the opportunists. They may come from an outgrowth of a species in the patient's indigenous flora

normally held back by their inability to compete with existing organisms, or they may be acquired from other patients or hospital personnel. Candidal stomatitis, disseminated candidiasis, staphylococcal pneumonia, staphylococcal enteritis, pseudomembranous enterocolitis, gram-negative septicemia, and *Pneumocystis carinii* pneumonia are just a few of the leading examples illustrating the consequences and complications of superinfections.[51]

DRUG RESISTANCE

Effective antimicrobial chemoprophylaxis and chemotherapy are often limited because drug-resistant cell lines arise in a relatively short time from previously sensitive cell populations. The incidence and frequency of resistance varies as a function of the specific antibiotic or a series of related antimicrobials, but in each well documented situation it seems that the greater the general clinical usage, the faster higher levels of resistance are seen in patient isolates as well as in the flora of the community population. The persistence of infectious diseases depends partially on this great propensity for microorganisms to circumvent the inhibitory action of initially very useful chemotherapeutic agents.

One necessary, indirect means of dealing with drug resistance involves selecting or finding another agent(s) to which the microbe or target cell line is susceptible. From one point of view, combination chemotherapy can be considered a variant of this approach based partially on the thesis that the probability of drug-resistant mutant selection is greatly minimized by the product of these rates of the individual drug. Nonetheless, substitute drug selection does not alter the basic problems of drug resistance or enlighten us as to its genesis or mechanisms.

Clinically virulent resistant strains among populations that were once sensitive arise by: (1) mutation and selection; and (2) genetic exchange.[50] In the former case random mutants with altered susceptibility to the drug may be selected from single colonies by the selective effect of the antimicrobial. In such cases the increase in level of resistance may be a single-step process with relatively high frequency or a multistep, slow process in which the virulence of the strain may or may not be changed.

The recent observation that drug resistance

in bacteria may arise by transfer of genetic material has far-reaching clinical implications. Genetic information that controls bacterial drug resistance occurs both in the bacterial chromosome and in the extrachromosomal elements—plasmids and episomes. When the resistant trait is passed via an episomal element from a resistant cell to a susceptible one it may transfer resistance not only to a single drug but also to several agents. Transfer is now known to occur between all of the Enterobactericeae and members of the genus *Pseudomonas*. To date, the drug-resistant determinants found to be transmitted in this manner include those for sulfonamides, chloramphenicol, gentamicin, tetracycline, neomycin, kanamycin, ampicillin, and streptomycin. There is every reason to believe that this list will be extended in the future. Environmental exposure of the normal intestinal flora to antibiotics favors the growth of organisms that carry the transfer (R) factor. Following infection with pathogenic species, these drug-resistant saprophytes can transmit resistance to cells of the sensitive pathogens, which may then, if antibiotics are used in the treatment, completely replace the initially drug-sensitive organism. There is evidence that the transfer of drug resistance of this type occurs within the human intestinal tract.

Because of the changing patterns of drug susceptibility on the part of microorganisms, it is recommended that the laboratory routinely document the antibiotic susceptibility patterns of their organisms and make these data available to the entire staff. One such profile is shown in Table 4. This allows the clinician to know, at the time he plans therapy, both the specific and the overall antibiotic status of the type of organism(s) he must deal with. Experi-

ence has shown that no two hospitals have identical antimicrobial susceptibility patterns. Excluding inherent variation in the technical aspects of susceptibility tests from one laboratory to another, individual and groups of strains may arise in a single institution which are not isolated in a nearby hospital. There are many reasons for this. The amounts and kinds of antibiosis used throughout the hospital, the nature of the patient population, the individual microflora of the personnel, and the level and quality of hospital surveillance and housekeeping are all contributing factors.

VIRUSES ASSOCIATED WITH BLOOD AND BLOOD COMPONENTS

A justified increasing concern over the occurrence and control of hospital-related viral infections has been kindled by the increased transmission of the agents of cytomegalic inclusion and hepatitis B (serum hepatitis) via blood and blood components used in hospitalized patients, i.e., plasma, fibrinogen, convalescent serum, washed cells, etc. All personnel face greater risk of infection in areas where blood is a common component of the environment, such as in surgery, renal dialysis, and the laboratory. Although major routes of infection are not always established in outbreaks, personnel may be exposed by direct contact with contaminated blood or by inapparent parenteral inoculation, ingestion, or inhalation of blood aerosols.

Cytomegalovirus infections have usually been associated with severe generalized congenital disease or with an acquired infection that is frequently hepatic in nature. The patient with either congenital or acquired disease

TABLE 4. Bacterial Susceptibility Profile

Organism	No. Tested	Percent Susceptible									
		Am	Chlor	Col	Gm	Kan	Sm	Tet	Cep	Pen	Meth
E. coli	376	69	92	98	99	89	63	68	83	—	—
Ent. cloacae	129	14	93	82	99	95	92	87	9	—	—
Kl. pneumoniae	278	5	90	98	94	89	86	82	88	—	—
Ser. marcescens	68	1	67	4	89	79	75	49	0	—	—
Ps. aeruginosa	193	0	7	97	93	8	11	14	0	—	—
Staph. aureus	158	18	—	—	—	96	85	78	99	18	96
Enterococcus	101	98	—	—	—	30	2	17	54	23	11

Am, ampicillin; Chlor, chloramphenicol; Col, colistin; Gm, gentamicin; Kan, kanamycin; Sm, streptomycin; Tet, tetracycline; Cep, cephalothin; Pen, penicillin; Meth, methicillin.

is known to excrete the virus via the pharynx or urine for an extended period and is infective for contacts throughout this period.

A posttransfusion mononucleosis syndrome[26] associated with cytomegalovirus may occur in patients receiving large volumes of blood. The disorder is characterized by fever, splenomegaly, and atypical lymphocytes in the peripheral blood several weeks after receipt of fresh whole blood. There is little lymphadenopathy or liver involvement, and the heterophile test remains negative. In most cases the illness is self-limited, but more serious consequences occur in patients with severe underlying disease.[20]

The problem of viral hepatitis is of greater magnitude because of the high virus carrier rate. It has been known for some time that hepatitis B is transmitted parenterally via inoculation of contaminated blood, *viz.*, blood transfusion, accidental needle puncture, percutaneous drug use, tatooing. The infectious agent associated with type B hepatitis is relatively resistant to disinfection and sterilization. Except for heat sterilization, no established procedure has been demonstrated to be effective in rendering the agent noninfectious.[18] The absence of a convenient demonstrably effective means for sterilizing environmental surfaces and apparatus that does not tolerate heat sterilization necessitates vigorous efforts to avoid contamination. The following recommendations[13] should be considered if this does occur:

1. If possible, disposable supplies should be used where contact with blood occurs. Products marketed as disposable should not be reused, even after sterilization or disinfection.
2. Nondisposable medical apparatus should be sterilized between use; steam autoclaving is preferable to ethylene oxide sterilization, but either is preferable to liquid sterilization.
3. When liquid agents must be used, aqueous 40 percent formalin, activated glutaraldehyde, or hypochlorite are probably the agents of choice; prolonged contact with the active agent is necessary.

Certain personnel practices are also recommended[13]:

1. Personnel having contact with blood products should wear protective clothing (laboratory coats for laboratory and venipuncture personnel); scrub suits or gowns for dialysis personnel); such clothing should be changed immediately if contaminated with blood. Protective clothing should not be worn outside work areas and should be discarded before eating, drinking, or smoking.
2. Personnel having direct contact with specimens known to be HBAg-positive or with blood from high-risk sources should wear protective gloves. Masks and gowns may offer additional protection if blood is likely to be aerosolized—as during certain laboratory procedures or manipulation of arteriovenous shunts.
3. Personnel with cuts or abrasions should wear gloves at the time of any potential contact with blood.
4. Personnel should wash hands vigorously after any direct contact with blood or blood products.
5. Eating, drinking, and smoking should be prohibited in areas where blood contamination occurs.
6. Personnel exposed to HBAg disease should not receive standard immune serum globulin since there are no conclusive data to support its efficacy; specific hepatitis B immune serum globulin shows prophylactic promise but is currently available only on a research basis.
7. There are insufficient data to recommend that personnel who are chronic carriers of HBAg be removed from any routine hospital job.

MICROBIAL COLONIZATION AND CLINICAL SUPERINFECTION

Chemoprophylaxis to circumvent surgical wound infection is influenced by a set of complex factors and is faced with serious risks that may outweigh its considered usefulness. Despite its continued application in some areas of surgery based on clinical impression or custom, definitive data showing that this modality effectively shields the patient from microbial invasion of the operative site before, during, or after surgery are controversial. There are specific circumstances when antibiotic prophylaxis targeted at a single sensitive organism is effective and indicated, but these are limited at best (Table 5).

To understand the special nature of the surgical wound and circumstances which lead to its inoculation with pathogenic organisms, it must be recognized that no single mechanism of infection is wholly culpable. The type of operative procedure itself is an important determinant.[45] A "contaminated" colon resection is 10- to 20-fold more likely to engender infection than an uncomplicated herniorraphy, which should virtually never be infected. Low pelvic anastomoses have been reported to have a leak of some sort in about 70 percent of these operations.[25] Exogenous or endogenous sources of wound contamination may occur during clean or dirty surgery. The nature of the organisms may be influenced by the flora of the patient, the surgical personnel or the envi-

TABLE 5.   Chemoprophylaxis of Infections

Disease or Organism	Drug
Usually Effective	
Group A streptococcus (rheumatic fever)	Penicillin G, sulfonamides
Neisseria meningitidis	Rifampin, minocycline
N. gonorrheae (ophthalmia)	Penicillin, silver nitrate
Enteropathic *Escherichia coli* diarrhea	Neomycin, kanamycin
Streptococcus viridans (SBE)	Penicillin, vancomycin
Congenital syphilis	Penicillin
Tuberculin contacts	Isoniazid
Sometimes effective	
Shigellosis	Ampicillin, neomycin
Gonococcal urethritis	Penicillin
Chronic bronchitis *(Hemophilus influenzae* or *Diplococcus pneumoniae)*	Ampicillin, tetracycline
Prolonged labor	Ampicillin, tetracycline
Short-term urethral catheterization (<24 hours)	Ampicillin, tetracycline
Cardiac surgery	Methicillin
Large-bowel surgery (preoperative)	Neomycin, kanamycin
Cystic fibrosis	Tetracycline
Ineffective	
Viral respiratory diseases	
Viral exanthems	
Clean abdominal surgery	Penicillin and streptomycin
Gynecologic surgery	
Burns	
Coma	
Shock	
Congestive heart failure	
Prematurity	
Prolonged urethral catheterization (>24 hours)	
Prolonged intravenous catheterization	
High-dose steroid therapy	

From Harrison's Principles of Internal Medicine, 7th ed, 1974. Courtesy of McGraw-Hill.

ronment at any given time. The size of the offending microbial inoculum delivered to the wound site varies in each case. Host status and degree of tissue trauma are never the same from one operation to the next. The wound may be infected after it is closed via unsterile manipulation of drains, tubes, or the wound itself. Often overlooked as a deterrent to the use of prophylatic therapy to avert infection in a surgical patient are nonmicrobial effects such as untoward drug reactions and idiosyncrasies. By no means the least danger is the emergence of drug-resistant populations described previously.

There is another aspect related to the usage of antibiosis that has not been given adequate consideration among the hazards of therapy: the phenomenon of superinfection.[36] Superinfections are secondary infections that occur during a course of antimicrobial therapy administered either for prophylactic or therapeutic purposes. The real extent of superinfection is not known, but it is estimated that it is seen in at least 2 percent of all patients treated with antibiotics.[27] With antimicrobial therapy in cancer patients using ampicillin, tetracyclines, and various combinations including gentamicin colonization occurred in 24.7 percent of the patients and superinfection in 8.2 percent.[32] Superinfections are certainly more common when antimicrobials are given in large doses or when combinations of drugs or broad-spectrum antibiotics are used. Presumably the incidence varies depending on the presence of factors predisposing to microbial colonization during the period of therapy. In this regard early diagnosis becomes a very important consideration in order to reduce morbidity and mortality.

It is important to distinguish clinical superinfections from simple colonization or mere overgrowth of potentially virulent organisms, since antibiotics used unsuccessfully for benign colonization may result in further superinfection and other complications. A normal ecologic change in flora of the host's tissues and organs accompanies all antimicrobial therapy. The number of resident microorganisms is reduced and the etiologic agent may even be eliminated, but then the normal flora is replaced by resistant endogenous strains and less commonly by exogenous organisms. Although these changes often involve small increases in numbers and are of no clinical significance, such colonization is a prerequisite for secondary infection. When the number becomes unusually high and host conditions are favorable, serious and lethal disease can ensue. Trauma incident to a surgical procedure and the effect it may have in reducing the ability of tissues to resist bacterial or fungal invasion is a factor that may play a role in the pathogenesis of this phenomenon. Most of us are familiar with preoperative bowel "sterilization" leading to pseudomembranous colitis, staphylococcal diarrhea, *Candida* infection of the bowel, or even systemic candidiasis. The poor prognosis in many instances is related to several factors, including drug resistance of the secondary organisms, pathogenicity of the microorganisms themselves once they are in a milieu that provides them the opportunity to multiply and invade tissues, and the underlying diseases so often present in these patients.

Once superinfection occurs, the course may be so rapid that treatment may not prevent a fatal result. It is essential that the clinician recognize patients who are most likely to develop colonization or superinfection, monitor these regularly with smears and cultures in order to diagnose early, and then rapidly institute appropriate therapy based on careful antibiogram data from the laboratory regarding the susceptibility of the organisms present.

STERILIZATION AND DISINFECTION

Certain terms warrant definition because they are often used erroneously or as synonyms, or they are used inappropriately to refer to procedural activities.

1. **Sterilization.** This is the process employed to destroy all forms of living matter—vegetative microorganisms, spores, fungi, protozoa, and viruses. Few if any chemicals, as used in practical disinfection, are actually sterilizing agents. It is essential that all materials which are to make direct or indirect contact with vital cavities such as the peritoneum, bladder, joints, etc. be sterile.
2. **Disinfection.** This is the process, physical or chemical, producing destruction of all vegetative (pathogenic) organisms but not spores or other resistant nonpathogenic organisms. This process is sufficient for many items of equipment used in situations where spore-formers are of no pathogenic significance. Anesthetic and respiratory apparatus and urinary tract endoscopic equipment fall in this category. Disinfection must also suffice for the human skin for which sterilization would be preferred but is not possible.
3. **Disinfectant.** This is any chemical substance used on inanimate materials capable of producing disinfection. Some agents can function as a disinfectant and as an antiseptic, e.g., 70 percent ethyl alcohol.
4. **Antiseptic.** This is any chemical agent that is usually applied to living tissue which renders microorganisms harmless by either killing them or preventing their growth or reproduction.
5. **Chemosterilizer.** This is any chemical compound that destroys all forms of microbiologic life including spores of pathogenic clostridial or aerobic bacilli, tubercle bacilli, fungi, and viruses. This term contrasts with "antiseptic" and "disinfectant," both of which should have the same capability by definition but in practice do not.[10]
6. **Chemical cleanliness.** An item may be sterile but not chemically clean, i.e., free from all organic or inorganic soil. The presence of pyrogenic protein and traces of detergent and other residual chemicals on instruments may elicit an untoward reaction in spite of sterility.
7. **Bacteriostat.** This is a chemical that retards or inhibits bacterial growth.
8. **Bactericide.** This is a chemical agent that kills bacteria.
9. **Germicide.** This is a substance that kills microorganisms.

METHODS FOR STERILIZATION AND DISINFECTION

The methods for sterilization and disinfection generally used in hospitals for controlling microbial contamination are, in order of dependability and effectiveness:

1. Autoclaving (steam under pressure)
2. Gaseous exposure (ethylene oxide or formalin)
3. Chemical treatment (soaking with activated glutaraldehyde)

Other forms of sterilization have been attempted (e.g., irradiation) but have limited usefulness in hospital procedures. It is most important to recognize that each acceptable method has its own appropriate applications, advantages, and disadvantages, so that selection of a specific technique in one situation may not prevail for another. Also it is axiomatic that one method not be substituted for another, particularly one that is less dependable, unless there is no other possible choice available or there is a definitive reason. Several excellent guides and manuals are available for consultation and reference.[1,6,16,33]

Autoclaving

Autoclaving (temperature 121 to 123 C; pressure 19 to 10 psi; time 30 minutes) effectively sterilizes most surgical materials. All bacteria, viruses, fungi, and even dry, resistant spores are destroyed. This is the most dependable method and is used whenever possible. The all-metal, rigid, classic proctoscopes and sigmoidoscopes may be autoclaved. The major limitations of autoclaving lie in the fact that it cannot be used for materials that are not easily permeable to steam (e.g., anhydrous oils, powders, greases) or are adversely affected by heat and water. Unfortunately the very useful modern flexible fiberscopes with their delicate mechanisms, coherent (image) and incoherent (illumination) bundles, and optical components cannot be autoclaved without damage. Rigid telescopes can be autoclaved with extreme care (delayed cooling period), but even so the life expectancy of these expensive items is shortened.

Gaseous Chemosterilizers

Ethylene Oxide. The usual equipment necessary for gaseous ethylene oxide sterilization consists of a closed sterilizing environment with controls for the entire cycle of the process. Factors that affect sterilization are humidity (25 to 50 percent has the greatest effectiveness); temperature (38 to 60 C; the exposure period can be reduced with a rise in temperature); gas concentration (450 to 760 mg per liter of chamber space); and the exposure period (dependent on temperature and concentration). Several commercial models are available, and new types are being engineered. Sterilization with gaseous ethylene oxide is a dependable method for numerous heat-labile materials.[11] Gaseous ethylene oxide sterilization is the preferred method for flexible fiberscopes, and even rigid endoscopes can be treated in this manner. It is a better treatment process from a bacteriologic point of view than "soaking" procedures, e.g., glutaraldehyde or its companion cold disinfectants. Most important is that ethylene oxide, when used properly, is *effective in destroying all forms of microorganisms including spores and viruses.*

The process of ethylene oxide gaseous sterilization is not without limitations, however. The time cycle is slow, usually requiring 6 to 10 hours or more. Many polymers can absorb quantities of ethylene oxide and retain this gas for various lengths of time, e.g., nylon, rubber, polyethylene, polypropylene, and polyvinylchloride. Ethylene oxide gas residues must be eliminated by aeration before coming into contact with human tissue in order to avoid possible vesicant action. Furthermore, the lack of sufficient hydration of microbes during the sterilization process can be a limiting parameter in treating articles with ethylene oxide. Desiccated microorganisms are highly resistant to the action of ethylene oxide gas, and unless the microbes are hydrated they are not destroyed. Also, wrapping materials must be permeable to ethylene oxide. Craft paper, muslin, plastic films, and polyethylene are suitable. When in the range of 3.6 to 100 percent by volume, ethylene oxide is heavier than air and is an inflammable, highly explosive gas. It is supplied as a liquid under mild pressure. Diluted with carbon dioxide or chlorofluorohydrocarbons, the mixture become nonflammable. Inhalation toxicity is that of household ammonia.

Formaldehyde Gas. Formaldehyde gas is a bactericidal agent. It has been used as a terminal fumigant and is an effective method of disinfection although not used as much as formerly. Formaldehyde disinfection is obtained by vaporizing formalin in specially designed cabinets and maintaining a relative humidity of at least 70 percent and a temperature of at least 20 C. Vegetative bacteria are killed within an hour or two, although a longer period is required for spores. A low-temperature steam and formaldehyde process has been described for use in sterilizing heat-sensitive endoscopes.[2] The many disadvantages to this method have caused it generally to be replaced by other, more reliable procedures. The gas is unable to penetrate materials and to diffuse evenly to all surfaces. It has an irritating odor and requires high humidity and high temperatures. The exposure period is long, and it is difficult to remove the residual formaldehyde after exposure.

Chemical Soaking (Cold Disinfection)

Numerous liquid chemosterilizers have been used for treating medical instruments, but the absolute destruction of all organisms by any of the chemicals is not ensured. Some of the more common are the quartenary ammonium compounds, phenolics, alcohol, mercurials, halogens, and strong acids or alkalis. Many of the chemicals are bacteriostatic (e.g., mercurials) and not germicidal, or they destroy only vegetative bacterial fungal forms and have no effect on spores (e.g., alcohols). Viruses seem to vary in their resistance to chemical destruction, but it is clear that some viruses are not affected by exposure to chemical disinfection in the normally used concentrations. Cold disinfection should be used only when autoclaving or gaseous sterilization is not possible. Also, it cannot be stressed strongly enough that when any chemosterilizer or disinfectant is used the manufacturer's directions must be followed to the letter.

The use of activated glutaraldehyde (a saturated dialdehyde: $CHO-CH_2-CH_2-CH_2-CHO$) has gained wide acceptance in recent years for use as an instrument germicide, particularly for incorporating optical elements and metal instruments where heat or steam cannot be applied. A wide range of organisms are destroyed by 2 percent aqueous solutions of glutaraldehyde. Contact time for killing vege-

tative bacteria and fungal cells, *Mycobacterium tuberculosis,* and many viruses is 10 minutes. Ten hours is recommended to kill resistant spores. If used properly, glutaraldehyde does not affect the lenses or lens cement of endoscopic instruments, has no irritant action, is noncorrosive, and is nontoxic to personnel. Most mishaps with glutaraldehyde and other cold-type instrument disinfection brought to this author's attention have been clearly caused by misuse of the chemical agent, e.g., soaking for extended periods of time, using improper concentrations of disinfectant, soaking unclean instruments.

TECHNIQUES FOR STERILIZING ENDOSCOPES

A simplified outline guide to methods that are currently used most commonly to sterilize or disinfect endoscopes is given in Table 6. Other methods have been suggested but are

TABLE 6.   Guide to Disinfection and Sterilization of Endoscopes

Disinfection
Group A (vegetative bacteria and fungi, influenza viruses)
 1. Time: 10 minutes
 2. Solutions:
   a. Iodophor: 100 ppm iodine (1:10,000)*
   b. Phenolic solutions (1 percent aqueous)†
Group B (group A plus tubercle bacillus and enteroviruses)
 1. Time: 15 minutes
 2. Solutions:
   a. Aqueous formalin (20 percent)*
   b. Activated glutaraldehyde (2 percent aqueous)

Sterilization
Groups A and B (plus hepatitis viruses, bacterial spores, and some fungal spores)
 1. Time: 10 to 12 hours
 2. Solutions:
   a. Ethylene oxide gas‡
   b. Activated glutaraldehyde (2 percent aqueous)
   c. Aqueous formalin (20 percent)*

In all cases it is essential to remove all gross organic material first.
*Sodium nitrite (0.2 percent) should be present to prevent corrosion.
†Sodium bicarbonate (0.5 percent) should be presented to prevent corrosion.
‡Depending on the procedure, 3 to 12 hours may be needed; it is more rapidly bactericidal for group A and B microorganisms.
From data compiled by Spaulding and Mallinson: CDC, Atlanta.

not yet widely used.[2] Several factors must be considered when selecting a given technique.

The first consideration prior to sterilizing any endoscope is that it must be *meticulously cleaned*. Quite often failures are attributable to insufficient cleansing of the instruments to be disinfected. Adherent dirt, blood, grime, body secretions, sputum, and other extraneous materials inhibit the action of the disinfectant by mechanical blocking or a neutralizing effect. Most disinfectants cannot penetrate even small layers of organic matter even after soaking for long periods of time. The endoscope is dismantled (stopcocks should be opened, fiber light carriers removed, biopsy forceps taken apart, etc.) as far as the design of the instrument allows and rinsed liberally with warm water (80 C). If a mild detergent or soap solution is preferred as a vehicle for removing attached bits of tissue, blood, mucus, etc., it should be followed by a thorough rinse with warm water to remove any residual detergent or soap. Brushing is also a very helpful mechanical means of removing adherent materials. It is advantageous if the instrument is *dry* before any type of disinfection. Opinions vary on the need to disinfect any suspect or actually contaminated surgical equipment before it is washed and definitively sterilized in order to protect wash-up and sterilizing personnel. A warm water rinse for 2 to 3 minutes is sufficient at this point.

If the endoscope set consists of *only* metal parts (e.g., the traditional rigid proctoscope-sigmoidoscope or broncoscope), it can be autoclaved. When this type of instrument is used only on a once-a-day basis, it should be gas sterilized after cleaning. If a set is used more often because a number of successive cases require examination with a single endoscopy set, there is no other option than cold disinfection. In such cases of repeated examination with one endoscope set, the instrument is cleaned thoroughly after each use and then soaked for 10 to 30 minutes in 2 percent aqueous glutaraldehyde solution; more complete decontamination is obtained when equipment is soaked for 30 minutes. The scopes are transferred under sterile conditions to a water bath for 2 to 3 minutes of rinsing or submerging with sterile water to remove residual glutaraldehyde. Irritation or inflammation are not uncommon if this aspect is not observed. It is worthwhile to perform bacteriologic monitoring at predetermined intervals (e.g., monthly) to be sure that the soaking procedure is effective; this can be accomplished by taking cultures from the rinse water of these rigid instruments. Similarly, the same type of quality control of the sterile water stocks should be carried out. A log should be kept of bacteriologic results. It is equally important to record any corrective action required and taken. In addition, the sterile water and containers in which the soaking disinfectant is placed should be autoclaved, and instrument transfer forceps changed daily. It is also essential that the nursing personnel be trained and educated fully before the responsibility for handling these procedures is assigned to them.

The more recently developed flexible fiber endoscopes (e.g., fibergastroscope, esophagogastroscope, colonoscope) pose more complex infection problems and as yet unresolved cross-infection dilemmas than the rigid, all-metal types during their use; they also pose problems in sterilization methods.

Probably the most important is the sterilization procedure itself (Table 6). These costly instruments contain delicate movement mechanisms, lenses, cover glasses, lens cement, plastic inner tubes, etc., which are vulnerable to damage by heat and corrosive chemical action. Since they cannot be autoclaved, boiled, heated, or subjected to strong chemical disinfectants, the techniques left for their sterilization are less than optimal. Recent studies of bacterial pollution and disinfection of the fiber colonoscope[14,15] and gastrointestinal fiber endoscopes[5a] reinforce the basic facts related to techniques.

These studies demonstrated that, after appropriate cleaning, ethylene oxide gas was clearly the superior method for sterilizing these endoscopes. Tap water–detergent treatment followed by 70 percent alcohol wiping is definitely ineffective for disinfecting the fiberscopes. Serious pollution by gram-negative and gram-positive organisms occurred on the tip, tube, and operation panel of the fiber colonoscope after routine examinations. Colonic bacterial flora were found simultaneously on the examiner's hands and in the house dust during clinical examinations. Also, sterilization of the scopes was generally inadequate when such disinfectants as cresol, chlorhexidine, and benzethonium chloride were applied. The usual slow process of sterilizing with ethylene oxide

(6 to 10 hours) was considerably shortened by using the new G.S. 10 chamber.* This machine has two automatic cycles: "sterilization," which takes 64 minutes, and "disinfection," which takes 26 minutes. At the end of each cycle the endoscopes are either left in air for 24 hours or placed in the ACMI aerator for 2 hours. Such rapid gas sterilization promises to replace selection of bactericidal soaking (glutaraldehyde), which is potentially capable of damaging the costly endoscope. However, if several patients must be examined during a half-day session and the time available between cases is limited, glutaraldehyde disinfection is the method of choice.[5a]

Is there danger of induced septicemia (bacteremia) due to routine manipulation with flexible fiber endoscopes in vascularized anatomic sites with heavy mixed flora such as the gastrointestinal or respiratory tract? Albeit limited, the available data seem to indicate a very low risk situation. Bacteremia has been reported after a single sigmoidoscopy.[33a] In contrast, transient bacteremia did not occur after endoscopy of the upper gastrointestinal tract with the fiberoptic esophagoscope or gastroscope in 40 patients studied.[34] Additional study is needed to draw definite conclusions in this matter.

The incidence or level of risk of viral hepatitis cross-infection associated with endoscopic examination (upper or lower gastrointestinal tract) also has not been completely established. The following statement of the Committee on Viral Hepatitis of the Division of Medical Sciences of the National Academy of Sciences summarizes the most recent attitudes on hepatitis antigen in human blood:[13a]

A clearer definition of the significance of viral hepatitis type B as a clinical and public health problem has arisen from the discovery, development, and widespread application of various serologic tests for the presence of an antigen–hepatitis B antigen that is associated with the disease. The demonstration of the antigen in the blood of a patient or of an apparently healthy person raises questions not only of the presence of active liver disease, but also of the potential risk of transmission of the infection to others. It is now recognized that, in addition to the well established parenteral mode of transmission, viral hepatitis type B can be transmitted by other means.

On the basis of the information acquired from clinical and epidemiologic studies and from antigen testing programs, the Committee on Viral Hepatitis finds that:

a. *A confirmed positive test for antigen is indicative of acute or chronic viral hepatitis type B or of an asymptomatic carrier state.*

b. *The presence of the antigen in the blood of a patient with acute viral hepatitis type B is usually transient. If it persists for more than 3 months after the onset of the illness, the person is likely to become a chronic carrier of the antigen.*

c. *A chronic carrier of the antigen may or may not have demonstrable evidence of related liver disease.*

d. *The occurrence of acute hepatitis type B or an asymptomatic carrier state during pregnancy or even during the first 2 months post partum is frequently associated with later infection in the newborn infant.*

e. *There is clear evidence that carriers should be prohibited from donating blood for transfusion.*

f. *Although the infectiousness of patients with antigen-positive hepatitis apparently diminishes when the antigen is no longer demonstrable in the blood, they are currently not accepted as blood donors.*

g. *There is insufficient knowledge of the extent to which chronic carriers can transmit hepatitis type B by nonparenteral routes. However, close contacts of some categories of chronic carriers, such as renal dialysis patients, are at increased risk for hepatitis type B infection.*

h. *With respect to risk of transmission to others, there is no indication at this time that routine antigen testing of any specific professional or occupational group should be required.*

i. *Standard human immune serum globulin (ISG) is of no demonstrable value in the treatment of carriers.*

There is insufficient evidence on which to recommend the use of standard ISG for prophylaxis among contacts of hepatitis B patients or carriers. Studies of the possible prophylactic effect of hepatitis B hyperimmune serum globulin are currently in progress.

The Committee recommends that:

a. *Persons found to have a positive antigen*

---

*Manufacturer: American Cystoscope Makers, Inc. (ACMI), 8 Pelham Parkway, Pelham Manor, N.Y. 10803.

test in the course of diagnostic studies, blood donor testing, or testing after known exposure to infection with hepatitis type B be so informed and the test be repeated promptly; and persons with a confirmed positive test be evaluated for the presence of liver disease and followed to determine whether the antigen persists.

b. *Persons with antigen-positive hepatitis be considered infectious and control measures be taken with respect to potentially infectious materials, such as blood and blood-contaminated secretions.*

c. *Women found to have hepatitis during pregnancy or during the first 2 months post partum be tested for hepatitis B antigen and their infants be tested for hepatitis B antigen at monthly intervals for at least 6 months.*

d. *Testing for hepatitis B antigen be required of all blood donors.*

e. *Until more complete knowledge of the significance of the antigen carrier state is acquired, particularly as to its relation to communicability, only routine precautions, such as those applying to percutaneous routes of potential transmission, be initiated.*

f. *The effort to obtain more accurate and complete reporting of hepatitis cases—on the basis of serologic test results as well as epidemiologic characteristics—be intensified to improve surveillance on a national basis.*

In view of our current level of knowledge of the epidemiology of viral hepatitis and in accordance with the above statements of the expert committee, the endoscopist must be concerned with the potential risk of operative hepatitis B cross-infection. Despite the thousands of procedures performed without report of associated or attributable endoscopic transfer of hepatitis B, all measures to prevent viral cross-infection should be utilized to ensure that this situation prevails. Gloves are recommended for the examiner and nursing personnel while carrying out gastrointestinal endoscopy. The usual surgical aseptic conditions should be maintained during bronchial endoscopic examinations. It is advisable to gas sterilize the scope after any examination of an antigen-positive patient. Elective procedures in hepatitis B-positive patients might be seriously reconsidered and carried out only if the indication for endoscopy far outweighs the risk of viral transmission. Of course, whether these proposals are fully warranted awaits further investigation and documentation.

REFERENCES

1. A Guide to Chemical Disinfection and Sterilization for Hospitals and Related Care Facilities. Michigan Department of Health, 1963

2. Adler VG, Mitchell JP: The disinfection of heat sensitive surgical instruments. In DA Shapton, RG Board (eds): Safety in Microbiology. London, Academic Press, 1972

3. Altmeier WA, Culbertson WR, Hummel RP: Surgical considerations of endogenous infections—sources, types, and methods of control. Surg Clin North Am 48:227, 1968

4. Anderson ES: The ecology of transferable drug resistance in the enterobacteria. Annu Rev Microbiol 22:131, 1968

5. Andriole VT, Lyons RW: Coagulase-negative staphylococcus. Ann NY Acad Sci 174:533, 1970

5a. Axion ATR, Cotton PB, Phillips I, et al: Disinfection of gastrointestinal fibre endoscopes. Lancet, 1974, p 656

6. Bartlett RC, Hammond JB, Wichersham VR (eds): Hospital Associated Infections. American Society of Clinical Pathologists, Council on Microbiology, Chicago, 1971

7. Beazley RM, Polakavetz SH, Miller RM: Bacteroides infections on a university surgical service. Surg Gynecol Obstet 135:742, 1972

8. Bennett JV, Scheckler WE, Maki DG, et al: Current National Patterns, United States Proceedings, International Conference on Nosocomial Infections. CDC, Atlanta, Aug 3–6, 1970, p 42

9. Bernard NR, Cole WR: Bacterial air contamination and its relation to postoperative sepsis. Ann Surg 156:12, 1962

10. Borick P: Chemical sterilizers (chemosterilizers). Adv Appl Microbiol 10:291, 1968

11. Bruch CW: Gaseous sterilization. Annu Rev Microbiol 15:245, 1961

12. Burke JF: Clinical determinants of host susceptibility to infection in surgical patients. Proceedings, International Conference on Nosocomial Infections. CDC, Atlanta, Aug 3–6, 1970 p 169

13. Center for Disease Control: National Noscomial Infection Study Quarterly Report. First quarter 1972 (issued January 1973)

13a. Center for Disease Control: Morbidity and Mortality Weekly Report, 1974

14. Chang FM, Sakai Y, Ashizawa S: Bacterial pollution and disinfection of the colonfiberscope. I. An investigation of traditional sterilization methods. Dig Dis 18:946, 1973

15. Chang FM, Sakai Y, Ashizawa S: Bacterial pollution and disinfection of the colonfiberscope. II. Ethylene oxide gas sterilization. Dig Dis 18:951, 1973

16. Cleaning Disinfection and Sterilization. A Guide for Hospitals and Related Facilities. State of California, Department of Public Health, 1965

17. Coriell LL: Use of laminar flow in surgery. Proceedings, International Conference on Nosocomial Infections. CDC, Atlanta, Aug 3–6, 1970, p 225

18. Cossart YE: Epidemiology of serum hepatitis. Br Med Bull 28:156, 1972

19. Darlow HM: Safety in the microbiological laboratory. In DA Shapton, RG Board (eds): Safety in Microbiology. New York, Academic Press, 1972

20. Duvall CP, Casazza AR, Grimely PM, et al: Recovery of cytomegalovirus from adults with neoplastic disease. Ann Intern Med 64:531, 1966

21. Edebo L, Laurell G: Hospital infection of the urinary tract with Proteus. Acta Pathol Microbiol Scand 43:93, 1958

22. Eickhoff TC, Brachman PS, Bennett JV, et al: Surveillance of nosocomial infections in community hospitals. I. Surveillance methods: effectiveness and initial results. J Infect Dis 120:305, 1969

23. Elliott RH, Dunbar JM: Streptococcal bacteremia in children following dental extractions. Arch Dis Child 43:451, 1968

24. Finland M: Changing ecology of bacterial infections as related to antimicrobial therapy. J Infect Dis 122:419, 1970

25. Golligher JC, Graham ME, DeDombrae FT: Anastomotic dehiscence after anterior resection of rectum. Br J Surg 56:692, 1969

26. Hanshaw JB, Betts RF, Simon G, et al: Acquired cytomegalovirus infection: association with hepatomegaly and abnormal liver function tests. N Engl J Med 272:602, 1965

27. Harrison TR: Principles of Internal Medicine, 7th ed. New York, McGraw-Hill, 1974

28. Infection Control in the Hospital, revised edition. Chicago, American Hospital Association, 1970

29. Johnson WD, Kaye D: Serious infections caused by diphtheroids. Ann NY Acad Sci 174:568, 1970

30. Kass EH: Asymptomatic infections of the urinary tract. Trans Assoc Am Physicians 69:56, 1956

31. Kislak K, Eickhoff T, Finland M: Hospital acquired infections and antibiotic usage in the Boston City Hospital in January 1964. N Engl J Med 271:834, 1964

32. Klastersky J, Cappel R, Daneau D: Bacterial colonizaton and clinical superinfection during antibiotic treatment of infections in patients with cancer. Rev Eur Etude Clin Biol 17:299, 1972

33. Lawrence CA, Block SS (eds): Disinfection, Sterilization and Preservation. Philadelphia, Lea & Febiger, 1968

33a. LeFrock JL, Ellis CA, Turchik JB, et al: Transient bacteremia associated with sigmoidoscopy. N Engl J Med 289:467, 1973

34. Linneman C, Weisman E: Blood cultures following endoscopy of the esophagus and stomach. South Med J 64:1055, 1971

35. List PM, Harbison PA, Marsh JA: Bacteremia after urologic instrumentation. Lancet 8:74, 1966

36. Louria DB: Quantitative analyses of bacterial populations in sputum. JAMA 182:1082, 1962

37. Martin WJ: Bacteremia and bacteremia shock in surgical patients. Surg Clin North Am 49:1053, 1969

38. McDermott W: Microbial persistence. Yale J Biol Med 30:257, 1958

39. Mims CA: Aspects of the pathogenesis of virus diseases. Bacteriol Rev 28:30, 1964

40. Ogden AE, Rathmell TK: Infections and penzallronium solutions. JAMA 193:978, 1965

41. Opfell JB, Miller CB: Cold sterilization techniques. Adv Appl Microbiol 7:81, 1965

42. O'Riordan C, Adler JL, Banks HH: Wound infections on an orthopedic service. Am J Epidemiol 95:442, 1972

43. Phillips CB, Warshowsky B: Chemical disinfection. Annu Rev Microbiol 12:525, 1958

44. Pirtle JK, Monroe PW, Smalley TK, et al: Diagnostic and therapeutic advantages of serial quantitative cultures of fresh sputum in bacterial pneumonia. Am Rev Resp Dis 100:831, 1969

45. Polk JC, Lopez-Mayor JF: Postoperative wound infection: a prospective study of determinant factors and prevention. Surgery 66:97, 1969

46. Sanders CV, Luby JP, Johanson WG, et al: Serratia marcescens infections from inhalation therapy medications: nosocomial outbreak. Ann Intern Med 73:15, 1970

47. Scott CC: Laminar/linear flow systems of ventilation; its application to medicine and surgery. Lancet 1:989, 1970

48. Slotnick IJ, Mackey WF: Observations on anaerobic bacteria in the female urinary tract. Am J Obstet Gynecol 99:413, 1967

49. Slotnick IJ, Tulman L: A human infection caused by an Erwinia species. Am J Med 43:147, 1967

50. Symonds N: Antibiotic resistance in bacteria. Postgrad Med J 48:216, 1972

51. Tillotson JR, Finland M: Bacterial colonization and clinical superinfection of the respiratory tract complicating antibiotic treatment of pneumonia. J Infect Dis 119:597, 1969

52. Walker DL, Hanson RP, Evans AS (eds): Latency and Masking in Viral and Rickettsial Infections. Minneapolis, Burgess, 1953

53. Williams REO, Blowers R, Garrod LP: Hospital Infection: Causes and Prevention. London, Lloyd Lube, 1969

EDITORIAL COMMENT

From a practical point of view, sterilization of a busy endoscopic unit can create problems. Dr. Slotnick clearly outlined the fundamental aspects of the various modes of sterilization and the interaction of sterilization technique and infective agents. There are slight variations between institutions, but in general a consensus has formed over the years.

Steam (Autoclave) Sterilization

Autoclaving is the most efficient form of sterilization, but this system was designed for surgical hardware. The high temperature of 273 F (134 C) at a pressure of 20 pounds/sq inch (59 kg/cm²) can destroy an endoscope completely. Some of the rigid telescope manufacturers do not exclude steam autoclaving of the telescopes if it is done with meticulous care. The telescope must be wrapped loosely in a perforated container. After it is removed from the autoclave under sterile conditions, an extended time is required for cooling. This procedure cannot be expedited by rinsing it with cold sterile water because this has a damaging effect on the properties of different materials (e.g., metal and glass) that have been combined in the construction of the instrument. Even if it is done as recommended, the life of the telescope is shortened. The small objective lenses at the working end or the cover glass on the other end of the eyepiece are cemented at both ends to seal the glass components from the outside and the metal sheet. If this hermetic seal is broken, water enters the system. Flexible fiber endoscopes are destroyed if they are inadvertently steam sterilized.

Metal accessories of various endoscopes can be steam sterilized, but instruments made of metal and covered by plastic insulation—or, for example, trocars in which the sleeve is made of insulated material (plastic) but the rest of the cannula (valve) etc. is made of metal—can also suffer at the joint spaces of the two materials. The various shrinking and distention factors of the different materials during the heating or cooling process are responsible for this. We do not use steam sterilization for the more delicate parts (telescopes), insulated materials, and fiberscopes.

Rigid Endoscope System

There are two alternatives for sterilizing rigid endoscopes: cold or gas sterilization.

Cold Sterilization.   Each hospital, particularly the urology department, has its own established policy. Instruments must be carefully cleaned before they are put into the soaking fluid. The recommended time of this disinfectant immersion should be carefully followed. If this time is significantly extended, it can cause early damage on the vulnerable part of the endoscope. The rinsing time should also be observed. We prefer Cidex (aqueous glutaraldehyde).

Gas Sterilization.   If possible we use gas sterilization for our rigid instruments. If the instruments must be used in several urologic cases, after the first (gas sterilized) session the instrument is carefully cleaned and, because of the shortage of time, soaked in Cidex. Gas sterilization also requires that certain parameters be controlled: gas concentration, gas temperature, time of sterilization, humidity, and vacuum. If we have only one case per day, gas is the method of choice.

Flexible Fiber Endoscopes

We wash and clean flexible fiber endoscopes according to our policy described in Chapter 7. There are exceptions where these endoscopes must be sterilized, e.g., after use in patients with active tuberculosis, positive Australia antigen tests, or other infections. In these instances we are careful with the rinsing and cleaning (personnel should wear rubber gloves), and an attempt is made to dry the channels properly before gas sterilizing the instrument. Cultures are taken from rinsed channels if there is any doubt about the effectiveness of sterilization.

There were questions raised in respect to the transfer possibility of hepatitis virus. Despite the large number of upper and lower gastrointestinal examinations, we have little knowledge about reported infections that can be traced back to an infected scope. Therefore I assume that the risk is perhaps theoretical rather than practical. An asymptomatic bacteremia can occur after a simple rectosigmoidoscopy.

In cases of flexible fiber bronchoscopy, it is recommended that flexible fiber endoscopes be soaked if several cases are scheduled for the same day. This must be done with extreme care. The viewing end containing the control mechanism cannot be immersed in the disinfectant fluid.

If there is the slightest hint that a wound or other infection is related to an endoscopy procedure, the case should be followed up precisely by the nurse and doctor to make sure that it was caused by an infected instrument—and if so, how such an event can be avoided in the future.

The key point of sterilization and problems which can occur is the training and skill of the nurse in charge.

THE EDITOR

9

Training of Nurses

Margaret McQueen

The training of nurses should not be interpreted as mere task orientation. As with all professional activities the quality as well as the degree of education greatly affects performance.

The tremendous impact of endoscopy during the past decade has certainly demonstrated the need for specialized knowledge and skill in the area of surgical nursing. The issue of the nurse-generalist versus the nurse-specialist presents itself again in this day of apparently never-ending subspecialization. Whichever philosophical approach one prefers, the basic need for developing this service presents us with the facts that the generalist must be further trained in this area.

Along with the expansion of an endoscopic department comes the large inventory of costly instrumentation with an even larger number of accessories. The use and care of these instruments can hardly be committed to memory without a thorough understanding of the procedures.

It became necessary for us to have two or three individuals undergo this additional training initially. It involves a desire and commitment by the members of the team—nurses and physicians—as well as the nursing administration, to allow time for orientation to the various procedures and care of the instruments. It further required that assignment to this area would be constant, since development of the service greatly depends on the growth of its members. It is of paramount importance that each member of the team share and respect the knowledge and contributions of each individual.

The time involved in this training program comprises several months. The aim of the procedure, the steps, and the possible complications are emphasized. Complete familiarization with the instrumentation, including assembling, disassembling, maintenance, and repair, as well as cleaning, wrapping, sterilization, preparation, anesthesia, and administrative procedures of the endoscopic examination are covered. Communication must exist between the manufacturer's representative and these endoscopy specialists.

After the initial 4- to 5-month period additional nursing personnel are exposed to selected procedures. The nursing instructor is the ideal person to rotate through the endoscopy room until expertise is achieved. She may then assist in the general operating rooms in teaching the staff.

Since in our institution we currently perform an average of five colonoscopies per week (requiring two nurses) and an average of two laparoscopies per day in the general operating rooms, the obvious procedure for the staff to learn was laparoscopy. The purpose of the procedure with the various steps and the use of instrumentation was presented by the endoscopy specialists and the instructor. This was repeated to small groups of scrub and circulating nurses. Repeat demonstrations with verbal presentation of each step was required. Verbalization has proved valuable for learning, since usually only the operator has visual access to the field. The size of the group that seemed to work best comprised three or four students. The following day, or as soon as possible, the instructor and/or endoscopy nurses served as back-up people for the nurses involved with laparoscopies in the general operating rooms.

Complete care of the instruments still remains the responsibility of the nurses in the endoscopy room, and they are informed of problems or breakdowns that occur during the day. They are further responsible for taking the necessary action for correction, repair, and additional instruction when indicated.

Concurrently, we rotate nurses through the endoscopy room for a period of time to acquaint them with additional procedures and care of equipment under direct supervision. It is imperative that all staff members gain a high respect for these instruments, since the cost of loss or damage is prohibitively high and results in a lesser quality of service to the patients.

Our program is by no means complete. It must be considered an ongoing program to increase the level of expertise for all nursing personnel. It has been successful, however, in virtually eliminating the frustration felt when it is recognized during a procedure that certain vital parts are missing and not sterilized; significant time is wasted while the patient is anesthetized until the missing part is located or a problem in faulty assembly is corrected. Regardless of whether the system employed for handling the materials is centralized or decentralized, the responsibility for educating and training individuals involved in any way with endoscopy procedures and/or equipment must be given great thought and planning because the cost of loss is extensive and high.

10

Endoscopy Room

Margaret McQueen

In a hospital with the subspecialities gastroenterology, urology, and gynecology, to name a few, and where the endoscopic service is active, it is certainly desirable to have instrumentation with accessories that are as much alike as possible in order to facilitate interchangeability. This standardization approach to endoscopy instrumentation is greatly advantageous in the administrative, operation, and budgetary control of these great expenditures. Maintenance, repair, and replacement costs may be greatly affected and reduced if the personnel handling the equipment are completely familiar with it and recognize the similarities rather than having the additional burden of unnecessary differences. The *individual preference approach can be extremely expensive* in terms of the operation and life expectancy of the equipment. It therefore behooves the buyer to choose instruments carefully, with as much expert input during the evaluation prior to purchase as is possible.

ENDOSCOPY OPERATING ROOM

When surgical suites are centralized, it is advantageous to have a room in the same area designated for endoscopy. This arrangement has proved very safe and efficient for us. The endoscopy service is used by other subspecialities and is upgraded in quality as well as quantity because appropriate equipment as well as qualified personnel and additional resources are readily available for patients' needs.

Although not used for general surgery, the endoscopy room should contain wall outlets for suction, oxygen, and compressed air. The size of the room should be such that space is available to accommodate additional or auxiliary equipment in the room as well as the work space (Fig. 1). A minimum of 16×20 feet is advisable to provide comfortable working conditions.

We set up bench space in the room for cleaning, dismantling, and assembling equipment. This is ideal for the purposes of care and control of the equipment. The danger of costly endoscopic instruments being damaged by carelessness or by stacking large, not so delicate instruments on top of them is virtually eliminated. It is further helpful to the nursing staff to have these highly specialized instruments cleaned, assembled, and stored in this central area.

Adjacent operating rooms are used for those procedures that .require meticulous sterile technique and general anesthesia (i.e., laparoscopy, choledochoscopy, encephaloscopy, arthroscopy, etc.). Instrumentation is still distributed from and returned to the endoscopy room. The same applies for cystoscopy, which is performed in the cystoscopy room for which there are similar requirements.

As one may imagine, storage could well become a problem. We strongly advise that separate storage areas especially for endoscopy be identified. Within the room itself recessed cabinets (Fig. 1) are very helpful for storing of instruments. The see-through (glass) cabinets, although locked, allow easy visibility for locating the instruments (Fig. 2). Valuable floor space is not compromised when wall-mounted facilities are utilized. Even the electrosurgical unit may be wall-mounted (Fig. 3).

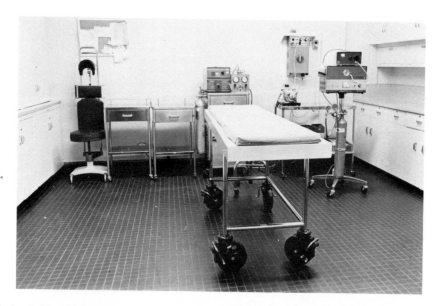

FIG. 1. A 16 × 20 foot area with a large amount of cupboard space on both sides. Recessed cabinets occupy one wall of the endoscopy room. Sufficient storage space is important.

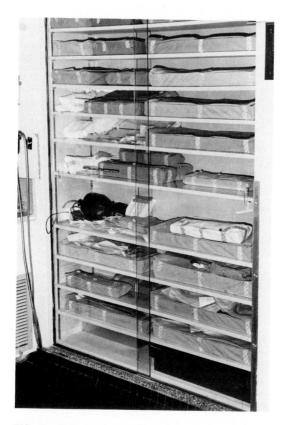

FIG. 2. See-through glass cabinets with locks allow easy location of prepared (sterilized) trays.

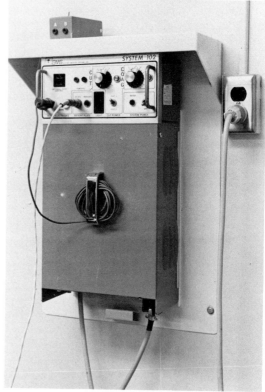

FIG. 3. The electrosurgical unit is wall-mounted, saving floor space.

A large amount of ancillary equipment is required during modern endoscopic procedures. X-ray apparatus with image amplification and television fluoroscopy are among the more common (Fig. 4) as well as among the most expensive. When damaged, the cost of repair or replacement may be exorbitant. This is one reason we recommend that a separate storage space be provided for this equipment alone. The traffic in and out of this area should be for the sole purpose of securing these items for endoscopy. It is essential that the personnel involved here be knowledgeable in the care and handling of these instruments.

Within the endoscopy room the surgical table must be radiolucent to fulfill the criteria for radiology. An x-ray viewing box is obviously needed. The lighting should be ceiling-mounted fluorescent tubes with a dimmer switch. Subdued illumination during certain examinations (e.g., gastroscopy, esophagoscopy, colonoscopy) may be necessary. Electrical outlets—one 220-volt plug (for a mobile or fixed-installation x-ray equipment)—and a sufficient number of 110-volt plugs (10 amp each) are necessary.

Some additional general aspects required in the endoscopy room are a separate suction unit with adequate (700 to 800 mm Hg) vacuum and light source(s) for the endoscopy instruments. We have found it satisfactory to keep these items on carts, which also facilitates mobility when needed in other rooms. Conductive floor tiles are not essential in this operating room provided a sign is clearly displayed on the door indicating that explosive anesthetics should not be used.

In addition to an emergency communication system, an intercommunication link with the central nursing station and a telephone with a light indicator is desirable. This reduces the time and motion required for nonemergency communication, and the light indicator on the telephone eliminates the startle reaction of patients under local anesthesia to a shrill bell.

In teaching institutions audiovisual intercommunication outlets (coaxial cables) are of great value. Postgraduate educational programs may be presented to large audiences by displaying the endoscopic procedures "live" via a black and white or color television chain; this provides ideal viewing without the disturbance of numerous observers in the room.

Procedures such an indirect laryngoscopy, esophagogastroduodenoscopy, colonoscopy with or without polypectomy, sigmoidoscopy, etc. are sometimes performed on an outpatient basis and are scheduled in the endoscopic operating room. In such cases facilities must be available to accommodate the outpatient's needs, such as a changing room, a couch, and toilet. It is

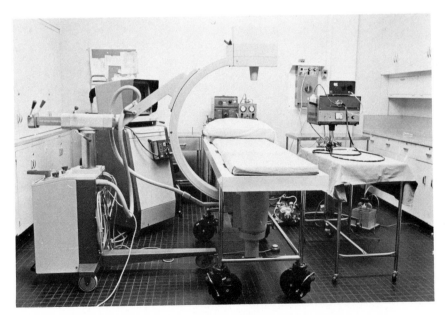

FIG. 4. Mobile image amplifier with television fluoroscopy. The top of the table is radiolucent. Stand-by fluoroscopy is a prerequisite for modern endoscopy. For details, see Chapter 17.

sometimes necessary to have the outpatient recover in this room, in which case nursing observation and care must also be provided.

One must always bear in mind that these examinations and treatments are never completely without risk. Awareness of the possibility of complications brings with it the responsibility for monitoring the patient's vital signs and immediate accessibility to equipment which may be required for any emergency (resuscitation). Cardiac or respiratory arrest protocol must be defined as in other operating rooms. An emergency signal to alert additional personnel is vital. The general operating room "crash" cart must be available for emergencies occurring during endoscopic procedures.

In addition to the routine paperwork of the operative procedure, we keep a separate log in the endoscopy room. We record every procedure performed in this area with the following data: continuous (chronologic) number; date; patient's name and hospital number, age, and sex; biopsy (yes or no); film (yes or no); in- or outpatient; examiner, assistant, and nurse;

remarks. From this log it is easy to establish a cross index of patients and procedures with corresponding pathology and operative reports, which are then available to staff members for statistical or other evaluations, preparation of publications, etc. The documentation on still or ciné strips are all provided with the corresponding log number, which facilitates identification of the patient and/or procedure, as well as the respective pathology. Fourteen types of endoscopic procedure are performed in our institution on adults and children. They amount to 15 to 20 percent of the total number of surgical procedures. As the service continues to expand, we are faced with the corresponding challenge to grow also.

Planning, organization, education, and supervision are directly related to the success of the service. By the same token, the hard work, dedication, and innovation required of medical and nursing staff are more than compensated for with the satisfaction experienced by these professionals in their continuous efforts to improve patient care.

11

Basic Principles of Ultrasound

Bodo Terhorst

In the field of urology methods have been devised by which stones in the kidney, ureter, bladder, and urethra can be dissolved without surgery, or disintegrated and removed transurethrally. While litholysis has been successful only with urate stones, the disintegration of bladder stones by means of electrohydraulic shock waves using a Russian URAT I device may be applied to all types of stones.[5] Its success in clinical application is inconstant, and the attendant dangers and complications are by no means negligible.

In 1953 Mulvaney[10] attempted for the first time to destroy urinary calculi by ultrasonic waves. More comprehensive were the experiments conducted three years later by Lamport and Newman[7] and Coats.[3] The latter tried unsuccessfully to destroy urinary calculi in a glass through the medium of water using ultrasound. After five minutes of ultrasonic treatment at 350 kilocycles/second (Kc/second) and 5 watts, a certain diminution in the resistance of the concrements occurred so that they could be crumbled between the fingers more easily.

Takahashi[15] and his team in 1964 were able to destroy urinary calculi in ultrasonic experiments at frequencies of about 20 Kc/second. Three years later Ouchi and Takahashi[11] reported on an ultrasonic device having a frequency of 29 Kc/second, an amplitude of 20 μm, and a power of 40 watts. In this device the sound conductor is connected at the end with a probe 70 cm long and 0.8 to 1.0 mm diameter. A ureteral calculus is trapped by a noose, the probe is placed near the concrement via a ureteric catheter, and the stone disintegrated. In spite of the intriguing concept there

are no definite clinical results as yet owing to the few and isolated applications of this technique.

Attempts to disintegrate bladder stones were made also in Italy by Pavone et al.[12] and Leone et al.[8] These authors noted that when an ultrasonic probe is advanced to the concrement any stone disintegrates, and they proved in animal experiments that ultrasound does not damage the wall of the bladder either macro- or microscopically.

Since 1968 physicians and technicians in the Federal Republic of Germany have been engaged in destroying bladder stones through ultrasonics, i.e., by "ultrasonic lithotripsy." Departing from the experience that the concrements can be disintegrated only if an ultrasonic probe is brought against the stone,[9] ultrasonic lithotriptors have been developed for the disintegration of bladder stones and have been clinically applied.[4,17,19] In spite of the reports by Ouchi and Takahashi,[11] attempts to disintegrate ureteral stones are still in an experimental stage.

PRINCIPLES OF ULTRASONIC WAVES

Acoustic frequencies beyond the range of audibility of the human ear are called ultrasonic waves. These are mechanical waves covering a frequency range of 20,000 to 10^{10} vibrations, or cycles. Being mechanical waves they cannot expand in a vacuum, only through a medium. This propagation occurs longitudinally in gases and liquids, and longitudinally and transversally in solid bodies.

Ultrasonic waves are generated in different ways.[1] They can be produced mechanically, thermally, electrostatically, magnetostrictively, and piezoelectrically. In practice, the magnetostrictive and piezoelectric ultrasonic transmitters are of principal importance. In the magnetostrictive effect the length of the metal rods is changed by magnetic energy, this magnetostriction causing ultrasonic waves. In the case of piezoelectric effect, high-frequency electric vibrations are converted into intensive mechanical vibrations. In ultrasonic lithotripsy the ultrasound is produced by the piezoelectric principle. The wavelengths of ultrasound are very small. This results in the following essential properties of ultrasound[13]: extremely high-energy densities may be produced to an extent far exceeding the range of audibility. Moreover, these short ultrasonic waves can be easily bundled so as to produce a radiation similar to that of light. These properties of concentrating high-energy densities to a small area suggested the possibility of disintegrating stones.

Technical Fundamentals

It had been known that the disintegration of urinary calculi by ultrasound in the bladder or ureter could be effected only by directly contacting the stone with a vibrating rod-shaped probe.[3,7,10,12] This probe transmits the impact forces to the stone. An abrasive ultrasonic treatment is achieved in the same way that hard, brittle materials are approached in the field of engineering.

To examine the drilling and disintegrating mechanism, the urinary calculus was forced by means of a lever having a certain contact pressure against the ultrasonic transducer, and the drilling path was measured by an inductive path recorder and recorded by a suitable device against time. It was found that constant abrasion could not be produced with a plain transmitting surface on the probe. The results improved when the ultrasonic transducer was designed as a tube (probe) whose working surface was provided with teeth to enter the concrement like a chisel.[14] The results showed, furthermore, that stones of different chemical composition can be disintegrated. Ultrasound-resistant urinary calculi were not encountered.[16]

The density of the stones examined varied between 1.5 and 1.8 g/cm³ with their hardness varying from 20 to 200 high frequency (HV) 0.025 (microhardness test on ground samples). The initial drilling speed was greater with soft than with hard stones; the speed decreased with both stones when the probe drilled deeper. The motional amplitude is dampened and the removal slowed down because of the diminishing relative movement between the drilling probe and stone. On the whole, the drilling speed was highest with phosphate calculi and average with lithic acid and cystine stones; calcium oxalate stones offered the greatest resistance to ultrasound.

The importance of selecting the proper contact pressure to obtain the optimal drilling speed became evident in further experiments. The ultrasonic effect is decreased when the contact pressure is excessive or too low. With low forces the ultrasound is rendered ineffective, and with excessive forces the ultrasonic probe is greatly dampened so that the relative movement between stone and probe is no longer maintained. The optimal contact pressure was found to be 20 g/mm length of the bit (Fig. 1), which in clinical application is currently applied by suction pressure.[14]

Examinations conducted on the pulse transmission of oscillating surfaces showed that the chatter vibrations of an elastic body may be utilized to increase the impact forces in the disintegration of urinary calculi. To do so, an impact body of hardened steel is inserted between

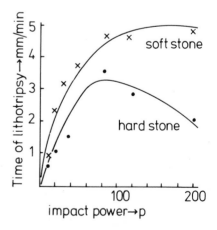

FIG. 1. Time of lithotripsy as a function of contact pressure of the probe against the stone.

the point of the probe and the urinary calculus, the body being firmly mounted on the probe point; owing to its relatively low contact pressure it is capable of considerably reducing the time required to disintegrate large urinary calculi.[2]

In summary, analysis of the experiments showed that the lithotripsy time is a function of such technical components as the ultrasonic probe itself, counterpressure, and stone-related factors, e.g., size of stone, as well as its density, hardness, and chemical composition.[16]

Biologic Fundamentals

Two probes were developed for ultrasonic lithotripsy: (1) a plain, hollow probe of monel; and (2) the impacted probe. As outlined above, the ultrasonic probe point was reinforced by an easily movable impact body. If a relatively light contact occurs between the probe point and the stone, the elastic impact body is rocked back and forth until its kinetic energy is sufficient to blow off a piece of the stone.

To determine any side effects produced by use of the two probes, 30 opened urinary bladders of rabbits were subjected to ultrasonic treatment. The amplitude, frequency, and probes were varied, and the perforations, temperature effects, epithelial changes, and impact and suction effects were studied.

The bladder wall was not perforated after application of conventional frequencies of 20

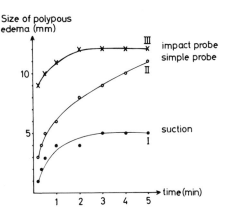

FIG. 3. Size of polypous edema as a result of ultrasonic and suction effects.

Kc/second and an amplitude of 15 to 20 μm, even when the bladder wall was subjected to the ultrasonic treatment for a period of 5 minutes (Fig. 2). Macroscopically, edema developed with surrounding hyperemia. If the amplitude was increased to 30 or 40 μm, perforations could be artificially produced, but these amplitudes are impracticable for clinical application. Such artificial perforations are more easily produced with the plain probe than with the impacted probe (Fig. 2) using the same amplitude, so that the more efficient probe also has a higher affinity for tissue.

Polypoid formations were observed as a function of the duration of the ultrasound and the suction effect (Fig. 3). Both probes produced such a change, which was attributed primarily to the suction mechanism of the ultrasonic lithotriptor. Histologically there was edema between the epithelium and muscularis submucosa, but no necrosis was observed. In general, the edema appeared, according to its extension, within six to eight days.[18,20]

The temperature of the bladder wall muscles was taken below the probe point as well as from an untreated place; these values were then plotted on a graph for comparison. In spite of the bladder surface being moistened with water, the temperature rose slightly. Following ultrasonic irradiation for 1 minute with the impacted probe the temperature increased 10 C, and that with the plain probe 31 C. On the whole, the impacted probe is more tissue-protective and efficient in lithotripsy than the plain ultrasonic probe.[18]

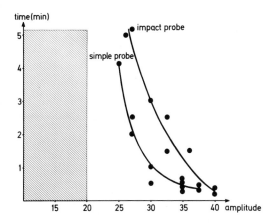

FIG. 2. Perforation of the urinary bladder as a function of the ultrasonic probe and the amplitude. Shaded area indicates the clinical range, no perforation.

REFERENCES

1. Bergmann C: Der Ultraschall. Stuttgart, S. Hirzel, 1949
2. Cichos M: Zum Mechanismus der Harnstein-zertrümmerung durch Ultraschall in Akutstik-und Schwingungstechnik. Berlin-Charlotten-burg, VDE-Verlag, 1972/1973
3. Coats EC: The application of ultrasonic energy to urinary and biliary calculi. J Urol 75:865–874, 1956
4. Gasteyer KH: Eine neue Methode der Blasen-steinzertrümmerung: die Ultraschall-Lithot-ripsie. Urologe [A] 10:30–32, 1971
5. Kierfeld G: Lithotripsie von Blasensteinen durch hydraulische Schlagwellenwirkung. Verh Bericht Dtsch Ges Urol 22, 1968
6. Knoch HG, Knauth K: Therapie mit Ultra-schall. VEB Gustav Fischer Verlag, Jena, 1972
7. Lamport H, Newman HF: Ultrasonic lithotresis in the ureter. J Urol 76:520–535, 1956
8. Leone G, Madonia S, Pavone-Macaluso M: Azione degli ultrasuoni sulla vesica. Arch Sici-liano Med Chir 6:1–8, 1965
9. Lutzeyer W, Pohlman R, Terhorst B, et al: Die Zerstörung von Harsteinen durch Ultraschall. I. Experimentelle Untersuchungen. Urol Int 25:47–63, 1970
10. Mulvaney WP: Attempted disintegration of calculi by ultrasonic vibrations. J Urol 70:704–707, 1953
11. Ouchi T, Takahashi H: Disintegration of uri-nary calculi by means of ultrasonic vibration. Presented to the 14th Internationale Gesellschaft für Urologie, München, 1967
12. Pavone-Macaluso M, Piazzi B, Pisani E: Ricer-che sulla litotrisia ultrasonica. Congr Padova 38:1–8, 1965
13. Pohlman R: Die Ultraschall-Therapie. Verlag Hans Huber, Bern, 1951
14. Pohlman R, Cichos M: Die Zertrümmerung von Harnsteinen durch Ultraschall. Presented to the Internatinal Congress on Acoustics, Budapest, 1971
15. Takahashi H, Ouchi T, Wagai T: Application of ultrasound in urology. Presented to the 13th Congress, International Urology Society, Lon-don, 1964
16. Terhorst B, Cichos M: Ultraschall zur Harn-steinzertrümmerung. Biomed Technik 16:106–108, 1971
17. Terhorst B, Cichos M: Ultraschall zur Harn-steinzertrümmerung. Biomed Technik 18:13–16, 1973
18. Terhorst B, Cichos M, Versin FJ, et al: Der Einfluss von Urat und Ultraschall auf das Uroepithel. Urol Res (in press)
19. Terhorst B, Lutzeyer W, Cichos M, et al: Die Zerstörung von Harnsteinen durch Ultraschall. II. Ultraschall-Lithotripsie von Blasensteinen. Urol Int 27:458–469, 1972
20. Versin FJ: Der Einfluss von Ultraschall und elektrohydraulischen Stosswellen auf das Uro-epithel. Inaugural Dissertation, Aachen, 1975
21. Wiedau E, Röher O: Ultraschall in der Medizin. Th. Steinkopf, Dresden-Leipzig, 1963

12

Clinical Applications of Ultrasound

Wolfgang Lutzeyer
Bodo Terhorst

Indications for ultrasonic lithotripsy are currently confined to calculi in the bladder, vesical diverticulum, and the urethra. The development of probes for application in the ureter are still in an experimental stage.

Ultrasonic lithotripsy is recommended for all bladder stones with a diameter exceeding 1.5 cm unless they can be simultaneously removed during an open suprapubic transvesical prostatectomy. Calculi having a diameter of less than 1.5 cm are more easily removed transurethrally by crushing forceps. All other concrements of any chemical composition can be destroyed by ultrasonics. This technique is recommended particularly if, at the same time or in a subsequent operation, the neck of the bladder is to be resected transurethrally.[3] Obstruction of the neck of the bladder (by the prostate, sclerosis of the sphincter) is the most common cause of bladder stone formation. Another possible application is lithotripsy of stones in the renal pelvis after a nephrostomy catheter has been introduced and if the ultrasonic probe can be approached through the stoma to the concrement.

Ultrasonic lithotripsy is contraindicated when there is urethral stenosis as this obstructs passage of the instrument into the bladder; the stenotic area should always be removed first. The procedure is also contraindicated during infancy and childhood since the urethra is too narrow for the instruments currently in use. A further relative contraindication may be found in *x-ray-negative* uric acid calculi in the bladder as they can be dissolved by alkalization of the urine. Owing to the invariably present concomitant infection, the obstruction of the passage at the bladder neck, and the associated increase in phosphate sedimentation, oral litholysis of urinary calculi is problematic.

If the patient is taking an anticoagulant it must be discontinued, lest the concomitant cystitis and impaired blood coagulation result in increased bleeding. Cystitis itself does not constitute a contraindication. After removal of the bladder stones, the infection heals with unimpeded passage.

ANESTHESIA

The criteria for operability are quite broad because general anesthesia is not required.[4,6] For nervous patients and those with contracted bladders we perform lithotripsy under spinal anesthesia; in other cases local anesthesia has nearly always proved sufficient. It is imperative, however, that premedication with a sedative and analgesic be applied.

TECHNICAL DESIGN

Ultrasonic Lithotriptor, "Aachen" Model

Following experimental investigations[2,5] and initial clinical tests with prototypes,[6] the ultrasonic lithotriptor, Aachen model, was developed in cooperation with the Storz Company* (Fig. 1A). The unit is composed of three

*Karl Storz Endoscopy Co., 72 Tuttlingen, Mittelstreet 8, West Germany. Distributor: K. Storz Endoscopy Inc. of America, Los Angeles, Calif.

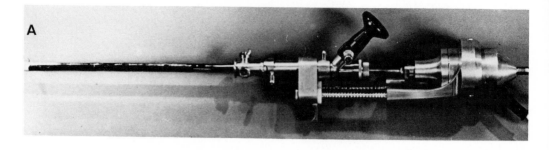

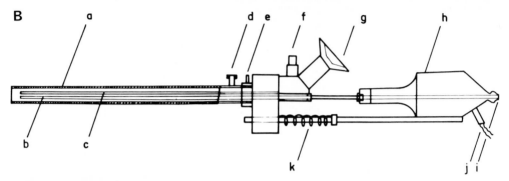

FIG. 1. **A.** Ultrasonic lithotriptor, Aachen type. **B.** Schematic view: a, Cystoscope shaft; b, Hollow ultrasonic probe; c, Telescope; d, Water inlet; e, Bayonet lock; f, Fiber light inlet; g, Eyepiece of optics; h, Ultrasonic transducer; i, Connection to suction; j, High frequency cord; k, Guide rail for transducer and probe movements.

elements: a conventional cystoscope, a piezo-electric ultrasonic transducer, and an interchangeable ultrasonic probe. An extremely short, light ultrasonic transducer was developed to facilitate manipulations. This piezoelectric transducer is subdivided for transformation of the motion amplitude. Its length is about one-third that of a conventional transducer of similar performance.

The ultrasonic transducer* is supplied from a radiofrequency alternator (Fig. 1B). The ultrasonic transducer is directly connected with the tubular ultrasonic probe, which slides through the cystoscope shaft.

The probe is made of a monel tube with an external diameter of 3.5 mm and a wall thickness of 0.3 mm. The free end of the probe is provided with teeth that are bent slightly inward; these serrations are designed to increase the surface pressure between stone and probe, thus producing a fine-grained dust capable of being aspirated. The cystoscope shaft may be separated from the ultrasonic unit by means of a bayonet lock. In a resting position the drilling probe is completely withdrawn in the shaft.

Laboratory of Ultrasonography, RWTH Aachen, Dr. R. Pohlman, 51 Aachen, West Germany.

During the operation the probe is advanced under visual control from the shaft toward the stone. Disintegration of the stone is observed through the cytoscope telescope; the generator is triggered by a foot switch. The hollow ultrasonic probe is connected to a suction pump via a hose to remove the minute stone fragments. Irrigation is performed through the cystoscope.

The piezoelectric ultrasonic transducer is operated at a frequency of 23 kilocycles (Kc) per second with a radiofrequency power input of about 30 watts. The vibration amplitude at the point of the drilling probe varies between 15 and 20 μm.

The ultrasonic lithotriptor developed by Gasteyer[1] has similar specifications, but without the features of simultaneous evacuation of the stone fragments and backward and forward movements of the probe.[1,2,4]

Bladder Stone Lithotripsy

The operation of the lithotriptor and performance of lithotripsy is so simple that its future application in urologic practice seems feasible. The patient is placed in the lithotomy position as for cystoscopy. No special preparation is required. A cystoscope shaft (Fr 24 or Fr 27) is first introduced into the bladder. After the obturator is removed, normal cystoscopy is performed. However, the ultrasonic probe with the attached ultrasonic transducer and telescope may also be introduced through the shaft at once. After the bladder is cleaned and distended, and the stone sighted, the probe is advanced until contact is made. When suction is started, the concrement usually adheres to the probe and is continuously reduced by the effect of the ultrasound. Additional pressure applied by the probe to the stone against the bladder wall increases the drilling speed. Irrigation and water drainage may be individually controlled. The loosened stone fragments are aspirated through the hollow probe, so that after the final lithotripsy the bladder is free of stones.

We normally proceed in such a manner that the probe is applied to a wide, flat surface of the concrement—if possible at a right angle in order to apply optimal suction and pressure. We always try in this fashion to drill a central hole into the stone (Fig. 2, Plate A*). The boundary areas are then quickly disintegrated and aspirated.

After the final stone remnants have been removed, a cystoscopy and/or x-ray film is made to make sure that all remnants have been removed. In many cases insertion of a postoperative indwelling catheter is indicated for 1 to 2 days. Antibiotics are administered and ample fluid intake prescribed to avoid an ascending pyelonephritis.

RESULTS

Since 1970, 237 bladder stones have been removed from 105 patients by ultrasonic lithotripsy, the concrements in question always having been 1 to 1.5 cm. The average age of the patients was 72 years (the advanced age possibly having contributed to the genesis of the bladder stones). In the majority of cases urinary passage had been impaired by an enlarged prostate or sclerosis of the sphincter, so that following lithotripsy we carried out a transurethral resection or freezing (cryosurgery) of the vesical cervix. Urethral stenoses

Note that all color plates appear together at the beginning of the book.

were first operated on, lanced, or treated with a bougie.

In agreement with our earlier experimental results, no ultrasound-resistant urinary calculi were found.[2–6] All stones could be disintegrated and aspirated. Infrared spectroscopic analysis of the stone crumbs revealed the composition to be magnesium-ammonium-phosphate in 50 cases (48 percent), oxalate-phosphate compound in 23 (22 percent), calcium oxalate in seven (6 percent), and uric acid in 25 (24 percent).

The time required for the entire lithotripsy procedure varied between 5 and 60 minutes. In regard to the litholapaxy time and the chemical stone composition, it was found that phosphate stones disintegrate most rapidly, followed by mixed stones and uric acid stones; pure oxalate stones resist ultrasonic treatment the longest.

The removed stone remnants consist of a fine grit with minute stone fragments (Fig. 3). With a large number of stones, the bladder must be rinsed thoroughly and care taken that the smallest stone particles have been washed out and the concomitant infection controlled. Often a permanent catheter is necessary.

COMPLICATIONS

The complication rate is remarkably low. In spite of the high average age of the patients, the primary mortality rate was only 0.8 percent. We encountered no operative or immediate postoperative mortality; one patient died on the seventh postoperative day owing to a severe, fresh myocardial infarction.

No perforations of the urinary bladder were observed.[3] Where the probe inadvertently irradiated the bladder mucosa, edema with surrounding hyperemia occurred after half a minute.

We often observed postoperative hematuria in patients with diffuse cystitis, but they never required a bladder tamponade or a blood transfusion. The bleeding usually stopped after 1 to 2 days.

The development of heat was low owing to the urine and water rinsing. Burns were not observed, even at the probe point, and a sensation of heat was never felt in the urethra either. With local anesthesia, pain registered only if the mucosa of the bladder was irradiated and subjected to suction. Care should

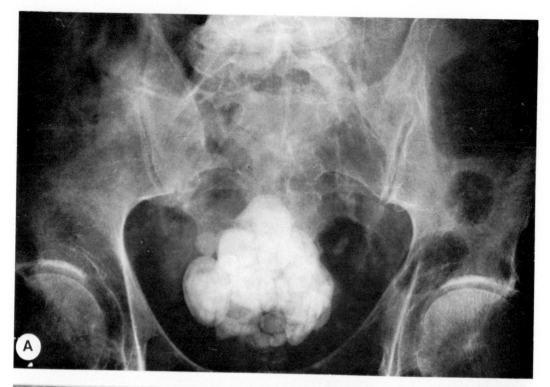

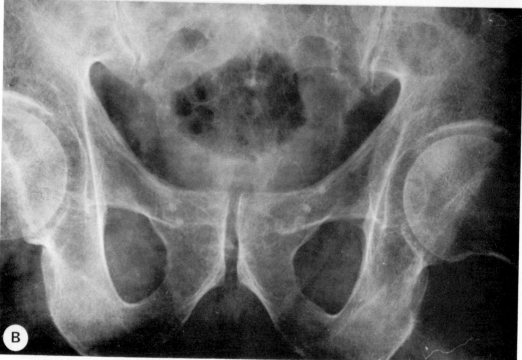

FIG. 3. **A.** Elderly (91-year-old) patient with bladder stones. Preoperative x-ray film showing multiple stones. **B.** Postoperative x-ray film from same patient without stone remnants. (Continued)

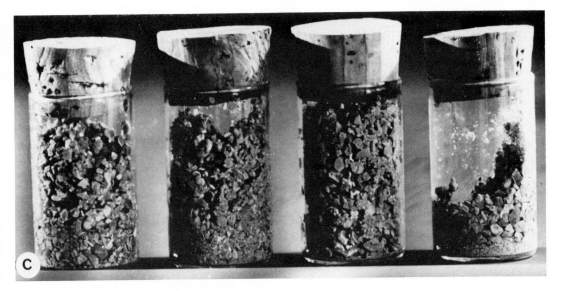

FIG. 3 (cont.). **C.** Aspirated stone fragments.

therefore be taken that the bladder is continuously filled with rinsing fluid, because an empty bladder carries the risk of bladder wall aspiration as well as increased risk of irradiation.

We occasionally found stone fragments on postoperative x-rays or endoscopic examinations that had escaped the 0-degree telescope vision. Complete removal of stones and restoration of a normal urethral passage are indispensable if recurrence of stones is to be avoided.[3]

SUMMARY

Ultrasonic lithotripsy offers a new possibility for treating bladder stones. The following advantages have been observed:

1. The risks of open surgery can be avoided.
2. Local anesthesia is usually sufficient, early mobilization is ensured, and the side effects of general anesthesia can be prevented.
3. The disintegration of stones is achieved under simultaneous visual control.
4. The backward and forward movements of the ultrasonic probe facilitate the localization and irradiation of bladder stones.
5. There is no risk of perforation to the bladder wall.
6. All types of stone can be disintegrated, even in the immediate vicinity of the wall and in diverticula.
7. No serious side effects have so far been observed.
8. Through the simultaneous aspiration of stone remnants, an additional, tedious rinsing operation may be dispensed with.
9. The outpatient treatment of suitable patients having small stones and without severe cystitis is possible.
10. Improvements in technical details suggest the possibility of ureteral application in the foreseeable future.

REFERENCES

1. Gasteyer KH: Eine neue Methode der Blasensteinzertrümmerung: Die Ultraschall-Lithotrypsie. Urologe [A] 10:30–32, 1971
2. Lutzeyer W, Pohlman R, Terhorst B, et al: Die Zerstörung von Harnsteine durch Ultraschall. I. Experimentelle Untersuchungen. Urol Int 25:47–63, 1970
3. Terhorst B: Blasensteinbehandlung durch Ultraschall. Dtsch Arzteblatt 71:519–522, 1974
4. Terhorst B, Cichos M: Ultraschall zur Harnsteinzertrümmerung. Biomed Technik 18:13–17, 1973
5. Terhorst B, Cichos M: Ultraschall zur Harnsteinzertrümmerung. Biomed Technik 16:106–108, 1971
6. Terhorst B, Lutzeyer W, Cichos M, et al: Die Zerstörung von Harnsteinen durch Ultraschall. II. Ultraschall-Lithotrypsie von Blasensteinen. Urol Int 27:458–469, 1972

EDITORIAL COMMENT

The use of ultrasound energy to disintegrate stones in the bladder is an interesting procedure. The incidence of bladder stones varies according to the differences in population, as well as to other factors.

It is difficult to transmit ultrasound through a flexible transmitter. Roger Goodfriend reported (Urology 1:260, 1973) his success in the experimental animal using a ureteral catheter containing an ultrasound probe with irrigation possibilities. The removal of stones from the ureter without surgical intervention will be an exciting approach.

THE EDITOR

13

Laser Energy Sources in Endoscopic Surgery

Thomas G. Polanyi

Surgery with lasers consists in directing laser energy, most often focused, on the tissue to be operated (Fig. 1). A practical system for clinical surgery requires additional features, such as variable control of the power of the laser and easy positioning of the laser beam onto the operating site. A carbon dioxide (CO_2) laser system for general surgery is shown in Figure 2.[18] The laser beam exits from the top of the free-standing rolling cabinet and is directed into a *beam-manipulating arm* furnished with multiple mirrors located in rotary joints. A lens located in the *hand piece* allows the surgeon to direct the focused beam at the operating site with good positional freedom. On the cabinet are power and timing controls which permit the surgeon to deliver appropriate laser energy dosages to the tissues. A foot switch controls the exiting of the beam either for a preset time interval or for continuous application. The surgical laser shown in Figure 2 has been used extensively in experimental and clinical surgery. The major results of these investigations, operative techniques, and areas of applicability were reviewed in detail by Stellar et al.[19,20] In summary, the following attributes of surgery with CO_2 lasers have been found.

1. Hemostasis. Excellent as far as capillary bleeding is concerned. In some cases vessels up to 2 mm in diameter can be sealed off.[19,20]
2. Tissue evaporation from a distance. Tissue removal by vaporization in thin layers or small volumes with good hemostasis and no contact with the tissues even from a distance is the most striking characteristic of CO_2 laser surgery. Large tissue volumes can be removed readily where difficulty of access would require extensive mechanical tissue manipulation with ordinary surgery.

3. Visual control of tissue removal. The rate of tissue removal is under the surgeon's visual control. The effects of the CO_2 laser beam are limited to the immediate visually observable effects.
4. Minimal damage to remaining tissues. Damage to tissues adjacent to those removed is minimal.[8,9,21] The damaged zone depends on the power and exposure times used. In many cases where low power is used, as in microsurgery, the damaged zone consists of only a layer(s) of a few cells.[22]
5. Healing. All clinical findings so far indicate that CO_2 laser-operated tissues, with the possible exception of skin,[8] heal promptly without complication and with improved postoperative patient comfort.[5a,13,22]
6. Precision and control. Volumes of tissues having the diameter of the (effective) spot size and much less depth can be removed by vaporization. Epithelial layers only a few cells thick or tissue volumes of a few cubic millimeters can be controllably removed. The problem of precision in CO_2 laser surgery is one of instrument design.
7. Sterility. The CO_2 laser beam sterilizes as it cuts, as well as sealing off capillary circulation. It appears possible to operate with less risk in necrotic and infected tissues such as one finds, for example, in decubitus ulcers.[19]

In endoscopy and microsurgery the attributes of CO_2 laser surgery is significant. Clinical applications in surgery of the respiratory-digestive tract[23] and in gynecology[2] support this view.

CHARACTERISTICS OF LASER LIGHT SOURCES

There are certain characteristics and mechanisms of laser light sources that make *selected* lasers useful in surgery.

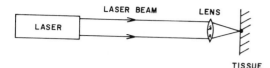

FIG. 1. Laser application.

Coherence of Laser Light

Laser light sources differ from other sources in that all the light they emit is coherent both spatially and temporally. This means basically that: (1) All the light emanating from a laser source propagates in a nearly parallel bundle; this is referred to as *spatial coherence.* (2) The wavelength spread of this light is narrow —much narrower than that of the best non-laser, monochromatic sources known; this is referred to as *temporal coherence.* Only in these quantitative ways does laser light differ from light from other sources.

For surgical applications the spatial coherence is the most important characteristic. It permits concentration of the entire energy emitted by the laser into the focal point of a lens. In the case of light sources that are not spatially coherent—all known nonlaser light sources—only a small fraction of the energy emitted can be concentrated in the focal point of a lens. Thus spatial coherence permits achievement of extremely high-energy density in a very small spot. The narrow wavelength spread of laser light is of little relevance in surgery. Of great importance, however, is the region of the spectrum in which the laser operates.

Time Behavior of Laser Emission

Laser light is emitted either in *pulses* or in a *continuous wave* (CW). The emission from solid lasers is typically in pulses lasting a fraction of a millisecond. A few solid lasers can be made to emit continuously at lower power. Gas lasers typically emit continuously, and their power output is generally better controlled. Currently only CW gas lasers are of importance in surgery.

Laser Devices

The basic phenomena that give rise to laser light are not discussed here as they are de- scribed in appropriate texts. A generalized laser device is shown in Figure 3.

Laser light—like all light—derives from selected systems of atoms, molecules, or ions. These can be in the gaseous, solid, or liquid state, and there are gas, solid, and liquid lasers.

A system of materials capable of producing laser light is referred to as a *laser medium.* Excitation energy must be supplied to the laser medium, and a fraction of this energy is re- turned by the laser in the form of coherent

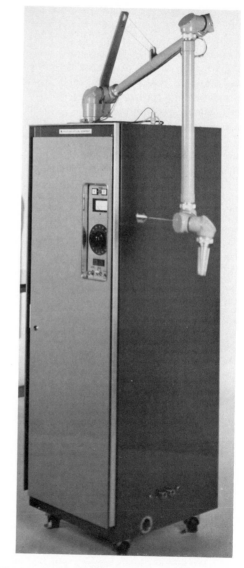

FIG. 2. Carbon dioxide laser system for general surgery. (Courtesy American Optical Corporation)

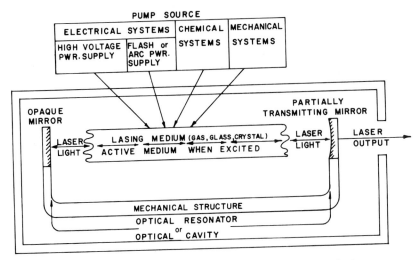

FIG. 3. Terminology and basic components of a laser device.

light. To supply energy is called *pumping the laser.* Usually in a gas laser the pumping energy derives from an electrical discharge through the gas; in a solid laser, energy derives from flashes of light, e.g., a xenon arc source. Chemical energy and electron bombardment are other possible pumping sources. When the laser medium is energized by pumping, it becomes an *active medium.* The laser medium generally has the shape of a narrow cylinder terminated at either end by mirrors, plane or spherical, having common axes coincident with the axis of the laser medium. The two mirrors and the mechanical structure keeping them in rigid alignment are referred to as the *optical cavity* or *resonator.*

Power Output. The laser medium within the optical cavity, activated by the pump energy, gives rise to laser radiation; this is emitted through one of the cavity mirrors, which is partially transmitting. The second mirror of the cavity is generally fully reflecting. The power output of a laser generally increases with the volume of the active medium and depends also on the pump intensity. The time behavior of the emission is characteristic of the laser medium and the pump. The degree of parallelism of the laser beam and its cross-sectional intensity distribution depend on the geometry of the optical cavity, i.e., the radii of curvature of the mirrors, their spacing, and the transverse dimensions of the mirrors.

Efficiency of Lasers. The ratio of the coherent power output of a laser to the pump power is the laser efficiency. It is important

because it gives an indication of the complexity and bulk of the total laser device. The higher the efficiency, the less complex the device.

Typical Laser Devices. Theodore Maiman set in operation the first ruby laser in 1959. Since then numerous other laser systems have been discovered, and today there are lasers in almost every region of the spectrum, from the near ultraviolet through the visible to the far infrared.

The power output of lasers covers the range from milliwatts to kilowatts in the CW mode and to megawatts in the pulsed mode. There are lasers that produce pulses as short as 10^{-12} seconds. However, *only rarely is it possible to find a laser operating in a selected wavelength region at a desired high power with a given time behavior of the emission.* The principal laser types of interest in surgery are as follows.

Ion Lasers. The active medium is a low-pressure ionized gas of the rare gas family or of a metallic vapor. The most used ones are the argon ion and krypton ion lasers. Each operates at several wavelengths of visible light: argon at 0.488 and 0.514 μ. The CW power output of commercial rare gas lasers can reach 10 to 15 watts. Their efficiency is low (0.1 percent or less), and so ion laser devices tend to be complex. For surgical purposes they are the energy source of choice for photocoagulation of the retina and blood vessel ablation in the eye.

Carbon Dioxide Lasers. The laser medium is CO_2 gas with nitrogen and helium added. These gas lasers operate in the infrared spectrum at several wavelengths around 10 μ

and have the highest practical efficiency of any known laser system (10 to 20 percent). Pumping is usually accomplished by an electrical discharge in the gas. For power outputs up to a few hundred watts or less, the gases are admitted from conventional high-pressure tanks to the discharge tube and exhausted to air continuously. In the discharge tube the pressure is between 10 and 60 torr. The power output is about 50 watts/meter of discharge length. A sealed tube containing the gases can be used at lower efficiency. It is currently the most useful laser for surgical applications other than ophthalmologic.

Solid-State Lasers. These lasers are mostly of historical interest in surgery:

1. Ruby laser. This is the first laser known. The laser medium is made up of chromium ions in a crystal of alumina. It operates at 0.69 μ, typically in the pulsed mode.
2. Neodymium in glass. This is one of the first lasers discovered. It operates at 1.06 μ in the pulsed mode.
3. Neodymium in yttrium-aluminum-garnet (Nd-YAG): This laser emits at 1.06 μ in the pulsed or CW mode. Pumping is through xenon arcs or tungsten iodide lamps. It has high efficiency, about 4 percent. Power outputs up to 200 watts have been reported.

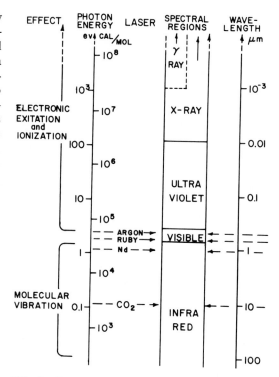

FIG. 4. Portion of the electromagnetic spectrum indicating major effects of radiation on matter and location of principal laser lines.

USE OF LASERS IN SURGERY

The use of lasers in surgery is based on: (1) the absorption properties of body tissues for electromagnetic radiation of certain wavelengths; (2) the high power density obtainable with focused laser beams; and (3) the existence of suitable-wavelength lasers having adequate power output. If the absorption of the laser energy in body tissues is sufficiently localized, at adequate power levels body tissues are vaporized—essentially reduced to steam at 100 C.[8,9] This is the basis of ablative surgery with lasers. The detailed process of tissue ablation is complex, but that tissue water limits the incision temperature to 100 C has been confirmed.[8,15,25]

Tissue-Radiation Interaction

The electromagnetic spectrum spans many orders of magnitude in wavelength. The major matter-radiation interactions that take place at an atomic or molecular level are illustrated in Figure 4. The magnitude of the interaction is measured by the amount of radiant power absorbed by a thin section of thickness t. In general the amount of radiant power incident and that exiting from a thin section are related by the expression

$$I = I_o e^{-\alpha t}$$

or the equivalent

$$I = I_o 10^{-t/L}$$

$I_o - I$ is the radiant power absorbed in the thickness t, α the *absorption coefficient; L*, the *extinction length,* the thickness of material in which 90 percent of the incident energy is absorbed. The larger the coefficient of absorption or the shorter the extinction length, the more *localized* the interaction. The coefficient of absorption alone gives no indication regarding the mechanism of the interaction. Absorption coefficients in vivo have been determined for only a few selected tissues, mostly skin and ocular media.

Energy, Absorption, and Power Requirements for Surgery

Ablative surgery is performed with the focused beam of a laser whose radiation is well absorbed by body tissues. Moving the focused spot along a line permits the excision or incision of tissues. This is how the "light scalpel" works. If the beam is made to cover progressively an extended area, a volume of tissue equal to the area covered multiplied by the depth of penetration is removed by progressive vaporization. To stop bleeding from large oozing surfaces, a broad beam with low power density is used.[6,7] The depth depends on the power density (power per unit area) of the beam and the absorption coefficient of tissues. Tissue removal should be fast enough (i.e., sufficiently high power should be used) to prevent heating healthy tissues by conduction and to afford reasonable operating speed compatible with adequate visual control. Assuming that tissues behave thermally like water and that the radiation used is fully absorbed, 2.5 joules is needed to transform 1 mm³ of water originally at 37 C into steam at 100 C; to accomplish this in 0.1 second requires a beam power of 25 watts. This simplified model is in good order of magnitude agreement with experience.

Time and power, and to a certain extent power density, can be traded within the limit of too much heat transfer to healthy tissues. Experimentally, for the microsurgical procedures explored so far, 10 to 25 watts in a 1 to 2 mm diameter spot is needed and for major surgery (e.g., burn debridement) up to 100 watts in a ⅓ mm diameter spot is appropriate.[14] Such power densities (300 to 15,000 watts/cm²) can be obtained only with laser energy sources.

The significance of the coefficient of absorption of tissues for the wavelength of the laser used is illustrated in Figure 5. The tissue is assumed to have thermal and absorption properties similar to those of water, and to be exposed to a laser beam having a gaussian cross-sectional intensity distribution, with a radius of 1.4 mm and a power of 5 watts. The increase in temperature (ΔT) at a level 100 μ below a surface that has been brought to 100 C is plot-

ted against the coefficient of absorption.[12] Tissue ablation takes place at 100 C ($\Delta T = 63$ C). The graph illustrates that the *localization* of tissue damage during ablation is a strong function of the coefficient of absorption.

Lasers Used in Surgery

Carbon Dioxide Laser. This is the only laser that so far has found application in clinical surgery, except ophthalmology where ion lasers and ruby lasers are used (vide infra). Its 10.6-μ radiation is strongly absorbed by body tissues (Fig. 6), which gives the absorption coefficient of water for radiations of 0.7 to 10 μ. Most cells have a large water content, and the absorption coefficient of water is a useful guide for that of body tissues. At the wavelength of operation of this laser, 90 percent of the energy is absorbed in a water layer 30 μ thick. Absorption data for tissues in vivo are generally not known. An extinction length for soft tissues of 100 and 200 μ agrees with experimental findings. Figure 4 indicates that the mechanism responsible for absorption is the excitation of vibrational levels. The effect of 10 μ radiation on tissues is purely thermal and highly localized. Macroscopically disruptive effects take place in tissues if energy is delivered in short pulses (less than a microsecond) typical of many solid-state lasers. This regimen of operation is not of interest in surgery. Figure 6 suggests that lasers operating at 3 or 6 μ might be even more effective than lasers at 10 μ. However, there are no lasers at this wavelength suitable for surgical experimentation. The absorption coefficient of all body tissues for 10 μ radiation can be expected to be uniformly high: *surgery with CO_2 lasers requires direct access of the laser beam to the tissues to be operated on.*

Ion Lasers. Argon ion lasers operating in the visible spectrum at 0.48 and 0.51 μ have a wavelength of operation ideally suited for retinal photocoagulation and blood vessel ablation through the *intact* ocular media, since for vision all tissues preceding the fundus must be transparent to visible radiation. In the fundus, however, visible radiation is absorbed. Blood also strongly absorbs in the blue-green region of the spectrum. An ion laser operating at 0.48 μ is well suited both for retinal photocoagulation and for the ablation of proliferating blood vessels. The CO_2 laser is totally unsuited for

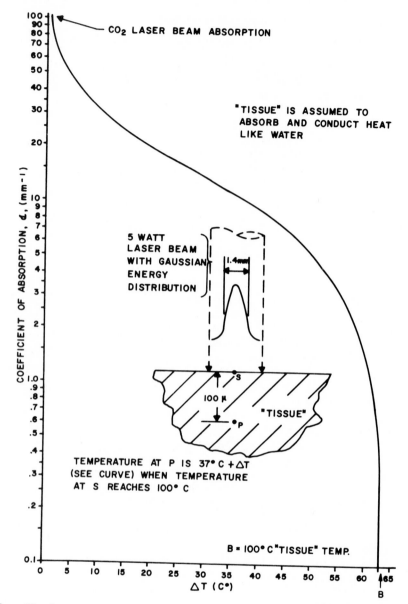

FIG. 5. A "tissue" having thermal and absorptive properties of water is exposed to a laser beam. The tissue point (S) exposed to the maximum intensity of the laser beam has just reached 100 C. The graph gives the rise in temperature (ΔT) at a point (P) 100 μ below S, as a function of the tissue coefficient of absorption (α) for the incident radiation. (From Johnson[12])

this task; its radiation would be absorbed at the cornea. The organ of vision is the only one in which it has been found possible to operate through intact tissue layers. It is likely to remain a unique case. Ion lasers so far have found surgical application only in the field of ophthalmology.

Solid-State Lasers. Of these, only the ruby laser is still used clinically for retinal photocoagulation. Experimental work is being

carried out with Nd in yttrium-aluminum-garnet.[5,16]

ENDOSCOPIC SURGERY WITH LASERS

The present use of lasers in endoscopic surgery is illustrated in Figures 7 and 8, slight modifications of Figure 1. The beam diameter

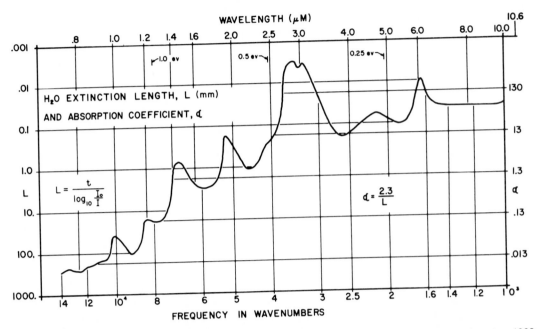

FIG. 6. Absorption coefficient of water between 0.7 and 10.0 μ. (From Bayly et al: Infrared Spectra, 1963. Courtesy of Pergamon Press)

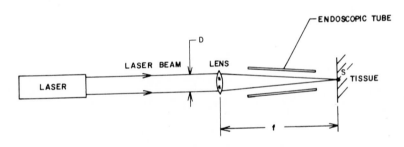

FIG. 7. Endoscopic surgery with lasers.

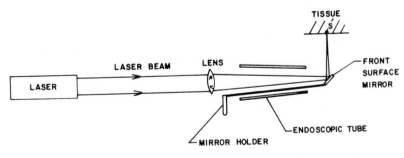

FIG. 8. Endoscopic surgery with lasers. Operative site is visualized via a mirror.

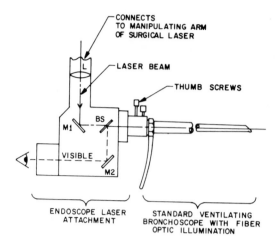

FIG. 9. Endobronchial surgery attachment to general surgery laser system seen in Figure 2. L, lens for 10.6 μ. M1, reflects 10.6 μ. BS, transmits 10 μ, reflects visible. (From Wallace and Pejchar[26])

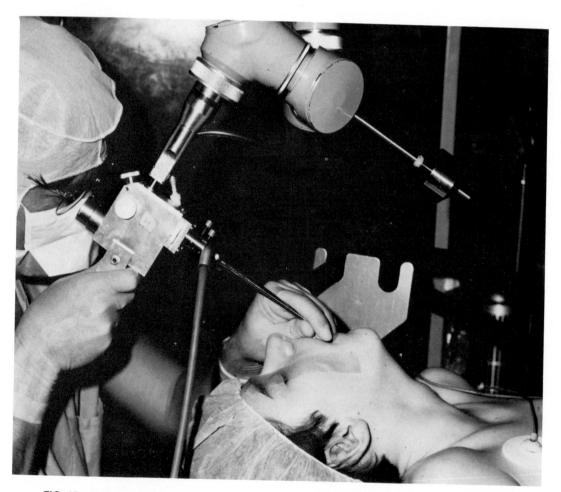

FIG. 10. Endobronchial surgery with attachment shown in Figure 9. (Courtesy of Dr. M. Stuart Strong, Boston University)

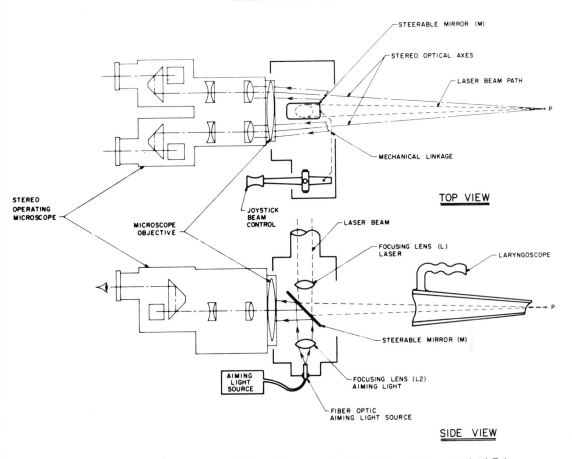

FIG. 11. CO_2 laser beam micromanipulator (heavy lines) for attachment to a standard Zeiss operating microscope. The manipulating arm of the surgical CO_2 laser shown in Figure 2 is attached as indicated.

(D) and the focal length *(f)* of the lens *(L)* are adjusted to allow focusing the laser beam through the endoscopic tube *(T)* onto the tissue site *(S)* seen either directly or via a mirror. The diameter of the focal spot *(s)* is limited by diffraction phenomena to the minimum value $s = 2\lambda f/D$, where λ is the wavelength used. In practical systems the spot size is generally larger than the theoretical minimum.

It would be desirable to transmit surgically effective laser beams through flexible fiber endoscopes.[16,17] The sole (and major) difficulty, as this author sees it, is that the only lasers available today for transmission through glass or quartz endoscopic fibers are ion lasers in the visible and the Nd-YAG at 1.06 μ. Goodale et al.[7] showed that hemostasis of bleeding stomach mucosa requires about 10 watts/cm^2 for 3 to 5 seconds of CO_2 laser radiation. The deeper penetration and smaller absorption by tissues for the visible radiation of ion lasers

and at the 1.06 μ radiation of Nd-YAG require the delivery of higher dosages with increased risk to underlying tissues. Tissue removal by vaporization with these lasers appears even more problematic.[5] Research activities in various laboratories will show whether these problems can be overcome or if we must wait for the development or the discovery of either an appropriate infrared laser whose radiation is well absorbed by tissues and is transmitted by glass or quartz, or a material suitable for flexible endoscopes and capable of transmitting both visible and CO_2 laser radiations.

Clinical Instruments for Endoscopic Surgery with CO_2 Laser

Monocular Endoscopic Instruments. One instrumental problem specific to surgery with a CO_2 laser beam is that the optical paths of this beam and of the light needed to vis-

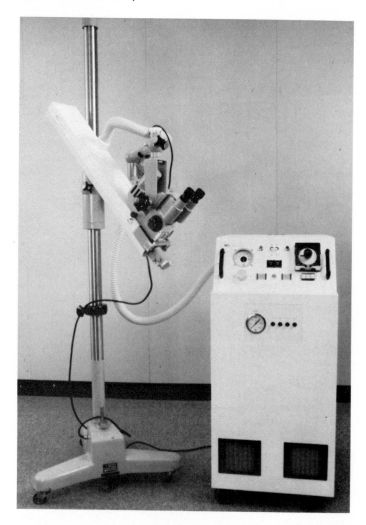

FIG. 12. CO_2 laser system for endoscopic microsurgery. Note the laser attached directly to the Zeiss operating microscope. (Courtesy of American Optical Corporation)

ualize the operating site cannot utilize the same optical elements throughout because materials transparent to both visible and the CO_2 laser radiation (and practical for surgical instruments) are not yet available.

Figure 9 shows the attachment to the laser of Figure 2[26] designed for endobronchial surgery. The different paths followed by laser and visible light are demonstrated. An experimental model in clinical use is shown in Figure 10. The articulated arm facilitates manipulation with a bronchoscope.

Binocular Endoscopic Microsurgical Instruments. In endoscopic laryngeal microsurgery the operative site is visualized by aiming the axes of a binocular operation microscope through an appropriate laryngoscope. The method shown in Figure 11 aims a CO_2 laser beam through the laryngoscope. The small rectangular mirror *(M)* located between the apertures of the binocular microscope and in front of the objective lens directs to the target tissue the laser beam focused by the lens *(L)*. The site is illuminated by fiber optical bundles located in the laryngoscope. An aiming light source *(S)* is projected by a lens *(L_2)* into the optical system of the microscope via a small mirror attached to *M*. The observer sees this point of light as located in *P*, onto which the laser beam is directed: it marks the site to be exposed to the laser beam when the surgeon actuates a shutter with a foot switch. A "joy stick" control permits fine positioning of the laser beam and marker in the visual field of the microscope by moving the mirror *(M)*. This *micromanipulator*[3] is attached to the microscope and connected to the articulated beam delivery arm of the surgical laser. This permits positioning of the operation microscope as needed.

The operating microscope, micromanipulator, and laser constitute an *endoscopic microsurgical laser* system. It was developed in the laboratories of the American Optical Corporation in collaboration with Jako.[11] Clinical experience with this system in laryngeal surgery is reported by Strong and Jako,[22] Strong et al.,[23] Andrews and Moss,[1] and in a chapter of this volume. Mounting the laser directly on the operating microscope (Fig. 12) leads to a more compact and versatile system. In this version of the microsurgical laser system, the operating microscope can be positioned as freely as without the laser. The laser has a power output of 25 watts, which is adequate for microsurgery.

APPLICATIONS OF ENDOSCOPIC CO_2 LASER SURGERY

The major clinical applications of endoscopic surgery with CO_2 lasers are currently in the larynx, bronchi, and other regions of the respiratory and digestive tracts.[1,5a,22,23,23a] These applications are reviewed in another chapter of this volume.

Promising initial clinical results have been obtained in gynecology for treating cervical erosion,[13] cervical intraepithelial neoplasia,[24] and vaginal adenosis.[2] Still in the experimental stage are applications to otology[27] and rectal[25a] and urologic[4,10a] pathology.

SAFETY AND HAZARDS

The CO_2 laser beam is potentially hazardous. It can ignite nonmetallic materials and cannot be used in explosive atmospheres. It is reflected by metallic objects. Ordinary plastic or glass spectacles absorb CO_2 laser radiation and in practice eliminate danger to the eyes. An understanding of the properties of this laser and of the potential hazards is necessary to make its use safe in operating rooms.

ACKNOWLEDGMENTS

I gratefully acknowledge the outstanding technical contributions by my colleagues Messrs. J. Pejchar and R. A. Wallace, and the invaluable technical assistance of Messrs. T. W. Davis and E. A. Goff.

I am most thankful to Messrs. W. M. Strouse and R. A. Wallace for their critical review of the manuscript and helpful suggestions, and Mrs. E. Phillips for her expert editorial assistance.

I would like to express my deepest gratitude to Dr. W. R. Prindle, Director of the American Optical Research Laboratories, whose help and encouragement made this project possible.

REFERENCES

1. Andrews AH, Moss HW: Experiences with the carbon dioxide laser in the larynx. Ann Otol Rhinol Laryngol 83:462, 1974
2. Bellina JH: Gynecology and the laser. Contemp Obstet Gynecol 4:24, 1974
3. Bredemeier HC: Stereo laser endoscope. US Patent No. 3,796,220, 1974
4. Ehrlich RM: Division of Surgery/Urology, University of California, Los Angeles. Private communication, 1974
5. Fidler JP: Department of Surgery, Cincinnati Medical Center. Private communication, 1974
5a. French RJ: Tonsillectomy with a carbon dioxide laser: alleviation of bleeding and pain. National Medical Association Meeting, New Orleans, 1974
6. Gonzales R, Edlich RF, Bredemeier HC, et al: Rapid control of massive hepatic hemorrhage by laser radiation. Surg Gynecol Obstet 121: 198, 1970
7. Goodale RL, Okada A, Gonzales R, et al: Rapid endoscopic control of bleeding gastric erosions by laser radiation. Arch Surg 101:211, 1970
8. Hall RR: The healing of tissues incised by a carbon-dioxide laser. Br J Surg 58:222, 1971
9. Hall RR, Beach AD, Baker E, Morison PCA: Incision of tissue by carbon dioxide laser. Nature 232:131, 1971
10. Hall RR, Hill DW, Beach AD: A carbon-dioxide surgical laser. Ann R Coll Surg Engl 48:181, 1971
10a. Hughes BF, Scott WW: Preliminary report on the use of a CO_2 laser surgical unit in animals. Invest Urol 9:353, 1972
11. Jako GJ: Laser surgery of the vocal cords. Laryngoscope 82:2204, 1972
12. Johnson JR: American Optical Corporation, Research Laboratories, Framingham, Mass. Private communication, 1974
13. Kaplan I, Ger R: The carbon-dioxide laser in clinical surgery—a preliminary report. Isr J Med Sci 9:79, 1973
14. Levine N, Ger R, Stellar S, et al: Use of a carbon dioxide laser for the debridement of third degree burns. Ann Surg 179:246, 1974
15. Mihashi S, Strong MS, Jako GJ, et al: Interac-

tion of CO_2 laser and soft tissue. Bioengineering Conference, Worcester Polytechnic Institute, 1974

16. Müssiggang H, Katsaros W: Laser in der operativen Medizin mit Möglichkeiten der Transmission über flexible Lichtleiter. Bruns Beitr Klin Chir 218:746, 1971

17. Nath G: Endlich das ideale Laser-Skalpell fur die Medizin aber auch zur Material-Bearbeitung. Laser Elektrooptik 1:49, 1972

18. Polanyi TG, Bredemeier HC, Davis TW Jr: A CO_2 laser for surgical research. Med Biol Engin 8:541, 1970

19. Stellar S, Meijer R, Walia S, et al: Carbon dioxide laser debridement of decubitus ulcers followed by immediate rotation flap or skin graft closure. Ann Surg 179:230, 1974

20. Stellar S, Polanyi TG, Bredemeier HC: In Wolbarsht (ed): Laser Applications in Medicine and Biology. Plenum Press, New York, 1974

21. Stellar S, Polanyi TG, Bredemeier HC: Experimental studies of the carbon dioxide laser as a neurosurgical instrument. Med Biol Engin 8:549, 1970

22. Strong MS, Jako GJ: Laser surgery in the larynx. Ann Otol Rhinol Laryngol 81:791, 1972

23. Strong MS, Jako GJ, Polanyi T, Wallace RA: Laser surgery in the aerodigestive tract. Am J Surg 126:529, 1973

23a. Strong MS, Vaughan CW, Polanyi T, Wallace Bronchoscopic carbon dioxide laser surgery. Ann Otol Rhinol Laryngol 83:769, 1974

24. Upton RT: Carbon dioxide laser surgery in the management of CIN. 6th Annual Meeting of the Society of Gynecologic Oncologists, Key Biscayne, Fla, 1975

25. Verschueren RCJ, Koudstaal J, Oldhoff J: The carbon dioxide laser; some possibilities in surgery. Acta Chir Belg 74:197, 1975

25a. Verschueren RCJ, Oldhoff J: The carbon-dioxide laser: a new surgical tool. Arch Chir Neerl 37:3, 1975

26. Wallace RA, Pejchar J: American Optical Corporation, Research Laboratories, Framingham, Mass. Private communication, 1974

27. Wilpizeski C, Reddy JB: Laser microsurgery: experimental middle ear procedures in monkeys. American Academy of Ophthalmology and Otolaryngology, 1974

EDITORIAL COMMENT

The author described the basic principle of laser energy and its application to medicine with emphasis on the CO_2 laser, which is one of his principal domains. The CO_2 laser beam cannot be transmitted through flexible media—only through rigid tubes. Corners can be bypassed or changes in direction of the beam achieved by special mirrors incorporated in articulated joints.

The introduction of flexible fiberscopes triggered the field of research for flexible laser transmitters, e.g., quartz fibers, plastic fibers, and flexible fluid transmitters (see Chapter 15). These flexible transmitters can be introduced through the biopsy channel of a fiber gastroscope, for instance, and the energy can be applied for coagulation from a distance. For these applications other types of laser energy were used, e.g., argon, neodymium.

The application of laser energy to achieve hemostasis through flexible endoscopes is in an experimental stage. Despite some sporadic previous reports appearing in the literature, we still do not have enough data to substantiate a correlation between the required energy output, beam-width, continuous or pulsed mode, and other physical parameter versus biologic effect. We need time, further simplification of instrumentation, and more biologic data to enable us to use it safely in our daily clinical work. However, it is an interesting new entity for hemostasis or dissection of structures during endoscopic or surgical procedures.

Kiefhaber recently reported the first successful treatment of GI bleeders with a Neodymium-Yag laser through a flexible scope.

THE EDITOR

14

Carbon Dioxide Laser Surgery: Endoscopic Applications

M. Stuart Strong

A carbon dioxide (CO_2) surgical laser was developed in the American Optical Gas Laser Research Laboratory in 1967, and it immediately became apparent that the instrument had potential for endoscopic application.[4] A prototype endoscope delivery system became available in 1968; it consisted of a cubical unit ($15 \times 15 \times 15$ cm) which contained the rotating mirror used to deflect the laser beam along the axis of the attached endoscope tube (20 mm $\times 30$ cm). This instrument demonstrated the feasibility of producing discrete lesions on the vocal cords of dogs.[3] Thereafter attention was devoted to the development and use of micromanipulator attachment to the Zeiss operating microscope (Fig. 1); using binocular visual control. Precise surgery could be carried out with the CO_2 laser on any tissue that could be viewed directly or indirectly in a mirror.

The animal experiments indicated that laser–soft tissue interaction had several desirable attributes: the target area was continuously under vision, bleeding was either minimal or absent, postoperative edema was conspicuous by its absence, the line of tissue destruction was clearly defined, healing was rapid, and postoperative scarring was minimal. These favorable attributes of laser surgery were immediately confirmed clinically in 1971.[5,6]

Experience was accumulated rapidly in the use of the micromanipulator laser attachment to the surgical microscope in the management of lesions of the nose, oral cavity, pharynx, and larynx. Involvement with cases of recurrent papillomas of the larynx that exhibited extension of the papillomas into the trachea and main stem bronchi indicated the need for a laser bronchoscope.

A standard Jackson-Pilling ventilating bronchoscope (5 mm $\times 30$ cm) was fitted to the original prototype laser endoscope attachment; it was found that the beam focused to a spot 2 mm in diameter at the end of the bronchoscope, and that it could be aimed adequately with the adjustment thumb screws.

Initial experience was gained by using the instrument in the canine trachea, using various mixtures of anesthetic gases including oxygen 100 percent, nitrous oxide 50 percent, and oxygen 50 percent with halothane and enflurane. It was found that these gases could not be ignited by the laser beam or its impact on the tracheal mucosa. The mucosa of the trachea could not be made to support combustion even in the presence of 100 percent oxygen. Occasionally if low power was used and a fragment of carbonized mucosa was allowed to dry out, an additional laser impact caused momentary incandescence of a tiny carbon particle in the presence of oxygen; if the carbonized fragment was moist, it did not glow after a laser impact.

With the availability of these additional data there appeared to be no contraindication to clinical application. This laser-bronchoscope assembly was used on 70 occasions during the management of various problems (mostly recurrent papillomas in 15 patients).[5] It was found that bronchoscopic laser surgery was associated with minimal bleeding, no visible postoperative edema, and rapid healing of the

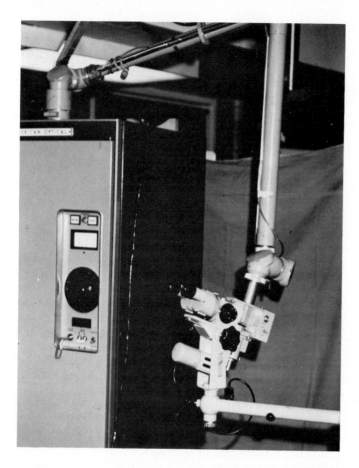

FIG. 1. Prototype CO_2 laser with the micromanipulator attachment to the surgical microscope.

mucosal defects. There were no complications directly attributable to the use of the surgical laser.

Because of this satisfactory experience, a second version of the laser endoscope delivery system was developed and became available in 1974. This attachment was small (3.5 × 7.0 × 7.5 cm), light (1 kg), and could be coupled very conveniently to the standard Jackson-Pilling ventilating bronchoscope (Fig. 2). The availability of the laser micromanipulator attachment to the Zeiss microscope and the laser endoscope attachment made possible a wide variety of endoscopic surgery with the CO_2 laser.

INDICATIONS FOR CO_2 LASER SURGERY

When *"nuisance" bleeding* is likely to obscure the field and make precise surgery difficult, surgery with the CO_2 laser should be considered. The capacity of this laser to main- tain hemostasis when dissecting mucosa, muscle, and fat is remarkable; only when a blood vessel measuring 0.5 mm or more is transected is the laser (using energy levels of 25 watts or less) inaffective in controlling bleeding.

Unwanted tissue destruction occurring coincidently with the removal of a lesion may impair function, e.g., of a mobile structure such as the vocal cord. CO_2 laser surgery allows precise removal of tissue and causes minimal unwanted heat coagulation of the walls of the surgical field; this may be as little as 50 to 100 μ depending on the power levels and time exposure.

Conventional surgical methods using diathermy or cryosurgery are often associated with *postoperative edema;* if postoperative swelling is likely to be a threat to the patient (e.g., in the airway) use of the surgical laser may be indicated. The lack of edema following CO_2 laser surgery is apparently related to the localized nature of the laser injury.

Inaccessibility of the surgical arena to ordinary surgical instruments may be an indica-

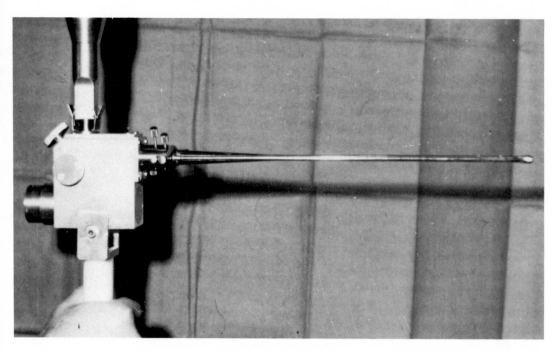

FIG. 2. A standard ventilating bronchoscope has been fitted to the laser endoscope attachment. An optional magnifying eyepiece can be fitted to the laser attachment. (From Strong et al.[7])

tion for the surgical laser if the target area is visible, either directly or in a mirror. Laser surgery allows controlled tissue destruction without placing the instrument in contact with the tissue.

CONTRAINDICATIONS TO USE OF A CO_2 LASER

Carbon dioxide surgery cannot be carried out in an *explosive atmosphere* because the effect of laser beam impact is entirely thermal. Combustible materials must be kept away from the target area. Fortunately the anesthesiologist now has no difficulty in maintaining anesthesia using noncombustible gases.

If the *lesion cannot be clearly seen,* surgery with the CO_2 laser may be either difficult or impossible. It is often possible to view an inaccessible area in a metallic mirror and to direct the laser with the same mirror.

When the *wound cannot be kept dry,* CO_2 laser surgery cannot proceed; in the presence of blood, cerebrospinal fluid, or urine, all of the laser energy is dissipated in vaporizing the liquid. With very high energy levels (100 watts), tissue destruction can proceed in the presence of blood, etc. (e.g., in experimental liver surgery).

Lack of difficulty with conventional methods of treatment is an indication that use of a CO_2 surgical laser is probably unnecessary. When the convenience of laser excision and conventional surgery are equal, the former offers the advantage that laser-induced wounds are associated with minimal discomfort.

ANESTHESIA

Surgical excision by a CO_2 surgical laser is achieved by vaporization and combustion of the tissues, which causes pain unless the area is anesthetized. Local anesthesia is entirely satisfactory when the exposure does not require general anesthesia; topical anesthesia with 4 percent cocaine may be adequate for a lesion of the nasal mucosa. In the oral cavity or on the skin, local anesthesia by infiltration with 1 percent lidocaine is usually entirely satisfactory. When general anesthesia is indicated, any type may be used provided the gases are noncombustible and there is complete control of the patient's airway.

If the CO_2 laser is to be used in the proximity

of an intratracheal tube, the tubes should be constructed of red rubber rather than polyethylene or Portex; red rubber tubes can be made to burn in the presence of oxygen, but much less readily than Portex or polyethylene. For intralaryngeal surgery the portion of the tube that lies within the larynx should be covered with a strip of self-adhesive aluminum; this affords complete protection of the tube from inadvertent laser impact (Fig. 3). The aluminum reflects the laser beam, and the convex contour causes diversion of the rays so that no significant damage to the adjacent soft tissues ensues.

TECHNIQUE AND EXPERIENCE

Nasal Cavity

Lesions accessible through the nostril or after lateral rhinotomy may be considered for laser excision if the usual methods of management are less than satisfactory. Recurrent papilloma (both squamous and inverted), cases of hereditary telangiectasia, and localized recurrence of adenoid cystic carcinoma have been managed with the CO_2 laser.

Anesthesia may be by infiltration if the lesion is on the skin of the nasal vestibule, or topical if it is on the mucosa; if lateral rhinotomy is needed for exposure, general endotracheal anesthesia is preferable.

The Zeiss surgical microscope is fitted with a 400-mm front lens and the micromanipulator laser attachment and is used to view the anterior one-third of the nasal cavity and vestibule. Exposure may be achieved with self-retaining or hand-held retractors. The microscope light provides marginal illumination at 400 mm from the target area, and this may need to be supplemented with light from a strategically placed fiberoptic light pipe.

In cases of hereditary telangiectasia the lesions on the anterior septum and anterior end of the inferior turbinates are first outlined with the laser using 10 to 15 watts of power; thereafter the lesion is excised down to the perichondrium without exposing the cartilage of the septum. Steam and smoke are removed from the operative field with a hand-held angled suction tube. Bleeding is either absent or trivial. If the patient keeps the nasal cavity moist, epithelialization takes place within 10 to 12 days without crusting.

Although inaccessible lesions in the depths of the nasal cavity are unaffected by this approach, all three patients so treated have had a marked reduction in the frequency and severity of epistaxis from the treated nostril. However, the follow-up period has been only 6 to 12 months, and it is impossible to know if telan-

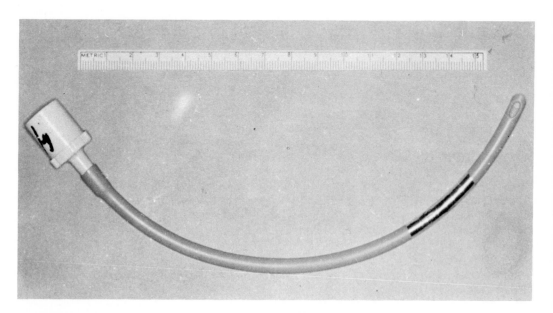

FIG. 3. A portion of the red rubber endotracheal tube has been covered with a strip of self-adhesive aluminum. (From Strong et al.[7])

giectactic lesions will recur in the excised areas.

Two cases of recurrent inverted papilloma localized to the anterior portion of the septum have been excised with the laser; in one case the resection included the septal perichondrium so that cartilage was exposed. The wound healed slowly over a 4-week period as a small area of cartilage was absorbed; no perforation developed. In the other case the cartilage had been removed by previous surgery and papillomas were growing on the contralateral perichondrium; a full-thickness resection of the septum was therefore carried out without bleeding to eradicate the papillomas. Healing of the perforation edges was prompt, and there has been no recurrence during the 12-month follow-up period.

One case of recurrent adenoid cystic carcinoma presented with tumor implants on the rim of a large septal perforation and on the lateral wall of the nasal cavity adjacent to the anterior end of the middle turbinate; a lateral rhinotomy had been done to expose additional disease in the frontal sinuses and on the anterior fossa dura. The lesions of the septum and lateral nasal wall were excised very conveniently with the laser with no bleeding.

Oral Cavity

Papillomas, extensive leukoplakia, and localized carcinomas have been managed with the CO_2 laser using the micromanipulator laser attachment and the surgical microscope. If the patient can provide adequate exposure by opening the mouth etc., local anesthesia by lidocaine infiltration has been used satisfactorily; in most cases general anesthesia with a standard endotracheal tube is used in order to provide maximal exposure. Self-retaining gags are utilized when possible to maintain exposure of the operative site. Most of the lesions are removed as a biopsy excision so the diagnosis can be verified and the margins checked for adequacy; in case of superficial leukoplakia that have been previously biopsied the tissue is destroyed by vaporization without further biopsy.

Lesions of the tongue, floor of the mouth, and buccal mucosa are outlined with the laser, transfixed with a suture, and placed on tension; the specimen is then excised with the laser with minimal bleeding unless a vessel greater than 0.5 mm is transected. These large vessels are either suture ligated or coagulated with a diathermy current. Steam and smoke can be removed through a suction tube. Marginal resection of the mandible can be carried out following excision of the soft tissue; 25 watts of power is needed to vaporize the organic constituents of the bone, following which the residual bead-like fragments of inorganic material can be removed with a curette.

Minimal postoperative edema develops, and the wound heals promptly within 1 to 3 weeks depending on its diameter; postoperative pain appears to be much less after laser excision than following other techniques. There is no contraction of the healed scar so that excellent mobility is maintained.

Laser excision in the oral cavity is particularly suitable for the management of multicentric disease or that subject to surface recurrence. Leukoplakia has not been seen to recur in areas of laser excision but sometimes appears on adjacent areas. Papillomas have not recurred in the oral cavity after laser excision in contrast to those occurring in the larynx; carcinoma in situ and verrucous carcinoma lend themselves to successful laser excision because their margins can be defined confidently.

Oropharynx and Nasopharynx

In the oro- and nasopharyngeal areas adenoids, tonsils,[2] papillomas, carcinoma in situ, and early invasive carcinoma have been successfully excised with the CO_2 laser using the microscope and the laser micromanipulator. Anesthesia should be general with an endotracheal tube to facilitate placement of appropriate mouth gags in order to provide adequate exposure of the oro- and nasopharynx. Dingman soft palate and Davis gags have been most useful.

Lesions of the soft palate, tonsil pillars and fossae, and posterior pharyngeal wall are outlined with an incision made with the laser, following which the lesion is put under tension and excised with the laser. Bleeding is absent or minimal; a 1-mm vessel in the tonsil fossa may require a suture ligation or diathermy coagulation. The wounds are relatively free of pain, and the healing is prompt with minimal scar contracture.

In the nasopharynx the tissues can be viewed in a front face metallic mirror (stainless steel); the same mirror is used to reflect the beam accurately onto the target site on the dorsum of the soft palate or in the vault of the naso-

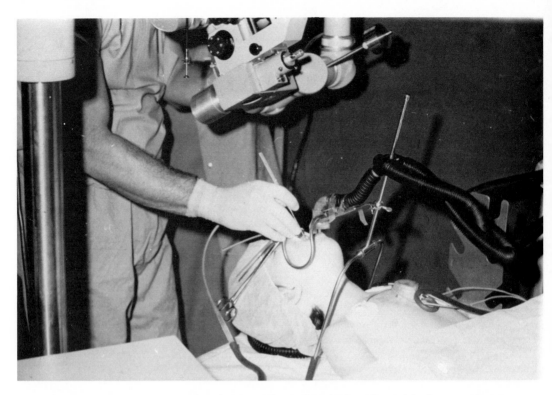

FIG. 4. A stainless steel mirror is being used to reflect the laser beam into the nasopharynx.

pharynx (Fig. 4). The palate may be retracted forward with a catheter passed through the nose and brought out through the mouth; steam and smoke are removed through a transnasal suction catheter. Biopsy, if indicated, should be carried out on all lesions prior to laser destruction because it is not possible to perform biopsy-excision in the nasopharynx. Papillomas and adenoids can be eliminated precisely with the laser; it is possible to carry out very precise dissection in the fossa of Rosenmueller without disturbing the eustachian tube orifices. This has been a striking application of the laser; it offers the possibility of a partial adenoidectomy in which the central mass of adenoid might be left in situ and only the lateral extensions toward the eustachian tubes removed. It is particularly suitable for secondary adenoidectomy in which the fragments are situated in the choanae and are inaccessible to the usual instruments.

Larynx

All mass lesions of the larynx and adjacent regions that can be well visualized and whose margins can be clearly defined are potential candidates for laser excision. A notable exception is probably a cavernous hemangioma, as it would be difficult to control bleeding with the laser from the large vascular spaces.

Anesthesia for suspension laryngoscopy should be general. If an endotracheal tube is used it should be small (6 mm for an adult) and made of red rubber, and the appropriate part of the tube lying adjacent to the vocal cord should be covered with a strip of self-adhesive aluminum to protect the red rubber from inadvertent laser impact.

The larynx is most often exposed with the Jako-Pilling laryngoscope and placed on suspension; this provides an excellent binocular view of the larynx through the Zeiss microscope (Fig. 5). Occasionally a small laryngoscope (e.g., a modified Hollinger anterior commissure laryngoscope) must be used to provide exposure; under these circumstances laser surgery can be carried out with monocular control although this is less than ideal. For lesions of the hypopharynx, the best exposure may be achieved with the Lynch suspension laryngoscope.

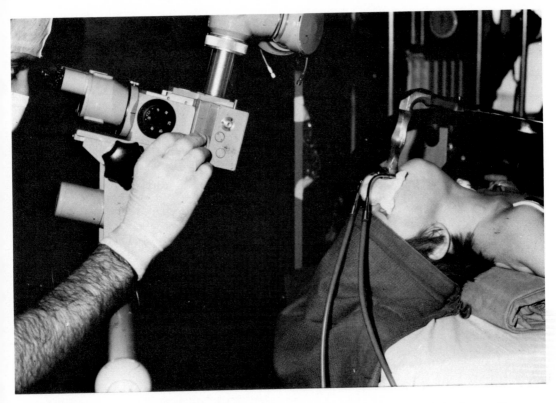

FIG. 5. Laser micromanipulator is being used to carry out microsurgery of the larynx. The large-bore fiberoptic bundles are attached to the Jako-Pilling laryngoscope and provide excellent illumination for surgery and photography.

Vocal cord nodules, polyps, granulomas, cysts, and keratoses are removed by grasping the lesion with a cup forceps and putting the lesion under tension; the surgical laser is then used to excise the mass without causing any unnecessary trauma to the adjacent tissues such as the vocalis muscle, etc. Steam and smoke are removed with the suction tube clipped to the wall of the laryngoscope. Papillomas are usually too friable to be handled in this fashion; after taking a biopsy the fronds of papilloma are vaporized until normal tissue is exposed. Care must be taken to avoid surgery on the anterior one-third of both cords at the same operation; if the lesion is excised simultaneously from each cord and the anterior commissure is involved, a webb can be anticipated. This can be avoided by using special retractors and operating on only one cord at a time.[1]

Carcinoma in situ and early invasive carcinoma of the membranous portion of the cord are carefully examined with the microscope, using retractors and mirrors to determine the exact extent of the lesion. Supravital staining (e.g., toluidine blue) is used to exaggerate the surface extent of the lesions. If it is felt that the exact extent of the tumor is known, the lesion is put on stretch and excised with the laser down to healthy tissue; the specimen is sent for histologic sectioning. If the lesion extends anteriorly to the commissure it is difficult to secure a margin of healthy, soft tissue; extension of invasive tumor to this area may contraindicate laser excision.

Although the laser wound is associated with no visible postoperative edema, if the manipulation with suction tips and probes etc. within the larynx has been excessive steroids may be used intravenously to prevent postoperative edema.

Tracheobronchial Tree

Most of the experience in the tracheobronchial tree area has been with papillomas, granulomas, and scar tissue using standard ventilating bronchoscopes and the endoscope laser attachment. Anesthesia for bronchoscopic laser surgery is usually general because the time required to complete the operation is often considerably more than a few minutes. Anesthesia is induced in the usual fashion using inhalation of nitrous oxide and oxygen in children, and thiopental and succinylcholine in adults; the patient is usually intubated (with a cuffed tube in adults and uncuffed tube in children), and anesthesia is maintained with noncombustible mixtures such as oxygen, nitrous oxide, halothane, and enflurane; ventilation is controlled manually while the patient is kept relaxed with succinylcholine. When anesthesia has been stabilized, the endotracheal tube is withdrawn and the appropriate bronchoscope (e.g., a 4-mm tube in a 4-year-old child or an 8-mm tube in an adult) is passed through the larynx into the trachea; ventilation is maintained through the side arm of the bronchoscope.

After the tracheobronchial tree has been inspected, biopsies are taken as indicated using a conventional cuff forceps. After bleeding has subsided, the bronchoscope is coupled to the laser endoscope attachment and laser excision is commenced (Fig. 6). It is usually advantageous to start peripherally in the trachea and main stem bronchi so the airway can be kept free at all times. The tidal flow of anesthetic gases keeps the airway free of smoke and steam. From time to time fragments of tissue may become detached by the laser or tip of the bronchoscope so that the bronchoscope must be uncoupled from the laser attachment and the fragments retrieved with a suction tip.

Dissection is continued until the desired amount of tissue has been ablated; there is no danger of inadvertent penetration of the tracheal wall because dissection continues in a controlled fashion until perichondrium or muscle appear. Penetration would be a danger if the lesion has destroyed the wall and extended outside the lumen of the trachea or bronchus.

In patients with a tracheostomy, if there is no disease in the upper trachea general anesthesia may be induced in the usual manner and the bronchoscope introduced through the stoma to expose the lower trachea and bronchi; anesthesia is maintained through the side arm

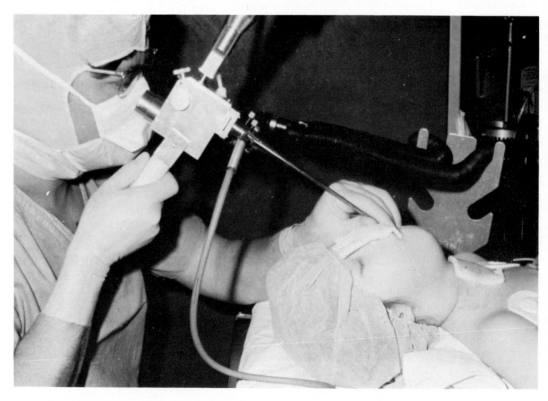

FIG. 6.   Laser endoscope-bronchoscope assembly is being used to ablate multiple papillomas of the lower trachea. (From Strong et al.[7])

of the bronchoscope while laser surgery is being completed.[7] Laryngectomies may not require general anesthesia; topical application of 4 percent cocaine is adequate to permit laser surgery in the lower trachea.

Recurrent papillomas can be removed conveniently from the trachea, carina, and main stem bronchi with the laser bronchoscope; bleeding is absent or minimal. Some patients with a presumed immune response to papillomas have gone into remission after three or four laser excisions, while in other patients without such host resistance there have been recurrences. Graulation with tracheomalacia can be removed with the laser in cases of post-tracheostomy stenosis; the tracheomalacia cannot be managed with the laser.

COMPLICATIONS AND PRECAUTIONS

There have been no complications specifically due to the laser. Several laryngeal webs have been caused by the overuse of laser excision on both cords simultaneously in the anterior commissure of the larynx in cases of papilloma; to avoid this, one cord is treated at a time when the anterior thirds are involved.

Noncombustible gases must be used during anesthesia and direct impact of the laser on the red rubber endotracheal tubes avoided. During intralaryngeal surgery the tube should be protected by a layer of soft adhesive aluminum tape. The patient's eyes are taped shut so that there is no chance of abrading the cornea or inadvertently reflecting the focused laser beam with a flat metal surface onto the eye.

FUTURE ENDOSCOPIC APPLICATIONS

The techniques described evolved during the management of more than 200 patients during a 3-year period. Many of the cases, particularly those with recurrent papillomas in the larynx, required repeated operations; more than 750 procedures were carried out.

There are several other areas where the CO_2 laser might be considered for endoscopic application. The urinary bladder could be drained of urine, expanded with an inert gas, and viewed through a modified cystoscope; the CO_2 laser would probably be most efficient in the management of recurrent papillomas and of localized, well differentiated carcinoma. The endoscope laser attachment could be fitted to a sigmoidoscope for the management of vascular polyps of the lower bowel, although free circulation of air would have to be ensured to eliminate the presence of combustible gas. Culdoscopy using the Zeiss microscope and laser micromanipulator would be an excellent method of managing lesions of the uterine cervix, and for superficial lesions the procedures could probably be handled on an ambulatory basis.

ACKNOWLEDGMENT

The author wishes to emphasize that this work is the result of a close collaborative effort between Thomas Polanyi, Ph.D., of the American Optical Corporation and Drs. Charles W. Vaughan and Geza J. Jako of the Department of Otolaryngology, Boston University School of Medicine.

REFERENCES

1. Andrews AH Jr: Experiences with the carbon dioxide laser in the larynx. Presented before the Annual Meeting, Laryngological Association, April 27, 1974, Palm Beach, Florida
2. French R: Personal communication
3. Jako GJ: Laser surgery of the vocal cords. Laryngoscope 82:2204, 1972
4. Polanyi TG, Bredemeier HC, Davis TW Jr: A CO_2 laser for surgical research. Med Biol Engin 8:541, 1970
5. Strong MS, Jako GJ: Laser surgery in the larynx. Ann Otol Rhinol Laryngol 81:791, 1972
6. Strong JS, Jako GJ, Polanyi TG, et al: Laser surgery in the aerodigestive tract. Am J Surg 126:529, 1973
7. Strong MS, Vaughan CW, Polanyi TG, et al: Bronchoscopic carbon dioxide laser surgery. Ann Otol Rhinol Laryngol. In press.

15

High-Energy Wave Guides

W. J. Mautner

For many years those projects that required the implementation of high-energy light sources were limited to optical line-of-sight applications. That is, either the source would be brought to bear directly on the target or it would be directed through one or more lenses and/or deflected by mirrors. However, the light could not be "bent."

Within the past several years, however, flexible fiberoptic bundles that can "bend" light have been constructed, able to transmit relatively high-intensity light. Endoscopy has been one of the chief beneficiaries of this development.

Actually, the field of endoscopy has very minimal specifications that must be achieved for successful illumination; however, procedures are facilitated by increased illumination. Specifically, the attenuation in typical fiberoptic bundles is approximately 65 percent for a cable 3.5 mm in diameter and 180 cm (6 feet) long. The color of the transmitted light from a standard endoscopic source (a 150-watt quartz Halogen bulb) is a pale but definite yellow, with transmission peaks at 595, 550, and 520 nm.

Sharp photographs have been difficult to achieve through fiberoptic bundles. The amount of light transmitted has been too low to allow shutter speeds that are fast enough to prevent the blurring caused by normal physiologic movements of the structures being photographed. Strobe units are being developed to facilitate endoscopic photography, but at present the fiber bundles cannot tolerate the continual high temperature at the input end of the cable without rapid deterioration.

Certain laser sources are now being considered for endoscopy, but the standard fiber cable cannot stand up to these energies either.

Before one can design the optimal light guide for endoscopy, the light sources to be implemented must be identified and characterized.

The most common light source for endoscopic examination is a 150-watt quartz Halogen bulb, mounted in a parabolic reflector that has been coated to reflect visible light efficiently and to transmit wavelengths beyond the range of visible light. This increases the relative amount of visible light at the focus of the reflector, which is approximately 1 cm in diameter. Since the quartz Halogen bulb has several spectral peaks, one of which is at 595 nm (yellow), the overall impression of the color of the light is definitely yellowish. Consequently, if "white" as opposed to "yellow" light is preferred, then the light guide selected to transmit such light should compensate for the spectral characteristics of the Halogen bulb.

Recently, the Eimac Division of Varian Corporation* has developed a series of xenon arc lamps from 150 to 1000 watts, depending on specific components. For example, in the focal plane, which is 4 mm in diameter, 4000 lumens are available from a 3000-watt lamp. This xenon source is employed in a new endoscopic illuminator† with the possibility of the added feature of being able to be pulsed for photographic applications. Experiments to strobe this source synchronously with a ciné-camera (1 pulse per frame) are in progress.

*Eimac, Division of Varian Corp., 301 Industrial Way, San Carlos, Calif. 94070.
†Storz Endoscopy America, Inc., 658 S. San Vicente Boulevard, Los Angeles, Calif. 90048.

Recent developments in the biomedical uses of laser energy, specifically in the area of hemostasis, have caused the argon laser to be considered as a potential energy source for endoscopy. This laser has several distinct spectral lines; the two primary lines are at 514.5 nm and 488 nm, although typically all lines are operating during laser photocoagulation in order to generate maximum energy. A good lightguide must have high transmissivity and little or no absorption at these wavelengths, if it is to be implemented for laser transmission.

The CO_2 laser has been used in laryngoscopy and surgery for tissue excision. However, at the moment, no flexible lightguide exists for this wavelength (10.6 μ).

Four distinctly different lightguides are available at this time:

1. The least expensive and least efficient is the plastic fiberoptic bundle. It is unacceptable for high-intensity illumination because it absorbs too much energy and soon melts at the end closest to the lamp.
2. The standard glass fiberoptic bundle has been the light guide of choice for some time, although some attractive alternatives are now being developed. It is very flexible, can be sterilized, and is reasonably priced. As previously mentioned, it lends a yellowish cast to the transmitted light. The attenuation in a fiber bundle 3.5 mm in diameter and 2 m long is approximately 65 percent. When this bundle is subjected to sufficient pulsed xenon arc for still photography, the epoxy cement between the individual fiber strands melts. Cinematography is also precluded. In either mode the temperature at the launching end exceeds the tolerance of the bundle, which breaks down. Fiber bundles, in general, have a lifetime in excess of one year. Ultimately, however, individual fibers in the bundle break, causing increasing attenuation of the transmitted light; eventually, the cable must be replaced.
3. A new and different type of waveguide has been developed and recently implemented in endoscopy; it is a liquid-filled, flexible waveguide, and it has several major advantages when compared with the standard glass fiber bundles.* Fundamentally, the advantages are as follows: The liquid-filled lightguide either transmits or reflects all light incident on its proximal tip that falls within its acceptance angle (no packing fraction loss); although some light escapes through the sidewall and some is shattered, essentially none is absorbed. Apparently, heat is dissipated by the waveguide as quickly as it is absorbed. The waveguide has not gotten hot even after it has been subjected to many different light sources, includ-

Manufacturer: Laser BioApplications, 4605 Lankershim Boulevard, Suite 515, North Hollywood, Calif. 91602. Patent pending.

ing xenon arcs and lasers. Some of the sources that have been successfully transmitted by the liquid-filled waveguide with no apparent difficulty or degradation in performance are as follows: a pulsed ruby laser (694.3 nm) with a 0.5-millisecond pulse width at 50 joules per pulse; a 7-millisecond pulse width, neodymium (1.06 μ) laser at 30 joules per pulse and 60 pulses per second; a continuous-wave neodymium-YAG (1.06 μ) laser at 18 watts for 30 minutes; a burst-pulse argon laser (514 nm) at 1.7 watts per pulse; and a Q—switched neodymium—YAG laser (1.06 μ) at 30,000 pulses per second, 40 to 50 Kw per pulse.

Conventional fiber bundles cannot withstand insults of this magnitude. They absorb heat at the input end of the waveguide. Either the cladding material or the epoxy between the fibers breaks down. At higher energies and short pulse lengths, the energy density within any individual fiber becomes so high that an impurity in the transmissive core of the individual fiber absorbs enough energy to cause the individual fiber itself to break at that point.

This last point illustrates another difference between the liquid and fiber waveguides. The liquid lightguide has a single, large transmissive core, whereas the fiber bundle has multiple small cores. The transmissive cores of the fiber bundle represent only 45 to 55 percent of the cross-sectional area of the bundle. It can be seen then that the cross-sectional area of the transmissive core of the fiber bundle increases at roughly one-half the rate that the area increases, or approximately $\pi r^2/2$, whereas the cross-sectional area of the single-core, liquid-filled waveguide increases directly with the area or πr^2. Obviously the difference is a factor of 2, such that as the diameter of the incident light beam in the plane of the launching end of the waveguide increases beyond approximately 1.5 mm, the disparity in transmissivity between liquid and fiber lightguides increases favorably for the liquid cable. The transmissivity of liquid and fiber lightguides is approximately equal when the diameter of the waveguide is 1.5 mm and the liquid waveguide gets relatively better with increasing diameter. Similar launching configurations will work for both types of waveguides when the spot size of the source is larger than approximately 1.5 mm.

Laser hemostasis through gastroscopes can be achieved with liquid bundles.

4. There is one case, however, when a single clad-glass fiber is used and when the formula pre-

sented above does not pertain. Corning Glass Co.* makes a highly transmissive glass fiber that has also been successfully used as an efficient laser transmitter. It does, however, require relatively sophisticated and expensive launching optics. The transmission through the complete system is on a par with the liquid system. Although the transmission through the fiber itself is greater than in the liquid system, the losses in the launching and termination optics are also greater, and both systems transmit about 70 percent of the incident light. Although the fiber is only on the order of 80 μ in diameter, it can be implemented for laser transmission because laser light is so well collimated that it can be focused to a very small spot size in order to be launched properly into such a small fiber. Even though this fiber has a relatively narrow acceptance angle (17°), rendering it of limited use for white light, a laser can easily be launched into it.

The liquid waveguide can be made with different components in order to optimize it for specific purposes. The parameters that can be selected for are color, transmissivity in the infrared region of the electromagnetic spectrum (greater than 700 nm), optimum transmissivity in the visible region as defined by the retinal response (CIE curve),† total transmissivity, temperature at the distal tip of the waveguide, and/or toxicity of the liquid material. Unfortunately, there are inverse relationships between some of the more desirable characteristics of this waveguide, particularly the color and the temperature at the distal tip. The waveguide can be made to modulate the light from either a quartz Halogen bulb or a xenon arc such that it appears absolutely "white" or colorless. Ordinarily, one is not aware of the overall effect introduced by the "yellowish" fiber bundle; however, when it is compared directly with the "white" waveguide, the difference is apparent. In its whitest configuration, the liquid-filled waveguide transmits light through a CIE filter (a filter designed to mimic the retinal response) approximately 10 percent better than the conventional glass fiber bundle. This configuration has a nontoxic filling material.

One significant difference between this waveguide and all others (including other configurations at the liquid waveguide) is that it stays much cooler at the distal tip than any

other waveguide tested so far, including the popular, conventional glass fiber bundles. This is significant during examination, but particularly so during photographic documentation, when very bright (hot) sources are used.

A second version of the liquid-filled waveguide, also nontoxic but slightly yellowish, can be constructed. It is approximately the same color as the glass fiber bundle. This waveguide is 33 percent more transmissive than the liquid "white light" or the conventional fiber bundles when read through a CIE filter. However, the temperature at the distal end is also higher than the "white" waveguide but not as hot as the fiber bundle.

A third configuration is also available. It is designed to transmit infrared wavelengths efficiently and to transmit "total energy"—that is, sensed by a silicon detector without a CIE filter—about 50 percent better than the conventional fiber. This waveguide is both yellower and hotter at the distal tip than the conventional fiber bundles, and the resulting compromise, which yields a yellow color and high temperature as well as a higher "total energy," does not seem to be a good one for endoscopic purposes.

DISCUSSION

A few subjective evaluations should be considered. The "white" light has been seen by many physicians. Independent of the fact that there is up to 50 percent more energy available from various other liquid waveguides, as measured both with and without the CIE filter, every physician preferred the cool, white light, rather than the palest yellow version, which gives 30 percent more light (according to a silicon detector) through the filter. The implication is obvious. Just because the CIE filter mimics the retinal response curve very accurately (± 2 percent of the integrated area under the curve), it does not mean that the light that is transmitted most efficiently through it will be selected as the most attractive to work with.

For photodocumentation, however, it may be a good choice to have a slightly yellowish light, if the reduction in shutter speed made possible by the additional light warrants the sacrifice of perfect color for sharp photos.

---

*Corning Glass Co.
†CIE: Commission Internationale de l'Eclairage (International Commission on Illumination).

EDITORIAL COMMENT

The invention of a more efficient flexible light-transmitting agent could be of great importance to endoscopy. If the present 60 to 70 percent absorption figures could be reduced and the disturbing yellowish color changed to a more optimal white light, it would add to the overall performance. Additional benefits in documentation (still photography, cinematography, or television) will also help in teaching and consultation.

We have tested a few prototypes, and the results are promising, although certain parts need improvement, e.g., flexibility. We do not have any figures or experience about their durability and cost. Only time will reveal the final outcome of this intriguing idea.

THE EDITOR

16

High-Frequency Electrosurgery

W. Rex Sittner
Jon K. Fitzgerald

Electrosurgery is a technique for surgical therapy whereby a high-frequency electrical current is caused to flow through the body in a carefully controlled manner to produce a therapeutic lesion or to control bleeding.

Electrosurgery is, perhaps surprisingly, one of the oldest applications of electronics in the medical field.[1] The oldest important use was in diathermy. Medical diathermy is based on the physical principle that alternating current of sufficiently high frequency can be passed through living tissue with no effects other than the production of heat. Nervous system stimulation results if a low frequency is maintained.[2]

When electrodes of large (normally more than 100 cm²) and near-equal sizes are used (as in medical diathermy), the current is quite evenly dispersed within the intervening tissue. This arrangement produces a corresponding temperature rise within the tissue which is adequate for diathermy. With diathermy there is no current concentration and therefore no cell destruction.

On the other hand, when one electrode is large and the other small (such as less than 1 cm² in contact area) the current is no longer evenly dispersed within the tissue. With this pattern there can be sufficient concentration at the small electrode to cause actual destruction of cells at the point where this electrode is applied to the tissue. The electrode arrangement and the current flow pattern for both cases are shown in Figure 1.

The nomenclature in electrosurgery is by no means standardized. Different names are used by different authors and users to describe the same piece of equipment.[6] In this chapter we refer to the small-area electrode as the *active* one, and the large-area electrode as the *patient plate*.

ELECTROSURGICAL PROCESS

High-frequency current flow for surgical therapy is an ideal tool for the surgeon. The characteristics of electrosurgery which lead to this are its: (1) ease of application; (2) sharp delineation of the lesion; (3) reproducibility; (4) speed; and (5) controllable hemostasis (from a pure cutting mode, through a mode of cutting with hemostasis, to a pure coagulating mode). Over the past 45 years these factors have resulted in electrosurgery becoming a universally used method and a standard tool in the operating room.

The electrosurgical process involves the formation of an electrical circuit in which the patient is the resistance to current flow (Fig. 2). For a better understanding of this process, the electrical characteristics of the therapeutic current are further discussed below.

Frequency

The therapeutic effect of electrosurgery is the result of the heat generated by a current passing through the tissue. Heat produced in this manner (by passing current through a resistance) is independent of the frequency of the current. However, for the following reasons only a rather restricted frequency range has been used in practice.

The lower frequency limit is set by the fact

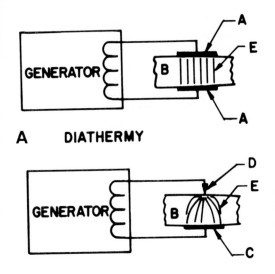

A   DIATHERMY

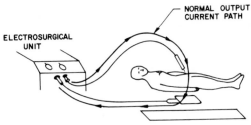

FIG. 2. Therapeutic current path.

B ELECTROSURURGERY

FIG. 1. Principles of operation of diathermy and electrosurgery. **A.** Large electrode. **B.** Patient. **C.** Patient plate. **D.** Active electrode. **E.** Current flow pattern.

that nerve cells respond to low-frequency currents and produce muscle contraction. The response of the human body to current at the power line frequency (60 Hz) is well known. In fact, the nerve response peaks near this frequency but decreases rapidly as the frequency of the electrosurgical current and all of the frequencies produced by any modulation of the current increases (Fig. 3). Electrosurgery should be performed at a frequency higher than that which causes neurophysiologic reactions, i.e., above 75 to 100 kHz.

The upper frequency value is loosely limited by the requirement that the therapeutic current be capable of flowing to and from the patient via metallic conductors. If the frequency is too high, the current *cannot be easily confined to the desired conductive path* because of capacitively coupled and radiated energy losses. Even at the frequencies used, these stray currents produce undesirable effects under certain circumstances. These effects are sometimes misinterpreted as "shocks" from power main current. In practical terms, the

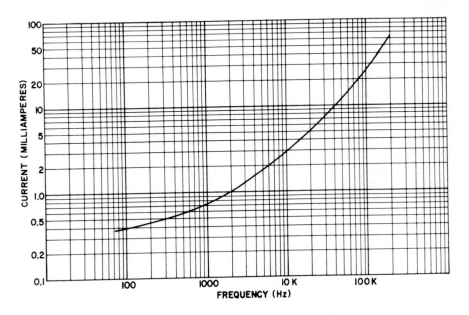

FIG. 3. Threshold of perception current versus frequency.

above criterion restricts the frequency of the therapeutic current to an approximate range of 350 to 2500 kHz.

Current Density

Current density is the measure of current concentration or, by definition, the current per unit area. The rate of heat generation and therefore the resulting therapeutic effect is a function of the current density. Current density in turn depends on the: (1) applied voltage; (2) resistance of the tissue; and (3) area of the active electrode in contact with the tissue.

The electrode contact area and the tissue resistance determine the resistance to current flow. The current flow pattern is determined by the small and large contact areas of the electrodes and their relationship to each other. (Note the differences in the current flow patterns in Figure 1.)

It is of course desirable to have a high current density at the active electrode in order to achieve the desired therapeutic effect. It is also desirable to have a low current density at the patient plate to prevent unwanted tissue destruction. This is achieved by giving the patient plate a large area of contact, thus minimizing current density and the possibility of burning the patient.

The therapeutic effects achieved by the high-frequency currents of electrosurgery are described by three terms: cutting, coagulation, and fulguration.

Cutting

In the cutting process the electrode is moved through the tissue in a manner similar to that used with the conventional scalpel. Parting of the tissue actually precedes the active electrode by a microscopic distance as it passes through the tissue. With the proper current density there is very little resistance to the cutting motion of the active electrode as it passes through the tissue; the cutting is essentially effortless. The very high current density at the leading edge of the electrode means that the power dissipated in the adjacent thin layer of tissue, where the resistance is concentrated, is very high. During cutting the water in the cells vaporizes and the proteinaceous materials in and of the cells are decomposed, producing a characteristic odor. In other words, a thin layer

of tissue evaporates.[3,5] Analysis and measurements show that the heat penetrates only a very short distance sideways if the electrode is moved rapidly through the tissue.[3] This accounts for the common observation that slow cutting leaves more destroyed tissue in the wound than does rapid cutting. Rapid cutting requires more power output from the electrosurgical unit. As one might expect, the nature of the tissue, the speed of the cut, and the cutting electrode surface area in contact with the tissue are important variables.

Coagulation

The coagulation procedure can be performed in either of two ways. In the first method the bleeder is grasped with a metal forceps, the active electrode is touched to the forceps, and current is applied until the tissue between the jaws of the forceps has been converted into a "plug" which seals the end of the bleeder. There is indeed a great variety of sizes and styles of forceps, including those constructed as a part of the electrosurgical active electrode. In this method of application, the current waveform (to be discussed later) employed is not important. It is necessary only that the energy "dose" given the bleeder is enough to produce the required physical changes within a convenient time. (Energy "dose" equals the product of the power dissipated in the tissue and the time of application.)

In the second method the surgeon is able to stop the bleeding more swiftly and often with less destruction of tissue than is associated with grasping each bleeder with a forceps or hemostat. This can be done by touching an electrode, often the side of the cutting electrode, to the bleeder *provided the coagulating current has the proper amplitude and waveform* (Fig. 4A). The requirements on the electrosurgical unit are quite different from the other method of coagulation with forceps because a coagulation effect without a cutting effect is needed. If a cutting effect is present, the pressure of the electrode against the tissue cuts the vessel or surrounding tissue instead of sealing the vessel. We will see later that the current waveform determines whether a coagulation effect or a cutting effect is produced.

Both of these methods for coagulation require an energy "dose" sufficient to cause the physical changes in the tissue. The area of the active electrode, the depth of coagulation needed, and the type of tissue determine the required energy "dose."

Fulguration

Fulguration is a method of coagulation wherein the active electrode is held some distance (viz., 1 to 10 mm) away from the tissue, and energy is dissipated in the area by means of sparking (Fig. 4B). Since the energy is applied to the tissue by means of an electrical spark, the entry point of the current at any given instant has an extremely small cross-sectional area. With all other factors equal, this small entry area produces very high current densities. Because of the high current density associated with each individual spark, fulguration is said to have greater depth of penetration and marked dehydration even to

the point of charring the tissue. The spark in this method has a tendency to play erratically about an area much larger than the cross-sectional area of the spark itself. Fulguration by its nature requires a relatively high applied voltage in order to ionize the gas between the electrode and the tissue and start the complex chain of events which occurs within a spark.[4] The previously discussed cutting and coagulating processes are different in their therapeutic effects primarily because of a difference in the current waveforms.

Cutting with Hemostasis (Modified Cut)

To add a hemostatic (coagulating) effect to the cutting effect, an interrupted current is generated. This is commonly called a *blended* current because early machine manufacturers actually combined (blended) the outputs of separate cutting and coagulating oscillators into a single waveform. This resulted in a current with an interrupted waveform which both cut and coagulated tissue simultaneously. The term "blended" continues to be commonly used even though the new solid state units have only a single oscillator to produce the interrupted waveform that both cuts and coagulates. In principle it is more correctly called a modified cutting current. However, the continued use of "blended" is still justified by many because of the blended effects (both cutting and coagulation) of this modified current.

It has been established that the fundamental characteristic of a current waveform which causes it to produce cutting alone, cutting with hemostatis, or hemostatis alone is the waveform.[8] A continuous uninterrupted waveform of high-frequency energy produces cutting alone. A waveform which is pulsed on and off, with the on times being one-fifth to one-tenth as long as the off times, produces coagulation only. Pulsed waveforms with longer on/off time ratios produce an intermediate effect called blend or modified cut.

Typical waveforms produced by classic vacuum tube–spark gap machines and the newer solid state units are shown in Figures 5 through 7. A study of these figures shows that the three modes of operation—pure cutting, modified cutting, and coagulation—follow the on/off ratio principle. The waveforms are quite different, which leads to differences in perfor-

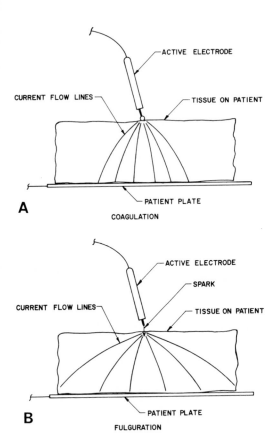

FIG. 4. Difference between coagulation (**A**) and fulguration (**B**).

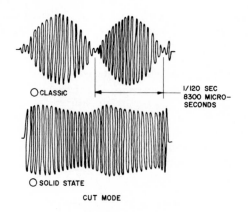

FIG. 5. Cutting current waveform for a classic machine and a solid state electrosurgical unit.

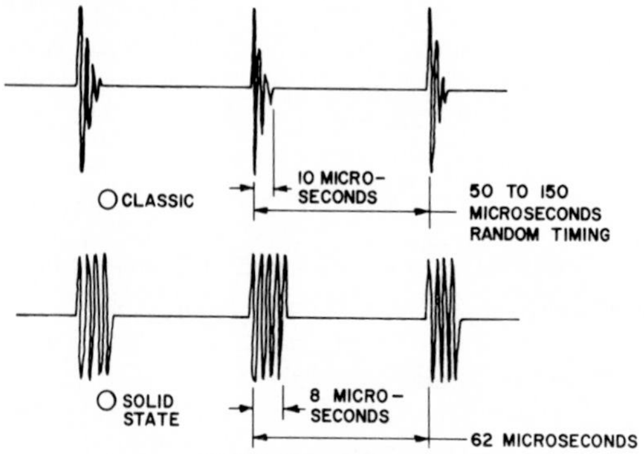

FIG. 6. Coagulation current waveform for a classic machine and a solid state electrosurgical unit.

mance and largely to advantages of solid state units *(vide infra)*.

ELECTROSURGICAL UNIT

The classic electrosurgical unit and the procedures for its use were developed concurrently in Boston during the late 1920s through the cooperative efforts of Dr. Harvey Cushing, a neurosurgeon with a keen interest in improving the procedures and apparatus used on his patients, and Professor William Bovie of Harvard University's Department of Physics, who was interested in the effects of high-frequency electrical currents on tissue. Their experiments were conducted at the Peter Bent Brigham Hospital.

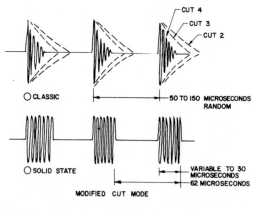

FIG. 7. Modified cutting current waveform for a classic machine and a solid state electrosurgical unit.

A close working relationship developed between these two men, and they discovered that a vacuum tube oscillator generating continuous high-frequency current would produce a cutting effect on tissue. In contrast, a spark gap oscillator producing a sharply damped intermittent high-frequency current pulse caused coagulation of the blood vessels with little or no tissue cutting.[1]

The original apparatus which evolved from this early effort consisted of two entirely separate high-frequency current oscillators installed in a single cabinet. Alternatively either of these oscillators could be operated, and the current produced was caused to flow between the two electrodes, which were applied to the patient.

The new electrosurgical apparatus was gradually accepted by surgeons. Over the years the acceptance has become quite general, with all surgeons in some specialties and most surgeons in all specialties using the equipment. This is true throughout the world wherever modern surgical theaters are available. The development of the equipment has proceeded somewhat differently in some countries outside the United States. For example, equipment built in the United Kingdom differs somewhat from that described above.[2]

As the large powerful apparatus were accepted in the operating theater for all major procedures, the need for specialized machines for particular surgical specialties was recognized and developed[7] (Figs. 8A, B). Smaller versions of the spark gap generator were developed for physicians' office and clinics, where

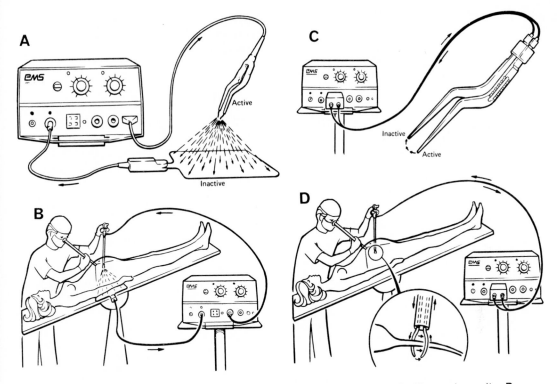

FIG. 8. Differences between monopolar and bipolar techniques. **A.** Monopolar unit. **B.** Monopolar endoscopy. **C.** Bipolar unit. **D.** Bipolar endoscopy.

they were used mainly for coagulation and fulguration. One of the important uses for the smaller coagulation machines was developed in neurologic procedures. A prime need of the neurosurgeon was the capability for extremely sharp delineation. This need was fulfilled by the development of a special handle which *had two active electrode tips instead of one* (Fig. 8C). Now, rather than current flowing from an active electrode through the patient and returning to the power unit by means of the patient plate, the current flows from one active tip to the other active tip. The current path is shown in Figures 8A–D. In other words, the current would flow only through the tissue between the two active electrodes. This procedure is called *bipolar electrosurgery*. If a patient plate is used, it is called *monopolar electrosurgery*.

Until 1968 only a few minor improvements were made in electrosurgical machines over those originally developed by Bovie and Cushing. By that time semiconductor technology had developed to the point whereby a solid state unit could be designed and built to provide all of the capabilities required by major surgical procedures. The result was a solid state unit with the following characteristics:

1. Small in size.
2. Light weight (20 to 30 pounds versus 150 to 200 pounds).
3. Cut and coagulation currents produced by a single generator instead of two separate ones.
4. Sufficient power capabilities for the most demanding surgical procedures.
5. Precisely controllable therapeutic effect.
6. Therapeutic effect reproducible within a single unit and between units day to day and year to year without adjustment.
7. Amount of hemostatic effect continuously adjustable from a pure cut to a pure coagulation.
8. Adaptable to the bipolar mode of operation.
9. Isolation from common ground. The benefit of this feature is the substantial elimination of patient burns. Such burns have been associated for decades with the operating room use of electrosurgical equipment.

The differences in therapeutic effect between classic and solid state units can be understood by studying the current waveforms shown in Figures 5 through 7.

From Figure 5 we see that the classic machine, in cutting, exhibits a sharp variation in output every 1/120 second. In contrast, the solid state units produce less hemostasis and less tissue destruction than do the classic machines. This is sometimes desirable and sometimes undesirable to the surgeon, depending on his technique.

As explained earlier, the "on time"/"off time" ratio in the solid state unit can in principle be varied continuously, smoothly, and controllably over a wide range. This enables the user to cut with precisely the amount of hemostasis desired for a particular procedure. We can expect more exploitation of this inherent capability of solid state electrosurgical units in the future.

The coagulation properties of the solid state unit are somewhat different because the waveforms are different (Fig. 6). A modern unit has a "pinpoint" capability—i.e., it is able to seal a bleeder while destroying an area of tissue around the bleeder smaller than that destroyed by the classic machine. This is possible for two basic reasons.

1. The current pulse of the solid state unit does not decay like that of the spark gap machine; hence the initial current of the pulse does not have to be nearly as high to provide the same overall result.
2. The tremendously great current in the initial part of the spark gap pulse results in spreading of the current paths over a larger area under the active electrode. This means that a larger area of tissue is destroyed, which is a substantial disadvantage of the spark gap coagulator.

The spark gap machines have greater fulguration capability than do the *present* solid state units for the same reason that they are inferior in coagulation. The very great initial current in the spark gap coagulation pulse implies a very high voltage output. This is especially true before the electrode contacts the tissue, i.e., in the "fulguration" situation. In this situation the spark gap machines generate 6000 to 8000 volts, and the most advanced solid state units develop 3000 volts. There may be a disadvantage to the patient when fulguration is used since a large amount of tissue is destroyed. It is expected that solid state units will gradually increase their coagulation voltage capability, and that surgeons will increasingly adapt to the advantages of bleeder contact and "pinpoint" coagulation. These changes have already created a trend toward replacement of the classic machine.

The fact that solid state electrosurgical units can be used readily in the bipolar mode will be of great importance in the future. Bipolar electrosurgery offers increased safety in the operating room as it virtually eliminates accidental patient burns and reduces internal organ damage due to reduced sparking. The bipolar mode permits therapeutic current to flow only in the localized area to be coagulated and consequently requires less energy. This mode of operation also permits finer resolution of coagulation power, increased isolation for patient safety, and low peak-to-peak voltages for safe tubal ligation (Fig. 8D).

Today bipolar techniques and accessories are being accepted and improved at a rapid pace for use in endoscopy. Accessories are now available for neurosurgery, plastic surgery, and many other general surgical procedures requiring coagulation only.

REFERENCES

1. Cushing H, Bovie WT: Electro-surgery as an aid to the removal of intracranial tumors. Surg Gynecol Obstet 47:751, 1928
2. Dobbie AK: The electrical aspects of surgical diathermy. Biomed Engin 4:206, 1969
3. Link WJ, Incropera FP, Glover JL: Development and Evaluation of the Plasma Scalpel: A Tool for Bloodless Surgery. Purdue University Press, August 1973
4. Loeb LB: Fundamental Processes of Electrical Discharge in Gases. New York, Wiley, 1947
5. Ning TC, Atkins DM, Murphy RC: Bladder explosions during transurethral surgery. Presented at the South Central Section of American Urological Association, Denver, September 1974
6. Oringer MJ: Electrosurgery in Dentistry. Philadelphia, Saunders, 1968
7. Petrone PJ, Dudzinski AF, Sittner WR: A new electrosurgical unit: report on clinical trials. J Urol 105:712, 1971
8. Sittner WR: Method and apparatus for high frequency electric surgery. US patent 3,675,655, July 11, 1972

EDITORIAL COMMENT

Unipolar Mode

The introduction of solid state electrosurgical units provided us with smaller and more compact machinery, as well as more efficient wave forms. Certain basic questions still remain unanswered, however. One of the major problems is the burn injury on the skin at the site of the patient's plate. It is true that the new units automatically shut off as soon as any mechanical fault occurs, completely disconnecting the patient plate during use. Unfortunately none of the units available have this automatic switch-off if only incomplete contacts or a reduced surface area is created. We should have some sort of alarm signal (or shutoff system). If for any reason during an operation this surface contact should decrease to the extent that, instead of conducting the current only, heat is created in excess resulting in a second- or third-degree burn on the patient's skin, we should be aware of this ahead of time.

There are other aspects that can be improved too, e.g., further reduction in the apparatus' weight and size, and a way to avoid the mixing of cutting current when the pure coagulation current is increased.

Bipolar mode

The introduction of new bipolar hand coagulation (hemostatic) instruments for general surgery with a built-in switch in place of the "burning stick" will be a great step forward. Its purpose would be to eliminate the use of the patient plate and to obtain more delineated hemostasis with less charring or a larger area of desiccation.

The bipolar mode in neurosurgery has been known for decades—gynecologic laparoscopy has already employed it. We hope that the flexible instruments will also be able to use flexible bipolar combined coagulation-suction cannulas introduced through a channel.

Progress has been made in that we can turn from the huge spark gap and tube current apparatus to the smaller, more efficient solid state units. However, some "homework" still remains to achieve further refinements.

THE EDITOR

17

Endoscopy and Radiology

George Berci

The number of recently introduced endoscopic examinations where simultaneous radiologic examinations with sophisticated x-ray equipment are required has increased significantly. This evolution poses several problems:

1. Capital outlay: Can we justify the purchase of this expensive equipment? The answer is yes. In those institutions where sophisticated (new) endoscopic examinations are performed, the number of cases referred for the procedures has increased significantly, providing the institution with added income. If this x-ray equipment can be utilized by other subspecialties as well, the investment is distributed to several areas, generating a larger fiscal income.
2. Organization and logistics of a modern endoscopy room: The x-ray equipment installed in an endoscopy room must be changed to suit our working conditions, which are different from those in a diagnostic x-ray room. If the operation of the endoscopy room is well organized, coordinated, and of high standards, close collaboration with a colleague from the x-ray department interested in some specific areas can be extremely fruitful. None of the interpretations of x-ray findings is taken away from the domain of the radiologist—the facilities have simply been topographically extended.

The conditions described are recommended primarily for medium-sized institutions where the endoscopic activities in terms of case numbers are largest among gastroenterologists, surgeons, gynecologists, urologists, and other subspecialty practitioners. The capital outlay for instruments to equip a modern endoscopy unit is not insignificant. Adding sophisticated x-ray equipment is also justified because (1) we are contributing to a higher diagnostic accuracy, therefore improving patient care; and (2) it pays off financially for the institution in the long run, with an increased number of patient referrals. If the investment can be defrayed and used as an interdisciplinary diagnostic tool, the capital outlay can be recouped from the x-ray charges within 2 to 3 years. The x-ray equipment can be employed in adjacent rooms (e.g., endoscopy and cystoscopy rooms, endoscopy and two or three operating or emergency rooms) and supplied with the same generator (time-sharing concept). With a minimum effort and coordination of scheduling cases, this can be achieved to everyone's satisfaction. The system of course must be "custom tailored" to the local conditions.

ENDOSCOPY WITH SIMULTANEOUS FLUOROSCOPY AND/OR RADIOGRAPHY

In order to combine endoscopy with a fluoroscopic or radiographic technique the endoscopic procedure must be performed in a diagnostic x-ray room, or a portable x-ray apparatus must be brought into the endoscopy room. If this is not possible, the procedures cannot be performed simultaneously and the endoscopic examination is referred to another institution.

Endoscopy in a Diagnostic X-Ray Room

Performing endoscopic procedures in the radiology department is inconvenient for a radiology department because this type of equipment is often in use or overbooked. The endoscopic procedure must be "squeezed in" during the normal busy function of the department.

In most cases the x-ray apparatus itself is adequate, but the x-ray tables (the older types) provide no movement, although some of the recent models move longitudinally. Using an image amplifier with a limited field, it is time-consuming and difficult to obtain lateral movement by moving the patient with the already positioned endoscope. The fixed arrangement of a diagnostic table, with its standard spot-film device, interferes spacewise with endoscopic manipulations. It is also inconvenient to wheel the endoscopic equipment with its auxiliary apparatus into this room.

Portable X-Ray Machines

Radiation dose to patient and personnel is high when employing portable x-ray machines for radiography only. The net result is that often x-ray films are exposed blindly. To know when the exposure is needed, we must be able to monitor dynamic events and to see them in consecutive order. The energy output of a portable x-ray machine is too small to obtain short exposures, and serial films cannot be taken in short time intervals (Fig. 1).

Portable Image Amplifiers

Mobile image amplifiers (IA) with an x-ray tube installed on a C arm can be used for fluoroscopy (Fig. 2). If an x-ray film is needed, costly time elapses before a film cassette can be placed in front of the image amplifier. The momentum to be recorded can be lost. These portable image amplifier units operate with a self-rectified x-ray tube where the energy output is small and extended exposure times are required; for instance, 1 to 2 seconds is needed to obtain a film of the abdomen. This is far too long to avoid movements such as respiration, peristalsis, transmission of aorta pulsation, etc., resulting in a blurred picture. The input screen of mobile IAs are only 6 to 7 inches. A larger one, 9 or 10 inches, is more convenient (e.g., colon, pancreas), reducing movements due to the smaller field.

Comment

Unfortunately there are a number of institutions which are small or located in an area

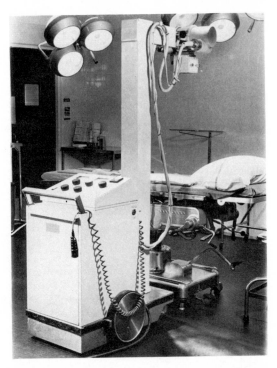

FIG. 1. Portable x-ray machine. The energy is limited by the small generator and tube. The average output does not exceed 200 to 300 ma. In case of an abdominal film, too-long exposure times are required. It can be additionally modified to be used for fluoroscopy as well, using an image amplifier underneath of the table, but the focal spot (1 to 2.0 mm) of this portable machine is not optimal for image amplification.

where few patients are referred for endoscopy, and so the investment is not justified. This produces an intricate question: Should a highly specialized examination be performed only in certain centers? It is clear that the practitioner who performs a large number of these special examinations in a well-equipped institution produces better results than the physician who has only occasional opportunities to do them with "second class" equipment. Before we introduce new examinations we must realistically assess the probability of case material in a particular area.

It is easier and faster to learn and to teach any procedure in a larger hospital that has up-to-date equipment and a well organized and conducted teaching program. This in turn allows a better education for those interested in learning. Sophisticated and difficult procedures should be evaluated first in those institutions where the conditions are optimal. If an exami-

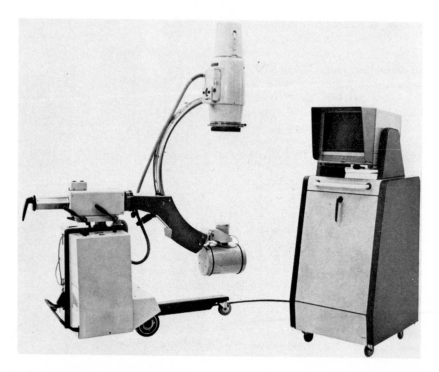

FIG. 2. Portable image amplifier. Assembled on a C arm for fluoroscopy. The size of the input screen varies from 6 to 7 inches. For colonoscopy or pancreatography the larger field (9 or 10 inches) is more suitable. The x-ray tube is small and a so-called self-rectified tube is used whereby the energy output is limited and extended exposure times are required (1 to 2 seconds) if a film is taken from a part of the body where larger radioabsorption is predictable. A film cassette can be inserted in the front of the input screen, but costly time elapses between insertion of the cassette, exposure of the machine, etc. (Courtesy of Siemens Co.)

nation proves to be successful, the method should be incorporated by other hospitals because the centers will be overwhelmed by referrals and unable to cope with the number of cases. From the patient's point of view, it is important that the distance traveled to receive treatment or undergo a special examination should not be far.

MODERN X-RAY EQUIPMENT FOR AN ENDOSCOPY ROOM

Fluoroscopy and aimed spot films are the basic components of modern radiology. Even during angiography the position of the catheter and the flow of the contrast material are first observed by fluoroscopy before the actual permanent (film) record is obtained. This becomes even more obvious during examination of the gastrointestinal tract. It is difficult to find any diagnostic x-ray room today where television fluoroscopy with the standard spot films is not available. It took us a long time to recognize that the same philosophy must be implemented in our field. Wherever x-ray techniques are employed to record the shape or outline of injected contrast material, the position of the endoscope should be first visually localized (by fluoroscopy) and the first drops of contrast material distribution well seen before a film is exposed. This concept was proved with several million examinations in the diagnostic x-ray field, thereby indicating the need for modern radiologic methods in the endoscopy and operating rooms.[2]

Endoscopy/X-Ray Table

It is true that many emergency surgical procedures have been performed under poor conditions, even on a "kitchen table"; however, an appropriate table designed for the purpose is preferred. If fluoroscopy or radiography is required, a radiolucent table top is a prerequisite. With the advent of modern radiology in surgery, tables have been developed by Kifa* and Maquet† that have a radiolucent top and provide various movements: up and down, lateral tilts, Trendelenburg and reverse Trendelenburg positions, etc. The same table can be obtained in several versions according to the application, e.g., endoscopy of the gastrointestinal tract, laparoscopy, urology, general surgery. The table must be designed to provide free space underneath to enable us to place an image amplifier (or the x-ray tube) in a fashion that it does not disturb any movements or procedures. This is its main advantage. It is of enormous help and expedites the examination if image amplification or television fluoroscopy can be used, and the tabletop with the patient can be moved with ease in a *longitudinal or vertical* "coordinate" fashion with the so-called floating top (Fig. 3). Every cardiac catheterization laboratory employs table tops designed to provide these coordinate movements. The table top with the patient's weight must be supported and fixed centrally to allow free space for the x-ray apparatus. To perform a variety of movements with safety, balancing can be achieved mainly by fixed installation of the main supporting table column. The advantages of this type of table far outweigh the disadvantages of a fixed, installed column. There is no additional gear obscuring the free space because all movements of the table are remotely controlled by compressed air or a mechanically driven gear box. All machinery required for the various movements are incorporated in the column. The table top can be exchanged according to the need of the subspecialty. In addition, these tops can be used as a stretcher top and the patient transported to and from the room. The top is also designed to accommodate single standard film cassettes.

X-Ray Generator

Radiophysics also contributed to the design of modern generators. We are anxious to reduce radiation and decrease the exposure time. In the case of a new installation a three-phase system is preferred.

Endoscopy and surgery were previously the collection places of out-dated x-ray equipment.

*Kifa Company, Stockholm, Sweden (represented by Affiliated Hospitals, St. Louis, Missouri).
†Maquet Company, Rastatt, West Germany (represented by Siemens Medical Company of America, New York, New York).*

There should be no difference in the film quality (information available) whether the abdomen is examined in the x-ray department or in any other area of the same hospital; the diagnostic accuracy should be equally excellent. In radiology our results depend largely on the performance of the equipment available.

If radiography is indicated during surgery the time required to obtain the actual radiologic information—fluoroscopic and spot films—does not exceed 2 to 3 minutes. If operations take several hours, I see no reason why the expensive but powerful generators cannot be (time) shared consecutively by adjacent rooms (e.g., for endoscopy) if the distance does not exceed 70 feet. This would make the investment in such equipment more economical. One generator can be used with ease in two or three adjacent rooms, employing image amplifier (fluoroscopy) and indirect radiography, or two or three rooms employing standard direct radiography only. If, for example, a lengthy endoscopy procedure (colonoscopy or endoscopic retrograde cannulation of the papilla of Vater) is interrupted for 2 to 3 minutes, this does not cause much inconvenience.

In photography today there are few cameras available in which an automatic exposure control is not incorporated. For similar reasons all modern x-ray equipment has built-in automatic exposure control for the standard x-ray film (cassettes) or small format films made through the image amplifier. Another aspect that needs consideration is the radiation dosage to patient or personnel. A recent development of having dosimeters in the collimator, counting the delivered roentgen dosage during the entire procedure (fluoroscopy and radiography), is a step forward. A hand stamp attached to the generator, detached after the procedure, stamps in the patient's chart the total delivered dosage. It is not an absolutely accurate system, but it is the first attempt to assess the dose rate during diagnostic procedures and to have some data on radiation exposure for that patient for future reference. These time-sharing generators have in each room a (slave) control console from which the main unit can be operated with a large variety of independent settings.

X-Ray Tube

The x-ray tube must be "matched" with the generator. It is worthwhile to invest in a larger generator only if the appropriate x-ray tube is

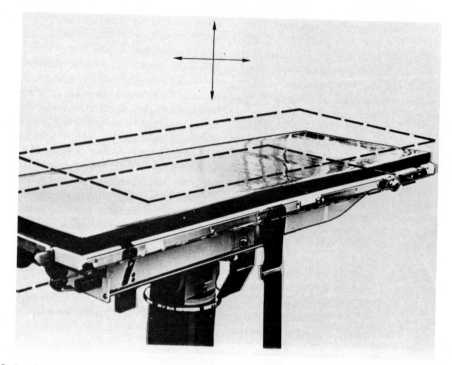

FIG. 3. A modern endoscopic-surgical operating room table. The table top is radiolucent and can be moved in both directions (longitudinally and laterally); this is the coordinate or floating top. The gear which operates the movement is installed into the fixed column. No handles or accessories obstruct the space underneath required for the x-ray machinery. Movements up and down, the Trendelenburg or reverse Trendelenburg positions, and lateral as well as coordinate movements are remote-controlled by a hand switch. The Kifa model uses compressed air, the Maquet model electric motors. If the bending or turning radius of the endoscope is in extreme position and the instrument cannot be turned or twisted further, the additional movement of the table "around" the scope facilitates better visibility of corners and parts of the organ, and can improve the position of the introduced instrument. Areas not seen, or only partially visible, can be made visible. The table tops are interchangeable and can be employed as transportation stretchers or carts. The interchangeability of the top makes this type of table versatile so it can be used by several subspecialities.

selected—one whose parameters are able to deliver certain amounts of energy within a particular (short) time without interfering with the so-called heat curve and other performance of the tube. Data (specifications) are available to radiologists from manufacturers. An automatic collimating system is preferred in order to avoid excessive radiation beside the object. Employing image amplification, a small but double focal spot tube (e.g., 0.6 to 1.2 mm) is desirable. These large-capacity tubes are heavy, however, so a suitable tube holder is required (Fig. 4). Recent new designs facilitate ceiling suspension from the side of the room with easy access, smooth movements, fast alignment, and a magnetic lock system to keep it in position (Fig. 5). In case of C-arm arrangements, the x-ray tube with the image amplifier is kept continuously in a fixed alignment. The entire structure is suspended from the ceiling (Fig. 6).

Image Amplifier

The invention of image amplification opened a new chapter in diagnostic radiology. Present-day fluoroscopy cannot be compared with earlier times when 20 to 30 minutes of accommodation was required, observing a low-light-level, yellow screen. Despite accommodation, our cone vision is immediately switched to rod vision, decreasing our visual acuity.

Coupling the bright-output screen of the image amplifier to a television camera, the optically visible image is picked up by a television camera, and the fluoroscopic image is seen on a television monitor, enlarged without the necessity of dark adaptation.

FIG. 4. Ceiling-suspended x-ray tube (old type). The high-tension cables are guided outside (arrow). This design is inherited from an x-ray department and does not suit modern concepts in avoiding the increased probability of contamination of clean areas due to increased movement of dust particles, etc.

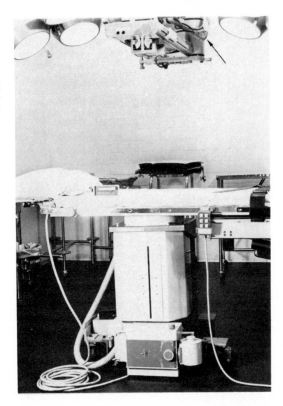

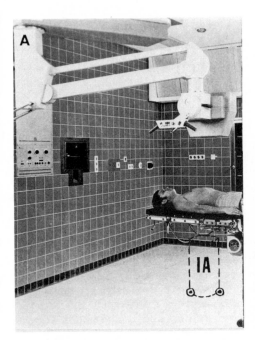

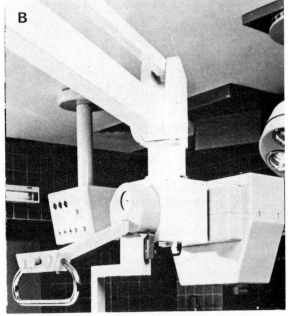

FIG. 5. New design of ceiling-suspended x-ray tube. **A.** A high-capacity x-ray tube is ceiling-mounted on a swivel arm and can be moved into position with ease. In this case the image amplifier (IA) is placed underneath. The high-tension KV cables are conducted *within* the column structure. If overhead tubes are employed, the image amplifier, on castors, can be wheeled from one room to another (adjacent) room, facilitating consecutive use of this expensive equipment. **B.** Close-up view of x-ray tube holder. (Courtesy of Philips Co.)

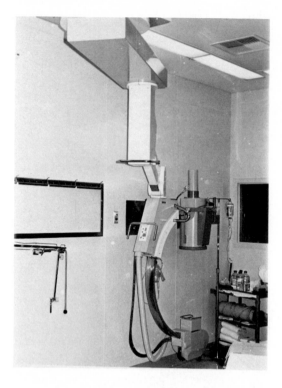

FIG. 6. X-ray tube and image amplifier with cameras (television and small-format spot films) are fixed, installed on a ceiling-suspended C arm. Oblique or lateral views can be obtained with this arrangement. During movement the axis of the x-ray beam with receptor (image amplifier) is maintained. With this installation the x-ray tube is placed underneath the table and the image amplifier with the camera above it. (Manufacturer: Philips Co.)

Recent improvements in image amplification (cesium, high-resolution tubes) closed the previous gap of direct and indirect radiography. Image amplifier technique is, practically speaking, introduced in every diagnostic field where radiology is employed. The larger-format image amplifier consists of a 9- or 10-inch input screen which can be electronically decreased to 5 or 6 inches. A beam splitter deviates the image into the television or into a small-format spot-film camera at will (Fig. 7). With the incorporation of automated brightness control, the x-ray energy is controlled by the light signal created at the output screen. In general, it is adjusted to a minimal radiation but sufficient image brightness. As soon as the brightness of the field is changing (e.g., shifting from the abdomen to the chest) the automatic brightness unit signals to the generator, and this in turn adjusts the x-ray energy output accordingly. The image amplifier reduces the radiation dose significantly compared with our old fluoro-screen technique or with standard radiography versus indirect radiography.

Recording of Fluoroscopic Images

The recording of fluoroscopic images can be achieved in various ways:

1. Continuous recording of the fluoroscopic image by means of a videotape recorder. In case of moving events, this is the matter of choice. The functional phenomenon can be studied on repeated reviews or analyzed in a slow motion replay. It is very important to select (specification) the proper recorder for this purpose.
2. In those cases where a single event or a still picture(s) suffices, a single-image storage device can be used. This picks up one frame and stores it (freeze-in) for any required time or automatically wipes and stores the next image during a preselected time interval, pulsing the x-ray tube.

Magnetic disk recorders or single-image electronic storage tubes are commercially available.[1]

Radiography

We must differentiate between two radiographic techniques:

Direct radiography—The x-ray film is positioned immediately under the object. This is also called standard radiography (Fig. 8A).

Indirect radiography—The film is exposed *through* an image amplifier, i.e., the image amplifier is placed underneath the object and the film is exposed directly from the output screen of this unit (Fig. 8B).

Indirect radiography gained wide acceptance with the recent improvements of image am-

FIG. 7. Mobile large-format 10-inch image amplifier with television camera and small-format spot film camera (SC). A beam splitter at the bottom (not seen) deviates the outcoming image from the output screen of the image amplifier to one or the other camera. Even during spot films employing a dichroic mirror (90/10 percent) a part of the image is directed (10 percent) into a television camera, allowing observation of the x-ray procedure during the actual film exposure. The size of the input screen (e.g., 9 or 10 inches) can be electronically decreased to a smaller format (e.g., 6 inches), producing an enlarged image from the object on the television monitor or on the small-format spot film. (Manufacturer: Siemens X-ray Co.)

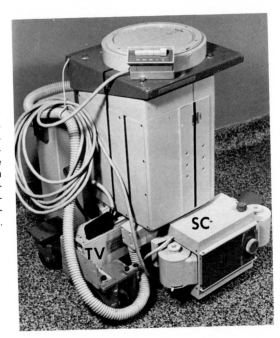

plification (increased resolution, brightness gain, contrast enhancement, etc.). This radiographic technique replaces standard radiography in many applications, e.g., for use in the gastrointestinal tract. It can be predicted that within the next few years the small-format spot films (indirect radiography; size: 4 × 4 inches or 100 × 100 mm) will replace the direct large-film format. Information obtained from the small-format spot films is compatible with that seen in the large ones in most cases.

The most important advantage of this small-format spot film is the significant reduction of radiation dose, which is approximately one-tenth to one-fifth that of the standard film dosage. Even in cases where more films are exposed, the end result is a smaller total radiation dosage.

If serial films are needed, no time is required for changing cassettes as it can be done by the press of a button. A magazine up to several hundred frames provides continuity. Immediate switching backward and forward for fluoroscopy versus radiography is possible. If movements or functional phenomena are to be recorded, up to six films per second can be exposed with this technique, displaying the minute changes in more detail. A certain reeducation is needed to interpret a small-film format, but this prejudice can be overcome.

FIG. 8. **A.** Standard radiography. X, x-ray tube. O, object. F, film cassette. **B.** Indirect radiography. X, x-ray tube. O, object. IA, image amplifier. SC, small-format (100 × 100 mm or 4 × 4 inches) spot film camera. The film is exposed from the image displayed on the output screen of the image amplifier. Advantages: reduction of radiation, complete automatization of exposure control and film sequences (up to six films per second).

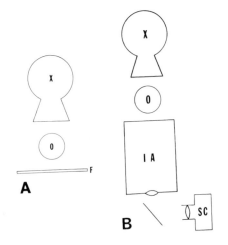

The readout can be simply accomplished by the naked eye, using the 100 × 100 mm film or a magnifying glass for the 70 × 70 mm film. These films can also be evaluated in a more sophisticated way using a closed circuit television setup (Fig. 9). The pictures can be sent from the endoscopy or operating room to the radiology department. Using television technique, the film is enlarged to the size of the monitor: 14 or 17 inches. Using television readout technique, the contrast can be enhanced or changed, the subtraction technique being employed, erasing the surrounding or underlying structures to emphasize the outline of the contrast material. The polarity can be changed (black to white or reversed). Using a zoom lens in front of the television camera and facing the processed dry film, certain suspicious areas can be optically enlarged. There are many modalities in television techniques which facilitate analysis of x-ray films and which should be considered.

The possibility of linking audio and visual apparatus in various remote areas of a hospital with the x-ray department is of immense value in communicating between those subspecialties which employ x-ray facilities outside the immediate radiology department area; this keeps these other areas in close contact with the radiologist, who does not have to waste time commuting between various locations, thereby making consultation and teaching much easier.

Storing or retrieving films is more convenient and economical using the small-format system. A contact print(s) can be inserted into the patient's chart, which eliminates the necessity of commuting to the x-ray area or going through a large number of films collected in several envelopes, looking for an x-ray viewer, etc.

CLINICAL APPLICATIONS

Bronchoscopy

Peripheral lesions that are out of reach, even for the fiber bronchoscope, are of special interest to the bronchologist. In 1961 Friedel reported his success in a series of 200 patients

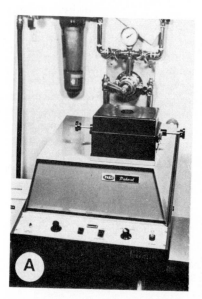
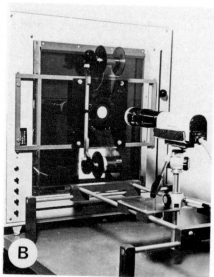

FIG. 9. **A.** Table top automatic processor. Develops within 5 minutes a number of small-format films, which are available as dry films, thereby avoiding the problems involved in reading wet films.   **B.** Television readout of small spot films. The television camera is facing an x-ray viewer with a zoom lens attached, scanning a roll of small-format spot films, frame by frame. The image is displayed and enlarged on a television monitor (14 or 17 inches). It can be sent to various places such as the endoscopy or operating room and the x-ray department. Using television readout technique, the contrast can be enhanced or changed, the subtraction technique employed, erasing the surrounding or underlying structures to emphasize the outline of the contrast material. The polarity can be changed from black to white or vice versa. Using a zoom lens in front of the television camera facing the processed dry film, suspected areas can be optically enlarged. There are many modalities where television techniques can help to analyze x-ray films and should therefore be considered.

with peripheral lesions; he introduced a guided radiopaque catheter into the periphery through a rigid bronchoscope under fluoroscopic control, and performed suction biopsies and selected bronchographies. He claimed a 90 percent diagnostic accuracy, histologically verified. Thus in one session he was able to perform bronchoscopy, catheterization of the peripheral lesion, cytologic studies, and selected bronchography.

Advancement of the fiber bronchoscope is limited by its diameter (5.5 mm). The majority of peripheral lesions are out of reach of even the fiber bronchoscope. In many fiber bronchoscopies, the cytology brush, biopsy forceps, or scraper is introduced through the biopsy channel far into the periphery, out of endoscopic control. In these cases fluoroscopy must be used to locate the instrument in relation to the target (lesion), and to perform manipulations under visual control.

An alternative can also be employed: The rigid scope (bronchoscope) is introduced and a radiopaque catheter* (Fr. 7, 2.3 mm) with remote (joy-stick) tip control is advanced toward the peripheral lesion. Suction cytology or brush technique is applied.

All these peripheral procedures require fluoroscopy. Routine utilization of fluoroscopic control increases diagnostic accuracy of the peripheral lesions and should be utilized whenever possible.

If contrast material is injected and distributed to the entire lung, the dye employed is diluted over a large area. In the case of selected bronchography, with the possibility of observing the inflow of the dye with aimed serial spot films, a large number of radiographs can be obtained showing minute details of the various filling stages. Much better contrast and sharper outlines are displayed, and a small volume of contrast material is distributed to a selected area only.

Thoracic surgeons who are interested in endoscopic exploration of the lung should not miss the opportunity to consider this additional diagnostic modality of selected bronchography in indicated cases. Fluoroscopy and indirect radiography can be very helpful in this application.

Cystoscopy

Retrograde pyelography is not frequently performed today because of the vast improvement in intravenous pyelography. However, there are still a number of cases when for one reason or another the kidney does not excrete and retrograde pyelography should be performed. There are several other indications also—e.g., difficult stone removal from the lower part of the ureter, differential diagnosis of a neurogenic bladder versus organic lesions—which demand fluoroscopy and radiography in the cystoscopy room. The urologic table has a built-in x-ray tube holder above and an x-ray cassette holder for standard radiography. A modern cassette holder should incorporate the automatic exposure control in order to ensure minimum radiation but appropriate exposure (not under- or overexposed films) with an appropriate generator and tube.

In a urology unit that uses two or more cystoscopy rooms, one room should be equipped with a built-in image amplifier and an indirect spot film device to enable the urologist to fluoroscope the patient before the permanent film records are taken. It is very helpful to see the tip or position when the ureteral catheter cannot be advanced further because of resistance. After 1 to 2 ml of contrast material is injected, we may receive valuable information about the nature of the stoppage with a glance at the television monitor.

Fluoroscopy is indispensable for studying the reflux mechanism, mainly in pediatrics, or for assessing functional disorders. The radiation dosage using *modern equipment* is minimal in terms of radiation hazard in pediatrics. The application of cinefluorography, where the dosage *must be increased*, can be substituted nowadays with a better image amplifier using *fluoroscopy only* but combining it with a videotape recording. The dose rate to a patient in this case is kept extremely low compared with cinefluorography. It is impossible to study functional disorders with static methods. The urologist is confronted with many functional disorders in the infant and adult. With proper equipment the endoscopic examination can be completed in one session in the cystoscopy room, without having to send the patient to the x-ray department for another procedure.

Colonoscopy

Colonoscopy should not be performed without having fluoroscopy available. In many instances the operator faces difficulties in advancing the scope after repeated attempts. It is an invaluable safety measure to be able to see

---

Manufacturer: Medi-Tech, Inc., 372 Main Street, Watertown, Massachusetts 02172.

the position, or the changing shape of the scope, during gentle advancement. It cannot be overstressed that the concept of "easy" introduction without standby fluoroscopy in those cases where the lesion is located in the sigmoid colon "only" is wrong. The sigmoid colon with its redundant configuration, various loops, diverticula, short mesocolon because of previous surgery, inflammatory process, or anatomic anomaly is extremely vulnerable to mechanical injury. The fluoroscopic image of a telescoping or curling scope is very useful in determining the next step if difficulties are posed during the passage. The recent complication figures[3] clearly indicate that "semiblind" attempts during manipulation constitute one of the main factors for perforation. Those hundred cases where everything went smoothly do not count if the hundred and first case has to be explored because of perforation. It is important to know that this perforation might have been avoided, thereby saving the patient from an unwarranted surgical intervention, had fluoroscopy been available.

On innumerable occasions we have had difficulty in passing the scope through the cecum, ascending colon, hepatic flexure, transverse, splenic flexure, or descending colon (Fig. 10). The straightening-out of overhanging transverse colon or the use of the outer stiffening tube in the case of a redundant sigmoid are examples where fluoroscopy is required. If a lesion is demonstrated on previous x-rays and the lesion cannot be located with the scope, it is important to compare the position of the scope with the x-ray film to make sure that the same area is being scanned. I am aware that there are a few outstanding "virtuoso" colonoscopists who probably can do well in the majority of cases without radiologic assistance and who perform a vast number of colonoscopies; I am referring, however, to those (majority) examiners who do not perform five or more cases per week.

Under certain conditions where a barium enema demonstrates a "lesion" in the cecum, ascending colon, or other delicate location, and colonoscopy does not reveal any abnormalities, during withdrawal a water-soluble contrast medium can be injected and a double-contrast

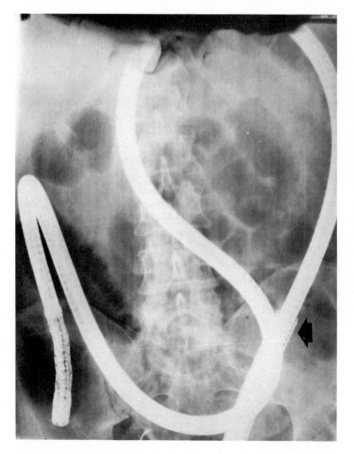

FIG. 10. Colonoscopy should not be performed without having fluoroscopy available. This is mainly true for the right colon, transverse, hepatic flexure, or redundant sigmoid colon. If a large sigmoid loop is formed, despite advancement of the scope in the sigmoid colon, the tip will not move forward and pain is produced when the mesocolon is stretched. The introduction of any stiffening device (arrow) requires careful fluoroscopic control. In elderly patients with a history of diverticula, inflammatory episodes, or pelvic surgery, a shorter fixed mesocolon cannot be excluded. In these cases manipulation must be performed very carefully. At present, the majority of complications (perforations) are due to manipulation. This risk could be decreased if simultaneous fluoroscopic observation is provided.

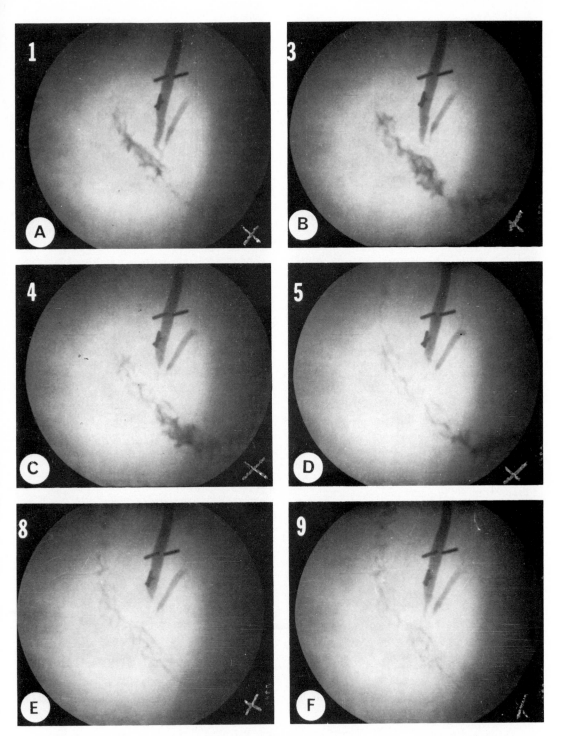

FIG. 11. Peroperative cholangiography. The sequence of the sphincter of Oddi functions are displayed. Dye was injected through the cannulated cystic duct, and 70-mm films were taken at 1-second intervals. Note the significant changes between the individuals films. The sphincter opens to the full width of the distal duct diameter and gives the impression of normal function. The numbers 1 through 9 indicate the number of seconds of sequential exposures. Time interval between films was 1 second. Films taken with 6-inch format (I.A.).

enema, with outstanding contours, can be recorded on a series of small-format spot films. This adjunctive procedure can contribute to clarification of the false-positive x-ray dilemma. Fluoroscopy (and indirect radiography) is of great help in facilitating the procedure and decreasing the risk to the patient.

Endoscopic Retrograde Cannulation of Papilla of Vater

Endoscopic retrograde cannulation of the papilla of Vater (ERCP) needs no supporting data to indicate the importance of having simultaneous radiologic services available. The resolution of the newer type of image amplifiers and the improved version of the television chains (less noise level, higher resolution) are required for this application. If a magnification technique is employed (switching from 9 or 10 to 6 inches), even 0.5 ml of injected contrast material can be observed. The problem is that we cannot clearly see the various filling stages. The small volume of the pancreatic duct system is injected under a relatively high pressure because of resistance of the small lumen of the tube (0.7 mm inside diameter). In this procedure improved visualization is of utmost importance. Furthermore, serial spot films would be required after small volumes (e.g., 0.25 to 0.5 ml per film), and would help to eliminate present discrepancies in the evaluation of pancreatograms.

Retrograde Cholangiography

Retrograde cholangiography has the same inherited problems as mentioned under retrograde pancreatography. In many cases the hepatic duct system is not visualized—partially because of drainage into the duodenum and partially because the film-recording procedure was performed as a completion cholangiogram rather than during the actual injection. If the cannulating tube is withdrawn or removed, the picture may be changed—as in the case of partial (obstruction) drainage—and only certain parts of the intra- or extrahepatic biliary system are displayed. An existing lesion or overlooked stone cannot be excluded with certainty.

Choledochoscopy and Peroperative Cholangiography

Choledoscopy is described in detail under that title. The combination of this endoscopic

procedure with operative cholangiography is important. Using the same (time-shared) x-ray equipment and a technique similar to that for operative cholangiography, we found that the function of the sphincter or changes in its appearance or shape can occur at very rapid intervals (Fig. 11). In another case we performed a cholangiogram with fluoroscopic control and serial films. One film of this series is depicted in Figure 12. If the same patient's operative cholangiogram had been performed using standard two- or three-film technique, and on one film the stoppage of dye inflow with this "thumbprint" had been observed (Fig. 12), a stone lodged in the distal end of the common bile duct or ampulla could not be excluded. Using fluoroscopy with serial films, however, this suspected configuration proved to be the functional appearance of the sphincter (Fig. 13).

Esophagoscopy

In organic or functional disorders the simultaneous observation of the scope in relation to the laryngopharynx, diaphragm, or other anatomic landmarks can be of great importance. Fluoroscopy is of immense help in the presence of dilatation of strictures. Appropriate

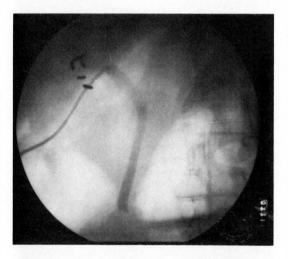

FIG. 12. Peroperative cholangiogram. Small-format film. The stoppage of the dye flow into the duodenum is visible with the characteristic thumbprint or half-moon configuration. When we perform routine cholangiograms with two or a maximum of three films—without fluoroscopy—before we close the abdomen (completion-gram) a picture such as this is not unusual. It is difficult to distinguish a retained calculus from a spasm if we have only one film to view. Size 1:1. Format: 70 × 70 mm.

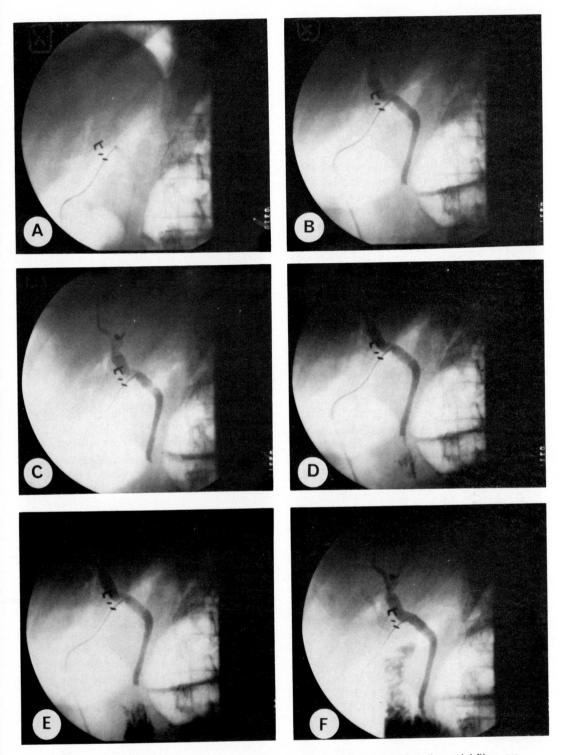

FIG. 13. Serial films from the same patient as in Figure 12, but this time the serial films are displayed. They were obtained with operative fluoroscopy and aimed spot film series. The spastic component of this configuration was visible on fluoroscopy. These functional changes were recorded on sequential films, and so the possibility of retained stones could be eliminated. For this and many other reasons, fluoroscopy and serial films are required in the operating room.

placement of the dilator or balloon and the magnitude of dilatation or extension is seen on the television monitor as well as on the pressure-indicating manometer. It is the greatest safety measure against the risk of perforation during dilatation.

Laparoscopy (Gynecologic) and Combined Hysterosalpingography

The use of combined laparoscopy and intraoperative salpingography employing television fluoroscopy with aimed spot films allows the most complete evaluation of uterine and tubal anatomy conducted during a single procedure (Fig. 14). It facilitates the study of some of the factors in reproduction, e.g., tubal spasm, cornual sphincter mechanisms, and the importance of endosalpingeal contour and function. It allows direct visual control of both intra- and extraluminal investigations. By using small increments of contrast medium, a more exact delineation of the lining of the mucosal pattern is possible; and the differential tubal filling rates show states of partial obstruction or tubal spasm. A preliminary report[4] was based on 45 patients performed with this simultaneous pro-

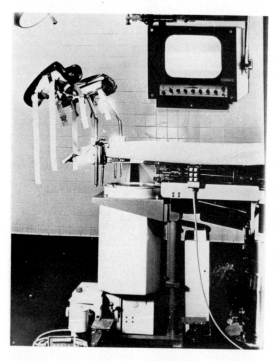

FIG. 14. Radiolucent coordinate table (Kifa) with image amplifier underneath and ceiling suspended television monitor prepared for combined laparoscopy and hysterosalpingography.

cedure. Significant benefit was obtained in almost every case. This single procedure offers the most complete evaluation of uterine and tubal anatomy. Figure 15 displays some examples of detail or information obtained.

The removal of intraabdominal foreign bodies such as a misplaced or perforating intrauterine device (IUD) via the laparoscope is sometimes troublesome. The IUD is often impossible to see because the omentum with its protective mechanisms wraps the foreign body. With simultaneous fluoroscopy, however, the radiopaque IUD can be located (Fig. 16). The atraumatic forceps is introduced through the second trocar, guided by fluoroscopy to this area, and the foreign body can be dissected and grasped. In our first study we reported on 16 misplaced IUDs (Lippes loops and Dalkon Shields) that were removed successfully without exploration.[5] Since then the number of removed intraabdominal foreign bodies has increased significantly, and fluoroscopy has proved very helpful.

Laparoscopy (Hepatology and General Surgery) with Cholangiography

Cholangiography is another interesting and promising approach for the differential diagnosis of "medical" and "surgical" jaundice. The key to the answer again is the information available on the cholangiogram (Chapter 29). The extrahepatic biliary system can be injected via a needle introduced under laparoscopic control through the liver parenchyma into the gallbladder; the indwelling Teflon catheter is left in the fundus of the bladder (Figs. 17 and 18), and the contrast material is injected under fluoroscopic control. The various filling stages are visualized and a number of aimed spot films exposed. The position of the patient and the injection pressure can be changed during the procedure to enhance the appearance, e.g., of the intrahepatic biliary duct system, sphincter and pancreatic duct junction (Figs. 19 and 20).

In cholecystectomized patients the right lobe cannot always be seen because of adhesions, but in the majority of cases the left lobe is free. Repeated punctures to find a dilated duct and aspirate bile can be attempted. In this case a percutaneous transhepatic cholangiogram is obtained but under laparoscopic control. More punctures can be performed because we are

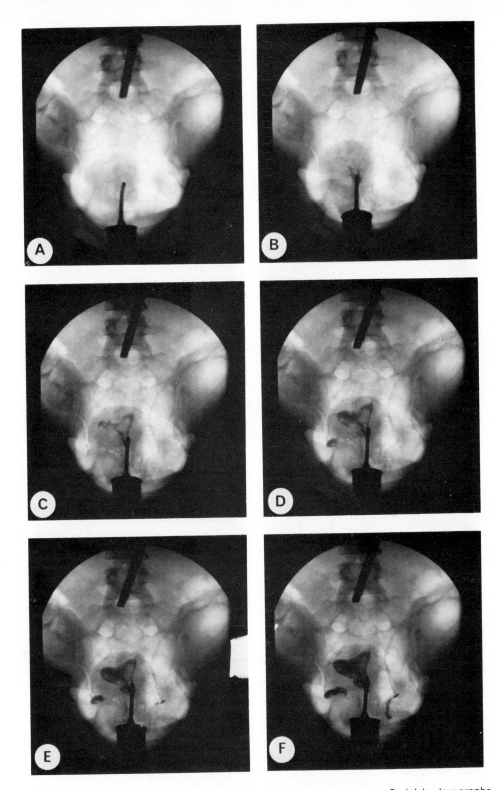

FIG. 15. Films taken during hysterosalpingography and laparoscopy. Serial hysterographs using 1- to 2-ml increments of dye, showing endometrial filling defects, patency of the left oviduct, and right hydrosalpinx. **A.** Scout film with cervical suction cannula and laparoscope in place. **B through F.** Dynamically changing appearance of the uterus, cornu, and oviducts. Note large filling defects within the uterus in films **C, D**, and **E**. Also note the distal enlargement of the right oviduct without apparent spillage of dye and the normal appearance with dye spillage on the left. (From Brooks et al: *J Reprod Med* 10:285, 1973)

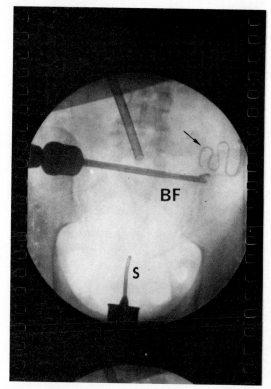

FIG. 16. Gynecologic laparoscopy combined with peroperative fluoroscopy. This IUD (arrow) was covered by omentum and was not seen using the introduced laparoscope. The biopsy forceps (BF) is advanced under fluoroscopic control. After a few gentle and careful dissecting movements over the locations indicated by fluoroscopy, the tip of the foreign body became visible through the scope, and further manipulation and removal were directed under visual control. S, suction cervical cannula.

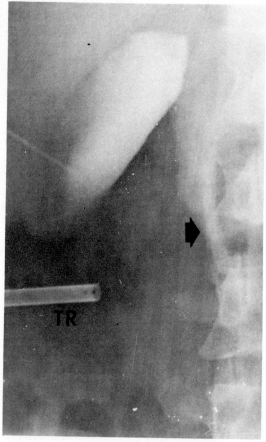

FIG. 17. Transhepatic cholecystocholangiography under laparoscopic control. Early filling stage. Teflon tube is in the gallbladder. Instrument trocar (TR) is seen at left. Paravertebral shadow (arrow) is air contrast of falciform ligament. No stones were detected in the gallbladder.

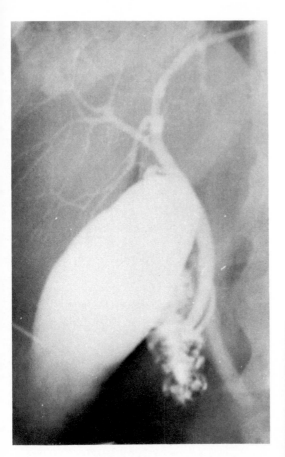

FIG. 18. Late filling stage in the same patient as shown in Figure 17. Normal-sized common bile and hepatic ducts. There is free drainage into the duodenum with reflux into the pancreatic duct. A total of eight films were taken.

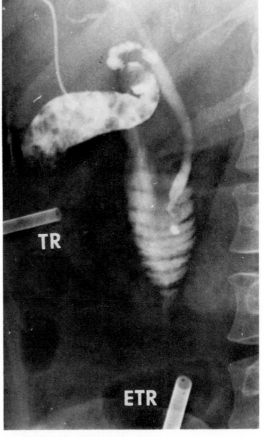

FIG. 19. Calculi in the gallbladder. Common bile duct is of normal size with free drainage into the duodenum. The examining trocar (ETR) and accessory or instrument trocar (TR) are visible.

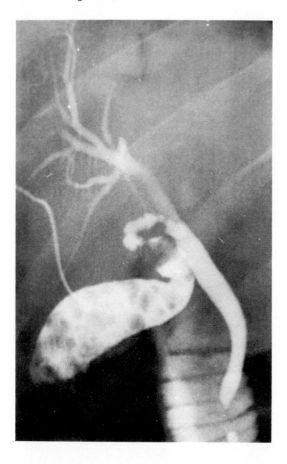

FIG. 20. Same patient as in Figure 19. Patient's position is changed to visualize the hepatic part. Normal-sized hepatic ducts. This patient had two distinct clinical entities: phenothiazine-induced icterus and nonobstructive cholelithiasis. Cholecystectomy was performed 2 months later when liver function tests returned to normal.

operating under visual control and the site of the needle entry can be observed. If bleeding or bile leakage accompanies the procedure the site can be coagulated, with the bleeding or leakage being brought under control by this "plugging" technique. Additional information is also available, e.g., the discovery of metastases and histologic identification (biopsy) of the lesion. If the obstruction is extrahepatic and this combined technique is performed in an operating room, immediate surgical exploration can follow endoscopy.

With greater experience a normal-sized intrahepatic duct can be found by careful needling and injection of a small amount of contrast material into the ductal system. The area is recognized immediately on the fluoroscopic screen and a cholangiogram performed. Wannagat[6] reported more than 2000 successful cholangiograms combined with laparoscopy, injecting the dye through the gallbladder or liver parenchyma with only three nonfatal complications (due to leakage) which were corrected by surgery.

CONCLUSIONS

Immediate visibility of an endoscope introduced into a body cavity and its configuration or position in relation to anatomic landmarks makes fluroscopy mandatory in conjunction with certain endoscopic procedures. If, in addition to fluoroscopy, contrast material is injected and radiographs are obtained, serial films can be exposed as aimed spot x-rays with small amounts of dye needed per film. Advantages of modern radiology include such factors as the possibility of changing the position of the patient, varying the injected volume as indicated by a fluoroscopic image, observing and recording various filling stages instead of making a "completion-gram," and documenting functional appearances because of the availability of dynamic recording techniques or serial films, with a general reduction in radiation dose to patient and personnel. These advantageous aspects in modern radiology should be considered with every endoscopic method where simultaneous x-ray procedures are to be employed.

Diagnostic radiology has undergone significant changes over the past 20 years. The introduction of image amplification with television fluoroscopy and aimed small-format film exposures have become a milestone in this diagnostic area.

When we introduce an endoscopic approach to unexplored areas we cannot overlook the progress in radiology, an integral part of our scoping procedure. The overall diagnostic accuracy, which is the final goal, can be improved if all existing new modalities are employed simultaneously.

Endoscopy has become more complicated because our tools are more sophisticated. This should not exclude or prevent us from going one step further and combining modern radiology with modern endoscopy—in one room.

REFERENCES

1. Berci G, Seyler AJ: An x-ray television image storage apparatus. Am J Roentgenol Radium Ther Nucl Med 90:1290, 1963
2. Berci G, Steckel R: Modern radiology in the operating room. Arch Surg 107:577, 1973
3. Berci G, Corlin R, Panish JF, et al: Complications of colonoscopy and polypectomy. Gastroenterology 67:584, 1974
4. Brooks P, Berci G, Adler D: The simultaneous and combined use of laparoscopy and hysterosalpingography using image amplification. J Reprod Med 10:285, 1973
5. Brooks P, Berci G, Adler D: Removal of intra-abdominal intrauterine contraceptive devices through the peritoneoscope with the use of intraoperative fluoroscopy to aid localization. Amer J Obstet Gynec 113:104, 1972
6. Wannagat L: Laparoskopische Cholangiographie. Radiologe 13:26, 1973

18

Permanent Film Records

George Berci
Gino Hasler
James G. Helmuth

VALUE, NEED, AND SHORTCOMINGS OF DOCUMENTATION

There have been a number of developments in instrumentation, illumination, and optics, but over the same period of time little has been done to design a recording apparatus to meet the needs of the practicing clinician. If we are to have a proper knowledge of pathology— be it a localized (stationary) or a functional disorder—the importance of having an objective permanent film record is self-evident. A slight deviation from normal is sometimes difficult to detect if the examiner's attention is divided in observing many facets of the investigation at the same time. It is hard to memorize and describe pathologic disorders if one has had only a fleeting glimpse of quickly changing events. With the help of a permanent film record, any deviation from the normal pattern can be reassessed at a later date and reviewed for an unlimited time without making further demands on the patient.

One of the factors responsible for the high level of diagnostic accuracy in radiology is the availability of the x-ray film, which can be scrutinized for a period of time. A lesion that may be overlooked on first inspection may be detected at a subsequent review. The possibility of comparing the findings at intervals during the patient's follow-up by means of a permanent film record is of utmost importance. Today we would hesitate to form an opinion or make a decision after reading *only* the description of a patient's fluoroscopic examination. We

are not satisfied unless we have a visual film record to supplement the typewritten report.

It is surprising that we have not developed analogous techniques for endoscopy. In the case of visual examinations, a permanent record would be of great value from diagnostic, consultation, and teaching aspects. A photograph or a film strip inserted into the patient's chart creates a much more objective, vivid, and effective impression than any description, however complete.

Every visual examination, in addition to a typewritten description, should be recorded and supported with an objective, permanent film. It is well known that on many occasions endoscopic examinations—not without risk—must be repeated because of a vague description. If the patient changes location or asks for a second opinion, it is highly unlikely that another doctor would create the same mental picture as the first examiner from a lesion with an unusual appearance. If a film in the form of a 35-mm slide, print, or movie film strip had been available, the progress or regress of the pathology could have been assessed with much greater accuracy, facilitating consultation and/or a final decision much more easily and objectively. Last but not least, many patients might escape an unnecessary additional examination.

Attempts to record endoscopic examinations were made as early as 1893 by Nitze.[13] A real impetus was given by Holinger, who showed his first endoscopic films in 1941.[8] Since then others have introduced alternative documentation techniques. Unfortunately, none of these methods gained wide acceptance because of the complexity and interference with the examination procedure.

Whenever we introduce a recording technique, we must keep in mind the following fundamental principles:

1. The operator must have complete control over the passage and manipulation of his instrument. He is largely dependent on sensation of resistance conveyed to his hand during such manipulation for the avoidance of dangerous pressure, risk of damage to mucous surfaces, or even perforation of the viscus. No restraint imposed by the recording apparatus must be allowed to interfere with this primary requirement. Even the best counterbalancing system imposes restrictions.
2. The examination time must not be considerably extended.
3. There should be no additional risk to the patient.
4. Equipment should be simple, easy to operate, and efficient in performance.
5. The capital outlay should be within the hospital budget.

A print inserted in the patient's chart and a photograph of the findings enclosed with the report to the referring doctor should be the scientific way of communication in our modern times of technologic achievements. Discrepancies between the clinical picture and the x-ray, endoscopic, and other findings can be discussed on ward rounds, grand rounds, clinicopathology conferences, and other meetings in a more meaningful way. There is no other or more convincing method to show minute lesions and pathologic functions than to display the actual visual findings as they were seen during the initial endoscopic examination. The value to consultation and teaching is self-evident.

Every endoscopist is conscious of these facts. The reason we are unable to employ this important adjunct routinely is that there is no simple, foolproof photographic equipment yet available to do the job. We need enthusiastic and knowledgeable doctors in photography, filming, and adjacent fields to accomplish this task. Every modern 35-mm still camera has built-in light meters and/or automatic exposure controls. Recent flash units meter the required discharge (output) for optimal exposure. These items are available commercially but are not designed or adaptable for endoscopy.

We have no chance to achieve our goal until we can fulfill the five criteria outlined above.

Our present problems and limitations in documentation are generally in these areas:

1. Loss in light transmission
2. Efficiency of light sources (flash and continuous)
3. Heavy cameras (still and movie)
4. Automatic light and exposure control

Loss in Light Transmission

Every endoscope (rigid or flexible) employs incoherent fiber glass threads for the transmission of illumination. The absorption is extremely high, approximately 10 to 15 percent per foot. The distinct yellowish color contributes to compression of the light red spectrum. Rigid telescopes are manufactured with fine fiber threads surrounding the optical system to provide illumination for examination. For this purpose the amount of light transmitted is sufficient. We are using large intensities (e.g., the condensed beam of a 150-watt quartz-Halogen lamp) where the overwhelming majority of brightness is lost in the 6-foot flexible fiber and at the connection on the other end to the fiber input of the surrounding fibers. Light is also absorbed in the tiny fibers around the optics.

Flexible Fiberscopes. The flexible fiberscopes eliminated the thread or other type of connections to the fiber optical compartment because an integral incoherent fiber bundle(s) is used. As an example, one 4 mm diameter bundle is guided in the "umbilical cord" (light, suction, water channel) to the eyepiece or operating handle of the scope, from where it is bifurcated into two smaller bundles to be conducted down to the working end. These bundles are very long (2730 to 3730 mm), and a huge amount of light is lost by traveling through these tiny fibers.

Rigid Endoscopes. The length of these telescopes is relatively short, but the absorption of light traversing the optical system—depending on the diameter, direction of view, etc.—is still significant. The most logical step was to place a filament globe at the end of the telescope (Fig. 1a).

Overburned Globes. This tungsten filament is originally made for 8 volts but was overburned for a fraction of a second with 24 volts, creating a flash[1] (Figs. 1b, c). It was difficult to procure this type of globe for straightforward (0-degree) telescopes. Most were made for lateral or forward-oblique optics

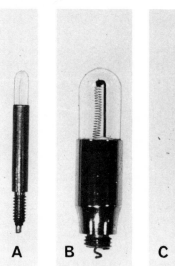 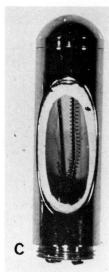

FIG. 1. **A.** Miniature electric globes were placed at the end of the endoscope beside the optic. It was most disconcerting if this globe burned out during the examination. The output was small, resulting in a dim image. This device was eventually replaced by glass fiber light transmitters. **B.** Six-volt filament globe which was overburned for a fraction of a second with 20 volts to create a large (flash) output for photography. The lifetime and the continuous output were unpredictable. **C.** Globe similar to that in **B** but with two filaments. The small one is for the examination and the large one for flash. The size of these globes precluded their use with smaller endoscopes.

and only for those of larger size. If this globe was overburned on repeated occasions, the heat production in respect to mucosal burns was in the danger zone. The lifetime was unpredictable, and after 10 to 20 overburned exposures the globe showed signs of "charring" with a significant decrease in output. Too-long exposure times (0.1 second) were needed.

Miniature (Distal) Flash. An excellent idea was the development of a miniature gas discharge flash tube.[9,11] Undoubtedly the results achieved were extremely good. The light source was near the object, and the color temperature of the flash discharge was ideal for a daylight film. These globes are large, and so their application is somewhat limited (today's smaller scopes or those used in pediatrics are excluded). The direction of illumination was also influenced by the direction of view —lateral or forward-oblique. During the discharge, heat as well as light is produced which requires that there be a mandatory distance from the object. The greatest concerns are those having to do with safety. Despite the fact that this system was widely employed in Europe without reported accidents, the possibility of an electric shock cannot be excluded. These globes work with an extremely high ignition voltage and amperage. The globe is held in position with a screw at the working end. If the scope is not kept under meticulous supervision, a faulty assembly, breakage of the insulating system due to an inadvertent knock, or substances such as soaking fluid damaging

the insulation and resulting in leakage can trigger irreversible cardiac irregularities. I doubt that this globe with its electronic design will fulfill the requirements of the present code.

Quartz Rod. Another worthwhile idea was the use of quartz glass rods.[7] Quartz has excellent light transmission characteristics in that it has minimal absorption and excellent color reproduction. The light source can be placed outside and therefore can be large. The disadvantages of a quartz rod are the diameter (2 to 3 mm), the extreme care needed in handling because of its fragile nature, and if light loss need be avoided the light source must be attached to the scope directly, which makes this assembly somewhat clumsy.

Fiber Glass. The use of fiber threads around the telescope, then, is our only choice. It can be shaped according to the configuration and the space allotted; even in a minute space beside the telescope enough fiber threads can be squeezed in to provide illumination (but only for examination).

In case of still photography or filming (or television) in larger cavities, the fibers around the telescope are far from sufficient to provide adequate light transmission. Therefore additional fibers are required. This setup can be achieved by a separate fiber shaft containing several square millimeters of fibers; alternatively a large number of fibers can be used in the form of an integral fiber bundle from the light source, several feet in length and extending beside the telescope up to the working end in one piece. This eliminates the joint spaces, e.g., fiber inlet of scope and fiber bundle (Fig. 2). Each fiber surface loosely attached (air space) is another source of light loss (15 to 20 percent). This loss does not interfere if it is used for examination only, but plays a role if photography is employed.

It was therefore necessary to use in larger adult scopes (broncho-, esophago-, laparo-, laryngo-, recto-, sigmoido-, and thoracoscopes) additional fiber threads in the form of a separate sheath; or they were incorporated within the telescope sheath in which case the outside diameter was enlarged. In these applications there is enough space to accommodate a larger telescope with more fibers.

In those fields where the diameter has a significant influence on the application (arthro-, cysto-, choledocho-, hystero-, rhino-, and transconioscopies, and pediatrics in general), the fibers around the telescope are the only ones that can be used for the transmission of flash or high-intensity illumination. In tubular organs like the urethra, flash photography meets the conditions; but if a photograph is to

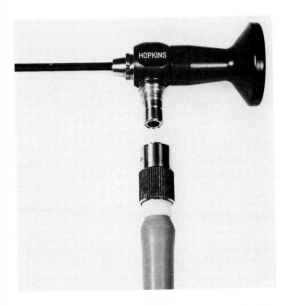

FIG. 2. If a fiberoptic light cable is connected to another fiber light guide by mechanical means (e.g., an attachment), light loss is encountered. For routine examination this can be compensated for; but for filming this estimated loss of 10 to 20 percent must be overcome by eliminating any interruptions of light transmission. Therefore integral fibers are employed which carry the light from the source, intact, to the working end of the scope.

be made, for example, with the cystoscope positioned at the bladder neck and the area to be recorded is the posterior wall of the bladder (object distance approximately 1.5 to 2 inches; 30 to 50 mm), it is difficult to reflect enough light for an exposure in depth. In smaller cavities (e.g., in pediatrics or arthroscopy), where white and good reflecting surfaces of near distances are present, we are dealing with better optical conditions.

Fluid Light Guide. This new invention (patent pending) is a flexible tube filled with an inert fluid. The refractory index between the wall of the tube and the fluid is optimal to guide light rays through, even in a bent position. Both ends are plugged with a special glass. When comparing a 6-foot fiber glass bundle with an identically sized fluid guide, the latter transmits more light. In addition, the yellowish tint or compression in the red spectrum is not apparent because of ideal color reproduction. We hope this will open a new chapter in light transmission.

Efficiency of Light Sources

Flash. We must use gas discharge flash globes to achieve a high output (watts per second) in order to keep the exposure as short as possible (1/30 or 1/60 second) to avoid a lack of sharpness caused by movement. The currently used flash globes are produced for other applications than endoscopy. The use of larger globes is most inefficient because it is difficult to condense a flash discharge to the small diameter of the fiber bundle (e.g., 4 mm). Therefore we utilize only a small percentage of the total output. The majority of light is wasted. The ideal is the point source flash globe *(vide infra,* pp. 256–59). Several problems must be overcome, e.g., heat production at the focal plane of the fiber, which is extremely high and difficult to cool because of the small duration (3 to 4 milliseconds). Smaller, more efficient, well designed flash tubes are needed. The development of the fluid fiber light guide is promising.

High-Intensity Light Sources. Continuous high-intensity light sources were needed for filming (or television), and it took us some time to realize that for our purpose a globe must be designed which will perform according to our specifications. Buying globes originally designed for 16-mm movie projectors (General Electric, Marc 300) is far from ideal. The frame of a 16-mm film is much greater than the diameter of a fiber bundle. More light also means more heat production. The transmission of wavelengths outside the visible range (ultraviolet and infrared) can result in tissue damage, especially if we are dealing with sensitive layers like the mucous membrane. We must be aware of existing limitations in technology; overlooking this aspect can result in a greater risk to the patient. Cold light does not exist; the terminology is a misnomer. The light source is extremely hot if we use a tungsten filament for the examination or an arc xenon for filming. In the first place, heat is absorbed by the length of the fiber bundle. We pay for this cooling effect with a minimal loss of 60 to 70 percent per 6 feet of the original output. With a xenon light source the heat is not negligible, even at the end of a 6-foot fiber bundle. Without getting involved with sophisticated temperature measurements, if you hold it to your wrist for a few seconds you can get some idea of the heat conducted inside the body cavity. An original design of an ideal light source for endoscopy with appropriate filtering may be the answer to our need.

Stroboscopic Flash. Strobing a flash globe synchronized with a movie camera shutter is a well known method. The shutter, if open, triggers the flash (duration: 2 to 4 milliseconds). The flash globe must be cycled according to the filming speed: 16 or 24 times/second. The maximum output of a flash globe with a short recharging time (e.g., 3 seconds) cannot be discharged with its full blast or output if the globe is triggered in this fast sequence. Consequently the output is decreased significantly. The electrodes and the cooling of the globe must be adjusted to withstand this big load. Another aspect which adds to the problems is the requirement of a point source, with an exit angle suitable for the admission of the light path or angle of the fiber. It seems to be the most ideal solution for filming because the present radiation and contact heat problems would be eliminated (*vide infra*, pp. 256–59). Colcher and Katz[5] cycled a tungsten filament globe to overcome the heat problems of a continuous, overburned distal globe. It also is questionable how the human brain will react to a prolonged flickering effect. It is difficult with present technology to manufacture a globe which, with this fast recycling time (24/second), will provide a continuous light between the cycles.

At this stage it is mainly the lack of a suitable flash globe which hinders the design of a strobounit with sufficient output for cinematography whose light is transmitted through a fiber or other type of light guide.

Flexible Fiber Endoscopes. There is no flash globe available at this stage that can produce sufficient energy at the end of a 2.5 to 3 meter long bundle to expose a 35-mm film with an acceptable displayed image size. Such a flash would be ideal because it would eliminate the use of continuous high-intensity light sources for still photography. Our present exposures are far too long (1/5, 1/8, and 1/10 second) to avoid movement. The absorption of the bundle is high. In order to photograph through a fiber bundle, a series of pictures is required to be sure that in a roll of 20 pictures we secure the important pathology or momentum within two or three frames. Making acceptable movie films through fiber bundles is easier than obtaining sharp still photographs.

Since the above was written, there has been made available a prototype of a flash unit with which we can provide examining light and a short, powerful flash burst through the fiberscope using an exposure time of 1/30 of a second to expose one 35-mm full frame. The initial results are promising.

Heavy Cameras

The size and weight of the camera, the dim image through the viewer, and the difficulties in manipulating with an attached camera, etc. made it necessary to develop cameras especially for our purposes. This applies to 35-mm still and 16-mm movie cameras, as well as to television cameras. The interposition of an image-transmitting medium (coherent fiber bundle or articulated optical arm) is cumbersome, deteriorates the image quality (fiber bundle), or is extremely delicate and expensive (optical arm). For our application we do not require sophisticated cameras. We need a small but light box, with a film-forwarding mechanism and a shutter with two or (maximum) three speeds. The lenses of existing cameras are designed for external photography; they have many features—e.g., absorption of more light and correction for peripheral distortion—that are not required in our application. In endoscopy the aperture is determined by the optical system of the telescope or fiberscope with its optical components on both ends. The exit angle of an endoscope is small. We utilize, at most, only the middle third of a photographic lens. For this reason simpler, less expensive lenses can be used. We cannot afford to focus continuously during our procedures, so we must compromise with a fixed-focus system during still and movie photography.

Automatic Light and Exposure Control

It is most disconcerting when effort and time are invested to produce a film record of an interesting event and the film turns out to be under- or overexposed. Even inexpensive 35-mm still cameras have built-in meters coupled to the exposure control. When we find something interesting or unusual during a procedure we concentrate on the actual event. We have no time to check the brightness of the picture, the needle position of the meter, etc. Our main concern is the patient.

One of the flexible fiber endoscope manufacturers advocated a high-intensity illumination source with an "automatic exposure control." This so-called automatization consists of a warning light which goes on only if the object distance is small. Could you image filming a polypectomy procedure in the colon, having one hand preoccupied with a 4- to 5-pound movie camera and the other trying to master the two knobs with four-way control, fighting the continuously appearing peristaltic wave and disappearing polyp, etc., etc.—and at the same time keeping an eye on the "on/off" red light? We need more freedom to operate our auxiliary apparatus, enabling us to concentrate, with less frustration and fewer distractions from our main commitment: patient care.

Simple electronic circuitries are needed for the already available automatic light and exposure controls. The controls have been used in industrial photographic applications for 5 to 10 years. The automatic brightness and density controls have also been adapted to diagnostic radiography.

Fifty years ago the radiologist, in close collaboration with radiophysicists, closed the gap between the visual observation and the lack of permanent records by developing modern radiographic techniques. Now it is up to the endoscopist and engineers to follow their lead.

George Berci

STILL PHOTOGRAPHY

35-mm Still Cameras

The models employed are mainly reflex (through the lens) viewing cameras with or without an automatic rewind mechanism, e.g., Olympus Pen-F, Robot, Honeywell-Pentax, Rollei, Endo-Storz (Fig. 3G). Practically speaking, any still camera can be coupled to an endoscope, but whether it is really convenient or useful for the purpose is another question.

Camera Body

We do not require an expensive and sophisticated camera body with many accessories (which are unnecessary for endoscopy). We do not need an iris in the lens because the aperture is determined by the endoscope. Using electronic flash, the built-in meters or even electronic shutters are of no help. All these accessories do is add to the cost and weight of the equipment. Full-frame bodies are preferred because the same camera can be used for large and small pictures.

Camera Attachment to Endoscope

There are a variety of coupling devices. Every manufacturer is anxious to produce a unique eyepiece and coupling device. The endoscope must be optically aligned with the camera lens and kept in this position. It must be firm and safe. The camera acts like a handle, and part of the weight and maneuvering of the scope during the photographic process is performed through the camera. Among the adaptors are the spring-loaded ball bearing (Figs. 3F, G) and the rotating "lock" type (Fig. 3A).

The rotating lock attachment (Olympus) is cumbersome. In a subdued light it is difficult to find the matching dots on the camera and eyepiece, and the thin tin blades can be bent over a period of time. The so-called automatic built-in exposure control is not necessary. Over the long run, a simple spring-controlled and finger-release double-blade system (Fig. 4) has proved most satisfying. It is easily attached and detached; it can be rotated around the telescope; and it keeps the camera well aligned with a firm grip. The double-blade system can be used with other endoscopes that have non-

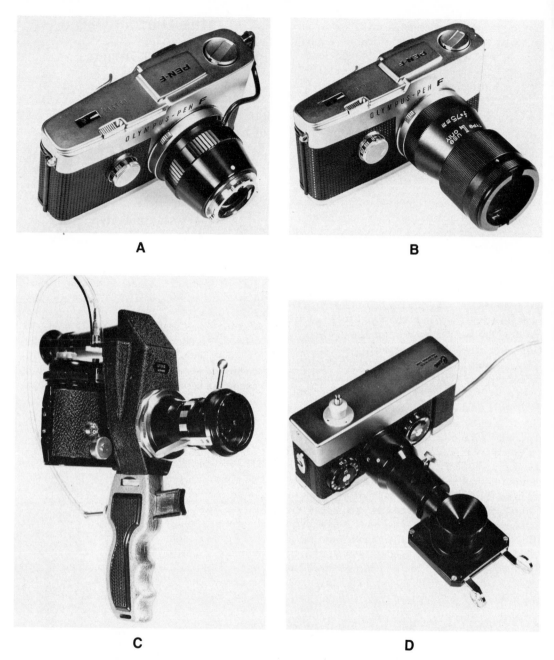

FIG. 3. A. Olympus Pen-F half-frame 35-mm camera without lens, with rotating lock adapter for Olympus fiberscopes. Size: 70 mm × 139 mm × 127 mm. Weight: 640 g (22 ounces). **B.** Olympus Pen-F half-frame 35-mm camera with Machida rotating lock adapter and 75-mm lens for Machida fiberscopes.   **C.** A 35-mm full-frame Robot body with (spring-loaded) automatic film advancement. Extended mirror reflex viewer and zoom lens (70 to 120 mm) made by Storz. Weight: 1060 g (37 ounces).   **D.** A 35-mm full-frame Rollei camera. Electric motor drive made and attached locally. Lens: 50 mm. Beam splitter: 15/85 percent with quick adapter. For weight and size see Table 2. (Continued)

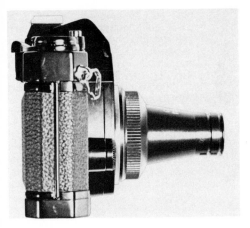

E

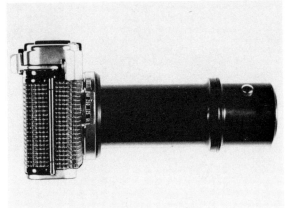

F

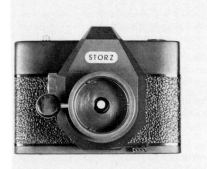

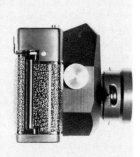

G

FIG. 3 (cont.). **E.** Honeywell-Pentax 35-mm full-frame camera with electronic shutter attachment to ACMI fiberscopes. For dimensions see Table 2. **F.** Olympus 35-mm half-frame camera with 80-mm lens attached to R. Wolf endoscopes. **G.** Endo-Storz 35-mm full-frame camera with low-voltage motor film drive, full-field clear viewer, and spring-loaded ball bearing attachment. Lens: 90 mm (can be interchanged to smaller focal length). Synchronous outlet to flash generator. This is currently the smallest full-frame camera with motor drive available. For dimensions see Table 2.

conventional eyepieces by using a simple adaptor (Fig. 5).

Size and Weight

Modern endoscopy employs delicate, lightweight, miniaturized instruments. The weight is crucial, providing the examiner with tactile sensation (which is conveyed to his fingertips by his instruments during manipulation). For example, if a pediatric endoscope (Table 1) is coupled to a camera weighing five times more than the scope, the important tactile sensation is lost. Table 2 gives the weight and size of various cameras.

Rewind Mechanism

A single exposure is generally not enough. The camera and endoscope are hand-held. Movement of a few millimeters on the proximal end or movement of the object itself is enough to lose the area of pathology to be photographed. To be on the safe side, several frames must be made. To rewind or push the film forward manually after exposure requires additional manipulation. This is enough to create disturbing movements, touching the mucosa with the distal end of the telescope, etc., spoiling a photographic moment. An automatic rewind mechanism when using rigid endoscopes is of paramount importance. Even when flexible fiberscopes are inserted, a slight twist at the eyepiece can cause the lesion to disappear. Good examples to illustrate the need for a "nontouch" photographic technique are organs with peristalsis or respiratory movements.

Exposure Time and Shutter

The various time exposures available on a camera are never used in our application. A camera with a maximum of three exposure times would meet our needs. With rigid tele-

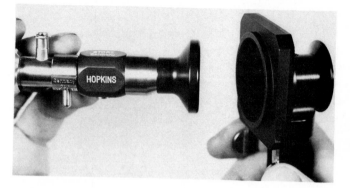

FIG. 4. Spring-controlled double-blade quick adapter. Easy to attach and detach. The telescope eyepiece can be rotated. This design keeps the endoscope (eyepiece) and camera well aligned with a firm grip. In this configuration a beam splitter is built into it, and the camera therefore is coupled at 90 degrees. Alternatively it can be directly attached to any camera lens. This attachment can be used with various brands of rigid endoscopes and ACMI fiberscopes. The same quick release is used with movie cameras for coupling to endoscopes.

scopes a short flash discharge is employed. Depending on the synchronization mechanism between the flash generator and the camera, an exposure time of 1/60 or 1/30 second is adequate. These short exposure times are ideal for avoiding disturbing movements like peristalsis, respiration, or transmission of the aortic pulsation, which can interfere with the sharpness of the picture. The actual time duration of the flash is 2 to 5 milliseconds (1/500 to 1/200 second). The extended exposure time is only a safety guard for the synchronization (1/30 = 33 milliseconds, 1/60 = 16 milliseconds).

With flexible fiber endoscopes (gastroscope or colonoscope) the integral incoherent light-

TABLE 1. Weight of Some Standard and Miniature (Rigid) Endoscopes

Endoscope	Weight (g)
Pediatric bronchoscope	132
Pediatric cystoscope	120
Adult cystoscope	155

If a camera is attached that is five times or more heavier than the endoscope, we lose the sensation in our fingertips that is so important during manipulations.

TABLE 2. Weight and Size of 35-mm Still Cameras

Camera	Weight*		Size†		
	Ounces	Grams	H ×	L ×	W
Olympus Pen-F	22	640	70	139	127
Honeywell Pentax	27	760	87	105	141
Rollei (motorized film advance)	21	590	65	137	120
Robot (motorized film advance)	37	1,060	114	218	115
Endo-Storz‡ (motorized film advance)	12	340	80	82	111

*Weight of camera with lens attached (without film).
†H, height. L, length. W, width. All in millimeters.
‡The Endo-Storz camera is the smallest and lightest 35-mm full-frame camera with motor drive available at this stage.

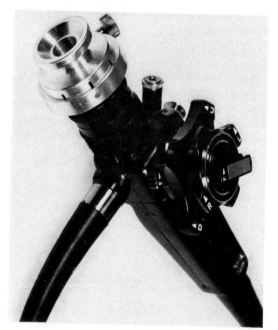

FIG. 5. A simple adapter can be employed in the case of a nonconventional eyepiece.

transmitting bundle is small and too long (2.7 to 3.7 meters) to transmit a flash discharge with sufficient illumination. In this group of instruments, therefore, high-intensity *continuous* light must be employed to obtain a still picture. In our experience the exposure time with a fiberscope is extended to 1/15 or even 1/8 second, resulting in an unsharp picture in most cases. We therefore need a camera with only three exposure times—1/15, 1/30, and/or 1/60 second—which cover the entire range of instruments. A simple shutter mechanism is just as good as the more expensive and delicate focal plane shutter.

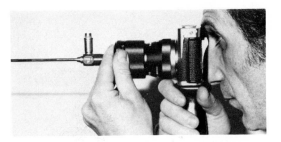

FIG. 6. The flat design of the viewer in this camera body is inconvenient.

Photo Lens

If standard (external) photography is performed, a good quality, multielement lens is required. In endoscopy, however, by coupling the camera with its lens to a telescope, the main objectives of image transmission are already completed by the optical system of the endoscope.

A lens for normal photography is designed for optical precision. The image quality or optical characteristics at the edge of the lens must be similar to those in the middle. In our applications (after coupling) we use only the middle portion of the lens. A simple (achromat) lens therefore suffices for us. If these simple lenses are properly selected and coated, they absorb less light than the multielement ones and are significantly less expensive and simpler to handle.

The focal length of the lens determines the size, diameter, or displayed image on the film, and is in proportion with the physical size (length) of the lens. The displayed image size determines the focal length.

Viewer

In attaching a standard 35-mm camera with a reflex (through the lens) viewer to an endoscope, the flat design of the camera body is inconvenient (Fig. 6). Some manufacturers therefore extended the viewing eyepiece, which gives the examiner more "breathing" space (Fig. 7). The standard coarse-grained viewer is disturbing, changing suddenly from a clear picture to a "fogged" one. Even using a clear glass viewing system produced a dim image due to the absorption of the multiple optical relay elements interposed between the telescope

eyepiece and the examiner's eye. Using larger cameras we found disturbing the sudden changes in the distance (which were due to the attached camera body plus viewing system), the changing appearance of the picture, and difficulties in manipulations.

For this reason we experimented with a beam splitter which deviates a part of the image to the examiner, the other part being directed into the camera. The viewer itself is the beam splitter. The camera is attached at a 90-degree angle to the endoscope (Fig. 8), and a simple fixed focal achromat lens is used as the camera lens. This arrangement offers the following advantages:

1. The distance between endoscope and examiner is not increased.
2. The same image that would be seen through the eyepiece is observed, with no changes in color, size, or magnification.
3. The camera is out of the way and can be used as a handle for supporting the instrument.

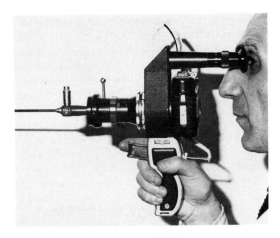

FIG. 7. An extended viewer system is practical, but if more relay elements are incorporated the system absorbs more light and the image is dim compared to the picture seen through the endoscope.

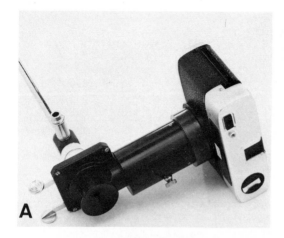

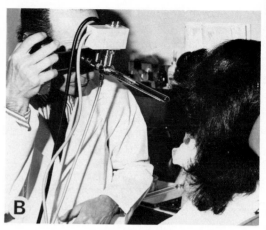

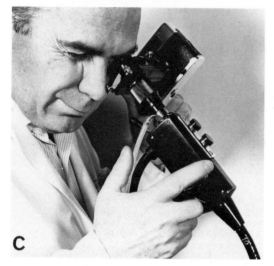

FIG. 8. **A.** A rigid endoscope is attached to the Endo-Storz camera via a beam splitter (15/85 percent). Camera lens: 80 mm. The endoscope-examiner eye distance is not increased, and the same image that we would see through the eyepiece directly is observed. The camera is out of the way and can be used as a supporting handle. The examining light is rarely used with maximum output. If the camera is attached, the examining light is turned to the maximum setting, which compensates for the light loss of the beam splitter. For flexible fiberscopes we use a high-intensity light source because flash discharge globes for this application are not available. **B.** Still camera attached through the beam splitter-viewer to a laryngoscope with an external flash. The entire apparatus is hand held by grasping the camera, leaving the other hand free for the introduction or manipulations. **C.** Same arrangements as in **B**, but this time attached to a flexible (ACMI) fiberscope. With a four-way control mechanism we need freedom to facilitate manipulation and documentation.

We found this arrangement in practice very efficient. It is true that the beam splitter decreases the light transmission to the camera by 10 to 20 percent, but with the improved optical and light-transmission systems in which light absorption is less we can afford this loss. Ten to twenty percent of the light is transmitted to the eye, and 80 to 90 percent to the camera. The examining light source, which is rarely used with maximum output for rigid endoscopes, can be increased. With fiberscopes a high-intensity light source should be used.

Displayed Image Size on Film

The size of the image exposed on the film is dependent on the optical parameters of the endoscope, the exit angle and enlargements of the ocular, the focal length of the photolens in the camera, and the available illumination. For instance, a 55-mm lens displays on the film a smaller but brighter image than a 70- or 90-mm lens (Table 3). As the displayed image on the film becomes larger, it requires the use of more light.

There is a trend which I call "unnecessary megalophotography." Overframing (Fig. 9) means that parts of the displayed image are cut and omitted from the picture. We can enlarge by this technique, but we cannot produce more details than are in fact available.

If the displayed and well exposed image is 10 to 20 mm in diameter (Fig. 9) we are more than happy. A slide with this size image can be copied or printed in a 3× to 6× enlargement with no difficulty, and our ultimate aim of plac-

TABLE 3. Displayed Image Size Versus Focal Length of Camera Lens in Various Rigid and Flexible Fiberscopes

Fiberscope	Image Size (mm) at Various Lens Focal Lengths		
	55 mm	70 mm	90 mm
Rigid telescope cystoscope (Hopkins)	7.4	10.0	12.5
Laparoscope (Hopkins)	13.5	18.2	23.3
Fiber colonoscope (Olympus)	6.9	8.7	11.0
Fiber gastroscope (ACMI)	12.0	15.6	20.5

The figures beside the actual image size indicate the diameter in mm. Several parameters play a role, e.g., light transmission of optical system, intensity of flash or continuous illumination, film speed. It is recommended that something be chosen that is between the extremes. Every large image on film needs more light.

ing quality prints in the patients charts from our endoscopic findings is fulfilled. If we overframe, from a 20-mm displayed image to a 30-mm diameter, we enlarge it but no more pathology is exposed.

We review our 35-mm slides by projection using a small room with a short distance (12 feet, 360 cm) and a 150-mm projector lens (smaller but brighter image). The displayed image on the 35-mm slide is 12.5 mm (0.5 inch) in diameter and the actual picture size on the screen is 337.5 mm (13.5 inches), which means it is enlarged 27× (Fig. 10). At longer distances and with different projector lenses this factor can be increased.

The size of the displayed image on film depends on a number of factors, e.g., size of telescope (or fiberscope) light transmission of optics, diameter of the light transmitter, light source, flash (rigid) or continuous (flexible fiber), exposure time, film speed. All these factors must be taken into consideration in order to select the proper focal length of the lens and displayed image size on the 35-mm film. The desire for a "king size" image on the 35-mm film should be kept within reasonable "diameters." It is senseless to use an extremely long focal length on the camera lens if under normal conditions the film cannot be adequately exposed. There are of course technical tricks: additional light guides, large telescopes, ultrahigh-speed films, forced processing, etc. The question which has to be answered is: Does this serve our aim—does it provide improved patient care with documentation but without a greater fuss?

Some Practical Hints (Focal Length)

A 50-mm lens is used for miniature (pediatric) endoscopes. For smaller telescopes (e.g., arthro-, cysto-, choledochoscope, etc.) where the flash discharge is transmitted only through the

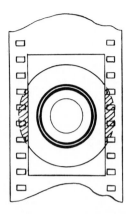

FIG. 9. Displayed image sizes on 35-mm film. Single circle represents 10 mm, and double circle 18 mm. We found the range 10 to 18 (20) mm most suitable for adult size scopes. If the image size is 30 mm, some parts of the picture are overframed, or cut (shaded areas). The 30-mm image gives no more information than does the 20-mm image, and it requires a longer (heavier) lens and much more light. The displayed image must be individually determined; for example, with pediatric (rigid) scopes we expose the film in a 5-mm circle. Frame size of 35-mm film: 24×36 mm.

examining-light-carrying fibers and no additional light-carrying fibers can be used, a focal length of 50 mm is recommended. For telescopes with additional photo (flash)-carrying fibers (broncho-, laryngo-, laparoscope, etc.), a focal length of 80 or a maximum of 90 mm is used. The displayed image size will be 15 to 20 mm. For flexible fiberscopes the focal length should be 50 mm.

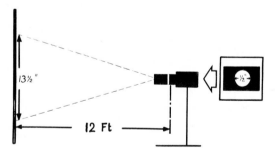

FIG. 10. For everyday use in a small room we analyze our slides from a 12-foot (3.6-meter) projector-screen distance (150-mm lens gives a small but bright image). The actual 0.5-inch (12.5 mm) displayed image on the transparency becomes as large as 13.5 inches (338 mm), which represents a 27-fold enlargement. This is sufficient for routine screening. For larger rooms or auditoriums the conditions of projection and screen size are adapted to the length of the room, etc.

From a practical viewpoint the entire range of endoscopic procedures can be covered with two simple interchangeable achromat lenses (50 and 90 mm), producing a good displayed image, taking the diameter, the required light, and the exposure time into account.

Discussion

Obtaining a good snapshot of the pathology without greatly extending the examining time, without increased risk to the patient, and with simple photography equipment is of utmost importance. The ultimate aim is to have a 35-mm slide in the file and a 4×5 inch (100×125 mm) print in the patient's chart or enclosed with the endoscopy report sent to the referring physician (Fig. 11).

In order to achieve this goal we must optimize several factors.

Illumination. A short flash is the method of choice for still photography. The efficiency of our present discharge globes is far from optimal. A new idea with better parameters is described in the section on flash systems. A proper flash has not been developed for use with flexible fiberscopes, so we must employ continuous illumination. The examining sources (150-watt Halogen-tungsten globes) are not suitable. The light output is not enough to compensate for the high absorption of the light by the image-transmitting bundles; therefore an extended exposure time (e.g., 1/5 second) must be used, resulting in an unsharp picture. The conditions can be improved by applying a high-intensity light source.

Light Transmission. Most of the transmitted light (flash) is absorbed in the light-carrying fiber bundle. The fibers surrounding the telescope comprise another limiting factor. In certain applications the instrument can be enlarged, adding more light-carrying fibers (laryngoscope, laparoscope, bronchoscope, etc.), but in those areas where miniaturization is imperative (pediatrics, and arthro-, cysto-, choledochoscope, etc.) we have to compromise with the small-diameter fibers. The invention of a new light-transmitting medium is promising where absorption is less and the color is more natural.

35-mm Camera. Previous 35-mm full-frame cameras were too heavy, and the viewer and lenses were not designed for our application. The new miniature lightweight 35-mm full-frame camera weighing only 12 ounces

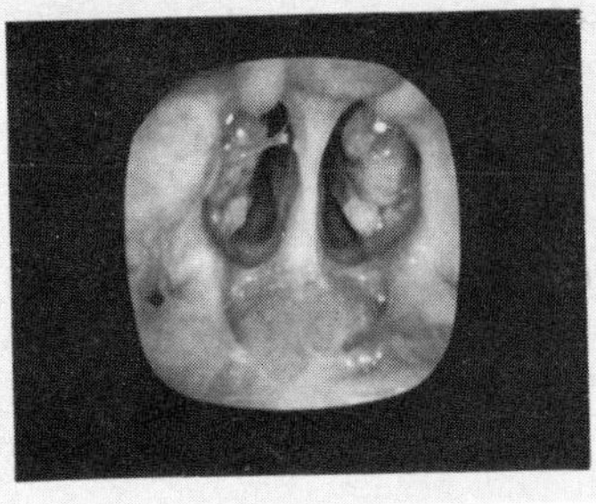

Mr. J. K. Blow M.64
J-324-568-90

DATE	Note progress of case, complications, consultations, change in diagnosis, condition on discharge, instructions to patient.
1.5.75.	Nasopharyngoscopy (J.McCallum,M.D,)
10 a.m.	History: Epistaxis for a period of one year. (Both nostrils).
	No family history of Ca. No prev.illness or common cold.
	Procedure: 5% Lidocaine spray was applyied in the posterior pharynx
	and in both nostrils. After 5 minutes apropriate topical
	anesthesia was achieved. The Hopkins-Storz 90° telescope
	with A.F.sheath was introduced. The wall of the post.naso-
	pharynx looked smooth. In both nostrils in depth in the vicinity
	of both inf.conchae a lobulated ½-1 cm polypoid appearance
	was found which on palpation seemed to be smooth and soft.
	Biopsies were taken from both lesions.
	The procedure took approx.:20 minutes
	No bleeding was observed. The patient left the Endo.O.R.
	in excellent condition.
	Photographs were taken from the findings and are enclosed below.
	J.McCallum,M.D.

FIG. 11. The typewritten descriptive report is supported by an enlarged color print from the original endoscopy slide. This size is large enough to display the pathology and to support our report in the patient's chart or file.

(340 g) and incorporating a clear viewer with 100 percent light transmission to the film (or with a beam splitter 85 percent) is a great step forward. In these (3 × 3 × 4.5 inches; 80 × 82 × 111 mm) a low-voltage driven motor is incorporated for automatic advancement of the film after exposure. This camera is small and compact enough to not interfere with our standard techniques.

Photo Lenses. An inexpensive, simple achromat lens is sufficient. The focal range must be adjusted (fixed) for the working range of the particular endoscope. If the endoscope ocular is properly designed it can be fixed at infinity. We found in many instances that the ocular system of the scope is different, and the lens must be adjusted according to the optical performance. This can be done with a minimal effort, the lens then performing optimally. There is no time to refocus if object distances are changing.

Automatic Flash Exposure. This idea is not new and has been applied in industrial photography for years. It should be used in endoscopy too, where the operator is involved in many more and important aspects of patient care. The operator's concentration should be devoted to the procedure rather than to measuring light, etc.

Film. Generally a daylight film with a 160 ASA speed is used. Technologic advances in emulsion chemistry have produced good films with excellent color reproduction and minimal grain. There are certain procedures in which there is enough light and in which we could afford to use a slower film speed, but in a hospital with a dozen different procedures the equipment and film material must be uniform to make it easier for the paramedical personnel who handle the maintenance, loading of films, etc.

Prints from Endoscopic Procedures. It is difficult to read a 35-mm slide, so a print with a 3× to 4× enlargement is preferable for insertion into the patient's chart. A recently employed material is mentioned in the section on instantaneous photography.

The reason photography has become extensively accepted by a large number of amateur photographers is the development of relatively inexpensive automatic cameras. The same goal must be achieved with endoscopic photography.

If the doctor is not particularly familiar with the technical aspects but is a good endoscopist, he should be able to make fast and reliable records of his findings.

George Berci and Gino Hasler

FLASH SYSTEMS FOR STILL ENDOSCOPIC PHOTOGRAPHY

General Illumination Requirement

Any photographic illumination system for endoscopy should provide sufficient light to (1) allow viewing of the object (pathology) before the film is exposed; and (2) expose the film.

Using medium or high speed (e.g., ASA 160) color film and large enough format (typically 35 mm) for good image resolution, the amount of continuous light required for a good exposure may be many times the amount necessary for observation, even with very slow shutter speeds. Of course a long exposure is undesirable since object and camera motion can blur the image. Also, a high level of continuous, high-intensity light may become harmful to the patient or mucous surface in terms of total energy (ultraviolet, visible light, and infrared/heat) exposure.

Flash photography is a realistic solution to the exposure problem. Since an enormous amount of light can be produced in a very short time, the film is exposed without problems of blurring. Because of the low total average power and less heat per unit light, risks due to excessive heat production are practically eliminated. As a bonus, the discharge of a flash tube color spectrum has much more blue content than light produced by most continuous sources, thus rendering better color contrast on the film.

Technical Problems

Because the endoscope has a very small entrance area for transmitting illumination (fibers), the source of light should be as small as possible. Light rays from a large source cannot be focused down into a small beam without proportional loss of total light. Conventional strobe (flash) sources are physically large and radiate relatively low light per unit area of their surface. In order to generate enough surface brightness, large peak power must be put into the strobe tube. In addition, it is required that coupling between tube and endoscope be very efficient to minimize loss of light.

Attempts have been made to insert a miniature (low power) flash tube directly into the body cavity[4] or built into the working (inserted) end of the endoscope.[10] Despite good results, the electrical danger of these systems is a very strong deterrent (see below).

Good results have also been obtained with a strobe tube mounted proximally at the entrance of the endoscope fiber illumination light input. The flash must be full power, however, to overcome the collection and transmission light losses. This method still involves electrical hazard to the patient and doctor[15] and has the further disadvantage of increased weight and bulk that must be supported during examination.

To discuss the danger factors one must be aware that strobe tubes are basically high-voltage devices in which the main flash may be produced by voltages in the range of 300 to 600 volts, and the flash is initiated by a trigger voltage on the order of 5000 volts! During the times of a flash (a few thousandths of a second), currents may pass through the tube on the order of 100 amperes! With all this electrical activity mechanically connected to the patient via the endoscope, the concern is obvious.[6] The size and weight factors arise from the fact that the strobe tube itself is physically large, and considerable electrical isolation of the tube and circuit from the endoscope is required.

As an additional problem, conventional strobes do not operate in a continuous-light-producing mode needed for viewing, so a separate source of steady light optically coupled to the endoscope is also required. This is normally done through the use of a fiberoptic bundle from an external (examining) light source to the strobe light housing—the light passing through the clear glass strobe tube and into the entrance port of the endoscope.

A final difficulty is obtaining correct control of the exposure. The variables are the flash intensity, effective aperture of the telescope, the distance of the working end of the endoscope to the object surface, and film speed. Thus typically several exposures should be made of a single subject to ensure a good exposure.

Using continuous (high-intensity) light as the source, exposure is controlled simply by changing shutter speed, and with motorized film winding a sequence of exposures is quickly made.

With strobe illumination exposure cannot be determined using the shutter because the duration of the strobe flash is far too short for the camera shutter to accept only a part of that time. The flash duration may be only a few thousandths of a second, so the camera shutter would have to be faster—a thousandth or less—to reduce exposure. Therefore the intensity of the flash (power to the strobe tube) is adjusted. This is conventionally done with a selector switch on the power supply of the strobe tube. The difficulty comes from the waiting period (recycle time) required between flashes (which may be as long as 5 to 10 seconds) for the strobe tube to cool and the power supply (condenser system) to recharge; thus the time to make a series of exposures can be quite long.

Future Improvements

Recently techniques have been developed to allow strobe flashing of "short-arc" xenon tubes (Fig. 12). These tubes have been used for many years to produce continuous light. Because of their extremely small source size and attendant high surface brightness:

1. Collection of light is very efficient.
2. A very bright beam or spot can be optically formed.
3. The optical system can be physically small.
4. The light is very "white."

When this tube is operated in a flashing mode, these benefits are retained.

With direct optical coupling to the illumination entrance of the endoscope fiber light-transmitting part, much more light can be obtained than is actually required. Therefore a convenient and safe (but somewhat inefficient) coupling such as a fiberoptic bundle may be employed between the flash and the endoscope, still providing enough flash illumination of the object.

With this "remote" positioning of the strobe tube from the endoscope, the potential hazards, the bulk and weight, have been eliminated. Since the fiberoptic bundle can be completely nonmetallic, there is no possibility of high voltage, current, or leakage endangering the patient, even in the form of a "microshock."

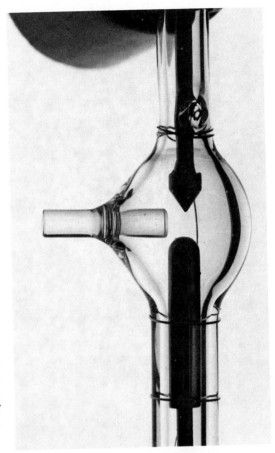

FIG. 12. Close-up of a short-arc xenon tube. Actual size of a rated globe: 150 watts/second: 80 × 15 mm. Because of their extremely small source size and high surface brightness, the collection of light is very efficient and a very bright spot (beam) can be formed; the optical system can be physically small, and the light is still very "white." The color temperature (K) is high. A quartz rod is inserted into the glass envelope and extends almost to the electrodes, thus facilitating optimal collection of energy output. Between flash discharges this globe produces continuous light for examination.

Another advantage of the short-arc tube is that it may be run in the conventional way so as to produce continuous (examination) light between flashes. Thus a separate viewing light source is not necessary. The color temperature (color balance) of the flash is somewhat more blue than the conventional strobe. Since light transmission in the endoscope tends to become slightly yellow due to the yellowish tint of the fibers, the final color balance of the illumination becomes more natural.

For control of flash exposure the electrical techniques have been well developed. A photocell in the camera produces an electrical signal proportional to the light falling on the film. This signal is integrated (produced of light intensity × time) to give a result proportional to exposure. This result may then be simply read on a meter (Fig. 13), and the intensity of flash output can be manually changed to bring the next flash reading to the desired value.

As an additional improvement, the result may instead be fed to circuitry, which computes the intensity required to give the desired exposure, and then this change is made automatically for the next exposure. However, in the best scheme (which is now available in commercial photography) the integration of the photocell signal during the flash is monitored, and when it reaches the desired result (the correct exposure) the flash is automatically stopped. Thus no trial flash need be made. There is no reason why this technique could

not be applied to endoscopic flash photography. When this is accomplished, the waiting time between flashes becomes unimportant since only one exposure of each region of interest need be made.

Current Status

At the time of this writing, a short-arc flash unit, as described above, has been undergoing evaluation for about a year. It has been found to be electrically safe and to produce sufficient light output in most applications. Effort is now being directed toward obtaining high-quality long-life short-arc tubes and fiber bundles for this special flash use.

This need arises from the method of light collection employed in the unit. The strobe tube is constructed with a quartz rod inserted into the envelope and extending almost to the electrodes. This rod acts as a light guide, collecting a large fraction of the light produced in the arc owing to its close proximity, and carrying this light out through the envelope. The input end of the fiber bundle is placed at the outside end of the quartz rod, and the light passes from the rod to the bundle. The bundle then carries the light to the illumination (fiber) input of the endoscope.

The energy level of the flash at the strobe tube is quite high in order to overcome these transmission and coupling losses, and some electrode deterioration occurs. The removed material (tungsten) redeposits on the tube envelope interior, causing the tube to darken quickly. The quartz rod, however, owing to its closeness to the high-energy arc, remains clear and there is no loss of light output as the tube ages.* However, as the electrodes wear, the continuous arc (for the examining light function) becomes flickery and unsteady, and is somewhat distracting to the viewer. Thus an improvement in materials and/or construction of the strobe tube is needed.

Also, because of the high-energy level of the flash, the input end of the fiber bundle is subjected to a very high instantaneous temperature. Even the so-called high-temperature bundles quickly burn and discolor at this end owing to the heat sensitivity of the cement used to bind the fibers together at the termina-

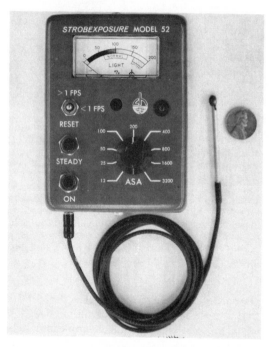

FIG. 13. Flash meter with a miniature photocell to record single or repeated (cycled) flash outputs. This photocell can be incorporated into the viewer of the still camera via a beam splitter; it indicates the amount of reflected light that goes through the endoscope. In the future the integration of the photocell signal *during the flash* can be monitored, and when it reaches the desired correct exposure the flash is automatically stopped.

Patent, United States and Europe: Chadwick-Helmuth Co.

tion. Bundles made using only glass as the end binder material have proved satisfactory, but currently production of such bundles appears difficult and expensive.

Hopefully these problems will be resolved in the near future, and this unit will be commercially available, opening a new chapter in still photography for endoscopic documentation. Laboratory tests of an automatic exposure control system have been initiated and have progressed to the point of producing a meter reading proportional to the integrated light (and thus to the resultant exposure).

James G. Helmuth

INSTANTANEOUS PHOTOGRAPHY

The introduction of immediately available prints through the development of Polaroid cameras and films made us very enthusiastic about being able to obtain a print of our findings during the endoscopic procedure. After employing this method our initial enthusiasm waned, however, for many reasons. The available Polaroid film packs were far too large and heavy. Furthermore, the cameras produced by some of the endoscopic manufacturers added to the weight and size. To be more economical with this large-film format, the back had to be rotated to place several small pictures on one film. The quality of the prints—for our application—leaves much to be desired. The information (resolution) available on a transparency (slide) is much greater than on a Polaroid film. The speed of the Polaroid film material is much too slow for our purpose. The color reproduction is also inferior compared with a reversal film. Instantaneous photography is extremely useful in innumerable industrial and other applications, but at this stage it cannot be recommended for direct endoscopic documentation. If further research results in a better and faster film material with instant developing features it will have its place.

We used the Polaroid CU-5 copying camera* to provide prints from endoscopic slides for insertion into the patient's chart. Using an x-ray viewer as a light source, the slide is placed on it with the camera (Fig. 14) and within 1 to 2 minutes the print is available. The maximum

Polaroid Co., 730 Main Street, Cambridge, Massachusetts 02139.

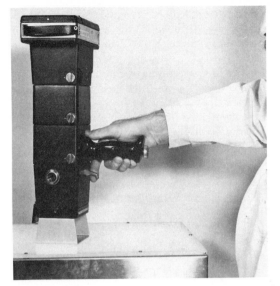

FIG. 14. The slide is placed on an x-ray viewer. The Polaroid CU-5 copying camera with three metal extensions is placed above this arrangement and exposed. A ×3 magnified print, obtained within 1 to 2 minutes, can be placed in the patient's chart. We found another technique (see text) more useful for enlarging endoscopic slides.

magnification with all the metal bellows attached is three times the original size of the image on the slide.

Another recent development is a material made by Kodak: RC copying reversal paper. The slide is inserted in an enlarger, and the paper is exposed. Using the RD processing kit, four 4 × 5 inch prints are obtained within 12 minutes, the cost ·of materials being only 20 cents per 4 × 5 inch print. The aim of this method is also to produce prints for the patient's chart from endoscopy slides. Enlargement of smaller images is not limited to the factor of three: up to a 10-fold enlargement can be produced. The color reproduction and information available on the print are better than those obtained with Polaroid film material.

Gino Hasler

CINEMATOGRAPHY

The problems in cinematography are similar to those for still photography. We use commercially available movie cameras. The size, weight, suddenly increased endoscope-examiner eye distance (Table 4), the change in image seen through the camera viewer, the limitations of a 100-foot magazine, the difficulties of maintaining sterile conditions if required, illumination, and heat production are the principal disturbing factors. The five criteria mentioned under *Value and Need of Documentation* are also valid here.

TABLE 4.   Movie Cameras: Endoscope-Examiner Eye Distance

Camera	Eye Distance	
	In	Cm
Arriflex	13	33
Beaulieu	9	22.9
Berci-Merei	4.5	11.4
Urban-Berci	0.8	2.2

The endoscope-examiner eye distance suddenly increases if a camera is connected. This interferes largely with the balance and routine of the examination.

Cameras

We started 17 years ago with a 16-mm Arriflex camera weighing 8.5 pounds (3.8 kg). A counterbalancing system was designed, but it still proved cumbersome. Despite the counterbalancing system the "feel" of the introduced endoscope—the sensation of resistance—was lost. We next used a Beaulieu 16-mm camera, which is smaller and somewhat lighter (4 pounds 8 ounces; 2.0 kg) but still too large. Filming during a gynecologic laparoscopic procedure requires that the operator be positioned practically at the position of the anesthesiologist. Because of the size of the camera coupled to a flexible fiberscope with its four-way controlled tip and continuous movements—leaving only one hand of the operator free—it became an almost acrobatic performance.

Filming was pioneered by a few skilled enthusiasts: Holinger,[8] Threthowan,[14] Montreynaud,[12] Berci.[2]

In trying to overcome these problems we developed a 16-mm movie camera in which we separated the heavy part (magazine, motor, clutch, etc.) from the actual gate. The film gate was designed with a 45-degree rotating mirror shutter and clear viewer (Fig. 15). This mechanism, including a 40-mm lens, was shaped in the form of grip and weighed only 1.8 pounds (0.8 kg). This "handle" was connected with the rest of the camera through a flexible film guide mechanism (Fig. 16) covered by a corrugated rubber tube. To the best of our knowledge this was the first remote camera with flexible film transport.[3] It functioned very well but proved to be too complicated in terms of production and service. We had to learn the difference between theory and practice, between the advantages of an institution with highly trained personnel and the need for a simple device in a community hospital. The Beaulieu camera became the "work horse" for many endoscopists (Fig. 17).

The question arose of how we could improve the conditions to make it acceptable to a larger number of endoscopists.

Camera Weight.   If we attach 4 pounds (2 kg) or more to the end of a scope it causes immediate problems. If the camera is too bulky or large it interferes with the routine of the examination.

Magazine.   We cannot afford to wait to rethread a 100-foot magazine if the film runs out in the middle of an interesting procedure. The additional weight of larger magazines excludes this proposition. There are no 16-mm cartridge cameras available.

Endoscopic Camera.   Among the cameras commercially available we found a 16-mm movie camera originally designed for the operating microscope* (weight: 2.2 pounds; 1 kg) that was approximately half the weight of the Beaulieu camera. The configuration is smaller partially because of the coaxial (side by side) film reel system (Fig. 18).

The shutter opening time is crucial for endoscopic filming. The time during which the film is stationary in the filmgate determines the exposure time. If it is long, the pull-down time must be faster. With the Beaulieu at 16 frames/second the individual frame exposure is 1/40 second (25 milliseconds) and at 24 frames/second it is 1/60 second (17 milliseconds). The above-mentioned microscope camera has a 270-degree shutter opening. This means that the frame is stationary for a long time in

Urban Engineering Co., 111 Buena Vista Avenue, Burbank, Calif.

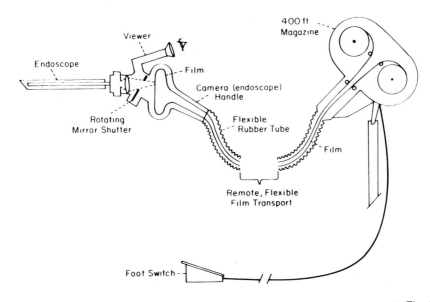

FIG. 15. Berci-Merei 16-mm endoscope camera. The first remote film transport. The heavy part of the camera (film with magazine), motor, clutch, etc. are located behind the examiner on a stand. The actual film gate was designed in the form of a hollow grip, which contains the film pull-down mechanism, a 45-degree rotating mirror shutter, the lens, and the endoscope adapter. It could be used as a handle for manipulation when the endoscope is attached. A clear, slightly tilted viewer facilitates continuous observation during filming. This (gate) handle is connected to the magazine through a flexible film guide mechanism covered by a corrugated rubber tube in which the film runs. (Courtesy Med Biol III 16:37, 1966)

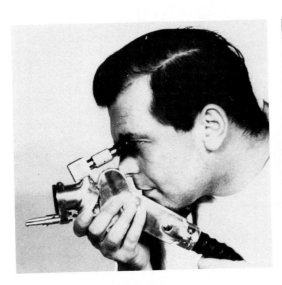

FIG. 16. The camera can be held with ease in the hand (1.8 pounds; 800 g) with a clear view. Film format: 16 mm. Film transport is covered with a corrugated rubber tube. (From Berci et al[3])

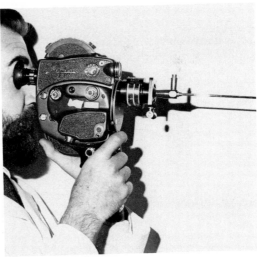

FIG. 17. The 16-mm Beaulieu has served us for more than a decade. It is the smallest commercially available camera on the market, but unfortunately is still too heavy (4.8 pounds, 2000 g). The eyepiece-examiner distance is long, and the viewer (optical relay) absorbs light, creating a dim image (e.g., with small endoscopes or fiberscopes). If the 100-foot magazine runs out during the procedure, reloading requires too much time.

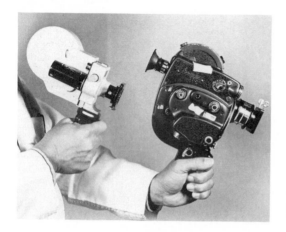

FIG. 18. The 16-mm Beaulieu camera with a Schneider 38-mm lens and quick adapter, compared to the Urban-Berci magazine loaded 16-mm camera, a simple 40-mm (achromat) lens and quick adapter.

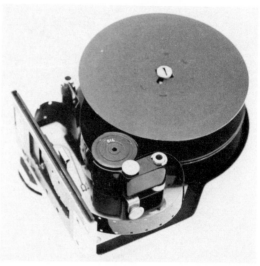

FIG. 19. The magazine with the precision gate open can be loaded in daylight using daylight reels. The film reels are positioned side by side instead of above and below.

the gate, which provides a long exposure time per frame, resulting in 16 frames/second, each with a 1/25-second, exposure (40 milliseconds). This is a very advantageous factor. The camera is driven by a low-voltage motor, the power supplied through a transformer.

The 100-foot film magazine is interchangeable within seconds, and several others can stand by preloaded (Figs. 19 and 20). Thus the unpleasant event of running out of film during the examination can be eliminated (Fig. 21).

This camera underwent modifications to suit

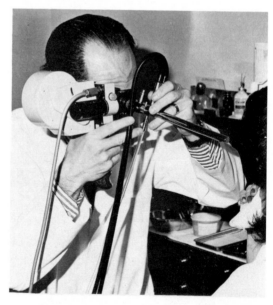

FIG. 21. This is the same camera shown in Figures 19 and 20, attached to a (Hopkins-Storz) laryngoscope through a beam splitter. The endoscope eyepiece-examiner distance is increased only with the size of the beam splitter (0.8 inches; 22 mm). The image seen is the same that is observed through the endoscope. A film counter and a warning light (only 5 feet left) with the electric motor is seen. The motor is triggered by a foot switch. The endoscope is held through the camera handle, leaving the left hand free for positioning and manipulations.

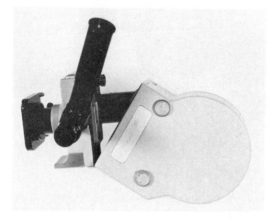

FIG. 20. There are several 100-foot preloaded magazines available. They can be interchanged within seconds and can be used with a side viewer or a beam splitter. The shutter opening is 270 degrees, which gives the individual frames a longer exposure in the gate during the stationary period. Lens: 40 mm with a quick adapter.

the needs of endoscopy. A photocell is available to measure light and trigger the light source through a controller (Table 5).

TABLE 5.   Comparative Dimensions of Beaulieu and Urban-Berci Endoscope Cameras

Camera	Weight		Size (mm)		
	Lb	G	H ×	L ×	W
Beaulieu	4.8	2,000	197	167	100
Urban-Berci	2.4	1,019	118.7	170	90.6

H, height; L, length; W, weight.

Displayed Image on Film

The size of a well-exposed image on the film is determined by several factors.

Illumination.   A new high-intensity light source has been developed with better efficiency than the previous one. However, we are at a point where the trade-off (more light–more heat) cannot be further enhanced at this stage in the development of light engineering.

Light Transmission. The high absorption of flexible glass fiber bundles has been mentioned. The number of fibers can be increased in larger instruments, but there are limitations. Some filming scopes evolved into much larger instruments, a trend not completely neutral to our concepts of improved patient care. With smaller instruments (pediatrics) we face the limitations of light-carrying fibers, the limitations imposed by the diameter of the endoscope. I have used several types of adult filming laparoscope models with various filming fiber sheets. The heat at the end (near the telescope) is very high. It is true that we are working in a cavity, but it is undesirable to manipulate "with a glowing soldering iron in the belly." Perhaps a new light-transmitting medium with much less absorption will help to overcome this obstacle.

Shutter Opening. The design of the shutter influences the exposure of the film. The film is momentarily stationary in the gate for the exposure before it is pulled down for the next frame. If the opening time of the shutter is longer, the pull-down time of the film must be shorter. The opening of the shutter is expressed in degrees. The new camera described above has a shutter with a 270-degree opening. The actual exposure is longer than with other cameras and therefore advantageous because in endoscopic filming more light is always desirable. The longer the film stays in the gate, the better it is exposed.

Film Speed. We use a daylight 160 ASA film, which has proved over the years to be the most suitable film (speed versus grain) for color reproduction, etc. Film speed can be "pushed" by processing but has several disadvantages.

Filming Speed. We use only the 16-mm format. The filming speed can compensate for the lack of light in certain instances. If the speed is slower (frames per seconds) the frame is better exposed but can create a "jumping" impression if a low filming speed (e.g., 8 frames/second) is displayed with a 24 frame/second projection. In general 16 frames/second is suitable for most endoscopic procedures and can be used in both the smaller and larger scopes.

Camera Lens. The focal length of the lens also influences the size of the displayed image. We believe that if the frame is filled vertically (7 mm) this is sufficient to enlarge it adequately at projection (Fig. 22). In general, taking all scopes (including flexible fiberscopes) into consideration, a 40-mm lens is the most appropriate.

Optical System. The transmission parameters of the rigid or flexible optical system can also influence the end results. The consensus is that if we use small or miniature

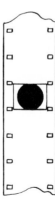

FIG. 22. A 16-mm film format (7 × 10 mm). With a displayed image size of 7 mm the format and the projection screen will be filled properly. Overframing creates illumination problems and does not produce more details.

rigid or flexible endoscopes the size of the image and light transmitters decreases proportionally. There are more light problems with small instruments than with large ones.

16- or Super 8-mm Film Format

The discussion over using Super 8-mm film is not new. There are several factors which lead us to use 16-mm instead of 8-mm film. It is true that the Super 8-mm format (Fig. 23) is somewhat larger than the standard 8 mm, but the displayed image is smaller than the 16-mm format image; therefore less light is required. However, the same high-speed film material is used for 8-mm as for the 16-mm format. Therefore the ratio of existing grain to displayed image is greater in the Super 8-mm than in the 16-mm format.

Every hospital has a 16-mm movie projector, but only a few have an 8-mm one. If an 8-mm projector is used, the illumination of the projector limits the projection in a large lecture room, or (if used) the projected image size on the screen will be too small for convenient viewing. If the film is reprinted from 8 to 16 mm, time and money are wasted because of the additional loss in the picture quality. For example, one frame from a 16-mm strip with an image size of 7 mm is large enough to use as a slide (transparency) or, if enlarged three times, as a print. The quality is somewhat inferior to that of a still photo of the same subject but can be useful and is economical. The same procedure cannot be done with one Super 8-mm frame having a displayed image size of 4.0 mm. Using an analytic projector for slow, forward, reverse, or even frame-by-frame analysis is essential for evaluating function. These projec-

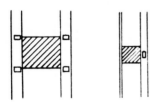

FIG. 23. A 16-mm (left) versus a Super 8-mm (right) film format. With a 7-mm displayed image we can fill out the 16-mm format in the vertical diameter using a 40-mm lens, providing good exposure in adult-size endoscopes. See test for details. Size: 1:1.

tors are hard to come by in an 8-mm format, and so we have chosen to stay with the 16-mm film format.

Conclusion

Filming endoscopic procedures, manipulations, operations, or functional disorders is of great importance. Many quickly changing events or deviations from normal anatomy can be overlooked when we are performing difficult procedures or when we can observe an area with rapid movements for only extremely short periods. It is impossible to memorize and to compute slight changes during speedy events. Furthermore, the communication problem encountered when trying to describe them in a way that another examiner can picture them is almost insurmountable.

The opportunity of having a film strip so that we can sit down at a convenient time and inspect the anatomy or pathology with others either for consultation or teaching is invaluable. This aspect of endoscopic diagnosis has been partially overlooked or only partially developed because of the extreme difficulty of obtaining ideal tools for this purpose. The major drawback is the (expensive) clumsy, complex gear involved, which interferes with the actual endoscopic procedures.

We have come a long way since pioneers Nitze and Holinger, among others (see the history of endoscopy, pp. xv–xix) under much more difficult conditions than we have today, tried to show us the direction in which to proceed. Smaller cameras that are easier to operate with better illumination, improved flexible light-transmitting media, new optical systems, and automatic controls are at our disposal. It is a matter of understanding the importance of these techniques and then coordinating the available equipment and methods so they are palatable to the practicing endoscopist.

The future looks bright for this developing field. It appears that in the following years a permanent movie film record will be an essential part of our diagnostic armamentarium, similar to the progress made in cardiology where cinefluorography became indispensable to understanding the hemodynamic changes in the heart.

George Berci and Gino Hasler

ILLUMINATION FOR CINEMATOGRAPHY

The illumination for cinematography is still a "dark spot" in our endoscopy armamentarium. With the introduction of incoherent fiberoptic light transmission, the illumination problems during a routine endoscopic examination improved. We could place a much larger light source outside the body at a convenient distance and could afford to lose 60 to 70 percent of the light output of the source, still ending up with a much brighter image inside the cavity than had been produced with the unreliable distal miniature electric globes. However, these units are not bright enough nor do they produce enough intensity to be employed for filming purposes. For cinematography we need a much more powerful, higher-intensity light (to compensate for the absorption that takes place in the light-transmitting and optical image relay systems) to expose a film.

The significant light loss due to high absorption in the fiber bundle cannot be compensated for by increasing the energy or light of a source without impunity. There are a number of light-generating sources commercially available with the required output, but accompanying these systems are other factors, e.g., enormous heat, and ultraviolet and infrared production.

The urge to document moving events triggered the need to use high-intensity light units which were originally manufactured for other applications. The unit available to us was large, complicated, unsafe, and expensive (Figs. 24 through 26). Manufacturers "custom tailored" the fittings for their own fiber bundle, and we were unable to interchange endoscopes of different makes.

We ended up at this stage with a xenon arc light source (Chapter 3); this provides adequate brightness density with a high color temperature (5000 to 6000 K), which is ideally suited for daylight film. A bluish tint is helpful in compensating for the yellowish hue of the fibers.

To collect the beam of a small light spot, matching the entrance angle of a fiber bundle is less complicated if the distance between the electrodes is small. The proper direction of the beam can be improved by specially designed mirrors or condensor lenses. These globes were originally earmarked for use with movie pro-

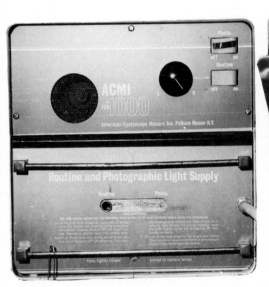 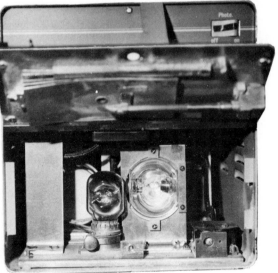

FIG. 24. ACMI filming unit. Type number: 1000. This employs two globes: one for examination, and another high-intensity globe for filming. Left: Unit with controls and sliding fiber attachment: for examination or cinematography. Right: General Electric Marc-300 quartz globe (cover lifted). This globe produces a tremendous amount of heat. The lifetime is only 25 hours and declines gradually. The same globe is available in a newly designed smaller unit with improved electronics.

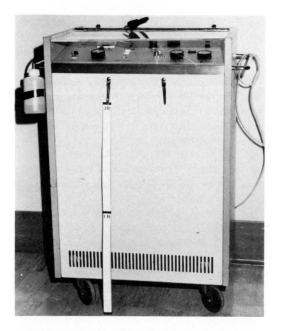

FIG. 25. Olympus CLX filming unit. It is 2.5 feet high and employs a quartz glass high-pressure xenon globe inserted in a special mirror.

dangerous in case of an explosion. For this reason the globe manufacturers recommend the use of a special safety helmet if the globe has to be replaced. Being a point source illuminator, the alignment in relation to the bundle is crucial. Slight misalignments can result in underexposure. At the beginning we were enthusiastic, but during years of use we became skeptical after seeing the problems, risks, and hazards involved. These factors exclude this globe from practical use, necessitating that it be handled by a doctor, nurse, or even a hospital electrician.

We collected more basic data to determine the limitations, and to determine if a required light output within safety margins can be developed. In a joint venture with a group of physicists we aquired a new type of xenon

jectors in large auditoriums. Because the format of a 16-mm film is larger than the diameter of the fiber bundle, the optical or mirror system had to be changed to provide better conditions for the recipient fiber light guide. Placing a condensor in front of a beam improves the light density and angle, but the heat production increases significantly.

We must deal with contact heat in the focal plane—where the recipient end of the fiber light guide is placed—and radiated heat (e.g., infrared) at the other (working) end of the fiber. Employing high-intensity units, the enormous heat factors caused us some concern. For instance, the heat in the focal plane of some of these units where the fiber is inserted was 400 to 500 F (200 to 250 C). To test the physiologic parameters on the working end of a 6-foot bundle (4 mm diameter), without going into sophisticated temperature measurements, we held the end of the bundle to our wrist. After a few seconds we felt a painful, burning sensation.

These xenon arc light electrodes are placed in a quartz glass envelope under high pressure. The pressure increases even further if the globe is burned and more heat is generated. These quartz glass globes can be extremely

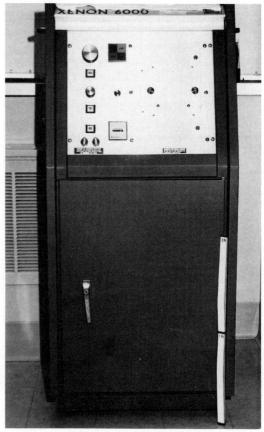

FIG. 26. Storz xenon 6000 filming unit, built with a storage cabinet. The dimensions are approximately the same as those of the Olympus CLX, employing also a quartz glass xenon high-pressure globe.

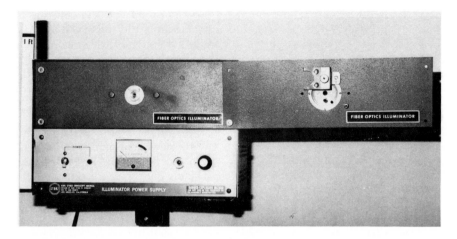

FIG. 27. Prototype I of the new illuminator. The new explosionproof miniature xenon globe is used. On the right is a separate frontplate with different fittings that can be interchanged with the existing one so as to accept different endoscopes.

globe that is compact (Chapter 3), explosion-proof, and easier to handle; its output is more than adequate, and the entire unit is built according to the hospital safety code. The unit is much smaller than its predecessors, and various endoscopes can be coupled to it (Fig. 27). With further experimentation the size of this unit was reduced (Fig. 28).

At the time of writing this chapter, ideal illumination for cinematography is still in its developmental stage. We must wait for some time to pass before we can recommend it for wider use. There is no doubt that we need a universal filming unit to which any type of endoscope or fiberscope can be connected. We must be very careful with our codes and testing

programs, not to block an important diagnostic aid from being used. On the other hand we cannot employ light units in the endoscopy or operating room which, practically speaking, need a steel-armored cover, or with which the light transmitted through the light guide can cause severe burns.

The development of a high-output stroboscopic light unit with which, for instance, 100 to 150 watts/second can be achieved in a 4 mm diameter at the end of the fiber bundle, recycling it at 24 times/second is not available yet. Another interesting aspect must be considered: How long can the brain tolerate the flickering effect? A powerful strobelight, synchronized with the camera shutter, would be ideal if we

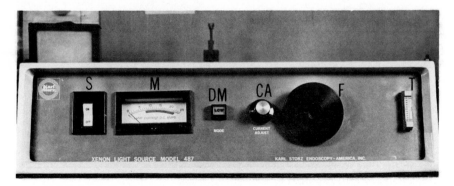

FIG. 28. Improved version (II) of prototype I shown in Figure 27. S, On and off switch. M, Meter to control current adjustment. DM, Dual mode switch (low or high). CA, Current adjustments. F, Connection to fiber cable. This adaptor can be exchanged according to the various types of fiber bundles. T, Timer to measure the lifetime of the globe and indicate replacement. Size: 450×300×150 mm (18×12×6 inches). (Type no. 487. Manufacturer: Storz Co.)

could achieve the required output and simultaneously provide continuous light between the strobe discharges.

Taking all the pros and cons into consideration, we feel that the recently developed universal high-intensity light source is a step forward in endoscopic cinematography. We must keep in mind, however, that illumination is only one aspect of the procedure, and what we gain with more light we lose by generating more heat. Moreover, we lose more than half the light during transmission. We hope that a new development in light transmission, in conjunction with this new filming light source, will overcome the present physiologic and technologic problems.

George Berci

AUTOMATIC EXPOSURE CONTROL FOR ENDOSCOPIC CINEMATOGRAPHY

General Control Requirement

The human eye can accommodate a very wide range of illumination levels: close to a million to one ratio. This is accomplished through two mechanisms: (1) the pupil-iris dilation and contraction in response to changing light levels; and (2) mental adaptation or latitude. The iris adjustment is a fairly slow process, taking seconds or sometimes minutes for full compensation, whereas the adaptation process is almost instantaneous.

Unfortunately cameras used in endoscopic photography have neither of these mechanisms. Due to the given aperture (iris) of the attached telescope, no adjustable iris (f/stop) can be used, and the film has very little latitude for reasonable detail and color balance. For best results, an illumination ratio of perhaps 2:1 or 3:1 should not be exceeded, unless the exposure time can be changed.

Technical Problems

This illumination ratio requirement presents two problems to the doctor. He must first visually estimate image brightness in the camera viewfinder and then manually set the exposure time (via framing rate, shutter angle) or the light source intensity. Unfortunately, the visual adaptive process works against the ability to estimate brightness, unless the change of brightness is large.

To compound this difficulty, as the subject distance from the end of the scope changes the illumination tends to change with the square of the distance (e.g., twice the distance gives one-fourth the illumination). Since the working distance from the endoscope exit to the object is small, even slight motion can change the brightness significantly.

Some cameras provide a light meter visible in the viewfinder which indicates the image brightness, thus theoretically solving the first problem: The exposure time or light intensity is simply adjusted to give a constant desired meter reading. The essence of cinematography, however, is motion, motion of the object or viewer (working end of the endoscope) or both in order to give spacial (three-dimensional) information about the subject from the change of perspective and/or lighting. Thus with the image brightness constantly changing, maintaining a constant meter reading becomes very difficult or impossible.

Automatic Control: Various Methods

Work has been done on automatic exposure control for movie cameras. The small-film format (16 mm) and high-power light source (500 watts) yield good exposure at reasonable maximum working distances (Fig. 29).

The camera is equipped with a photocell that senses the average light falling on the film.

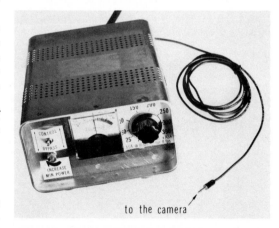

to the camera

FIG. 29. Light controller (prototype: Chedwick-Helmuth Co.). This light intensity control system triggers the power (output) of a 500-watt xenon short-arc lamp. The photocell output of the movie camera was made available to this controller. Response time was optimized at about 1 second for the greatest change between the lowest and highest light intensity output of the source of illumination.

The photocell produces an electrical signal proportional to the light intensity. In one method this signal is wired to a controller, which in turn automatically adjusts the light source intensity so as to maintain the photocell signal *constant*. Thus if the intensity tends to become greater, the controller reduces the light as required to prevent the increase.

In another method of control the photocell output commands a variable neutral density filter placed before the photocell and film. This system then acts in the same way to maintain constant average light on the cell and film. However, the variable filter is a mechanical device, adding weight and size to the camera. Furthermore, full light input to the subject is always present even at very close working distances, creating the possibility of tissue damage; the intensity control method reduces the light input under these conditions and provides full light output only at maximum working distances.

The intensity control adjustment may be done in two ways: (1) changing the power input to the light sources; or (2) employing constant (full) power to the source by changing the transmission of the optical system via a variable neutral density filter or iris diaphram.

The power control method (1) may be accomplished all-electronically, while the transmission method (2) must be mechanical unless very inefficient elements (e.g., Kerr cell) are used. Mechanical devices, apart from the disadvantages of high cost and maintenance and low reliability (compared to today's solid state technology), are inherently slow compared to the essentially instantaneous response of electronics.

As a practical consideration, the power control method may be used with existing light sources with very little if any modification to the unit. One difficulty with the power control method is that the light source must maintain reasonably constant color balance as its intensity is changed. Thus a tungsten light source is not very suitable and sources such as the xenon short-arc lamp must be used.

Current Status

An intensity control system based on the power control method has been built and tested in actual use. A Beaulieu 16-mm movie camera (which already contains a photocell light sensor) and a 500-watt xenon short-arc light source were used. A jack was mounted on the camera to make the photocell output available to the controller, and the light was wired so that the main power to the lamp power supply passed through the controller (without changing the power to the lamp cooling system).

Response time of the controller was experimentally optimized at about 1 second (for greatest change in light intensity); a slower speed gave noticeable segments on the film of under- or overexposure, whereas a faster speed began to affect system stability. This controller unit should be available commercially in the near future at a relatively low cost.

James G. Helmuth

CONCLUSION

Documentation of endoscopic findings in the form of a permanent objective record is of utmost importance. We have come a long way with the introduction of the rod-lens system and coherent fiber bundles in image transmission. There has also been considerable improvement in the incoherent flexible fiber threads for transmitting light from an external source. With the help of these inventions the endoscopes were improved, new investigative instruments created, and unknown areas explored. Unfortunately the last step to enable us to preserve the findings or to reproduce them at will has not been developed to the extent that the practicing endoscopist would like.

Our results will gain even further acceptance if we can support our diagnoses with stored data. In cases with disputable diagnoses the value of a permanent record for consultation, repeated reviews, and teaching cannot be overlooked.

The currently available photographic methods are in a stage of experimentation. Every day during the most common procedures we face sudden critical situations due to the patient's poor general condition or unexpected complications with which we must cope and be able to resolve immediately. Under such conditions we cannot afford to turn our concentration from the patient to the operation or supervision of a complex mechanism, and therefore simple and reliable protocols and equipment must be developed.

The recording cameras must be designed to be compatible with our lightweight endoscopes and not vice versa. The first 35-mm miniature, full-frame camera with motor drive and a small 16-mm movie camera are already available.

The new light-transmitting system will probably help to eliminate our present high absorption figures (60 to 70 percent per 6-foot fiber cable) and contribute to a more powerful flash or continuous light transmission without attendant increases in heat production source power requirements.

A high-intensity light source is also under construction according to our specifications. These systems should be safe, efficient, and universal in the sense that they can be interchanged with several types of endoscopes, especially since the cost of some of these units is astronomical.

Industrial photography introduced automatic brightness (flash and continuous) exposure controls and has proved its usefulness and reliability over the years. The time has now come for the manufacturers and the medical profession to recognize the facts: documentation is now possible. Our decisions for further treatment must be based on visual findings and permanent records. The technologic prerequisites are available. Again let me draw attention to the enormous progress in radiology with the introduction of radiography and cinefluorography.

Histologic slides or x-ray films are sent out for consultation when an opinion or final diagnosis cannot be reached by one person. We are unable even to scratch the surface of our endoscopic "gold mines" in this regard and so far have had no opportunity to compare similar cases or to teach ourselves or others.

If we can generate more interest and understanding for this important and at this stage neglected adjunct, scientific communication and interpretation of endoscopic pathology will take a new course and will be shared with much more enthusiasm by our referring colleagues and students.

George Berci

REFERENCES

1. Berci G: Peritoneoscopy. Br Med J 1:562, 1962
2. Berci G: Advances in endoscopy. Med J Australia 2:653, 1962
3. Berci G, Merei F, Kont LA: A new approach to clinical film recording with special reference to endoscopy. Med Biol Illus 16:37, 1966
4. Calame A: Laparoscopic photography. Med Biol Illus 6:148, 1956
5. Colcher H, Katz GM: Cinegastroscopy. Am J Gastroenterol 35:518, 1961
6. Dalziel CF: Electric shock hazard. IEEE 9:50, 1972
7. Fourestier M, Gladu A, Vulmiere J: Perfectionnements à l'endoscopie medicale. Presse Med 60:1292, 1952
8. Holinger PH, Brubaker JD: The larynx, bronchi and esophagus in Kodachrome. J Biol Photogr Assoc 10:83, 1941
9. Lent H: Die Entwicklung der Photolaparoskopie mit dem Electronblitz. Acta Hepatosplen (Stuttg) 9:195, 1962
10. Lindner E: Fortschritte, der Photolaparoscopy. Med Welt 27:3, 1956
11. Lindner H: Peritoneoscopic photography with intra-abdominal electronic flash. Med Biol Illus 15:146, 1965
12. Montreynaud DJM, Bruneau Y, Jomain J: Traite pratique de photographie et de cinématographie medicales. Paris, Montel, 1960
13. Nitze M: Zur Photographie der menschlichen Harnrohre. Berl Med Wochenschr 31:744, 1893
14. Threthowan JD: Experiments in endoscopic photography. J Photogr Sci 4:145, 1956
15. Walter CW: Electrical Hazards in Hospitals. National Academy of Science, Washington DC, 1970

19

Television and Endoscopy

George Berci

A still considerable shortcoming in endoscopy is the restriction imposed by using a small eyepiece. The discovery of television was therefore of great interest to those concerned with the improvement of documentation, communication, and teaching. It offers the following *advantages* over the standard viewing methods:

1. The image can be viewed immediately and observed with both eyes (binocular) from a convenient distance.
2. The image is significantly enlarged, depending on the size of the television monitor.
3. The image can be seen by several observers in different locations simultaneously, thus facilitating consultation and teaching.
4. The image can be corrected on the spot by appropriate adjustment for brightness and contrast.
5. The image can be recorded and replayed instantly with a video tape recorder or recorded directly from the television screen using a synchronized movie camera (kinerecording).

Disadvantages to the procedure are:

1. The image quality is inferior to a 16-mm movie or a 35-mm still film.
2. Operation of the equipment requires certain skills and technical assistance, especially if you intend to televise in color.

Despite the advantages of using television, progress in applying it in medicine, especially endoscopy, has been slow. The debut was a televised bronchoscopy reported by Soulas in 1957.[11] A studio camera (image Orthicon) was employed for the first closed-circuit televised endoscopic procedure. The weight (180 pounds) and size of the camera excluded its practical application.

McCarthy and Ritter[8] used a Vidicon industrial television chain for displaying the inside of the urinary bladder in 1957. Use of improved Vidicon camera chains was reported by Montreynaud et al.[10] in 1960. Such cameras, however, were still too heavy (4 to 10 pounds) to allow gentle, accurate handling.

We became aware of the problems[1] involved with the weight and size of the camera and so developed our first miniature television camera in 1958, reporting our clinical experience 4 years later.[2] The camera was 45 mm (1.8 inches) in diameter, 120 mm (4.8 inches) in length, and 350 g (12 ounces) in weight. Our miniature camera was built around a 0.5-inch Vidicon tube. To decrease the size and weight of the image pickup system many components were removed from the camera to the control unit (Fig. 1). Resolution did not exceed 350 television lines (3.5 MHz). The sensitivity of this 0.5-inch tube 12 years ago was less than that of the new generation of similar Vidicon tubes available today.

Our miniature system was first employed for televising bronchoscopies and laryngoscopies to a large audience during meetings or for teaching students.

Anyone who intends to use any type of television system must be aware of two major problems: (1) sufficient illumination must be provided, significantly more than the standard examining light source gives; and (2) the television camera must be properly attached to the endoscope. The latter problem can be dealt with in several ways:

1. Direct attachment of the camera to the eyepiece of course provides the best image because the light loss is minimal except for the absorption

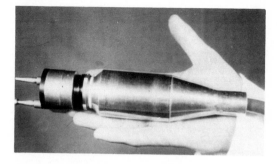

FIG. 1. Miniature television camera (black and white). Diameter 45 mm (1.8 inches); length 120 mm (4.8 inches); weight 350 g (12 ounces). Developed at the University of Melbourne in Australia. (From Berci and Davids: Br Med J 1:1610, 1962)

factors of the camera lens. On the other hand, if the camera is large, it disrupts the routine of the examination. It is most inconvenient and can interfere with important manipulations during any endoscopic procedure and lessen the needed sensations in the fingertips. Manipulating the instrument that has a weight attached to the eyepiece so that undue pressure on the mucosa (or even perforation) is avoided requires skill.

2. A coherent image-transmitting bundle can be interposed between the eyepiece and the television camera. In this case the camera is located remotely and a beam splitter is attached to the eyepiece, deviating a great percentage of the image into the camera. This arrangement permits more free movement than if the camera were attached directly, but it must be kept in mind that

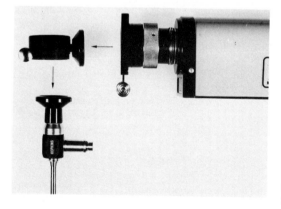

FIG. 2. The telescope (choledochoscope) is coupled to the television camera via a beam splitter. Fifteen percent of the image (light) is directed to the examiner and 85 percent to the television camera. If the camera is not too heavy this is a better approach than direct attachment. The examiner has an unobstructed view, and the camera is out of the way or can be used as a handle to support the endoscope and camera.

the coherent bundle in rigid telescopes diminishes the image quality and contributes to further light loss. With flexible fiber endoscopes the "mix-match phenomenon" (Chapter 4) also contributes to loss of resolution.

3. A better solution is to attach the camera (if not too heavy) directly to the endoscope via a beam splitter (Fig. 2). This system affords the examiner an unobstructed view. In televising procedures there are many instances when the object is too near or too far, thereby "washing out" the picture or making it too dark. Certain details cannot be seen with the resolution available. For this reason provision of the normal endoscopic view is of great importance. We must increase the illumination for television anyhow, and therefore a beam splitter (15/85 percent) provides enough illumination for the examiner. Fifteen percent loss of light into the television camera can be compensated for in most adult (large) rigid and flexible scopes.

4. The articulated optical arm is a better solution than a coherent bundle. The image quality and color reproduction are the same as seen through the endoscope. The beam splitter transmits an image into the camera (85 percent) and to the examiner (15 percent). Using a high-intensity light source the 15 percent suffices the viewing conditions. The image is relayed by a rigid optical system connected by optical joints, which allow circular or angled movements. This system produces a better image than the coherent bundle.[5–7,12] At this stage there are only a few prototype optical arms available. They are very delicate and expensive (Fig. 3).

BLACK AND WHITE TELEVISION

There is no argument that a display of any televised endoscopic object in the color identical to that of the original would be ideal. There are many advantages and disadvantages that have to be carefully weighed before a decision is made in favor of a black and white or a color system. We are particularly used to color display, and therefore expect to see the television picture or photograph in color. Interestingly the same desire is not expressed for a radiograph (e.g., to see a chest x-ray film in full color). There are still several drawbacks with regard to a color display: The contrast ratio of existing color films is relatively small, usually 1:4 or 1:5, compared to that of a black and white television screen, which can be 1:10 or even more. Another aspect for consideration in endoscopy is that the color of the objects is almost entirely within the red part of the spectrum. To demonstrate this we performed bronchoscopies in an experimental animal (the dog)

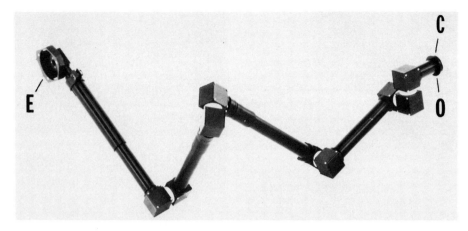

FIG. 3. The articulated optical arm consists of a beam splitter (E) which deviates part of the image (10 percent) to the examiner; approximately 70 percent is received by the camera. Twenty-thirty percent of the light is absorbed by the optical elements of this transmitting system, which consists of five rigid optical relay systems connected to each other by rotating prisms or mirrors. The heavy camera can be placed on a tripod at a distance that facilitates free movement of the scope. The image quality is superior compared with a coherent fiber bundle. The absorption is high (25 to 30 percent) but can be compensated for (adult scopes). The arm is delicate and fragile, and so needs extreme care in handling. Only prototypes are available for evaluation. E, Quick adaptor to the endoscope. C, Camera, or O, Observer. (Courtesy of J. Landre)

in which we had partially occluded venous return to the lung, causing congestion. This was recorded through the bronchoscope simultaneously in black and white and in color. There was a striking degree of venous engorgement that was no less evident from a black and white photograph made from the television screen than from the color picture itself.

Movements of the vocal cords, the bronchial tree, otologic procedures, and certain tumors or protruding lesions can be very well seen and assessed from a monochrome picture. Inflammations are not reproducible, however, and so color is required, although subtle changes in the red spectrum are not easy to display even using color television. Even a television engineer needs time "to tune" his red shades or mix his colors to represent the actual situation. Television can be more easily adapted to our standard methods of endoscopy when employing a black and white television system.

The following specifications should be kept in mind:

1. The weight and size of the camera should be small enough that the camera can be coupled directly to the endoscope.
2. It should be simple enough to be operated by untrained or paramedical personnel.
3. Its use should not be time-consuming and should be without any risk to the patient.
4. It should be financially feasible, both in its capital outlay and its running cost, keeping in mind that it must be operated within the restrictions of a hospital budget.
5. The displayed image quality should be sufficient for the purpose.

Our first miniature television camera was improved by our Mark II model.[4] This model is

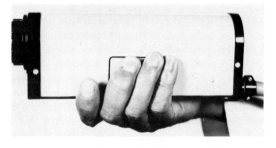

FIG. 4. Mark II miniature high-resolution black and white camera: weight 860 g (1 pound 14 ounces); length 170 mm (7 inches); width 50 mm (2 inches); height 60 mm (2.25 inches). Horizontal resolution: More than 900 television lines. The number of scanning lines can be changed from the conventional 525 to 1023, depending on the application. Its small size and light weight facilitate coupling and maneuvering with an endoscope.

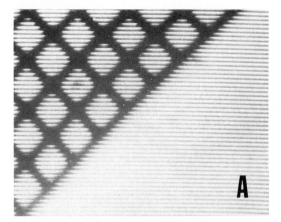

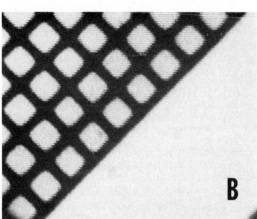

FIG. 5. **A.** Test pattern televised with 525 scanning lines. Photograph obtained from the television monitor. **B.** Same test pattern but scanned with 1023 lines. The edges of the line pattern are sharper, and the entire image appears smoother.

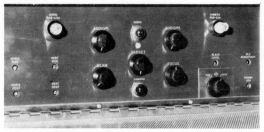

FIG. 6. Camera control of the black and white miniature high-resolution television chain. It is simple to operate. Two audio channels are also incorporated.

(Fig. 5). On the other hand, the normal standard 525 scanning line is a prerequisite for versatility and recording. The camera control unit is easy to operate (Figs. 6 and 7) and incorporates an automatic target, brightness control, and two audio channels.[4]

The same television chain can be used for scanning x-ray films (Chapter 17) because the wide contrast range is important in the display of a radiograph, where sharp differentiation of the various gray scales is required.

slightly larger than the Mark I but weighs only 860 g (less than 2 pounds). It measures 170 mm (6.8 inches) in length, 50 mm (2 inches) in width, and 57 mm in height. It employs a 1-inch Vidicon image tube (Fig. 2). It can be hand held, and a simple 40- to 50-mm achromat C-mount lens is placed in front of the beam splitter. The camera itself could be used as a handle of the endoscope. The beam splitter provides a clear view through the endoscope eyepiece (Fig. 4) with the television camera attached at the side.

The double scanning line system (525 versus 1023) can be changed by flipping a button on the control unit and switching on the monitor. Sometimes the visible 525 scanning line can be disturbing when trying to see minute detail

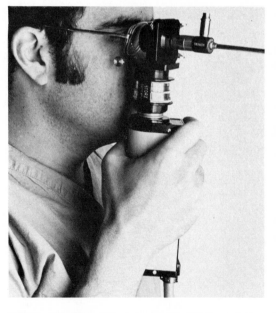

FIG. 7. Miniature black and white high-resolution television camera coupled via a beam splitter to a telescope. The camera is used as a handle. There is an unobstructed clear view through the beam splitter.

COLOR TELEVISION

Progress in technology is practically infinite. There is no doubt in my mind that if we observe an object in color through the endoscope then our mind is "tuned" to the natural display. At the time of this writing the market is saturated with relatively inexpensive ($6,000 to $8,000) color television chains whose operation is claimed to be "simple." The color cameras available can be classified in two large groups: the single tube (stripe—Vidicon) camera or the multiple (two or three) tube (Vidicon) camera. The weight and sensitivity, which are important aspects and problems in endoscopy, vary, and instruments are chosen taking into consideration their performance versus the capital outlay.

We have come a long way from the first Orthicon (three-tube) system, where approximately six times as much illumination was required as was needed for the black and white system, but there is still a "soft spot." The signal created on the Vidicon front-plate is proportional to the intensity of the image brightness traveling through the telescope and camera lens to the receptor.

When scoping a viscus, the examiner is eager to see as much as possible with the best image quality obtainable. Coupling the scope to a still or movie camera ensures that the same information obtained through the telescope or fiberscope is preserved on film. A great deal of this information is lost by attaching a color camera.

On the other hand when teaching endoscopic procedures to several students it is sometimes very difficult to hand over the teaching attachment from one observer to the other. Moreover, the examination time is significantly extended. Certain examinations (e.g., using rigid scopes to examine the larynx,

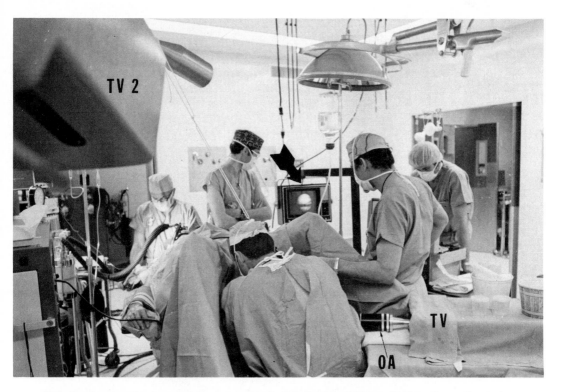

FIG. 8. Transurethral resection of prostate is televised and transmitted to the audience by microwaves a few miles from the operating room. The SEC camera (TV) is coupled to the resectoscope via an optical articulated arm (OA). The image could be observed through the beam splitter or directly from the television monitor (large arrow). Two-way audio communication was established with the auditorium. The procedure was displayed with a color television projector on a large screen. A second television camera (TV 2) surveys the procedure. (Courtesy of Professor J. J. Kaufman)

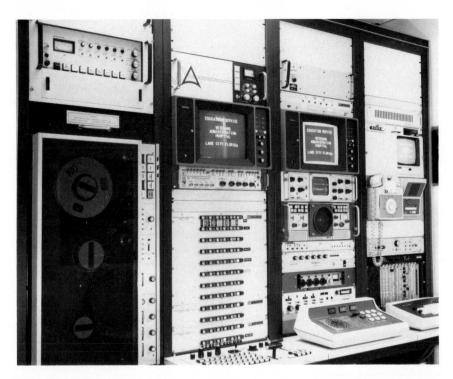

FIG. 9. Control room for closed circuit color television equipment used for endoscopy. (Courtesy of Dr. J. Rayl)

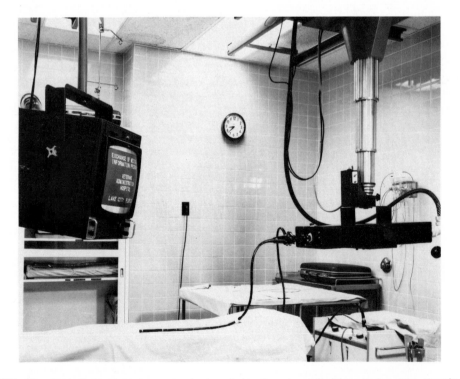

FIG. 10. Operating room for use of closed-circuit color television endoscopy showing ceiling-mounted Conrac television monitor (at left) and head of CEI-410 color television camera (at right). Olympus FIG-D2 gastrofiberscope with Olympus xenon CLX light source is attached to the camera. (Courtesy of Dr. J. Rayl)

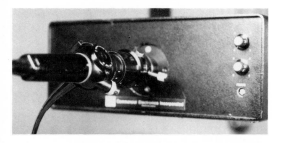

FIG. 11. Olympus BF-B2 bronchofiberscope is attached with C-mount adaptor to the CEI-410 color television camera. Yoke for ceiling suspension system is seen in the background (upper right). (Manufacturer of CEI-410 and CEI-435 color TV chains: Commercial Electronics, Inc., Mountain View, California) (Courtesy of Dr. J. Rayl)

nasopharynx, bronchial tree, or esophagus; or with flexible fiberscopes for gastroscopy and colonoscopy) are better suited to teaching than are procedures where miniaturization (pediatrics) or other applications create limitations in illumination, despite the availability of low level television chains (SEC camera).

During a urologic seminar[6] a transurethral resection was performed and transmitted live to a large audience via color television with audio communication using an SEC camera, 40 pounds in weight, placed several feet from the scope and coupled by an optical articulated arm to the camera itself (Fig. 8). The response of the audience was extremely good. The cost of this camera chain is high (approximately $40,000 to $60,000), and operation of the equipment is not simple. If we employ a more sophisticated color television chain it cannot be operated by a nurse or doctor. The various color levels must be constantly adjusted and checked to maintain ultimate performance.

A closed-circuit color television system should be considered in those institutions where large teaching programs are scheduled. Some loss of image quality must be taken into account if video tape recording is included (Figs. 9 through 12).

Recently we used a small color television chain (MV 9265 type with one stripe Vidicon; manufacturer: Circon Corp.). This relatively inexpensive set was tested in various endoscopic procedures. It is simple to operate, and the image quality is in proportion with the capital outlay. Further miniaturization of the camera will make it more attractive for endoscopy (Figs. 13 and 14).

RECORDING TELEVISION PICTURES

It is very helpful if interesting parts of the televised procedure can be displayed immediately. If there are no movements, the object can be documented with a still image storage device.

The simplest and best method is to photograph the image from the monitor or record the moving events with a kinecamera. The disadvantage is the delay in being able to review it due to processing. For documentation, an instant replay of a still image, electronic charge storage tubes, or magnetic disks are available.[3] The video tape recording machines available can perform only with 525 scanning lines. The band width of the disk is limited to approximately 4.5 MHz. In case of functions, a dynamic record is the method of choice. Inexpensive video tape recorders operate with band widths between 2.5 and 4 MHz. The studio quality video tape recorder is beyond our financial means.

If high-quality documentation is required,

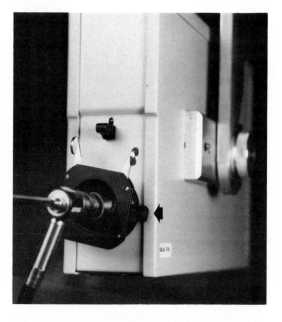

FIG. 12. Hopkins rod-lens forward telescope is attached to the CEI-435 television camera. A quick connect-disconnect adaptor and a focusing device (arrow) are features of a fabricated endoscope lens. The attached yoke (center of camera) is part of a ceiling counterbalance system that provides a weightless, freely moving camera head. (Courtesy of Dr. J. Rayl)

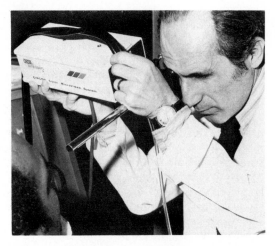

FIG. 13. MV-9265 color video camera with a built-in microphone attached through a beam splitter to an indirect laryngoscope, with Hopkins rod-lens system. The operation of this color TV chain is relatively simple and does not require complicated control mechanisms. There are 525 scanning lines; automatic gain control circuitry (AGC) compensates light level changes from 10 to 1.

ture depends partly on the progress in technology and partly on economics. The first steps have already been taken in the United States by Rieder (gastroenterology), McDonald (urology),[9] Rayl (bronchology), and Berci (gastroenterology, urology, and broncholaryngology), who employ color television for teaching or demonstrations. Even the best equipment, however, is in its infancy in respect to a high-quality natural color image display. If more sophisticated color television chains are used, the complicated design makes it necessary to employ trained personnel. A simpler and less expensive version can perhaps be run by the operator or nurse.

I am sure television techniques will improve during the next few years, with better image quality, increased sensitivity, smaller cameras, and overall improved color display. In endoscopy we are dealing mainly with the red spectrum. The color contrast is not very great here, and the different shades (from light pink to dark red) must be differentiated, which is still

kinerecording is optimal. This means that the television monitor is filmed directly with a 16-mm camera synchronized with the electronic circuit of the monitor.

Each piece of electronic equipment interposed results in some degree of loss in the image quality. Video tape recording is relatively simple and convenient because of the possibility of immediate display and for analyzing functions in a slow motion replay. If complete programs have to be arranged, editing the tapes requires special equipment, time, and personnel. Storage of video tapes is expensive. The transfer of tapes (black and white or color) to 16-mm film is a somewhat better solution.

CONCLUSION

The television display of an endoscopic procedure is an intriguing entity and is the next logical step to avoid looking with one eye through the small exit pupil of an endoscope. The inside of the viscus can be seen enlarged, observed most conveniently with both eyes, recorded simultaneously, and displayed in full color at a number of locations to be seen by several persons. It should be our final goal. Whether we can reach it in the foreseeable fu-

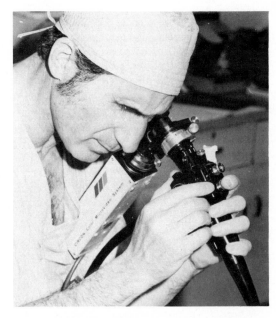

FIG. 14. Recent, improved version of the camera shown in Figure 13, with similar, but smaller, operational parameters. Diameter 2 × 2 inches (50 × 50 mm); length 8 inches (200 mm); weight only 1.5 pounds (680 g); can be easily attached through a beam splitter to provide unobstructed view for the examiner, in this case using the Olympus flexible gastroscope. (Manufacturer: Circon Corp., Santa Barbara, California)

difficult today. Teaching institutions should include basic television research activities in their programs because this field has great potential, especially for use in endoscopy.

REFERENCES

1. Berci G: Medicine and television. Med J Aust 2:1005, 1961
2. Berci G, Davids J: Endoscopy and television. Br Med J 1:1610, 1962
3. Berci G, Seyler AJ: An x-ray television image storage apparatus. Am J Roentgenol Radium Ther Nucl Med 6:1290, 1963
4. Berci G, Urban JC: A miniature black and white television camera for endoscopy and other medical applications. Biomed Engin April:116, 1972
5. Hopkins HH: Personal communication, 1973
6. Kaufman JJ: UCLA urology seminar, Los Angeles, 1972
7. Landre F: Personal communication, 1974
8. McCarthy JF, Ritter JS: Black and white television of the human urinary bladder. J Urol 78:674, 1957
9. McDonald HP: Personal communication, 1972
10. Montreynaud JM, Bruneau Y, Jomain J: Traite Pratique de Photography et de Cinematography Medicales. Montel, Paris, 1960
11. Soulas A: Televised bronchoscopy. Presse Med 64:97, 1956
12. Wittmoser R: Fortschritte der Farbfernseh-Endoskopie. Forschritte der Endoskopie 2:47, 1970

Part II
CLINICAL
APPLICATIONS

20

Choledochoscopy

J. Manny Shore
George Berci

Since the first choledochotomy by Thornton in 1889, surgeons have been frustrated by their inability to consistently clear all bile ducts of calculi by instrumental manipulations. This limitation is essentially "built into" the operative procedure because of its blind nature. The true incidence of retained stones could be assessed only following the introduction of postoperative cholangiography during the 1930s. The disappointingly high failure rate revealed by such examinations has continued to haunt biliary surgeons throughout the world.

The persistence of this problem appears more astonishing in view of the early introduction of biliary endoscopy by Thornton during the third recorded choledochotomy.[23] Failure of surgeons to adopt this direct method for the diagnosis and retrieval of biliary calculi must be attributed to technologic inadequacies over the intervening years.

The primitive instrument described by Bakes[2] was simply an illuminated speculum without an optical or irrigating system. The design of McIver's contribution in 1941[25] was more appropriate for the task, but the concept was overshadowed by the advent of operative cholangiography. It remained for Wildegans[41] in 1953 to popularize biliary endoscopy in Europe with the introduction of a satisfactory instrument.[11,13,19,20,22,28,30,35,41,42]

Extensive clinical trials with the rigid Wildegans scope[3] and the flexible fiber endoscope at this institution[33-36] have made us keenly aware of the technical limitations of these instruments and have helped to explain the reluctance of other surgeons to use this technique.[7] With the advent of the Hopkins optical system,[4] however, a new compact rigid choledochoscope has been developed.[26,37] Experience with this improved instrument over the past 4 years has convinced us of its superiority and general applicability to the longstanding problems of extrahepatic biliary exploration.[5]

INSTRUMENTATION

The right angle choledochoscope* with the Hopkins rod-lens optical permits miniaturization, so that the 40 mm long exploring horizontal limb, incorporating optical, lighting, and irrigating systems, measures only 5 × 3 mm (Fr 15 × Fr 9) in cross section. The right angle construction and compact design eliminate technical difficulties encountered with the bulkier Wildegans scope and overcome manipulation problems associated with the flexible fiberoptic instruments (Chapter 5).

Optical System

The image is transmitted from the exploring tip along a series of rod lenses through a tiny prism housed in the angle of the instrument, another series of rod lenses along the vertical

---

Manufacturer: Karl Storz KG Instrument Company, 7200 Tuttlingen/Wurtt, Mittelstrasse 8, Postfach 400, West Germany. Distributor: Karl Storz Endoscopy-America, Inc., 658 South San Vicente Boulevard, Los Angeles, California 90048.

shaft, and an eyepiece. The wide viewing angle (90 degrees), increased light transmission, excellent resolution, extreme depth of field, and fixed focus of this system provide the exquisite image quality so essential for prompt endoscopic orientation, and permits mastery of the endoscopic technique with a minimum of training or experience.

Lighting System

Illumination is provided by means of any standard external light source, with a flexible fiberoptic cord attached to the miniature (1 mm) fiberoptic light-transmitting channel of the endoscope. Sufficient light is provided to examine the ducts even when they are markedly dilated.

Irrigation System

The Fenwal pressure-irrigation system,* commonly used for intraarterial infusion, provides the appropriate distention and clearing of the ducts required for inspection. For convenience, commercially available plastic containers preloaded with sterile normal saline† are placed within the Fenwal pressure bag. The saline is delivered to the irrigating channel of the scope by a series of sterile venous extension tubes. A bag pressure of 300 mm Hg ensures adequate delivery of perfusion fluid.

Accessories

An instrument channel can be attached to the scope for the introduction of a variety of flexible stone-retrieving instruments. The most useful of these is a flexible stone grasping forceps with alligator jaws (Fr 7). A new flexible four-wire, stone-retrieving basket can also be advanced through the guide channel for endoscopic removal of larger calculi. Other stone-retrieving devices that have been found useful are the Fogarty biliary catheter and the Dormier stone basket. In addition, Randall stone forceps can be introduced alongside the scope for stone extraction under visual control.

*Manufacturer: Travenol Laboratories, Inc., Morton Grove, Illinois.
†Variflex, 1000 cc. Manufacturer: Travenol Laboratories, Inc.

TECHNIQUE

Biliary endoscopy is performed following conventional choledochal exploration (Fig. 1). The horizontal limb of the choledochoscope is introduced through the choledochotomy incision after the lighting and irrigation attachments are made (Fig. 2). The procedure is best carried out from the left side of the operating table.

The common bile duct and ampulla are examined first (Fig. 3). The lumen is sought by tilting the vertical limb to an appropriate angle while guiding the angle of the scope with the right hand. Traction on the duodenum and liver by an assistant facilitates the procedure. Once the lumen is identified the scope is advanced under direct vision until the ampullary orifice is seen. Complete inspection of the distal duct is then carefully carried out while slowly withdrawing the scope toward the choledochotomy. When the duct is elongated, the angle of the instrument may be inserted within the lumen and the duodenum telescoped proximally for complete examination. Mobilization of the duodenum by the Kocher maneuver is usually not necessary. Examination may be hampered by inadequate duct distention when the common duct is markedly dilated and the sphincter is patulous. This may be overcome by: (1) closing the choledochotomy snugly around the scope with temporary sutures; (2) maintaining bag pressure on the infusion fluid at 300 mm Hg; (3) positioning a Fogarty biliary catheter via the choledochotomy into the duodenum, inflating the balloon, and withdrawing the catheter to engage and gently occlude the sphincter during endoscopic examination.

Excess fluid escaping through the choledochotomy is aspirated by suction. The bright image permits viewing from a safe distance without fear of contamination, while the operating room lights are left on. A teaching attachment can be used to permit simultaneous observation and instruction.

After satisfactory distal endoscopy, the instrument is withdrawn and reinserted toward the hilum of the liver (Fig. 4). Once the lumen of the common hepatic duct is identified, the scope is advanced to the bifurcation. The instrument is then threaded along the lumen of each division as far peripherally as possible.

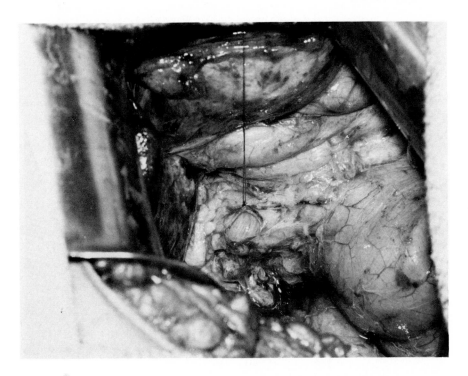

FIG. 1. Common bile duct is open and a stay suture applied.

Once again, precise anatomic definition is best achieved by inspection during slow withdrawal of the scope toward the choledochotomy.

Retained stones found by endoscopy can usually be retrieved by conventional instrumentation. This is always followed by completion en-

doscopy to ensure ductal clearing. Occasionally one must resort to lithotomy under endoscopic control. The most efficient instrument for this purpose is the flexible (Fr 7) stone-grasping forceps with alligator jaws passed through the instrument guide channel (Fig. 5). Stone-

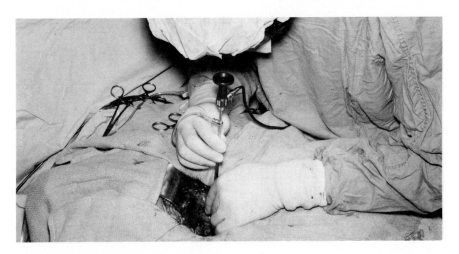

FIG. 2. The choledochoscope is connected to the irrigation (Fenwal) system and to the light source. The assembled scope with running irrigation fluid is inserted. The operator should keep a safe distance from the eyepiece.

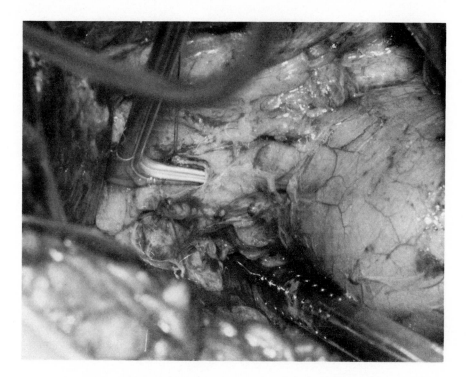

FIG. 3.   Scope introduced to visualize the sphincter region.

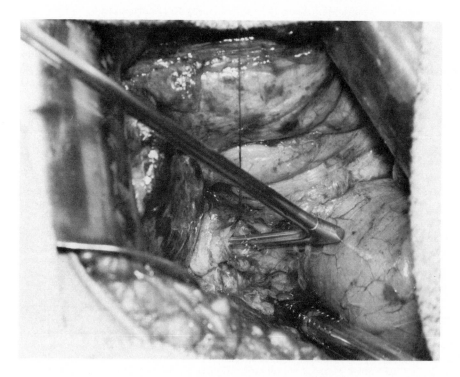

FIG. 4.   Choledochoscope advanced into the hepatic duct system.

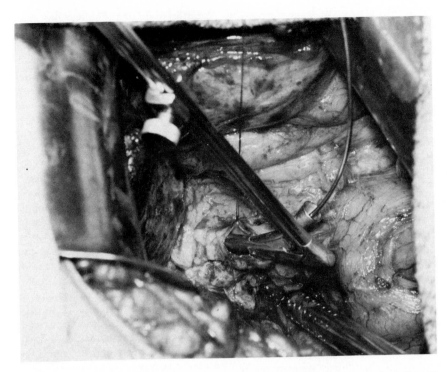

FIG. 5. If stones are located the additional instrument guide channel is attached, the alligator stone forceps inserted, and the scope reintroduced. Stones can be removed under visual control. The stone forceps can be replaced with a Fogarty catheter.

retrieving baskets can also be positioned through the instrument channel for the removal of larger stones under visual guidance. A Fogarty biliary catheter can be advanced beyond a nonimpacted calculus and used to recover the stone by traction after inflating the balloon. Markedly dilated ducts permit the passage of Randall stone forceps alongside the endoscope for choledocholithotomy under direct optical control. Rarely a calculus visualized by endoscopy defies removal by all available techniques and must be managed by a biliary bypass procedure.

ENDOSCOPIC FINDINGS

Normal

The mucous membrane of the distal common bile duct has a pale, glistening, pinkish yellow appearance and is raised into longitudinal folds, which are ironed out by the pressure of the irrigating fluid. A delicate, submucosal vascular reticulum is usually visible. As the ampulla is approached, the duct becomes narrower and funnel-shaped, coursing toward the right and slightly anteriorly. The ampulla itself has a characteristic appearance which must be identified endoscopically to ensure complete distal examination. The ampullary orifice is seen outlined against the dark void of the adjacent duodenal lumen. Its outline is usually stellate but may appear fish-mouthed, triangular, pinpoint, or patulous. The mucosa at this point becomes coarser and is raised into papillary folds, often covered by flakes of fibrinous exudate. Failure to visualize this structure clearly precludes any diagnostic conclusions regarding the status of the distal duct. The orifice of the pancreatic duct is rarely visualized endoscopically.

The bifurcation of the common hepatic duct is readily recognized as a carina, similar to the bronchial bifurcation. The right hepatic duct shortly divides into two segmental divisions, whereas the left duct usually has no major visible tributaries. The mucosa is paler than that of the distal duct and has a distinctive yellowish cast. Variations in hepatic ductal anatomy are common. The segmental divisions of the right hepatic duct may join the left duct at the same level, having the appearance of a trifurcation endoscopically. The junction of the right and left ducts may occur at a wide angle, limiting visualization of the left duct orifice to an en face view. Under these circumstances, it may not be possible to inspect the left duct for more than 1 or 2 cm. The ducts may be markedly dilated, allowing examination of the tertiary (subsegmental) hepatic ducts. In such cases accurate identification of the major carina is mandatory to ensure complete hepatic duct visualization.

Pathology

Cholangitis. Cholangitis of varying degrees is often encountered in ducts harboring calculi and may vary from mucosal congestion and edema to marked ulcerative cholangitis with fibrinopurulent exudate. Inflammatory changes become progressively more marked toward the ampulla of Vater. At times examination of the ampulla is obscured by inflammatory exudate which accumulates in this region. Removal of this debris with stone forceps after temporary withdrawal of the scope is frequently rewarded by improved visualization. These changes are far less conspicuous in the hepatic ducts.

Calculi. Intraductal calculi are easily identified by endoscopy. They are usually free-floating and roll around under the pressure of the irrigating fluid. Not uncommonly a calculus comes in direct contact with the scope, limiting image definition to a colored blur. When this occurs, withdrawal of the instrument usually leads to spontaneous evacuation of the calculus by the irrigating stream. At times a stone is found impacted in the orifice of a hepatic duct or at the ampulla, partly embedded in the duct wall or hidden in a diverticulum of the distal duct. Multiple calculi and biliary mud are not infrequently found behind a large presenting calculus. Repeat endoscopic examination is required to ensure their complete removal.

Ampullary Stenosis. The normal ampulla appears soft and pliable endoscopically and can often be seen to yield to the pressure of the irrigating stream. A stenotic sphincter presents as a fixed circular pinpoint opening at the end of an easily distended common duct "tunnel" resembling an esophageal stricture endoscopically. This picture, however, is not diagnostic, since it may be mimicked by spasm of the sphincter of Oddi, not infrequently encountered during choledochal manipulations. Definitive diagnosis of ampullary stenosis must still be relegated to radiologic and histologic criteria.

Neoplasms. Papillary tumors protruding into the biliary lumen are rarely visualized endoscopically. They can be readily biopsied with the flexible forceps passed through the instrument guide channel. Partial or complete extrinsic duct obstruction by carcinoma of extraductal origin (pancreas, metastatic carcinoma to periductal lymph nodes, lymphoma, carcinoma of the gallbladder) are more commonly encountered. The endoscopic appearance is usually one of sudden, complete occlusion of the duct lumen through which the scope cannot be advanced. The tumor itself can rarely be visualized for biopsy. Extrinsic compression of the distal common bile duct by an inflammatory mass in the head of the pancreas is generally indistinguishable endoscopically from that due to carcinoma. Lesser degrees of narrowing of the distal common bile duct by pancreatitis may permit cannulation of the stenotic segment by the endoscope.

Other Lesions. Lesions rarely seen endoscopically include benign tumors of the common bile duct, diverticula of the distal duct, congenital webs, foreign bodies (e.g., food particles, particularly following biliary-intestinal anastomosis), and parasites.

CLINICAL EXPERIENCE

Operative biliary endoscopy was performed during the course of 315 choledochotomies at the Cedars-Sinai Medical Center between 1960 and 1974. The total experience with this procedure is shown in Table 1. While preliminary experience with the Wildegans endoscope was satisfactory,[3,35] operational limitations result-

TABLE 1. Experience with Biliary Endoscopy, 1960–74

	Choledochotomy	
	Primary	Secondary
Wildegans scope (rigid), 1960–64	54	5
Fiberoptic scope (flexible), 1965–70	160	20
Hopkins-Storz scope (rigid), 1970–74	70	16
Total	284	41

TABLE 2. Experience with Hopkins-Storz Choledochoscope

Findings	Number
Primary choledochotomy	
Calculi found	47
No calculi found	11
Stenosis, sphincter of Oddi	6
Carcinoma, biliary tract	3
Stricture, biliary tract	3
Total	70
Secondary choledocotomy	
Calculi found	16
Total endoscopic exploration	86

TABLE 3. Value of Biliary Endoscopy in 47 Primary Choledocholithotomies

Procedure Result	No.	%
Detection of calculi missed by exploration*	17	36
Aid to operation	10	21
Endoscopic removal of calculi	5	—
Assisted in operative decision	3	—
Cholangiogram unavailable†	2	—
Aid to interpretation of cholangiogram	11	25
Evaluation of nonemptying	5	—
Evaluation of filling defects	4	—
Technically inadequate	2	—
No value	9	18

*Endoscopy performed prior to completion cholangiogram.
†Dye sensitivity, 1; pregnancy, 1.
‡In the remaining nine cases endoscopy did not contribute to the management of the patients.

ing from faulty design led to consideration of other technical options. A flexible fiber choledochoscope, which overcame many disadvantages of the Wildegans scope, was introduced in 1965.[34] Favorable results in 100 choledocholithotomies were reported in 1970.[36] Despite this, the procedure failed to gain popularity, since the optical qualities were not optimal and considerable experience was required to gain expertise.

The recent invention of the "rod-lens" optical system by Hopkins permitted the design of a new rigid choledochoscope,[37] which has been evaluated during the past 4 years. Because of its superior performance, this instrument can now be considered the definitive diagnostic tool for biliary endoscopy. The total experience with the new choledochoscope at this institution includes 70 patients undergoing primary choledochotomy and 16 patients subjected to secondary exploration (Table 2). In each case the ducts were explored by conventional methods until the surgeon was satisfied he had cleared them of calculi. Operative biliary endoscopy was then carried out. Overlooked calculi detected by endoscopy were usually readily removed with standard common duct instruments; occasionally removal under direct endoscopic control was required (Table 3). Completion operative cholangiograms were obtained on all patients. The final status of the biliary tract was assessed by routine postoperative T-tube cholangiography.

RESULTS

The results in 70 primary choledochotomies are shown in Table 4. Routine postoperative cholangiography revealed that the ducts were cleared of all calculi in 46 of 47 patients by exploration, endoscopy, and cholangiography. In only one patient (2 percent) undergoing primary choledocholithotomy was a stone overlooked at operation. Calculi were retained in 2 of 16 patients (12 percent) subjected to secondary choledocholithotomy.

Biliary endoscopy was of benefit to the surgeon in the majority of cases (Table 3). In 17 patients (36 percent) calculi missed by standard exploration were found by endoscopy. Many of these would undoubtedly have been discovered by operative cholangiography as well. In 10 patients (21 percent) endoscopy served as an aid to operation, since the precise information provided by direct visualization led to prompt, definitive management. In five of these cases calculi visualized by endoscopy could be removed only by stone forceps or the Fogarty biliary catheter under endoscopic control. In three instances the endoscopic findings provided the basis for proper surgical management without operative delay. These experiments are briefly summarized.

TABLE 4. Results of Exploration, Endoscopy, and Cholangiography in 70 Primary Choledochotomies

Results	Number
Calculi found	47
All calculi removed	46
Calculi not removed	1
Nonremovable	0
Overlooked	1
No calculi found	23
Total	70

Case 18

In a 65-year-old man undergoing cholecystectomy the initial operative cholangiogram revealed good emptying, no calculi, and a "halo" surrounding the choledochoduodenal junction. No stones were recovered by common duct exploration, and a Fogarty catheter (Fr 5) could be passed into the duodenum. Biliary endoscopy revealed two small calculi in the distal common bile duct as well as a stenotic sphincter. The endoscopic findings supported the clinical suspicion of ampullary fibrosis, and a primary transduodenal sphincteroplasty was performed. The diagnosis was confirmed histologically. The patient has remained asymptomatic over a 3-year follow-up period.

Case 56

A firm mass was palpated in the head of the pancreas of an 80-year-old cholecystectomized man undergoing emergency choledochotomy for acute obstructive cholangitis. The initial operative cholangiogram revealed a filling defect with obstruction of the distal common bile duct. Exploration yielded purulent bile under pressure. Choledochoscopy revealed extrinsic compression of the common duct, but no calculi were visualized. The decision to perform choledochojejunostomy could thus be made without hesitation. The patient has remained well during the past 9 months.

Case 64

No stones were recovered from the markedly dilated biliary tree of a 65-year-old cholecystectomized woman undergoing choledochotomy for recurrent biliary colic and jaundice. A Fogarty catheter (Fr 5) could be advanced into the duodenum. Endoscopic visualization of a pinpoint ampullary orifice, which did not yield to the pressure of the irrigating fluid, confirmed the diagnosis of stenosis of the sphincter of Oddi. The indication for a biliary bypass procedure was thus precisely and promptly identified.

Comments

Problems with interpretation of operative cholangiograms usually relate to the presence of filling defects, to nonpassage of contrast medium, or to technically inadequate studies. Nonemptying is usually considered due to

sphincter spasm if a probe or catheter has been advanced into the duodenum.[32] Endoscopic visualization of a normal sphincter confirmed this interpretation in five patients, thus avoiding operative delay from repeated cholangiograms or unnecessary transduodenal exploration. Biliary endoscopy was also of value in the interpretation of filling defects, where appropriate treatment requires differentiation between calculus, blood clot, exudate, bubble, neoplasm, or artifact. In all four cases the cause of the filling defect was identified by endoscopy, leading to proper and efficient operative management.

COMPLICATIONS

Complications possibly related to the use of biliary endoscopy are listed in Table 5. Significant infection was encountered in 2 percent of the patients. This incidence is within the range usually reported for choledocholithotomy without endoscopy. There were no intraoperative injuries to the bile ducts, duodenum, or liver due to endoscopy. Mild postoperative pancreatitis occurred in three patients (4 percent). Two patients had prolonged postoperative drainage which resolved spontaneously. Such complications occur occasionally without endoscopy and cannot be directly attributed to this procedure. There were no deaths in this series in which the use of endoscopy could be justifiably faulted.

DISCUSSION

The incidence of retained calculi following common duct exploration by instrumental manipulation alone is approximately 20 percent.[14,15] With the use of routine operative

TABLE 5.   Complications Possibly Related to Biliary Endoscopy

Complication	Number of Cases
Infection	5
Main wound	1
"Stab" wound	3
Subhepatic abscess	1
Pancreatitis postoperative (mild)	3
Prolonged drainage (biliary or pancreatic)	2
Missed ampullary carcinoma	1

TABLE 6. Results of Biliary Endoscopy

Author, Date	Choledocho- lithotomy (No.)	Calculi Missed (%)	Calculi Visualized but Not Removed (%)
Wildegans 1960	143	1	2
Schein, 1969	43	2	0
Wiechel, 1969	233	1	2
Shore, 1970	100	2	1
Shore, 1974	47	2	0

cholangiography the results can be improved to a varying degree.[1,6,10,12,14–18,21,24,27,31,38,39] Nevertheless, overlooked stones are still detected postoperatively in approximately 10 percent of choledocholithotomies.[36] Other ingenious devices, such as the Fogarty biliary catheter[9] and the ultrasonic probe,[8] have failed to reduce the incidence of missed stones significantly beyond that of cholangiography. Operative biliary endoscopy, however, has been found consistently to decrease the number of retained calculi to 2 to 3 percent of the choledocholithotomies performed[29,33,40,42] (Table 6). Only 1 to 2 percent are truly overlooked, since the remainder, which are visualized but not removable, can be treated definitively by primary duct drainage procedures. Although these calculi may be retained, their discovery by endoscopy has led to prompt corrective surgery, thereby eliminating the probability of symptomatic recurrence.

The incidence of retained stones with the Hopkins-Storz choledochoscope in 47 primary choledocholithotomies was 2 percent. This figure varies, depending on how it is calculated (Table 7). Most series express the frequency of retained stones as a percent of all choledochotomies. As a result, comparison of experience from different institutions may not be meaningful owing to the variation in the number of negative and secondary choledochotomies included. A preferable reporting method would standardize the data by separately itemizing the results, as shown in Table 7. The benefits derived from various technologic and instrumental innovations could thus be assessed more accurately.

The precise observation provided by cholangioscopy has been of value in many ways. Removal of calculi localized by direct inspection has been facilitated. This has occasionally been possible only under endoscopic guidance. The definitive information provided by direct inspection can promptly indicate appropriate operative strategy, e.g., the decision to perform transduodenal exploration or a biliary-intestinal bypass procedure. The proper interpretation of doubtful or suspicious cholangiograms has on several occasions shortened operative time by eliminating the need for repeat cholangiograms, reexploration, or unnecessary duodenotomy.

The major application of this diagnostic tool is in the surgical treatment of choledocholithiasis. Tumors of the biliary tract have been visually identified and biopsied, but they are rare. The differential diagnosis of distal duct obstruction due to carcinoma of the head of the pancreas versus chronic pancreatitis has not been materially aided by this technique.

The technique of biliary endoscopy can be readily learned. The important anatomic landmarks are easily identified. Unlike endoscopic examination of other organs, there is no complex endoscopic anatomy to master, and the changes to be recognized are limited to calculi in the majority of cases. The atraumatic nature of the choledochoscope is demonstrated by the absence of injury to the ducts and the low incidence of postoperative infection and pancreatitis.

TABLE 7. Variation in Incidence of Retained Calculi

Method of Calculation	No. of Cases	Retained Stones No.	Retained Stones (%)
Negative choledochotomy	20	0	0
Primary choledocholithotomy	47	1	2
All choledochotomies	83	3	4
All choledocholithotomies	63	3	5
Secondary choledocholithotomy	16	2	12

SUMMARY AND CONCLUSIONS

1. The history of biliary endoscopy is briefly reviewed. While the concept originated with the inception of choledochotomy, it is only in recent years that technology was able to meet the task suitably.
2. The definitive choledochoscope with the Hopkins-Storz system is described. Revolutionary advances in optics have led to the construction of this compact, right angled, rigid endoscope.
3. The technique of biliary endoscopy is outlined. The rapidity, ease, and safety of the examination are stressed.

4. The endoscopic anatomy and pathology of the biliary tract are documented. Key anatomic landmarks such as the sphincter of Oddi and the hepatic duct bifurcation are easy to recognize after a minimum of experience. The presence of calculi or other changes within the biliary tree can be clearly and readily identified. The technique of choledocholithotomy under endoscopic control with a variety of stone-retrieving instruments is described.

5. Experience with biliary endoscopy during the course of 325 choledochotomies during the past 15 years is discussed.

6. The results of choledochoscopy in the current series of 70 primary choledochotomies are reviewed in detail.
   a. Of 47 patients undergoing primary choledocholithotomy, the ducts were cleared of all calculi in 46 and a small retained stone was found by postoperative cholangiography in only one (2 percent).
   b. Biliary endoscopy was of benefit to the surgeon in the majority of cases: In 17 patients calculi missed by standard exploration were detected; on five occasions calculi were retrieved under endoscopic control; in three instances operative strategy was clarified; and in 11 cases interpretation of operative cholangiograms was aided.

7. The use of biliary endoscopy did not increase the postoperative morbidity or mortality rates beyond those usually encountered in choledocholithotomy.

8. Current experience indicates that the new choledochoscope overcomes the limitations of previous endoscopes and should serve as the definitive diagnostic tool for operative biliary endoscopy. Addition of this technique to the armamentarium of the biliary surgeon will play a significant role in overcoming the age-old problem of the retained common duct stone.

REFERENCES

1. Allen KA: Routine operative cholangiography. Am J Surg 118:573, 1969
2. Bakes J: Die Choledochopapilloskopie nebst Bemerkungen über Hepaticusdrainage und Dilatation der Papille. Arch Klin Chir 126:473, 1926
3. Berci G: Choledochoscopy. Med J Aust 2:861, 1961
4. Berci G, Kont L: A new optical system in endoscopy with special references to cystoscopy. Br J Urol 41:564, 1969
5. Berci G, Morgenstern L, Shore JM: Endoscopic inspection of the biliary system: choledochoscopy. In Nyhus LM (ed): Surgery Annual 1973. New York, Appleton-Century-Crofts, 1973, pp 222–24
6. Colcok BP, Perry B: Exploration of the common bile duct. Surg Gynecol Obstet 118:20, 1964
7. Custer MD Jr: Inhibitions concerning the choledochoscope. Surg Gynecol Obstet 117:110, 1963
8. Eiseman B, Greenlaw RH, Gallagher JQ: Localization of common duct stones by ultrasound. Arch Surg 91:195, 1965
9. Fogarty TJ, Krippaehne WM, Dennis DL, et al: Evaluation of an improved operative technique in common duct surgery. Am J Surg 116:177, 1968
10. Glen F: Common duct exploration for stones. Surg Gynecol Obstet 95:431, 1952
11. Griesmann H: Experiences with choledochoscopy. Beitr Klin Chir 195:251, 1957
12. Griffin TFR, Wild AA: The case for peroperative cholangiography. Br J Surg 54:609, 1967
13. Guderley H: Endoscopy of the deep bile duct. Zentralbl Chir 83:263, 1958
14. Harvard C: Non-malignant bile duct obstruction. Ann R Coll Surg Engl 26:88, 1960
15. Hicken NF, McCallister AJ: Operative cholangiography as an aid to reducing the incidence of "overlooked" common bile duct stones. Surgery 55:753, 1964
16. Hight D, Lingley JR, Hurtubise F: An evaluation of the operative cholangiogram as a guide to common duct exploration. Ann Surg 150:1086, 1959
17. Isaacs JP, Daves ML: Technique and evaluation of operative cholangiography. Surg Gynecol Obstet 111:130, 1960
18. Jolly EC, Baker JW, Schmide HM, et al: Operative cholangiography: a case for its routine use. Ann Surg 168:551, 1968
19. Kolder LJ: Biliary tract surgery, choledochoscopy and radiomanometry in a number of European clinics. Sinai Hosp J (Balt) 11:81, 1963
20. Leslie D: The use of choledochoscope: or, leaving no stone unturned. Med J Aust 49:235, 1962
21. Letton AH, Wilson JP: Routine cholangiography during biliary tract operations: technique and utility in 200 cases. Ann Surg 163:937, 1966
22. Lortat-Jacob JL: First findings on endoscopy of the bile ducts. Arch Mal App Dig (Paris) 46:856, 1957
23. Madden JL, McCann WJ, Kandaloft S, et al: Considerations in surgery of the common bile duct. Curr Probl Surg 1968
24. Madsen CM: Routine or elective cholangiography during cholecystectomy. Acta Chir Scand [Suppl] 283:247, 1961
25. McIver MA: An instrument for visualizing the interior of the common duct at operation. Surgery 9:112, 1941
26. Morgenstern L, Shore JM, Berci G: Potentials of a new miniature optical system (endoscope) as a diagnostic aid. Am Surg 38:312, 1972
27. Neinhuis L: Routine operative cholangiography: an evaluation. Ann Surg 154 (Suppl):192, 1961
28. Richard C: La choledoscopie. Rev Med Chir Mal Foie (Paris) 34:55, 1959
29. Schein CJ: Biliary endoscopy: an appraisal of its value in biliary lithiasis. Surgery 65:1004, 1969
30. Schein CJ, Stern WZ, Jacobson HE: The Common Bile Duct. Springfield, Ill, Charles C Thomas, 1965
31. Schulenberg CAR: Operative cholangiography: 1000 cases. Surgery 65:723, 1969

32. Senter KL, Berne CJ: Significance of non-passage of radiopaque medium through ampulla of Vater during operative cholangiography. Am J Surg 112:7, 1966

33. Shore JM, Berci G: The clinical importance of cholangiography. Endoscopy 2:117, 1970

34. Shore JM, Lippman HN: A flexible choledochoscope. Lancet 1:1200, 1965

35. Shore JM, Lippman HN: Operative endoscopy of the biliary tract. Ann Surg 156:951, 1962

36. Shore JM, Shore E: Operative biliary endoscopy. Ann Surg 171:269, 1970

37. Shore JM, Morgenstern L, Berci G: An improved rigid choledochoscope. Am J Surg 122:567, 1971

38. Smith RB III, Conklin ES, Porter MR: Five year study of choledocholithiasis. Surg Gynecol Obstet 116:731, 1963

39. Smith SW, Engle C, Averbrook B, et al: Problems of retained and recurrent common bile duct stones. JAMA 164:231, 1957

40. Wildegans H: Die operative Cholangioscopie. Munich, Urban & Schwarzenberg, 1960

41. Wildegans H: Endoskopie der tiefen Gallenwege. Langenbecks Arch Klin Chir 276:652, 1953

42. Wiechel KL: Results of choledochoscopy in routine use in biliary tract surgery. Proceedings 1st European Congress of Digestive Endoscopy, Prague, 1968. Karger, Basel, 1969

EDITORIAL COMMENT

Common bile duct exploration for stones has always been a blind procedure. Surgeons attacking this problem have been plagued by the insoluble question of retained stones. Despite the introduction of various specially designed instruments and routine operative cholangiography, stones are still missed following choledochotomy in approximately 10 percent of cases.

With the advent of proper biliary endoscopy it has become possible to improve our results significantly. Following our initial clinical trial, a cooperative multi-institutional study was launched in 1973. The figures in the table include the participation of surgical residents and represent the initial experience of all participants. Nevertheless, the overall results of 2.7 percent retained stones in 326 primary choledochotomies indicate the value of operative biliary endoscopy.

Since the submission of this chapter, 25 additional patients have undergone choledochoscopy. In none of these cases have calculi been overlooked.

Date Through	P. CBD. E.	Stones	O.S.
Tompkins et al, University of California, Los Angeles			
2/75	27	18	1*
Dorazzio et al, Kaiser Permanente, Los Angeles			
9/74	23	10	2†
Warshaw et al, Massachusetts General Hospital, Boston			
2/75	80	60	1
Silen et al, Beth Israel Hospital, Boston			
2/75	28	25	4†
Wilson et al, Milwaukee County and VA Hospital			
2/75	42	16	0
Nora, Columbus-Cuneo Hospital, Chicago			
9/74	19	10	0
Shore and Berci, Cedars-Sinai Medical Center			
6/75	87	56	1
Norton, Denver General Hospital			
2/75	20	20	0
Total	*326*	*215*	*9 (2.7%)*

P. CBD. E., *number of primary common bile duct explorations.* **Stones,** *number of cases with stones.* **O.S.,** *number of stones retained.*
Stone seen at surgery could be removed.
†*Performed by surgical residents.*

A 16-mm color sound motion picture entitled "Precise Biliary Exploration" has been completed. This film is available from the authors or from the Motion Picture Library, American College of Surgeons.

THE EDITOR

21

Colonoscopy

Joel F. Panish

The first prototype colon fiberscopes were produced and tested by various Japanese workers from 1963 to 1966.[2,6,7,18] At the same time in the United States Overholt was working with American manufacturers on the development of a fiber sigmoidoscope.[9] One of the earliest clinical reports of successful colonoscopy in the United States was by Dean and Shearman.[2] Although the instrument* was quite flexible, there was only a two-directional controllable tip. Frequently after negotiating a tight sigmoid curve, the ability to rotate and flex the tip of the instrument was greatly diminished. Thus the instrument could not be advanced while the lumen of the bowel was being visualized. Following this Overholt suggested that the instrument could be advanced without visualizing the lumen by exerting gentle pressure, which was safe so long as the mucosa could be seen to "slip by" the viewing surface.[8] The bowel lumen could then be visualized very well on withdrawal of the instrument.

Various techniques of introduction and passage were then reported which involved the passage of a guiding or pulling catheter or thread. Once the patient swallowed it and it passed through the anus, it was attached to the tip of the colonoscope, which was then pulled through the colon to the cecum.[4,13]

Olympus Model CF-SB, Olympus Corporation of America, 2 Nevada Drive, New Hyde Park, New York 11040.

INSTRUMENTATION

In 1971 a greater degree of flexibility and tip control was established with the appearance of the four-way tip deflection with proximal control. Manufacturers (AMCI, Olympus, and Machida*) offer fiberoptic colonoscope instruments with features mentioned above (Chapter 6).[12]

INDICATIONS

Indications for performing colonoscopy include:

1. A questionable lesion seen on barium enema
2. Lower gastrointestinal bleeding when the barium enema (x-ray) is negative
3. Biopsy of questionably malignant lesions, especially in poor-risk surgical patients
4. Stenotic lesions of the colon
5. Presence of polypoid lesions that appear to be removable by cautery snare
6. Unexplained diarrhea
7. Unexplained lower abdominal pain
8. Differential diagnosis of chronic inflammatory bowel disease
9. Removal of foreign bodies

ACMI: 8 Pelham Parkway, Pelham Manor, New York 10803. Olympus Corporation of America: 2 Nevada Drive, New Hyde Park, New York 11040. Machida: Manabu Medical Instrument Co., Ltd., 10–8 Honkomagome 5-Chrome, Bunkyo-Ku Tokyo, Japan.

PREPARATION OF PATIENT

Our usual preparation consists of putting the patient on a 72-hour clear liquid diet. When the polyp is in the mid or distal sigmoid, it sometimes suffices to have the patient on a 48-hour clear liquid diet. Diagnostic colonoscopy patients are examined as outpatients. Polypectomy patients are admitted to the hospital. At 4 PM on the day preceding the examination the patient is administered a laxative. The type does not seem to be important, as we have had success with various agents. On the morning of the examination the patient is given cleansing tap water enemas approximately 3 hours before colonoscopy is undertaken. This time interval is important as it allows the colon to be emptied completely of liquid material preceding the examination and visualization is much easier and better. It is unwise to plan colonoscopy within a week of the administration of barium, either for barium enema or upper gastrointestinal x-rays. This is particularly true in older patients for it may take 1 to 2 weeks for barium to clear the lower intestinal tract despite numerous attempts at laxation and cleansing enemas. The presence of barium in the colonic lumen makes evaluation at the time of colonoscopy impossible.

We have had limited experience with the examination of patients with acute colonic hemorrhage. In these few patients we found that despite numerous attempts to cleanse the colon with enemas, there is still too much blood present to allow adequate examination. Unlike the stomach, which can be expanded to a degree which permits observation of most of the interior even though blood is still present, the normal colonic lumen is too narrow to permit this distention and even the retention of minor amounts of blood can obscure the visual field.

PREMEDICATION

We have found it necessary to premedicate most of our patients. A combination of demerol and diazepam (Valium) intravenously is administered and titrated to a point where the patient is comfortable and drowsy but not somnolent. On the average approximately 50 mg demerol and 5 mg diazepam was sufficient. Even in some very cooperative patients it was impossible to carry out the examination without premedication. An antispasmotic is not routinely employed.

TECHNIQUE

All examinations are begun with the patient in the left lateral position. One author stated that he begins all examinations in the right lateral position and feels that this allows him to pass the instrument through the sigmoid curve more easily.[5]

The anal area is prepared by applying a small amount of anesthetic lubricant. We lubricate the scope with mineral oil. If examination is going to include the right side of the colon, we begin with the longer colonoscope and with the stiffening sheath in place on the outside of the proximal part of the scope.

We found fluoroscopy to be extremely helpful when attempting to examine the colon beyond the splenic flexure. Fluoroscopy can also be helpful in a sigmoid colon that is difficult to navigate.

The scope is inserted into the rectum, and under direct vision a small amount of air is used to insufflate the rectum and to find the lumen. In a great number of cases it is a fairly simple task to advance the tip of the scope under direct vision, following the lumen throughout the sigmoid colon. If the lumen disappears from view, it is safe to advance the scope by exerting gentle pressure as long as the mucosa easily slips by the lens and does not "blanch." If there is undue resistance, the mucosa blanches, or the patient complains of pain, the scope must be withdrawn slightly and rotated to various positions to see if it advances easily in some other direction. The so-called alpha maneuver consists of rotating the scope in a counterclockwise fashion while advancing it, thus changing the configuration of the sigmoid colon into the shape of the Greek letter α, which usually permits easier passage of the scope through the sigmoid colon. If the scope still cannot be advanced, the patient may be placed in the supine and/or the right lateral position in an attempt to pass the instrument through the sigmoid into the descending colon.

At times, after having successfully passed through the sigmoid colon and entering the descending colon, with the lumen of the descending colon clearly visible, further advancement of the scope only brings a complaint of pain from the patient. At the same time the lumen of the descending colon is seen to recede from view. The problem here is that the tip of the scope has been hooked into a sharply angulated junction of the descending and sigmoid colon, and further introduction of the scope results only in a widening of the sigmoid loop. This stretches the mesentery, is painful to the patient, does not advance the tip, and may result in perforation. Under these circumstances it is best to wait, turn the patient to a supine position, and check the position of the scope by fluoroscopy. If the above described configuration is present, it can usually be overcome by hooking the tip of the scope as much as possible into the descending colon and then pulling the scope back while rotating it very slowly in a clockwise fashion. This usually straightens the sigmoid colon and results in advancement of the tip of the scope up the descending colon. Once one is familiar with this maneuver and has observed it on fluoroscopy, it can usually be attempted successfully under direct vision and fluoroscopic control becomes less necessary.

At times even this maneuver has failed and we have given the patient glucagon (1 mg I.V.) or propantheline (Probanthine; 15 to 30 mg I.V.) in an effort to relax any colonic spasm. This is sometimes successful in aiding passage of the scope through a hypertonic sigmoid colon.

If one fails to navigate the sigmoid colon after all these maneuvers it is usually best to terminate the procedure. These unsuccessful introductions become quite rare as the examiner gains experience and are usually limited to those patients who have had prior inflammatory bowel disease or pelvic surgery and/or irradiation. The sigmoid colon becomes fixed, and not enough mobility remains to allow manipulation of the scope through the sigmoid colon.

Once in the descending colon it is usually quite simple to advance the tip of the scope rapidly under direct vision to the splenic flexure. About half the time the splenic flexure can be navigated under direct vision and the tip of the scope passed into the transverse colon. However, once the tip of the scope is hooked into the splenic flexure, it is not unusual to encounter the same situation as occurred in the sigmoid colon. That is, further insertion of the scope results only in enlarging

the sigmoid loop, and the lumen of the transverse colon recedes from view. When this occurs it is necessary to employ fluoroscopic control, hook the tip of the scope into the splenic flexure, and straighten out the sigmoid colon by pulling back on the scope and rotating it in a counterclockwise fashion. Following this the scope may once again be successfully introduced, but if the sigmoid loop again tends to re-form the stiffening sheath should be used.

Once the sigmoid colon is straightened in this fashion, the stiffening tube, after having been well lubricated, is introduced into the anus over the colonoscope and then guided under fluoroscopic control into the sigmoid colon, thus stiffening and keeping the sigmoid colon straight. *This maneuver must be done under fluoroscopic control.* If one does not make sure that the sigmoid colon is as straight as possible and tries to pass the stiffening tube around a more than slightly curved colonoscope, one can either tear the outer skin of the colonoscope or engage mucosa between the stiffening tube and the scope, running a high risk of bleeding or perforation.

Usually the scope can then be advanced rapidly across the transverse colon to the hepatic flexure. However, in some cases there is a deep transverse colon that reaches down into the pelvis. When this occurs the tip of the scope no longer advances, but instead a large splenic flexure loop is formed. The patient begins to complain of discomfort, and one either sees a receding lumen through the lens or loses complete sight of the lumen. This difficulty is overcome by hooking the tip of the scope superiorly as far as possible, usually with the aid of fluoroscopic control, and then pulling back on the scope. This has the effect of raising the transverse colon back into the upper abdomen and at the same time advancing the tip of the scope into the hepatic flexure.

The last maneuver that may entail some difficulty is passage of the tip of the scope from the hepatic flexure into the ascending colon and cecum. Under direct vision the ascending colon is entered and the scope is passed into the cecum with good visibility. Most of the time, however, it is quite helpful to have fluoroscopy available so that the tip of the scope can be visualized on the fluoroscopic screen and tilted downward in the direction of the ascending colon. The scope may then be advanced directly; if this produces a deeper transverse colon loop then once the tip of the scope is hooked into the ascending colon, withdrawal rather than advancement of the instrument results in straightening of the transverse colon and rotating (flipping) the tip of the scope into the cecum. At times it is necessary to put the patient in either a left or right lateral position to facilitate entrance into the cecum. Sometimes palpation of the abdominal wall can be helpful in guiding the scope into the cecum, as well as when other difficult areas are encountered in passing the scope.

We have encountered no difficulties in the passage of polypectomy snares. However, on several occasions we encountered great difficulty in the passage of biopsy forceps when the instrument was sharply angulated. There are times when the lesion to be biopsied cannot be kept in view while the biopsy forceps is being passed. To overcome this, the tip of the scope is unlocked, straightening it as much as possible (which probably means losing sight of the target), and then the biopsy forceps is pushed through. One other useful maneuver to help passage of the biopsy forceps is to lubricate the forceps and the biopsy channel with mineral oil.

DIAGNOSTIC COLONOSCOPY RESULTS

Aside from colonoscopic polypectomy, the most valuable information was obtained in the differential diagnosis. This examination has a high diagnostic accuracy of chronic lower gastrointestinal bleeding. We have diagnosed polyps that have not been evident on x-rays. Carcinomas not evident on barium enema were found in three cases: two in the cecum and one in the sigmoid colon. We have also demonstrated in a number of cases that colitis in uremic patients is a cause of significant lower gastrointestinal bleeding.

We have confirmed the presence of malignant lesions by biopsy and have differentiated stenotic lesions of the colon by biopsy, classifying them either as malignant or benign, secondary to inflammatory bowel disease (Fig. 1, Plate A).* In some cases of unexplained diarrhea and negative barium enema findings, we have established early phases of inflammatory bowel disease. It can be discovered by

All color plates appear in the front of the book.

superficial, serpiginous ulcerations scattered throughout the colon. In two cases granulomatous colitis was found, the classic appearance of which showed up on the x-ray films taken at a later date. We removed foreign bodies successfully—a part of a thermometer that had been swallowed in one case, and in another an entire thermometer that had become located at the rectosigmoid junction.

Our experience with the colonoscope for diagnosing acute lower gastrointestinal bleeding has been unrewarding because we have been unable to clean the colon of blood adequately during the acute episode. At the present time we advocate waiting until the acute episode has ceased, then clean the colon and perform colonoscopy prior to barium enema.

COLONOSCOPIC POLYPECTOMY

The efficacy and safety of cautery snare removal of colon polyps through the colonoscope now appears well established.[1,10,11,16,17] The location and size of the lesions are relatively unimportant, since even the cecum is accessible and large polyps can be removed in sections. Even lesions that are sessile have been removed safely. Multiple polypectomies at one session are not unusual.

We are summarizing here a series comprised of the first 100 consecutive patients during the first year of our experience with colonoscopic polypectomy. We utilized the Olympus CF-LB fiberoptic colonoscope, ACMI light source FO-1000, Storz cautery snare, and EMS* electrocautery surgical unit in 82 procedures. In 29 colonoscopic polypectomies the Olympus CF-LB colonoscope was utilized with the CL-3 light source and the Cameron-Miller† electrosurgical unit.

The criteria used for performing colonoscopy and polypectomy included the appearance on barium enema of one or more polypoid lesions in the colon measuring over 1 cm in diameter, or any polypoid lesion regardless of size if there was a prior history of colonic polyps, colonic carcinoma, or a family history of colonic polyps or carcinoma.

*Storz Endoscopy America, Inc., 658 South San Vicente Boulevard, Los Angeles, California 90048. Electro Medical Systems, Inc., Building 43, Denver Technological Center, Englewood, Colorado 80110.
†Cameron-Miller Surgical Instruments Co., 329 South Wood Street, Chicago, Illinois 60612.*

The patients were prepared with a 3-day clear liquid diet, laxative at 4 PM the day prior to the polypectomy, and cleansing tap water enemas 3 hours prior to the procedure. Most patients were admitted to the hospital the afternoon prior to the procedure and discharged 24 hours after the procedure. A few patients with long pedunculated sigmoid colon polyps have been operated on on an outpatient basis. In those cases where there is no fear of bleeding or perforation, normal diet was resumed immediately following the procedure. The patients resumed sedentary work within 48 hours of the polypectomy and began engaging in all normal physical activity within 5 days.

The average time spent performing the procedure has been approximately 45 minutes. The length of time was related to the anatomic configuration of the colon, the number and position of polyps, and the experience of the examiner.

When there is a definite stalk present (Fig. 2, Plate A), we usually try to snare the polyp at the midportion of the stalk, close the snare loop around it lightly, give a short burst of coagulation current, then tighten the snare completely and continue to coagulate.

The settings on the various electrosurgical units are quite variable, and anyone performing this procedure should thoroughly familiarize himself with his own unit by testing its ability. This can be done using surgically resected material or even meat to ascertain what setting is necessary to coagulate approximately 5 mm tissue thickness.

We used coagulation current almost exclusively when using the EMS electrosurgical unit. In rare instances when we have not been able to sever the polyp stalk by coagulation alone we used short bursts of cutting current. It is much safer to use very short (0.5- to 1-second) bursts of coagulation current at repeated intervals than to apply coagulation current for a prolonged length of time. The latter method appears to result in a more extensive burn and necrotic area. Once the stalk has been quite carefully coagulated it is usually possible to draw the stalk up tightly against the tip of the colonoscope and sever the stalk without significant bleeding (Fig. 3, Plate A).

When the polyp appears to be somewhat sessile we try to snare it close to the adenomatous portion, taking as little normal mucosa as possible. This is to prevent deep coagulation necrosis and the probability of late perforation. In those few instances where more than the usual amount of bleeding is observed, one can attempt to electrocoagulate the bleeder by means of a combined suction cautery probe catheter. We have found this fairly effective. Small sessile polyps—which probably could be referred to as mammilations and which measure less than 3 to 4 mm in diameter—we treated first by biopsy and then fulguration with the suction cautery probe.

Although our experience in this series was limited to the Storz snare we have utilized snares manufactured by ACMI, Cameron-Miller, and Olympus, and have found that all of these seem adequate for the required task. We have found the newer instruments (i.e., Olympus colonoscope with the larger channel and the double-channel instrument of ACMI) to be helpful during polypectomy when accummulation of fluids begins to obscure the vision and suction can be applied at the same time that the cautery snare is also introduced. The lack of a double channel is a drawback in the older models, but it is not insurmountable. There are certain conditions when a double channel is helpful, e.g., in the case of a mobile polyp which can be immobilized by holding it with a forceps through one channel while snaring it with the cautery snare through the other. The increase in size and number of channels in the new scopes makes them thicker and less flexible. This may make manipulation more difficult and increase the possibility of perforation.

We have not found hyperperistalsis to be a great problem, but in certain cases it is helpful to administer either propantheline 30 mg I.V. or if the patient is an elderly male and prostatitis may be a problem we prefer glucagon 1 mg I.V. Both these medications produce colonic hypomotility for 5 to 10 minutes and greatly enhance the ease of polyp removal when the colon is irritable.

The results of our series are as follows: There were 68 males and 32 females. The age range of the men was 44 to 88 years (average 66.9), and that of the women 36 to 83 years (average 59.2). A total of 100 patients underwent 111 colonoscopies, 92 patients having one colonoscopy, five patients two colonoscopies, and three patients three colonoscopies each.

A total of 183 polyps were removed; 81 percent (148/183) of the polyps were recovered from the entire series, but this percentage increased from 76 percent in the first 50 patients to 94 percent in the second 50. Of the 35 polyps lost, 22 were estimated to be under 0.5 cm in diameter and 13 were under 1.0 cm. The difference in the recovery rate between the first and second group of 50 patients was due to the fact that we did not recognize in the first half of this study that many of the polyps which we thought were being lost in the colon lumen were actually being suctioned back through the channel of the colonoscope into the collecting bottle in fragmented form. When we began to look for these polyps at the end of the procedure, filtering the vacuum container, our recovery rate improved significantly. It should be observed that all polyps which were not recovered were under 1 cm in size, two-thirds of them being under 0.5 cm. Almost all of these were polyps incidentally discovered at colonoscopy and had not been seen on barium enema. These incidental polyps were not the prime indication for the colonoscopy.

The vast majority of polyps were found and removed from the sigmoid with the number decreasing as inspection proceeds proximally in the colon (Table 1). Histologic classification of the removed polyps revealed that the vast majority were benign adenomas (Table 2). In six polypoid lesions only a part of the benign adenoma showed carcinomatous changes. Similar pathology was found in two polyps which indicated the presence of both villous adenoma and carcinoma. Two of the three lipomas had

definite stalks. These polypoid lesions are usually distinguishable because the "head" of the polyp is much softer and more friable than in the ordinary adenoma (Table 2).

Almost half of the polyps were 1 to 2 cm in size (Table 3). The distribution of the number of polyps per patient is shown in Table 4. Thirty percent more polyps were found during colonoscopy than had been discovered by barium enema.

TABLE 3.   Colonoscopic Polypectomy: Polyp Size

Size (cm)	No.	%
<0.5	11	6.0
0.5–0.9	40	21.8
1.0–1.9	87	47.5
2.0–2.9	27	14.7
3.0–3.9	9	4.9
4.0–4.9	4	2.3
>5.0	5	2.8

TABLE 4.   Colonoscopic Polypectomy: Polyps per Patient

Polyps	Patients
1	66
2	18
3	9
4	3
5	1
6	1
10	2

TABLE 1.   Colonoscopic Polypectomy: Polyp Location

Polyp Location	Number
Sigmoid	105
Descending colon	33
Transverse colon	30
Ascending colon	8
Cecum	7

TABLE 2.   Colonoscopic Polypectomy: Pathology

Pathology	Lesions	Patients
Adenoma	129	67
Villous adenoma	5	5
Typical adenoma	1	1
Carcinoma in adenoma	6	6
Carcinoma in villous adenoma	2	2
Lipoma	3	3
Inflammatory	2	2

COMPLICATIONS

Bleeding occurred in two patients. One patient had arterial bleeding at the site of polypectomy and required 2 units of blood. We believe that administration of intravenous vasopressin (Pitressin) was helpful in arresting this arterial bleeder. The second patient showed a blood loss of 200 cc per rectum 72 hours after the polypectomy. He was observed and required no treatment.

No perforations were encountered in this series. However, perforations do occur, as shown by a review of the literature.[14,15-17] Table 5 summarizes the complications of bleeding and perforation. The complication rate is much less than the morbidity and mortality when one performs laparotomy and colotomy for removal of a colonic polyp.[18]

TABLE 5.   Bleeding and Perforation After Colonoscopic Polypectomy

Authors	Colonos-copies	Polypec-tomies	Bleed-ing	Perfo-ration
Wolff and Shinya[16,17]	2,000	499	1	1
Hedberg[3]	—	123	4*	2
Schrock[3]	300	70	1	0
Sugar-barker[3]	355	109	1	2
Rosecrans[14]	627	49	3	5
Total	3,282	850	10	10

One bleeder was due to splenic rupture.

Eight malignancies were encountered in this series (one malignant polyp was discovered in each of eight patients). Therefore the incidence of malignancy is 8 percent of the total number patients in the group, although only 5.7 percent of the total number of polyps (143) were recovered from these patients. No malignancy was encountered in any polyp under 1.2 cm in diameter. There was no relationship to position in the colon or the number of polyps. Half the malignant lesions were sessile, the other half pedunculated. Pathologically seven malignancies were of the variety wherein carcinoma occurred in an adenoma (Table 6). One was a carcinoma in a villous adenoma.

Six of the patients had surgery. In four of these cases no residual malignant lesion was found in the resected specimen; even though the stalk showed invasion, it seemed to us to be cleared at the time of cautery snare removal through the colonoscope. In one explored patient a residual tumor was revealed, but adjacent lymph nodes were free of malignant invasion. One patient with carcinoma occurring in a villous adenoma exhibited a microscopic focus of carcinoma in the submucosa, but the nodes were free of disease.

Two patients refused surgery; one of these was recolonoscoped 6 months after removal of a polyp through the colonoscope where malignancy had invaded the stalk but had been believed cleared; no lesion was observed on the repeat examination. The other patient who refused surgery was recolonoscoped 3 months after partial polypectomy and fulguration. The lesion had recurred and was coagulated again. This patient continues to refuse surgery, and further follow-up is planned.

COMMENTS

We have found colonoscopic polypectomy to be a safe and efficient procedure that is well tolerated even by elderly high-risk patients. The procedure can sometimes be difficult and time-consuming. We advise that only those ex-

TABLE 6.   Colonoscopic Polypectomy: Analysis of Malignant Polyps

Date	Size (cm)	Location of Polyp	No. of Polyps in Patient	Location of Malignancy Gross	Location of Malignancy Microscopic	Follow-up
4/72	1.5	Descending colon	1	Stalk	Ca in adenoma; superficial	Surgery: no lesion
6/72	4.0	Sigmoid	10	Sessile	Ca in adenoma; not cleared	Surgery: tumor left, no nodes
9/72	1.2	Sigmoid	1	Stalk	Ca in adenoma; stalk invaded but cleared	Surgery: no lesion
9/72	1.3	Descending colon	1	Stalk	Ca in adenoma; stalk clear	Surgery: no lesion
3/73	1.5	Descending colon	1	Stalk	Ca in adenoma; stalk invaded but cleared	Recolonoscoped at 6 mo: no lesion
8/73	5.0	Transverse colon	2	Sessile	Ca in adenoma; stalk invaded, ? cleared	Surgery: no lession
8/73	1.5	Descending colon	1	Sessile	Ca in adenoma; ? cleared	Recolonoscoped at 3 mo: recurrent lesion

aminers who have had fiberoptic endoscopy experience should undertake this procedure.

Our findings are similar to other reports regarding size, location, pathology, complications, and incidence of malignancy in colonic polyps. It is too early to ascertain whether complete removal of a malignant adenomatous polyp by means of the colonoscopic cautery snare will prove to be a curative procedure. At the present time we advise that patients with malignant changes undergo laparotomy and segmental resection, particularly if the lesions are sessile. Longer follow-up in a large number of cases is needed to show whether localized carcinoma in pedunculated adenomatous polyps can be cured by colonoscopic polypectomy alone.

Colonoscopic polypectomy offers some very positive advantages over surgery. The average duration of the hospitalization was 36 hours, and the time lost from work 48 hours. The patient was able to resume regular activity within 72 hours. A normal diet is started on the first postpolypectomy day. The cost to the patient and/or insurance carrier is reduced by approximately 75 percent.

SUMMARY

We reviewed our experience with diagnostic and therapeutic colonoscopy, including colonscopic polypectomy. The procedure is a difficult technique for an individual to learn, even though he has had prior endoscopic experience with fiberoptic equipment. Therefore we advise that only those who have had some experience in fiberoptic gastrointestinal endoscopy perform this procedure, although some individuals are probably talented enough so that in the absence of any prior experience they will be able to learn the technique of colonoscopy after adequate exposure and teaching.

The technique for the most part is extremely safe and without major complications except in an extremely small percentage of cases. The diagnostic and therapeutic value of this procedure has been established.

REFERENCES

1. Berci G, Panish J, Morgenstern L: Diagnostic colonoscopy and polypectomy. Arch Surg 106: 818, 1973
2. Dean AC, Shearman DJ: Clinical evaluation of a new fiberoptic colonoscope. Lancet 1:550, 1970
3. Hedberg, Schrock, Sugarbarker: Cited from discussion of Wolff and Shinya's presentation. Ann Surg 178:377, 1973
4. Himtsuke S: Technique for insertion of colon fiberscope by means of intestinal guide string. Gastrointest Endosc (Tokyo) 12:209, 1970
5. Howard JE: Personal communication, 1973
6. Nagasaka T, Yamagata S, Miure S, et al: Description of fibercolonoscope VII. Gastroenterol Endosc (Tokyo) 12:218, 1970
7. Oshiba S, Watanabe A: Endoscopy of the colon. Gastroenterol Endosc (Tokyo) 7:400, 1965
8. Overholt BF: Technique of flexible fibersigmoidscopy. South Med J 63:787, 1970
9. Overholt BF: Clinical experience with the fibersigmoidoscope. Gastrointest Endosc 15:27, 1968
10. Panish J, Berci G: 100 consecutive polypectomies. West J Med In press
11. Panish J, Berci G: Colonoscopy and polypectomy. Surgery Annual 1973. New York, Appleton-Century-Crofts, 1973, pp 211–214
12. Panish J, Berci G: Suggestions for a better colonoscope. Gastrointest Endosc 19:38, 1972
13. Provenzale L, Revignas A: An original method for guided intubation of the colon. Gastrointest Endosc 16:11, 1969
14. Rosecrans DM: Report from San Diego. Gastrointest Endosc 20:36, 1973
15. Turell R: Diseases of Colon and Rectum, 2nd ed, Vol. 1. Philadelphia, Saunders, 1969, p 359
16. Wolff WI, Shinya H: A new approach to colonic polyps. Ann Surg 178:367, 1973
17. Wolff WI, Shinya H: Polypectomy via the fiberoptic colonoscope. N Engl J Med 288:329, 1973
18. Yamagata S, Oshiba S, Watanabe H: New fiberendoscope and its application to the colonic diseases. Proceedings of the 1st Congress of the International Society of Endoscopy, Tokyo, 1966, p 431

EDITORIAL COMMENT

Within a few years colonoscopy has established its clinical merit as an endoscopy method. It is more difficult to acquire the skill or perform it than, for example, an upper gastrointestinal examination. This then brings up the following questions.

How to Teach?

It would be advantageous if the candidate would have some experience in gastro-enterology or endoscopy (Gastroenterology Fellow), or have some familiarity with colon surgery (Fellow in Surgery). We should have some centers in the country with well defined programs that provide opportunities to gain experience in colonoscopy under the aegis of expert teachers. It is difficult to establish exactly the primary requirements because of the large individual variations between students; however, in my experience the procedure becomes interesting after the first 20 cases, and some experience and confidence has accumulated after 50 cases. This again, though, can vary from one individual to another.

We must be able to provide our colleagues—through a program in gastroenterology or colon surgery and a certain number of cases—with facts and figures on indications and contraindications, as well as a chance to gain experience in the performance of the method.

Postgraduate courses help to provide the elementary technical hints and other academic aspects of the procedure (e.g., pathology and sequelae), but they cannot substitute for practice. It is up to the various colleges, endoscopy societies, and medical schools to find a modus vivendi to include this important subject in the official teaching programs.

Complications

We call our method noninvasive, which is true. In cases of polypectomy the morbidity and mortality figures are significantly lower than those associated with surgical intervention (see table). There is a minimal but existing risk, however, which decreases with time and experience. Perforations in the overwhelming majority of cases were caused by manipulations and not by the polypectomy procedure itself.

Fluoroscopy should be available. The interior or lumen appearance and the length of scope introduced can be misleading. In many occasions it is advanced with ease, and the appearance and length would give the impression that we are in the descending colon. However the picture seen on the T.V. screen would indicate that we still are in a stretched redundant sigmoid loop. Large diverticula, misread as the lumen, produce a sudden resistance against further introduction. The elderly patient after pelvic

Group	Colonos-copies	Perfo-ration	Deaths	Morbidity (%)	Mortality (%)
Southern California Endoscopy Society, 1973[1]	3,850	7	1	0.25	0.26
Southern California Endoscopy Society, 1974[2]	4,246	13	2	0.35	0.05
American Society of Gastro-intestinal Endoscopy, 1974[3]	25,298	55	2	0.22	0.008
Chabanon[4]	11,288	27	10	0.24	0.09

1. Berci G, Panish JF, Shapiro M, et al: Complications of colonoscopy and polypectomy. Gastroenterology 67:584, 1974.
2. Survey of the Members of the Southern California Society Gastrointestinal Endoscopy Society, Colonoscopy Postgraduate Course, Los Angeles, January 1975.
3. Rogers G, et al: Analysis of the 1974 survey conducted by the American Society of Gastrointestinal Endoscopy. J Gastrointest Endosc 22:73, 1975
4. Chabanon R: Accidents of coloscopy. Acta Endoscopica 5:63, 1975.

surgery, for example, could be a problematic colonoscopy case; in such cases fluor-oscopy could be helpful in analyzing the situation, obviating the risk that would accompany further unnecessary or critical manipulations.

Facilities and Trained Personnel

The room where colonoscopy is performed should be adequately equipped, including apparatus to deal with emergencies (Chapter 10). In our experience of approximately 2,000 upper and lower gastrointestinal endoscopies, we have been confronted with three instances in which we required such equipment. One incident occurred toward the end of the procedure and one immediately after injection; the latter was a case of severe hypoxemia or respiratory depressive reaction, probably due to diazepam (Valium) effects. The immediate availability of resuscitation equipment and trained personnel was necessary for successful resuscitation in our premedication, respiratory, or cardiac complications. We employ one trained technician at the side of the operator, assisting or helping him, while the nurse continuously observes the patient, skin color, pulse, blood pressure, and electrocardiograph monitor. An inserted intravenous line is recommended. It is possible that our organizational framework for colonoscopy is perhaps overcautious, but we believe it is justified after noting our success in those cases in which we needed it and it was there.

Malignant Changes in Polyps

We can see and remove more polyps since colonoscopy has become available; therefore the incidence of finding unexpected malignancies is higher than it once was. Surgery is recommended for carcinomas with an invasive character. Pedunculated polyps are sometimes smaller than 1 cm in diameter, the stalk is free of malignant cells, and the carcinomatous changes in the head are confined to histologic boundaries. With these lesions the question arose concerning the method of treatment. The Southern California Gastrointestinal Endoscopy Society established a polyp registry among its members to collect a larger group of cases. The patients are categorized in two major groups: those who undergo surgery postpolypectomy and those treated by conservative measures. The last group is determined by the pathologist's description, the visual findings, and the patient's age and general condition.

We need five and perhaps ten years to define the proper treatment and to support our thesis of noninvasive treatment of certain types of well defined and localized carcinoma in pedunculated polyps.

Instrumentation

Instrumentation for colonoscopy is still in a developmental stage. The fact that new types of scopes (short, medium, or long; one channel, two channel, etc.) are constantly being marketed clearly indicates that we have not defined our requirements. The constantly rising cost of these expensive items and the significant number of repairs with its "side effects" ("off time" of equipment and expenses) are problems that must be dealt with.

THE EDITOR

22

Duodenoscopy: Endoscopic Retrograde Cannulation of the Papilla of Vater

László Sáfrány

The first phase of the history of duodenoscopy is identical with the history of fibergastroscopy, differing from it only during the late 1960s. McCune et al.[10] in 1968 were the first to cannulate the papilla of Vater by means of endoscopic visualization. Prior to this in 1965 Rabinov and Simon[14] introduced a catheter into the papilla under a fluoroscopic screen and performed cholangiopancreatography. Based on these early attempts Japanese investigators[5,6,11,12] elaborated a practicable diagnostic method, which soon became popular in Europe and the United States.

Endoscopic examination of the duodenum is practiced in two ways. The first method is visualization of the first portion of the duodenum, chiefly the duodenal bulb; this is usually performed in association with study of the esophagus and stomach, i.e., *esophagogastrobulboscopy.* The device used for this purpose is equipped with prograde optics, and the chief aim of the investigation is detection of the source of upper gastrointestinal bleeding.

The other method, often referred to as *deep duodenoscopy,* is undertaken with a fiberscope provided with side-view optics, allowing easy visualization of the entire duodenum. Duodenal diseases like duodenitis, ulcers (Fig. 1, Plate A),* diverticula (Fig. 2, Plate A), polyps, and benign neoplasms, as well as malignant

All color plates appear at the front of the book.

tumors (Fig. 3, Plate A) can be readily recognized. However, the study is undertaken most frequently to cannulate the papilla of Vater thereby allowing radiologic visualization of the biliary system and the pancreatic ducts by retrograde filling with contrast medium (endoscopic retrograde cholangiopancreatography: ERCP).

INDICATIONS AND CONTRAINDICATIONS OF DUODENOSCOPY AND ERCP

Duodenoscopy is usually aimed at clarification of duodenal diseases by means of endoscopy and biopsy. *Retrograde cholangiography* is indicated whenever conventional techniques, primarily excretion cholangiocholecystography, fail to clarify the origin of complaints and symptoms related to the biliary system.[17] This is the case in disorders of bile excretion due to primary liver disease or secondary to longstanding biliary obstruction.

Retrograde pancreatography is undertaken if some pancreatic disorder is suspected clinically or to define accurately the nature of an already known pancreatic disease.[4] Detection of morphologic abnormalities of the pancreatic duct belongs to up-to-date clinical investigation of the pancreas. This is amply demonstrated by the fact that radiologic detection of ductular changes (e.g., stenotized segments in chronic

305

pancreatitis) provides the basis for a rational surgical approach (demonstrated in Figure 33, below).

The examination is *contraindicated* in all kinds of infectious diseases owing to the danger of contamination with an instrument that cannot be sterilized, in patients with poor general health, and if therapy is not available regardless of the diagnostic information obtained. Drug idiosyncrasy, either to the compounds used for premedication or to the radiologic contrast medium, constitutes a relative contraindication of ERCP. ERCP must not be performed in acute pancreatitis.

DEVICES

ERCP studies were started with the Machida FDS-LB and the Olympus JF-B duodenoscopes. At present the Olympus JF-B II is the most widely used instrument. ACMI recently constructed a similar endoscope, but experiences with this device are lacking and some technical refinement seems necessary.

The Olympus JF-B duodenoscope (Fig. 4) is a highly flexible device with a diameter of 1 cm. The end portion is movable in four directions. In the axis there is a tunnel for the introduction of biopsy forceps or cannula. The cannula can be directed under vision. Automatic air insufflation, water flushing, and suction of secreta are additional facilities.

TECHNIQUE OF ERCP

Premedication

The patient fasts overnight and receives 0.5 mg atropine and 100 mg pethidine (Demerol) intravenously. Some authors prefer the use of diazepam (Valium). Glucagon has been used recently for duodenal paralysis with excellent effect. The pharynx is anesthetized with a lidocaine (Xylocaine) spray.

Endoscopy

The duodenoscope is introduced as far as the pylorus in the same way as the gastroscope. Passing the pylorus is usually easy, requiring very little practice. The picture of the *pylorus* is adjusted into the center of the visual field, and the tip of the duodenoscope is then angulated upward while the device is pushed forward into the duodenal bulb. Usually the optic touches the wall of the bulb and the picture disappears. The device is then rotated *clockwise,* air is insufflated, and the duodenoscope is passed into the first portion of the duodenum. After having reached the upper duodenal angle, the second portion of the duodenum can be visualized, often in its entire length (Fig. 5, Plate A). The papilla of Vater can be found on the medial wall, at the proximal end of a longitudinal fold running perpendicularly to the cir-

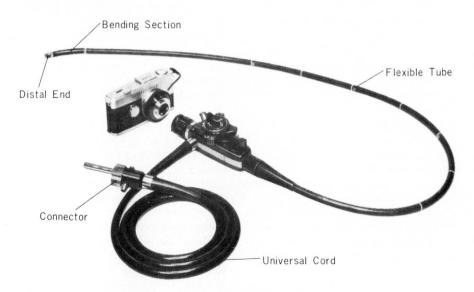

Bending Section

Flexible Tube

Distal End

Connector

Universal Cord

FIG. 4.   Olympus JF-B fiberduodenoscope.

cular folds of the duodenal mucosa (Fig. 6, Plate A). Due to the special importance of the papilla of Vater in ERCP, its morphology is discussed in detail.

The most important part of the examination comes now. The duodenoscope is manipulated so that the papilla, which is usually seen side-faced, lies opposite the optic since the cannula can be introduced into the orifice only in this position. Cannulation is sometimes a simple procedure, but it can be also a highly difficult task, the rules of which cannot be defined exactly. The rate of success of cannulation increases with the practice and skill of the examiner, the success rate being over 90 percent in the hands of experts. Similarly, the duration of the procedure can be reduced to 10 minutes.

The cannula previously filled with *contrast medium* rather frequently slips into the pancreatic duct. In cases where visualization of the pancreatic duct seems necessary, pancreatography is made with 2 to 6 ml of the medium; if unnecessary the cannula is withdrawn from the papilla, then reinserted and passed in another direction to fill the biliary ducts. In 42 percent of cases both the pancreatic and biliary ducts are filled simultaneously through the common channel, usually when the cannula is introduced shortly into the ampulla of Vater several millimeters from the orifice. The bile ducts are visualized with 10 to 50 ml of radiopaque medium. Various water-soluble contrast media have been tested with equally satisfactory results.

Roentgenologic Examination

Valuable information can be obtained even during injection of the contrast medium, since the pancreatic and biliary ducts are satisfactorily visualized on the television screen. Nevertheless, diagnosis must be invariably based on the analysis of serial roentgenograms taken during the procedure. In some cases detailed study of several roentgenograms is necessary for the exact diagnosis. For instance too-dense opacification may mask even huge gallstones (Fig. 7).

In certain patients ERCP may require *special techniques*. It may be difficult to find the papilla of Vater in patients previously subjected to surgery of the stomach, particularly after Billroth II operation. Cholangiodigestive anastomoses require cannulation of the bile ducts via the stoma as suggested by Classen et al.,[3] which again may be found with difficulty. In such cases administration of 25 mg indocyanine green (Cardiogreen) 1 hour prior to the study may be helpful in searching the stoma.[15] Since this dye is excreted by the liver, appearance of the intensely green-stained bile guides the examiner to the stoma. This method is helpful in searching the orifice of the bile duct in cases where the anatomy of the papilla of Vater is atypical, e.g., in cases of double orifice.

ENDOSCOPIC MORPHOLOGY OF THE PAPILLA OF VATER

The papilla of Vater is the most prominent part of the second portion of the duodenum and is usually the ultimate goal in duodenoscopy. Therefore its morphology and endoscopic appearance seem to deserve special attention.

The fold proximal to the papilla and which frequently covers it is called the covering fold (Fig. 8, Plate A); sometimes it is referred to as preputium. On the medial duodenal wall a longitudinal fold runs perpendicularly to the circular folds (Fig. 8). It is very helpful in finding the papilla; if it is short, it may be called frenulum. The papilla is usually protruding into the lumen of the duodenum. Kozu et al.[6] distinguished three types according to the shape: papillar, hemispherical, and flat. In our view this classification is not warranted since the shape of the papilla depends largely on the angle and direction of viewing; furthermore, owing to alterations in the tone of the rich and intricate musculature of the papilla, it may change its appearance even during the investigation.

The orifice usually can be detected on the tip of the papilla, and it is frequently surrounded by a crown of white fimbria. It usually looks like a reddish erosion but is sometimes pale compared to the adjacent mucosa. The two duct systems normally unite and form a common channel with a single orifice; however, separate orifices are sometimes seen, or only the pancreatic duct opens on the papilla and the bile duct has a separate orifice nearby. Accessory papilla is seen in about 40 percent of cases. It contains the orifice of the duct of Santorini, the cannulation of which is difficult and has no practical value.

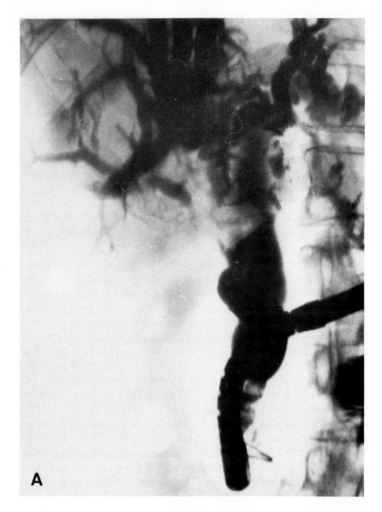

FIG. 7. A. Huge stones in the extremely enlarged bile ducts. (Continued on facing page.)

TABLE 1. Results of 366 Endoscopic Retrograde Cholangiographies

Diagnosis	No. of Cases
Normal bile duct system	48
Intrahepatic cholestasis	13
Primary biliary cirrhosis	22
Papillary stenosis	22
Benign stricture of the bile ducts	27
External compression of the bile ducts	4
Primary sclerosing cholangitis	2
Caroli's syndrome	1
Gallbladder stone	8
Bile duct stone	108
Carcinoma of the papilla of Vater	10
Carcinoma of the bile ducts	18
Carcinoma of the head of the pancreas	24
Pancreatic fibrosis	9
Normal cholangiodigestive anastomosis	23
Narrowed or excessive cholangiodigestive anastomosis	9
Alterations due to juxtapapillary diverticulum	18
Total	366

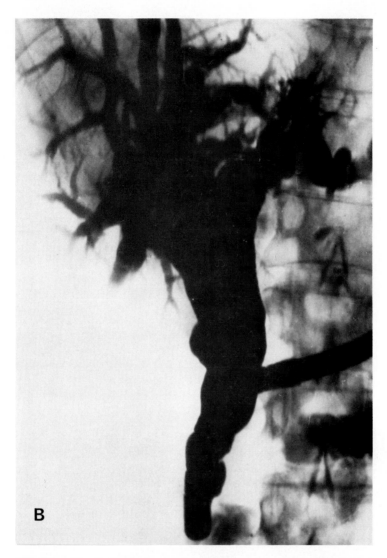

FIG. 7 (cont.). **B.** Stones become masked after too-dense opacification.

ENDOSCOPIC RETROGRADE CHOLANGIOGRAPHY (ERC)

The importance of ERC in the diagnosis of biliary diseases is demonstrated by our experience with 366 examinations performed within a period of 3 years (Table 1). If several abnormalities were found in the same patient, the one that was most significant was considered.

The *normal biliary tree* is characterized by homogenous filling of the extrahepatic bile ducts, gallbladder, and intrahepatic arborization. The contours are regular and sharp (Fig. 9). In *cholecystectomized* patients the bile ducts are frequently enlarged, but a diameter of the

common bile duct over 1 cm is not considered pathologic (Fig. 10).

Intrahepatic cholestasis is established if extrahepatic obstruction is excluded on the basis of a normal biliary system in patients with cholestatic jaundice (Fig. 11). Similarly the diagnosis of *primary biliary cirrhosis* is based on the exclusion of mechanical obstruction in the biliary tree. Narrowing, irregular distribution, disruptions of the intrahepatic ducts, and caliber variations of the common bile duct could be revealed (Fig. 12), although in several patients no abnormality was detected at all.

Papillary stenosis is characterized by homogeneous filling of the entire enlarged biliary

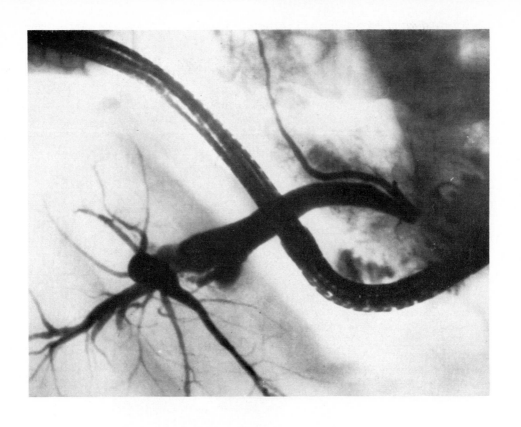

FIG. 10. Enlarged but normal bile ducts in a cholecystectomized patient.

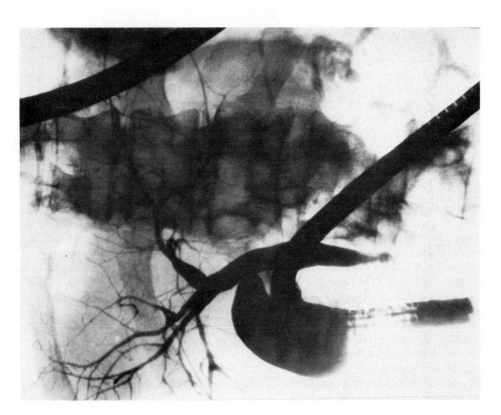

FIG. 9. Normal cholangiogram.

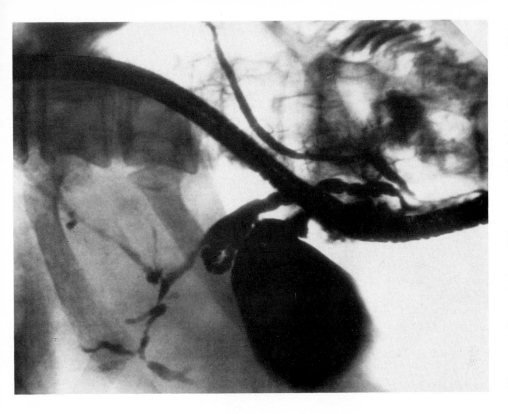

FIG. 12. Caliber variations of the common bile duct and irregular distribution and disruptions of the intrahepatic ducts in primary biliary cirrhosis.

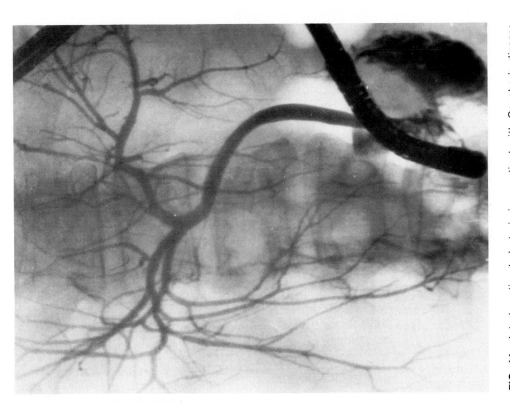

FIG. 11. Intrahepatic cholestasis in a patient with Gaucher's disease. There is no mechanical obstruction in the bile ducts. The liver is extremely enlarged.

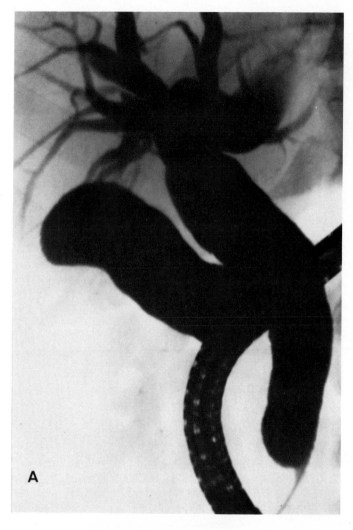

FIG. 13. Papillary stenosis. **A.** Homogenous filling of the whole dilated biliary system. (Continued on facing page.)

A

system (Fig. 13A). The pathognomonic findings are retention and the remarkably slow flow of the contrast medium through the narrowed ampullary segment into the duodenum (Fig. 13B).

Benign stricture of the common bile duct is detected in patients with previous abdominal (mostly biliary) surgery, presumably resulting from surgical injury to the bile duct. The typical finding is a short cicatricial narrowing and prestenotic dilatation at the level of the cystic junction in a patient with previous cholecystectomy (Fig. 14). If obstruction is complete, the radiograms do not significantly differ from those obtained in tumorous obstruction.

External compression of the bile ducts is caused predominantly by lymph nodes, retroperitoneal tumor, or pancreatic cysts. The extremely rare *primary sclerosing cholangitis* and

Caroli's syndrome are characterized by grossly narrowed bile duct and primary cystic dilatation of the intrahepatic bile ducts, respectively.

The astonishingly low number of patients with *stones* exclusively in the *gallbladder* indicates that the stones are readily demonstrable by orthodox cholecystography and usually do not require retrograde filling of the biliary system (Fig. 15).

Common bile duct stone is the most frequent finding, and 86 of our 108 patients had been previously subjected to cholecystectomy or even repeated biliary surgery. Stones of excessive variability of size and localization caused a variety of clinical signs and symptoms (Figs. 16 through 18). Recognition of stones underlying a complete or incomplete biliary obstruction is of prime importance from the viewpoint of effective treatment.

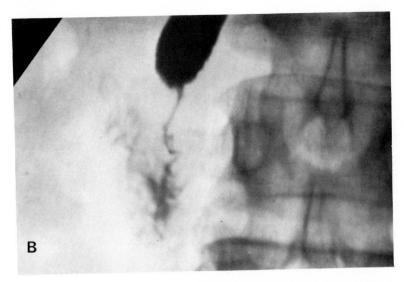

FIG. 13 (cont.).   **B.** Slow outflow through the narrowed ampullary segment into the duodenum.

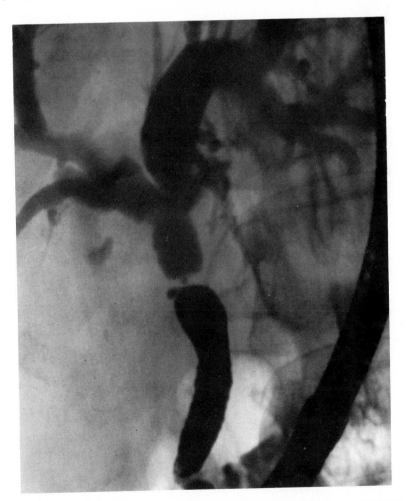

FIG. 14.   Gross narrowing at the level of cystic junction after cholecystectomy.

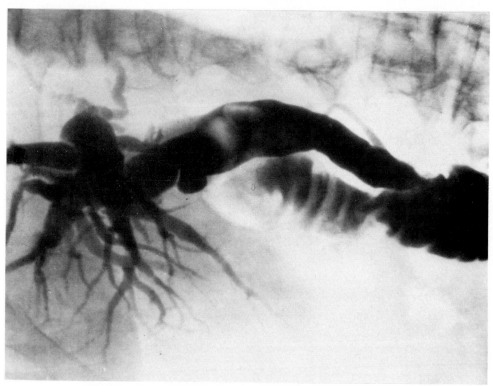

FIG. 16. Two bile stones in the dilated common bile duct.

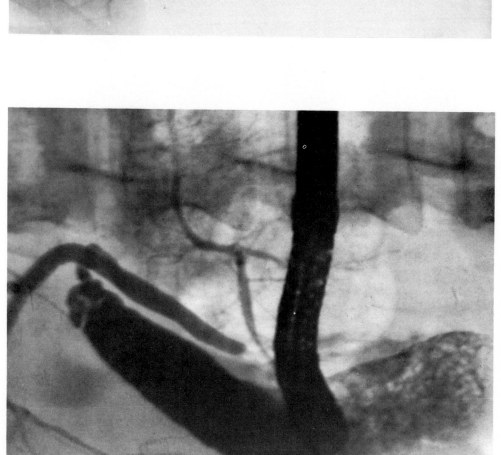

FIG. 15. Gallbladder stones.

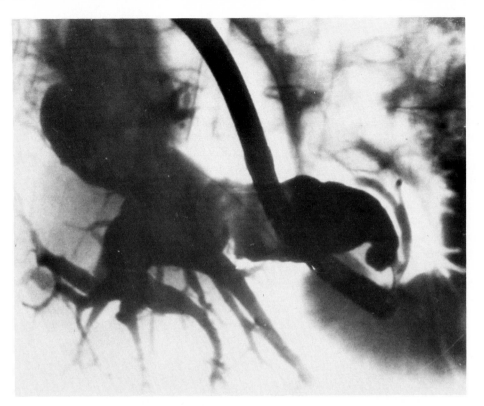

FIG. 18. A solitary stone is built around an unabsorbed suture causing extreme dilatation.

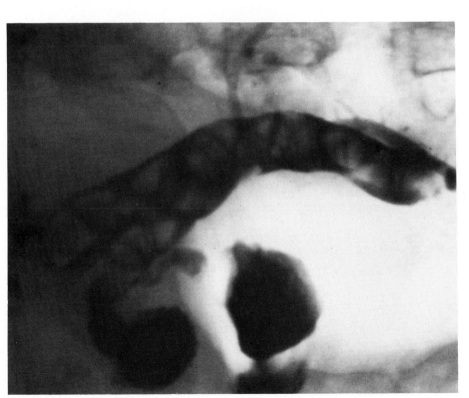

FIG. 17. Almost the entire biliary system is filled by a cast of stones.

According to Oi et al.[12-13] diagnosis of *cancer of the papilla of Vater* is based on endoscopic and biopsy findings. However, the orifice of the duct systems can be easily recognized even on the tumorous papilla, and the bile duct can be easily cannulated. Retrograde filling may be helpful in establishing the extension of the tumor (Fig. 19).

In *primary carcinoma of the bile duct* the abnormalities of the radiogram can be summarized as follows: (1) In a case of partial obstruction the involved segment of the bile duct is narrowed, with an irregular, rat-gnawed margin (Figs. 20 and 21). Below the narrowing the duct has a normal appearance, while there is marked dilatation of the ducts, including the intrahepatic branches, proximal to the tumor (Fig. 22). In the case of complete biliary ob-

struction the narrowing has an irregular contour; the pitch of the narrowing usually has an eccentric position and occasionally may have a long "moustache" (Fig. 23).

Cancer of the head of the pancreas can be diagnosed both by cholangiography and pancreatography. The most characteristic finding on the cholangiogram is the irregularly shaped narrowing of the common bile duct along its intrapancreatic segment (Fig. 24).

In the case of *pancreatic fibrosis* the mechanism of obstruction is similar to that observed in patients with cancer of the head of the pancreas, differentiation between the two relying on the simultaneous pancreatographic study or the presence of calcified areas, typical for fibrosis (Fig. 25).

Abnormalities of cholangiodigestive anasto-

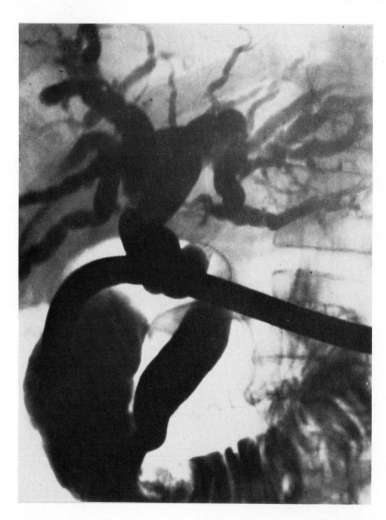

FIG. 19. Enlarged biliary system above the tumorous papilla of Vater.

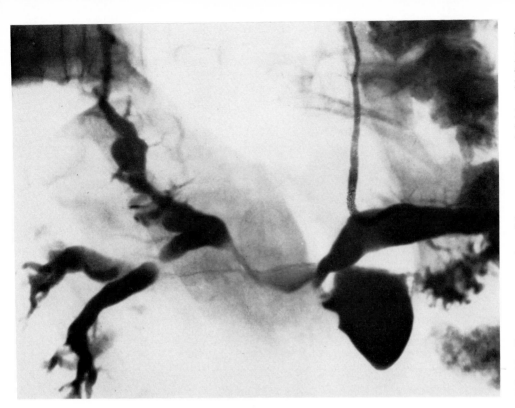

FIG. 21. Tumorous narrowing of the common and right and left hepatic ducts.

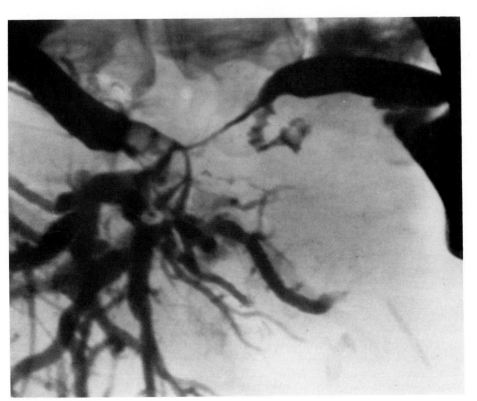

FIG. 20. Carcinoma of the bile duct causing partial obstruction at the level of the common hepatic duct, resulting in dilatation of the intrahepatic branches. Two small stones are in the left intrahepatic duct.

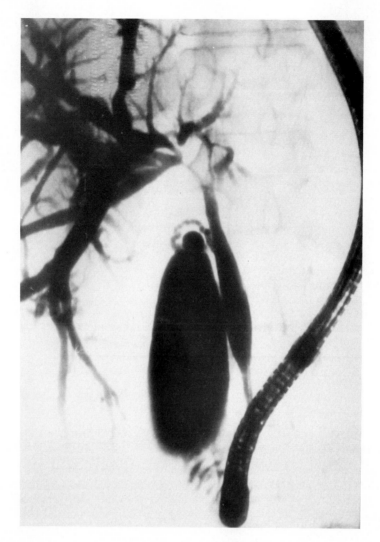

FIG. 22. Primary cancer of the bile duct at the hepatic porta obstructing the left hepatic branch completely, with an absence of filling in the left lobe. The right hepatic duct is narrowed, while ducts in the right lobe are dilated.

mosis (e.g., cicatricial narrowing or obstruction caused by local tumor recidivism, or ampulla-like dilatation filled with food remnants) can be detected first by endoscopy. Nevertheless retrograde filling of the bile ducts through the stoma may provide additional information in assessing abnormalities in this region. Stones can thus be detected both distal and proximal to the stoma (Fig. 26).

Juxtapapillary diverticulum is a frequent cause of recurring biliary disease. Cannulating the papilla of Vater located in or at the edge of a juxtapapillary diverticulum (Fig. 2, Plate A) often reveals dislocated, enlarged bile ducts,

and not infrequently stones as well (Figs. 27 and 28). It is important to establish an accurate diagnosis prior to surgery, since the method of choice in such cases is removal of the diverticulum together with papilloplasty; otherwise the recurrence of jaundice is highly probable.

Several disorders of the biliary system occasionally are demonstrated in the same patient. Thus gallstones are frequently found both over and below cicatricial or even neoplastic narrowings (Fig. 20). If concrements are present in the bile ducts they are often accompanied by secondary papillary stenosis. Three causes of

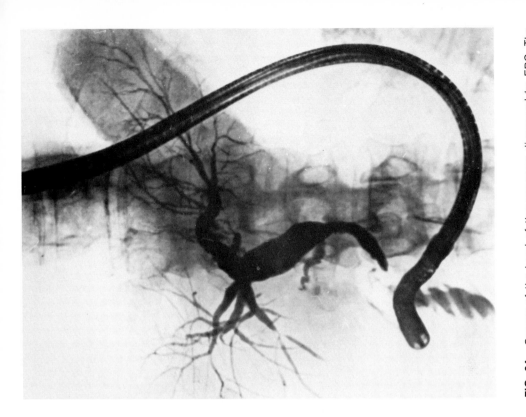

FIG. 24. Cancer of the head of the pancreas diagnosed by ERC. The common bile duct is irregularly narrowed along its intrahepatic segment.

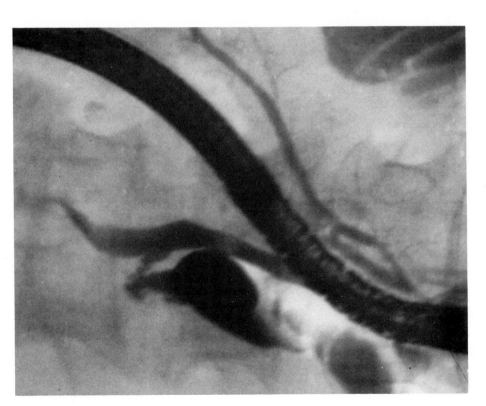

FIG. 23. Fusiform narrowing of the common hepatic duct due to bile duct cancer, maintaining complete obstruction.

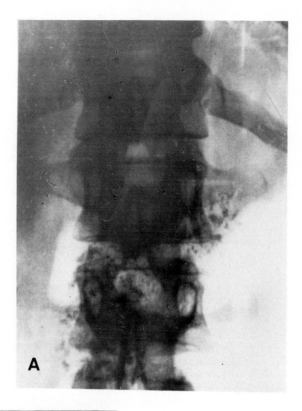

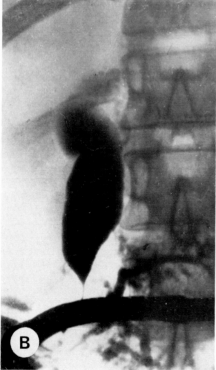

FIG. 25. Pancreatic fibrosis. **A.** Calcified areas in the pancreatic region. **B.** Clear-cut gross narrowing of the pancreatic segment of the common bile duct.

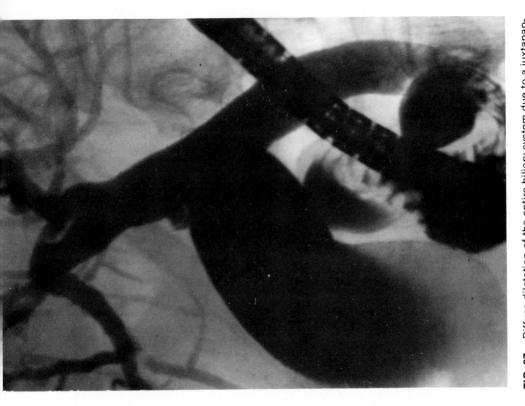

FIG. 27. Diffuse dilatation of the entire biliary system due to a juxtapapillary diverticulum. The displaced and compressed distal end of the bile duct contains several small bile concrements.

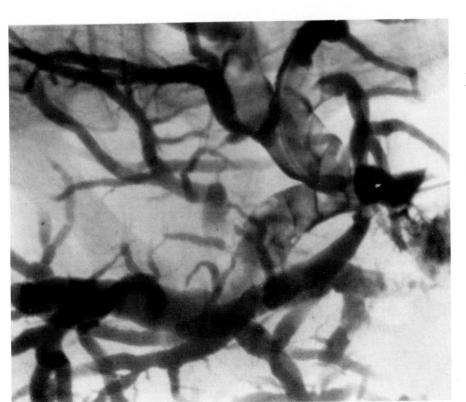

FIG. 26. Several intrahepetic stones above a narrowed stoma.

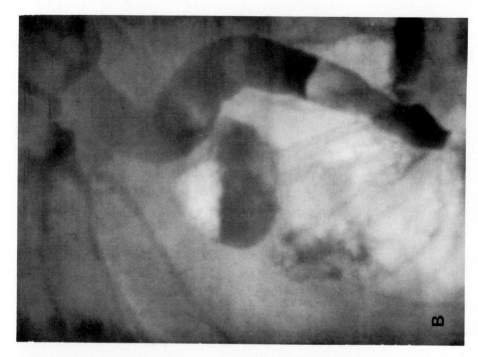

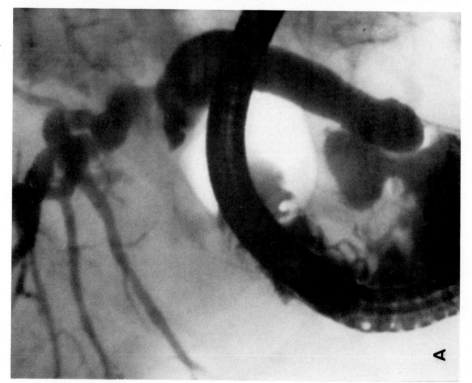

FIG. 28. A. Juxtapapillary diverticulum underlies recurrence of biliary stones. B. After dilution of contrast medium stones become visible.

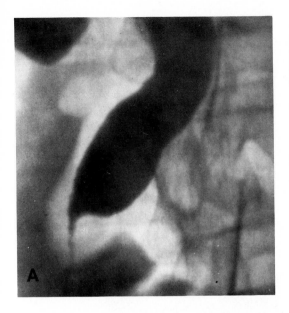

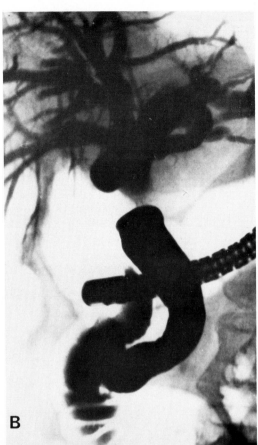

FIG. 29. Three causes of jaundice in one patient. **A.** Papillary hypertrophy and stenosis. **B.** Stricture of the common bile duct. Three causes of jaundice in one patient. **C.** A stone above the stricture in the common hepatic duct.

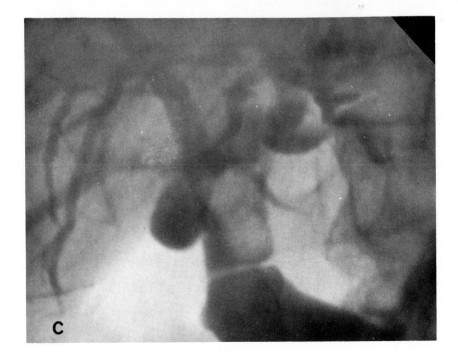

recurrent jaundice were found in one of our patients: papillary stenosis, stenosis of the common bile duct, and a stone in the common hepatic duct above the stricture (Fig. 29).

ENDOSCOPIC RETROGRADE PANCREATOGRAPHY (ERP)

Depending on the amount of the injected contrast medium, the main pancreatic duct is depicted (2 to 6 ml, Fig. 30), or the main duct plus its side branches (4 to 9 ml, Fig. 31), and even the acini and parenchyma as well (8 to 18 ml, Fig. 32). Table 2 summarizes the diagnoses established on the basis of our 506 pancreatographic studies.

The *normal pancreatogram* shows considerable individual variations; therefore it is difficult to establish criteria of the normal pancreatic duct system. Kasugai et al.[5,6] distinguished ascending (Fig. 30), horizontal, sigmoid (Fig. 31), and descending variants. In our view such a classification is unnecessary for there are numerous intermediate patterns; furthermore the pancreas, particularly the tail, may undergo substantial changes both in shape and position in the same patient during the course of investigation.

Chronic pancreatitis is perhaps the most

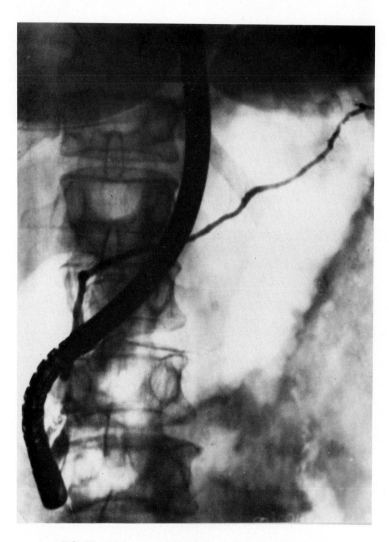

FIG. 30. Main pancreatic duct of the ascending type.

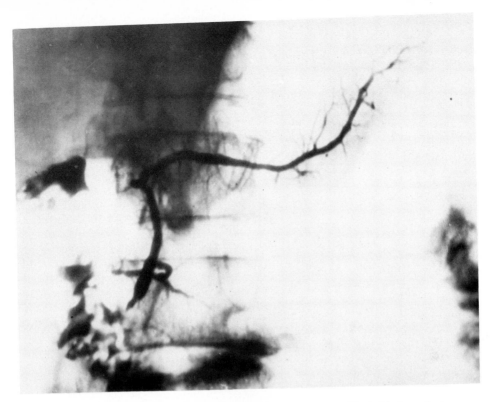

FIG. 31. Normal pancreatogram of the sigmoid type with filled side branches.

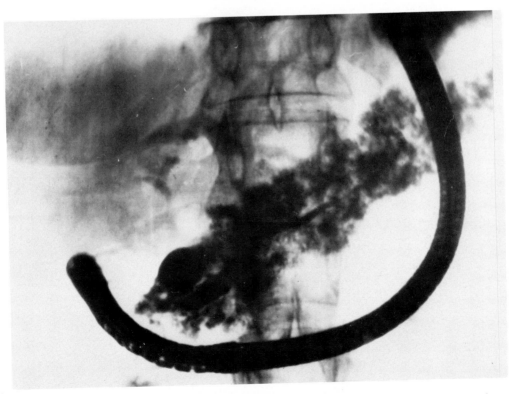

FIG. 32. Parenchymal filling in a patient with chronic pancreatitis. Cyst formation in the head.

TABLE 2. Results of 506 Endoscopic Retrograde Pancreatographies

Diagnosis	No. of Cases
Normal pancreatogram	324
Chronic pancreatitis	114
Pancreatic cyst and pseudocyst	21
Pancreatic abscess	3
Peripancreatic tumor	2
Pancreatic tumor	32
Carcinoma of the papilla of Vater	10
Total	506

difficult to diagnose by means of retrograde pancreatography. This is due to the scarcity and vagueness of clinical criteria of the disease. Anacker et al.[1] suggested that dilatation and stenosis of the main and smaller pancreatic ducts (i.e., changes in the caliber of the ducts; Fig. 33), the presence of clubby side branches, and further premature filling of the parenchyma (Fig. 32) with the contrast medium are the most characteristic abnor-

malities of the pancreatogram in chronic pancreatitis. Kasugai et al.[5,6] believe that the tortuous appearance of the main pancreatic duct, irregular branching, and cystic dilatation of the secondary ducts (Fig. 33) are important radiologic findings as well. In our own material variation of the caliber of the main pancreatic duct was the most frequently encountered sign, and in several cases single or multiple stenoses were found as well (Fig. 33). The latter sign is interpreted mostly as a sign of pancreatic cancer. The difficulties in differentiation are discussed later.

Pancreatic pseudocyst may cause abruption or tapering of the main pancreatic duct (Fig. 34), but can be diagnosed unequivocally if the cavity communicates with the duct system, i.e., when it is filled with the contrast medium (Fig. 35). Purulent infection is possible in cases where the cyst is filled directly; therefore in such cases surgery must be performed.[18] When a good outflow of dye from the cyst is visible, urgent operation is not necessary.

Pancreatic abscess does not differ radiomor-

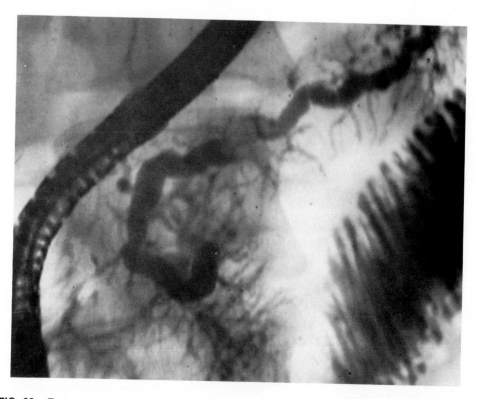

FIG. 33. Tortuous main pancreatic duct with caliber variations, irregular distribution of side branches, and a solitary area of stenosis in the head region. The pain disappeared after surgery (Wirsungoplasty).

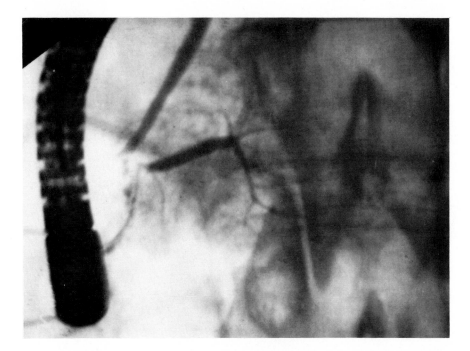

FIG. 34. Abrupt amputation of the main pancreatic duct in the head region. Instead of a suspected type 3 tumor, the surgery revealed a pancreatic pseudocyst.

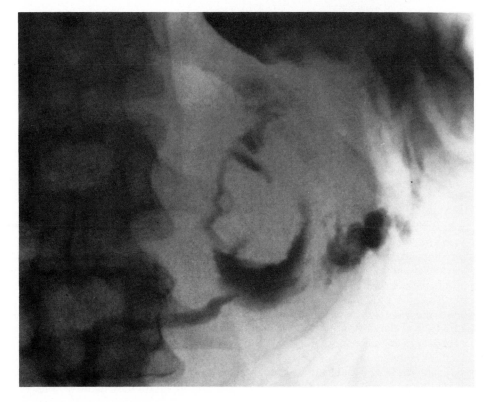

FIG. 35. Pseudocyst is filled at the tail of pancreas, dislocating the lesser curvature of the stomach.

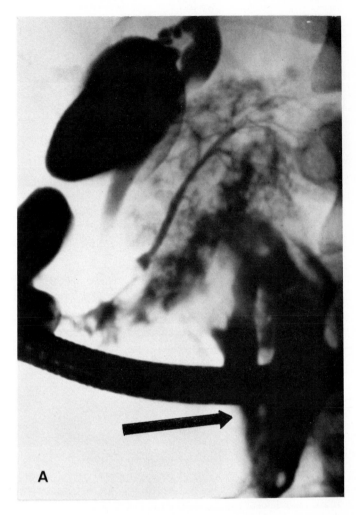

FIG. 36. **A.** Pancreatic abscess (arrow) is filled below the atrophic pancreas. (Continued on facing page.)

A

phologically from the cyst. Figure 36A shows an abscess filled at ERCP, which was diagnosed by the duodenoscope introduced through a cystogastrostomy opening, allowing a biopsy to be taken from the wall of the abscess (Fig. 36B).

Peripancreatic tumor may be revealed by dislocation of the pancreas, as shown in Figure 37, where a calcified carcinoma metastasis of unknown origin replaces the tail of the pancreas downward. Recognition of *pancreatic tumors* is perhaps the most important achievement of ERP. Large tumors may dislocate the stomach and the duodenum to such an extent that intubation of the duodenum is impossible. The tumor may penetrate the duodenum and be recognized both by endoscopy and biopsy.

Ogoshi and Hara[11] classified the characteristic pancreatographic abnormalities of pancreatic neoplasm in three fundamental types. Type 1 is recognized by the narrowing of the main pancreatic duct with prestenotic dilatation and is termed the stenosing type (Fig. 38). The rare tapering type, type 2, is characterized by the rigidity and gradual tapering of the main pancreatic duct, showing an irregular margin. The narrowing is relatively diffuse, and branches are lacking in such portions. It has been suggested that acinary adenocarcinoma arising from the parenchyma usually presents with this type of pancreatogram. The third obstructed type is recognized on the basis of abrupt amputation of the pancreatic duct (Fig. 39). We suggest the distinction of a fourth, "cavernous" type, where a tumorous prestenotic cavity may be filled (Fig. 40).

In patients with *cancer of the papilla of Vater* the pancreatograms show excessive dilatation

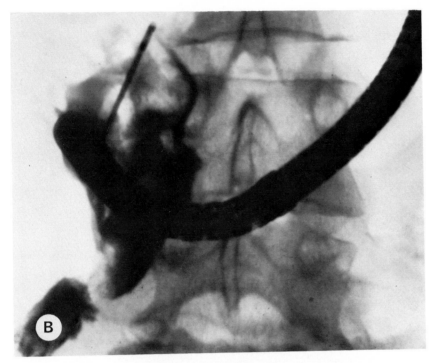

FIG. 36. (cont.).   **B.** Biopsy from the abscess wall with the scope introduced through a pre-formed cystogastrostomy opening.

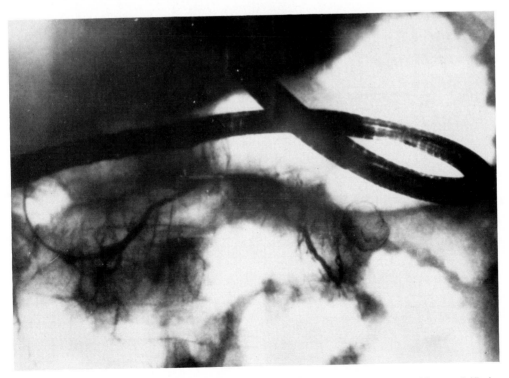

FIG. 37.   Peripancreatic tumor. The tail of the pancreas is dislodged downward by a calcified mass.

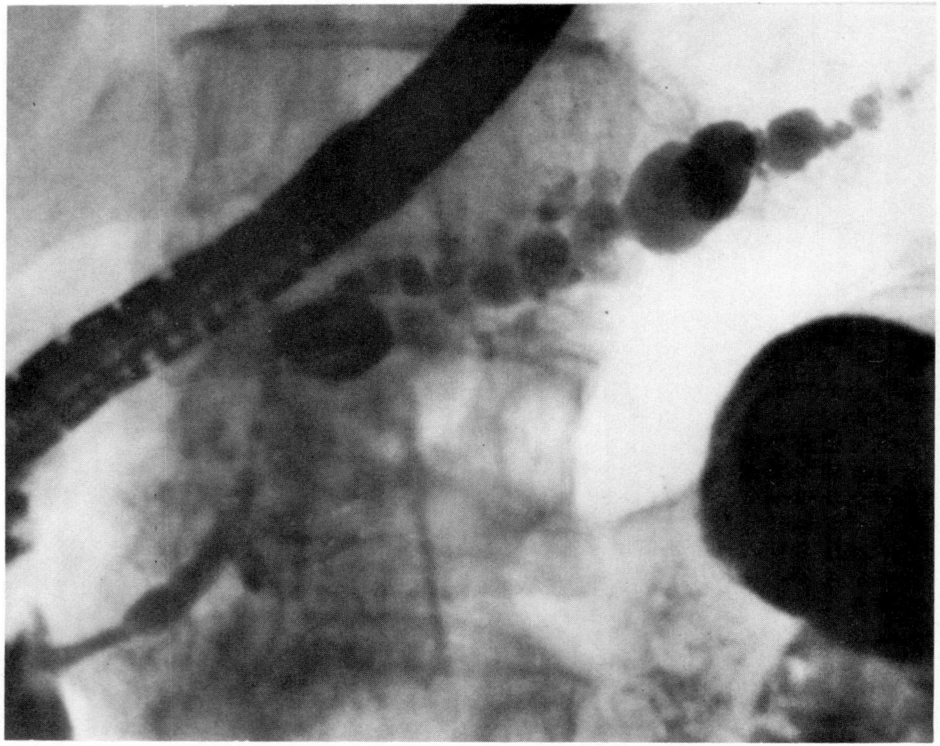

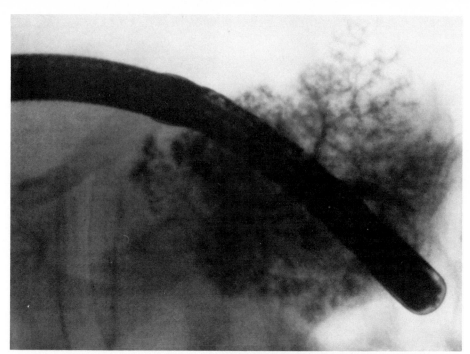

FIG. 38. Pancreatic tumor of stenosing type (type 1) with marked prestenotic dilatation.

FIG. 39. Pancreatic obstructed-type (type 3) tumor. There is no filling in the body and tail. Remarkable parenchymal filling of the head indicates an organic cause of the filling defect.

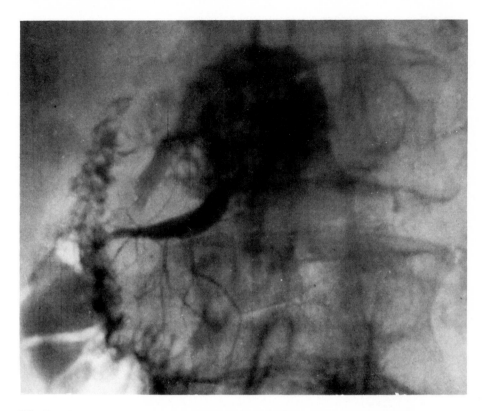

FIG. 40. Pancreatic cavernous-type (type 4) tumor. A tumorous prestenotic cavity is filled.

of the entire pancreatic duct (Fig. 41A). The examination is helpful in determining the extension of the tumor (Fig. 41B).

DIFFICULTIES IN INTERPRETATION OF PANCREATOGRAMS

It should be emphasized that *all* the signs of tumor (e.g., stenosis, tapering, obstruction, and cavity formation) may be present, although this occurs infrequently; in patients with chronic pancreatitis or pancreatic neoplasms, however, subsequent surgery and histologic studies often fail to confirm the endoscopic finding. Evaluation of the changes found on a pancreatogram is one of the most difficult tasks in endoscopic radiologic diagnosis. Cooperation between groups of workers internationally seems a desirable way to improve the diagnostic success rate, mainly by examining a large number of pancreatographic findings in different centers and comparing them to each other as well as with surgical and autopsy data (Fig. 42).

HAZARDS OF DUODENOSCOPY AND ERCP

The complications of duodenoscopy and ERCP are in part the same caused by other fiberendoscopic procedures; from a practical point of view, however, these hazards are not significant. Other adverse sequelae are due to the filling of ducts under fluoroscopic screen. Thus unsatisfactory sterilization of the catheter (i.e., conditions of cannulation may cause hepatitis) and the x-ray load received by the patient may be significant.

The most important hazard of ERC is cholangitis, usually caused by gram-negative organisms and leading to septicemia. Several fatalities have been reported. It appears that the patient with mechanical obstruction is at the highest risk. The use of broad-spectrum antimicrobial agents has been advocated as a preventive measure, but there is no completely safe treatment.

The main hazard of ERP is the transient pain reminiscent of acute pancreatitis, as well as some laboratory findings pointing to pan-

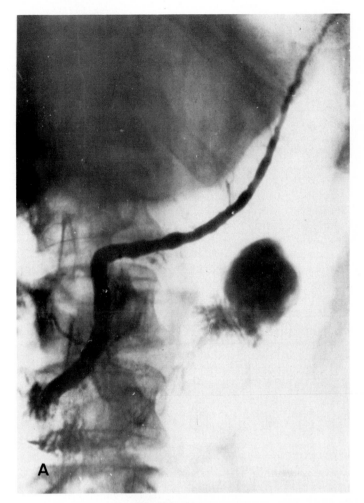

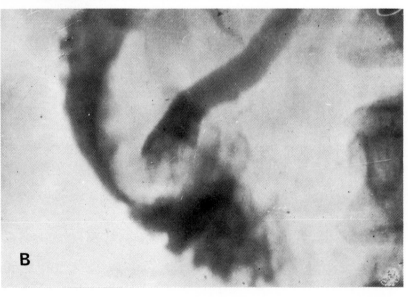

FIG. 41. **A.** Excessive dilatation of the entire pancreatic duct above the tumor of the papilla of Vater. **B.** The cancer protrudes into the duodenal lumen.

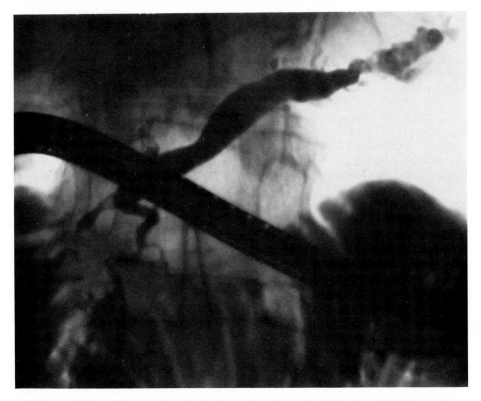

FIG. 42. Features of the stenosing type tumor are mimicked by a surgically confirmed abscess.

creatic involvement.[4–6·19] The symptoms and signs soon disappear, however, and pancreatic lesions of longer duration have not yet been observed in our series. Tamás and Sáfrány[19] believe that elevation of serum amylase levels seems to be the most constant finding, occurring in 76 percent of their patients. The rise is a function of the amount of injected contrast medium and the pressure under which the substance was injected, but is independent of the quality and concentration of the employed medium. Prior administration of trypsin inhibitors (Trasylol) failed to prevent the rise in amylase activity in our cases.

Considering the diagnostic value of ERCP, the hazards noted above are rare and mild enough to be outbalanced by the quality and quantity of the information obtained.

SUMMARY

Duodenoscopy is a suitable method to establish diagnoses of diseases of the duodenum. *Endoscopic retrograde cholangiography* is a highly effective method for visualization of the bile duct system and exploration of even the most complicated causes of jaundice. In the majority of cases *endoscopic retrograde pancreatography* proved to be of great diagnostic importance as well, although correct interpretation of the pancreatograms at times can be difficult.

EPILOGUE:
ENDOSCOPIC PAPILLOTOMY
AND REMOVAL OF GALLSTONES
BY NONINVASIVE TECHNIQUE

Complete or partial biliary obstruction due to papillary stenosis or stones in the common bile duct represent an indication for surgery. The aim is to establish normal drainage of the bile ducts. The endoscopic visualization with cannulation of the ampulla of Vater of the common bile duct, as well as the development of a suitable papillotome, made endoscopic papillotomy possible.[2·7·8·16]

Patients, Instruments, and Methods

Endoscopic papillotomy was attempted in 71 patients and completed in 60; of these, 15 were male and 45 female. Their ages varied from 28 to 86 years (average 64). The indications were organic papillary stenosis and common duct stones (for criteria and description see earlier material in this chapter).

Endoscope: The Olympus JF-B2 duodenoscope was used, as in ERCP.

Papillotome: A high-frequency diathermy catheter developed by Demling and Classen[2] was used. It consists of a wire fixed at the tip of a plastic catheter which can be passed through the instrument channel of the duodenoscope and acts as a cutting knife. The catheter is bent by pulling the wire, making it taut.

Energy source: The Olympus PSD diathermy unit was used.

Stone extractor: A Dormia catheter consisting of a wire basket was inserted into the bile duct in a closed position. During slow withdrawal it opens to collect and extract stones.

Papillotomy Technique

The anatomy of the pancreatic and common bile ducts is demonstrated during ERCP by radiography *(vide supra)*. When the papillotome is introduced into the common bile duct its position is confirmed by fluoroscopy and radiography. The wire is pulled taut, and current is applied intermittently under continuous visual (radiologic) control (step 2–3 of cutting current of PSD unit). We cut the roof of the papilla and the major duodenal fold covering the papilla. After the incision (15 to 25 mm long) is made the yellow mucosa of the bile duct can be observed through the enlarged opening.

As a rule there is little or no bleeding. Gallstones can be extracted by using the Dormia basket. For this purpose the Dormia catheter is inserted above the stone. After pushing the wire through the catheter the basket opens and an attempt is made to catch and remove the stone under fluoroscopic control. At the beginning we favored stone removal immediately after papillotomy. We later found that after a papillotomy of adequate size the calculi pass spontaneously. Lately we attempt mechanical stone extraction only if a residual stone is still present at the follow-up examination at 1 week.

Results

In 12 of 16 patients with *papillary stenosis* improved emptying of contrast material from the bile duct was observed after papillotomy. At the control examination after 1 week, the signs of cholestasis disappeared. Restenosis of the papilla developed in three patients, and they were later subjected to surgery. In one patient a perforation occurred which is described below.

The stones of the common bile duct disappeared in 37 of 44 cases. The stones passed spontaneously after papillotomy in 24, while extraction of the stones was successfully achieved in 13.

The patients tolerated papillotomy well; they felt no pain at the time of incision, and only five noted a sensation of heat during application of diathermy. Papillotomy is only a slightly more extensive procedure from the viewpoint of the patient than ERCP alone.

Complications

One patient developed a perforation at the junction of the common bile duct and the duodenum. After papillotomy, air and contrast material could be visualized retroperitoneally. The defect was repaired surgically, and the patient made an uneventful recovery. In one patient the Dormia basket containing a huge stone was wedged into the bile duct and had to be removed surgically. Bleeding was observed in one patient 2 days after papillotomy and was controlled by blood transfusion. There were no lethal complications. Koch[8] described acute pancreatitis after papillotomy with a complete recovery.

Discussion

Endoscopic papillotomy is always successful when the papillotome can be inserted into the common duct. This was achieved in 60 of 71 patients (84 percent), which corresponds to the rate of success for diagnostic biliary cannulation.

In 50 of our 60 papillotomized patients cholecystectomy had been undertaken previously. We consider papillotomy to be indicated also in noncholecystectomized high-risk patients with or without evidence of gallbladder stones if papillary stenosis and/or choledocholithiasis is present.

Contraindications for endoscopic papillotomy are as follows: (1) long stenosis of the common bile duct, spread over the intraduodenal segment of the duct; (2) a papilla situated in a duodenal diverticulum; (3) if the ideal position of the papillotome in the common duct is not confirmed fluoroscopically or radiographically; (4) if the papillary stenosis and/or the choledocholithiasis are not the only causes of cholestasis (e.g., if postoperative stenosis of the common duct is also present).

We failed to remove stones in seven cases. It is remarkable that the jaundice in four patients with retained stones also disappeared after papillotomy. A free flow of bile was observed once papillary stenosis was relieved despite the residual stones. Four patients with residual stones, three with restenosis after papillotomy, and two with complications were successfully operated later.

Conclusions

Endoscopic papillotomy and extraction of gallstones from the common bile duct is a relatively safe (and in a high proportion of cases an effective) method in the treatment of biliary stasis due to papillary stenosis and/or choledocholithiasis. A successful procedure results in a complete cure and was achieved in 82 percent of our series. A failed intervention does increase the difficulty of later open surgery, however.

REFERENCES

1. Anacker H, Weiss H-D, Wiesner W: Das pankreatographische Bild der entzündlichen Pankreasprozesse. Fortschr Roentgenstr 117:418, 1972
2. Classen M, Demling L: Endoskopische Sphinkterotomie der Papilla Vateri und Steinextraktion aus dem Ductus choledochus. Dtsch Med Wochenschr 99:496, 1974
3. Classen M, Frühmorgen P, Kozu T, et al: Endoscopic-radiologic demonstration of biliodigestive fistulas. Endoscopy 3:138, 1971
4. Cotton PB: Cannulation of the papilla of Vater by endoscopy and retrograde cholangiopancreatography (ERCP). Gut 13:1014, 1972
5. Kasugai T, Kuno N, Kizu S, et al: Endoscopic pancreatocholangiography. I. The normal endoscopic pancreatocholangiogram. Gastroenterology 63:217, 1972
6. Kasugai T, Kuno N, Kizu S, et al: Endoscopic pancreatocholangiography. II. The pathological endoscopic pancreatocholangiogram. Gastroenterology 63:227, 1972
7. Kawai K, Akasaka Y, Murakami K, et al: Endoscopic sphincterotomy of the ampulla of Vater. Gastrointest Endosc 20:148, 1974
8. Koch H: Endoscopic papillotomy. Endoscopy 7:89, 1975
9. Kozu T, Oi I, Suzuki T, et al: Fiberduodenoscopic observation on the dynamics of the duodenal papilla. Endoscopy 2:99, 1970
10. McCune WS, Shorb PE, Moscovitz H: Endoscopic cannulation of the ampulla of Vater: a preliminary report. Ann Surg 167:752, 1968
11. Ogoshi H, Hara Y: Retrograde pancreatocholedochography. Jap J Clin Radiol 17:455, 1972
12. Oi I, Kobayashi S, Kondo T: Endoscopic pancreatocholangiography. Endoscopy 2:103, 1970
13. Oi I, Takemoto T, Nakayama K: "Fiberduodenoscopy"—early diagnosis of cancer of the papilla of Vater. Surgery 67:561, 1970
14. Rabinov KR, Simon M: Peroral cannulation of the ampulla of Vater for direct cholangiography and pancreatography: preliminary report of a new method. Radiology 85:693, 1965
15. Sáfrány L: Endoscopic visualization of bile flow using indocyanine green. Endoscopy 5:18, 1973
16. Sáfrány L: Endoskopische Papillotomie und Gallensteinentfernung. In: II European Congress of Endoscopy, Konstanz, West Germany, 1975, p 36
17. Sáfrány L, Tari J, Barna L, et al: Endoscopic retrograde cholangiography. Gastrointest Endosc 19:163, 1973
18. Seifert E, Stender HS, Sáfrány L, et al: X-ray findings of pancreatic cysts diagnosed by endoscopic pancreatocholangiography. Endoscopy, in press
19. Tamás G, Sáfrány L: Blood glucose, insulin and amylase levels in pancreatic lesion due to pancreatography. Acta Diabetol Lat 10:518, 1973

EDITORIAL COMMENT

ERCP became very well accepted as one of the most useful noninvasive diagnostic tests in the problematic jaundiced patient. In small pancreatic lesions without icterus the situation is somewhat different. If there are no gross changes (e.g., dilated duct with a stop of contrast material, narrow parts, or succular dilatations) it is difficult if not impossible to differentiate an inflammatory process from a malignant one. Perhaps an additional aid would be if more x-ray films could be taken with less amount of contrast material per film (Chapter 17).

The value of ERCP in diagnosing early pancreatic lesions has yet to be demonstrated. If pancreatic secretion could be collected for cytology more readily than it is done today, the diagnostic value of ERCP may be enhanced.

Noninvasive Sphincterotomy

For noninvasive sphincterotomy the instrumentation and technique became an extension of the method of cannulation. A coagulation snare is made by fixing a small wire at one end of a plastic tube (Fig. 1A) and is advanced through the sphincter. By pulling the end of the wire, a free loop is created (Fig. 1B). By applying pulling action and coagulation current simultaneously, the sphincter of Oddi can be transected. A minimum incision length is 10 mm, but 20 mm is recommended.

The procedure is done mainly to remove or facilitate spontaneous passage of retained biliary calculi. Those who undergo it are from the group of postcholecystectomy patients whose clinical signs and symptoms indicate the presence of (retained) stones.

There are many requirements for this procedure: An excellent high-resolution image amplifier with spot films is essential in order to see precisely the positioning of the thin wire before electric current is applied to cut and/or coagulate the sphincter. This fine wire is so thin that it is sometimes difficult to visualize it on the fluoroscopy screen. Even small amounts of contrast material injected through this tube are hard to recognize. The position of the wire must be clearly identified because the cut has to be performed in an 11 o'clock position (Fig. 2), otherwise injuries of the entrance portion of the pancreatic duct can be anticipated.

In a symposium on this topic at the Second European Congress of Endoscopy in Konstanz in 1975, the presented data were as follows:

Total sphincterotomies: 135
Total perforations requiring exploration: 6
Fatalities: 2

Here are some preliminary reports from two institutions:

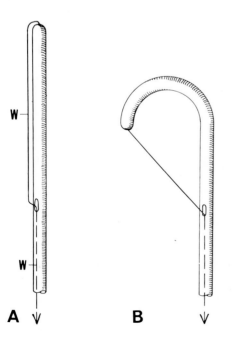

FIG. 1.A. Papillotomy snare. A thin wire (W) is secured at the tip of a plastic tube, approximately 2 inches (50 mm) from a hole through which it is threaded, leading into the lumen. **B.** The wire is advanced through the sphincter; when the wire is pulled, a loop is formed. Applying (unipolar) current, the wire with its loop is withdrawn through the sphincter (coagulation-cutting action).

A   B

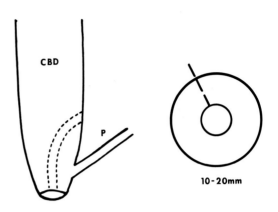

FIG. 2. The position of the wire and its cutting direction has to be precisely identified. *Left:* CBD, common bile duct; P, pancreatic duct. Anatomic variation of pancreatic duct drainage (dotted line) is not uncommon. (See Kune G: Current Practice of Biliary Surgery. Boston, Little, Brown, 1972.) *Right:* Schematic display of proposed division (11 o'clock); this has to be carefully observed to avoid complications. Recommended length: 20 mm.

Institution A
  Total cases: 30
  Unsuccessful cases (problems in cannulation): 5
  Perforation (exploration): 1
  Restenosis of sphincter: 5
Institution B
  Total cases: 50
  Perforations requiring surgical intervention: 2
  Cases in which stones were retained after the (too small?) sphincterotomy: 2
  Restenosed sphincters seen on repeated ERCP: 2

In eight cases there were difficulties entering the common bile duct.

Sometimes it is possible to introduce a Dormier basket (if the incision is long enough) to retrieve the stone. In other cases the incision alone is sufficient for spontaneous passage of stones.

Dr. Sáfrány, who is one of the pioneers in this procedure, reported 71 attempts, in 60 of which he successfully cannulated the common bile duct (CBD). He claims 84 percent success. His data included:

Attempts to cannulate the sphincter: 71
Successful cannulations: 60
Stones in the CBD: 44
Spontaneous passage: 24
Extracted: 13
Failure to remove: 7
Surgical interventions required: 9
  Residual stones after sphincterotomy: 4
  Restenosis of sphincter: 3
  Complications requiring exploration: 2

There is no mention as to the fate of those 11 cases where the indications of retrograde sphincterotomy were sound but the cannulation maneuver was unsuccessful. If these patients in addition to the stones were also icteric, they probably underwent surgery. This means that of 71 cases, despite the attempt, approximately one-third underwent surgery.

Stenosis of the papilla is a very interesting entity. In Dr. Sáfrány's epilogue it is not clear whether these stenoses were secondary to stone disease—which is understandable—or if they represent a primary sphincter of Oddi stenosis without jaundice. "Hypertony" or "hypertrophy" have been of extreme interest during the last three decades. What were the criteria with which this diagnosis was established?

The impact of vastly improved intraoperative procedures (choledoscopy and cholangiography) and the first results of a multiinstitutional prospective study (Shore et al:

Surg Gynecol Obstet 140:601, 1975) showed a significant reduction of the overlooked stones during primary choledocholithotomy (2.7 percent). We believe that appropriate treatment of biliary stone disease during the first (surgical) session is the answer, and that the number of cases requiring retrograde sphincterotomy today will thus be reduced to a minimum.

If a perforated biliary or pancreatic system must be corrected, the surgeon has to enter an already operated area, which sometimes can be extremely difficult and time-consuming. Opening the common bile duct and drainage, if required, add to the risk of morbidity and mortality. Furthermore, every opening of the common bile duct with drainage can result in a small but existing number of complications, including biliary duct stricture formation.

With further experience I am sure the complication rate will be reduced. I also have no doubt that this procedure should be performed only by highly skilled endoscopists in well equipped institutions. This method of noninvasive stone removal needs very careful and accurate follow-up of patients before we can recommend it on a wider scale.

THE EDITOR

23

Icterus: Differential Diagnosis, Noninvasive and Invasive Methods

Leon Morgenstern

Modern endoscopic techniques have added a new dimension to the differential diagnosis of jaundice. In the past, weeks of observation were necessary to provide the answer to two cogent problems in every jaundiced patient. The first problem is to determine if the jaundice is due to some hepatocellular dysfunction and thus amenable to medical management, and the second is to see if it is due to a surgically remediable obstructive mechanism so that the subsequent surgical procedure can be more carefully and properly planned.

It has been customary to state that "medical" and "surgical" jaundice could be differentiated accurately by indirect means in approximately 85 percent of all jaundiced patients. In the remaining 15 percent no end of sequential laboratory tests could provide the ultimate answer, and eventually laparotomy would be required. Six weeks was the customary time limit imposed on the observation period, this being the arbitrary time after which irreversible liver changes were to be expected. Such long periods of observation were disadvantageous on several counts. They were inordinately expensive, mentally and physically debilitating, and in cases of malignant obstruction possibly lethal. The advent of newer diagnostic techniques, among them modern endoscopy, has changed the waiting period from weeks to days. It should now be possible to make an accurate diagnosis of the etiologic mechanism of jaundice in over 95 percent of patients within 5 to 7 days after admission to the hospital.

STANDARD INVESTIGATION OF THE JAUNDICED PATIENT

The history should include the mode of onset of jaundice, presence or absence of pain, exposure to infectious hepatitis, record of drug ingestion, and the presence or absence of known biliary tract disease. Additional clues to the nature of the jaundice may also be anorexia, itching, malaise, fever, increasing acholia of stools, and progressive choluria. Since the number of icterogenic drugs is large and ever increasing, it is sometimes helpful to have the patient bring all of his medicine for direct inspection, rather than trusting his memory or description of drugs currently being ingested. The history of alcohol ingestion should be precise.

The physical examination should give the examiner a rough estimation of the degree of jaundice. In good daylight minimal jaundice is detectable at a serum bilirubin level of 2.0 mg percent. Easily detectable jaundice in skin and sclerae generally means that the serum bilirubin is above 3.0 mg percent. Cutaneous stigmata of hepatocellular disease—e.g., spider angiomas, malar telangiectasia, palmar erythema, caput medusae, and scattered ecchymoses—are easily detectable. Abdominal examination should yield information about the size of the liver and spleen, liver tenderness, abdominal masses, presence or absence of ascites, and presence or absence of a palpable gallbladder.

Fever, chills, and hypotension comprise the only triad which lends extreme urgency to the decision-making process in the jaundiced patient. This triad leaves little time for procrastination, since it generally means ascending cholangitis with gram-negative sepsis. Although the fever is generally high and septic in character, it may be low grade in the very elderly or debilitated patient. This complex of signs and symptoms, especially in the patient with known biliary tract disease, usually demands prompt surgical intervention for biliary decompression, unless response to appropriate antibiotic therapy is prompt and dramatic.

Laboratory investigation should establish not only a base line of the most useful liver function tests but also the trend or evolution of such tests. Tests should include bilirubin (with direct/indirect fractionation), alkaline phosphatase, SGOT and SGPT, prothrombin time, and serum albumin. Generally it requires 5 to 7 days to establish a trend which may alter the nature of the subsequent investigations. The initial level of bilirubin, with a high component of the direct fraction, may be suggestive but is certainly not diagnostic of an etiologic mechanism. A constantly rising direct hyperbilirubinemia of 1 to 2 mg percent per day is suggestive but not diagnostic of extrahepatic biliary obstruction. Waxing and waning hyperbilirubinemia is suggestive of choledocholithiasis. An initially high bilirubin may fall to below 2.0 mg percent within this period of observation. At this level and below it is advisable to perform intravenous cholangiography. Above 3.0 mg percent the yield is too small to justify this procedure.

The alkaline phosphatase likewise is not infallibly useful in differentiating the anatomic or functional level of cholestatic disorders. High and increasing levels of alkaline phosphatase reflect obstruction, but this may be on the hepatocellular or extrahepatic level. The higher values are generally seen with mechanical obstruction.

The SGOT and SGPT may be very high (up to 1,000 units) in cases of acute biliary tract obstruction, especially when associated with severe inflammation. However, such high values usually drop rapidly to normal or moderately elevated levels even when the obstruction persists. When these enzyme levels remain high and continue to rise, they suggest hepatitis rather than mechanical obstruction.

The values for prothrombin time and serum albumin should be normal in patients whose jaundice is of short duration when the etiology of the jaundice is mechanical obstruction. Low values on initial and early sequential examination should suggest hepatocellular damage rather than mechanical obstruction.

Other blood tests yield little or no additional useful information. The complete blood count is of course routine, and observations such as anemia, leukocytosis, relative lymphocytosis, or abnormal white cells may provide some helpful clues in establishing the diagnosis.

A simple test which is often done late or omitted is the direct observation of stool color. An acholic (white) stool does not tell whether cholestasis is at the cellular or ductal level, but it does establish that there is an obstruction to the delivery of bile. More often than not the acholic stool is due to complete or near complete mechanical obstruction in the extrahepatic biliary tree. Likewise a brown stool does not rule out intermittent mechanical obstruction, but it is more suggestive of dysfunction on the cellular level. In the opinion of this author, direct observation of the stool over a period of 5 to 7 days gives the same information as the radioactive rose Bengal test, at vastly less cost.

A word of caution is in order regarding overzealous serial blood tests, which only help deplete the patient, especially if for any reason the period of observation extends beyond a period of days into weeks. Significant blood loss may occur with daily "bloodletting" for the panel of liver function tests as well as others which may be performed concomitantly. To establish the trend as described above, testing is necessary at 2- or 3-day intervals, not daily.

There is not complete unanimity of opinion as to when the more "invasive" of investigatory procedures should begin in the jaundiced patient who still remains a diagnostic enigma. It is this author's opinion that a period of observation of 5 to 7 days is indicated in most cases unless there is more urgency for diagnosis (e.g., with known history of biliary tract disease, diabetes of recent onset, presence of Courvoisier gallbladder, etc.). Examination of the gastrointestinal tract using barium should not be done before endoscopic examination, since interference with radiography of the biliary tree may result. Likewise liver biopsy is not conclusive and may be dangerous in the presence of mechanical obstruction; hence it should not precede endoscopic investigation.

ENDOSCOPIC INVESTIGATION OF THE JAUNDICED PATIENT

Endoscopic Retrograde Cholangiopancreatography

The first of the endoscopic procedures that should be utilized in the differential diagnosis of jaundice is endoscopic retrograde cholangiopancreatography (ERCP). There may be circumstances in which laparoscopy may be preferred as the first procedure—e.g., the presence of multiple abdominal masses, a strong suspicion of hepatic metastases, or the presence of a lower abdominal mass in association with jaundice. Generally, however, ERCP is the first of the direct approaches to diagnosis.

The technical details pertaining to the technique and instrumentation of ERCP are described elsewhere in this book (Chapter 22). It is an endoscopic procedure that requires consummate skill; but once this skill has been acquired, it should be possible to cannulate the papilla of Vater in 85 percent of attempted cases.

ERCP offers the following diagnostic possibilities. Intrinsic neoplasms of the stomach and duodenum are ruled out in transit toward the papilla of Vater. Effacement of the duodenal mucosal pattern or narrowing of the duodenal lumen may suggest extrinsic pressure by neoplasm. Once the papilla is visualized, specimens of the effluent may be obtained for cytology, cholesterol crystals, electrolytes, pancreatic enzymes, and carcinoembryonic antigen. Brushings of the papilla itself may be taken for cytologic study. Once the ampulla is cannulated, it may be possible to collect specimens for study from either the bile duct or the pancreatic duct.

The most direct aid afforded by ERCP in the diagnosis of jaundice is the radiographic visualization of the biliary and pancreatic ductal systems. In the bile ducts it is possible to delineate calculi, narrowing by neoplasm or pancreatitis, and biliary ductal strictures. Cannulation and radiographic visualization of the pancreatic ductal system may reveal stenosis, obstruction, irregularity, compression, deviation, and calculi. Alone or in combination these findings may suggest the diagnosis of pancreatitis, pancreatic neoplasm, or pseudocyst, all of which may be associated with cryptogenic jaundice. Thus a wide variety of lesions which may cause extrahepatic mechanical biliary obstruction are discoverable by ERCP. Conversely, normal biliary and pancreatic ductal systems place the etiology of jaundice on the hepatocellular level.

ERCP is not without its drawbacks. Cannulation of the papilla may be made difficult or impossible by the condition responsible for the jaundice. A stone impacted in the ampulla can render cannulation impossible. Edema secondary to pancreatitis or marked deviation or obstruction secondary to pancreatic neoplasm may also preclude successful cannulation. However, these difficulties in themselves are suggestive or indicative of mechanical obstruction and should weight judgment in that direction when encountered.

The most common sequela of ERCP is pancreatitis. This is usually mild but in some cases may be moderate or severe. Clinically there is left upper quadrant pain and tenderness, generally lasting 24 to 72 hours. The serum amylase may rise to levels as high as 1,000 units, and a transient hyperbilirubinemia may occur.

The most important complication of ERCP is cholangitis. Fevers, chills, and abrupt hyperbilirubinemia herald this complication. Associated hypotension implies gram-negative septicemia, the condition most frequently responsible for the lethal complications of ERCP. In the University of Oregon study of 10,000 cases of ERCP[2] 0.8 percent of the patients experienced this complication, and of these 10 percent had a fatal outcome. Four severe septic complications were described by Davis et al.,[4] including gallbladder empyema, purulent cholangitis, and conversion of a pseudocyst into a pancreatic abscess. Since the majority of organisms in the obstructed biliary tree are of the gram-negative variety, pretreatment with a broad-spectrum antibiotic such as ampicillin has been recommended and practiced by some. Others have added an antibiotic such as chloromycetin to the radiopaque dye. It is this author's opinion that adequate blood levels of ampicillin should be achieved for at least 24 hours before, during, and at least 48 hours after ERCP. No controlled study exists to date to prove the effectiveness of such a regimen, but extrapolation from studies in analogous situations in surgery tends to support this approach.

Less frequent complications of ERCP are drug reactions to sedatives or contrast agents (0.6 percent), pancreatic sepsis and pseudocyst abscess (0.3 percent), and instrumental injury (0.2 percent). Of these latter complications, pancreatic sepsis and pseudocyst abscess are clearly the most serious and have been associated with appreciable mortality.

In summary, ERCP, when successful, offers a direct visual approach to the biliary and pancreatic ductal systems without breaching the hepatic or pancreatic parenchyma. It can establish rapidly and with minimal risk the presence and site of mechanical obstructive mechanisms. Its principal disadvantages are the technical difficulties in cannulating the papilla, difficulties in visualizing the entire biliary tree radiographically, and the possibility of sepsis in the biliary tree or pancreas. As a diagnostic tool it is firmly established as an excellent means for the earlier diagnosis of cryptogenic jaundice.

Laparoscopy

The indications for laparoscopy have already been briefly alluded to in the foregoing section on ERCP. Restated they are: (1) obvious mass lesions within the liver or remote from the liver within the peritoneal cavity; (2) strong suspicion of peritoneal carcinomatosis or intrinsic liver disease; and (3) failure of ERCP to establish an etiologic basis for jaundice. The technique and instrumentation are described in detail in Chapters 29 and 30.

Laparoscopy with modern improved optical systems provides an excellent view of the peritoneal cavity. Probably the best visualized organ during this procedure is the liver; three-fourths of its surface area may be inspected. The appearance of the liver itself offers an important clue to the etiology of jaundice. A turgid, enlarged, greenish parenchyma is indicative of extrahepatic obstruction. A flabby, reddish brown, soft parenchyma favors hepatocellular damage. Primary neoplasms such as hepatoma or cholangiocarcinoma may be readily visible; and the presence and extent of metastatic involvement, when present, is easily discernible. Such neoplasms may be biopsied under direct vision, an infinitely better method than the percutaneous blind biopsy in

terms of diagnostic yield and hemostatic control. In cases of suspected hepatocellular disease, a generous biopsy may be taken under direct vision with hemostasis achieved by electrocautery. Naturally when there is a strong suspicion of mechanical obstruction based on the appearance of the liver, biopsy should not be performed because of the high risk of bile leakage and peritonitis. Under these circumstances transhepatic cholecystocholangiography is indicated, a procedure described in Chapters 17 and 29.

It is also possible to assess the appearance of gallbladder during laparoscopy. A tense, inflamed gallbladder or a distended, hydropic gallbladder clearly implicates the biliary tract in the etiology of jaundice. A collapsed gallbladder indicates obstruction of the bile duct proximal to cystic duct entry or hepatocellular dysfunction.

Extrahepatic masses may also be visualized during laparoscopy. Unfortunately the pancreatic head, body, and tail are not readily visible, lying covered by the gastrocolic omentum in the lesser sac. Some laparoscopists have devised means of entering the lesser sac by manipulation and perforation of the gastrocolic omentum, but the safety and diagnostic yield of these methods remain to be proved. Secondary evidence of neoplasm or pseudocyst of the pancreas may be seen as protruding masses from the retroperitoneum, or in cases of malignant neoplasm as intraperitoneal metastases. Primary and secondary ovarian, colonic, and retroperitoneal tumors are among those which have been seen and biopsied in cases of cryptogenic jaundice.

The drawbacks of laparoscopy are: (1) discomfort when done under local anesthesia, and the anesthetic risk when done under general anesthesia; (2) occasional cardiac arrhythmias with induction of pneumoperitoneum; (3) inability to visualize retroperitoneal structures; and (4) inability to palpate or see in those recesses where rigid instruments cannot penetrate.

Laparoscopy with Transhepatic Cholecystocholangiography

Transhepatic cholecystocholangiography is a technique whereby contrast medium is introduced into the gallbladder for the purpose of visualizing the biliary ductal system. The gallbladder is punctured under direct vision through the laparoscope, traversing overlying hepatic parenchyma so that the needle enters the fundus of the gallbladder through the liver substance. The hazards of bile leak from the gallbladder are avoided by entering the gallbladder through hepatic parenchyma. The hepatic puncture site is sealed by electrocautery. This technique is described in detail in Chapter 29 and by Berci et al.[1]

To the diagnostic advantages of laparoscopy are thus added those of radiographic visualization of the biliary ducts. Unlike transhepatic percutaneous cholangiography, success with this method does not depend on dilatation of the ductal system, nor does the method carry the inherent risk of leakage of bile and blood into the peritoneal cavity. This risk is minimized by the tamponade effect of the overlying hepatic parenchyma. Used in conjunction with image amplification, fluoroscopy, and other modern radiographic techniques, a dynamic, functional assessment of the biliary ductal system can be obtained as well as a precise anatomic delineation.

This method has been used successfully to demonstrate calculi in the biliary system, obstructive neoplasms, and nonobstructive hepatocellular cholestatic disorders (Figs. 17 through 20 in Chapter 17). It has a high diagnostic yield with relatively small risk, as compared to percutaneous cholangiography and laparotomy. Obviously it cannot be used in the absence of the gallbladder, but this disadvantage should be present in a relatively small number of patients presenting with cryptogenic jaundice.

Sepsis has not been a problem to date in those cases in which this technique has been used. Sepsis seems a more likely complication when dye is introduced under pressure into the relatively nondistensible common duct as compared with the readily distensible gallbladder. Nevertheless, it seems a wise precaution to pretreat patients with potential sepsis in the same manner as was described in the section on ERCP.

The relative advantages of ERCP versus transhepatic cholecystocholangiography and the advisability of employing one method over the other depends on the individual case. Generally ERCP is preferable as the initial diagnostic technique since it is noninvasive and can be done without general anesthesia. It is also the obvious method of choice when the gallbladder is absent. However, if there are indica-

tions for laparoscopy as described above, or if ERCP has failed, transhepatic cholecystocholangiography is a reasonable and effective alternative.

Choledochoscopy

Choledochoscopy implies that laparotomy has been necessary to establish the cause for jaundice, and within the content of this chapter the procedure is mentioned only as an adjunct in differential diagnosis. Even with the abdomen open and the extrahepatic biliary tree exposed, there still remains a fraction of cases in which the etiology of a ductal obstruction is unclear. In these instances choledochoscopy, using the modern choledochoscope is of inestimable value.[9] With the choledochoscope it is possible to differentiate between functional disorders of the sphincter of Oddi and the presence of a calculus or neoplastic obstruction. It is also possible to visualize calculi, strictures, cholangitis, and intraductal neoplasms. Under direct vision the latter may be biopsied or specimens taken for cytologic examination.

Choledochoscopy is best performed with the rigid choledochoscope, which offers tremendous advantages in terms of definition, depth of focus, and wide angle of view. It is not recommended for ducts that are under 1.0 cm in diameter, but for dilated ducts the diagnostic merits of its use are unquestionable. It should be part of the surgical armamentarium wherever biliary tract surgery is performed.

Other Ancillary Techniques, Used with or without Endoscopy

Since this chapter stresses endoscopic techniques in the differential diagnosis of jaundice, only brief mention has been given to other techniques and some have not yet been mentioned at all. They are deserving of mention since they may supplement endoscopic methods and at times provide clues to diagnosis where endoscopic methods fail.

Hypotonic duodenography, by its precise delineation of duodenal anatomy, may localize small neoplasms extrinsic to the duodenum which might ordinarily be missed on routine endoscopic examination. Early lesions of the head of the pancreas, tumors of the ampulla, and duodenal lesions distal to the ampulla are examples of pathology well shown by hypotonic duodenography.

Selective visceral angiography examines those viscera supplied by the celiac and superior mesenteric arteries. It can be of value in the differential diagnosis of jaundice by delineating the vascular architecture of the liver, gallbladder, pancreas, and associated structures. Characteristic vascular patterns indicative of neoplasm may establish the diagnosis of intrahepatic or pancreatic neoplasm. For detailed descriptions of technique and interpretation of findings, the reader is referred to several excellent articles on this subject.[3,5,13]

Transjugular transhepatic cholangiography entails the passage of a catheter through the right internal jugular vein, superior vena cava, right auricle, and via the inferior vena cava into the hepatic vein. By means of a needle passed through this catheter, the hepatic parenchyma is penetrated and radiopaque dye slowly injected as the needle advances until a biliary radicle is entered. It is then possible to obtain a cholangiogram and with the same needle to obtain an aspiration biopsy of the liver. Proponents of this technique[7,11] claim a high degree of success with reasonably low risk. The main advantage is the minimal invasiveness of the technique, thereby eliminating the risks of bile peritonitis and bleeding. Its main disadvantage is the reported occurrence of sepsis since in essence an iatrogenic biliary-venous fistula is created, albeit a temporary one. This method depends somewhat on the dilatation of the intrahepatic bile ducts, much as the percutaneous cholangiogram does. Also obtainable by this ingenious method are wedge hepatic vein pressure, a reflection of portal venous pressure. This method is an alternative when ERCP has failed or is contraindicated for any reason.

Finally, laparotomy is the method of last resort for purposes of differential diagnosis. Even if any or all of the foregoing techniques have been unsuccessful in establishing the exact diagnosis, they at least suggest some diagnoses and help rule out others. The least of the operative procedures, a "minilap," is a limited exposure of the liver through a small upper midline incision under local anesthesia.[10,12] It permits wedge and needle liver biopsy under direct vision, transhepatic cholangiography, and umbilical vein catheterization for portal venography. To this might be added the use of the laparoscope to visualize those surfaces of the liver not visible through this limited incision. This procedure is well tolerated and en-

tails minimal operative risk, but it does represent a major entry into the peritoneal cavity and hence should not be undertaken lightly. Finally, when all else fails, formal exploratory laparotomy is indicated. Although it may imply admission of failure on the diagnostic level, it may also hold promise of solution to the problem on the therapeutic level. To be avoided at all costs is prolonged, meddlesome exploration in cases of hepatitis or hepatocellular disease. Once it is established that no ductal obstruction exists (e.g., by simple cholecystocholangiography), a judicious retreat from further exploration is advisable.

Postoperative Jaundice

Jaundice following major operative procedures may be due to a multiplicity of factors, and the diagnostic dilemma may be no less challenging than jaundice occurring without operation.[6] Among the etiologic factors that may be added by operation are hepatotoxic anesthetic agents, hypotension, transfusions, sepsis, hemolysis, hemoperitoneum, retroperitoneal hematoma, and others. The most worrisome but probably the least frequent of the etiologic mechanisms is injury to the extrahepatic biliary tract if the operation has been in this area. This is the only etiologic mechanism that would warrant early operative intervention.

Since most of the more severe cases of postoperative jaundice fall within that well described but ill understood entity "benign postoperative cholestasis,"[8] it is well to delay any kind of diagnostic intervention save for sequential testing of hyperbilirubinemia and liver function. These cases are generally associated with major operative procedures and prolonged anesthesia, multiple transfusions, hypotension, and sepsis. The cholestatic syndrome may be severe, with bilirubin values as high as 25 mg percent, and the course may be prolonged for as long as 3 weeks. Since all the aforementioned endoscopic procedures would entail maneuvers not well tolerated during the early postoperative period, it is best to delay any such procedure in the case of postoperative jaundice until 3 or 4 weeks have elapsed. At that time ERCP would be the first of the diagnostic measures indicated. An exception to this rule would be those cases in which bile duct injury is strongly suspected—cases in which early diagnostic and therapeutic intervention are indicated. For the majority, however, watchful waiting has its rewards in yielding the least morbidity and mortality compared with any other approach.

REFERENCES

1. Berci G, Morgenstern L, Shore JM, et al: A direct approach to the differential diagnosis of jaundice. Am J Surg 126:372, 1973
2. Bilbao MK, Dotter CT, Lee T, et al: Personal communication, 1974
3. Boijsen E, Reuter SR: Combined percutaneous transhepatic cholangiography and angiography in the evaluation of obstructive jaundice. Am J Roentgenol Radium Ther Nucl Med 99:153, 1967
4. Davis JL, Milligan FD, Cameron J: Septic complications following endoscopic retrograde cholangiopancreatography. Surg Gynecol Obstet 140:365, 1975
5. Katon RM, Bilbao MK, Rösch J: Algorithm for an aggressive diagnostic approach to obstructive jaundice. West J Med 122:206, 1975
6. Morgenstern L: Postoperative jaundice: an ap-
proach to a diagnostic dilemma. Am J Surg 128:255, 1974
7. Rösch J, Lakin PC, Antonovic R, et al: Transjugular approach to liver biopsy and transhepatic cholangiography. N Engl J Med 289:227, 1973
8. Schmid M, Hefti ML, Gattiker R, et al: Benign postoperative intrahepatic cholestasis. N Engl J Med 272:545, 1965
9. Shore JM, Berci G, Morgenstern L: The value of biliary endoscopy. Surg Gynecol Obstet 140:601, 1975
10. Strack PR, Newman HK, Lerner AG, et al: An integrated procedure for the rapid diagnosis of biliary obstruction, portal hypertension and liver disease of unknown etiology. N Engl J Med 285:1225, 1971
11. Weiner M, Hanafee WN: A review of transjugular cholangiography. Radiol Clin North Am 8:53, 1970
12. Wexler MJ, McLean APH, Skinner GB, et al: "Minilap": an accurate, rapid and safe approach to the diagnosis of liver disease and jaundice. Ann Surg 178:736, 1973
13. Young WB: Obstructive jaundice—the radiologist, the surgeon and the patient. Am J Roentgenol Radium Ther Nucl Med 119:4, 1973

EDITORIAL COMMENT

I had many reasons for asking Leon Morgenstern to elaborate on the differential diagnosis of jaundice.

First, he had spent significant time in researching and collecting data on the complexity of the pre- and postoperative jaundice problems and had accumulated experience in assessing the various differential diagnostic dilemmas.

Second, I wanted attention to be drawn again to the fact that in the problematic, icteric patient, it is imperative to keep the workup period to a minimum.

Third, I wanted an objective evaluation of the various methods of approaching jaundice problems from someone who is not an endoscopist but who is very much interested in the problem and the solution.

Recently, Okuda and co-workers (Am J Dig Dis 19:21, 1974) introduced an improved technique of percutaneous transhepatic cholangiography. A fine, 15-cm needle (0.7 mm OD, 0.5 mm ID) is introduced percutaneously under the guidance of a high-quality image amplifier with a spot film device, connected to a syringe with contrast material. If the needle enters the liver parenchyma in a certain direction (for detailed technique, see the references), contrast material is slowly injected and observed on the television monitor for resemblance to the extrahepatic biliary system. The needle can be moved under constant slow injection until the aimed duct system is entered. Favorable results are already reported in the United States.

Being partial to laparoscopy, I am inclined to perform this technique under visual control to obtain more information than would be obtained by a cholangiography alone, but I must admit that in certain circumstances the needle technique is simpler than an elaborate method such as laparoscopy. Further time and experience will make clear the value of this improved percutaneous cholangiography, if a larger number of investigators will report their results.

I believe that the needle technique will be the greatest competitor of the more complicated, presently employed ERCP, and that in the future it will obtain results superior to those obtained by retrograde cannulation of the extrahepatic biliary system. If dilated, the hepatic ducts can be displayed more easily by injecting from above than they can by injecting from below.

However, the technique should be included in our armamentarium of tools to help us to unravel the controversial aspects of jaundice, an important and serious entity.

THE EDITOR

24

Pediatric Esophagoscopy

Stephen L. Gans
Dale G. Johnson

The first real esophagoscopy was performed by Kussmaul in 1868. He selected a professional sword swallower for his subject and passed an open tube into the gullet, using for illumination the reflected light of a gasoline lamp. Except for improvements in lighting, the hollow tube remained the basic instrument for esophagoscopy for the next hundred years. This arrangement was reasonably satisfactory for examining adult patients, but when its size was reduced for pediatric use the viewing angle became very small and the image dim.

Recent advances in optical image transmission and illumination (Chapter 5) have made it possible to miniaturize all endoscopes and at the same time provide a vastly improved view and increased capabilities. The instruments were redesigned, and in 1971 the first report of their clinical application in infants and children was published.[3]

INDICATIONS

Endoscopy is quite indispensable for the management of many esophageal conditions, for it provides diagnostic information and a method of treatment unattainable in any other way. Table 1 lists the indications gathered from our experience. There is obvious overlapping, such as the evaluation of corrosive effect and treatment of its secondary stenosis; or pain, bleeding, and even obstruction all due to reflux esophagitis sometimes associated with hiatal hernia.

CONTRAINDICATIONS

Esophagoscopy is well tolerated by all pediatric patients except those in severe states of debility due to overwhelming general problems. Local contraindications may include conditions which render the esophagus susceptible to rupture, e.g., acute severe esophagitis from corrosives or infection. Inasmuch as these may be just the conditions where direct inspection might be useful, experience and good judgment should prevail, and sometimes a limited examination is better than none.

ANESTHESIA

Esophagoscopy can be performed either with or without a general anesthetic. We prefer general anesthesia because the procedure is easier for the surgeon as well as the patient. There is also less likelihood of trauma to the esophagus, and the examination can be carried out more thoroughly. The use of an endotracheal tube is an additional safety factor in preventing respiratory obstruction by pressure from the instrument in the neighboring esophagus. The same advantages are even more prominent in the removal of esophageal foreign bodies.

INSTRUMENTS

For most purposes the Storz rigid esophagoscope with the Hopkins rod-lens telescope pro-

TABLE 1.   Indications for Esophagoscopy

Indication	No.
Intrinsic obstruction	
Congenital	
Webs	1
Stenosis	1
Upper pouch atresia—? upper fistula	4
Acquired stenosis	
Postoperative (plus differential diagnosis)	44
Caustic ingestion (plus dilatation)	15
Stricture secondary to gastroesophageal reflux	8
Stricture secondary to foreign body perforation	4
Neurogenic	
Swallowing incoordination (plus differential diagnosis)	8
Cardiospasm	3
Gastroesophageal reflux evaluation —? esophagitis	52
External obstruction (cyst, tumor, vascular ring)	2
Evaluation of chemical burns	11
Differential diagnosis of fistula or diverticulum	21
Foreign body removal	15
Pain	1
Bleeding	
Differential diagnosis (no findings)	14
Varices	5
Esophagitis secondary to reflux (see above)	
Evaluation of trauma	4

vides a brilliant wide-angle view and the capability of instrumental manipulation in the direct magnified sight of the telescope. When larger instruments must be passed through the lumen, the same esophagoscope sheath can be used without the telescope and with proximal illumination.

Flexible esophagoscopes are also available, *but the image quality is not comparable to that of the rod-lens telescope.* Furthermore, when miniaturized for pediatric use, both image and maneuverability suffer further reduction. These instruments are advantageous, however, in examining a tortuous or curved and bent structure, such as may occur after operations for esophageal replacement with colon or gastric tubes (Chapter 27). The flexible instrument is essential for examining the gastrointestinal tract below the esophagus. The flexible scope also provides controls for inflation, suction, and lens washing during examination. The inflation-suction feature is particularly useful in examining the function of the gastroesophageal junction.

PROCEDURE AND TECHNIQUE

With few exceptions, examination of the esophagus by direct vision is preceded by radiographic studies. These should include an anterior-posterior chest film and a lateral neck and chest x-ray, taken in such a way as to reveal the pharynx, larynx, and the retropharyngeal and retroesophageal spaces. Cinefluorography is particularly advantageous in evaluating function and sometimes in locating a fistula.

After adequate sedation and immobilization, or preferably endotracheal general anesthesia, the patient is placed supine on the operating table. The head of the table is dropped or removed and the patient positioned with the neck flexed on the chest and the head extended on the neck. The upper alveolar ridge or the upper teeth are retracted with the fingers of the left hand and the distal portion of the esophagoscope grasped with the left thumb and forefinger in a manner similar to that used while grasping a pool cue for a shot near the cushion. The proximal esophagoscope is manipulated with the right hand holding it as one would a pen or pencil. The tip of the scope is thus advanced along the right lateral border of the tongue and passed laterally to the epiglottis into the right pyriform sinus. The larynx is lifted forward by the lip of the advancing esophagoscope to reveal the entrance of the esophagus. This may be clearly visualized after a few moments of observation, and the esophagoscope is then inserted into the cervical esophagus. If this anatomy is not quite clear, *very* gentle probing with the tip may reveal it and allow introduction of the scope. However, it must be remembered that the most common site of perforation occurring during esophagoscopy is the posterior portion of this field, and forceful manipulation is contraindicated. Instead, a small woven bougie or even a rubber tube can be passed through the esophagoscope and the cricopharyngeal sphincter which forms this anatomic constriction, and then into the proximal esophagus. The scope is further advanced over this "lumen finder" under direct vision, and as the esophagus is entered the guide is removed. Inspection continues, keeping the lumen in view as the head is rotated posteriorly.

The method and technique of examining the rest of the esophagus depends on the type of pathology expected. Advance through the cardia may be facilitated by first inserting a guide tube or bougie into the stomach and passing the scope over it. Manipulation of the instrument into the lower one-third of the esophagus is also facilitated by having an assistant place both hands beneath the patient's lower chest to elevate and straighten the curvature in the dorsal spine.

Postoperatively the patient is checked for signs and symptoms of esophageal perforation, such as fever, pain in the chest or upper abdomen, cervical subcutaneous emphysema, mediastinal emphysema, or pneumothorax. In the absence of these, a liquid diet is permitted, with progression to normal diet and activity.

CLINICAL EXPERIENCE

Experience with traditional esophagoscopes has been widely described. There have been only a few reports involving use of the new telescopic endoscopes.[3,4] The technical advances in these instruments have so improved and changed methods and results that this discussion involves only material from this new era of endoscopy (Figs. 1–3, Plate A).*

SPECIFIC INDICATIONS

Difficulty in swallowing (dysphagia) is the most common indication for esophagoscopy and may be due to mechanical obstruction, neurogenic obstruction, or pain (Table 1).

Congenital stenosis of the esophagus may be a diaphragm-like web or may consist of a short or long segment of the esophagus itself. Congenital stenoses are less common than formerly supposed. Many of these stenoses in the lower third of the esophagus are in fact secondary to reflux esophagitis, even in infants. The entity formerly called congenital short esophagus probably does not exist. This lesion in our experience has proved to be an advanced form of reflux esophagitis with stricture and shortening. *Webs* may be incised by electrocautery through the instrument channel under direct telescopic control if their treatment with dilatation is difficult or must be repeated.

Acquired stenosis is either postoperative or the result of caustic or corrosive ingestion. The former is most often a complication of surgery for esophageal atresia and is usually managed

by retrograde dilatation with Tucker dilators, pulled through a gastrostomy by a swallowed string. When gastrostomy is not present, dilatation is carried out by gentle bouginage with an assortment of dilators. If the stricture does not respond to this treatment, the esophagoscope is used as a dilator or as an aid in passing a bougie or string through a very small opening. This can be a very trying and prolonged effort because the view through a standard open-tube esophagoscope is difficult enough without further obstructing it with an instrument in the lumen. When using the new esophagoscope with telescope, however, several advantages become readily apparent. Even a tiny opening can be entered with ease by a Fogarty catheter (2 or 3 Fr.) passed through the instrument channel in full view of the telescope. The balloon itself can be used to start progressive retrograde dilatation. If a gastrostomy is present the catheter can be directed through the structure and into the stomach, where a string is attached. The string is then drawn back through the narrowed esophagus for conventional dilatation with Tucker dilators. Ashcraft and Holder[1] treated children with persistent strictures by injecting triamcinolone into the area endoscopically, followed by dilatation.

Neurogenic or physiologic obstructions are usually related to incoordination of the swallowing mechanism. The role of esophagoscopy is to rule out mechanical obstruction or fistula, inasmuch as the symptomatology may be very similar. *Achalasia*, or *cardiospasm*, is generally considered to be a failure of coordination of the mechanism at the cardia, which results in a physiologic obstruction with proximal dilatation and hypertrophy of the esophagus. Treatment varies from simple dilatation of the spasmodic ring, to esophagoscopic dilatation, to forceful stretching with pneumatic or mechanical devices, to esophagogastric surgery.

The diagnosis of *external obstructions* usually involves other modalities. Esophagoscopy is occasionally useful for differentiation from internal obstructions, observing esophageal irritation or infiltration, or demonstrating localized compression or pulsation as from a vascular ring.

Part of the past difficulty and controversy in the treatment of *chemical burns* of the esophagus has come from an inability to assess and evaluate accurately the nature and extent of the injury. Also there has been a reluctance to

All color plates appear at the front of the book.

examine an esophagus with potential serious damage. With the new telescopes, rapid atraumatic orientation is obtained, decisions for continued advancement are more properly made, and the condition of the esophagus is more accurately noted and documented (by photography). The latter is of particular value for secondary review, later comparison, and teaching.

The diagnosis of recurrent *tracheoesophageal fistula,* or *H fistula,* is best made by bronchoscopy, where the opening can be seen with great clarity and even cannulated. The fistula may also be seen in the esophagus, particularly after flattening any folds by inflation through the antifog tube. If there is any doubt, methylene blue can be dropped in the trachea and then quickly spotted entering the esophagus.

Endoscopic removal of *foreign bodies* is sometimes quite troublesome, the difficulty stemming from the fact that the small lumen of the pediatric esophagoscope becomes even smaller in terms of vision when a grasping forceps is inserted down the middle. With the new esophagoscope a grasping forceps can be introduced through its instrument channel, and manipulations and removal can be carried out with direct visual control. Hard, smooth objects are very difficult to grasp, and they try the skill and patience of the endoscopist. We have successfully and quickly removed such foreign bodies by directing a well lubricated Fogarty catheter beyond the object and, after slight inflation, drawing the catheter and object out together. For simple cases involving smooth objects that have not become embedded in the esophageal wall (e.g., a recently swallowed coin) this balloon catheter technique can be used safely under fluoroscopic control without the need for esophagoscopy.

Pain may be due to esophagitis, hiatal hernia, foreign body impaction, cyst, tumor, or cardiospasm. We have already commented on all but the first two lesions, which frequently appear together. Demonstration of esophagitis or ulceration may well influence the course of therapy for the associated hiatus hernia.

Mild *esophagitis* may be difficult to recognize even with the magnified sharp image through the esophageal telescope, and mucosal biopsy may be necessary to detect the very early changes secondary to gastroesophageal reflux. As this lesion progresses, however, inspection by esophagoscopy reveals a reddened blush progressing to friability and bleeding on con-tact, dull granularity of the surface, and in severe cases frank mucosal ulceration.

Esophagoscopy can demonstrate the presence of gastroesophageal incompetence and free reflux, but cinefluoroscopy and particularly continuous esophageal pH measurements are much more accurate techniques for quantitative reflux. Esophagoscopy is more accurate in evaluating esophagitis as a complication of reflux. Photography allows for a genuine comparison or reevaluation at a later date.

Esophagoscopy is also of considerable value in the diagnosis of upper gastrointestinal *bleeding.* It can rule out the esophagus as a site of bleeding or it may demonstrate hiatus hernia, esophagitis or ulcer, esophageal varices, or a bleeding tumor. Usually these diagnoses can be made radiologically. However, as many as 20 percent of varices are not demonstrated by x-ray alone, and esophagitis is even more elusive, particularly in evaluating its appearance and extent.

COMPLICATIONS

Perforation is by far the greatest hazard of esophagoscopy and its associated procedures. It happens in fewer than 0.5 percent of all examinations, but it is much more frequent with dilatation and other operative events. Perforation may be associated with manipulation in a dimly illuminated area that is not clearly visualized and not adequately evaluated as to the condition of the esophageal wall.[2] We have observed no complications from esophagoscopy or associated manipulative procedures since we have been using the new telescopic endoscopes. No doubt the incidence of these problems is reduced by better vision and by maneuvers carried out in full view.

REFERENCES

1. Ashcraft KW, Holder TM: The experimental treatment of esophageal strictures by intralesional steroid injections. J Thorac Cardiovasc Surg 58:685, 1969
2. Bill AH, Mebust WK, Sauvage LR: Evaluation of techniques of esophageal dilatation in relation to the danger of perforation. J Thorac Cardiovasc Surg 45:510, 1963
3. Gans SL, Berci G: Advances in endoscopy of infants and children. J Pediatr Surg 6:199, 1971
4. Gans SL, Berci G: Inside tracheoesophageal fistula. J Pediatr Surg 8:205, 1973

25

Esophagoscopy with Rigid Instruments

Angelo E. Dagradi

The earliest attempts to inspect the interior of the upper gastrointestinal tract by means of instruments utilized hollow metallic tubes. The esophagus, being the most proximally located structure, and because of its relatively straight course, was readily adaptable to examination with such instruments. Although these were originally developed by nonsurgeons, esophagoscopy became an expertise performed by surgeons and especially by those practicing the specialty of ear, nose, and throat.

It was mainly through the studies and efforts of Rudolf Schindler[4] that "medical esophagoscopy" (i.e., the performance of esophagoscopy by the gastroenterologic internist) came into being. This derived from his development of an "optical esophagoscope," which was introduced into the esophagus blindly by the so-called palpatory technique. This instrument consisted of a hollow metallic tube 40 cm in length and with an internal diameter of 9 mm. It was provided with a removable internal obturator having a soft rubber fingertip at its distal end which protruded from the esophagoscope. This permitted its introduction to be performed easily and safely because it enabled the cricopharyngeal sphincter to be disengaged gently. This principle of construction was adapted from Schindler's previously developed "flexible" gastroscope. Following introduction of the instrument into the esophagus, the obturator was removed from the esophagoscope and was replaced by an internal telescope, which provided an excellent view of the interior of the organ. A modification of this telescope was provided with biopsy forceps, which permitted specimens of tissue to be obtained for microscopic examination. Visualization was contingent upon distention of the esophagus with air, insufflated through an air channel by means of a hand-bulb attachment.

Shortly thereafter Hufford[2] devised a modification of the open-tube esophagoscopes of the Jezberg and Jackson types, providing them with the principle of the internal obturator with leading rubber fingertip construction devised by Schindler. This instrument is manufactured by the Eder Instrument Co. and is known as the Eder-Hufford esophagoscope; it replaced the Schindler instrument and became generally accepted by the gastroenterologist-endoscopist. This instrument has been used extensively and has proved its worth. It possesses capabilities the fiberoptic instruments lack.[1] The advent of use of the latter instruments to the exclusion of the former has occasioned the development of a generation of endoscopists described as "autocastrated esophagologists."[3]

The Eder-Hufford esophagoscope is 50 cm long and is calibrated at intervals of 5 cm. (We subcalibrated ours by notchings spaced 1 cm apart.) The calibration is of value for measuring the longitudinal extent of lesions and for locating them during subsequent examinations. The instrument has an external diameter of 13 mm and an internal diameter (for visualization and operation) of 9 mm. The field of vision is magnified ($\times 4$) by a proximally attached telescopic eyepiece, and is illuminated by an incandescent bulb located at the distal end of a light carrier introduced through a specially constructed channel. A fiberoptic light carrier is available and may be used in place of that with the incandescent bulb. Although the former provides more intense illumination, the "softer" quality of light produced by the incandescent bulb is more desirable to many people. The intensity of illumination is controlled by a rheostat. A suction channel for removing secretions from the field of vision is also incorporated in the instrument and is ordinarily adequate for its purpose. However, copious or thick and viscid secretions (especially blood and clots) may be more difficult to remove satisfactorily by this means. These may be evacuated by means of a metallic suction tube of larger diameter introduced through the lumen of the instrument. (For detail see Chapter 5.)

TECHNIQUE

Preparation of the average patient for esophagoscopy is similar to that used for upper gastrointestinal endoscopy. It includes a period of fasting, generally overnight, administration of parenteral medication to relax the patient, and topical medication for local anesthesia of the pharynx, mouth, and tongue.

The stomach must be empty to prevent regurgitation and possible aspiration; the former is annoying because it obscures the visual field and requires removal by suction; the latter may occasion pneumonia, or the patient may expire from asphyxia or cardiac arrest. In selected instances, especially in patients with gastric retention and in those with longstanding achalasia, a clear liquid diet may be prescribed for a period of 2 days and the stomach or the esophagus thoroughly lavaged with a lukewarm solution of sodium bicarbonate (5 percent) prior to esophagoscopy to remove retained food material and secretions.

Satisfactory relaxation of the patient is achieved by intramuscular administration of sodium phenobarbital 120 mg and atropine sulfate 0.4 mg 1 hour prior to the examination, and meperidine hydrochloride 50 to 125 mg one-half hour before the procedure. Topical anesthesia to the mouth and throat is produced by administration of a local agent such as lidocaine hydrochloride (2 percent viscose solution) just prior to instrumentation. Following removal of loose dentures, the patient is instructed to swallow one teaspoonful of this mixture and then alternately to gargle and swish around in his mouth, on eight to ten separate occasions, each of two subsequently administered teaspoonfuls.

The esophagoscopic examination is performed with the patient placed in the standard left lateral position, i.e., lying on his left side with knees flexed and drawn up to his chest. He is instructed to permit his head to hang loosely. It is held and its movements are controlled by the endoscopic assistant.

During the initial introduction of the instrument the head (and chin) of the patient is thrust forward from his body, analogous to the posture of a "craning bird," and his mouth is allowed to fall open. The left index finger of the operator is inserted into the mouth of the patient, and the tip of the instrument is introduced alongside it to the back of the tongue. The rubber leading tip of the obturator is deflected downward by the operator's left index finger, and the instrument is advanced. As it passes through the posterior pharynx and the cricopharyngeal sphincter, the head-holder senses its advance and slowly but progressively extends the patient's head to assist the progress of the instrument.

It is mandatory that the instrument be introduced with the distal beveled surface facing cephalad relative to the patient. This permits it to slide along the arch of the posterior pharynx. If it is introduced in any other position, the bending of the internal obturator creates a hiatus between it and the lip of the distal end of the instrument. When, during advance of the esophagoscope, the two become again opposed after the curve has been traversed, mucosa may be pinched between them. Further advance of the instrument eventuates in avulsion of a strip of mucosa of the posterior pharynx and of the esophagus of varying lengths. The bleeding which ensues may be severe.

Another point of importance is the necessity for maintaining the tip of the instrument in the midline of the patient as it is advanced, as well as for handling the patient and the instrument gently in order to avoid traumatic perforation. Use of force, especially if the tip of the instrument has entered and lodged in a pyriform sinus, can occasion pharyngeal perforation.

When the instrument tip has passed through the cricopharyngeal sphincter, the obturator is removed, the instrument attached with a rubber tube to a suction pump, the light carrier introduced through its proper channel, and the eyepiece loupe magnifier ($\times 4$ magnification) deflected into the viewing position and focused. The instrument is now insinuated distally along the esophagus under direct inspection. As it is advanced the esophageal lumen must be maintained constantly in the center of the visual field. The examiner's left thumb and index finger hold the instrument close to but not touching the incisor teeth (or upper gum in their absence). This functions in the manner of a fulcrum on which the instrument is balanced. Deflection of the instrument to permit a better view in any direction is occasioned only by moving the patient's head. In response to instructions to the head-holder by the examiner, the head is displaced in the various planes depending on the location of the view desired. Thus the upper half of the visual field is observed when the assistant is instructed to displace the head toward the left shoulder of the patient, the lower half by bending it toward the right shoulder, the posterior half by bending (flexing) it forward, and the anterior half by bending (extending) it backward.

In general, the main initial emphasis is to obtain full introduction of the instrument, inspection for diagnosis being accomplished during its withdrawal. The lower segment of the esophagus deviates to the left and anteriorly to approach and traverse the esophageal hiatus of the diaphragm and to enter the gastric fundus. In the patient with a normally positioned stomach (absence of esophageal hiatus sliding hernia), the assistant must be instructed to extend the patient's head backward and to flex it toward the right shoulder as the instrument is advanced to and through the hiatal orifice. It is usually quite helpful to have the patient inspire deeply at this point. This depresses the diaphragm, straightens the lower esophageal segment, and permits the tip of the instrument to advance easily into the stomach.

The gastric mucosa, with its orange-red color and rugal folds, is identified, and as the instrument is slowly withdrawn the esophagogastric mucosal junction comes into view. The margination between the yellow-pink of the esophageal mucosa and the orange-red gastric mucosa is sharply distinctive and readily apparent. The distance of this junction point from the incisor teeth, as a point of reference, should be measured by the calibrations on the instrument. In the normal adult this junction is found at a level of 40 cm or greater. Esophagoscopic examination is not considered complete unless the esophagogastric mucosal junction has been identified. Proximal withdrawal of the instrument demonstrates a pulsating imprint on the anterior wall of the esophagus created by the aortic arch, generally located at the 25 cm level from the incisor teeth. Continued withdrawal of the instrument demonstrates the esophagus to terminate at the 15 cm level from the incisor teeth, the cricopharyngeal sphincter closing over it as it enters the posterior pharynx and is removed.

INDICATIONS FOR ESOPHAGOSCOPY

The competent upper gastrointestinal endoscopist must be experienced in the use of the metallic, open-tube instruments as well as the newer fiberoptic ones. Even though the future of the latter instruments is secure, the capabilities of the endoscopist untrained in the use of the former ones is severely limited. In competent hands esophagoscopic examination performed with the open-tube instrument is equally safe and no less comfortable for the patient than is examination accomplished with the fiberoptic ones.

Esophagoscopic examination is mandatory when symptoms suggest a disorder of the esophagus but the radiologic examination gives negative findings.

1. Foreign body: This includes not only radiolucent objects but radiopaque ones as well, for they too can be overlooked on radiologic examination. A dramatic example was encountered several years ago which emphasized the tragic consequences of failure to perform esophagoscopic examination. A young male accidently swallowed a solitary prosthetic tooth while drinking water. Subsequently he noted mild substernal distress during the act of swallowing and reported the occurrence to his physician. Radiologic studies were made but failed to demonstrate any abnormality of the esophagus. Shortly thereafter the patient's symptoms subsided, and he offered no further complaints. Eighteen months later, however, he suddenly vomited a massive quantity of blood and expired. Autopsy was performed and demonstrated a radiolucent (plastic) tooth to have eroded through the esophagus and into the aorta, causing the exsanguination.

   It is not too uncommon for radiopaque foreign bodies to lodge in the esophagus and to escape detection during radiologic examination. This applies especially to the accidental ingestion of such common objects as fish and chicken bones.
2. Esophagitis: Esophageal mucosal inflammatory disorders, even when severe and extensive, are demonstrated infrequently by x-ray examination.
3. Esophageal hiatus sliding hernia: This disorder, because of its inherent proclivity to occur inter-

mittently, may escape detection on radiologic study. Esophagoscopic examination is frequently of great value in demonstrating this abnormality and its complications.

4. Early carcinoma of the esophagus: Small lesions may produce symptoms but fail to be demonstrated on x-ray examination. They may be readily apparent on esophagoscopic study.
5. Esophageal varices: These submucosally located structures are diagnosed by esophagoscopy with a much higher degree of accuracy than by x-ray examination. In comparison with the former, the latter fails to demonstrate 40 percent of the largest varices.
6. Hemangiomas and lesions of hereditary telangiectasia are easy to visualize during esophagoscopy but are not demonstrable by radiographic methods.

Esophagoscopy permits clarification of the etiology of radiologically demonstrated abnormalities.

1. An x-ray defect that is questionable may be confirmed to be a specific lesion by esophagoscopic inspection.
2. A radiologically demonstrated abnormality may be demonstrated during esophagoscopy to have been a spurious, nonexistent lesion.

Esophagoscopy is indicated for the diagnostic evaluation of patients bleeding from the upper gastrointestinal tract. Use of x-ray for this purpose, in general, represents an exercise in educated guesswork. Esophagoscopic inspection, when accomplished during the phase of active bleeding, readily discloses the bleeding source, which most commonly originates from esophageal varices, erosive esophagitis, or esophageal ulcer.

Esophagoscopy is necessary to establish the presence or absence of injury to the esophagus in patients who have ingested corrosive chemicals by accident or intent. This documentation is all-important for proper management of the patient. The general trend has been to supplant use of the open-tube esophagoscopes by fiberoptic ones, and a complacency has developed in the community of endoscopists relative to this occurrence. While use of the fiberoptic instruments provides satisfactory results in many of the examinations performed for the indications outlined, there are specific instances in which use of the open-tube instruments is indispensible. The latter provide advantages which are lacking in the former.

To the uninitiated the rigid esophagoscopes are undoubtedly formidable in appearance and may seem to be extremely difficult and dangerous to introduce into the esophagus. Actually, however, their construction makes them somewhat safer than their much more flexible fiberoptic counterpart. This derives from the fact that the leading tip of these instruments is tapered, is made of soft rubber, and is more readily controlled by the examiner during its passage through the pharynx and into the esophagus. On the other hand, the leading end of the fiberoptic instruments is blunt and flat, and is consequently not physiologically adapted to disengage a sphincter in gentle fashion. We have encountered instances from time to time where the open-tube instrument could be easily passed into an esophagus when several preceding efforts to introduce a fiberoptic one had failed.

In the presence of active bleeding from the esophagus it is usually impossible to clear the blood from the distal viewing surface of the fiberoptic instruments, rendering the examination of little or no value. The open-tube instruments permit ready identification of the bleeding source, since blood can be rapidly cleared from the field of vision by means of a large-bore metal suction tube introduced through the lumen of the instrument while the latter is insinuated distally to the bleeding source. The field of vision can also be cleared by instilling ice water through the tube via a bulb syringe and removing it by suction. Furthermore, the mucosal surface can be wiped clean with cotton applicators introduced into the esophagus, and packing can be used to assist in the control of bleeding.

The open-tube instruments can accommodate the passage of biopsy forceps of decent size. This permits tissue specimens to be obtained for microscopic examination that are much larger and more adequate for diagnosis than those obtainable through the fiberoptic instruments. Moreover, the specimens can be secured and removed under clearer conditions of observation, since the examination is not hampered by the need to continuously clear blood from the distal viewing surface as is necessary when fiberoptic instruments are used.

Foreign bodies lodged in the esophagus usually can be removed readily via the open-tube esophagoscopes. As a general rule, the fiberoptic instruments are not only inadequate for this purpose but can cause injury to the patient.

When severely narrowed esophageal strictures are encountered during examination, their dilatation can be initiated immediately if the open-tube instrument is used by successively introducing filiform Jackson-type bougies (up to 28 Fr) through its lumen. This is not possible if fiberoptic instruments are used.

The calibrations on the rigid esophagoscope permit accurate localization and mensuration of the longitudinal extent of lesions (varices, ulcer, esophagitis, neoplasms, etc.) by reference to the incisor teeth or front upper gum of the patient. Because of the flexibility of the fiberoptic instruments, there is a variable degree of accuracy in localizing a lesion by use of their calibrations.

The identification of esophageal varices is more accurate when observation is made through the open-tube instruments. This is due to several factors operating alone or in combination. Of great importance is the factor of intraesophageal pressure. When the open-tube instruments are used, the pressure exerted on the wall of the esophagus (and hence on the submucosally located varices) is constant (atmospheric pressure) since the cricopharyngeus sphincter is kept open by the instrument. When examination is done with fiberoptic instruments, the esophagus is a closed tube and the insufflated air causes the intraesophageal pressure to vary greatly, even exceeding 25 mm Hg. This pressure compresses the varices, reduces their size, and can even cause them to become ablated if its degree of magnitude exceeds that of their internal pressure. Another important factor is the intensity of illumination. A bright light such as that provided by the fiberoptic instruments can "burn out" the color characteristics of varices, rendering them less conspicuous. The same applies to the mucosal changes occurring in esophagitis. These are more readily apparent when viewed through the rigid instrument and are more prone to escape detection when the fiberoptic instrument is used.

Another advantage of the metallic esophagoscopes is the fact that they are much more easy to sterilize between examinations than are the fiberoptic instruments. They can be subjected to temperatures of sufficient magnitude to destroy disease-producing organisms. This is impossible with the more delicate fiberoptic instruments. For this reason, their potential for transmitting diseases such as viral hepatitis is a source for great concern among gastrointestinal endoscopists.

The construction of the open-tube instruments is so simple that they are practically indestructible; very little of a mechanical nature can go wrong with them. We have used the same esophagoscope for many thousands of esophagoscopies over a period exceeding 15 years. The only structural damage sustained by the instrument during this time was the creation of a tiny hole in the aspirating channel when a patient bit into it. This was easily repaired with a bit of solder. When the fiberoptic instruments are used, however, even when reasonable care is exercised, periodic repairs at the factory are unavoidable, involving expense as well as loss of the use of the instrument for varying periods of time.

Finally, training endoscopists to develop an expertise in the use of the open-tube instruments provides them with an invaluable ability to sense the mechanics of the posterior pharynx and cricopharyngeal sphincter and to develop the respect, familiarity, and touch so essential for the easy and safe introduction of instruments along this delicate region.

CONTRAINDICATIONS

There are few contraindications to the use of endoscopic instruments for examining the esophagus and certainly none which favor the use of fiberoptic over open-tube instruments. The contraindications were categorized originally as being either absolute or relative. The accumulation of experience over the years has served to eliminate almost all of the absolute contraindications. Esophageal varices were considered to be in this category at one time because it was feared that instrumentation would cause them to rupture and bleed seriously. However, when it became apparent that untoward reactions seldom if ever occurred during such examinations in patients having previously unsuspected large and extensive esophageal varices, the absolute contraindication to the use of these instruments was accordingly modified. Today an experienced examiner can perform esophagoscopic examinations in patients having huge esophageal varices without fear of any serious consequences from the procedure. As a matter of fact and as previously mentioned, the esophagoscopic method is so much more highly reliable than the radiologic method for demonstrating esophageal varices that the suspicion of their existence in a given patient is sufficient indication to warrent esophagoscopic examination.

Similarly, the patient unable to cooperate was once considered to represent an absolute contraindication to esophagoscopic examination. However, the development of relatively simple methods for performing this procedure under general anesthesia and, more recently, adoption of the use of Valium administered intravenously have succeeded in eliminating this type of patient from the list of absolute contraindications.

The *absolute contraindications* to esophagoscopy are:

1. Patients with large Zenker's diverticulum. These outpouchings occur just below the cricopharyngeal sphincter and are thin-walled (consisting only of mucosa and submucosa). They are easily perforated during blind introduction of instruments because as they enlarge the diverticular sac displaces the esophagus forward while it assumes a position of alignment with the pharynx such that instruments, as well as ingested food, enter them directly. These diverticula have been perforated by as innocuous an item as an 18 Fr soft rubber nasogastric tube.
2. Patients with large aneurysms of the thoracic aorta. Instrumentation may cause traumatic rupture of such lesions when they are large and thin-walled.
3. Acute pharyngeal inflammation of infectious origin. Instrumentation in such cases may occasion aggravation and spread of the infection and should be postponed until the inflammation has subsided.

The *relative contraindications* to esophagoscopy include such conditions as acute myocardial infarction, peripheral vascular collapse states, psychosis, severe dyspnea, etc.

COMPLICATIONS

The hazards and danger associated with esophagoscopic instrumentation include perforation and reactions to the premedications. In our experience instrumental perforations have been quite rare (Table 1). They are produced in one of three areas. The most frequent site for

TABLE 1. "Open-Tube" Esophagoscopy

Parameter	No.
Examinations	9,000 (approx.)
Perforations	6 (0.007%)
Location of perforations	
Cervix (hypopharyngeal)*	3
Distal third of esophagus*	2
Gastric fundus	1

Operated and survived.

the occurrence of this mishap is the hypopharynx; less common in occurrence is perforation of the distal third of the esophagus; and least common is perforation of the stomach. The occurrence of such an accident is usually apparent as soon as it is produced. It occasions pain of varying degree, at times associated with peripheral vascular collapse, and is followed shortly thereafter by the finding on physical examination of crepitations in the skin of the neck and upper thorax and/or pneumomediastinum, pneumothorax, or pneumoperitoneum produced by the escape of air into the tissues from the site of perforation.

Gastric perforation may be treated successfully by nonsurgical means, including administration of antibiotics and decompression of the stomach with a nasogastric tube. Hypopharyngeal and distal esophageal perforations, however, are most properly treated by surgical intervention, suturing the perforation and instituting drainage of the injured site. Since the advent of antibiotic drugs, mortality is rare when such mishaps occur and morbidity is generally mild.

Reactions to the premedications are a matter of individual susceptibility and are treated as they occur.

REFERENCES

1. Dagradi AE: In defense of the flexirigid (open-tube) esophagoscope (editorial). Gastrointest Endosc 17:101, 1971
2. Hufford AR: Flexirigid optical esophagoscope. Gastroenterology 12:779, 1949
3. Palmer ED: Commentary. JAMA 227:511, 1974
4. Schindler R: A safe diagnostic optical esophagoscope. JAMA 138:885, 1948

26

Flexible Fiberoptic Esophagoscopy

Melvin Schapiro

Flexible fiberoptic esophagoscopy is an outgrowth of the technical advancements of fiberoptic gastroscopy. The first successful esophagoscope was described in 1881 by Mikulicz.[18] This open metal tube instrument has undergone a variety of modifications by many prominent endoscopists and remains in use today.

Hirschowitz in 1962, 5 years after his demonstration of the side-viewing, flexible fiberoptic gastroscope,[11] introduced a forward-viewing fiberoptic esophagoscope.[10] This instrument lacked flexibility of the tip and could not negotiate the normal distal esophageal angle. LoPresti and Hilmi soon modified this instrument by changing the lens system, producing the "foreward oblique" fiberoptic esophagoscope.[15] The Olympus model EF esophagoscope introduced in 1969[21] had the short flexible tip controllable from the proximal end, enabling direct advancement along the esophageal lumen. The addition of fingertip control for suction, air insufflation, and water injection greatly facilitated the endoscopic procedure. It was not long before this basic design was lengthened for a forward-viewing evaluation of the stomach and duodenum creating the pan-upper gastrointestinal endoscope of today.[16,17]

The 35-degree field of view of the original fiberscope has been increased to 70 degrees. The tip is capable of deflection in four directions up to 180 degrees, allowing a satisfactory intragastric turnaround view of the cardioesophageal junction. Light transmission is of such caliber as to allow high quality still and motion picture photography. Channels for passage of forceps, snares, brushes, loops, and electrocautery tubes have been improved, allowing an ever-increasing number of operative techniques.

FLEXIBLE FIBEROPTIC ESOPHAGOSCOPY

Fiberoptic endoscopes designed primarily for esophageal examinations are available but for practical purposes have been replaced by the fiberoptic pan-upper gastrointestinal endoscope (Chapter 28). This instrument differs from the fiberoptic esophagoscope primarily in having a greater length. With it, a complete examination of the esophagus from the cricopharyngeus to the cardia, including both the esophageal and gastric sides, is possible in nearly all patients (Fig. 1).

The main advantages of these flexible fiberoptic instruments are the high frequency of successful intubation, completeness of esophageal examination, increased patient comfort compared to the rigid esophagoscopes, and low incidence of complications.[13]

Fiberoptic esophagoscopy requires a sacrifice in capability of working through the larger passageway of the open rigid endoscopes. The channel for suction of the fiberoptic instruments allows passage of biopsy forceps, cytology brushes, and guide wires for esophageal dilators. Biopsy specimens, however, are smaller and more superficial. Multiple specimens therefore are required to sample an area adequately. Strictures cannot be dilated with direct vision; and foreign body removal—though performed with increasing efficiency

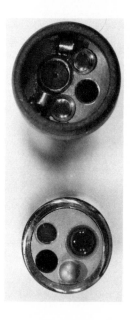

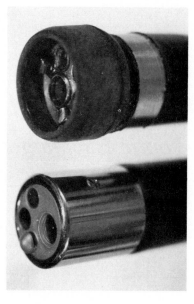

FIG. 1. Tip of flexible fiberoptic pan-upper gastrointestinal endoscope. Top, Olympus GIF-D. Bottom, ACMI F-8.

with newer forceps, loops, and graspers—is often more practical with the larger open-channel, rigid instruments. Some doubt exists about the ability to perform a satisfactory evaluation for esophageal varices with fiberoptic instruments.[22] The characteristic variceal appearance identified with open esophagoscopes is modified by the fiberoptic bundle. The additional examination time, more comprehensive evaluation of esophageal motility and folds, as well as the awareness of the color changes produced by fiberoptic bundles may more than compensate and allow for accurate diagnosis.[4,32]

Technique

Before beginning intubation the fully connected instrument should be checked for satisfactory function of the light, tip deflection, air, suction, and water channels. A bite guard should be slipped over the instrument for the patient with teeth. The biopsy forceps should be checked and the appropriate materials for biopsy and cytology collections made ready.

The first stage of passage of fiberoptic endoscopes is a blind intubation of the instrument through the cricopharyngeus. This blind passage may be initiated with the patient in the sitting position or lying on either side. The index and middle fingers of one hand are inserted into the mouth and depress the tongue far forward. The instrument is guided over and

between these fingers down to the cricopharyngeus, and the patient is instructed to swallow. Intubation through the cricopharyngeus is often easier with the patient swallowing in a sitting position. However, the effects of premedication, tendency for less apprehension while lying comfortably, and elimination of an extra movement to lie the patient down has made intubation in the lateral position a common procedure. An occasional intubation through the cricopharyngeus is not possible in this position.

Although intubation in the sitting position may be successful, a few patients still exhibit failure to relax the cricopharyngeus. Additional intravenous medication may be administered and the instrument passed to the area of hold-up. The spastic opening of the cricopharyngeus may be visualized and negotiated with gentle pressure while waiting and watching for a swallow.[28] Alternatively, a forceps or wire guide may be passed through the suction channel of the instrument and introduced through the cricopharyngeus as the patient swallows. The instrument may then be passed over this guide using steady, gentle pressure. Direct visualization may be used while passing through the cricopharyngeus.[8] When it is apparent that these maneuvers are not successful the procedure should be terminated and the patient studied again with x-ray to look for an unsuspected lesion. Diverticula and high stenosing lesions are the most frequent causes for unsuccessful intubation. Failure of passage of the pan-upper gastrointestinal fiberoptic endoscope in the absence of a defined lesion occurs in less than 1 percent of the cases.

Once passage is accomplished beyond the cricopharyngeus the bite guard, if necessary, is brought into position. In some patients there is a tendency to bite down immediately on intubation. The danger to both the endoscope and the examiner's fingers may then require that passage through the cricopharyngeus be done with the bite guard in place.

The instrument is guided with direct vision, usually keeping a full view of the esophageal lumen, by controlling the tip. Enough air is insufflated to maintain distention of the lumen, though constant air insufflation is to be avoided. Mucus and other fluid material may be removed through the suction channel, and if necessary the lens cleared with a jet of fluid. Occasionally the lumen is not seen well, but the mucosa is noted to glide by easily as intubation is continued with gentle pressure. This forward passage may be continued for a short distance and then reversed. With additional tip deflection the lumen often appears promptly.

The instrument is advanced either to the area in question or to the cardiac sphincter, usually at a level of 40 cm from the teeth. The cardiac opening may vary in size but in the absence of such conditions as achalasia is rarely closed. An appreciation of the color change from the glistening pink of esophageal mucosa to a slightly duller orange of gastric mucosa is readily observed. A more satisfactory examination of the esophagus is possible later when withdrawing the instrument. In the absence of endoscopic change at the cardioesophageal junction the instrument is advanced into the fundus of the stomach by bringing the opening of the cardiac sphincter into direct view and exerting gentle pressure.

The endoscope is turned around in the stomach so that a view of the cardioesophageal junction from the gastric side is obtained (Chapter 28). The mucosa is inspected, folds suggestive of gastric varices examined, and the diameter of the cardioesophageal opening compared to that of the instrument.

The instrument is again straightened and, while carefully inspecting, slowly withdrawn through and to an area just above the cardiac sphincter. At this point esophageal motility at the sphincter may be appreciated.

Further withdrawal gives a view of the tubular esophagus with an excellent appreciation of the symmetry of the walls. The longitudinal mucosal folds with varying degrees of prominence are seen and may form a rosette pattern. Peristaltic activity may best be studied with this tubular view. A pulsatile extrinsic pressure defect on the left anterior wall at 20 to 25 cm is frequently seen and represents the aortic arch.

Visualization of the nondilated esophagus is complete, without blind areas, from the cardioesophageal junction through the cricopharyngeus. Although examination of the distal pharynx above the cricopharyngeus is difficult, visual inspection of this area is frequently continued as the instrument is withdrawn from the patient.

A lesion or esophageal mucosal surface chosen for biopsy is brought as close to on-face view as possible and held in view by locking the controls. Any mucus or exudative material obscuring the area may be washed and aspirated with the water and suction controls of the instrument, or a catheter may be passed through the suction channel and direct lavage carried out.

The biopsy forceps with jaws closed is passed through the suction channel, and when in view the jaws are opened. The forceps are pressed firmly against the area, closed, and removed. This effects a mucosal tear or superficial surface biopsy. Because the shallow biopsy specimen rarely returns submucosal tissue, attempts are made to sample mucosal areas showing visible change. Multiple biopsies (frequently eight to ten) are taken from a lesion in question.

Material for cytologic studies may be obtained by direct washings through a polyethylene catheter passed through the suction channel. We have found, however, that this is a cumbersome procedure with relatively poor return of the washing fluid. A more productive technique is passage of the cytology brush through the suction channel and directly brushing the area at the termination of the procedure. The brush is withdrawn just into the tip of the instrument but not deeply into the channel. The instrument with brush in place is removed from the patient and the brush immediately streaked on the prepared cytology slides. If the brush is withdrawn through the channel before the slides are prepared, there is a loss of cytologic material and contamination with cellular material present from the esophageal aspirations.

Indications

The two primary indications for esophagoscopy are to evaluate upper gastrointestinal bleeding and to establish the malignant or benign nature of a defect. Despite the fact that endoscopic diagnostic procedures and cytology collections are easily and accurately performed, most patients with esophageal malignancy present at an advanced stage and so with a poor prognosis. Any esophageal symptom (particularly dysphagia) present for 7 to 10 days, even in the face of a "normal esophagram" should be evaluated with endoscopy.

Esophageal varices are most frequently diagnosed by endoscopy, and the emergent endoscopic evaluation for gastrointestinal bleeding requires accurate esophageal inspection. Additional indications include operative endoscopic techniques such as foreign body removal, passage of wires through strictures, fracture of webs or rings, cauterization of polypoid or bleeding lesions, injection of sclerosing solutions into esophageal varices, injection of chemotherapeutic agents into neoplasms, and coagulation loop polypectomy.

Although motility disorders of the esophagus are diagnosed more satisfactorily by manometric and ciné radiologic studies, endoscopic examination of these conditions not infrequently reveals significant pathology. Esophagitis with esophageal spasm, and the unsuspected esophageal carcinoma in the patient with achalasia, are experiences encountered by most active esophagoscopists.

Contraindications

The problems of mouth size, kyphosis, and vertebral spurring that relate to the passage of rigid esophagoscopes have been considerably reduced with the advent of the fiberoptic instruments. Old age is no longer a contraindication.[1] Fiber bundles of very small diameter have been constructed into pediatric endoscopes. In addition to their use in children, these pediatric-type instruments may be tried in special circumstances in the adult when some compromise of lumen size precludes use of standard instruments.[19] The presence of known esophageal varices does not represent a contraindication to esophagoscopy, as variceal rupture and subsequent bleeding has been shown not to be a complication of the endoscopic procedure.[14]

The contraindications to fiberoptic esophagoscopy are in general relative ones and related to the value of the potential information to be obtained in view of the patient's clinical condition. Medical problems such as pneumonia, peritonitis, or acute myocardial infarction should be cared for first, and esophagoscopy carried out electively. Not infrequently, however, the urgency of the situation (e.g., acute gastrointestinal bleeding without obvious cause) requires esophagoscopy in the presence of these medical conditions. The risk to the patient is increased, but rarely enough to contraindicate the endoscopic procedure.

An additional relative contraindication is a hypopharyngeal or Zenker's diverticulum because of the tendency on blind intubation to pass the instrument into the thin-walled diverticulum and bring about its rupture. Optimal care is taken on intubation to avoid pressure. The cricopharyngeus may be passed using a string or wire guide without the use of air insufflation. In this fashion intubation may be accomplished safely in most patients with these diverticula.

Esophageal diverticulum beyond the area of blind intubation should not be a contraindication. Direct visual passage is done with care to see that the instrument does not engage the diverticulum sac with subsequent blind pressure against its wall.

A thoracic aortic aneurysm has been an absolute contraindication to rigid esophagoscopy because of the risk of rupture. These aneurysms still represent a relative contraindication, although with proper sedation to avoid undue retching and with the smaller-diameter pediatric-type endoscopes esophagoscopy might be attempted under special circumstances.

Recent abdominal surgery represents a relative contraindication because of the tendency for the insufflated air to bring about organ and abdominal distention with separation of suture lines. When necessary esophagoscopy may be carried out by applying an abdominal binder and exercising care in the amount of insufflated air.

The question of performing endoscopy on a patient with a positive test for hepatitis-associated antigen (HAA) is by no means settled. The determination of HAA is not a regular preendoscopic procedure, and there is no controlled clinical or experimental evidence documenting transmission of hepatitis in this fashion. Theoretically the possibility exists, however, and in view of the inability to sterilize the instruments rapidly against HB virus, it is best to try to avoid the procedure when the patient is known to be HAA-positive.

Preparation of Patient

Wherever possible, barium radiologic studies should be performed and reviewed before all endoscopic examinations. The endoscopist then can concentrate on areas of radiologic concern while performing the general endoscopic survey. In addition, unexpected pathology requiring special care in passage of the instrument will be known.

Emergency upper gastrointestinal endoscopy in the bleeding patient is frequently performed without radiologic studies. Washout of the stomach to clear blood clots and slow bleeding is often performed through a large-bore nasogastric tube while the patient and instruments are being readied. Although direct examination of the esophagus rarely requires washout of blood clots, the endoscopic procedure is carried on to include the stomach and duodenum. A satisfactory turnaround examination is not possible when the gastric side of the cardioesophageal junction is obscured with blood.

Since routine esophagoscopy with gastric turnaround views requires an empty stomach, patients are kept fasting after a regular diet on the evening before the examination. When difficulty in gastric emptying is suspected, clear liquids are utilized for 24 to 48 hours prior to the examination. If the examination is to be delayed until the afternoon, a clear liquid breakfast is allowed and the patient kept fasting thereafter. The general details of the procedure—its indications, potential complications, and possible alternatives—should be discussed with the patient by the endoscopist on the day before the procedure and a signed consent obtained.

A pharmacologic program depends on the medical status of the patient. Some young, apprehensive individuals who have been exposed to a number of drugs in the past, may require very large doses of analgesic and sedative drugs to reach the level of desired sedation. Other individuals, particularly the aged, are easily oversedated with small doses of parenteral drugs.

Generally 180 to 300 mg sodium luminal combined with 50 to 100 mg meperidine administered by injection 20 to 30 minutes before the procedure is sufficient. Intravenous diazepam, administered slowly while continuously talking to the patient, is very helpful in titrating to a level of desired sedation. The endpoint is a drowsy state with thickness of speech and delayed response to questions. The average dose is 10 to 15 mg; however, extreme sedation and apnea may be encountered in older individuals, even without prior medication.

Since the use of intravenous diazepam has become so commonplace, we have not found the need for pharyngeal swabbing, spraying, or gargling with tetracaine or similar topical anesthesia. A gargle with a small amount of 0.5 percent tetracaine may be helpful in occasional apprehensive patients. When the endoscopist reassures the patient and explains the procedure in detail, the level of anxiety is frequently diminished and the premedication dosage considerably reduced.[12]

Anticholinergics (e.g., atropine) may be included in the premedication program in an attempt to decrease salivary secretion. Whether there are additional benefits to the cardiocirculatory system through its action on the vasovagal reflex is debatable. Contraindications to the use of these drugs are well known, and in general we have not found their routine use particularly beneficial.

Esophagitis

Inflammation of the esophageal mucosa and submucosa is not reliably diagnosed endoscopically in the absence of mucosal ulcerations or erosions. The color change of the esophageal mucosa from that of pink-yellow to deeper red, suggesting erythema, occurs not only with esophagitis but also with ectopic columnar or gastric-type epithelium and depends on the variability of the light. For these reasons the diagnosis of nonerosive esophagitis depends on mucosal biopsy. The optical system of the fiberoptic endoscopes allows very close inspection of the fine detail of the esophageal mucosal surface. This surface normally appears with a vascular network of fine red lines.[9] Loss of this fine pattern—associated with erythema, erosions, ulcerations, or nodularity—is found with varying degrees of esophagitis.

When the mucosa bleeds easily on contact with the endoscope or forceps, biopsy usually reveals esophagitis. The most characteristic appearance of chronic reflux esophagitis is that of white plaques of various configurations surrounded by an erythematous border and frequently in a longitudinal distribution on the esophageal folds. Acute erosions and ulcerations may be lacking in exudate and reveal only a friable erythematous base (Figs. 2 and 3, Plate B).*

A cobblestone appearance of the mucosa often associated with a patchy erythema and adherent mucus may be seen with the inflammation of Crohn's disease affecting the esophagus. This endoscopic picture is by no means characteristic and is more frequently found with reflux esophagitis. Further, granulomatous esophagitis may be associated with a normal endoscopic appearance and therefore requires biopsy for diagnosis. The usual superficial biopsy specimens are frequently of insufficient depth to sample the area satisfactorily for the characteristic granulomas. Multiple specimens are taken, and when necessary deeper specimens are obtained using larger forceps through open, rigid instruments or with blind biopsy capsules under fluoroscopic guidance.

Neoplasms of the Esophagus

Most esophageal lesions are highly suspect as carcinoma from the clinical and radiologic presentation. The role of esophagoscopy for these lesions is primarily to obtain tissue for verification of the diagnosis.

The endoscopic appearance of carcinoma of the esophagus is usually that of a friable, occasionally ulcerating, polypoid lesion. A nodular, friable, eroded, and stiffened mucosa is usually seen with submucosally stenosing carcinomas. A stenosing carcinoma may, however, appear endoscopically as a benign stricture. The surrounding mucosa frequently reveals the gross and biopsy appearance of esophagitis. Multiple biopsies taken by passing the forceps into the stricture frequently reveal the tumor tissue, as the surface mucosa is more apt to be eroded within the stricture. Cytologic brushing of friable nodular areas, as well as within the stricture itself, increases the yield of positive diagnosis significantly. Occasionally stenosing carcinomas have an entirely submucosal infiltrating appearance. Here superficial esopha-

gitis occurs frequently and often obscures the diagnosis. Multiple biopsies and cytologic studies are usually negative for tumor cells. When the clinical or radiologic appearance is suspicious, additional deeper biopsy material should be obtained with the open esophagoscope or blind biopsy capsules.

Submucosal neoplasms, often arising in the fundus of the stomach, may infiltrate the cardioesophageal junction and present clinically and endoscopically as achalasia. The cardioesophageal junction appears closed with prominent mucosal folds, often as a rosette. Mucosal change, when present, suggests esophagitis, and biopsies are usually negative for malignancy. The instrument can usually be passed through the junction into the fundus of the stomach; but unlike achalasia, where resistance to passage through the junction is minimal, there is an elasticlike resistance often felt with submucosal tumor infiltration. The turnaround maneuver should be performed and any suspicious areas of the fundus of the stomach biopsied. Deeper biopsies, however, are usually required for diagnosis.

Benign esophageal leiomyomas, lipomas, or neurofibromas may be seen as smooth, round or irregular polypoid lesions, often submucosal with normal movable overlying mucosa. The biopsy forceps may freely move the mucosa over the surface of the tumor. Biopsy reveals only normal esophageal tissue. When the lesion protrudes extramucosally into the lumen or is an adenomatous polyp, biopsy is possible though the superficial tissue usually requires that multiple or deeper specimens be obtained for more accurate diagnosis.

Esophageal cysts appear as benign submucosal tumors. A cystic feel and indentation may be found by probing it with the biopsy forceps.

Stricture

Benign compromise of the esophageal lumen may involve any area of the esophagus. When the segment involved comprises several centimeters the endoscopic picture is that of a funnel-shaped narrowing with a smooth, rounded orifice of variable diameter relating to the severity of the stenosis.

The surrounding mucosa above the peptic stricture of gastroesophageal reflux frequently reveals changes of erosive esophagitis (Fig. 4,

All color plates appear at the front of the book.

Plate B). The mucosa, however, may appear endoscopically quite normal, especially when associated with the presence of columnar or ectopic gastric-type epithelium below the area of narrowing (Fig. 3, Plate B). These strictures are frequently located in the mid to upper third of the esophagus. An irregular fingerlike color change from glistening pink to dull orange or red may be seen above the orifice of the stricture and represent a transition from squamous to columnar mucosa. More frequently the orifice is a smooth, shiny, thin, white ring. Biopsy of this ring may reveal both squamous and columnar epithelium representing the junction.

Stenosis of the esophagus related to previous lye ingestion or to irradiation appears endoscopically identical to that of reflux esophagitis. The mucosal appearance relates to the interval of healing from the irritating agent.

Very thin, sometimes irregular or eccentric ringlike narrowings are not uncommonly seen in the terminal esophagus at the junction of the gastric and columnar epithelium. The degree of narrowing may be high grade, and the surrounding mucosa may show evidence of esophagitis. When the degree of lumen compromise is enough to promote clinical dysphagia, the ring frequently appears as a thin, shiny, white fibrous band (Fig. 5, Plate B).

Esophageal webs are not often visualized intact with the endoscope, as their usual occurrence, high in the esophageal inlet, is associated with their fracture or intubation. The remnant may be seen on withdrawal of the instrument as a thin, superficial erosion or hemorrhagic tag with normal surrounding mucosa.

Carcinoma may submucosally infiltrate and stenose the esophagus with an endoscopic appearance indistinguishable from that of a benign stricture. Diagnosis depends on appropriate biopsy and cytologic techniques (*Neoplasms of the Esophagus,* above).

Esophageal Varices

Submucosal veins of sufficient prominence to elevate the esophageal mucosa are identified radiologically and endoscopically as esophageal varices (Fig. 6, Plate B). Peristaltic activity produces folds of varying prominence that may be confused with esophageal varices. During the performance of fiberoptic esophagoscopy, the nearly constant insufflation of air distends the esophagus and compresses the mucosa thereby tending to obscure the smaller varices that may be more frequently identified with open-tube esophagoscopy. In addition, the color transmission of the fiber bundle tends to attenuate the natural bluish hue of prominent varices, producing an orange-red coloration resembling that of normal mucosal folds.[4] The magnified image produced by the fiberoptic endoscope is not uniform and depends to a large extent on the distance of the image from the instrument. Folds lying close to the instrument tip may appear quite prominent and tortuous, giving the appearance of varices.

However, the overall quality of the image, clarity of the total view, and the additional time allowed for study with the use of fiberoptic endoscopes allows for the diagnosis of varices with an accuracy of about 85 percent, a figure that compares well with that of open-tube endoscopy in experienced hands.[4,32]

Dagradi et al.[5] described criteria for the endoscopic differentiation of esophageal varices from esophageal folds (Table 1). These criteria are of value for both fiberoptic and open-tube endoscopes though in their hands seem somewhat more accurate in individual cases using open esophagoscopes.

Hiatus Hernia

Sliding-type hiatal hernias are identified with a high degree of accuracy with flexible fiberoptic endoscopes.[30] The diagnosis of a hiatus hernia by open-tube esophagoscopy depends almost entirely on the distance from the incisor teeth. Their detection with fiberoptic instruments is facilitated by the ability to identify accurately the indentation produced by the diaphragmatic hiatus.

When the mucosal change identifying the esophagogastric junction is seen to lie above the diaphragmatic hiatus impression, a hiatus hernia is present. This occurs less than 38 cm from the teeth, and with moderate to large hernias is associated with visualization of a portion of the hernia pouch. Although identification of a hiatus hernia is frequently made on intubation and the initial approach to the diaphragmatic hiatus, accuracy is considerably increased by inspection on withdrawing the instrument.

The intragastric turnaround maneuver usu-

TABLE 1.   Endoscopic Criteria Differentiating Esophageal Varices from Esophageal Folds

Criterion	Esophageal Varices	Esophageal Folds
Tortuosity	Present	Absent
Nodularity	Present	Absent
Caliber	Diminishes progressively in orad direction	Usually unchanged and terminates abruptly
Color	May be off-colored gray or bluish	Color of esophageal mucosa
Mucosal crinkling	Present	Absent
"Cherry spots"	Present in largest varices	Absent
Cross esophageal-gastric junction	Yes	No
Esophageal peristalsis	Persist	Ablate
Deep inspiration	Persist	Ablate
Valsalva	Intensify	Do not
Air distention	May or may not ablate	Ablate

From Dagradi et al: Am J Gastroenterol 60:240, 1973.

ally visualizes the cardia satisfactorily with the end-on-viewing pan-upper gastrointestinal endoscopes, although the view is sometimes more satisfactorily obtained with the 90-degree viewing gastroscope.

The gastric mucosa of the cardia normally surrounds the endoscope snugly as it exits from the esophagus into the stomach. The presence of a hiatus hernia is indicated by a widened opening having a variety of shapes with a total diameter exceeding twice the diameter of the endoscope as it passes through the cardia.[26]

Upon completion of the turnaround evaluation, the instrument is slowly withdrawn above the diaphragmatic indentation, where in the presence of a hiatus hernia the continuation of gastric-type mucosa is appreciated. The margin of the hernia is seen as a semilunar curve of gastric mucosa that descends with inspiration and rises with expiration. Additional air insufflation generally allows inspection of the hernia sac at this time.

Demonstration of a paraesophageal hiatus hernia is not possible on routine esophagoscopy but may be made at the time of the intragastric turnaround study. This is accomplished by identifying an additional pouch separated by a mucosal bridge from the cardia containing the exiting endoscope.

Esophageal Diverticulum

Smooth, rounded, saclike openings with necks of varying sizes may be found at any level of the esophagus. The mucosal appearance reflects that of the surrounding mucosa, though occasionally large sacs with superficial erosions or ulcerations are seen. Small, narrowed neck diverticula are frequently missed as the openings are visualized tangentially and tend to be lost among folds or obscured by contraction waves.

Hypopharyngeal or Zenker's diverticula are rarely visualized with blind intubation of the flexible esophagoscope. When their presence is ascertained by preendoscopic radiologic studies, esophagoscopy may be contraindicated for fear of perforation (*Contraindications,* above).

Motility Disorders

The disorders of esophageal motility (including esophageal spasm, scleroderma, achalasia, and allied disturbances of cardioesophageal sphincter function) are rarely diagnosed by esophagoscopy without associated radiologic or manometric studies. Factors such as air insufflation, psychologic status, and premedication so vary esophageal peristaltic activity that normal patterns are rarely identified.

A dilated esophagus is easily identified regardless of its cause. Normally as the instrument approaches the cardioesophageal junction, the sphincter is open allowing a view of the gastric mucosa with its characteristic color change. The association of dilated esophagus with a closed sphincter whose folds converge in a rosette pattern and require gentle pressure on the instrument for passage through the cardioesophageal junction is highly suspicious of achalasia (Fig. 7, Plate B). Retention of food particles, mucosal erythema, and superficial erosions of esophagitis are frequent accompaniments in longstanding cases.

The presence of an unsuspected ulcerating or polypoid carcinoma in the esophagus of achalasia occurs with such frequency as to require a careful cleaning and examination of the entire dilated esophagus. Endoscopic examination of the markedly dilated "sigmoid" esophagus for carcinoma is frequently inadequate and capable of revealing only the larger advanced polypoid carcinomas.

Vigorous nonprogressive high-pressure waves characteristic of esophageal spasm may occasionally be visualized in both normal individuals and patients symptomatic of esophageal spasm. The irregular distribution of the muscular contractions may distort the mucosa, producing a pseudodiverticular appearance with sacculations appearing in constant location but tending to flatten or disappear between contractions.

The endoscopic appearance of scleroderma of the esophagus is not specific, though it may resemble achalasia when the motility disorder affecting relaxation of the cardiac sphincter occurs. The mucosal appearance is usually normal, though subtle changes in coloration secondary to submucosal infiltration or associated esophageal irritation and esophagitis may occur.

Esophageal Bleeding

Emergency endoscopy for upper gastrointestinal hemorrhage includes inspection of the esophagus. Use of the pan-upper gastrointestinal fiberscope in most cases avoids the need for multiple instruments, though occasional cases of brisk hemorrhage from the esophagus or cardia of the stomach require open esophagoscopes to handle better the blood clots that tend to fill the field of vision.

The bleeding lesions of esophageal carcinoma, esophageal ulcerations, or erosive esophagitis are readily recognized. Esophageal varices may be identified by the usual criteria (*Esophageal Varices*, above); however, their coincidental presence with an additional source of upper gastrointestinal hemorrhage (e.g., gastritis or peptic ulceration) in the alcoholic patient requires additional observation for the source of blood loss.

Nonbleeding esophageal varices may be confused as the source of blood loss when active gastroesophageal reflux of bloody gastric contents covers the field and coats the varices. A discrete blood clot, often with a surrounding ooze of fresh blood and frequently associated with changes of erosive esophagitis over the nodular varices, is compatible with variceal bleeding.

When the endoscopic procedure is performed in the bleeding patient following intubation with a tube that effects cardioesophageal tamponade, superficial oozing mucosal tears are often identified at the region of previous pressure. These lesions, occurring on folds or actual esophageal varices, should not be taken as the primary source of bleeding without further exclusion. Prolonged nasogastric tube intubation also frequently produces an associated erosive esophagitis. This lesion alone is often the primary source of blood loss but must not be considered as such until other sites are excluded. Acute nasogastric intubation for gastric lavage prior to the endoscopic procedure is rarely associated with endoscopic esophageal change but may produce superficial gastric erosions, including some at the cardia of the stomach. For this reason we prefer to initiate the emergency endoscopic examination without prior gastric lavage whenever possible.

The esophagus is grossly examined to the cardioesophageal junction. Note is made of the presence or absence of blood and, if present, its relationship to possible reflux. When no bleeding lesions are identified the instrument is passed through the cardia, carefully evaluating the junctional ring and proximal gastric mucosa for erosive gastritis or cardioesophageal tears (Mallory-Weiss lesion). When the stomach is found to contain excessive quantities of blood and clots not allowing for satisfactory additional gastroduodenoscopic examination, including turnaround views, the instrument is removed and gastric intubation carried out with an appropriate large-bore gastric tube followed by ice water lavage.

The endoscopic demonstration of blood loss from a hiatus hernia depends first on the demonstration of the hernia (*Hiatus Hernia*, above). During the course of active bleeding the diagnosis of a small hiatus hernia is frequently missed. Large hernia sacs, however, should be insufflated and the mucosa inspected. Direct endoscopic washings within the sac may be necessary to remove confusing retained blood or demonstrate the mucosal pathology. When possible the instrument should be advanced into the stomach and the turnaround maneuver performed looking for the ooze of fresh blood flowing through the widened hernia orifice down the gastric wall.

The bleeding of the Mallory-Weiss syndrome arises usually from one, though occasionally two or three, mucosal tears occurring at the cardioesophageal sphincter. The laceration characteristically runs parallel to the long axis of the esophagus and may involve the mucosa of both the esophagus and the gastric cardia as a bridge; more frequently, however, it occurs alone on the gastric side just below the esophageal gastric junction. A clot with oozing edges is often adherent to the tear. The surrounding mucosa often reveals superficial gastritis. Esophagitis and esophageal varices are likewise frequent accompaniments, probably due to the higher frequency of this lesion in the alcoholic population. An oozing Mallory-Weiss tear may therefore be confused with a bleeding varix when esophageal varices are also identified.

Operative Endoscopy

Foreign body removal has traditionally required the open esophagoscope and appropriate graspers. However, small and soft foreign bodies may be removed with the fiberoptic endoscope by advancing the tip to the object and activating the suction channel. The image is seen to red out partially or completely, and while maintaining suction the instrument and object are removed.

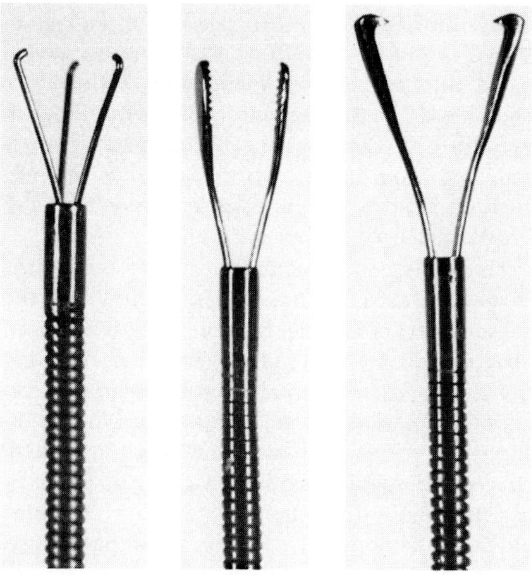

The development of wire loops and forceps of special design, capable of passage through the suction channel of the fiberoptic instruments, has enabled the removal of harder and larger foreign bodies. These special forceps (Fig. 8) include variously shaped tips designed to fit the foreign body and strong enough to hold a weight of 1 kg. In addition, the wire loop designed for lassoing, cutting, and coagulating polypoid lesions through fiberoptic instruments may be used to lasso and hold larger and irregular foreign bodies. When tightened snugly about the object, the loop is usually easily removed along with the endoscope, guided by direct vision.

Additional operative procedures that may be carried out with the fiberoptic esophagoscope include polypectomy (Chapter 21), passage of wires through strictures for the purpose of dilatation,[25] injection of sclerosing agents into esophageal varices or chemotherapeutic agents into tumor tissue, electrocoagulation of bleeding points, and removal of retained sutures.[7] Special loops, injection needles, and suture removal forceps are available for passage through the suction channel, and the appropriate procedure is carried out under direct visual control.

Complications

Accidents that occur with fiberoptic esophagoscopy are those seen in general with fiberoptic endoscopy of the upper gastrointestinal tract. The complication rate of perforation with fiberoptic instruments (0.093 percent) is only slightly more favorable than with the open-tube metal esophagoscopes (0.11 percent).[13] This survey was conducted early in the development of fiberoptic instruments and may not be a true reflection of the present status of safety. A recent survey has revealed a perforation rate of 0.03 percent of all cases of pan UGI endoscopy.[27]

When esophageal perforations occur with fiberoptic endoscopes they are often large linear tears that are usually treated with immediate surgery.[31] The marked flexibility of the fiberoptic instruments allow for excellent intragastric turnaround views of the cardioesophageal junction. This maneuver is not without potential problems, however. Impaction of the instrument in the stomach and

FIG. 8.   Special tipped graspers for fiberoptic endoscopic foreign body removal.

esophagus may occur and require surgical exploration for relief, though a technique for nonsurgical removal has been suggested.[2,23]

Gastrointestinal bleeding as a consequence of fiberoptic esophagoscopy or endoscopic biopsy is rarely seen. Prior correction of alteration in clotting factors should be attempted wherever possible. Bleeding, when it occurs, generally stops with supportive therapy and correction of clotting abnormalities.

Additional complications include salivary gland swelling,[29] severe abdominal distention from air insufflation,[24] and rarely myocardial infarction.[20] Electrocardiographic changes are not uncommon during upper gastrointestinal endoscopy but are rarely of clinical significance.[6]

Premedication programs occasionally result in prolonged apnea, even with the use of small amounts of diazepam. However, for the most part complications associated with diazepam premedication are minor and well tolerated.[3]

REFERENCES

1. Anselm K, Schuman BM, Cook CA: Fiberoptic esophagoscopy in geriatric patients. J Am Geriatr Soc 19:167, 1971
2. Barrett B: New instruments, new horizons, new hazards. Gastrointest Endosc 16:142, 1970
3. Castiglioni LJ, Allen TS, Patterson M: Intravenous diazepam: an improvement in preendoscopic medication. Gastrointest Endosc 19:134, 1973
4. Conn HO, et al: Fiberoptic and conventional esophagoscopy in the diagnosis of esophageal varices. Gastroenterology 52:810, 1967
5. Dagradi AE, et al: "Open-tube" vs fiberoptic esophagoscopy for evaluation of esophageal varices. Am J Gastroenterol 60:240, 1973
6. DeMassi C, Akdamar K: Electrocardiography during upper gastrointestinal endoscopy. Gastrointest Endosc 16:33, 1969
7. Endo M, Nakayama K: Removal of a foreign body from the esophagus using oesophagofiberscope: urgent endoscopy of digestive and abdominal diseases. In: International Symposium Praque, Carlsbad, 1971. Basel, Karger, 1972, pp 150–152
8. Giulimi E, et al: A "tip" on passing the scope. Gastrointest Endosc 19:199, 1973
9. Hattori K, Winans CS, Archer F: Endoscopic diagnosis of esophageal inflammation. Gastrointest Endosc 20:102, 1974
10. Hirschowitz BI: A flexible fiberoptic oesophagoscope. Lancet 2:388, 1963
11. Hirschowitz BI, et al: Demonstration of a new gastroscope, "the fiberscope." Gastroenterology 35:50, 1958
12. Johnson JE, Morrissey JF, Leventhal H: Psychological preparation for an endoscopic examination. Gastrointest Endosc 19:180, 1973
13. Katz D: Morbidity and mortality in standard and flexible gastrointestinal endoscopy. Gastrointest Endosc 15:134, 1969
14. Lopez-Torres A, Waye JD: The safety of intubation in patients with esophageal varices. Am J Dig Dis 18:1032, 1973
15. LoPresti PA, Hilmi AM: Clinical experience with a new foroblique esophagoscope. Am J Dig Dis 9:690, 1964
16. LoPresti PA, Cifarelli PS, Dixit N: Successful examination of the esophagus and stomach with a new fiberoptic instrument. Gastrointest Endosc 17: 103, 1971
17. Ludwig RN, Sullivan BH Jr: Esophagoscopy and gastroscopy with a single instrument: experiences with a fiberoptic esophago-gastroscope. Gastrointest Endosc 17:173, 1971
18. Mikulicz J: Über Gastroskopie und Esophagoskopie. Zentralbl Chir 43:673, 1881
19. Miwa T, Sakita T: Esophago fiberscope for screening. Gastrointest Endosc 19:70, 1972
20. Morrissey JF: Progress in gastroenterology, gastrointestinal endoscopy. Gastroenterology 62:1241, 1972
21. Morrissey JF, Koizumi H, Sultan MN: Clinical use of the Olympus fiberesophagoscope. Gastrointest Endosc 16:207, 1970
22. Palmer ED: Today's esophagologist, autocastrated. JAMA 227:511, 1974
23. Parker LS: Impacted fiberscope in the esophagus. J Laryngol Otol 83:1123, 1969
24. Rastagi H, Brown CH: Pseudo acute abdomen following gastroscopy. Gastrointest Endosc 14: 16, 1967
25. Rockman S, Morrissey JF, Koizumi H: A simple approach to narrow esophageal strictures. Gastrointest Endosc 16: 212, 1970
26. Schachter H, Kobayashi S: The gastroscopic retroflexion method in the diagnosis of sliding esophageal hiatus hernia. Gastrointest Endosc 17:78, 1970
27. Silvis S, et al: Endoscopic complications. JAMA 235:928, 1976
28. Sivik MS Jr, Sullivan BH Jr: Visually guided insertion of endoscope. Gastrointest Endosc 20:77, 1973
29. Slaughter RL, Boyce HW: Submaxillary salivary gland swelling developing during peroral endoscopy. Gastroenterology 57:83, 1969
30. Trujillo NP, Slaughter RL, Boyce HW Jr: Endoscopic diagnosis of sliding-type diaphragmatic hiatal hernias. Am J Dig Dis 13:855, 1968
31. Youngs J, Nicoloff D: Management of esophageal perforation. Surgery 65:264, 1969
32. Zimmon DS, Tesler MA: A controlled comparison of rigid and fiberoptic esophagoscopy. Gastrointest Endosc 14:220, 1968

27

Flexible Endoscopy in Infants and Children

Stephen L. Gans

Gastroduodenoscopy has become almost routine in adult patients with upper gastrointestinal disease, and by using colonoscopy the advantages of sigmoidoscopy, including tissue biopsy and polyp removal, are now being extended all the way to the cecum and even the terminal ileum. However, flexible endoscopy in infants and children is still uncommon. One apparent reason for this is the serious problem in miniaturization. In adult-sized fiberscopes the image quality is obtained by the large number of threads incorporated into the system. By decreasing the diameter for pediatric use, the resolution drops considerably, in proportion to the number of threads eliminated. In addition, space is needed for remote control of the tip, suction, air insufflation, and instrument channel. Thus the smaller diameter results in a smaller image of lesser quality and also eliminates some of the functions and versatility of the adult-sized instruments.

INSTRUMENTS

In 1971 we started using an adult flexible *fiberbronchoscope* (Olympus model BF, type 5B2) for gastroduodenoscopy in infants and children, and at present still use this instrument for neonates and small infants. It does not have the view and maneuverability of larger fiberscopes, and air and water injection and suction are somewhat cumbersome. However, such compromises are necessary to gain the advantages of a very small flexible endo-

scope. Since 1973 we have been using a prototype pediatric flexible fiberendoscope (Olympus) with a much better view and greater versatility. We have also used a pediatric model (Olympus model GIF, type P) already generally available but with somewhat lesser capabilities. Comparative specifications are shown in Table 1. Finally, the usual adult sizes are available for larger pediatric patients.

INDICATIONS

Endoscopy with flexible fiberscopes was carried out 92 times in 84 patients ranging in age from 3 weeks to 15 years. The upper gastrointestinal tract was examined 65 times. Indications for this study were hematemesis and/or melena, abdominal pain and/or vomiting, evaluation and biopsy of tumor, and removal of a foreign body. In all patients adequate radiologic and other studies had been previously done, except in two infants in whom gastroscopy was done first.

Colonoscopy was performed on 18 occasions. Indications were blood in the stools, diagnosis and/or removal of polyps, and the evaluation of ulcerative colitis. A further indication would be to biopsy a tumor, but we have not as yet had this opportunity in the pediatric age group.

Other indications include examination of an esophageal replacement segment that has become too tortuous for the conventional rigid instrument. We also examined a bleeding ileal loop and the jejunal limb of a cutaneous portoenterostomy.

TABLE 1. Comparative Specifications of Three Fiberendoscopes

Parameter	BF Type 5B2: Fiberbronchoscope	GIF Type P: Gastrointestinal Fiberscope	Prototype: Gastrointestinal Fiberscope
Outside diameter			
Tip	5.2 mm	7.2 mm	11.0 mm
Tube	5.7 mm	6.8 mm	8.5 mm
Working length	600 mm	1100 mm	1050 mm
Viewing direction and angle	Forward viewing 72°	Forward viewing 65°	Forward viewing 65°
Bending angle of tip	130° up, 30° down	150° 2-way, each way	120° 4-way, each way

CONTRAINDICATIONS

Contraindications include patients with hepatitis A and B, unruly patients (inadequate sedation or anesthesia), and unavailability of an experienced endoscopist. Severely diseased organs should be approached with great caution if at all.

ANESTHESIA

In infants and children we prefer to use general anesthesia for gastroduodenoscopy. Without it cooperation is questionable at best, and with it the procedure is easier on both patient and surgeon. In addition, respiratory problems due to pressure of the instrument in the esophagus against the adjacent airway are avoided by tracheal intubation. As experience increases we may elect to forego general anesthesia in selected cases at both ends of the age spectrum.

For colonoscopy we also prefer general anesthesia to secure maximum efficiency and safety. One must keep in mind that under general anesthesia the patient does not always empty his overdistended bowel of insufflated air, so this must be carried out from time to time by the operator using the suction channel.

PROCEDURE AND TECHNIQUE

Gastroduodenoscopy

After adequate sedation and immobilization, (or preferably endotracheal general anesthesia) the scope can be passed blindly but gently over the back of the tongue into the esophagus; or it can be guided under direct vision. Orientation and examination of the esophagus is usually rapid and without difficulty. Once the stomach is entered, manipulation with suction, air insufflation, water injection, movement of the endoscope tip, and rotation of the patient are carried out to gain a clear view and complete examination. Brief fluoroscopy with image amplification can be of considerable help in orientation and further advancement of the scope.

Colonoscopy

For colonoscopy, the patient is prepared by 3 days of liquid or elemental diet, cathartic the day before, and enemas at least 3 hours prior to the examination. With the anesthetized patient supine on the x-ray table, the scope is introduced as far proximally as possible under direct visual control. When further passage does not proceed easily, the scope position is checked by fluoroscopy with image amplification; further progress continues with tip manipulation, turning and twisting the scope, and checking by fluoroscopy as necessary. Considerable patience, deftness, and dexterity are required, and gentle handling of the scope is mandatory. In some instances the scope can be passed around to the cecum, but this is not always possible and advancement frequently stops short of this, depending on the experience and ability of the operator.

RESULTS

Gastroduodenoscopy

In patients with upper gastrointestinal lesions radiologic examination more often than not failed to establish a diagnosis. Many lesions missed by x-ray were demonstrated by direct examination with a flexible fiberscope. We have seen shallow acute ulcers, chronic deeper ulcers, and gastritis in patients with negative radiologic studies. Even when radiologic diagnosis was established, endoscopy often expanded the available information by direct inspection and by biopsy. In two instances the papilla of Vater was catheterized in search of pancreatic ductal lesions.

After 65 upper gastrointestinal examinations we conclude that endoscopy is a meaningful extension of radiologic and other studies. The procedure is safe and uncomplicated, the only danger being the risk of anesthesia.

Colonoscopy

We are very careful in the selection of cases for this examination. In all 18 patients radiologic studies and proctosigmoidoscopy were done first. Polyps were found by x-ray in only two patients; but by endoscopy of the same group polyps were found in five. In one instance a polyp was found by barium studies but could not be found at colonoscopy. One patient suffered a perforation at the time of polyp removal. Punctate isolated ulcerations were seen in two bleeding patients with negative x-rays. Three patients were studied to determine the extent and severity of ulcerative colitis. The rest were negative examinations.

COMPLICATIONS

There were no complications in our series of upper gastrointestinal studies. The only complication of colonoscopy occurred while removing a polyp with an adult-sized colonoscope. The perforation was immediately recognized, and after a temporary colostomy (1 month) the patient made an uneventful recovery.

28

Gastroscopy

Basil I. Hirschowitz

Endoscopy of the upper digestive tract serves not only as a means of resolving or amplifying diagnoses made by indirect means (e.g., history, physical examination, or radiology) but also as the primary diagnostic procedure for conditions not otherwise diagnosable in the intact patient. As such its advantages and limitations should be familiar to any physician concerned with gastrointestinal diagnosis.

Radical technologic innovations during the last 15 years have changed gastroscopy from an occasional optional procedure to one that is now widely available, commonly performed, and considered essential in the proper diagnosis of upper gastrointestinal disease.

In one form or another endoscopy of the esophagus and stomach has been practiced since 1880, but the first practical semirigid gastroscope was introduced only in 1932.[21] Until recently the instruments used have depended on vision through straight tubes for the esophagus or on a system of lenses for the gastroscope, limiting the instrument's shape to a virtually straight rod. Because the upper digestive tube is not straight, passage of those instruments required great skill and subjected the patient to much discomfort and risk of injury. Rigidity of the instrument prevented visualization of certain blind areas of the stomach—the fundus, the posterior wall, and frequently much of the antrum and pylorus.[1]

Supported by funds from the USPHS (grants AM04978 and TIAM5285) and from the Wappler Foundation.

Furthermore because of the limited illumination afforded by the miniaturized incandescent lamp carried into the stomach and the high rate of light loss in the multiple lens system, mucosal detail was not always well perceived, and even limited photography could be performed only with specially modified instruments.

With the introduction of the fiberoptic gastroscope by me and my colleagues in 1957[9-11,13,14] and the rapid evolution of fiberscopes since then, intubation and endoscopy of the esophagus, stomach, and duodenum has become easy and the risk of injury much less. Additionally the value of these instruments has been extended by the capacity to perform biopsies, obtain brushings or washings for cytology, pass catheters under direct vision, and obtain photographic or television records with unmodified instruments. Very recently it has also become possible to remove polyps safely by snare cautery through the instrument.[4]

INDICATIONS

Since intubation with the flexible fiberoptic instruments is not subject to such contraindications as a short or fixed neck, small mouth, obesity, or kyphosis, the indications for endoscopy are based on the ability of the examination to make or clarify a diagnosis. The only definite contraindications are a totally uncooperative patient (where necessary, general anesthesia may be used), a recent ulcer perforation, and the acute phase after corrosive ingestion.

Except in emergency situations (e.g., bleeding) it is always preferable to x-ray the esophagus, stomach, and duodenum first. Radiology serves to focus attention on particular lesions or areas and also may give warning of potentially troublesome anatomic problems such as esophageal diverticulum or obstruction, parahiatal hernia, and any unusual configuration of the stomach. Although this may be counsel of perfection, any lesion of the upper gastrointestinal tract shown by x-ray should be directly visualized by endoscopy and, if indicated, further clarified by biopsy or cytology. Furthermore symptoms such as dysphagia, x-ray negative dyspepsia, persistent vomiting, upper gastrointestinal bleeding, and any symptoms after gastric surgery provide clear indications for endoscopy. In 843 symptomatic patients with negative x-rays Schuman[22] found 160 normal stomachs, 59 with ulcer, and 4 with cancer. Gastroscopy is recommended as a screening procedure in patients at high risk for gastric cancer (e.g., those with pernicious anemia), in the follow-up to gastric ulcer healing, and late after gastric surgery to determine the state of the gastric mucosa.

It may be argued that there is no real indication which limits the endoscopy to the stomach (i.e., gastroscopy in its refined sense) except when because of disease it is not possible to see beyond the pylorus. With current instrumentation it is possible with one procedure to inspect the esophagus, stomach, and duodenum, and therefore no examination for either a lesion or a symptom can be considered reliable or complete unless adjacent areas have been inspected for the presence of related or unrelated disease. Some of the related disorders may be anticipated—e.g., esophagitis in patients vomiting because of pyloric ulcer or stenosis, duodenal ulcer in a significant number of patients with gastric ulcer or pyloric stenosis, esophageal varices in patients with gastric varices, and esophageal invasion with fundic carcinoma. However, because of the organization of this book, most of the discussion here is limited to the stomach, even if it is implicit that most times as a routine, and always when indicated, adjacent structures are examined at the same procedure.

INSTRUMENTS

Fiberoptic Bundle

The image-transmitting element of the fiberscopes[9] is a bundle of 200,000 or more glass-coated fibers, each about 5 to 10 μ in diameter, each going from end to end and so arranged that the spatial orientation of the fibers at each end of the bundle is the same. The fibers are permanently bonded to each other at the ends but are free in between so that the bundle is completely flexible. There is no distortion of the transmitted image by any degree of bending or flexion between the fixed ends. Each fiber transmits a minute part of the image as a separate spot of light and contains it within the glass core of the fiber by a phenomenon known as total internal reflectance.[25] The image, or picture, at the other end, is made up of these individual spots of light, so that the quality of the picture depends on the exactness of the orientation of the fibers to each other. Compared with a multiple lens system of equivalent length, fiber bundles transmit more than 20 times the light. Fiber bundles are also being used to transmit large amounts of light from external high-intensity light sources to supply brilliant, cold illumination and have replaced the distally placed incandescent lamp in all types of endoscopes.

Fiberscopes

There has been a profusion of newly developed instruments over the last few years with a strong tendency to make multipurpose instruments.*[18] These are of essentially similar basic design, all using fiber bundles of 1.5 to 3 mm diameter for illumination, and 2- to 5-mm optical bundles for image transmission. At the distal end the image is focused on the optical-image fiber bundle by a lens system that has a fixed-focus arrangement in some instruments and a variable, externally controlled focusing system in others. There are essentially two types of instruments, distinguished by whether the distal lens looks straight ahead (esophagoscopes and esophagoduodenoscopes) or side-

---

The three major manufacturers are American Cystoscope Makers, Inc. (New York, New York) and Olympus and Machida (both in Tokyo, Japan).

ways (gastroscopes, gastroduodenoscopes). In all the latest instruments the distal 7 to 15 cm is more flexible than the rest of the instrument and the curvature of that segment controllable in one plane or in all directions from the external end by a single control or pair of controls. The degree of flexion from the longitudinal axis varies from 80 to 170 degrees, the latter forming a J or U configuration.

PREPARATION OF THE PATIENT

Most persons gag or retch while swallowing tubes, especially when anxious, so that premedication should be used routinely. The patient has the procedure explained to him and is told why it is to be done. Since the stomach is ideally as empty as possible, the patient fasts 8 to 12 hours. It is seldom necessary to empty the stomach additionally by Ewald tube before endoscopy as most of the normal fasting gastric contents can be aspirated through the fiberscope during examination. Both barium sulfate and aluminum gel antacids cling to the surface of the stomach in patches, making it difficult to exclude discrete lesions such as ulcers. These antacids are thus not given within 10 hours of examination, and barium within 18 to 24 hours of endoscopy.

The patient is generally sedated, though cautiously if he has been bleeding and is hypotensive or is subject to respiratory depression or insufficiency. Meperidine (50 to 100 mg I.M. or 25 to 50 I.V.) or diazepam (Valium, 5 to 10 mg I.M. or I.V.) are the drugs most commonly used today, either alone or in combination. All removable dentures or bridges are removed before proceeding. A surface anesthetic is applied to the throat either by gargling or by a spray-nebulizer. We have used 0.5 percent dyclonine (Dyclone) for more than 6,000 examinations without a single reaction. The amount used by spray is very little; onset of anesthesia is within 30 seconds, and it lasts about 1 hour —all advantageous for endoscopy.

Using too much drug by either spray or gargle, however, may also anesthetize the larynx and upper trachea, allowing inhalation of saliva or regurgitated gastric contents. If this happens the patient is encouraged to cough immediately after the procedure with postural drainage, i.e., head down.

PASSING THE FIBERSCOPE

After this preparation the fiberscope may be passed with the patient sitting and the neck slightly flexed, or lying either supine or on the left side. While an assistant holds the head of the instrument, the distal tip is guided over the back of the tongue by the left index finger and the patient is asked to swallow. When the tip is in the esophagus it is steadily pushed into the stomach.[25] If there is undue resistance, pain, difficulty in breathing, cyanosis, coughing, or marked patient agitation during the initial part of the intubation, the instrument is withdrawn and a fresh start made as it most likely had been passed into the trachea. The instrument may be badly damaged by a hard bite, and various types of guards are available, the best being the short flanged tube. In a pinch, a cut-off 10- or 15-ml plastic syringe barrel suffices.

RISKS

There is a small risk of anaphylactic reaction to various premedications, although in 6,000 examinations in our experience none has occurred. Each patient should be questioned regarding allergies before any drug is administered.

Because upper gastrointestinal endoscopy is now very widely practiced, and not always by persons properly trained or qualified, some accidents unavoidably occur. The more manipulative procedures such as biopsy polypectomy and cannulation of the ampulla of Vater add to the risk.

The major risk of intubation is perforation of the esophagus, which may occur in the neck or at the site of stricture (twice in 6,000 examinations, both with stiffer, earlier gastroscopes), severe esophagitis (once in 6,000 patients), or diverticulum. Perforation of the stomach may occur at the site of a recently sealed-off perforated ulcer; in our series this happened once. Patients with esophageal varices are at risk especially from suction or ill-advised biopsy, but this condition is not normally a contraindication to endoscopy.

Inhalation of regurgitated gastric contents may occur if too much surface anesthesia has been used, if the patient has been oversedated, or if inadequate suction is applied to keep the mouth clear of fluid (especially if the patient is vomiting large amounts of blood). Inhalation of blood can cause troublesome pneumonia and should be anticipated by appropriate measures.

The diameter of the instruments is 7 to 12 mm. The instruments may also be distinguished by their working length, varying from 65 to 105 cm. The shorter, forward-viewing instrument is useful only for the esophagus and stomach; it is too short to enter the duodenum. The 75- to 90-cm side-viewing instruments are essentially gastroscopes only; they are confined to routine use for examination of the stomach and occasionally provide the only means of examining the lesser curve of the antrum. The 105-cm instruments are of two types. The end-viewing instrument is the commonest now in general use for examining the esophagus, stomach, and duodenum. The side-viewing instruments of similar length are of use only in the stomach and duodenum. These are the only instruments which allow intubation of the ampulla of Vater and in certain cases provide better visualization of the duodenal bulb.[2] The eyepiece of the instruments consists of a lens for enlarging the image from the proximal end of the image bundle, connections for air and water, and controls for image focusing and control of the distal flexible tip.

Biopsy and Cytology

All the instruments incorporate an open channel for air or water to distend the organ and wash the lens; the same channel may be used for aspiration in most instruments, and in some is also used as a biopsy channel. The more satisfactory arrangements with the forward-viewing instruments is that in which one channel is used only for insufflation of air or water to wash the lens and a second, open channel is provided for aspiration, biopsy forceps, cytology brushes, or for the introduction of fluid to wash the mucosa or obtain material for cytology. Biopsy capacity has broadened the scope of the fiberscopes, and though they are small (1 to 3 mm) they are usually adequate. Some instruments have additional distal controls to make the siting of biopsies more precise. In all cases, however, biopsy and brushing or jet washing for cytology is done under direct vision.

Photography

Light transmission through the optical bundles of the length used is high enough for adequate photography especially with the ability to introduce much more light using fiber bundles. With optical resolution of the bundles in the range of 40 lines/mm, still or moving pictures in color can be taken at normal speeds with standard camera equipment requiring only a built-in light meter for proper exposure and a simple clamp to attach the camera to the eyepiece of the fiberscope. By the same token, there is enough light for television photography in black and white or in color.[9]

By a marriage of the fiberscope and the gastrocamera, some instruments take direct photographs in the stomach under endoscopic visual control. These instruments have a much longer rigid portion and are limited to use in the stomach.[18] These are more difficult to pass and thus more hazardous than either alone.

Teaching Fiberscope

The teaching fiberscope is a separate device that can be attached to the eyepiece of the instrument being used for normal endoscopy; it consists essentially of an image-splitting prism and a 1-meter fiberoptic bundle. Using this device allows the examiner to do a normal examination and the student to see the field at the same time.

Since there is enough light for adequate viewing by two persons at the same time, the second viewer can be a valuable assistant during biopsy, cytology, and operative endoscopy including polypectomy and retrieval of foreign bodies. Furthermore with two trained endoscopists looking at the same time, there is less chance of overlooking or mistaking an endoscopic view.

INSPECTING THE STOMACH

In the stomach there are several landmarks that should be observed, including the angulus, the gastroesophageal junction, and the pylorus. Note that the false pylorus (proximal antral spasm) may be misleading and look like a pylorus; it can be eliminated by an anticholinergic, e.g., atropine. With the newer instruments in which the distal end is very flexible and controllable, it is essential to develop a systematic routine for gastric inspection. This differs according to the instrument used to inspect the stomach.

The gastroscope (side-viewing) is designed primarily to visualize the stomach and is still used by many for gastroscopy. Before passing it the examiner should know the direction of the view related to an external landmark, as well as the plane(s) and extent of flexion of the distal end, also related to an external landmark. Once the instrument is in the stomach the examiner must know he has fully inspected the pylorus and antrum, which may be paralyzed by probanthine or atropine or, more recently described, by intravenous injection of glucagon.[19] He should also be sure about the greater and lesser curves, the fundus, and the esophagogastric hiatus. Because the instrument is lateral-viewing it must be rotated in the vertical axis to see all walls. The anterior and posterior walls can be identified by starting from the angulus and turning the instrument in the appropriate direction. The lesser curve is often difficult to be sure about, and since many lesions occur at or near the angulus it sometimes helps to have the instrument bent in a J, looking up from below the angulus. The reverse J allows inspection of the whole lesser curve; and the L or reverse L position allows inspection of the fundus and the hiatus. Under those conditions the shaft of the instrument can be seen issuing from the hiatus.

More and more, however, multiple purpose instruments are being used. These are generally forward-viewing instruments that can inspect esophagus, stomach, and duodenum. Even though the viewing angle is 60 to 70 degrees they have a relatively small field especially in close-up, thus making it even more important to be systematic when examining the stomach. When this instrument is used, the esophagus is inspected both going in and coming out; the stomach is also inspected on the way to the duodenum and upon returning. The same landmarks are used, but because the instrument is end-viewing the tip must be bent a further 90 degrees to accomplish the same as the gastroscope, e.g., a U shape instead of an L shape is necessary to inspect the fundus and a b shape to look at the whole lesser curve.[6]

SPECIFIC APPLICATIONS OF FIBEROPTIC ENDOSCOPY

Several conditions seen by gastroscopy are illustrated in Figures 1–6, Plate B.*

Upper Gastrointestinal Bleeding

Any patient who presents with acute upper gastrointestinal bleeding is a potential candidate for emergency operation. Should surgical intervention be necessary, it is self-evident that foreknowledge of the lesion to be dealt with offers the surgeon and consequently the patient a considerable advantage. The commonest lesions responsible for significant bleeding are chronic or acute gastric or duodenal ulcers, while other lesions such as esophageal or gastric varices, tears at the cardio-esophageal junction (Mallory-Weiss syndrome), benign or malignant tumors, and acute hemorrhagic gastritis together are responsible for about 15 to 20 percent of cases, thus forming a significant fraction of the differential diagnoses.

The value of endoscopy rests principally on its ability to localize the source and nature of bleeding early in the course, and thus to determine in part subsequent treatment.[3,14] As soon as resuscitative measures have been instituted—securing an intravenous line for infusion and measurement of central venous pressure, blood sampling for typing and cross-matching and for blood count and chemistry, and institution of intake-output measurement—the stomach is gently lavaged and aspirated with an Ewald tube to free it of as much of its bloody contents as possible. With appropriate sedation the fiberscope is passed without moving the patient. It is unusual not to obtain an adequate endoscopic view except in cases of massive bleeding.

Since the endoscopist has only the history to guide his examination, he should systematically examine as much of the esophagus, stomach, and duodenum as possible. It is thus a matter of choice which instrument to use. In most cases it is preferable to start with a long, forward-viewing fiberscope with which it is possible to do a comprehensive examination of the esophagus, stomach, and duodenum. Be-

All color plates appear at the front of the book.

cause of the direction of view and the relatively small field, the body and fundus of the stomach are less certainly fully examined than the other areas; and if the diagnosis is not clearly established by this instrument, a gastroscope (i.e., a lateral-viewing fiberscope) is then used. A minimal amount of air should be used as massive air distention of the intestine may make closure of the abdomen in subsequent operation more difficult.

The first objective is to determine how much if any blood is in the stomach and then to attempt to localize the anatomic site of origin of any fresh blood. Bleeding at the cardia is most often caused by varices (which should be suspected from the prior history and physical examination) or by a Mallory-Weiss tear, which can usually be positively diagnosed by endoscopy but rarely by x-ray study. In fact, many cases of hematemesis after heavy drinking are due to this lesion rather than to so-called alcoholic gastritis. The Mallory-Weiss lesion may also occur in other instances when vomiting has preceded bleeding.[17] Esophagitis is also a possible cause for bleeding.

In the body of the stomach, diffuse mucosal bleeding can be readily appreciated, and although an infrequent cause of massive bleeding it occurs in uremia, in blood dyscrasias, and occasionally with no antecedent cause. The commonest sources of bleeding in the stomach are chronic and acute ulcers (i.e., acute gastric erosions),[15] the latter accounting for almost 30 percent of all cases of upper gastrointestinal bleeding, including patients with coexisting chronic ulcers in the stomach or duodenum.[3,14] Bleeding from acute ulceration is self-limiting in most cases.

Gastric tube suction may produce lesions of the mucosa often indistinguishable from acute ulcers or erosions. However, they are usually multiple, occurring in rows of three or four, and on careful inspection are seen to be small hematomas. Twenty-four to 48 hours later, however, they may slough, leaving small ulcers. It is highly desirable therefore to examine the stomach before vigorous suction has been applied.

Tumors of the stomach that may bleed include leiomyoma or leiomyosarcoma and carcinoma, both of which can be readily distinguished from other lesions by endoscopic examination. Together they account for 2 to 3 percent of patients with massive hematemesis.

Duodenal ulcers account for about 20 to 40 percent of patients with massive upper gastrointestinal bleeding. With the new fiberscopes it is now possible to examine the duodenum much more easily and comprehensively than before.[2,3] Even if the duodenum cannot be entered, it is usually enough to see fresh blood returning through the pylorus to diagnose duodenal ulcer. The mere presence of a duodenal ulcer or deformity on x-ray does not automatically implicate duodenal ulcer as a source of bleeding: 30 percent of our bleeding patients who had duodenal deformity on x-ray were found to be bleeding from other lesions, especially acute erosions in the stomach.[14] It is thus important to make a positive diagnosis of the site of bleeding by direct inspection.

If surgical intervention is not immediately necessary and the patient may be moved safely, *x-ray examination* of the upper tract should logically follow endoscopy. However, in many cases the site and source of bleeding is so clearly identified by endoscopy that x-ray can be delayed until the acute problem has subsided.

Although chronic persistent occult bleeding from the gastrointestinal tract is generally caused by the presence of malignancy, especially of the colon (now also amenable to fiberoptic endoscopy), the stomach occasionally is the seat of the responsible lesion. Such gastric lesions include leiomyoma, lymphoma, carcinoma, and vascular anomalies such as hereditary telangiectasia and hemangioma as well as unsuspected aspirin-induced erosive gastritis. The postgastrectomy stomach is also quite commonly responsible for persistent or repetitive occult bleeding. In our experience hiatus hernia is not a source for such bleeding. Finding a number of stools containing blood should ultimately be an indication for gastroscopy if other sites, especially the colon, have been exonerated.

Cancers and Ulcers

Gastric Ulcers.   One of the major applications of gastroscopy is finding and clarifying the status of gastric ulcers. Since many gastric ulcers, especially the small or superficial ones seen at endoscopy, are not found by x-ray, endoscopy has become the principal basis for rational treatment of ulcer disease.

Gastric ulcers range from acute superficial lesions to penetrating chronic ones. *Acute ulcers* are generally small (1 to 3 mm diameter), and although most often confined to the antrum, especially the distal antrum, they may occur anywhere in the gastric mucosa. These are met with in several situations. In stress situations (e.g., uremia or after shock) there are usually multiple erosions; many are bleeding and scattered throughout the gastric mucosa, often being more numerous in the fundus. The mucosa is frequently congested and friable at the same time. It is important to distinguish artificial acute ulcers caused by suction from nasogastric tubes. These are most commonly arranged in lines of three or four, and some at least may be seen to be small hemorrhagic bullae.

The typical acute ulcer, such as that caused by aspirin, occurs singly or in groups of two or three, most commonly in the antrum; it is 1 to 3 mm in diameter, is surrounded by a narrow ring of erythema, and looks very much like aphthous ulcers of the mouth. These ulcers may bleed and be hidden by a small clot. If an ulcer is suspected underneath a clot the lesion should be washed by a jet of fluid; an adherent clot usually indicates an ulcer, and not infrequently a small part of the white slough in the base appears. Since these ulcers are small and can easily be hidden in the folds of the pylorus, the pylorus should be inspected through at least three or four cycles of contraction. These ulcers are a cause not only of bleeding but of ulcer dyspepsia, which may be undiagnosed unless gastroscopy is done.

Chronic gastric ulcers are here meant to include intermediate ulcers which are superficial but larger than the typical 1 to 3-mm round acute aspirin ulcer. These may be overlooked at x-ray, and not infrequently may be seen a short distance away from a chronic ulcer (satellite ulcer). When chronic ulcers heal to the point where they are too shallow to be seen on x-ray, they can still be seen by endoscopy for as long as 6 to 8 weeks. Such ulcers may break down before complete healing, and treatment should therefore more logically depend on endoscopy than on x-ray. During this phase of healing such ulcers resemble subacute ulcers but may be distinguished by the mucosal contraction or puckering present.

Finding an ulcer by x-ray is an indication for endoscopy, which adds several dimensions to the diagnosis. These include its size and depth, as well as the state of its base.

Since almost all gastric ulcers occur in patients who secrete acid and pepsin, the base is clean without loose debris or clots. This contrasts with the typical malignant ulcer where there is not enough digestive juice and the ulcer looks dirty. Thus the base of the benign ulcer consists of a white adherent slough and is smooth. When recent bleeding has occurred the slough may be stained brown in patches, and the tip of the blood vessel which has bled may be visible. The edge of a benign ulcer may be flat with surrounding mucosa but can be so edematous as to form a doughnut around the ulcer base, usually when most active. The healing gastric ulcer shows a pink edge extending onto the base and composed of growing capillaries which can be seen when the field is in sharp focus. This finding is seen only with benign ulcers. Part of an ulcer may have been cut off by this healing, leaving an island of slough, usually superficial, beyond the edge of the ulcer. This too is seen only with benign ulcers.

Benign chronic gastric ulcers usually occur from the angulus down to the pylorus and vary from 5 to 125 mm, though most are 1 to 2 cm in diameter. When in the pylorus they are usually smaller but with edema on the ulcer sufficient to occlude the lumen partially. Few stomachs contain more than one chronic ulcer, though one or two subacute satellite ulcers may be seen near the primary ulcer. The gastric ulcer may coexist with a duodenal ulcer. The distortion in the gastric wall induced by an ulcer usually results from contraction during healing; after healing has occurred the contraction, especially on the angulus, may remain, but generally both the mucosa and the wall are fully restored. Occasionally a flat scar remains after a gastric ulcer, and cytology or biopsy of such a scar would avoid missing a carcinoma. However, a biopsy here can activate a chronic ulcer, and if the ulcer was shown to be benign while active it may not be necessary. A biopsy specimen of the underside of the edge and material for cytology (preferably by brush and also from the edge) should be obtained from each gastric ulcer while it is active in order to exclude carcinoma (see below).

Gastric Cancer. Although most gastric tumors present as a mass rather than as an ulcer, it is always possible that any ulcer crater, regardless of size, shape, or location, may actually represent a cancer. Consequently gastroscopy is essential in the differential diagnosis of every gastric ulcer shown on x-ray. Diagnosis of malignancy can usually be readily made by inspection alone, and in our experience only 5 of 110 gastric cancers were not recognized visually. These were in patients who had normal or high gastric secretion and in whom the ulcer-cancers looked clean, i.e., there was an absence of debris at the edges and in the base.

With improved instrument capacity for biopsy and cytology (jet, washing, or brush), and with specimens collected under direct vision, borderline diagnoses can be resolved in many cases. Hermanek[8] collected a number of studies totaling 1,643 patients with gastric cancer; among these, gastric biopsy was positive for cancer in 87 percent, though individual studies varied from 40 to 92 percent. It is thus important not to be misled by a negative biopsy and to develop appropriate histologic techniques for the small (2 mm or less) biopsies. When the appearance suggests cancer, even though the biopsy is negative, laparotomy is indicated.

Much has been written (especially in the Japanese literature, by Kawai et al.[16] and Kuru[8]) about early gastric cancer and its classification by endoscopy and histology. In actual practice in the United States, few gastric cancers are sought or seen before symptoms occur, and at that time the cancers are usually readily diagnosable by endoscopy, biopsy, or cytology. Additional value of endoscopy in gastric tumor diagnosis is to determine its extent, location, and spread; if it ulcerated or is bleeding; and after surgery, if it has recurred.

Other Tumors. Other solid tumors of the stomach and of adjacent organs protruding into the stomach need to be distinguished from gastric carcinoma. These include both benign tumors—e.g., adenomatous polyps (present in 1 to 3 percent of stomachs being gastroscoped), ectopic pancreas, leiomyomas—and malignant tumors, including sarcomas, lymphoma (which may be hard to distinguish from Menetriere's disease), and metastatic melanoma. Often the tumor proper is deep to the mucosa, and the superficial biopsy, which is all that can be obtained, is inadequate to make a definitive diagnosis. Whenever feasible, polyps should be removed by snare cautery,[4] but otherwise appropriate surgery is recommended for further diagnosis and treatment.

Deformity of the Antrum

Antral deformity presents a special diagnostic problem. It is usually found by x-ray in patients with chronic peptic ulcer disease and often raises the possibility of malignancy. It is usually possible to resolve the question endoscopically since the mucosa is often diffusely gastritic but free of tumor and the antrum pliable. This can be confirmed by palpation from the outside while watching through the gastroscope and by seeing symmetrical motility throughout. In such cases atropinization reduces motility and makes it more difficult. Routine atropinization should thus be avoided.

Pyloric Stenosis

Pyloric stenosis may be recognized endoscopically when the orifice is small, fails to open with antral contraction, and does not allow the instrument to pass. Such a diagnosis can often be made long before x-ray evidence becomes positive. Adult hypertrophic pyloric stenosis may be distinguished from tumor by finding a normal mucosa and a symmetrical ring intruding into the lumen.

Diffuse Mucosal Lesions

Diffuse superficial lesions of the esophagus or gastric or duodenal mucosa are not detectable by x-ray, and several details of mucosal appearance should be carefully considered.[20] Gastritis may be classified either on histologic or endoscopic grounds. The histologic criteria are adequately dealt with elsewhere.[21-24] The endoscopic appearance does not always correlate with that seen histologically.[23] I therefore make no attempt to anticipate the histologic diagnosis and consider endoscopically diagnosable gastritis in two groups. In one there is increasing degrees of inflammation represented by degrees of redness with, successively, petechiae, friability (hemorrhagic gastritis[15-21]), and exudate and pus in the lumen (phlegmonous gastritis). Involvement of the mucosa may be patchy or diffuse, and it may be confined to the antrum or to the body. Another classification is described by the degree of mucosal atrophy, which may be of all degrees up to complete loss of mucosal thickness such as that seen in pernicious anemia. In the latter the underlying vascular pattern is clearly visible, as in the fundus of the eye. Atrophy may be patchy, and even in pernicious anemia the antrum is almost always spared. Gastritis (inflammation) and atrophy should be clearly considered separate. Even though atrophy can and probably does result from gastritis, the two do not always coexist an any one time.

Other superficial mucosal lesions not amenable to x-ray diagnosis include vascular anomalies such as telangiectasia (Osler-Weber-Rendu), blue rubber blebs, gastric varices, and arteriovenous malformations, all of which may be the cause of bleeding.

Gastroesophageal Junction

Examination of the gastroesophageal junction is included in both gastroscopy and esophagoscopy. Because the lower 5 cm of esophagus curves to the left, it is as reasonable to make the diagnosis of hiatal hernia with the lateral-viewing instrument (gastroscope) as with the forward-viewing one. In fact with the stomach distended with air and the gastroscope being withdrawn, conditions are right to uncover a hiatal hernia, diagnosed by seeing a complete pouch of gastric mucosa above the diaphragm. Hiatal hernia may also be diagnosed by a retrograde view of the hiatus from within the stomach; the bell-shaped protrusion of gastric mucosa through the diaphragm can often be seen, although the direct view from above is the most reliable.[26]

Other pathology in this area includes hard-to-diagnose infiltrating carcinoma, often presenting with dysphagia, and Mallory-Weiss tears as discussed above.

Postgastrectomy Stomach

It is in the patient after gastric surgery that endoscopy provides information not obtainable by any other means.[12] During a period of 12 years we have examined 691 patients complaining of one or more of the following symptoms: pain, vomiting, anorexia, bleeding and anemia, dumping, weight loss, and diarrhea. The distribution of symptoms is given in Table 1. Most patients had undergone surgery for duodenal ulcer, and about one-third of these for bleeding. All types of surgery in vogue over the past 30 years were represented in this group, and no particular symptom or abnormality occurred predominantly with any one operation. The lesions diagnosable by endoscopy are summarized in Table 2 and may be conveniently grouped under anatomic headings as follows.

Gastric Stump. Gastritis of some degree is present in about two-thirds of patients

TABLE 1. Symptom Distribution in 691 Patients After Gastric Surgery

Symptom	Percent
Pain	63
Vomiting	47
Bilious vomiting	19
Weight loss (>3 kg)	36
Dumping	32
Bleeding	27
Anemia	16
Diarrhea	17
Anorexia	15

Most patients had two or more symptoms.

after gastric resection and is marked in 14 percent where it is usually the only finding. No consistent symptom complex can be ascribed to this gastritis, although some patients have pain after eating and some bleed from hemorrhagic gastritis. In addition about 10 percent have atrophic gastric mucosa, in some cases advanced enough to have lost intrinsic factor secretion in all cases, indicating the need for vitamin B_{12} therapy. Atrophy may be the end-stage of gastritis. By contrast with the gastritis usually seen, the Zollinger-Ellison stomach mucosa is very healthy looking and may be seen to be actively secreting gastric juice. Other mucosal lesions include vascular anomalies such as hereditary telangiectasia, which

TABLE 2. Distribution of Endoscopic Diagnoses in 691 Patients Symptomatic After Gastric Surgery for Ulcer

Diagnosis	Percent
Normal	14
Hiatal hernia	10
Gastric mucosal disease	
Gastritis	14
Atrophy	10
Stomal disorders	
Stomatitis	27
Stomal stenosis	6
Double barrel stoma	10
Sutures	5
Chronic ulcer	
Marginal ulcer	17
Gastric ulcer	2
Jejunal ulcer	3
Jejunitis	5

Some patients had two major diagnoses.

may be responsible for chronic bleeding and not diagnosed before or at surgery.

Disorders of the Stoma.   Chronic Marginal Ulcer.   This lesion was found in 17 percent of the symptomatic patients and could be visualized by endoscopy in 9 of 10 cases, whereas only 50 percent of marginal ulcers were correctly diagnosed radiologically. The difficulty of radiologic diagnosis in an area distorted by surgical manipulation is not hard to understand. Many a surgical tuck has been read as a crater, especially since the stoma is relatively inaccessible to palpation, being generally above the costal margin. Consequently an almost equal number of ulcers diagnosed by x-ray were not in fact present. If for no other reason then, endoscopy is essential in the symptomatic postgastrectomy patient. In addition there were 18 patients with jejunal and 12 with gastric ulcers for a total of 149 patients with chronic recurrent peptic ulcer (22 percent of the total sample).

Stomal Inflammation.   Stomatitis (superficial ulceration, edema, redness, and exudation of the stomal margins) was seen in 27 percent of patients and was the only lesion in almost 20 percent. These findings were often associated with pain and were sometimes the only abnormality in patients presenting with bleeding or anemia. Stomatitis may represent a lesser variant or interval stage of chronic marginal ulcer; several of these patients had demonstrated ulcers at other admissions.

While stomal edema is common early after surgery, this may be the only finding in patients long after surgery who are complaining of pain or bleeding and may thus be hiding small ulcers, or in some cases extruding nonabsorbable sutures. It is more commonly seen in Billroth I anastomoses. A late result of stomal inflammation or ulceration is stomal *stenosis,* which may cause persistent vomiting and is easily diagnosed endoscopically.

Foreign Body.   Not infrequently nonabsorbable surgical suture material is seen at the anastomosis, and quite commonly it causes ulceration through which it is extruding into the lumen.[7] It is now possible and advisable to remove these with the biopsy forceps under direct endoscopic vision. Suture material may also cause localized edema or mucosal hyperplasia, sometimes enough to obstruct the stoma.

Double Barrel Stoma.   This is a disorder of stomal anatomy in which both afferent and efferent loops present side by side in the stoma, separated by a bridge of jejunal mucosa at the same level as the gastric margins of the stoma. This abnormality was found in about one gastrojejunostomy in 10.[5] In these patients several significant difficulties arise: The bridge of mucosa is frequently traumatized and bleeds as a result; ulceration of the bridge and of either loop occurs in over 50 percent. The afferent loop fills easily from the stomach and often produces afferent loop stasis. Almost all the afferent loop syndromes are found in this group of patients.[27] Since the afferent loop secretions must enter the stomach first, with this disorder gastritis and bilious vomiting are frequent. When found, this disorder should be surgically corrected, preferably by conversion to Billroth I.

Size and Motility of the Stoma.   When the stoma is small and the gastric resection 50 percent or less, the stoma generally retains circular contractions on the gastric side. Large stomas (over 3.5 cm) with high resections usually have abortive or no gastric contractions and never close. Vagotomy reduces or eliminates these contractions. Dumping, when present, is found five times more frequently with large nonclosing stomas than with those that are small and closing.

Jejunal Disorders.   The jejunum may suffer from jejunitis, jejunal ulceration, stenosis of the efferent limb due to stricture or twist with proximal dilatation, and stasis in the afferent limb. These can all be visualized endoscopically. Furthermore material for culture as well as biopsies can be obtained under direct vision.

CONCLUSIONS

Although special consideration must be given to the stomach as the seat of most of the upper gastrointestinal disease requiring endoscopic diagnosis, it is not justified to consider gastroscopy in isolation. Inspection of the stomach should form part of a comprehensive endoscopic examination of esophagus, stomach, and duodenum in each patient.

REFERENCES

1. Allegra G, Macchini M, Andreoli F: Gastroscopy With the Fiberscope. Padua, Piccin Medical Books, 1971

2. Belber JP: Endoscopic examination of the duodenal bulb—a comparison with x-ray. Gastroenterology 61:55, 1971

3. Cotton PB, Rosenberg TM, Waldran RP, et al: Early endoscopy of oesophagus, stomach and duodenal bulb in patients with haematemesis and melaena. Br Med J 2:505, 1973

4. Curtiss LE: High frequency currents in endoscopy: a review of principles and precautions. Bull Am Soc Gastrointest Endosc 20:9, 1973

5. Demaret AN, Hirschowitz BI, Luketic GC: Double barrel gastrojejunal stoma and its complications in 38 patients. Scand J Gastroenterol 6:77, 1971

6. Demling L, Ottenjann R, Elster K: Endoskopie und Biopsie der Speiseröhre und des Magens. Stuttgart, Schattauer Verlag, 1972

7. Gear MWL, Dowling BL: Suture-line ulcer after gastric surgery caused by non-absorbable suture materials. Br J Surg 57:356, 1970

8. Hermanek P: Gastro biopsy in cancer of the stomach. Endoscopy 5:144, 1973

9. Hirschowitz BI: Fiber optics in modern medicine. Med Biol Illus 15:224, 1965

10. Hirschowitz BI: A fiber flexible oesophagoscope. Lancet 2:388, 1963

11. Hirschowitz BI: Endoscopic examination of the stomach and duodenal cap with the fiberscope. Lancet 1:1074, 1961

12. Hirschowitz BI, Luketic GC: Endoscopy in the postgastrectomy patient—an analysis of 580 patients. Gastrointest Endosc 18:27, 1971

13. Hirschowitz BI, Curtiss LE, Peters CW, et al: Demonstration of a new gastroscope, the "fiberscope." Gastroenterology 35:50, 1958

14. Hirschowitz BI, Luketic GC, Balint JA, et al: Early fiberscope endoscopy for upper gastrointestinal bleeding. Am J Dig Dis 8:816, 1963

15. Katz D, Siegel HI: Erosive gastritis and acute gastrointestinal mucosal lesions. In Glass JB (ed): Progress in Gastroenterology. New York, Grune & Stratton, 1968

16. Kawai K, Akasaka Y, Misaki F, et al: Gastrofiberscopic biopsy on early gastric cancer. Endoscopy 2:82, 1970

17. Miller AC, Hirschowitz BI: Twenty-three patients with Mallory-Weiss syndrome. South Med J 63:441, 1970

18. Morrisey JP: Gastrointestinal endoscopy. Gastroenterology 62:1241, 1972

19. Paul F, Misaki F, Seifert E: Crystalline pancreatic glucagon—a new spasmolytic agent. Endoscopy 5:199, 1972

20. Petersen H, Myren J: Gastroscopy in the estimation of maximum acid output. Endoscopy 5:194, 1973

21. Schindler R: Gastroscopy, 2nd ed. Chicago, University of Chicago Press, 1950

22. Schuman BM: The gastroscopic yield from the negative upper upper gastrointestinal series. Gastrointest Endosc 19:79, 1972

23. Taylor KB: Current concepts: gastritis. N Engl J Med 280:818, 1969

24. Wood IJ, Taft LI: Diffuse Lesions of the Stomach. Baltimore, Williams & Wilkins, 1958

FILMS

The author has made three 16-mm sound films in color which illustrate and amplify the material in this chapter. These films can be borrowed from the National Medical Audiovisual Center, Atlanta, Georgia 30333.

25. The principles of fiberscope construction and of gastroscopy are illustrated in a 10-minute film: Fiberscope Endoscopy of the Upper G.I. Tract. NMAC Cat. No. M-1164.

26. Many of the common lesions of the stomach are illustrated in a 20-minute film: Common Gastric Lesions. NMAC Cat. No. M-2836.

27. A third film illustrates the lesions found in the postgastrectomy stomach in 500 symptomatic patients: The Symptomatic Postgastrectomy Patient. NMAC Cat. No. M-1714.

29

Laparoscopy in General Surgery

George Berci

The procedure of laparoscopy is more than 70 years old. Credit must be given to Kalk, who advocated it in Europe and produced the largest series, 2,000 cases, without fatality.[16] He emphasized its value in liver disease and the value of biopsy under visual control. Ruddock, in the United States, published his first experience of 500 cases in 1937.[28]

Despite the fact that the diagnostic accuracy in general surgery and hepatology has been well established, there is still some reluctance to use this procedure to evaluate difficult abdominal diagnostic problems. Reliance is generally placed on clinical findings, biochemical assays, roentgenographic studies, radioactive scans, lavage, or even finally on a diagnostic laparotomy.[3,5,6]

Although the dilemma of differential diagnostic problems or the differentiation between medical and surgical jaundice can be frequently resolved by laparoscopy, the procedure is not utilized to its fullest extent. This examination has been "rediscovered" in the field of gynecology, and during the past 4 years the reported number of cases performed in the United States is 230,000.[37]

The development of a new image-relaying system permitted the design of a markedly improved instrumentation (Chapter 5) in both adult and pediatric patients.[4] This should give us courage to reevaluate this important examination. There is nothing that provides more accuracy than actually seeing a lesion and performing a target biopsy. The question should not be: laparoscopy or diagnostic laparotomy. This procedure is the final step before a diagnostic exploration and should be performed as another but important diagnostic method. The dome of the liver is never seen as well, even during exploration, as through a scope. During surgery we are using our hand or fingertips to slide over the liver surface, to palpate any irregularities, but the actual palpated area cannot be properly visualized.

From the hepatology point of view, the risk of a blind biopsy is just the same as, if not greater than, the biopsy under visual or laparoscopic control in experienced hands. The large percentage of false-negative tissue samples in cirrhotic patients[34] or even a greater number of false-negative results in hepatic cancer[40] clearly indicates the preference for this procedure.

It is true that it requires certain skill and training, but this can be acquired with ease within the framework of an established program. If laparoscopy is performed properly with sound indications, in the overwhelming majority of cases it can save an unnecessary exploration with high morbidity and mortality figures, and/or the diagnosis can be established with histologic proof.

INDICATIONS

Laparoscopy is indicated to evaluate liver disease: cirrhosis, suspected hepatoma, suspected metastases, or hepatomegaly. It is also useful for solving abdominal diagnostic problems, such as in cases of a palpable mass, ascites, jaundice, gallbladder disease, staging malignancy prior surgery, mesentary vascular insufficiency, or a second look after treatment of malignancy.

CONTRAINDICATIONS

Inflammatory and/or infectious diseases, general peritonitis, mechanical or paralytic ileus, blood dyscrasias, nonresponding coagulopathies, and a large hiatal hernia are contraindications to laparoscopy.

Cardiovascular or respiratory insufficiency does not in general represent a contraindication, but the creation of a pneumoperitoneum must be performed with extreme care in this group of patients. Existing dyspnea, cyanosis, or cardiac failure requires careful individual evaluation.

Previous explorations do not constitute a contraindication, but the technique and knowledge of where to insert the pneumoneedle and trocar necessitate judgment and experience on the part of the operator.

GENERAL ASPECTS PRIOR TO THE PROCEDURE

After carefully checking the various laboratory and other routine examinations, blood typing and cross matching is performed. The patient should be aware of the remote but existing possibility of complications. They should be discussed with the patient and the relatives if necessary. The properly phrased consent should include "possible laparotomy." This helps to protect the operator in disputed cases.

Exploring the upper abdomen is a different situation. Patients with suspected or existing malignant disease or jaundice belong to a different group from those who undergo gynecologic laparoscopy for sterilization, infertility problems, or chronic pelvic inflammatory disease.

PATIENT PREPARATION

We use the same standard skin preparation as is applied for any surgical abdominal procedures.

ANESTHESIA

The majority of patients referred to us are severely ill, have unsolved diagnostic prob-

lems, or are in a cachectic state and sometimes not able to withstand the risks of a general anesthesia. Laparoscopy can then be performed under local anesthesia with premedication. General anesthesia is used in other situations.

Local Anesthesia

After a complete work-up the patient arrives in the endoscopy or operating room with an intravenous line in place. We inject diazepam (Valium) and meperidine (Demerol) very slowly. The dosage must be titrated individually to produce a relaxed state but no somnolence. Diazepam can cause respiratory depression if it is not administered slowly and with care. Oxygen administration, as well as complete resuscitation equipment, should be at hand. In high-risk patients local anesthesia is the method of choice, but the manipulations require experience and skill. Every touch with the instrument or accessories (biopsy forceps) on the parietal peritoneum can cause pain. The area of needle or trocar insertion is infiltrated with 1 percent local anesthetic.

General Anesthesia

The majority of gynecologic cases are performed with general anesthesia. This group of patients is comprised mainly of young, healthy females. General anesthesia provides greater safety because if arrythmias or respiratory or other complications occur they can be controlled more easily in the intubated patient. Muscle relaxants are not necessary but are helpful for the inexperienced operator.

The risk of general anesthesia, the problems of a sore throat, and other existing sequelae of intubation must be taken into account. The choice of anesthesia has to be custom-tailored to the patient's condition and the skill of the examiner.

STERILIZATION OF INSTRUMENTS

We use gas to sterilize the instruments because it is bacteriologically more reliable than soaking (Chapter 8). The laparoscope can be soaked between cases but must be meticulously cleaned before and rinsed after soaking to avoid contamination or transfer of the highly concentrated cleansing chemicals into the abdominal cavity, since they can cause irritation or local peritonitis. The metal parts can be autoclaved. The type of sterilization is dependent on the number of cases performed per day, institutional policy, etc. We prefer gas sterilization and thus have acquired several sets of instruments so as to perform three cases simultaneously per day if necessary.

PNEUMOPERITONEUM: AIR OR GAS?

Early in the history of laparoscopy room air was used for pneumoperitoneum, but there were some cases of air emboli reported with a fatal outcome.[10] If high-frequency electrosurgery current (coagulation) is employed the combustion problem also poses a high risk. These factors influenced us to change from air to gas.

CO₂ or N₂O?

CO_2 is safe from the point of solubility, fast absorption, and avoidance of air emboli if only small amounts enter the bloodstream. After desufflation the retained minimal amount is absorbed from the abdominal cavity within approximately 30 minutes, without after effects. It appears that with local anesthesia insufflated CO_2 causes a central stimulation for which the patient compensates with moderate hyperventilation. The reports in the literature are somehow contradictory in respect to favoring CO_2 or N_2O.[13,17,20,21,23,24,30,31,46] A recent study by Stephens and Thompson,[35] who placed the patients into one of two groups (CO_2 and N_2O) is of interest. The procedure in both groups was performed under local anesthesia. No significant differences between the two gases with respect to Po_2 and Pco_2 and respiratory volume was noted. More than 2,000 laparoscopies were performed in our endoscopy department during the last 4 years. CO_2 was administered in all cases, and we saw no reasons to indicate that CO_2 is more hazardous or that we should change to N_2O.

TECHNIQUE

The most important step for a successful laparoscopy is the performance of a sufficient pneumoperitoneum. The insufflation of air or gas into the abdominal cavity was started in a large series during the 1930s—as an outpatient procedure—for the treatment of lower-lobe tuberculosis. When laparoscopy took its place room air was employed at first, later to be changed to gas (CO_2 or N_2O). The pneumoneedle was introduced by Veress[41] in 1938 and was first designed for the creation of pneumothorax; he advocated that it also be used for pneumoperitoneum. It incorporates a spring-loaded blunt stylet in a larger injection needle. The idea is that as soon as the thorax or abdominal wall is penetrated and the needle enters an empty cavity, the spring pushes the blunt stylet forward because there is no resistance. Its aim was to avoid injuries to the lung and abdominal organs during further manipulation. A side hole in this stylet facilitates insufflation (Chapter 5).

Insertion of the Needle

Kalk taught that the lateral third between the iliac crest and umbilical line (Fig. 1) is a safe area for insertion; it was later replaced by the umbilical fold below the umbilicus in the midline. After the needle is in position, a syringe containing saline is attached and aspirated to make sure that a vessel is not punctured.

If previous abdominal operations have been performed, there should be assessment for possible adhesions. If a right upper abdominal scar is present (which there is in the majority of the cases) the lower midline can still be used. Adhesions can be expected in the right upper quadrant; even if they are massive or cannot be safely dissected or penetrated with the telescope through an empty, free area, the left upper abdomen or the left lobe of the liver is free and can be approached. If the left upper quadrant shows scars, the needle again can be introduced in the same position as mentioned above and the right upper quadrant examined. If the right upper and lower quadrants were previously explored for one reason or another, the needle should be inserted into the left lower quadrant. It is not advisable to go in above the umbilicus in the midline because injury to the falciform ligament can cause bleeding.

Technique of Pneumoperitoneum

After the needle is in position it is connected to a insufflation apparatus (Chapter 5). It is very important to observe the intraabdominal

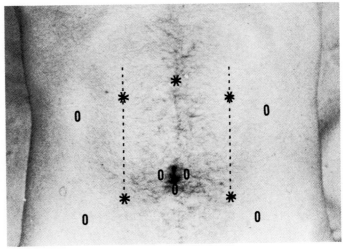

FIG. 1. Preferred areas for introducing the pneumoneedle or trocar (0). Areas marked with (*) are dangerous or not recommended.

pressure at the onset of insufflation. If this pressure is low (in the vicinity of 8 to 10 mm Hg), we can assume the instrument is in the abdominal cavity. Sometimes the mesocolon is pierced and the needle lies between the two leaves of this fine structure. Unfortunately the pressure in this position does not always show significant increase, i.e., the dial would not indicate higher pressure or resistance. We saw several cases where 1 or 2 liters of gas was insufflated in this space, the two layers were dissected with ease, and a pneumomesocolon was created. The gas can spread also into the retroperitoneal space. For this reason we change the needle position after 1 or 2 minutes, when a small cushion has been created. It is therefore important to relocate or check the position of the needle after a short period of insufflation. A "false" pneumoperitoneum can also occur if adhesions are present. We found in several patients who had never been operated on before that the needle became entangled within adhesions and formed an insufflated sac containing CO_2. Movements of the pressure gauge needle following inspiration and expiration, palpation, assessment of the symmetry of the distended abdomen, and percussion are important clinical tests which should not be overshadowed by automatic gadgetry. If gas inflow is higher (more than a liter per minute) sudden distention can cause arrythmias or respiratory problems. The electrocardiograph apparatus should always be attached to the patient, even when local anesthesia is used, and the audible sign switched on. The rhythm changes can warn the operator in time. If irregularities occur repeatedly, the outside sheath of the needle is left in position, the (inside) blunt stylet

unscrewed and pulled out, and the patient desufflated. At the same time oxygen should be administered if local anesthesia has been used. If cardiac arrythmias occur at a later stage, when the trocar is already inserted, partial desufflation is advisable.

Insertion of Examining Trocar

After the pneumoneedle is withdrawn the needle puncture is slightly enlarged by a scalpel (blade No. 11), only enough to accommodate the trocar sleeve. It is essential that the skin incision not be large or deep, otherwise leakage can occur. There are many topographic variations where the trocar or needle can be inserted, depending on the conditions, e.g., several scars due to previous surgery, extension of a palpable mass, etc. If the pneumoneedle is inserted in the lateral third of the umbilicus-iliac crest line it can be left there, but care should be taken that during the procedure it is not accidentally removed and the trocar placed in the midline or other positions. After we are satisfied that the abdominal wall is properly tight due to the pneumoperitoneum, the trocar is inserted with a drilling-pressing action. The trocar is held in one hand, while the other hand (thumb and index finger) holds the sleeve. I found this to be a safety measure in thin patients. If the trocar drilling-pressure is high and the abdominal wall does not present great resistance, the instrument can suddenly slip into the abdominal cavity, hitting an underlying bowel segment or mesenteric vessels, even rupturing or puncturing great vessels. The thumb and index finger can act as a sensor to this sudden move and act as a "break." Some laparoscopists advocate lifting the abdominal wall with one hand while the penetrating maneuver is performed. If the patient is a female with a flaccid, slightly obese abdomen, we are lifting mainly subcutaneous fat. Even if the rectus muscle can be elevated partially, the parietal peritoneum can be left behind. Under local anesthesia the patient can be asked to lift his head to tighten the rectus muscles, producing firmer resistance and allowing easier penetration. After the cannula is in position a hissing noise indicates the escape of gas through the side hole at the tip of the stylet. With other types of cannulas momentarily opening the trumpet valve displays the same hissing noise of escaping gas. Semm[32] recommended the Z (zigzag) insertion of the trocar through the muscle layer to avoid herniation at a later stage. In our series of 1,800 gynecologic laparoscopies we never came across this complication. Frangenheim[10] also found this approach of penetration unnecessary. The trocar should never be inserted if you are hesitant about the completeness of the pneumoperitoneum. A small, longer needle attached to a syringe with saline can be inserted through the abdominal wall and aspirated with only slight suction applied on the plunger to see if air bubbles are returned.

The majority of surgical traumas or organ injuries are caused by inappropriate trocar insertion. We prefer the smallest available trocar (7 mm outside diameter). If a trocar is larger (wider), the length of the sharp tip of the stylet must be longer. A shorter tip (5 to 6 mm) or a smaller sleeve makes a significant difference in the ease of penetration and the distance between the entered sharp tip and underlying organs (Chapter 5). Despite our protective gas cushion this distance is decreased remarkably during the drilling-pressing action. The recent improvements in optics provide a telescope with 5 to 6 mm outside diameter including light transmission which produces a superb image quality. There is no need for the giant 10- to 11-mm trocars. If a pneumoperitoneum does not incorporate the entire peritoneal cavity, a larger pseudosac is formed.

Always observe the early introduction through the endoscope. The walls of the cannula should be seen as soon as the sleeve is exited. You may immediately discover that the instrument is between adhesions, or you may see the fine fibers between the peritoneum and the posterior sheath of the rectus muscle. *Never insert the telescope without looking through at the same time.* If the trocar is in the peritoneal cavity the stylet is withdrawn. In the case of a thin abdominal wall, the trocar sleeve is advanced further, parallel to the abdominal wall, in order to avoid injuries with the sharp edges of the sleeve. The site above the trocar insertion is inspected first to make sure that the area below the penetration is intact. This maneuver is repeated at the end of the procedure. If an area of pooling blood is seen, the accessory trocar is inserted (see below), and the origin and nature of bleeding must be determined. Usually the vessels of the mesenterium are severed. If a collection of venous blood is seen the site is dissected gently with the suction-coagulation cannula and hemostasis can be attempted. Coagulation must be performed carefully to avoid burning adjacent bowel. In the case of an arterial bleeder coagulation is tried, but valuable time should not be wasted if bleeding is vigorous and difficult to localize or to arrest. Immediate arrangements should be made for appropriate surgical management. If costly time has not elapsed, sometimes one stitch or suture through a smaller laparotomy avoids complications such as shock or other irreversible sequelae in high-risk patients.

After the procedure is completed the trocar penetration area is observed before complete withdrawal. Sometimes signs of injury are not seen at insertion but become visible later on. If damage to the bowel mucosa is recognized, it is observed for some time in a close-up position to determine if the dehiscence is superficial or if there is leakage of bowel content. This determines whether the lesion should be treated conservatively or surgically.

Introduction of Telescope and Inspection

Three directions of view are available: 0 degrees (straightforward), 30 degrees (forward oblique), and 90 degrees (lateral). The 0-degree view is used mainly for gynecology in conjunction with the single-puncture approach, using one combined instrument (Chapter 5). I do not advise the single-puncture approach for upper or abdominal (liver) diagnostic procedures but recommend the instrumentation available with two (trocar) puncture approaches only.[2,9,36] It is safer and easier to manipulate with this double approach during the procedure, as well as when taking a biopsy or controlling bleeding.

Examination of the upper abdomen is much more difficult than the pelvic area because of its peculiar anatomic configuration. A good example is the dome of the liver, which cannot be seen properly with a 0-degree straightforward view. We use a telescope with a wide angle (70 degrees), a 30-degree forward oblique direction of view. This allows easy orientation, a "bird's-eye" view from above as well as a close-up view with sufficient magnification. The recent development of the Hopkin's Mark II enlarging laparoscope* resolves from a 15 mm object distance 37.5 μ, which is sufficient to see minute lesions, small vessels, or lymph channels. We must draw the line between microscopic and macroscopic inspection. This type of scope combines the wide-angled view with a greater enlargement in the ocular; therefore a larger and brighter image is displayed to the eye and to the film (Fig. 2). The minute details that are revealed assist in the decision of tissue sampling. The magnifying lupe telescope described by Lent and Jansen[18] and Lindner[19] is questionable as a diagnostic aid.[47] With the new Hopkins telescope enlarged lymph vessels or other changes can be seen very well without sacrificing the wide angle, which is so important for easy and fast orientation. If further magnification is applied—but still in the macroscopic range—this does not add to better assessment of a progressive or regressive stage in liver disease, nor is it of help prognostically.

The 30-degree direction of view gives us the opportunity to slide the telescope over the liver and inspect the upper surface, the dome, and down to the diaphragm. Rotation of the telescope facilitates scanning of "hidden" areas.

The telescope is kept on the instrument table in a hot saline container and is prewarmed to a temperature slightly higher than that of the abdominal cavity to avoid fogging. After its insertion through the trocar we immediately start observation while the telescope is still in the sleeve.

First the area above the trocar insertion is inspected; then the trocar is turned with the optic cranial to locate the falciform ligament for orientation. Once this landmark is found we can then try to obtain an impression of the general area or the positions of certain organs

Manufacturer: K. Storz Endoscopy Co., Tuttlingen, West Germany. Distributor: K. Storz Endoscopy Company of America, Inc., 658 S. San Vicente Boulevard, Los Anglees, Calif. 90048.

in the cavity. For instance, if a retroperitoneal mass is present the stomach and liver may be displaced anteriorly.

Under normal conditions the undersurface of the liver cannot be seen unless it is pushed forward by a retroperitoneal mass, an intrahepatic lesion, or a large, distended gallbladder. The falciform ligament is yellowish and fatty in appearance. The vessel architecture of the ligament should be carefully observed, as well as the parietal peritoneum above and around the liver lobes. If a distended, tortuous venous system is present, it indicates that venous return to the portal system is blocked. This picture is often seen in portal hypertension. The parietal peritoneum can be better inspected by turning the telescope 180 degrees.

Small, whitish nodules can be discovered in the case of metastases (e.g., in carcinoma of the pancreas, hepatocellular carcinoma, or tuberculotic dissemination). Approaching the right lobe, the telescope must be turned downward. When inspecting the liver edge, the gallbladder (with its smooth, shiny, greenish, thin wall) is brought into view. If the wall of the gallbladder is thick, it may not have the usual greenish tint—it may appear whitish. If adhesions are around or heading to the gallbladder, or if this part of the edge of the right lobe of the liver is fixed by adhering omentum, cholecystitis could have been the cause. Sometimes the fundus of a normal gallbladder can be seen only if the right lobe is elevated. The appearance of a normal liver is generally reddish brown, with a smooth, shiny surface (capsule). The telescope can be glided over the dome, keeping close to the parietal peritoneum, looking down over the curved upper surface to the back of the liver, and observing the fine structure of the parenchyma. The impression of the smoothness of the capsule, the appearance of fibrotic or fatty infiltration—or in cases of liver disease, the various changes of the liver architecture or nodularity—can be discovered (Chapter 30). There are intrahepatic lesions which appear as a bulging lump from the liver. It is uncommon that intrahepatic lesions do not become obvious, i.e., distorting the liver's contour, etc. If such a lesion is anticipated, several needle biopsies are indicated. After inspection of the right lobe the telescope is withdrawn almost into the sheath. It can be sometimes directed underneath the falciform ligament toward the left lobe. If the ligament appears like a curtain, dividing the upper abdomen, the instrument

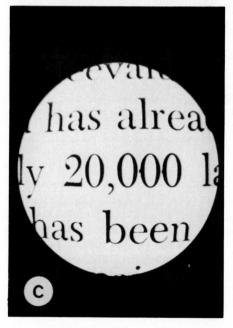

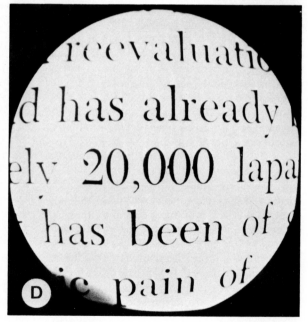

FIG. 2.   A. View with a standard telescope with Hopkins optics. Viewing angle is 60 degrees. Ojbect distance is 40 mm.   **B.** View with an enlarging telescope. Outside diameter of standard examining trocar is 7.0 mm. The Mark II Hopkins optics has a viewing angle of 70 degrees but a larger back (ocular) enlargement. The size of the displayed image on film is also enlarged. The slight aberration at the edges (in cases of flat objects as it is seen here) does not interfere because the abdominal organs are not displayed in one plane and the resolution at the edges is excellent. Even minute changes in the normal anatomy can be discovered. Direction of view is 30 degrees (forward oblique). The color reproduction is superior. Wide-angled view is of utmost importance from the point of view of fast and accurate orientation. Object distance is 40 mm.   **C.** View with a standard Hopkins telescope. Object distance is 15 mm.   **D.** View with an enlarging telescope with Hopkins optics. Object distance is the same as in **C.**

must be rotated counterclockwise to the pelvis and then brought back toward the left hypochondrium. The left lobe is inspected in the same way as the right lobe.

Information about the edges, the general appearance, size (large or small), the under-surface (can you see it?), the smoothness or nodularity, color, architectural changes, vascularity, lymph vessels, symmetry and size of lobes, etc. can add to the overall impression of the status of liver parenchyma and function.

The spleen cannot be visualized under normal conditions. If it is enlarged then the lower pole is seen first. To observe a normal spleen, the patient must be positioned in a steep, reversed Trendelenburg position, rotated to the extreme lateral right. If the stomach in front of the liver is distended or if the small bowel obscures the view, a reversed Trendelenburg position helps to keep these organs in a more caudal position owing to gravity and the liver is more easily seen. If the patient is in the normal horizontal position both gutters are observed for fluid. Sometimes small amounts of ascitic fluid can be discovered that are not detected by physical examination. This can follow inspection of the anterior wall of the stomach. Turning the instrument counterclockwise under constant visual control, the ascending colon can be seen, and lifting the cecum with a probe brings the appendix, pelvic organs, uterus, ovary, bladder, sigmoid colon, etc., into view. Before completing the examination do not forget to observe the site of the trocar insertion below, making sure that there were no accidental injuries during penetration with this dangerous, sharp tool. When the telescope has been withdrawn, the valve is opened and the abdominal cavity desufflated. The incision is closed with clips or skin sutures.

Accessory Trocar Insertion

The second trocar is smaller (5 to 5.5 mm) and is necessary for introducing the manipulating or operating instruments. If a lesion is located, if there are suspicious changes requiring histological clarification, or if organs are to be moved, use of the second accessory trocar is the method of choice. The location and selection of the site is determined by the topography assessed through the telescope. The distance between the trocar to be inserted and the lesion can be determined by pressing the index finger against the abdominal wall above the selected site. The indentation is observed through the telescope, and then this point of reference and the anatomy (cave superior epigastric artery) correlated with the lesion. Once the site has been selected, the local anesthetic is injected (if local anesthesia is to be used). A small stab incision is made and the second trocar introduced *under visual control*. This is a safer procedure than penetration with the examining trocar, which is done blindly. Here you can see the piercing tip of the sharp stylet. If there is not enough gas cushion, wait and increase the amount of gas. If the trocar must be introduced near the rib cage, try to direct the trocar tip toward the telescope to avoid injury to the (enlarged) liver, which is immediately underneath. After the trocar is inserted and the stylet withdrawn, the next important tool is the palpation probe. This is a solid rod with centimeter gradations. It can be tremendously helpful in moving organs (bowel) that obscure the view or gently lifting the liver edge to visualize the gallbladder. It is important to see the undersurface of the liver since in some cases the upper surface can be free of disease while the undersurface contains metastases.

The probe is used an an "extended finger." The sensation gained by palpating a cystic or solid organ is transmitted to the fingertips and gives us a hint about the consistency of the tissues in question.

Biopsy

The first step in biopsy is to introduce the accessory trocar. It is important to locate the entrance of penetration in proper relation to the biopsy site. You must determine, by palpating or depressing the abdominal wall with the fingertip, the relation of this identation (seen through the telescope) to the area to be biopsied. The operating instruments are long enough so that if two biopsies are desirable —from both liver lobes—they can be done from one approach. In the case of a cirrhotic liver or a malignancy I always use the biopsy forceps with a sharp tip and edge. Before introducing or inserting the biopsy forceps, its proper operation is tested. It must be rotated sometimes to avoid obstructing the view. During liver biopsies, if done under local anesthesia, the respiration must be taken into account. If you work fast the procedure can be done with little difficulty. Ask the patient to withhold breathing during a deep inspiration, insert the forceps into the liver in an open position, close it, and withdraw it quickly.

Always have the suction-coagulation probe at hand. If you believe that bleeding or oozing might be a problem, or if it is profound, introduce the suction-coagulation probe into the wound produced by the biopsy forceps; with short periods of suction, depressing the trumpet valve, create a dry field. It is very important to remove oozing and pooling of blood to achieve coagulation. Before starting make sure that the foot switch is nearby so you are ready at any time to start coagulating. This must be well coordinated and fast. The quantity of tissue removed from the liver with the biopsy forceps must be sufficient to obtain tissue from below the capsule. If the liver does not show any changes in the architecture macroscopically and you regard it as a normal liver, and if previous examinations (angiography or scan) showed filling defects that now you cannot recognize even after careful palpation or by lifting the edge of the liver, a liver biopsy with any type of needle is sufficient. For lesions on the parietal peritoneum or in a location which comes into a tangential view, use of the punch biopsy forceps (Chapter 5) is the method of choice. If there is the slightest doubt in respect to solid or cystic appearance, palpation with the probe is of importance before taking a biopsy. If the lesion looks cystic and you have the same impression after palpation, you may aspirate if spillage of toxic or infected material can be avoided. If needle biopsy must be performed, the laparoscopy is advantageous in that it allows repeated attempts at several sites. There is also complete visual and hemostatic control.

If biopsies must be taken from lesions in the pelvic area in the female, the suction cannula should be inserted through the vagina and onto the cervix. It is a great help in elevating the uterus, testing the mobility, and keeping the genital organs (tube, round ligament) in a stretch position. Female patients are catheterized on the table; in males the bladder should be empty. Preventive catheterization is necessary when there is pathology in the pelvic area. Before inserting the second trocar under visual control, observe the relation of your fingertip indentation and the bladder, and make sure that there is enough protective gas

cushion. The intraabdominal pressure should be approximately 25 mm Hg. If the cushion looks too small or shallow, refill and start the drilling-pressing action with the trocar tilted toward you (telescope) in an oblique fashion to avoid injury to the underlying organs.

Biopsy of the ovary is sometimes tricky. This organ is very mobile, and if a deep biopsy is to be obtained (e.g., from the medulla) and bleeding occurs, the organ must be fixed. There is a special drill biopsy forceps available (Cohen-Palmer) for this purpose, but I prefer to introduce a third trocar. Small trocar incisions do not cause any increased morbidity as long as it is done under visual control. First the ovary is fixed or held in position with a grasping forceps. Then a biopsy forceps is advanced through the second trocar to take multiple biopsies (if required). It is advantageous to have this mobile organ stabilized in a position during various manipulations. If bleeding occurs the organ is fixed, and the bleeding can be arrested with the suction-coagulation cannula. If blood is found in the abdominal cavity at the end of the procedure, it is evacuated and observed for further accumulation, if any, before completing the examination.

Ascites

If the patient has obvious ascites, do not insert the examining trocar immediately. It is advisable to start with the pneumoperitoneum needle and aspirate fluid. Measure the intraabdominal pressure and insufflate gas to create a small cushion. Do not exceed 30 mm Hg pressure, and penetrate the abdominal wall very carefully. Make sure that the skin incision is small enough to ensure a tight fitting. In ascitic patients the bowel is floating on the top of the fluid. The concept that it is safer to puncture an abdomen with ascites is untrue. The danger of bowel perforation is just as great if it is performed without precaution. Therefore a small pneumoperitoneum should be produced. Introduce the telescope in a relatively parallel line to the abdominal wall in order to avoid immediately diving into the fluid. In the majority of cases the liver is under water, and even with positioning (reversed Trendelenburg) the visibility can be far from ideal. The second accessory trocar is introduced under visual control and the suction cannula advanced to aspirate ascitic fluid under continuous observation. A sterile sampling tube for cytology or bacteriology studies can be inserted into the suction line and a certain amount of fluid slowly removed. The fluid must be replaced by gas, which is maintained through a link of the examining trocar and the insufflation machine. This provides a clear vision. The color of the fluid provides some hints (clear, opaque, hemorrhagic, etc.). Before starting the visual or instrumental manipulation, make sure that sufficient fluid is removed. Check the patient's vital signs continuously. Do not remove more fluid than is required for observation and manipulation.

CHOLANGIOGRAPHY AND SPLENOPORTOGRAPHY DURING LAPAROSCOPY

The combination of visual observation, tissue sampling, and various radiologic examinations are helpful because they can be performed at a single session.

Differential Diagnosis of Jaundice

A diagnostic dilemma is presented in approximately 20 percent of icteric patients. The critical differentiation between medical and surgical jaundice must be resolved. After a judicious period of observation these patients are subjected to exploration. This approach necessarily subjects a certain percentage of patients with hepatocellular disease to the increased morbidity and mortality (12 to 19 percent) of diagnostic laparotomy.[1]

In recent years a number of new diagnostic modalities have become available that can be used for the preoperative evaluation of jaundiced patients. These procedures are all based on the principle of direct cholangiography using a variety of approaches. The radiopaque material is introduced directly into some portion of the biliary system so that it can be visualized despite the presence of jaundice. With the exception of endoscopic retrograde cannulation of the papilla (ERCP) via the duodenoscope, these methods generally depend on the presence of a dilated intrahepatic bile duct, and this has inherent limitations.

This disadvantage can be overcome by selecting the gallbladder as the injection site. Guidance is readily provided by means of the laparoscope. Direct injection into the gallbladder fundus was advocated by Kalk and Bruhl,[16] Royer et al.[27] The risk of bile leakage was overestimated. Wannagat[45] performed more than 2,000 cases, among which only three were associated with bile leakage, which was corrected at surgery and without fatal outcome.

Rosenbaum[26] advocated the transhepatic approach. This has the advantage of tamponade of the gallbladder puncture by the liver to prevent bile extravasation. In fact, it is a percutaneous transhepatic cholecystocholangiogram, but using double guidance. (See also Chapter 17.)

Technique

The procedure is reserved for those jaundiced patients in whom the diagnosis could not be established after 7 to 10 days of hospital observation and investigation. It also depends on whether a surgeon or gastroenterologist performs the procedure. In the case of surgeons, the patients are prepared for possible laparotomy should a surgical lesion be demonstrated. This also decreases hospitalization time if a surgical procedure can be helpful and performed in the same session with the diagnostic one. Appropriate systemic antibiotics are administered prior to the procedure. The studies are performed in the operating room using a special operating table equipped with a radiolucent coordinated-movement tabletop. A large-field amplifier with a television linkup is placed beneath the operating table. The fluoroscopic image is displayed on a television monitor. Simultaneous display in the x-ray department is possible. Roentgenograms are readily obtained at the appropriate time with reduced risk of radiation dosage using the indirect radiographic technique but serial films (Chapter 17).

The procedure can be performed under local or general anesthesia depending on the general condition of the patient and the circumstances. The patient is positioned obliquely with the left side elevated 15 degrees. After the laparoscope is introduced, a general survey of the abdominal cavity is performed. It is the great advantage of this technique that the abdominal organs can be observed at the same time. In case of malignancy dissemination can be detected and biopsied, and the malignant process can be staged. Special attention should be paid to the right upper quadrant. The gross appearance of the liver and gallbladder is noted. Diagnosis is readily made with liver metastases or carcinomatosis. In the majority of instances the diagnosis may be inferred by the appearance of the liver and gallbladder; however, definite diagnosis requires supplementation of the endoscopic examination with direct cholangiography. The smaller accessory trocar is inserted in the right upper quadrant. A palpation probe is advanced for elevating the right lobe of the liver. This permits observation of the undersurface and facilitates inspection of the gallbladder. It also provides stabilization of the liver during cholangiography. With this technique the gallbladder can be visualized in most patients, even in those in whom only a small number of adhesions were found.

A site is then chosen for percutaneous puncture. Under visual guidance a 20-gauge 8-inch Longdwel needle* is inserted through the abdominal wall, the appropriate intercostal space, or the midclavicular line. The needle is directed toward the hepatic surface of the gallbladder by traversing the right lobe of the liver. An appropriate angle is chosen so that the liver is entered approximately 2 to 4 cm from the anteroinferior margin. Once the liver parenchyma is entered, the stylet is withdrawn and the needle advanced until the gallbladder is entered and bile is aspirated. The needle is then withdrawn from the system and the Teflon catheter left in positon in the gallbladder. The catheter is then anchored to the skin at the exit site of the suture. A bile specimen is sent to the laboratory for bacteriologic and cytologic studies.

An air-free system of 50 percent Hypaque in a 50-ml syringe attached to a venous extension tube is prepared. The contrast medium is injected slowly under fluoroscopic control. As soon as the dye appears in the gallbladder the first film is exposed. Serial films are obtained as the entire biliary system is outlined by continuous injection. If the gallbladder looks distended through the telescope and no dye enters the common bile duct, it is advisable to wait 1 or 2 minutes, observing on the fluoroscopic screen the gallbladder contraction or dyestuff appearance in the extrahepatic system. Rapid runoff into the duodenum is readily recognized and permits the table to be repositioned for the

filling of hepatic ducts. This is very important because it is a great help to know in stone disease whether the calculi are located in the distal duct only or if there are suspicious filling defects in the hepatic part also.

Before the procedure is completed the gallbladder or hepatic duct system is aspirated, removing the contrast material, and decompressed. The puncture site is observed for bile leakage or bleeding, and if required a "plug" is created with the coagulation-suction cannula.

Appropriate display of the hepatic biliary system is very difficult, as in case of retrograde cannulation. With this method we have complete control about the various filling stages. By obtaining serial films, minute changes can be analyzed from film to film.[6]

A videotape can be added to the television system and replayed for immediate review while the x-ray films are being processed. After satisfactory x-ray interpretation, the biliary system is decompressed, the catheter withdrawn, and the puncture site in the liver observed through the laparoscope. A follow-up survey film of the abdomen is taken 2 hours later to exclude leakage of contrast material from the gallbladder. Liver biopsy is obtained under visual control. Figure 3 illustrates the puncture approach.

In cases of previous cholecystitis or other inflammatory process, the gallbladder and the liver edge can be covered with adhesions that are difficult to dissect or which can cause bleeding. In jaundice the liver can be enlarged, with a characteristic dark greenish appearance. The liver parenchyma can be punctured several

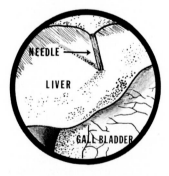

FIG. 3. Laparoscopic approach of percutaneous transhepatic cholecystocholangiography. The needle is directed toward the hepatic surface of the gallbladder by traversing the right lobe of the liver. The liver parenchyma is used as a tamponade against bile leakage.

*Burton, Dickinson Co., Rutherford, N.J.

times until bile is aspirated from a dilated biliary duct.

For direct punctures of a nonicteric normal-looking liver, a long narrow needle (1 mm OD) is employed. Wannagat[44,45] proved in a large series that even normal-sized biliary ducts can be punctured and a cholangiogram obtained.

In jaundiced patients with previous cholecystectomy the left lobe must be approached because the right one is obscured owing to adhesions. Again, the advantages of puncturing the liver under visual control are obvious: the ability to select the site and seeing accurately how deeply the parenchyma is penetrated. If it is done gently and with continuous injection and/or suction, several attempts can be made to find even a small duct.

Visualization of the enlarged or collapsed gallbladder; the appearance, size, and color of the liver; the indirect signs of blockage of return of portal blood to the liver (portal hypertension); the anterior displacement of the stomach or duodenum; and a large spleen or metastases can guide us in the direction of etiology and treatment.

Splenoportography

Hemodynamic investigations in the diseased liver has its own merits. Laparoscopy again offers the help of visual control. With meticulous technique the spleen can be punctured, and manometry and splenoportography performed. According to Wannagat the function of the outlet sphincter of the spleen sometimes interferes with the recorded pressure, especially if it is measured when the sphincter is contracted, indicating a higher pressure than the existing one. After the needle from the spleen is withdrawn very slowly and just enough to achieve spontaneous arrest of bleeding from the splenic pulp, the liver parenchyma is punctured and the needle advanced or relocated under aspiration until portal blood is withdrawn. Injection of a few milliliters of contrast material immediately shows the portal tree if the needle is correctly positioned. The pressure is recorded and a portogram obtained through a T-tube connection. With this combined technique the splenoportogram displays the anatomy and flow pattern, and the splenic pulp and portal pressures in the liver are assessed. Direct pressure measurements of the portal system and aimed portography with separate splenoportog-

raphy is advantageous over the "one shot" technique. If this procedure is performed with skill, appropriate indication, and the proper equipment, then as far as the hemodynamics and flow pattern of the portal system are concerned this method can be valuable diagnostically and prognostically in the various stages of portal hypertension.[4a,45]

PERMANENT FILM RECORDS

The need for documentation as evidence with its various aspects were detailed in Chapter 18. Laparoscopy is perhaps the most difficult endoscopic procedure with which to perform photography or filming (Fig. 4). The abdominal cavity presents longer object distances and more light-absorbing objects with disturbing reflecting surfaces, mainly in the upper abdomen. The light-carrying fibers incorporated in the telescope are not enough to transmit a flash of sufficient intensity or continuous illumination to expose a high-speed (160 ASA) film.

We never know in advance whether the ex-

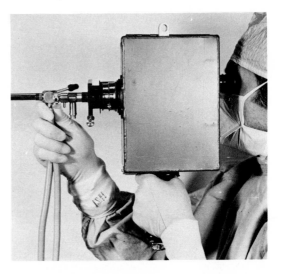

FIG. 4. One (difficult) way to do cinematography. The telescope is inserted into the filming (more fibers) sheath. The 16-mm Beaulieu camera is inserted in a sterile case. The camera lens is gas-sterilized. The camera is triggered remotely via a gas-sterilized electric cord. The distance between telescope eyepiece and the examiner's eye is disturbingly long. Holding the camera for a long period of time without losing the object is difficult as the instrument is heavy. Performing a biopsy or other manipulation during filming requires an acrobatic performance.

amination will reveal normal or abnormal
anatomy. Our examining trocar is 7 mm in
diameter, and a telescope with its fibers inserted through this cannula transmits only
enough light for examination. The idea for inserting a flash tube separately[7a] or attaching a
small flash globe in front of the telescope [17a]
provided adequate intensity for still photography but carries too much risk in case of
failure (Chapter 18). Whenever light is transmitted from outside (external source) intensity
is lost through the transmission system. Consequently this loss has to be compensated for
using more fibers surrounding the optic with a
larger total diameter. This results in a 10- to
11-mm trocar. Introduction of this "king-sized"
trocar with a longer, sharp stylet can carry a
higher risk of injury.

Still Photography

An additional fiber sheath packed with more
light-carrying fibers (Figs. 5 and 6) is used for
still photography. The external flash tube is attached to the sheath or to the end of the larger

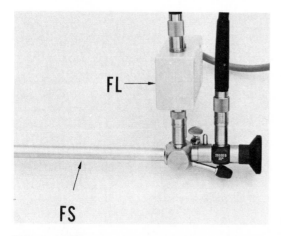

FIG. 5. Additional photofiber sheath with telescope. Trocar diameter is 10.5 mm. The flash tube is
encased in a plastic housing and attached outside.
A bifurcated fiber light cable is attached to the telescope and to the back of the flash tube. The still
camera is coupled (omitted from the picture) to the
eyepiece. The camera is synchronized with the flash
generator. FL, (sterilized) flash tube in plastic housing. FS, additional fiber (flash-transmitting) sheath.
The same or similar flash tube can be placed at a
distance and connected to the photofiber sheath via
an integral fiber bundle. The main disadvantage of
this arrangement is that a much larger trocar must
be inserted if permanent documentation of the
pathology is desired.

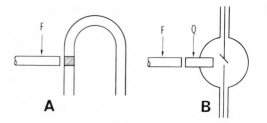

FIG. 6. Basic principles of flash transmission.
A. The flash globe (U-shape) is connected via a
quartz rod or fiber light (F) cable to the endoscope.
In this case only a fraction (shaded area) of the entire output of the flash tube is collected. Even with
the help of condensor lenses the efficiency is poor
and the loss is significant. (Estimated collection:
10 to 20 percent of total output.) **B.** An arc strobe
tube is employed, but a quartz finger (Q) is inserted
into the glass envelope of the tube near the source.
This finger permits maximum collection and transmission of the total energy output, so the efficiency
is much greater. A fiber or fluid fiber light guide can
be attached for transmission (Chapters 15 and 18).

fiber bundle (Fig. 7). Light transmission with a
0-degree straightforward exit is easier to manufacture, and it provides better illumination
than one with, for example, a 30-degree forward oblique direction of view. In hepatology
the 0-degree view has its limitations. The combined light and image transmission in one
sheath has the advantage that the beam to illuminate the object is aligned with vision. On
the other hand, it is a much larger instrument
and is inconvenient.

Separated Light (Flash) Transmission for Photography

Difficulties are encountered as follows: (1) It
is necessary to document interesting lesions,
but we never know in advance if we will find
pathology at all. (2) An examining trocar (7
mm) is used, and we must be able to obtain
photographs without increasing the trocar size
or interfering with the routine. These aspects
gave us the impetus to consider another approach.

We use the standard 7-mm examining trocar
and telescope. If a lesion is observed the second
accessory trocar is introduced. A previously
gas-sterilized (external) flash tube with a
4.5-mm quartz rod in a metal cover, but fully
insulated from the plastic housing inside, is
inserted through the accessory trocar (Fig. 8).
Quartz is an excellent light transmitter—bet-

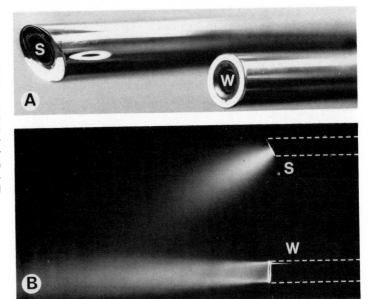

FIG. 7. Top: Storz (S) photofiber sheath with the laparotelescope inserted. Direction of view is 30 degrees. Wolf (W) photolaparoscope with fibers arranged in a circular shape. Direction of view is 0 degrees, straightforward. The oblique view is more suitable for examination of the liver and other upper abdominal organs. Both are integral photofiber sheaths. Bottom: Light pass of Storz (S) and Wolf (W) scopes.

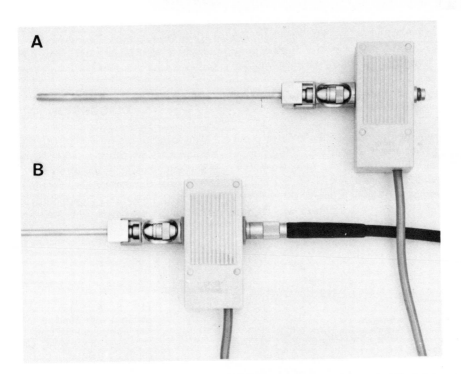

FIG. 8. A. A quartz rod (diameter 4.5 mm) is placed in front of the flash tube. Flash tube and quartz rod are gas-sterilized. **B.** A light guide (fiber) cable is attached to the back of the tube. Illumination is transmitted through the flash tube and quartz, and serves as a spotlight to indicate the proper direction of the flash. Quartz is a better light transmitter than glass fibers. In most cases we introduce the accessory trocar. This quartz rod can also be advanced through the same separate trocar; larger trocars are unnecessary. A standard examining set is employed.

ter than glass fibers. The large exit angle of this quartz rod permits wide areas to be covered. A bifurcated fiber cable, with one end coupled to the telescope to provide examining light, is attached on the other end to the back of the plastic housing of the flash tube. The continuous light through the flash globe and quartz rod give us an indication (spotlight) where the flashlight will be directed. With a minimum of maneuvering, the spotlight through the flash is aimed to the middle of the pathology, the camera connected to the telescope and flash generator. The generator is synchronized with the camera. With this arrangement we can obtain excellent pictures from the pelvic area. The liver, being a protuberating organ, requires that the operator have somewhat more experience to illuminate the proper area, but it can be done. Further refinements are under development. The new stroboflash system (Chapter 18) provides continuous illumination and flash with a single globe-placed remote apparatus (Fig. 9). This arrangement eliminates the need for changing trocars, introducing larger ones if photography is needed. It does not interfere with the routine procedure.

Cinematography

Filming in the upper abdomen creates problems. The liver absorbs or reflects light in a different way than does, for example, the pelvic area, parietal peritoneum, etc. To film through the laparoscope and to see properly through the camera viewer, or even to manipulate, is one of the most difficult and clumsy endoscopic

filming procedures (Fig. 4). At this stage of development this problem will very likely remain in the hands of a few skilled enthusiasts.

TELEVISION

It is relatively easy to televise the pelvic areas. The upper abdomen again needs more light to expose, for example, the liver and diaphragm "in one shot." We use the same light and light-transmission system as described above for filming. Two years ago we conducted a postgraduate course in tubal sterilization. The entire procedure was performed by the operator in the operating room and was displayed via the television screen to a large audience located seven floors below. This can be done but requires elaborate preparation—technicians on the controls of the television systems, etc.—and is very expensive. The details obtained, for example, from a color videotape are inferior to the quality achieved with a 16-mm film. The advantages and limitations of television must be weighed (For details see Chapter 19.)

DISCUSSION

The surgeon may resent infringements on his territory by the laparoscopist, particularly if the endoscopist is an internist. One way to avoid this unpleasantness would be for the surgeon to reevaluate laparoscopy and become more familiar with it. The majority of skepticism and negativistic approach originates in

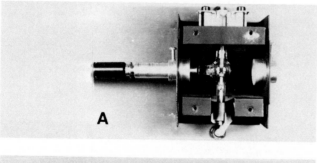

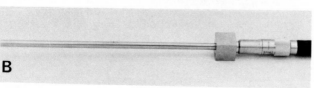

FIG. 9. A. Flash tube (100 watts/ second) with quartz finger and flexible light guide. Front cover is removed. (Courtesy of Chadwick-Helmuth Co.) **B.** Light guide is attached to quartz rod. In this version the high-efficiency flash tube is placed remotely, and the flash discharge is transmitted via a flexible fiber (or fluid guide) to the quartz rod and finally into the abdominal cavity. Loss is minimal compared with systems displayed in Figures 7 and 8.

unfamiliarity or misinformation about the procedure. A good example of this is gynecologic laparoscopy. This procedure was not recognized by the obstetrics-gynecology profession until recently in the United States, when it was suddenly rediscovered on a large scale.

The surgeon has other advantages. If he prepares the patient for diagnostic laparotomy, laparoscopy can first confirm and support his assumption, and he can then perform the surgical intervention during the same session. On the other hand, if the laparoscopic findings are clear and definite he may be able to avoid an unnecessary, costly, and risky operation. Furthermore, in those few patients in whom complications occur the surgeon can correct them immediately and appropriately. The mortality of diagnostic laparotomy in patients with liver damage is high: 12 to 19 percent.[8,22] The diagnostic accuracy of laparoscopy is over 90 percent (see *Discussion,* below) for intraabdominal lesions of unknown origin, liver disease, and differential diagnosis of jaundice.

The limitations of this procedure are partially due to the anatomy. For instance, retroperitoneal organs or lymph nodes are not accessible. In a few exceptions a large mass can bulge into the abdominal cavity, displacing the bowel or other intraabdominal organs. This could be assessed or even biopsied, but otherwise these areas are blind spots.

If other operations precede laparoscopy, in many cases the procedure can still be performed with proper judgment and skill. There are great variations among adhesions. If they are curtainlike, large, thick, or strongly adherent to the parietal peritoneum or liver edge, it is difficult to dissect or lyse them, a procedure that is often not without risk owing to the possibility of bleeding. It is very difficult to arrest bleeders from adhesions or omentum, because as soon as they are divided they retract and it is not easy to find these bleeders.

In general, this procedure provides the opportunity for a clear intraabdominal look, one that is familar to a surgeon but this time is seen through a stab incision. The small accompanying morbidity and mortality figures speak for themselves compared to those associated with a diagnostic surgical intervention. Even if the surgical exploration is a "quick in and out" one, the patient's recovery and hospitalization time is much longer than after laparoscopy, where the patient usually can leave the hospital on the following day.

RESULTS

Some data about the value of diagnostic accuracy are displayed in Table 1. One of the greatest assets of laparoscopy is that we can obtain tissue samples to verify our findings histologically. This is important in liver disease where false-negative needle biopsies are not uncommon in cirrhotic patients. These negative results (using blind needle biopsy) increase significantly where there are metastatic lesions of the same organ.

TABLE 1. Data on Diagnostic Accuracy

Author	Year	Diagnostic accuracy (%)
McHardy et al.[22]	1947	96
Shackleford[33]*	1947	94
Anderson et al.[1]	1950	94
Kalk and Bruhl[16]	1951	90
Zoeckler[50]*	1958	96.3
Ruddock[29]	1957	96
Herrera-Llerandi[12]*	1961	97
Wildhirt[48]	1970	97.3
Rivera and Boyce[25]	1972	94.6
Berci et al.[5]	1973	92

Collected series.

Among 254 cirrhotic patients Vido and Wildhirt[42] found a correlation between the visual findings and the histology in only 68.6 percent, and claimed superiority of the macroscopic appearance and target biopsy in view of prognosis. A diagnostic accuracy of over 90 percent is a great contribution to our existing diagnostic modalities compared with biochemical assays, isotope scans, and radiologic examinations.

Figures 10–12, Plate B* show laparoscopic findings of metastatic lesions. These photos were taken through the standard examining trocar and telescope (7 mm). Flash illumination was transmitted through an accessory trocar and quartz rod.

COMPLICATIONS

The incidence of complications is higher during the laparoscopist's learning period and de-

All color plates appear at the front of the book.

clines as he gains experience. If the procedure is soundly judged to be indicated and is performed with appropriate technique, the risk involved is minimal. The complications can be classified in four major groups:

1. Creation of pneumoperitoneum. The needle is inserted into the wrong place, perforating a viscus, or gas is insufflated in viscera, tissue, or bloodstream. This can be avoided if precautionary measures are strictly followed.
2. Insertion of the trocar. If the pneumoperitoneum is not complete, an inadequate gas cushion cannot prevent perforation of underlying organs or vessels. It is of paramount importance to ensure that the pneumoperitoneum is sufficient.
3. Bleeding from the biopsy, puncture site, or after adhesiolysis.
4. Inadequate monitoring of the cardiac or respiratory system.

There is no question that accidents can occur, even with the most careful technique. Their number can be kept very low, however, and accepted as a minimal but calculated risk.

Statistics available from the literature provide some indications of risk but not a clear picture because some reports contain collective figures and some are personal series. Certain reports include gynecologic cases or patients with a variety of indications. These different groups are not comparable. The risk factor in a patient with treated or untreated cancer, severe liver damage, or jaundice is different from that in the patient, for example, in whom tubal sterilization is performed. Table 2 displays collected figures from four series. The mortality rate (0.07 percent) in Table 2 would probably be slightly different if the various diseases, age groups, etc., breakdown were available by subgroups. It seems that even in this "package deal" presented, however, it is acceptable. Wildhirt[47] reports one death per 5,250 lapa-

TABLE 2. Mortality with Laparoscopy

Author	No. of Cases	Mortality		
		No.	%	Rate
Bruhl (1966)[7]*	63,845	19	0.029	1/3,000
Wildhirt (1969)[47]	10,500	2	0.02	1/5,250
Horwitz (1972)[14]*	35,368	66	0.18	1/530
Cedars (Berci) (1975)*	2,000	1	0.05	1/2,000
Total	111,713	88	0.07	1/2,670

Collected series.

TABLE 3. Mortality with Liver Biopsy

Author	No. of Cases	Mortality		
		No.	%	Rate
Blind liver biopsy				
Volwiler (1947)	174	2	1.1	1/87
Terry (1952)[38]*	10,600	13	0.12	1/815
Zamcheck (1953)[49]*	20,016	34	0.17	1/588
Thaler (1964)[39]*	23,382	4	0.017	1/5,845
Liver biopsy during laparoscopy				
Kalk and Bruhl (1951)[16]	900	0		
Wildhirt (1969)[47]	8,500	3	0.03	1/2,800

Collected series.

roscopies performed, predominantly in liver disease.

Blind liver biopsy, apart from its shortcomings in patients with cirrhosis or malignancy, must be separated according to the technique. The risk is smaller if the biopsy is done with a Menghini needle (pure aspiration) than when performed with a drill core method (e.g., Vim-Silverman, etc.). Table 3 displays the range of mortality reported by several authors, ranging from 1/87 to 1/5,845.

If liver biopsy is added to the laparoscopic procedure, it increases the risk. Kalk and Bruhl[16] performed 900 biopsies under visual control without mortality, and Wildhirt[47] 8,500 cases with only three fatalities—still within acceptable limits.

The morbidity (patients required exploration because of perforation of bleeding post laparoscopy) varies from 0.1 to 0.8 percent. In our own gynecologic series of 2,000 cases (Table 2), where tubal sterilization is included, the morbidity was 0.3 percent and the mortality 0.05 percent (one death).

In our series of 200 patients with upper abdominal diagnostic problems we saw subcutaneous emphysema, which absorbed spontaneously, in three cases. Transient arrythmias occurred in six cases but disappeared after desufflation. No death was recorded in this high-risk group of patients.

The competence of the examiner is one of the most important factors in keeping the complication rate at an acceptable level. Well organized training programs help the laparoscopist acquire the needed experience.

REFERENCES

1. Anderson HR, Dockerty MB, Waugh JM: Peritoneoscopy. Proc Mayo Clin 25:601, 1950
2. Berci G, Brooks PG: Diagnostic techniques in laparoscopy. Paper presented at the International Congress on Gynecological Laparoscopy, New Orleans, 1973. New York, Stratton, 1974
3. Berci G: Peritoneoscopy. Br Med J 1:562, 1962
4. Berci G, Gans SL: Peritoneoscopy in infants and children. J Pediatr Surg 8:399, 1973
4a. Berci G, Allcock, EA, Ewing, MR: The diagnosis of portal hypertension. Aust NZ J Surg 28:300, 1959
5. Berci G, Morgenstern L, Panish JF, et al: The evaluation of a new peritoneoscope as a diagnostic aid to the surgeon. Ann Surg 178:37, 1973
6. Berci G, Morgenstern L, Shore JM, et al: A direct approach to the differential diagnosis of jaundice. Am J Surg 126:372, 1973
7. Bruhl W: Zwischenfaelle und Komplikationen bei der Laparoskopie. Dtsch Med Wochenschr 91:2297, 1966
7a. Calame A: Laparoscopic photography. Med Biol Ill (London) 6:148, 1956
8. Cayer D, Sohmer MF: Surgery in patients with cirrhosis. Arch Surg 71:828, 1955
9. Frangenheim H: Chronic pelvic diseases of unknown origin. Paper presented at the International Congress on Gynecological Laparoscopy, New Orleans, 1973. New York, Stratton, 1974
10. Frangenheim H: Laparoscopy and Culdoscopy. Stuttgart, Thieme, 1972
11. Haubrich WS, Uhlich GA: Current status of upper abdominal laparoscopy. Hosp Pract July:79, 1973
12. Herrera-Llerandi R: Peritoneoscopy. Br Med J 2:661, 1961
13. Hodgson C, McClelland RMA, Newton JR: Some effects of the peritoneal insufflation of carbon dioxide at laparoscopy. Anesthesia 25:382, 1970
14. Horwitz TS: Laparoscopy in gynecology. Obstet Gynecol Surv 27:1, 1972
15. Jacobeus HC: Kurze Ubersicht uber meine Erfahrungen mit der Laparoskopie. Munch Med Wochenschr 58:2017, 1911
16. Kalk H, Bruhl W: Leitfaden der Laparoskopie und Gastroskopie. Stuttgart, Thieme, 1951
17. Kunzel W, Kastendieck E, Ferneding L: Der Saure-Base-Status und die Ventilation waerend gynekologischer Laparoskopien. Anesthetist 21:294, 1972
17a. Lent H: Die Entwicklung der Photolaparoskopie mit dem Elektronenblitz. Acta Hepatosplen 9:195, 1962
18. Lent H, Jansen HH: Die Beobachtung der Leberoberflache mit dem Photo-laparoskope. Dtsch Med Wochenschr 83:1, 1958
19. Lindner H: Fortschritte der Photolaparoskopie. Med Welt 27:3, 1965
20. Lode H, Huttemann U, Wolff C: Der Einfluss endoskopischer abdomineller Untersuchungen auf die Atmung. Respiration 29:61, 1972
21. Marshall RL, Jebson PJR, Davie IT, et al: Circulatory effects of carbon dioxide insufflation of the peritoneal cavity for laparoscopy. Br J Anaesth 44:680, 1972
22. McHardy G, Browne DC, Edwards E: Peritoneoscopic and biopsy evaluation of hepatic disease. Gastroenterology 9:682, 1947
23. Morley TR: Cardiac arrythmias during laparoscopy. Br Med J 2:295, 1972
24. Peterson EP: Anaesthesia for laparoscopy. Fertil Steril 22:695, 1971
25. Rivera RA, Boyce HW: Peritoneoscopy. Am J Gastroenterol 58:594, 1972
26. Rosenbaum FJ: Die Laparoskopische Cholangiography. Klin Wochenschr 33:39, 1955
27. Royer M, Mazure P, Kohan S: Biliary dyskinesia studied by means of the peritoneoscopic cholangiography. Gastroenterology 16:83, 1950
28. Ruddock JC: Peritoneoscopy. Surg Gynecol Obstet 65:623, 1937
29. Ruddock JC: Peritoneoscopy: a critical clinical review. Surg Clin North Am 37:1249, 1957
30. Scott DB: Cardiac arrythmias during laparoscopy. Br Med J 2:49, 1972
31. Seed RF, Shakespeare TF, Muldoon: Carbon dioxide hemostasis during anesthesia for laparoscopy. Anaesthesia 25:223, 1970
32. Semm K: Weitere Entwicklung in der gynekologischen Laparoskopie. In H Schwalm and G Doderlein (eds): Gynecology and Obstetrics. Vienna, Urban and Schwartzenberg, 1970
33. Shackelford RT: Peritoneoscopy. Surgery 10:742, 1947
34. Soloway RD, Bagenstoss A, Schoenfield LJ, et al: Observer error and sampling variability tested in evaluation of hepatitis and cirrhosis by liver biopsy. Am J Dig Dis 16:1082, 1971
35. Stephens H, Thompson W: Lecture at the Symposium on Gynecological Laparoscopy[37]
36. Steptoe PC: Laparoscopy in Gynecology. Livingstone, Edinburgh, 1967
37. Symposium on Gynecological Laparoscopy. American Association of Gynecological Laparoscopists, Anaheim, California, 1974 (in press)
38. Terry R: Risk of needle biopsy of the liver. Brit Med J 1:1102, 1952
39. Thaler H: Uber den Vorteil und Risiko der Leberbiopsie nach Menghini. Wien Klin Wochenschr 76:533, 1964
40. Uhlich GA: Liver biopsy in the diagnosis of hepatic cancer. Gastroenterology 63:208, 1972
41. Veress J: Neues Instrument zur Ausfuhrung von Brust-oder Bauchhohlenpunktionen. Dtsch Med Wochenschr 41:1480, 1938
42. Vido I, Wildhirt E: Korrelation des laparoskopischen und histologischen Befundes. Dtsch Med Wochenschr 94:1, 1969
43. Villardel F, Seres I, Marti-Vincente A: Complications of peritoneoscopy. Gastrointest Endosc 14:178, 1968
44. Wannagat L: Die Segmentoportography und die transhepatische Cholangiography mit laparoskopischer Technik. Verh Dtsch Ges Inn Med. Munich, Bergmann, 1966, p 72

45. Wannagat L: Laparoskopische cholangiography. Radiologe 13:26, 1973

46. Wheeless CR: Anaesthesia for diagnostic and operative laparoscopy. Fertil Steril 22:690, 1971

47. Wildhirt E: Abgrenzung der Indikation zur Laparoskopie. Med Klin 64:287, 1969

48. Wildhirt E: Laparoskopie und Leberbiopsy. Wien Med Wochenschr 120:66, 1970

49. Zamchek N: Needle biopsy of the liver. N Engl J Med 249:1020, 1953

50. Zoeckler SJ: Peritoneoscopy. Gastroenterology 34:969, 1958

EDITORIAL COMMENT

Since this chapter was written, a new idea was introduced by Dr. Frangenheim for measuring the intraabdominal pressure during pneumoperitoneum more accurately. As mentioned in the chapter, the pneumoperitoneum needle consists of a blunt stylet, which is spring-loaded with a side hole. After passing any resistance (muscle layer or peritoneum) the blunt stylet is pushed forward into the abdominal cavity to avoid injuries. What we measure today in one channel is the inflow pressure, the resistance of the needle where the diameter of the needle plays a significant role, and the abdominal pressure.

The new Veress-Frangenheim needle (figure) is a triple-lumen cannula instead of the previous double-lumen cannula; one channel is completely free, and one end is in

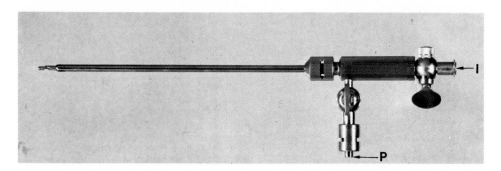

Verress-Frangenheim pneumoperitoneum needle, a triple-lumen cannula. I, channel for gas insufflation. P, separate channel for abdominal pressure measurements only.

the cavity and the other is connected to the pressure gauge. Through this channel no gas is inflated under pressure. The abdominal cavity is directly connected to a pressure gauge. (This is a preliminary report, courtesy of Dr. Frangenheim.)

THE EDITOR

30

Laparoscopy in Hepatology

Richard C. Cammerer
Daniel L. Anderson
H. Worth Boyce

Laparoscopy has been used in the evaluation of liver disease for over 60 years. The procedure was first performed on a dog early in the twentieth century[3] and had gained some measure of popularity in the United States by 1934.[15] Subsequently, interest in laparoscopy declined in this country, but in Europe its use was expanded and it became a well accepted investigative procedure. Following the development of improved instruments with "cold" fiberoptic light transmission and excellent photographic capability, there has been renewed interest in the application of laparoscopy to the diagnosis of liver disease in the United States.

INDICATIONS

Indications for the use of laparoscopy include the spectrum of liver disease. Besides allowing multiple direct-vision biopsies of specific areas in both the right and left lobes of the liver, laparoscopy provides additional information about the liver, biliary system, and portal circulation unobtainable by blind needle biopsy alone. In brief, laparoscopy should be considered whenever there is an indication for liver biopsy. In acute viral hepatitis and in other diffuse inflammatory processes, blind needle biopsy of the liver is usually reliable. Laparoscopy, however, provides additional pertinent information in many cases of chronic liver disease such as metastatic carcinoma to the liver, chronic active hepatitis, postnecrotic cirrhosis, unexplained hepatic scintiscan defects, hepatoma, alcoholic liver disease, and diagnostic problems characterized by cholestasis. The laparoscopic findings in each of these conditions is reviewed here.

CONDUCT OF EXAMINATION

Once the laparoscope is introduced into the peritoneal cavity and an unobstructed field of view obtained, a brief survey of the upper abdomen and identification of the ligamentum teres helps orient the examiner before a systematic examination is undertaken. The liver, gallbladder, and anterior surface of the stomach are visualized best with the patient in a supine position or with the head of the table up 15 to 20 degrees. Visualization of the spleen in this position suggests the presence of splenomegaly. Omentum and loops of bowel which occasionally cover these organs slide inferiorly when the head-up position is assumed. Occasionally a gentle, side-to-side shaking motion is needed to move the omentum off the liver or spleen. A palpating probe also may be used for this purpose. Turning the patient into a left lateral decubitus position permits visualization of the lateral aspect of the right lobe of the liver. Rotating the patient into a right decubitus position often brings the spleen into view for close inspection. The greater curvature aspect of the stomach, the splenic flexure of the colon, and the phrenicocolic ligament also are well seen with the patient in this position. The peritoneum covering the anterior half of each hemidiaphragm is also visualized optimally in the head-up position and should be examined for deformities, inflammatory lesions, and metastatic nodules before the instrument is rotated into the lower quadrants. Positioning the patient in the Trendelenburg position allows the bowel loops to fall out of the pelvis and permits an optimum view of the structures in both lower quadrants.

Auxiliary instruments (Fig. 1) used for manipulation or biopsy purposes are inserted through a second puncture, usually in the right upper quadrant when the liver is being examined. The palpating probe is extremely helpful in performing a more complete examination of the liver and gallbladder. Appropriate use of this instrument permits palpation of liver surface lesions, elevation of the right or left lobes of the liver for inspecting their inferior surfaces, elevation of the right lobe for inspecting the gallbladder, and indirect palpation of the gallbladder. A biopsy needle or biopsy forceps can also be introduced under direct vision for biopsy of the liver or peritoneum.

LIVER BIOPSY

Laparoscopy with direct-vision needle biopsy of the liver offers significantly greater diagnostic capabilities than blind or closed needle biopsy.[9-11] The ability to diagnose focal diseases (e.g., granulomatous liver disease) and neoplastic processes of the liver is greatly enhanced when the biopsy needle can be directed to areas most representative of the underlying pathology. Additionally, laparoscopy enables the examiner to direct the needle away from lesions such as cysts, abscesses, blood vessels, dilated bile ducts, and atypically located gallbladders which would be hazardous to punc-

ture. Passive congestion of the liver, cholestasis secondary to extrahepatic obstruction, and extensive amyloidosis also can be recognized laparoscopically; and biopsy, which could result in excessive loss of blood or bile, can be avoided.

A new disposable needle (Travenol Tru-Cut model) with a 15.2-cm cannula and a 20-mm specimen notch has been used effectively for obtaining adequate specimens during laparoscopy (Fig. 1). A subcostal site for a second puncture is selected by applying external abdominal compression with a finger and observing the relationship of the abdominal wall indentation to the area to be biopsied. An intercostal approach may result in pneumothorax and usually should be avoided. Selection of a site below the xiphoid permits biopsy of lesions involving the left lobe of the liver and areas which should not be investigated by a blind biopsy. When a specimen is needed from a site close to the liver margin it is wise to use a tangential approach to the liver surface. Elevation of the margin also may be used to prevent puncture damage of adjacent organs if the needle should pass entirely through a thin hepatic lobe.

Introduction of biopsy forceps into the abdominal cavity through a separate cannula permits punch biopsies of lesions on the liver surface and along its thin inferior margin. Ability to recognize and control excessive postbiopsy bleeding is another advantage of this procedure.

NORMAL LAPAROSCOPIC ANATOMY

Round and Falciform Ligaments

The falciform ligament may vary in appearance from a thin, veillike structure that is

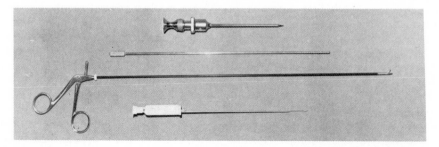

FIG. 1. Auxiliary instruments. From top to bottom: cannula with trocar for introduction of probe and forceps, palpation probe, biopsy forceps, Travenol Tru-Cut biopsy needle.

slightly opaque to a thick, yellow membrane due to heavy fat infiltration. The vascular pattern throughout this structure usually consists of scattered fine red vessels without tortuosity or apparent distention. The round ligament located along the caudad margin of the falciform ligament is usually fatty in appearance with a few fine vessels running along its length. In the very thin individual the round ligament contains minimal fat and the falciform ligament contains no visible fat at all. In the patient with severe fatty metamorphosis or gross obesity, the round ligament typically is distended with fat.

Hepatic Lobes

The normal liver is reddish brown or a mahogany color with a smooth, shiny surface and relatively sharp margins along the lateral aspects of both lobes. The medial aspect of each lobe often is slightly rounded as it approaches the interlobar notch or fissure. The capsule of the liver may show varying degrees of capsular thickening and subcapsular fibrosis with slight retraction or thickening of the capsule that may be patchy or diffuse. A diffuse homogeneous thickening of the capsule may be seen in individuals with past surgery, peritonitis, or ascites. Occasionally small (1 to 2 mm) cream colored to white nodule(s) may be noted on the liver surface without surrounding increased vascularity or other abnormality. These lesions are called mesothelial pearls and are simply focal accumulations of mesothelial and collagen tissue.

In normal individuals the round ligament exits the interlobar notch at a point about even with the medial aspect of the inferior margins of the two liver lobes. When the hepatic lobes extend more than 2 cm caudad to the exit point of the round ligament, the liver is considered enlarged. In a tall person the right hepatic lobe is somewhat elongated and may extend well below the right costal margin in the flank. This hepatic contour often creates concern because of a questionable hepatic mass, but palpation of this tonguelike projection of liver down the right anterior-lateral lumbar area in the presence of no other evidence of hepatic abnormality and a normal-sized left lobe should raise the suspicion that this is simply a structural variation considered to be within normal limits.

The surface appearance of the left lobe should be similar to that of the right lobe, except that the inferior and lateral margins of the left lobe often are very thin, being only 3 to 4 mm thick, for a distance of 1 or 2 cm cephalad. In a tall person the left hepatic lobe may be quite small, but in short stocky persons the left lobe is relatively more prominent.

Gallbladder

The normal gallbladder in a fasting patient appears slightly tense with multiple, small, slightly tortuous blood vessels over its surface. The bile showing through the normal gallbladder wall gives it a robin's egg blue color. In those individuals who have had ascites, cholecystitis, or right upper quadrant peritonitis from some other cause, the gallbladder wall may appear opaque and pale. Any adhesions about a gallbladder with an opaque color should suggest the presence of cholecystitis. The student must recognize that the surface appearance of a colonic haustrum may be similar to that of the gallbladder if only a small area is seen. Use of a probe is helpful here to ensure accurate organ identification.

Stomach

In most individuals the anterior wall of the body and antrum of the stomach can be seen as it protrudes below the left lobe of the liver. The gastroepiploic vessels can be seen along the greater curvature to run anteriorly and superiorly over its surface. In the fasting patient the stomach appears relatively flat and does not elevate the left hepatic lobe. However, in some individuals with aerophagia, there may be rather remarkable distention of the stomach. Peristaltic waves can be seen to originate in the body of the stomach and sweep gently down through the antrum to the pylorus.

Peritoneum

The undersurface of the anterior and lateral aspects of the diaphragmatic parietal peritoneum are easily seen. Usually several sets of arteries and veins course across the undersurface of the diaphragm. In this area it is common to see a single bright red artery running between dark blue veins on each side. This vascular pattern of a central artery with two closely adjacent, parallel veins is peculiar to the undersurface of the diaphragm. Muscular ridges running from anterior to posterior along the undersurfaces of the muscular portion of both sides of the diaphragm are seen occasionally. Rarely a large muscular ridge(s) protrudes inferiorly from the diaphragm. Such a ridge may produce a deep furrow or indentation across the dome of the right lobe (Zahn's indentation). This indentation may simulate a filling defect on liver scan. The point of insertion of the caudad extension of the diaphragmatic muscle fibers on the abdominal wall may be seen in the anterior and lateral aspects of both upper quadrants. In general, it is considered best to stay below the caudad extent of these muscle fibers when doing guided liver biopsies by a second puncture. A biopsy above this level may be transpleural, and in the presence of a pneumoperitoneum may result in pneumothorax.

Left Upper Quadrant

Ordinarily the haustra of the distal transverse colon and splenic flexure may be seen directly or by contour change under a thin veil of omentum. The phrenicocolic ligament extends from the anterolateral wall of the left upper quadrant to the splenic flexure. This peritoneal reflection, a normal structure, is often interpreted by the neophyte as an adhesion. When portal hypertension develops, extensive portal collaterals can be seen in and about this ligament.

Spleen

The normal spleen usually is not visible with the patient in the supine position. If it is visible, it may be seen only as a slight elevation of the omentum just cephalad to the phrenicocolic ligament. Occasionally a small portion of the uncovered inferior pole of a normal spleen may be detected. If the patient is rolled to the right decubitus position, with the left side elevated approximately 40 to 60 degrees, the inferior pole of the normal spleen can be seen in most patients. This maneuver should be a routine part of the examination. Typically the spleen appears cyanotic or bluish brown. It is usual for a small globule of fat to be seen attached to the inferior pole of the spleen. Occasionally there are several notches or crenna along the medial margin of the spleen; these are much more pronounced when the spleen is enlarged.

Omentum

The size and extent of the omentum seems to correlate directly with the patient's body weight and habitus. Individuals with severe fatty metamorphosis of the liver often have quite thickened falciform and round ligaments, as well as a large omentum, referred to as a "sea of omentum." A thin or emaciated patient may have very little omentum visible, and even that which is present is very thin and transparent in many areas because it has little fatty tissue.

DISEASES OF THE LIVER

Cirrhosis

Laparoscopy is particularly helpful in evaluating patients with suspected cirrhosis.[11] Inspection of surface morphology alone often permits definition and even classification of the underlying disease process. Macronodular (postnecrotic) cirrhosis, as its name implies, is characterized by coarse nodularity of the liver surface (Fig. 2, Plate C).* The grossly irregular surface, typical of well established macronodular cirrhosis, results from the development of smooth-surfaced regenerative nodules of varying sizes. Progression of the cirrhotic process results in an indurated, stiff-appearing liver which often projects rigidly into the air-filled peritoneal cavity. The inferior surface of the liver in this instance is exposed and can be examined without excessive manipulation. The cirrhotic liver may be pale in areas of collapse with fibrous tissue. Reddish coloration of the normal or regenerating liver parenchyma is due to blood-filled sinusoids. Additionally, neovascularization of the liver surface, manifested by fine, tortuous vessels which extend over the surface, can be identified in well established cirrhosis, particularly when active parenchymal inflammation and/or portal hypertension are also present. Multiple pinhead-sized, round, elevated, glossy white lesions frequently are seen on the surface in advanced cirrhosis with portal hypertension and ascites. These represent lymphatic blebs. The liver in the late stages of macronodular cirrhosis usually is shrunken, hard, and coarsely nodular.

All color plates appear at the front of the book.

Multiple regenerative nodules of varying size surrounded by deep, broad bands of scar tissue are typically present. Macronodular cirrhosis associated with a bluish gray mottling of the liver surface, particularly in a young individual, should suggest the possibility of Wilson's disease.

The importance of laparoscopic diagnosis of cirrhosis is emphasized by reports indicating that blind or closed needle biopsy of the liver is unable to document the presence of a macronodular cirrhosis in 50 to 60 percent of cases.[20] Gross inspection of the liver surface alone often permits greater diagnostic accuracy than blind needle biopsy.[11]

Micronodular cirrhosis is characterized by diffuse, uniform, monotonous, coarse granularity or fine nodularity of the liver surface (Fig. 3, Plate C). In some cases the contour of the liver surface is undulating and on first glance may be interpreted as macronodular. True regenerative macronodules have a smooth surface in contrast to the apparent macronodules in micronodular cirrhosis, which have a granular surface. Fatty metamorphosis manifested by a mottled yellowish discoloration of the liver surface frequently accompanies the micronodular changes when the disease is related to alcohol. Prominent surface vascularity and dilated lymphatic ductules also may be seen in well established micronodular cirrhosis. Blind needle biopsy of the liver, while more accurate in confirming the presence of micronodular than macronodular cirrhosis, nevertheless falls short of the diagnostic capabilities of laparoscopy combined with guided needle biopsy.[11] Although micronodular cirrhosis is a sequela of alcoholic liver disease in most cases, hemochromatosis, primary biliary cirrhosis, and chronic passive congestion or cardiac cirrhosis in advanced stages should be considered in the differential diagnosis.

Neoplastic Disease

Suspected primary or metastatic neoplastic disease of the liver is a prime indication for laparoscopy. Liver function tests, liver scans, and even blind needle biopsies of the liver, although reasonably reliable in patients with extensive hepatic involvement, are unreliable in detecting the presence of early neoplastic lesions. Blind needle biopsies of the liver in one series yielded malignant tissue in only 39.5 percent of the patients.[9] Guided needle biopsy, on the other hand, yielded positive results in 69 percent of the cases. While both of these figures appear low in contrast to the frequently quoted 75 percent accuracy of blind biopsies,[14] it must be remembered that the latter were obtained in selected patients who had extensive neoplastic involvement of the liver. Early detection by laparoscopy not only may have significant therapeutic benefits but in the majority of cases may spare the patient an unnecessary laparotomy or other major extraabdominal procedure.

Metastatic disease of the liver may be suspected by visualization of an isolated yellowish orange or cream-colored nodule at or just beneath the liver surface, multiple nodules, or diffuse infiltration of an entire lobe. The presence of a round, well circumscribed, firm, elevated nodule with central umbilication resulting from necrosis of the underlying tissue and with marginal neovascularity is characteristic of a hepatic metastatic lesion. Telangiectatic-like proliferation of vessels surrounding these nodules and scattered zones of retracted scar tissue over the surface of the liver resulting from a compromised vascular supply with small infarcts also may be seen. Occasionally involvement is so extensive that normal liver tissue is difficult to identify between the metastases. Color changes in the liver surface with metastases may be due to their secondary effects on blood vessels and bile ducts. The white-to-orange metastases stand out in some areas against the dark green patches of focal cholestasis or the cyanotic areas due to venous obstruction.

Although the majority of metastatic nodules are yellowish orange to creamy white, the typical metastatic lesions of malignant melanoma are deep brown or black. Amelanotic metastases of this tumor are seen occasionally. Inspection of the diaphragm and the available peritoneal surface for metastatic nodules should be routine for all examinations. A punch biopsy of peritoneal metastasis is safer and eliminates the need for liver biopsy.

Primary carcinoma of the liver often is unifocal and either infiltrating or nodular in appearance. Carcinoma developing in an otherwise normal liver is usually grossly nodular. Hepatomas more than several millimeters below the capsule may produce an alteration in surface contour without color change. Since hepatomas have an excellent blood supply, the central umbilication noted in metastases usually is not present. Hepatic cell carcinomas arising in cirrhosis are less likely to present as large nodular tumor masses but instead diffusely infiltrate the liver. Recognizing these tumors in the presence of advanced cirrhosis is often difficult. Guided biopsies with touch cytology must be relied on to establish the diagnosis.

Laparoscopy has also been utilized to stage patients with Hodgkin's disease.[5] The presence of splenomegaly, tumor nodules within the parenchyma or on the surface of the spleen, hepatomegaly, or tumor nodules in the surface of the liver in a patient with Hodgkin's disease confirm metastatic disease. Naturally biopsy is required for definitive diagnosis, since granulomatous diseases of the liver, spleen, and peritoneum can mimic the gross changes of metastatic malignancy.

Chronic Hepatitis

Chronic active liver disease (CALD) is a term used to describe a group of diseases which share certain clinical, biochemical, and immunologic features.[6-19] Differentiation generally can be made only by examining the histologic features of the disease process. Chronic persistent hepatitis, subacute hepatitis, and chronic active hepatitis are the three disease processes most often considered in the differential diagnosis of chronic hepatitis. Primary biliary cirrhosis and Wilson's disease,[18] particularly in the early stages, however, may be difficult to distinguish from other forms of chronic hepatic inflammation. Since therapeutic regimens for each of these diseases have been recommended, establishment of an accurate diagnosis is imperative. The histologic appearance of the liver appears to be the most relevant and sensitive method of judging response to treatment. Although blind needle biopsy of the liver is capable of establishing the diagnosis of hepatitis in 90 percent of cases, the presence of cirrhosis in patients with CALD is confirmed in only 33 percent of the cases.[17] Considering this large sampling error and the therapeutic and prognostic implications of determining the presence or absence of cirrhosis, blind needle biopsy is less than optimal in the management of patients with these disease processes.

A diagnosis of chronic persistent hepatitis usually can be established reliably by blind needle biopsy; however, in cases which cannot be distinguished from early or mild chronic active hepatitis, laparoscopic examination is useful. The typical morphologic features of chronic persistent hepatitis include minimal swelling of the liver, a smooth somewhat erythematous surface, increased capsular vascularity, and occasionally minimal exaggeration of the lobular pattern resulting from portal inflammation. In this condition the inflammatory infiltrate in portal areas makes them paler, sometimes with a cream color, which provides sharp contrast with the red to brown surrounding hepatic lobules. Irregularity of the liver surface resulting from proliferation of underlying connective tissue, in addition to the other surface changes, is characteristic of advancing chronic hepatitis (Fig. 4, Plate C). More pronounced irregularity of the liver surface becomes evident as the disease progresses.

Subacute hepatitis, which is associated with a high mortality rate, is characterized initially by extensive areas of necrosis and collapse of liver tissue. Large depressed or retracted zones of liver lying between areas of parenchyma that are erythematous and swollen as a result of severe inflammation can be seen during the acute phase of the disease. These abnormalities may resolve completely or heal with only minimal residual scar formation. Progressive disease, on the other hand, is characterized by the development of broad areas of scar formation, persistent inflammatory changes, and masses of regenerative nodules over the liver surface.

Granulomatous Diseases

Although the differential diagnosis of granulomas in the liver can be extensive, the majority of cases are secondary to tuberculosis or sarcoidosis, or are idiopathic.[7] The diagnosis of granulomatous hepatitis is often suspected only by liver biopsy. Because of the focal nature of some of these diseases, laparoscopy with a guided needle biopsy may be necessary if a blind biopsy is negative. The frequent occurrence of surface lesions often permits the endoscopist to suspect the diagnosis of granulomatous disease by gross inspection. The biopsy obtained from an area of gross abnormality, however, is relied on for a definitive diagnosis.

Tuberculosis of the liver is characterized typically by hepatomegaly and the presence of numerous, uniform, small, white, miliary foci scattered over the surface.[2] These lesions may be difficult to distinguish from lymphatic cysts or mesothelial pearls. Although they are consistent with a diagnosis of tuberculosis, histologic examination of a biopsy specimen must be relied on for confirmation of this impression. Areas of capsular thickening (a nonspecific finding in a variety of liver diseases) may be quite marked in the presence of tuberculosis. However, adhesions between the liver surface and the dome of the diaphragm, also a nonspecific finding, may suggest the possibility of this form of granulomatous hepatitis. The parietal peritoneum also should be carefully evaluated for the presence of a miliary foci of tuberculosis, particularly in patients with chronic liver disease, ascites, and unexplained low-grade fever.

Sarcoidosis of the liver, present in at least 66 percent of the patients with pulmonary sarcoidosis, is characterized by elevated, whitish, isolated, single or multiple lesions scattered throughout the liver surface.[12] Occasionally the liver is so diffusely and uniformly involved that differentiation from a fatty liver may be quite difficult. The nodular form of sarcoidosis may be difficult to distinguish from metastatic carcinoma, although guided biopsy is a reliable method for establishing the diagnosis.

Hodgkin's disease of the liver, which has been discussed previously and which may present with surface lesions indistinguishable from tuberculosis or sarcoidosis, must be considered in the differential diagnosis of granulomatous hepatitis. Early cases of schistosomiasis may resemble sarcoidosis, but advanced cases demonstrate striking scarring and lobulation, typically without true regenerative nodules.

Infiltrative Disease and Hepatic Congestion

Infiltrative processes such as amyloidosis often produce no specific surface abnormalities. The liver is generally pale and enlarged with blunted edges and an irregular surface. Similar findings are present in neoplastic infiltrative diseases such as myeloid metaplasia and leukemia. In some cases the latter produces localized surface lesions.

Hepatic vein thrombosis is usually documented by techniques other than laparoscopy, but the gross hepatic appearance may provide a clue to the diagnosis. Hepatomegaly, patchy or diffuse cyanosis, superficial venous distention, and features of portal hypertension may be found. Early in this condition the liver may appear diffusely cyanotic, but as hepatic damage with fibrosis occurs the liver may be somewhat pale.

Chronic passive congestion due to right heart failure may produce a sequence of gross changes identical to those of hepatic vein thrombosis, eventuating in the classic "cardiac cirrhosis."

Cholestasis

The differential diagnosis of cholestatic jaundice is one of the more difficult problems facing the physician. Although the classic features of extrahepatic obstruction are well known, they may be closely simulated by drug-induced toxic hepatitis, cholangiolitic viral hepatitis, granulomatous hepatitis, some cases of postnecrotic cirrhosis, chronic active hepatitis, primary biliary cirrhosis, alcoholic liver disease, as well as primary or secondary malignancy. In the presence of jaundice the usual diagnostic techniques are compromised. Percutaneous transhepatic cholangiography is utilized in some centers but carries the risk of bile peritonitis and is usually done as a preoperative procedure. Endoscopic retrograde cholangiography is now recognized as the best technique for differentiating intra- and extrahepatic causes of jaundice.[16]

Laparoscopy with or without liver biopsy has been utilized with good success in the evaluation of cholestatic jaundice. Differentiation of intrahepatic cholestasis from extrahepatic obstruction depends on the appearance of the liver and the gallbladder.

The laparoscopic index of cholestasis is a gray greenish to green black discoloration of the hepatic surface (Fig. 5, Plate C). Surprisingly, this does not necessarily correlate with the level of serum bilirubin. A dark green liver may be seen when the bilirubin is only mildly elevated, and the reverse may also be true. Although a green liver establishes the presence of cholestasis, it does not localize the site unless dilated surface biliary radicals, diagnostic of extrahepatic obstruction, can be identified. Examination of the gallbladder often provides the answer.

The finding of a normally filled or collapsed gallbladder strongly suggests cholestasis of intrahepatic origin. Obstruction of the common hepatic duct, however, may give an identical picture. In contrast, tense enlargement of the gallbladder indicates obstruction distal to the cystic duct, in the distal common bile duct of ampulla of Vater. This is the laparoscopic equivalent of Courvoisier's sign and is usually seen in the presence of malignant obstruction (Fig. 5, Plate C). Lesser degrees of gallbladder distention are not infrequently encountered in patients with alcoholic liver disease without obstruction. This phenomenon is termed cholecystocholestasis and must be appreciated lest too much significance be attributed to this mild to moderate, nonobstructive enlargement of the gallbladder.

Demonstration of a small, white, opaque gallbladder and a variable number of small surface vessels is strongly suggestive of chronic cholecystitis. Frequently adhesions to surrounding structures are present. These findings in conjunction with cholestatic changes in the liver suggest extrahepatic obstruction due to choledocholithiasis.

A small collapsed gallbladder may be misleading. When seen in a patient with a greenish liver, an empty gallbladder suggests obstruction above the cystic duct most often due to intrahepatic cholestasis or hepatic duct carcinoma. In addition, the collapsed gallbladder may be a physiologic phenomenon, resulting from contraction and emptying prior to or even during laparoscopy. From a negative standpoint, a collapsed but otherwise normal gallbladder provides strong evidence against distal common bile duct obstruction.

The simple principles outlined above are quite useful in differentiating intra- from extrahepatic cholestasis. In addition, laparoscopy often provides specific etiologic information about the source of cholestasis. A classic example is the finding of scattered hepatic or peritoneal metastases plus the findings of extrahepatic obstruction.

It is well known that patients with alcoholic hepatitis occasionally present a cholestatic clinical picture which must be distinguished from obstruction.[13] Laparoscopy has been performed early in the hospital course of five of our patients during the past 3 years. Closed liver biopsy was considered hazardous because of the question of extrahepatic obstruction. Laparoscopy demonstrated a fatty liver and/or cirrhosis. The associated features of cholestasis and a normal gallbladder provided the neces-

sary data for diagnosis of alcoholic hepatitis with intrahepatic cholestasis. This was then confirmed by direct-vision needle biopsy of the liver. The subsequent courses of these patients were characterized by prolonged jaundice, pruritus, and an elevated serum alkaline phosphatase; however, because of early laparoscopy and guided biopsy the possibility of obstruction was excluded.

Primary biliary cirrhosis is another disorder in which extrahepatic obstruction may be difficult to exclude by usual clinical and biochemical methods. Laparoscopy in these patients often shows few of the nodular surface changes expected in other forms of cirrhosis. The greenish discoloration of an irregular hepatic surface, a normal gallbladder, a direct-vision biopsy, and a positive antimitochondrial antibody[10] determination adequately eliminate the need for laparotomy in most cases.

Several ancillary techniques to discern the cause of cholestasis have been used in conjunction with laparoscopy. In several European centers contrast medium was injected into the gallbladder under direct vision, and excellent cholangiograms were obtained.[8] This procedure, however, carries the risk of bile peritonitis and should be followed by insertion of a drain into the right upper quadrant.

A less aggressive, but nevertheless helpful ancillary measure is insertion of a palpating probe to determine the mobility, thickness, and turgidity of the gallbladder, as well as the presence of stones.

Alcoholic Liver Disease

Although closed liver biopsy is much more reliable in alcoholic liver disease than in other forms of chronic liver disease,[4] laparoscopy provides the clinician with additional information with which to formulate his diagnosis and prognosis. Not infrequently extensive cirrhotic changes are noted, although the biopsy (even under direct vision) reveals only fatty change and/or alcoholic hepatitis. Conversely, the significance of a biopsy diagnosis of finely nodular cirrhosis is uncertain when the laparoscopist knows that the usual surface changes characteristic of advanced cirrhosis are minimal.

The classic hepatic findings in alcoholic liver disease are finely nodular cirrhosis and/or fatty infiltration (Figs. 3, 6, Plate C). The cirrhotic changes are generally seen as a fine nodularity covering the surfaces of both liver lobes. Close examination of the surface of such nodules frequently demonstrates a fine proliferation of tiny vessels, sometimes telangiectatic and reminiscent of the neovascularity seen in hepatoma. Although the "cobblestone" liver with its uniform finely nodular surface pattern is typical of Laënnec's cirrhosis, rarely are large regenerative nodules encountered as are seen in postnecrotic or macronodular cirrhosis. Such regenerative nodules may be confused with hepatoma and should be biopsied for clarification.

Fatty infiltration of the liver is easily appreciated if it is of moderate extent. In these instances the liver is almost always grossly enlarged, particularly the left lobe. We have found that the size of the left lobe in alcoholic liver disease (for unknown reasons) is relatively more increased than the right lobe and serves as a clue to the etiology of hepatomegaly in these cases. Fatty change per se is manifested by a glistening liver surface with a yellowish hue (Fig. 6, Plate). The liver edges are blunted, and the surface contours of both lobes may be slightly irregular, although these changes are not specific enough for a diagnosis of alcoholic hepatitis. Cholestatic changes as described above are frequently noted. The value of laparoscopy in alcoholic hepatitis lies in the exclusion of other processes which may be confused with this diagnosis (e.g., hepatoma or cholecystitis). Also the extent and severity of associated cirrhosis may be assessed.

One finding associated with alcoholic liver disease, although mentioned previously, deserves further emphasis. The gallbladder in many of these patients is large and moderately distended. This phenomenon has been called cholecystocholestasis. It is important to recognize that moderate enlargement of the gallbladder may occur here so that an incorrect diagnosis of a Courvoisier gallbladder due to obstruction of the common bile duct is avoided. Although the gallbladder is large in cholecystocholestasis, it is not tense, and the vessels coursing over the surface retain their tortuous, irregular path. Conversely, a Courvoisier gallbladder is characterized by marked distention, with stretching and straightening of its serosal vessels.

Laparoscopy also provides the examiner with an opportunity to evaluate the presence or absence of portal hypertension, the severity of liver damage, and the occurrence of complications such as hepatoma and rarely the presence of associated tuberculous peritonitis in patients with alcoholic liver disease.

Portal Hypertension

Laparoscopy provides an excellent opportunity for qualitative assessment of portal hypertension. Although nonspecific, the presence of splenomegaly suggests an elevated portal pressure, which is then confirmed by evaluating the vascularity of other intraperitoneal structures. In portal hypertension a profuse network of small veins is seen within the round and falciform ligaments (Fig. 7, Plate C). A profusion of small peritoneal vessels in the falciform ligament, serosal surfaces, and parietal peritoneum may be found in patients with a recent history of peritonitis. The vascular changes with portal hypertension are characterized by distention, tortuosity, and in severe cases sharp angulations which give the vessels a nodular appearance. A distended umbilical vein may appear as a bluish nodular mass in the ligament and must not be confused with metastatic carcinoma, which can involve the same area. Distention of the gastroepiploic veins over the greater curvature of the stomach and the omental veins are also pathognomonic of elevated portal pressure.

Adhesions between visceral and parietal peritoneal surfaces are a favorite site for the development of natural portosystemic collaterals. Collaterals are seen around and within most adhesions in well developed portal hypertension.

A final index of portal hypertension is the presence of ascites. Although small amounts of fluid may be found in the pelvis in normal individuals, the demonstration of larger amounts of ascitic fluid, sufficient to obscure inspection of pelvic organs or to fill the paracolonic gutters, provides strong evidence of portal hypertension. This conclusion must be predicated on the examiner's failure to demonstrate another cause of ascites (e.g., metastatic carcinoma of the peritoneum, ovarian neoplasm, peritoneal tuberculosis) and the finding in most instances of chronic liver disease.

Dilated hepatic lymphatics *(vide supra)* are also a manifestation of portal hypertension.

Although unusual, portal hypertension may exist with none of the intraperitoneal findings described above. Thus laparoscopy cannot absolutely exclude the presence of elevated portal pressure. Nonspecific postinflammatory changes in the peritoneum, gut serosa, and falciform ligament may be misinterpreted as indicative of portal hypertension when distended, tortuous veins are not considered as an essential criterion. Quantitative measurement and radiographic demonstration of the portal venous system may be obtained by performance of splenoportography at the time of laparoscopy.[1] Although we have not employed this technique, others reported its use and pointed out that it allows direct-vision splenic puncture and accurate assessment of splenic bleeding after removal of the needle and catheter.

REFERENCES

1. Beck K: Diagnose und Differential diagnose des Pfortaderhochdruckes im laparoskopischen Bild. In L Wannagat (ed): Leber und Milz. Stuttgart, Thieme, 1967
2. Beck K: Schaefer HJ: Color Atlas of Laparoscopy. Stuttgart, Schattauer Verlag, 1970, p 58
3. Bernheim BM: Organoscopy cystoscopy of the abdominal cavity. Ann Surg 53:764, 1911
4. Czaja AJ, Steinberg AS, Saldana M, et al: Peritoneoscopy; its value in the diagnosis of liver disease. Gastrointest Endosc 20:23, 1973
5. DeVita VT, Bagley CM, Goodell DA, et al: Peritoneoscopy in the staging of Hodgkin's disease. Cancer Res 31:1746, 1971
6. Geall MG, Schoenfield LJ, Summerskill WHJ: Classification and treatment of chronic active liver disease. Gastroenterology 55:724, 1968
7. Guckian JC, Perry JE: Granulomatous hepatitis. Ann Intern Med 65:1081, 1966
8. Henning M, Demling L, Sigglberger H: Uber die laparoskopische cholecysto-cholangiographic. Munch Med Wochenschr 94:830, 1952
9. Jori GP, Peschle C: Combined peritoneoscopy and liver biopsy in the diagnosis of hepatic neoplasm. Gastroenterology 63:1016, 1972
10. Klatskin G, Kanter IS: Mitochondrial antibody in primary biliary cirrhosis and other diseases. Ann Intern Med 77:533, 1972
11. Lindner H: Why laparoscopy? Gastrointest Endosc 19:176, 1973
12. Maddrey WC, Johns CJ, Boitnott JK, et al: Sarcoidosis and chronic hepatic disease: a clinical and pathologic study of 20 patients. Medicine (Balt) 49:375, 1970
13. Mikkelsen WP, Turrill FL, Kern WH: Acute hyaline necrosis of the liver. Am J Surg 116:266, 1968
14. Nelson RS, Salvador DSJ: Percutaneous needle biopsy in malignant neoplasm with special reference to myeloid metaplasia. Ann Intern Med 53:179, 1960
15. Ruddock JC: Peritoneoscopy. West J Surg Obstet Gynecol 42:392, 1934
16. Safrany L, Tari J, Barna L, et al: Endoscopic retrograde cholangiography. Gastrointest Endosc 19:163, 1973
17. Soloway RD, Baggenstoss AH, Schoenfield LJ, et al: Observer error and sampling variability tested in evaluation of hepatitis and cirrhosis by liver biopsy. Am J Dig Dis 16:1082, 1971
18. Sternlieb I, Scheinberg IH: Chronic hepatitis as a first manifestation of Wilson's disease. Ann Intern Med 76:59, 1972
19. Summerskill WHJ: Chronic active liver disease re-examined: prognosis hopeful. Gastroenterology 66:450, 1974
20. Vido I, Wildhirt E: Correlation des laparoskopischen und histologischen Befundes der chronischer Hepatitis und Leberzirrhose. Dtsch Med Wochenschr 94:1633, 1969

31

Laparoscopy in Infants and Children

Stephen L. Gans
Dale G. Johnson
George Berci

Improvement in the technique of laparoscopy (peritoneoscopy) led to its widespread use in a number of adult abdominal and pelvic conditions. However, it is rare to find mention of the procedure in the pediatric literature, or use of the method in pediatric treatment centers of the world. No doubt this is due to the fact that when conventional instruments were miniaturized for pediatric use the view was so poor they were relatively useless.

In recent years development of the rod-lens optical system by Hopkins made possible miniaturization of telescopic endoscopes with a wide-angle view, increased transmission of light, fine resolution, and an overall brilliant image. After our initial experience with these new instruments, we reported our results and a technique for pediatric peritoneoscopy, the first such reports in the literature.[4,5]

TECHNIQUE

Laparoscopy (peritoneoscopy) is the visualization of the contents of the peritoneal cavity by means of a small telescope introduced through the anterior abdominal wall after establishment of a pneumoperitoneum (Fig. 1). Although this procedure can sometimes be done under local anesthesia in adults, general anesthesia with controlled respirations is necessary in infants and children because pneumoperitoneum significantly inhibits diaphragmatic movement.

When indicated cleansing enemas are given the night before, and the stomach is emptied with a nasogastric tube if the upper quadrants are to be examined. Under anesthesia the bladder area is carefully palpated and the bladder emptied if necessary when the lower abdomen or pelvis is to be entered. The skin is prepared and draped for the appropriate site of entrance, which depends on the area to be examined. However, the smaller the infant, the wider is the area that can be covered from any entrance site. In the infant it is usually best to enter just lateral to the umbilicus, penetrating the most medial portion of the rectus muscle. Care must be taken not to penetrate the muscle more laterally than this because of the danger of hitting the epigastric artery. In the older child the midline just above or below the umbilicus is satisfactory. Needless to say, the umbilicus must be scrupulously cleansed.

Pneumoperitoneum is initiated with a spring-controlled, blunt stylet which springs forward when the peritoneum is pierced, thus protecting the abdominal contents from injury by further advancement. If the tip of the needle can now be moved to and fro, it probably is properly placed inside the peritoneal cavity. With a syringe attached to the needle, cautious and gentle aspiration is attempted before and after injection of a few milliliters of normal saline as a precaution and warning of possible entrance into a blood vessel or viscus.

Carbon dioxide (CO_2) is then introduced through the needle from a gas cylinder by

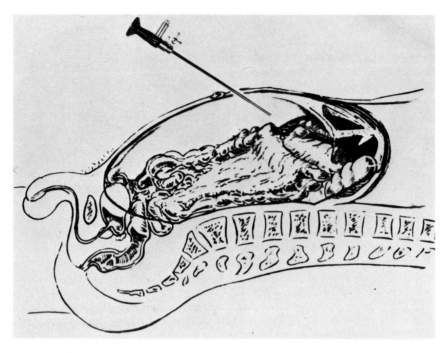

FIG. 1.   The telescope is introduced through a cannula inserted through the abdominal wall. The pneumoperitoneum protects the underlying viscera and provides a space for the examination. The telescope is connected to a fiber light source, and there is an insufflator for maintaining the pneumoperitoneum.

means of an insufflating device that has a reducing valve, flowmeter, and continuous-pressure meter. With this apparatus any pressure can be preselected, and as soon as the intraabdominal pressure reaches the set level it automatically shuts off. If the pressure then drops, the valve automatically opens and refills until the given pressure is again reached (Chapters 5, 29). Our experience has indicated that with proper precautions and careful monitoring, as well as cooperative collaboration of the anesthesiologist, pneumoperitoneum does not impose undue strain on the respiratory or cardiovascular systems. Intraabdominal pressure in an infant should not exceed 15 to 20 mm Hg, and this restriction must be carefully coordinated with the patient's general condition, as observed by the anesthesiologist. In neonates it is very important that the insufflation proceed slowly and that the lower figure should not be exceeded. CO_2 is chosen because it is rapidly absorbed and excreted, and it does not support combustion.

When the pneumoperitoneum is adequate, the needle is removed. A tiny skin incision, only large enough for a 4- or 5-mm (OD) can-

nula, is made with a pointed scalpel, and a cannula with a trocar is gently drilled through the abdominal wall and into the air cushion. The trocar is withdrawn and replaced with a miniature telescope (Fig. 1). CO_2 does not escape because of a valve in the cannula. Inspection of the peritoneal contents may then begin.

Biopsy needles or needles for injection can be inserted through the abdominal wall in direct view of the telescope. For more involved manipulation a second, smaller (4 mm OD) cannula is introduced separately through the abdominal wall. Through this cannula a palpating probe, biopsy forceps, and grasping forceps can be used, and suction, electrocoagulation, or dissection can be accomplished, always under direct telescopic view.

INDICATIONS

It should be made clear at the onset that laparoscopy is indicated for diagnosis only when more simple studies are not adequate or definitive, and when exploratory surgery would therefore be considered. It is indicated for therapy only when such a procedure can be carried out safely without laparotomy. *The advantage of this technique is that it either avoids laparotomy altogether, or it establishes the need and plan for operation.* A list of specific indications is shown in Table 1.

TABLE 1. Indications for Laparoscopy in 43 Pediatric Patients

Indication	No.
Hepatobiliary conditions	20
Metabolic or inflammatory disease	2
Hepatomegaly	8
Hepatosplenomegaly	2
Jaundice	8
Neonates	7
Infants and children	1
Ascites	1
Abdominal cysts and tumors	8
Primary	3
Metastatic	4
"Second look"	1
Status of pelvic genitalia	11
Intersexuality	2
Precocious puberty	2
Primary and secondary amenorrhea	1
Gonadal dysplasia	4
Ovarian cysts and tumors	1
Congenital virilizing adrenal hyperplasia	1
Occult abdominal pain	2
Removal of foreign bodies	1
Abdominal trauma	0*
Total cases	43

This is a suggested indication, but there is no clinical evidence to date.

CONTRAINDICATIONS

Peritoneoscopy is contraindicated in infants and children for whom general anesthesia is contraindicated. It is further contraindicated in conditions where puncture of the abdominal wall might be hazardous: peritonitis, intestinal obstruction, or where extensive scarring or adhesions may be present from previous surgery.[2]

CLINICAL EXPERIENCE AND RESULTS

This report concerns all cases performed by the authors at the Cedars of Lebanon Hospital (S.G. and G.B.), the Children's Hospital of Los Angeles (S.G.), and the Primary Children's Hospital of Salt Lake City (D.J.). The number of combined cases follows each indication on Table 1.

Hepatobiliary Conditions

Under the main heading of hepatobiliary conditions are found a group of categories with a wide variety of patients who, after thorough study, may still require tissue sampling for accurate diagnosis. This has most frequently been done by blind needle biopsy or open surgery. Direct-vision liver biopsy by means of peritoneoscopy has distinct advantages. The appearance of the liver and gallbladder may be significant in giving a presumptive diagnosis. The color, size, structure, and feel can be evaluated; and the presence of cysts, hemangiomas, nodules, tumors, or diffuse hepatic involvement can be noted before the biopsy needle or biopsy forceps is directed under clear vision into the most promising areas. Focal or nodular lesions can be missed by blind needling, and direct observation is a safety factor in preventing penetration of vascular or other potentially harmful targets. Lesions of pinhead size can be accurately biopsied with ease. If bleeding or leakage of bile persists after biopsy, it is readily observed and controlled by electrocoagulation. The diagnosis was correctly established in all patients in this group. We feel that open surgery for the sole purpose of liver biopsy is now an obsolete procedure, except in those situations where larger amounts of liver tissue are required, such as for histochemical studies.

Metabolic or Inflammatory Disease. An example is the case of a 21-month-old female who was being investigated for a possible glycogen storage disease. Three attempts at percutaneous blind needle biopsy of the liver had failed to provide the diagnosis. Peritoneoscopy and forceps biopsy of the liver were accomplished, providing adequate tissue to conclude the study accurately.

Hepatomegaly. This common problem has a multitude of causes most of which can be determined in the usual manner. In some, however, a look at the liver itself is helpful, and a tissue sample is mandatory for diagnosis. Such a case was that of an asymptomatic 7-year-old boy found to have a large right upper quadrant mass during a routine school examination. The diagnosis remained in question until peritoneoscopy revealed an enlarged nodular liver and biopsy confirmed the diagnosis of advanced cirrhosis.

Hepatosplenomegaly. The addition of an enlarged spleen to the above group provides further differential diagnostic problems. Not only can the liver be observed and biopsied, but the spleen can be demonstrated and examined for characteristic findings. An example from our series was a 3.5-year-old child whose liver was seen to have a characteristic mottled yellowish appearance. The enlarged spleen was coarsely granular and involved with omental adhesions. This was the picture of Gaucher's disease (Fig. 2, Plate C)* and was confirmed by liver biopsy.

Jaundice. An old and difficult problem is distinguishing between neonatal hepatitis and biliary atresia—or to put it in another way, to determine which infants should undergo open surgery for attempts at corrective procedures. There are several laboratory methods, none of which is entirely satisfactory; new ones are being developed and investigated at the present time. In addition, the whole problem of biliary atresia is under intensive scrutiny as to definition, etiology, methods of treatment, and prognosis.

We are investigating an endoscopic approach to diagnosis. The liver and gallbladder are first inspected through the peritoneoscope. If the gallbladder is absent, the procedure is terminated and laparotomy is performed in an effort to do definitive corrective surgery for biliary atresia. If the gallbladder is indeed present and distended, and the liver is dark green, a distal common duct obstruction is presumed to be present. Again laparotomy is indicated. If the gallbladder appears normal but is collapsed, the liver is biopsied for study of permanent sections and the procedure is terminated. This procedure is short and, in our small series, safe and accurate. The diagnosis was correctly established in six patients, the four with hepatitis being spared a laparotomy. We are fully aware of the difficulties with microscopic anatomic diagnosis in many cases, and further investigation and study are necessary. Attempts at percutaneous transhepatic cholangiography (Fig. 3) under direct telescopic view have thus far been unsuccessful in such pa-

*All color plates appear at the front of the book.

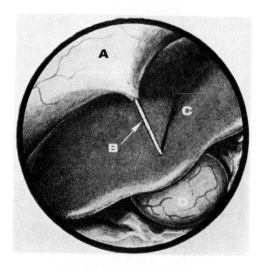

FIG. 3. Percutaneous transhepatic cholangiography. The needle with Teflon catheter passes through the liver and into the gallbladder. When the catheter is removed, the liver tamponades the hole in the gallbladder and prevents leakage. A. Parietal peritoneum. B. Needle. C. Liver. D. Gallbladder.

tients, but further attempts will be made. Such roentgenologic demonstration of an open ductal system would preclude the necessity of laparotomy.

The differential diagnosis of jaundice in older infants and children can be made in most instances by evaluating history, symptoms, signs, laboratory tests, and special diagnostic studies. It is in the remaining small number of cases that peritoneoscopy should be considered. The important features of this procedure include evaluation of the appearance of the liver and gallbladder, direct-vision liver biopsy, and the addition of percutaneous endoscopically guided transhepatic cholangiography when appropriate. An example in this series is a 5-year-old girl with deep jaundice of several months' duration. She had been treated for hepatitis, with no response. Finally, changes in her laboratory studies indicated a possible extrahepatic obstruction, and she was referred for surgical exploration. However, laparoscopy was performed and revealed a liver of relatively normal color but with somewhat rounded edges. The gallbladder was empty and collapsed. Liver biopsy revealed hyperplastic cholangitis. The patient was spared a laparotomy and subsequently made a slow but complete recovery.

Ascites

A 1-day-old female presented with an enlarged, fluid-filled abdomen, so large that the obstetrician reported related difficulty in delivery. Paracentesis showed that the fluid was not chyle, bile, pus, or intestinal contents. CO_2 was introduced through the same needle, and peritoneoscopy ruled out hepatic, urologic, ovarian, or neoplastic etiologies. Indigo carmine injected intravenously appeared in the urine but not in the ascitic fluid. This 4-pound neonate is probably the youngest and smallest human to undergo this procedure, and a bright, clear, accurate view was obtained with no detectable harmful effect on the patient. No lesion was found, and the ascites cleared after three aspirations. Subsequent roentgenologic investigations for genitourinary lesions were negative.

Abdominal Cysts and Tumors

Because the variety of malignant, benign, and inflammatory cysts and tumors is so great, and many of them are so bizarre, all must be considered malignant until proved otherwise. Adequate proof that such a lesion is not malignant can be obtained only by direct inspection and through microscopic study of the tissue. In addition, almost all such nonmalignant lesions can and frequently do produce trouble by pressure on neighboring structures, by rupture or leakage, and occasionally by producing harmful chemical or hormonal products. For these reasons all suspicious abdominal masses should be identified and treated. Advice that the lesion should be watched in the hope that it will disappear should never be given or followed.

Almost all except retroperitoneal masses can be inspected and biopsied by means of laparoscopy when indicated. Identification of an inflammatory lesion may indicate a retroperitoneal approach. Obviously benign lesions such as cysts or hemangiomas may permit election between surgical removal and nonoperative observation. An important occurrence is the demonstration of peritoneal and/or omental seeding of metastases and/or liver metastases because this finding may spare the patient a laparotomy. A limited "second-look" procedure can be equally useful.

Status of Pelvic Genitalia

Eight patients were investigated for such problems as intersexuality, precocious puberty, primary and secondary amenorrhea, gonadal dysplasia, and ovarian cysts and tumors. Pelvic anatomy is particularly clearly visualized by laparoscopy, and biopsy can be done where indicated. We believe that laparotomy for this purpose is now an obsolete procedure. Cognat et al.[1] described the use of laparoscopy in 60 infants and adolescents with gynecologic conditions.

In addition to using the usual technique, we passed the laparoscope through a hernia sac to inspect the pelvis of an apparent female infant having hernia surgery in which a testis had been found in the groin, a case of testicular feminization.

Occult Abdominal Pain

Laparoscopy may be appropriate in the child with repeated severe abdominal pain in whom all other nonsurgical modalites for diagnosis have been exhausted. In two such instances negative examination was at least reassuring to the parents and the referring physician, and was a reasonable substitute for negative laparotomy.

Removal of Foreign Bodies

In one instance we were asked to remove a piece of a Raimondi tube which had broken off from a ventriculoperitoneal shunt and settled in a pelvis full of adhesions secondary to rectovesical surgery. Under direct-vision laparoscopy, using the telescope itself as a dissecting instrument, adhesions were carefully separated and the tube was visualized and removed.

Abdominal Trauma

In most instances the diagnosis of traumatized intraabdominal organs can be made in the usual manner. At least the decision to operate can be made using acceptable criteria. In a few cases the decision is difficult, and sometimes the affected organ is not known. Some recommend peritoneal needle or tube tap and lavage as an aid in this problem. Doletsky et al.[3] showed that laparoscopy not only demonstrates which organ is affected but often determines its status in regard to the severity and activity of bleeding, permitting abstinence from laparotomy in selected instances. Although we independently considered this approach, we have not used it to date.

COMPLICATIONS

There have been no complications in this series. A detailed discussion of complications in adults is given by Cohen,[2] Mosenthal,[6] and elsewhere in this book (Chapter 29).

SUMMARY

Laparoscopy in infants and children is a safe procedure which provides a clear view of the peritoneal cavity and its contents, and offers a satisfactory means of biopsy and other manipulations under direct vision. Details of the technique are provided. Indications and contraindications are listed. Clinical experience includes 43 cases. There were no complications.

REFERENCES

1. Cognat M, Rosenberg D, David L, et al: Laparoscopy in infants and adolescents. Obstet Gynecol 42:515, 1973
2. Cohen MR: Laparoscopy, Culdoscopy and Gynecography. Philadelphia, Saunders, 1970, pp 41, 42
3. Doletsky SY, Okulov AB, Shpringvald-Udris SI: Laparoscopy in closed injury of the abdomen in children. Khirurgiia (Mosk) 42:112, 1971
4. Gans SL, Berci G: Advances in endoscopy of infants and children. J Pediatr Surg 6:199, 1971
5. Gans SL, Berci G: Peritoneoscopy in infants and children. J Pediatr Surg 8:399, 1973
6. Mosenthal WT: Peritoneoscopy. Am J Surg 123:421, 1972

32

Proctosigmoidoscopy

Thomas T. Irvin

Proctosigmoidoscopy is the endoscopic examination of the distal sigmoid colon, rectum, and anal canal, and it is a routine procedure in the clinical examination of all patients presenting with anorectal or colonic symptoms. It is a simple diagnostic examination which requires relatively inexpensive equipment, and without question it is the most important endoscopic procedure in the investigation of the large intestine.

It also has a significant role in the treatment of neoplasms of the distal colon and rectum. Before introduction of the fiberoptic colonoscope the endoscopic resection of polyps and neoplasms by diathermy electrosurgery was a procedure performed entirely by proctosigmoidoscopy, and this technique retains a significant place in proctologic surgery.

INSTRUMENTATION

The term proctosigmoidoscopy actually refers to two examinations—proctoscopy and sigmoidoscopy—and a variety of instruments are currently used. Unfortunately the names attached to the different instruments are somewhat misleading in that the sigmoidoscope is used for the examination of the rectum in addition to the distal sigmoid colon, and the proctoscope is used only for the examination of the anal canal and the lowermost part of the rectum. The instruments were described in Part I of this volume, and particular emphasis is given here only to those instruments which the author uses.

Diagnostic Proctosigmoidoscopy in the Office

A small trolley of equipment should be available for proctosigmoidoscopy in the office. A suitable arrangement is shown in Figure 1 and includes the following:

- Two sigmoidoscopes (one large, one small)
- Eyepiece and air-insufflation attachments for sigmoidoscope
- One proctoscope
- High-intensity light source with fiberoptic connection for sigmoidoscope and proctoscope
- One sigmoidoscopy alligator-type swabbing forceps
- One sigmoidoscopy alligator-type biopsy forceps
- One nontoothed dissecting forceps for proctoscopy
- Two syringes for hemorrhoid injection
- One kidney dish with gauze swabs and cotton wool
- One kidney dish for dirty swabs
- One jar of lubricant

A suitable examination couch and movable spotlight are essential; a bucket is required for the disposal of used instruments; and additional equipment such as probe-pointed directors for the examination of anal fistulas and specimen containers for bacteriologic and pathologic examination should be available.

Diagnostic Sigmoidoscope. The conventional diagnostic sigmoidoscope is a rigid, tubular instrument measuring 25 to 30 cm in length. It is used for examination of the distal sigmoid colon and the rectum, and instruments of different internal diameter are available. One of the most important features of the in-

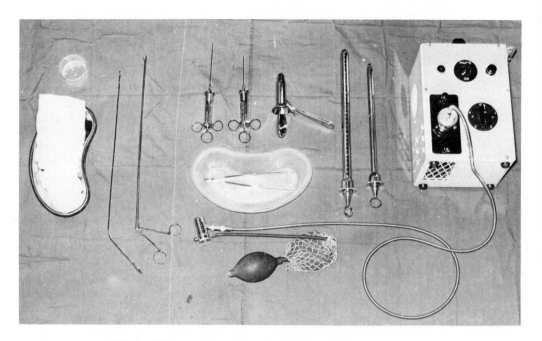

FIG. 1.   Office equipment for diagnostic proctosigmoidoscopy.

strument, however, is the method of lighting used. There are essentially two types of lighting. In the Strauss type of sigmoidoscope the light is placed toward the distal end of the instrument; until recently this was mounted on a light carrier which traversed the lumen of the sigmoidoscope. In the other type of instrument the light is located at the proximal end of the instrument, and this has proved to be a more acceptable arrangement since distally placed lights have a tendency to become obscured by fecal material. However, recent improvements in the methods of distal lighting—by the use of high-intensity light transmitted along the wall of the sigmoidoscope—have largely resolved the problems of the Strauss type of instrument. A new Strauss diagnostic sigmoidoscope* has a plastic obturator and a high intensity light delivered by a fiberoptic system to the distal end of the instrument.

I use the Lloyd-Davies type of sigmoidoscope, which has proximal lighting. The diagnostic instrument comes in two sizes (Fig. 1). The larger model measures 30 cm in length and has an internal diameter of 13 mm. The smaller instrument is generally more acceptable for routine diagnostic use. The larger model causes

more discomfort in the conscious patient, but its wider lumen proves more satisfactory when rectal or colonic biopsies are required. Both instruments have metal obturators and a single eyepiece which incorporates a magnifying lens and an attachment for the manual insufflation of air. The proximally mounted light was recently improved by the use of high-intensity light delivered by a fiberoptic system from a distant source.

When using the sigmoidoscope it is frequently necessary to swab the lumen of the bowel or the instrument to remove fecal material, which is achieved either by the use of cotton wool held in a long alligator-type sigmoidoscopy forceps (Fig. 1) or specially designed, disposable swab sticks.* In certain circumstances, when there is profuse discharge from the bowel or when the feces are very liquid, a long suction tube is helpful in clearing the bowel lumen.

Biopsies are taken through the sigmoidoscope with a long alligator-type forceps. In general, instruments with small blades are desirable for diagnostic biopsy, and I use a forceps based on the Lloyd-Davies design (Fig. 1).

Diagnostic Proctoscope.   The standard proctoscope is a rigid, tubular instrument. It is

Manufacturer: Welch-Allyn, Skaneateles Falls, New York.

Fuller Pharmaceutical Co., Minn.

used for examining the anal canal and lower rectum; a number of different types of instrument are available. I use the Milligan-Morgan instrument, which is shown in Figure 1. It measures 7 cm in length and has an internal diameter of 22 mm at the distal end and 32 mm at the proximal end or base. Proximal lighting is provided by a light source inserted through a tunnel in the handle of the instrument; in the newer model this is a fiberoptic attachment relaying high-intensity light from a distant source.

During proctoscopy the lumen of the anal canal and rectum is swabbed with gauze or cotton wool held in a pair of nontoothed dissecting forceps. Biopsies may be taken with the same alligator forceps used in sigmoidoscopy, or a shorter instrument with rather larger blades can be used, e.g., a Hartmann conchotome.

It is often desirable to treat any internal hemorrhoids found in the course of an otherwise negative proctoscopic examination. For this purpose I routinely provide two Gabriel syringes charged with 5 percent phenol in almond or arachis oil (Fig. 1).

Operative Proctosigmoidoscopy Equipment

Special instruments are desirable for therapeutic endoscopic procedures.

Operating Sigmoidoscope. The removal or destruction of rectal or distal colonic neoplasms by electrosurgery is an important aspect of proctosigmoidoscopy, and for this a sigmoidoscope larger than the conventional diagnostic model is usually required.

I find the Aylett sigmoidoscope and other instruments designed on the Strauss pattern (with distal lighting) unsatisfactory for electrosurgical procedures, and so I use a large version of the Lloyd-Davies instrument with proximal high-intensity lighting. This instrument measures 15 cm in length and 30 mm internal diameter; it has a detachable eyepiece with a magnifying lens, an attachment for the manual insufflation of air, and a suction tube attached within the lumen of the sigmoidoscope.

Operating Proctoscope. Excellent exposure is required for endoscopic operations on the anal canal and lower rectum, and this is best achieved with a bivalve speculum. I use the Goligher pattern of bivalve speculum,

which has a detachable third blade. This instrument provides excellent exposure during operations for anal fissures and fistulas, excision of hypertrophic papillae, fulguration or excision of low rectal neoplasms, and cryosurgical treatment of hemorrhoids. It is also a useful diagnostic instrument since it permits detailed inspection of the anal canal, crypts, and lower rectum. However, the instrument is not tolerated well by unanesthetized patients, and with the exception of those undergoing cryosurgical treatment of hemorrhoids I tend to use it only in anesthetized subjects.

INDICATIONS FOR PROCTOSIGMOIDOSCOPY

Proctosigmoidoscopy is indicated in any patient complaining of anorectal or colonic symptoms, or any symptom which may indicate the presence of disease implicating the lower alimentary canal.

Disturbance of Bowel Habit

An alteration in bowel habit may be caused by changes in diet, emotional factors, or intercurrent viral, bacterial, or parasitic infections of the alimentary tract; it is a presenting symptom of many diseases of the large intestine, including colonic or rectal cancer. The change in bowel habit may take the form of constipation or diarrhea, or a combination of both. Any change in bowel habit—whether intermittent, continuous, or progressive—warrants thorough investigation.

Bleeding

Passage of blood in the stool is an alarming symptom and one which tends to cause patients to seek early advice. The commonest source of rectal bleeding is internal hemorrhoids, but rectal bleeding is also a common presenting sign of a rectal or distal colonic cancer, and it always requires thorough investigation.

Passage of Mucus

The passage of mucus or slime in the stool cannot be regarded as a normal occurrence. It may signify the presence of a neoplasm, proctitis, or proctocolitis; and in such cases it is frequently accompanied by rectal bleeding. In other cases the patient complains of a mucous discharge that soils his underclothing, which is very suggestive of an anal disorder. Anal fistulas, fissures, condylomas or warts, neoplasms, and prolapsing internal hemorrhoids can also cause mucous soiling. Occasionally thorough investigation of this complaint reveals no obvious lesion.

Pain

A number of different types of pain and pain distribution may be associated with disease arising from or implicating the large intestine. Hyperactive peristaltic contractions of the colon may result from obstruction of the intestinal lumen, irritation due to inflammatory disease, or the effects of drugs or emotional stimuli. The pain which results from such colonic activity is a lower abdominal colic, and it is usually relieved by defecation unless the lumen of the intestine is obstructed.

Localized abdominal pain and tenderness may occur in the presence of inflammatory, ischemic, or neoplastic disease of the intestine. This pain is probably caused by stimulation of the parietal peritoneum overlying the diseased intestine, and it is frequently a prominent feature of diverticular disease of the left colon.

Perineal pain may be directly related to disease of the anal canal or referred from disease of the rectum or other pelvic organs. Anal pain is aggravated by defecation. It is a prominent feature of anal fissure, perianal hematomas, intermuscular abscesses, and prolapsed thrombosed hemorrhoids; and it is frequently a feature of anal neoplasms. Perineal pain is a feature of anorectal abscesses, and it may be referred from a rectal or pelvic neoplasm owing to involvement of sacral nerve roots. In the latter instance the pain may also be present in the sacrococcygeal region and referred along the distribution of the sciatic nerve in the leg.

Pain localized to the rectum or perineum may result from inflammatory conditions of the prostate or seminal vesicles, as well as pelvic endometriosis. In some cases, however, there is no apparent cause for this symptom.

Prolapse

The patient may complain that something prolapses through the anus on defecation. The most common explanation for this symptom is prolapsing internal hemorrhoids, but a similar complaint occurs in partial or complete prolapse of the rectum, prolapsing hypertrophic anal papillae, and occasionally with pedunculated anorectal polyps. Some patients may give a graphic account of the size and appearance of the prolapsed tissues.

Pruritus

Itching or perianal irritation is a very common symptom, and one for which no apparent cause is found in the majority of cases. Occasionally irritation results from disorders causing excessive mucous discharge, or from dermatologic diseases affecting the perianal region.

Incontinence

True incontinence is an uncommon symptom, but patients frequently refer to this term when they are actually suffering from an anal or perianal discharge. Incontinence of feces or flatus is a feature of complete prolapse of the rectum, congenital or acquired megacolon, or scarring of the anal canal or sphincteric musculature as a consequence of surgery. Incontinence is not uncommon in the very elderly, in whom it may be a result of fecal impaction.

GENERAL ASPECTS OF EXAMINATION

A standard procedure of assessment and investigation is used in all patients presenting with anorectal or colonic symptoms, and a proctosigmoidoscopic examination is one part of this procedure. A careful history is obtained first, and the patient is then given a routine general physical examination which includes a careful examination of the abdomen.

A rectal examination and proctosigmoidoscopy are then performed. The anus is inspected first for evidence of disease or any condition which might make proctosigmoidoscopy a difficult or painful procedure. Digital examination of the rectum is then performed followed by proctosigmoidoscopy. The digital examination should never be omitted for it may yield valuable information in addition to proctosigmoidoscopy. It may reveal the presence of a palpable extrarectal pelvic mass that is not apparent on endoscopy, and it is of great importance in the assessment of rectal neoplasms. This is particularly true in the case of papillary adenomas, for the appearance of these lesions on endoscopy is frequently less helpful than the findings on simple palpation in differentiating benign and malignant tumors.

In a number of cases further investigation is required to determine the cause of the patient's symptoms. Frequently a barium enema examination is required; and in a few patients investigation of the small intestine by a small bowel barium study or endoscopic examination of the proximal colon by fiberoptic colonoscopy may be required to establish a final diagnosis.

DIAGNOSTIC SIGMOIDOSCOPY

A complete sigmoidoscopic examination involves examination of the rectum and distal sigmoid colon for a distance of 25 to 30 cm from the perineal skin.

Surgical Anatomy

The sigmoid colon is a loop of intestine of variable length and position which connects the iliac colon with the rectum. It is enclosed in peritoneum and suspended on a mesentery, the latter largely accounting for its variable position.

The rectosigmoid junction arises at the level of the third piece of the sacrum, and the rectum follows the curve of the sacrum downward. The rectum ends several centimeters distal to the coccyx by turning sharply backward as it passes through the musculature of the pelvic floor to become the anal canal. The rectum also has three lateral curves in its course through the pelvis: the upper and lower curves are convex to the right, and the middle curve is convex to the left. The extent of these curves or angulations is quite variable. At sigmoidoscopy the rectosigmoid junction is encountered at 13 to 16 cm from the perineal skin, and the anorectal junction at about 4 cm from the perineum.

The most important anatomic feature of the rectum in relation to sigmoidoscopy is its peritoneal attachment. The upper third of the rectum is completely covered with peritoneum, except for a small area posteriorly; but the peritoneal attachment becomes progressively less as the rectum descends in the pelvis. The peritoneum is finally reflected forward off the front of the rectum at the bottom of the rec-

tovesical or rectouterine pouch on to the seminal vesicles and the base of the bladder in the male, and the vagina and uterus in the female. The lower part of the rectum is thus completely devoid of a peritoneal coat. The level of the peritoneal reflection is by no means a fixed landmark. It is generally about 8 to 9 cm from the perineal skin in the male, and about 5 to 8 cm in the female.[19] The importance of the peritoneal attachment of the rectum in sigmoidoscopy arises if there is trauma to the rectal wall. Perforation of the rectum resulting from passage of the endoscope is uncommon, but damage or perforation of the rectum is a recognizable complication of rectal biopsy or polypectomy. When the intraperitoneal rectum is perforated in this way (Fig. 2) fecal peritonitis ensues unless the injury is immediately recognized and repaired.

Preparation

No special preparation of the bowel is required for ordinary diagnostic sigmoidoscopy. Some proctologists routinely prepare the bowel for diagnostic endoscopy,[40] but in my experience this is unnecessary and undesirable. Enemas or rectal washouts administered shortly before the examination may hinder rather than help the sigmoidoscopy owing to

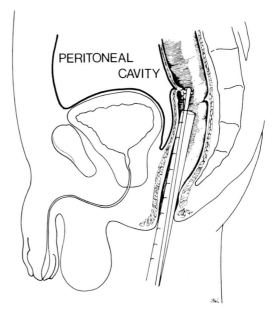

PERITONEAL CAVITY

FIG. 2.   Damage to the rectal wall during biopsy or removal of lesions in the intraperitoneal rectum may result in perforation and fecal peritonitis.

the presence of retained fluid and liquid feces. On the rare occasions when there is significant fecal loading of the rectum two glycerine or bisacodyl (Dulcolax) suppositories are quite effective in preparing the bowel for sigmoidoscopy.

Intestinal preparation is desirable as a prelude to operative sigmoidoscopy for several reasons. First, the electrosurgical treatment of polyps or adenomas must be performed with precision, and it is an advantage to have the intestine well prepared. Secondly, there is a small risk of intraluminal explosion resulting from endoscopic electrosurgery[17] and caused by the presence of flammable gases in the bowel lumen, some of which are derived from feces. Finally there is a slight risk that endoscopic surgery may perforate the bowel, and it is clearly advantageous to have minimal fecal leakage should this complication arise. Preparation should be thorough, for ineffective preparation is often worse than no preparation at all. I admit the patient to the hospital two nights before surgery. The dietary intake is restricted to fluids; four Senokot tablets are given on the night of admission; a soap and water enema is administered the next morning; and two oxyphenisatin (Veripaque) enemas are given, one on the evening before operation and one on the day of surgery.

Anesthesia

In most patients no anesthesia is required for diagnostic sigmoidoscopy. However, the presence of a painful anorectal condition such as an abscess or anal fissure precludes a sigmoidoscopic examination without anesthesia, and in such cases I perform the endoscopy under a general anesthetic in conjunction with the surgical treatment of the anorectal lesion.

In some patients psychologic factors may prevent an adequate sigmoidoscopy without anesthesia. These problems can be avoided to some extent by establishing a good rapport with the patient before and during the examination. The patient is naturally apprehensive and fearful of rectal examination, and it undoubtedly helps to have these fears allayed. It also builds the patient's confidence if the proctologist carefully explains the symptoms and discomfort which may occur during the examination. There is no point in pretending that the procedure is totally free of discomfort, when in fact some discomfort is likely to be experienced.

A gentle technique accompanied by suitable reassurance regarding the symptoms the patient may experience usually result in a satisfactory endoscopy.

When a satisfactory examination is not possible because of discomfort or apprehension I repeat the endoscopy under general anesthesia or with sedation. Suitable sedation can be achieved with diazepam (Valium), 10 to 20 mg by intravenous injection, and this can be supplemented with an analgesic such as pethidine, 50 to 100 mg by intramuscular injection.

Some form of anesthesia or sedation is essential for operative sigmoidoscopy. I prefer a general anesthetic for this procedure, but intravenous sedation with diazepam supplemented with an analgesic such as pethidine is quite acceptable.

Technique

Positioning the Patient. Positioning the patient for sigmoidoscopy is a critical factor in the performance of a complete examination. Two positions are commonly used. The knee-shoulder position is popular among North American proctologists and is particularly a suitable position for proctoscopy.[19] It has the disadvantage that it is a somewhat uncomfortable posture for the patient to maintain, and it may also seem somewhat degrading, particularly for female patients. It is not a position that is commonly used for sigmoidoscopy in England, where most proctologists tend to use the left lateral or Sims' position. In the Sims' position for sigmoidoscopy (Fig. 3) the patient lies on his left side in a semiprone position; the hips and knees are flexed, and the left hip is elevated on a sandbag so that the buttocks project beyond the edge of the examination table.

Inspection of the Anus. After the patient is correctly positioned the anus and perianal region are displayed by elevating the right buttock. Good lighting is required, preferably a spotlight, and the anus is carefully examined.

Any abnormality such as a prolapsed hemorrhoid, fistula, fissure, skin tag, tumor, or perianal abscess, or the presence of dermatitis or pruritic changes in the perianal skin can be observed. It is particularly important to determine if the patient has a painful anal condition which might prevent digital examination of the rectum and sigmoidoscopy. The tone of the anal sphincters is assessed by determining if the

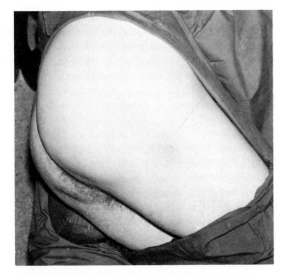

FIG. 3. Diagnostic sigmoidoscopy. The patient is placed in the left lateral position.

anal orifice is closed or patulous, and if it remains closed when the buttocks are retracted.

Digital Examination. The gloved and lubricated index finger of the right hand is gently inserted through the anus, the patient having been warned in reassuring terms that this part of the examination is about to commence. Any induration and tenderness in the anal canal is noted. Some discomfort and apprehension are commonly experienced by the patient, but the operator quickly discovers if there is a painful condition of the anal canal. Painful conditions such as an abscess or anal fissure are associated with intense spasm of the anal sphincters, which prevents adequate digital palpation of the anal canal.

In the normal anal canal the anatomic groove marking the lower edges of the internal and external sphinters, and the anorectal ring at the upper end of the anal canal, can be clearly palpated. The anorectal ring is formed by the puborectalis muscle, and this band of tissue is clearly palpable on the posterior and posterolateral aspects of the anorectal junction. In incontinent patients and especially in those with complete prolapse of the rectum the sphincters and puborectalis sling may be lax and poorly defined.

The examining finger is advanced into the rectum. The fecal content is noted and the rectal mucosa thoroughly examined. A proctitis seldom produces mucosal changes which can be detected by digital examination, but the presence of strictures, tumors, and pseudopolyps is readily determined. The consistency of a tumor should be carefully assessed. Carcinomas may be ulcerative or proliferative lesions, but they always feel hard. Benign tumors, whether sessile or pedunculated, feel soft on palpation. The position of a tumor in relation to fixed anatomic landmarks such as the prostate or uterine cervix and the anorectal ring should be determined.

Digital examination may also reveal the presence of an abnormality outside the rectum. A not infrequent finding in proctologic clinics is a mass anterior to the rectum in the recto-uterine or rectovesical pouch. This may be due to pathology affecting the sigmoid colon, uterus, or ovary; or it may represent peritoneal deposits from a carcinoma elsewhere in the abdomen. On completion of the rectal examination, the examining finger is inspected for the presence of mucus, blood, or pus.

Sigmoidoscopy. I use the small Lloyd-Davies instrument for routine diagnostic sigmoidoscopy (Fig. 1). The instrument is tested before use to ensure that the obturator can be withdrawn with ease. It is lubricated along its length, and the patient is warned that a small instrument is about to be passed.

The sigmoidoscope is taken in the right hand with the obturator held firmly in position; the right buttock is elevated, and the tip of the instrument is inserted into the anal canal (Fig. 4). Unless a gentle technique is used at this stage of the examination the patient may experience pain, and his confidence in the operator rapidly disappears. The initial reaction of the anal sphincters is to contract when presented with the tip of the endoscope, and the operator should avoid undue haste in inserting the instrument through the anal canal until some degree of sphincter relaxation occurs. The tip of the instrument is directed along the long axis of the anal canal toward the umbilicus, and gentle pressure is maintained until the operator experiences a reduction in the resistance to the instrument. The sigmoidoscope is then advanced through the anal canal, and the direction of insertion is altered when it enters the rectum. The instrument is angled backward toward the concavity of the sacrum, and the obturator is removed.

The eyepiece is attached, complete with fiberoptic light attachment and bellows apparatus for the insufflation of air, and the instrument is then advanced only under direct

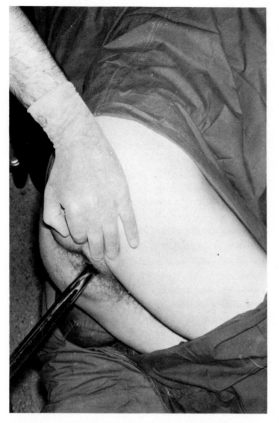

FIG. 4. Diagnostic sigmoidoscopy. The right buttock is elevated, and the sigmoidoscope is inserted through the anus.

vision (Fig. 5). Movement of the instrument is controlled with the left hand. The bellows are held in the right hand, and air is gently introduced to distend the rectum. The patient should be warned that he may experience a slight "windy" sensation and a desire to defecate, and that he should not be embarrassed by the passage of flatus around the instrument. The operator should avoid introducing too much air as this causes significant discomfort. The direction of insertion of the instrument in the rectum is upward and backward along the hollow of the sacrum. Any difficulty encountered at this stage of the examination is usually due to poor positioning of the patient, most often resulting from the patient's feet being too close to the operator.

The presence of feces in the rectum is seldom a nuisance. It is usually possible to manipulate the endoscope around any solid fecal material, but if the view is obscured by feces the eyepiece is detached and cotton wool held in an alligator

type of sigmoidoscopy forceps is used to swab the lumen (Fig. 6). When the examination is made difficult by the presence of liquid feces, mucus, or purulent discharge, use of a suction tube is helpful in obtaining adequate visualization.

The rectosigmoid junction is reached at about 12 to 15 cm from the anal verge, and the operator then attempts to advance the endoscope into the distal sigmoid colon. This is undoubtedly the most difficult part of the examination, for the rectosigmoid junction may form quite an acute flexure, and the manipulation required to advance the sigmoidoscope may cause discomfort to the patient. At this stage of the examination the patient is warned that he may experience some discomfort or colicky pain in the lower abdomen. The instrument is moved slightly backward and forward until the lumen is found; this is aided by the gentle insufflation of air, and it soon becomes apparent that the correct direction through the rectosigmoid flexure is quite sharply forward and to the left. Once the sigmoid colon has been entered the instrument can usually be advanced with great ease to its full length with-

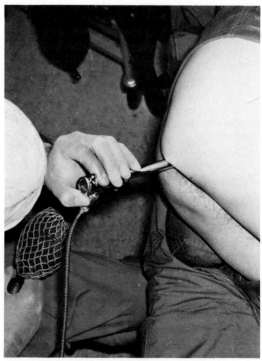

FIG. 5. Diagnostic sigmoidoscopy. When the instrument enters the rectum, further insertion is performed only under direct vision.

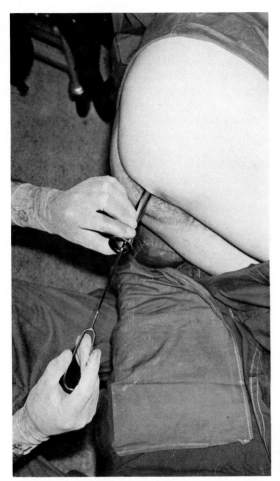

FIG. 6. Diagnostic sigmoidoscopy. An alligator type of sigmoidoscopy forceps is used to swab fecal material from the lumen of the endoscope.

out encountering any further bends in the lumen of the intestine.

In the course of the examination the mucosa is inspected on all aspects of the bowel, during both the insertion of the instrument and its withdrawal. A gross lesion such as proctitis or carcinoma is usually quite readily appreciated during the introduction of the instrument, but less conspicuous lesions such as polyps or solitary ulcers may be missed unless the bowel is carefully examined both on insertion and withdrawal.

Biopsy. Biopsies are obtained with an alligator type of sigmoidoscopy biopsy forceps. Biopsy is technically easier with a large-caliber diagnostic sigmoidoscope, but it can be achieved with a small instrument. The magnifying lens of the eyepiece is detached, leaving the light and rest of the eyepiece attached to the sigmoidoscope; the lesion is then biopsied under direct vision (Fig. 7).

The risks associated with biopsy are hemorrhage and damage to the rectal or colonic wall. In practice hemorrhage is a rare complication, although very occasionally a significant and persistent hemorrhage may cause alarm and may even require blood transfusion. Damage to the wall of the bowel is of importance chiefly if it arises in the intraperitoneal rectum or colon. A full-thickness injury or perforation of the intraperitoneal intestine results in fecal peritonitis. Great caution should thus be exercised in biopsying lesions of the intraperitoneal rectum and colon, and it should be remembered that the peritoneal attachment on the anterior rectal wall may extend down to within 8 or 9 cm of the perineal skin in the male, and 5 to 8 cm in the female. It is a golden rule therefore that biopsies obtained at a level which may involve the intraperitoneal rectum or colon should be taken only under direct vision and with great care. The biopsy should not extend deeply into the submucosa; and the specimen should be gently detached from the bowel wall. Specimens may be detached in two ways: first,

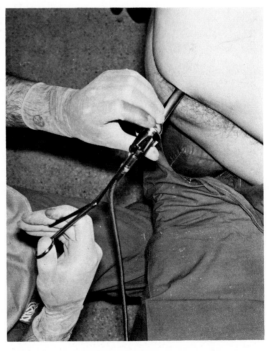

FIG. 7. Diagnostic sigmoidoscopy. Biopsies are obtained under direct vision with an alligator type of biopsy forceps.

by simply avulsing the specimen from the intestinal wall; and second, by twisting the biopsy forceps until the specimen is torn from the surrounding mucosa. The second method is less traumatic to the bowel wall and is recommended for biopsying flat, nonneoplastic mucosa. The avulsion technique is suitable for biopsy of proliferative neoplasms where there is little risk of avulsing part of the normal intestinal wall. There is never any difficulty in biopsying carcinomas since the biopsy forceps cuts through the carcinomatous tissue like a knife through butter.

It may be difficult to obtain good visualization with the sigmoidoscope for biopsying lesions that are very low in the rectum. If the lesion lies within a few centimeters of the anorectal ring, a better and more accurate biopsy may be obtained through a proctoscope. A relatively blind biopsy through the sigmoidoscope is permissible, there being no real risk of serious damage to the rectal wall, but clearly there is a chance that a biopsy attempted in this way may miss the lesion.

Following a rectal or colon biopsy the patient should be informed that he may experience slight bleeding when he next opens his bowels, but that he should report back if bleeding continues or if he experiences any abdominal discomfort.

FINDINGS ON DIAGNOSTIC SIGMOIDOSCOPY

Normal Features

The normal rectal and colonic mucosa is pale pink with a slightly orange tinge. It is smooth and glistening, and the submucosal vessels show clearly beneath the mucous membrane. The normal mucosa is supple. It moves easily against the end of the sigmoidoscope and distends when air is introduced into the lumen of the bowel.

The presence of obvious mucus on the surface of the bowel is abnormal. This may be due to an underlying pathology, or it may be the result of preparation of the bowel with enemas or cathartic agents. The presence of blood in the lumen of the bowel is almost always a finding of pathologic significance. However, slight bleeding occasionally occurs as a result of trauma to the anterior rectal wall immediately above the anorectal ring during insertion of the sigmoidoscope.

Proctitis and Proctocolitis

Inflammation of the colon or rectum is a common abnormality and has a wide variety of causes. It may be due to a specific infection such as a bacillary dysentery or a gonococcal infection; it may be caused by ischemic disease; or it may be a nonspecific inflammation caused by ulcerative colitis or Crohn's disease.

In many cases, irrespective of the cause, the sigmoidoscopy features are entirely nonspecific and simply those of an inflammation; and determination of the cause of a proctitis or proctocolitis may involve a process of detection which includes careful evaluation of the history, bacteriologic studies, sigmoidoscopy and rectal biopsy, and a barium enema examination. In every case of proctitis or proctocolitis a biopsy should be obtained for histologic examination.

There is a tendency for physicians to diagnose proctitis or colitis more frequently than it actually occurs, and the endoscopist should take care to be as objective as possible in his assessment of the sigmoidoscopic findings. Clinical studies have shown that considerable observer error is possible in interpreting the features of mild inflammation at sigmoidoscopy. Signs such as excess mucus, edema, congestion, and granularity of the mucosa may be interpreted differently by different endoscopists.[47] The classic features of proctitis or proctocolitis are loss of normal submucosal vessel pattern due to thickening and inflammation of the mucosa, and the presence of contact bleeding when the mucosa is touched with the endoscope or when the mucosa is swabbed. In more severe cases the diagnosis is simple for there may be spontaneous bleeding and a mucopurulent discharge from the intestinal mucosa.

Ulcerative Colitis. Ulcerative colitis is a nonspecific inflammation affecting the mucosa of the large intestine. It is classically a chronic, relapsing condition, although a small proportion of cases may present with an acute, fulminating diarrheal illness. In about 20 percent of cases the disease affects the rectum alone and in 30 percent the whole of the large intestine; in the remainder there is a variable degree of partial involvement of the colon.

The symptoms of ulcerative colitis include the passage of blood and mucus in the stool, tenesmus, diarrhea, colicky lower abdominal pain, and in some cases anemia and general malaise of variable severity depending on the extent of colonic involvement. In a minority of patients other systemic features may occur, including skin lesions such as erythema nodosum and pyoderma gangrenosum,[14] arthritis,[7] and eye complications such as iritis and episcleritis.[6] Patients with ankylosing spondylitis have an increased incidence of ulcerative colitis.[50]

Examination of the anus and perianal region may reveal evidence of anorectal suppuration or an anal fissure, but such findings are more common in Crohn's disease. Digital examination of the rectum is usually normal, although in longstanding cases of ulcerative colitis the mucosa may feel roughened and granular and there may be a palpable rectal stricture.

The inflammatory features on sigmoidoscopy may be mild, moderate, or severe. Some evidence of inflammation in the rectum is present in almost every case of active ulcerative colitis. A segmental colitis which spares the rectum[37] is usually found to be caused by Crohn's disease.[19] Mild inflammation is apparent as loss of the normal submucosal vessel pattern, with or without contact bleeding. Contact bleeding is apparent in areas where the endoscope touches the mucosa and when the intestinal mucosa is swabbed. In severe inflammation the extent of the contact bleeding is more gross, there may be spontaneous bleeding from the mucosa, and there is often a mucopurulent exudate in the rectal lumen and lining the intestinal mucosa. Ulcers are not evident as macroscopic sigmoidoscopy features of ulcerative colitis. The ulcers are very small, and they are apparent only on histologic examination of biopsy material or in a barium enema examination.

In longstanding cases of ulcerative colitis inflammatory polyps or pseudopolyps may be found on endoscopy, usually in the upper rectum. These pseudopolyps may have an epithelial covering, but they are composed of granulation tissue or fibrous tissue. They often appear in closely packed clusters in the upper rectum and are usually readily distinguishable from true adenomatous polyps by their multiplicity and the inflammatory changes in the surrounding mucosa.

Other endoscopic features of a longstanding ulcerative colitis are stricture formation and carcinoma of the colon or rectum. Although benign strictures may occur in ulcerative colitis, any stricture should be regarded with suspicion. Patients with longstanding ulcerative colitis affecting the whole colon are prone to develop carcinoma,[14] and the tumor may have atypical features often leading to confusion with benign strictures. Any stricture should be carefully examined and biopsied.

Repeat sigmoidoscopy examinations are required in the follow-up of patients with ulcerative colitis; the response of the disease to medical treatment is assessed by this means. The patients are seen at intervals of several weeks while the disease remains active, as judged by sigmoidoscopy findings, and in the quiescent phase at intervals of 6 months or 1 year. The patients who must be followed up with the greatest care are those who have had disease involving the whole colon because of their increased risk of carcinoma. The risk of carcinoma arises chiefly in those who have had symptomatic disease affecting the whole colon for 10 years or more, and these are difficult patients to manage. Repeat sigmoidoscopy examinations do not alone provide adequate information regarding the malignant potential of the colorectal mucosa. It was suggested by Morson and Pang[35] that patients at risk of developing carcinoma may show epithelial dysplasia or precancerous changes in rectal biopsies, and that repeat rectal biopsies in patients at risk might give an early warning of cancerous change elsewhere in the colon. Recent evidence suggests, however, that rectal biopsies alone are a poor guide to the potential for malignant change elsewhere in the colon, and if biopsy information is to be a helpful guide in monitoring patients with total colitis it appears that this would involve fiberoptic colonoscopy and multiple biopsies throughout the colon.[39]

Crohn's Disease. Crohn's disease, classically a disease of the small intestine, may also affect the colon; and in some cases the colon is the only site of the disease. In about 65 percent of cases of Crohn's disease there is some degree of involvement of the colon, and in 15 percent of cases the large intestine is the only site of the disease.[20] It differs from ulcerative colitis in that it is typically a transmural disease characterized by the presence of granulomas or sarcoid foci. Nevertheless, there are similarities between ulcerative colitis and Crohn's disease in their clinical presentation, and in a minority of cases the pathologist may find it difficult to distinguish the two on histologic examination. The prognosis of Crohn's disease, however, is quite different from that of ulcerative colitis. The latter generally responds well to medical treatment, whereas the results of medical treatment in Crohn's disease are frequently disappointing, and there is a significant incidence of recurrence of the disease after surgery.[11]

Like ulcerative colitis, Crohn's disease tends to be a chronic relapsing condition, although a small proportion of cases present as an acute fulminating illness. In most cases the symptoms of Crohn's disease are not unlike those of ulcerative colitis. The patients present with diarrhea, and the passage of blood and slime in the stool. However, rectal bleeding is often a less prominent feature in Crohn's disease, and anal lesions and symptoms occur more frequently than in ulcerative colitis. Patients with disease involving much of the colon may be quite ill. Anemia, malaise, weight loss, and abdominal pain are prominent features in such cases; and when there is additional small-bowel involvement there may be malabsorption and significant cachexia. Crohn's disease also mimics ulcerative colitis in that eye complications, arthritis, and skin lesions are also found.[22,46]

Abdominal examination is likely to reveal some abnormality in patients with Crohn's disease more frequently than in cases of ulcerative colitis. An abdominal mass may be apparent, often located in the right iliac fossa.

Anal examination in Crohn's disease reveals the presence of disease in a high proportion of cases, particularly in patients with disease involving the colon or rectum.[34] The most common anal lesion is a fissure. Abscesses and fistulas are frequently encountered, but the most characteristic lesions in Crohn's disease are anal or perianal ulcers.[27] These are edematous, indolent, undermined lesions of variable size; and they are never found in ulcerative colitis. Digital examination of the rectum may reveal no abnormality or a rough, thickened mucosa and a palpable stricture.

The findings on sigmoidoscopy examination are variable. The rectum is unaffected in about 50 percent of patients with Crohn's disease of the large intestine. In the remainder in whom the rectum is involved, the sigmoidoscopy features may be like those of ulcerative colitis: loss of vessel pattern, granularity and contact bleeding, mucopurulent discharge. Not infrequently, however, the rectal involvement is of a patchy nature. The loss of vessel pattern and contact bleeding may have a patchy distribution, with apparently normal areas of rectal mucosa; there may be localized, raised papules or areas of polypoid mucosa, and discrete ulcers

may be seen. Strictures are more commonly seen than in ulcerative colitis. In cases with no rectal involvement similar changes may be found in the distal sigmoid colon if it is possible to proceed with the sigmoidoscopy examination to this level. Biopsy of mucosal lesions may reveal typical features of Crohn's disease, but in a number of cases typical sarcoid or granulomatous lesions are absent on histologic examination and a definite diagnosis may prove difficult.

It is apparent that sigmoidoscopy may be less helpful in establishing a diagnosis in Crohn's disease than in ulcerative colitis. In Crohn's disease a firm diagnosis may be possible only after barium enema examination or fiberoptic colonoscopy.

Infections.   The specific dysenteries are a very frequent cause of proctocolitis. Such cases present acutely with diarrhea, passage of blood and mucus in the stool, and a variable degree of malaise, pyrexia, and systemic upset.

Bacillary infection is common in temperate climates. The sigmoidoscopy features of this disease resemble those of ulcerative colitis and are quite nonspecific. The diagnosis is established by bacteriologic culture of the stool and serum agglutination tests, which become positive within a few days of the onset of the illness.

Amebic dysentery is common in tropical and subtropical climates, and it is often associated with typical sigmoidoscopy features. In the acute infection numerous tiny ulcers surrounded by areas of inflammation are seen on sigmoidoscopy. The intervening rectal mucosa may appear quite normal, or there may be submucosal hemorrhages. The diagnosis is made by obtaining material from the surface of an ulcer for immediate microscopic examination. Chronic amebic infection may occur in the large intestine, and it most frequently affects the right colon. These cases present with diarrhea and right-sided abdominal signs suggestive of either appendicitis or carcinoma of the right colon. Occasionally the rectum and distal colon are affected, and in these cases multiple small rectal or colonic ulcers may be found on sigmoidoscopy.

Bilharzial infection is endemic in Egypt, Japan, and certain parts of Africa and South America. It may present as an acute dysentery, with inflammatory features on sigmoidoscopy which are entirely nonspecific. In the subacute or chronic infection there may be much fibrosis and stricture formation in the rectum and colon, and anorectal fistulas are common. Adenomatous and papillomatous neoplasms occur in the rectum, but unlike bilharzial infection of the urinary bladder bilharziasis of the rectum and colon does not predispose to carcinoma. The diagnosis of bilharzial infection is established by demonstrating the ova (usually *Schistosoma mansoni*) in feces or in rectal biopsy specimens.

Various venereal infections may cause proctitis or disease of the anal canal. Gonococcal proctitis is becoming increasingly prevalent. In the male it results from homosexual anal intercourse, and in female patients it is often associated with a genital infection. Jensen[23] found that a gonococcal proctitis was present in 31 percent of his female patients presenting with genital gonorrhea. The infection may spread directly to the anus or rectum in the female, or it may result from heterosexual anal intercourse with an infected partner. The condition may cause little or no discomfort, or it may result in tenesmus and anal pain. Sigmoidoscopy shows the features of an inflammation in the lower rectum: loss of the normal vessel pattern, contact bleeding, and a mucopurulent discharge. The diagnosis is made by bacteriologic examination and culture of mucopus obtained at sigmoidoscopy or proctoscopy.

A syphilitic infection of the rectum is less common than a gonococcal proctitis. Syphilitic lesions are more frequently found in the anal canal and perianal region, where primary infection manifests as an ulcer or chancre, and secondary infection presents with anal condylomas or warts. Occasionally, however, a primary chancre may occur in the lower rectum,[26] usually following homosexual anal intercourse. The sigmoidoscopy diagnosis of this lesion may prove difficult unless the possibility of syphilis is considered. The lesion is typically a localized ulcer with a surrounding proctitis. The diagnosis is established by obtaining material from the surface of the ulcer for immediate bacteriologic examination.

Lymphogranuloma venereum is a venereal infection with a worldwide distribution, and it is especially prevalent in colored races. It is characterized by genital infection and infection of the regional inguinal lymph glands. Suppuration and extensive tissue destruction are prominent features of the condition. Anorectal involvement may occur in either sex,[5] resulting in a proctitis which may spread into the distal sigmoid colon. The sigmoidoscopy findings at this stage are quite nonspecific and simply those of a granular proctitis. Chronic or subacute infection results in fibrosis and stricture formation. The diagnosis of lymphogranuloma infection is made by serologic tests and the Frei intradermal test.

Tuberculous disease and actinomycosis of the rectum are very rare and seldom produce recognizable abnormalities on sigmoidoscopy. Both infections, however, are recognized causes of anorectal abscesses and fistulas.

Irradiation Proctitis. A proctitis frequently follows pelvic irradiation, and in some cases the radiation injury to the rectum may be severe enough to produce long-term damage. Various forms of pelvic irradiation are commonly used in the treatment of advanced carcinoma of the urinary bladder, carcinoma of the cervix and body of the uterus, and other forms of pelvic malignancy.

Symptoms of proctitis are frequently encountered during such therapy: diarrhea, tenesmus, and the passage of blood and slime in the stool. Sigmoidoscopy reveals the nonspecific features of a proctitis, but the lower third of the rectum is often unaffected. Usually these symptoms and changes clear spontaneously when radiotherapy is terminated.

Long-term changes are infrequently encountered with modern techniques of radiotherapy. In chronic cases the sigmoidoscopy features are variable. In some cases a proctitis is evident; in others there may be frank ulceration of the rectum; and some cases progress to stricture formation or fistulation into the vagina. Usually the diagnosis is simplified by the history of previous radiotherapy, but rectal strictures and ulcers must be carefully examined and biopsied, for only in this way can a diagnosis of carcinoma be confidently excluded.

Ischemic Colitis. Ischemia of the colon may follow ligation or occlusion of the inferior mesenteric artery, sometimes as a complication of reconstructive surgery of the abdominal aorta. However, ischemic colitis may occur spontaneously, either as a consequence of atheromatous occlusion of a major arterial trunk such as the inferior mesenteric artery[29] or in association with disease of the small colonic vessels.[30]

Colonic ischemia may be mild, moderate, or severe; and the clinical presentation and sequelae are closely related to the severity of the disease. Severe ischemia may result in gangrene or full-thickness necrosis of the colon; and such cases present as acute abdominal emergencies, often with perforation and fecal peritonitis. Most cases are less severe and present with diarrhea, pyrexia, and abdominal pain and tenderness, sometimes accompanied by the passage of blood and mucus in the stool.

The rectum is not commonly affected in this disease, and sigmoidoscopy usually shows no abnormality or blood and mucus descending from a higher level in the colon. Occasionally the lower limit of the ischemic lesion is encountered on sigmoidoscopy; and granularity of the mucosa, contact bleeding, and a mucopurulent exudate are found in the upper rectum and distal sigmoid colon. In a few cases similar changes are encountered in the rectal ampulla.[10]

Roentgenologic studies, including a barium enema examination, may be required to establish the diagnosis of ischemic colitis when sigmoidoscopy is normal; but when disease is encountered on sigmoidoscopy a rectal or colonic biopsy often shows characteristic features. The presence of hemosiderinladen macrophages in a mucosal biopsy is strongly suggestive of ischemic disease.[29]

Nonspecific Ulceration. Nonspecific ulcers, usually solitary, may occur anywhere in the large intestine, but about 50 percent are found in the cecum.[2] A minority occur in the rectum and sigmoid colon. The etiology of this condition remains uncertain, but there is no evidence that it predisposes to carcinoma.

Nonspecific ulcers in the rectum are usually solitary, and they present with symptoms of a proctitis:[28] tenesmus and the passage of blood and mucus in the stool. Sigmoidoscopy usually shows an ulcer located in the anterior wall of the middle third of the rectum. The ulcer has a purulent base, and the surrounding mucosa may appear edematous and elevated. Biopsy of the edge of the ulcer may show characteristic features; there is obliteration of the lamina propria by fibroblasts, and the epithelium may show a reactive hyperplasia. Multiple biopsies may be required to exclude other conditions such as carcinoma or Crohn's disease.

Proctitis Autophytica. Ulceration and inflammation of the lower rectum may result from self-inflicted trauma. The extent of the rectal changes depends on the nature and frequency of the trauma, but the changes are usually localized. A variety of phallic objects may be inserted through the anus for erotic stimulation. It may prove difficult to elicit a history of self-inflicted trauma, and the proctologist must be extremely careful to exclude other causes of rectal ulceration or proctitis.

Tumors

A variety of tumors occur in the large intestine. The most important of these is carcinoma, but several types of benign tumor are encountered and it is important to recognize them. Some are harmless lesions; some are not strictly tumors in a pathologic sense; while others are associated with an increased susceptibility to carcinoma of the colon, or they may themselves undergo malignant change.

The symptoms associated with neoplasms of the large intestine are variable and depend on the site of the lesion and its nature. Benign polyps may be asymptomatic, or they may cause occult or overt blood loss, alteration of bowel habit, or abdominal pain due to intussusception or obstruction of the intestinal lumen. Malignant tumors may produce symptoms akin to those of benign lesions, but the symptoms are usually progressive in their severity and they may occur because of the extension of the growth beyond the bowel wall.

Benign Tumors.   Epithelial Tumors. The majority of benign tumors of the large intestine are adenomas arising from the mucosal epithelium; like tumors of glandular epithelium elsewhere, they are commonly referred to as polyps.

At sigmoidoscopy adenomatous polyps vary in size from minute lesions to large exuberant tumors: they may be sessile or pedunculated, the latter having a well defined pedicle. The surface of the adenoma is smooth or only slightly irregular. The color of the tumor is variable, some having an appearance similar to normal colonic mucosa while others are dark red.

The papillary adenoma or villous papilloma is an adenomatous polyp with a rather different appearance at sigmoidoscopy. This is a sessile lesion of variable size and ill-defined edges. It may implicate a wide area of intestinal mucosa. It has an irregular polypoidal surface, and its color is usually darker than that of normal colonic mucosa.

The majority of polyps are found in the sigmoid colon or rectum. Ordinary adenomatous polyps are more common in the sigmoid colon, and the papillary adenoma occurs more frequently in the rectum.[21]

The importance of these lesions, apart from the symptoms they may cause, is their relation to carcinoma of the colon or rectum. Benign adenomatous tumors are found in a significant proportion of resected specimens of colon in operations for carcinoma. In the experience of Goligher[19] benign tumors may coexist in about 30 percent of cases of colonic carcinoma. *Whether benign adenomas undergo malignant change or start out as malignant lesions is a question surrounded by considerable controversy.* The important practical lesson, however, is that invasive carcinoma is present in about 3 percent of apparently benign adenomatous polyps and *in 32 percent of papillary adenomas.*[21]

It follows, therefore, that patients with adenomatous tumors found on sigmoidoscopy must undergo a thorough assessment both of the lesion itself and of the remainder of the large intestine in view of the tendency for such lesions to be multiple and because of their association with carcinoma. All patients must have a sigmoidoscopy and a barium enema examination. The latter should be a double-contrast type of examination as described by Welin.[48] Further examination of the colon by fiberoptic colonoscopy may be necessary in a number of cases, and this type of endoscopy may be required for the removal of suitable lesions.

The important question regarding the polyp found on sigmoidoscopy is whether it is benign or malignant. The macroscopic appearance of the tumor may not be a useful guide, and biopsy may not be helpful. Areas of cellular atypism with hyperchromatic, pleomorphic nuclei are not infrequently found in biopsies of benign tumors, but a diagnosis of carcinoma cannot be made with certainty unless there is demonstrable invasion of the muscularis mucosa.

In the case of the papillary adenoma the risk of malignant change is very great, and the proctologist should not be reassured by the absence of invasive carcinoma in serial biopsies, particularly if the tumor is large. The findings on digital palpation of a papillary adenoma are frequently more useful than visualization of the lesion at sigmoidoscopy or biopsy in determining whether the tumor is benign or malignant. A benign papillary adenoma should feel perfectly soft; the presence of any induration in such a lesion is strongly suggestive of malignancy. When the suspicion of malignancy arises, the operation for removal of the tumor should be planned as a radical cancer operation rather than a local excision or an electrosurgical procedure. When a papillary adenoma occurs high in the rectum or out of reach of the examining finger, it is safer to assume that the lesion is malignant than to rely on repeated inspection and biopsy.

The risk of malignancy is less of a problem with the ordinary adenomatous polyp. Carcinoma is rarely encountered in small polyps less than 1 cm in diameter.[21] Such polyps can be left alone unless they can be removed with ease and safety. Polyps judged to be more than 1 cm in diameter should be removed because of the risk of malignancy. The removal of these lesions has been simplified by the introduction of the fiberoptic colonoscope, which can be used for the removal of polyps that are beyond the reach of the sigmoidoscope.

Patients who are found to have benign adenomatous tumors should be regularly followed up even if the initial lesion has been successfully treated. They should be sigmoidoscoped at intervals of 6 months to a year, and a double-contrast barium enema should be performed at intervals of 1 year or 18 months, either routinely or if colonic symptoms occur. In doubtful cases colonoscopy may be required. Such measures are necessary because of the increased potential for these patients to develop further benign tumors or colonic carcinoma.

The finding of multiple adenomatous polyps in the rectum and elsewhere in the large intestine should always suggest the diagnosis of familial polyposis coli. This hereditary condition is characterized by the occurrence of multiple adenomatous polyps in individuals carrying the dominant mutant gene, and there is an overwhelming tendency for affected subjects to develop carcinoma of the colon or rectum at an early age. In a variant of the condition, patients with polyposis coli also develop multiple sebaceous or dermoid cysts and connective tissue tumors.[18] The diagnosis is usually suggested by the large number of tumors found on sigmoidoscopy, and the multiple tumors elsewhere in the colon produce a striking appearance on a barium enema examination. The polyps vary in size and may be sessile or pedunculated. Biopsies of the polyps show the typical features of an adenoma. When the diagnosis is established, surgery is indicated in every case as prophylaxis against the development of carcinoma. In addition, the family history of the patient must be thoroughly investigated and all siblings examined for the disease.

A not infrequent and sometimes perplexing finding at sigmoidoscopy is the presence of multiple tiny mucosal protrusions which resemble very small adenomas. These are the so-called hyperplastic mucosal polyps which are not true adenomas, and they have no apparent association with malignant disease of the large intestine. Biopsy of these harmless lesions reveals mucosal changes that are quite different from those of true adenomatous tumors.[32]

Hamartomatous Tumors. Two types of hamartomatous polyp occur in the large intestine: the juvenile polyp and the polyps found in Peutz-Jeghers' syndrome. Juvenile polyps are found in infants and children. They may occur anywhere in the large intestine, but the majority are found in the rectum.[24] They are hamartomatous lesions composed of a cellular vascular tissue. In 30 percent of cases they may be multiple. At sigmoidoscopy the polyp appears as a smooth and often pedunculated tumor. The differentiation between this tumor and an adenomatous polyp is suggested by the age of the patient, and the distinction is readily made on biopsy. Symptomatic lesions should be removed.

The Peutz-Jeghers' syndrome is a familial condition characterized by the occurrence of multiple hamartomatous polyps throughout the intestine. A feature of the condition is the presence of a characteristic pigmentation of the buccal mucosa and the skin of the fingers and toes. The appearances of these polyps on sigmoidoscopy are indistinguishable from those of adenomatous polyps, and the condition may be confused with familial polyposis of the colon. The distinction between this condition and familial polyposis is important, for the malignant potential of hamartomatous lesions is much less than that of true adenomatous polyps.[33] The diagnosis is made by biopsy. Treatment is seldom indicated, except for the removal of symptomatic lesions.

Connective Tissue Tumors. Connective tissue tumors are rarely found in the large intestine, but they are apt to be confused with adenomatous tumors until the diagnosis is made by biopsy. The most common of the benign tumors is a lymphoma of the rectum, which appears on sigmoidoscopy as a reddish, purple, or gray polyp of variable size. There is no evidence that these tumors undergo malignant change,[43] but careful histologic assessment may be required to differentiate this lesion from a lymphosarcoma.

Leiomyomas and lipomas occur more commonly in the colon than in the rectum, and they present as submucosal lesions causing polypoidal distortion of the mucosa. The sigmoidoscopy features may thus be not unlike those of an epithelial tumor.

Hemangiomas are exceedingly rare tumors in the large intestine. Lesions which occur low in the rectum may also involve the anal canal.[4] Large lesions appear on sigmoidoscopy as reddish or purple tumors, and it may be apparent that the lesion is associated with dilated submucosal vessels.

Malignant Tumors. Carcinoma. Carcinoma is the most common malignant tumor in the large intestine. As a cause of death it is exceeded only by carcinoma of the bronchus in most western communities. According to Smiddy and Goligher[41] approximately 57 percent of these tumors occur in the rectum and 21 percent in the sigmoid colon, but this distribution varies somewhat in different races.[25]

The appearance of a carcinoma at sigmoidoscopy is variable. The tumor may be polypoidal or fungating. It may be an ulcerative lesion with raised, everted edges and a purulent base; or it may be an annular or stenosing tumor which causes a stricture of the colon or rectum of variable length. Sometimes a combination of these features is found. A less common type of tumor is the diffusely infiltrating type which produces much thickening of the mucosa over a wide area, with a limited amount of mucosal ulceration. This type is not uncommonly found as a complication of ulcerative colitis.

In most cases the sigmoidoscopy features of a carcinoma are quite characteristic and leave little doubt regarding the malignant nature of the lesion. Some idea of the fixity of the lesion may be gained at sigmoidoscopy, although in the case of low rectal tumors this is best appreciated by digital examination. Resistance may be encountered when the endoscope is gently pressed against the lower edge of the growth: The immobility of a fixed tumor feels quite different from the slight yielding sensation of an early mobile tumor. A further distinctive feature of carcinoma is the excessive friability encountered when the tumor is biopsied, and it is usually found that the biopsy forceps cut through the tumor with considerable ease.

When a carcinoma can be reached by the finger on digital examination of the rectum it is found to have characteristic features. The tumor feels indurated and may seem fixed. Exuberant growths are usually extremely friable and bleed readily on palpation. In some cases the tumor may not be directly palpable but can be felt through the rectal wall. This is frequently a feature of sigmoid tumors lying in the rectovesical or rectouterine pouch, and in these cases a hard mass may be felt through the anterior rectal wall.

For tumors out of reach of the sigmoidoscope a barium enema is required for diagnosis. Colonoscopy is rarely required except when atypical appearances or lesions resembling benign adenomatous tumors are found on barium enema.

Carcinoid. Carcinoid tumors are less commonly found in the large intestine than in the small bowel. The tumor may occur in the colon or rectum; and unlike the multiple tumors which tend to occur in the small intestine, tumors in the large intestine are usually solitary. Tumors in the colon have a greater potential for malignant change than tumors of the rectum.[16,43]

At sigmoidoscopy the carcinoid tumor may look very much like an ordinary adenomatous polyp; or if malignant change has occurred, it may be an ulcerated lesion similar in appearance to a carcinoma. The diagnosis is made by biopsy. Malignant lesions require a radical surgical resection of the affected bowel, but benign tumors can be treated by local excision, provided complete excision can be ensured. If the tumor has reached a size of 2 cm or more in diameter local excision is likely to prove inadequate.[36]

Lymphosarcoma. Lymphosarcoma is an extremely rare malignant tumor in the large intestine. The clinical and sigmoidoscopy features of this tumor may be indistinguishable from those of a carcinoma. In the early stages it may be apparent that the tumor is a submucosal lesion with an intact mucosal covering, but the majority have already ulcerated by the time the patient presents to the proctologist. Histologic confirmation of the diagnosis may prove difficult as the tumor can have characteristics similar to those of anaplastic carcinoma.[12]

Other Sarcomas. Other malignant tumors of connective tissue are even more uncommon than lymphosarcoma. Of these the most common is the leiomyosarcoma, which is found more frequently in the rectum than in the colon. Once again the sigmoidoscopy features of the tumor may resemble those of a carcinoma, except in the few instances in which the tumor has not yet ulcerated through the mucosa. The difficulty in histologic diagnosis in this case is in deciding whether the tumor is truly a sarcoma or a benign leiomyoma, as the appearances may be quite similar.

Extrarectal Tumors. Digital examination of the rectum may reveal a tumor mass outside the rectum. Anteriorly this may be a tumor arising from other pelvic organs or tumor deposits from a lesion elsewhere in the abdomen; posteriorly an extrarectal mass is frequently a benign or malignant tumor arising from the bony sacrum. Not all extrarectal masses are necessarily tumors. An anterior extrarectal mass may result from a pelvic abscess or diverticular disease of the sigmoid colon. Extrarectal tumors are not well appreciated on sigmoidoscopy unless there is considerable distortion of the rectal or colonic lumen, or infiltration of the bowel wall.

Pelvic endometriosis may affect the upper rectum and distal sigmoid colon, and it may be found as an extrarectal mass on digital examination or sigmoidoscopy. In some cases a considerable stricture of the intestinal lumen may occur, but it is apparent at sigmoidoscopy that the mucosa throughout the stricture is intact and unaffected.

Other Findings on Sigmoidoscopy

Diverticular Disease. The presence of diverticula in the sigmoid and descending colon is a common pathologic finding. However, although diverticular disease is a common cause of colonic symptoms and presentation in the proctologist's office, it is rare for the colonic lesion to be demonstrated by sigmoidoscopy. Indeed sigmoidoscopy is often incomplete in these patients owing to distortion of the sigmoid colon and rectosigmoid, and the openings of mucosal diverticula are rarely visualized at sigmoidoscopy.

Melanosis Coli. Melanosis coli is a condition characterized by pigmentation of the rectal and colonic mucosa. It results from the chronic ingestion of laxatives of the anthracene group, such as senna or cascara.

At sigmoidoscopy the rectal and colonic mucosa has a peculiar brown or black appearance. Close inspection reveals that the pigmentation is widespread but that it has a patchy distribution, separated by thin lines of normal mucosa. Biopsy shows that the pigmentation is located in macrophages in the submucosa. The condition is harmless, and it may gradually regress when the laxative is withdrawn.[42]

Pneumatosis Cystoides Intestinalis. In this rare condition multiple gas-filled cysts are found in the intestinal wall, either in the submucosa or the subserosa. The condition is commonly found in the small intestine, but the rectum and sigmoid colon are occasionally affected.

The majority of cases are discovered by chance, but symptoms may occur because of narrowing or obstruction of the bowel lumen. Careful inspection of the cysts at sigmoidoscopy usually reveals that they are submucosal translucent structures. Indeed the features are usually quite striking, but if doubt exists regarding the nature of the lesions the diagnosis is made by biopsy. The proctologist must be careful not to attribute symptoms to this condition when in fact there may be an alternative explanation, and symptomatic patients who are found to have pneumatosis coli at sigmoidoscopy should undergo a full investigation to exclude the presence of other lesions in the colon.

OPERATIVE SIGMOIDOSCOPY

Operative sigmoidoscopy is used in the treatment of benign adenomatous tumors of the distal sigmoid colon and rectum by electrosurgery. It may also be used as a palliative treatment of inoperable or recurrent carcinoma of the rectum or distal colon, and electrosurgery has recently been suggested as the treatment of choice for certain types of low rectal carcinomas.

Preparation and Anesthesia

Preparation of the intestine by purgation and enemas is desirable. Details of the methods of preparation were described in the section on diagnostic sigmoidoscopy.

I prefer to admit the patient to hospital for this procedure and to perform it under a full general anesthesia. Sedation with intravenous diazepam (Valium) supplemented with an analgesic is also acceptable, but I have no experience with this technique in operative sigmoidoscopy.

Electrosurgical Equipment

Diathermy Machine. A Bovie or spark-gap type of diathermy machine is most commonly used for electrosurgical procedures, although some surgeons now use solid-state, "cold cautery" units which are safer for the patient and operator.

The operator must consciously beware of producing accidental thermal injury to the bowel wall. This is particularly important in the treatment of tumors occurring above the peritoneal reflection of the rectum, since damage to the intraperitoneal rectum or colon may result in peritonitis. Thus the working potential of each diathermy machine should be known to the operator, so that the appropriate current is selected for each electrosurgical procedure. The principles and use of diathermy machines are well described by Swerdlow et al.[45]

Sigmoidoscopy Equipment. I generally use the large Lloyd-Davies operating sigmoidoscope for electrosurgery, although the ordinary diagnostic instrument is suitable for treating very small lesions.

Various snares, electrodes, and forceps are available for treating rectal and colonic tumors at sigmoidoscopy. The snare is a wire loop mounted in an insulated shaft and handle, and is used to remove pedunculated tumors. A common type is the Frankfeldt snare.[19] Sigmoidoscopy electrodes are usually of the button type, also mounted in an insulated shaft and handle, and are used for the electrocoagulation and destruction of sessile tumors. The sigmoidoscopy diathermy forceps may be used as an addition to the snare for removing pedunculated lesions. It is simply an ordinary alligator type of sigmoidoscopy forceps covered with some form of insulation along the shaft.

Scrupulous attention is required to ensure that the sigmoidoscopy equipment is properly insulated to protect the patient and the operator from accidental burns. With the Bovie type of instrument, the patient is placed on a ground plate attached to the diathermy machine. The diathermy snares, electrodes, and forceps must be carefully insulated so that short-circuiting of the current is avoided. The operator should wear gloves and rubber boots, and he should be careful to avoid facial contact with the sigmoidoscope when the diathermy is in use.

Intraluminal explosions have been described as a rare complication of sigmoidoscopy electrosurgery; when they occur they are due to the ignition of flammable gases in the bowel lumen, which is an argument favoring the use of carbon dioxide or nitrogen insufflation during electrosurgery. This is standard practice in colonoscopy electrosurgery[49] but is probably unnecessary in sigmoidoscopy if preoperative intestinal preparation is used.

Technique of Operative Sigmoidoscopy

The patient is anesthetized and placed in the left lateral position, as for a diagnostic examination (Fig. 3). The sigmoidoscope is introduced in the usual way, and the lesion is visualized.

Removal of Pedunculated Polyps. The snare is the ideal instrument for removing pedunculated tumors. The wire loop should be tested before use to make sure that it is not broken. It is then manipulated over the tumor and tightened around the stalk (Fig. 8), and the tumor is removed by applying the coagulating diathermy current. The diathermy usually

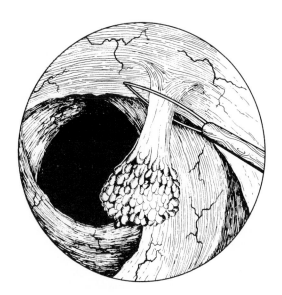

FIG. 8. Operative sigmoidoscopy. Technique of snaring pedunculated polyps.

cuts slowly through the pedicle until the tumor separates with little hemorrhage. The residual area of mucosal necrosis heals within about 2 to 3 weeks. If difficulty is encountered in placing the loop of the snare over the tumor, it is often helpful to grasp the tumor first with an alligator forceps before passing the snare over the polyp. Alternatively, when the pedicle of the tumor is well defined, it is often possible to remove the lesion simply by using an insulated alligator-type sigmoidoscopy forceps: The pedicle is seized with the forceps, and the diathermy current is applied directly to the handle of the forceps.

Minichan[31] recommended an alternative method of snaring pedunculated tumors. In this technique a rubber ring is placed over the tumor and applied to the pedicle; the tumor is excised with a biopsy forceps, leaving the hemostatic ring on the base of the pedicle. The equipment used is the same as that used for rubber ring ligation of hemorrhoids,[3] and the method avoids the risk of diathermy injury to the bowel. It is alleged that hemostasis is achieved more readily with this technique than with the diathermy snare, but hemorrhage is a rare complication of diathermy snaring when careful technique is used.

Another method recommended by Minichan[31] is injection of a vasoconstricting solution such as 1:50,000 epinephrine into the base of the polyp prior to its removal. The tumor is then removed either by the snare technique or after application of a rubber ring.

Removal of Sessile Polyps. The removal or destruction of sessile tumors by electrosurgery is more difficult. It may be possible to remove small polyps with the diathermy snare, but the method involves a greater risk of injury to the bowel wall than in the treatment of pedunculated tumors. The polyp is grasped with an alligator forceps so that the tumor is pulled away from the bowel wall on a false pedicle of mucosa; the wire snare is then manipulated over the tumor and tightened around the pedicle, and the coagulating current is applied to the snare. Care must be taken to avoid including more than the mucosa of the bowel within the snare; otherwise serious damage to the bowel wall may occur.

The snare technique is impracticable in the treatment of large sessile tumors such as papillary adenomas. The method of treatment used for these tumors is to apply the coagulating current to the surface of the lesion. An insulated button electrode (Fig. 9) or an insulated

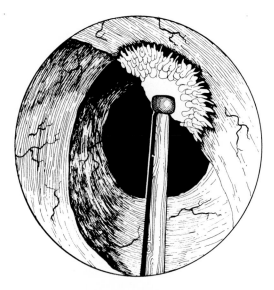

FIG. 9. Operative sigmoidoscopy. Technique of electrocoagulation of sessile tumors using the insulated button electrode.

alligator forceps is commonly used. There is undoubtedly a significant risk of injury to the bowel wall with this type of electrocoagulation, and while small tumors may be suitable for this treatment I avoid surface coagulation of large sessile tumors occurring above the peritoneal reflection of the rectum. An additional and important reason for avoiding conservative treatment of large sessile tumors in the upper rectum or distal sigmoid colon is the risk of malignancy in such tumors.

When large tumors are regarded as suitable for electrosurgical treatment—usually tumors in the middle or lower rectum—several sessions of electrosurgery may be required for their complete eradication. The operator should be quite conservative in the amount of electrocoagulation he uses at each session, for the amount of tissue destruction which results is often greater than it first appears. Excessive tissue destruction results in stricture formation.

Management of Polyposis Coli. The ideal treatment of familial polyposis of the colon is proctocolectomy and ileostomy, removing all the intestine which is at risk of malignant change. In practice, however, a colectomy and ileorectal anastomosis is usually preferred, at least in the first instance, as there is a risk that young patients may refuse an operation which involves the creation of an artificial stoma.

When the rectum is retained it must be examined repeatedly by sigmoidoscopy and rectal polyps treated by electrosurgery. Because of the multiple nature of the polyps, extensive diathermy fulguration may be required, and there is a risk of stricture formation, which may make further treatment and examination difficult. Treatment of the rectum is usually deferred until after the colectomy and ileorectal anastomosis. Sometimes there is a spontaneous regression of the rectal polyps following this operation, but the majority of patients require sigmoidoscopy electrosurgery.

Carcinoma. Diathermy electrocoagulation with the insulated button electrode is occasionally used in the treatment of low rectal carcinomas in poor-risk patients, and in the palliative treatment of inoperable tumors and tumors recurring after previous surgery. Crile and Turnbull[9] used this method as the treatment of choice in many patients with low rectal carcinoma as an alternative to abdominoperineal excision of the rectum, with impressive survival figures. I do not use electrosurgery for the treatment of carcinomas which are suitable for surgical excision.

Usually several sessions of electrosurgery are required in the treatment of carcinoma unless the tumor is very small. If this method is used as an alternative to surgical removal of potentially curable lesions, the patient must be followed carefully at frequent intervals to ensure that local recurrence is detected early.

DIAGNOSTIC PROCTOSCOPY

Proctoscopy is performed in all patients in addition to sigmoidoscopy, either before or after the sigmoidoscopy examination. I tend to perform the proctoscopy after the rectum has been thoroughly evaluated on sigmoidoscopy.

Surgical Anatomy

The anal canal measures some 3 to 4 cm in length. It is lined by the mucosa of the large intestine in its upper third and by skin in its lower two-thirds. The mucocutaneous junction is clearly demarcated by the anal valves, which produce a rather serrated appearance; and the mucocutaneous junction is commonly known as the pectinate or dentate line. Above each anal valve there is a tiny pocket known as the anal crypt, and each anal crypt contains the orifices of several anal intermuscular glands.

The anal canal is surrounded by the internal and external sphincter muscles. The lower edge of the external sphincter projects beyond the internal sphincter, thus forming an intersphincteric groove that is readily appreciated on palpation of the lower anal canal and may be seen on inspection of the anus. The disposition of the lower edges of the sphincter muscles is rather different in the anesthetized patient. Anesthesia causes relaxation of the external sphincter; this muscle is displaced laterally, and the lower edge of the anal canal is thus formed by the internal sphincter.

The anorectal ring is a band of muscle marking the junction of the anal canal and rectum. It is formed by the upper borders of the sphincter muscles, and on the posterior and lateral aspects by the puborectalis muscle. The identification of the anorectal ring is of paramount importance in operations for anal fistulas.

Preparation and Anesthesia

As in diagnostic sigmoidoscopy no special preparation of the intestine is required for a diagnostic proctoscopy, and anesthesia is not required for a routine examination unless the patient is suffering from a painful anal condition such as a fissure or abscess. Anesthesia is required for detailed inspection of the anal canal or lower rectum with the bivalve speculum, and I tend to use general anesthesia for such an examination. The need for this type of examination usually arises in patients who have intermuscular or intersphincteric anal abscesses or anal fistulas; and the proctoscopy examination with the bilvalve speculum is required for both diagnostic purposes and exposure of the anal canal during the surgical treatment of these conditions.

Technique of Diagnostic Proctoscopy

The examination may be conducted in the left lateral or the knee-shoulder position. The latter position has certain advantages for proctoscopy in that there is a tendency for the rectum to fill with air, thus enabling better examination of the lower rectal mucosa. In England the left lateral position is usually preferred.

When a digital examination of the rectum and sigmoidoscopy have been performed, the patient is informed that the final part of the examination is about to commence and that another small instrument is to be passed. It is often reassuring for the patient if he is informed that this part of the examination involves significantly less discomfort than the sigmoidoscopy.

I use the Milligan-Morgan type of tubular proctoscope with high-intensity lighting for diagnostic proctoscopy (Fig. 1). The instrument is tested first to ensure that the metal obturator can be easily withdrawn from the instrument. It is then lubricated and inserted through the anal canal in a similar fashion to the sigmoidoscope: The right buttock is elevated, and the tip of the proctoscope is gently pressed against the anus; if any resistance is encountered because of spasm of the anal sphincters the gentle pressure is maintained until relaxation occurs, and the instrument is passed upward and forward through the anus. When the proctoscope is judged to have reached the level of the anorectal ring, the axis of insertion is altered and the instument is passed backward toward the hollow of the sacrum as it enters the rectum. The instrument is inserted to its full length, the obturator removed, and the light source inserted through the handle of the instrument.

The rectal mucosa is inspected and the anal canal examined during withdrawal of the instrument. Biopsies may be obtained with an alligator type of sigmoidoscopy forceps or with short forceps such as a Hartmann conchotome. The cutaneous lining of the anal canal is endowed with a rich sensory nerve supply, and biopsies of this part of the anal canal cannot be obtained without some form of anesthesia.

For detailed examination of the anal canal under general anesthesia, the bivalve speculum is preferred. I use the Goligher speculum, and as the examination is often followed by surgical treatment of the anal disorder it is convenient to perform the examination with the patient in the lithotomy-Trendelenburg position. The instrument is lubricated and inserted into the anal canal. The anus is illuminated with a bright spotlight, and the blades of the instrument are gently separated, displaying the anal canal. The instrument is rotated so that all quadrants of the anal canal are inspected. For detailed inspection of any one area, the blades of the instrument may be locked in the open position, and the opposite wall of the anal canal may be retracted away with the help of an attachable third blade.

FINDINGS ON DIAGNOSTIC PROCTOSCOPY

The normal appearance of the rectal mucosa was described in the section on diagnostic sigmoidoscopy. At proctoscopy the rectum is not forcibly distended with air, the mucosa is not stretched, and the normal submucosal vessel pattern is frequently less obvious than it is at sigmoidoscopy.

After inspection of the rectal mucosa and the contents of the rectal lumen, the instrument is slowly withdrawn through the anal canal. As the proctoscope enters the anal canal, the mucosa at the level of the anorectal ring closes over the end of the instrument. The mucocutaneous junction is encountered as the proctoscope is further withdrawn, and the anal valves and crypts are inspected. Finally the cutaneous lining of the anal canal below the pectinate line is examined.

Abnormalities in the Rectum

Many of the abnormalities found at sigmoidoscopy may also be apparent on proctoscopy if the lower rectum is affected. In some instances pathology occurring in the lower rectum may be more readily examined with the proctoscope. This is particularly true of low rectal tumors and various types of nonmalignant ulcers. A more careful evaluation and accurate biopsy of these lesions may be obtained at proctoscopy.

The presence of intestinal parasites may be more readily appreciated at proctoscopy. Threadworm infestation is a common disorder, particularly in children, and the tiny worms are not uncommonly found in the rectum at proctoscopy.

Abnormalities in the Anal Canal

Hemorrhoids.   Internal Hemorrhoids. Internal hemorrhoids are an extremely common finding at proctoscopy. These mucosal swellings are caused by varicosities arising in the submucosal venous plexus of the upper part of the anal canal and the lower end of the rectum. In some cases these hemorrhoids enlarge progressively, and they tend to prolapse through the anal canal—at first only at defecation; later during coughing, sneezing, or other minor exertion. Finally, the hemorrhoids may remain permanently prolapsed. Apart from the symptom of prolapse, patients may experience bleeding, the discharge of mucus, or anal irritation. Pain is not a common feature unless strangulation and thrombosis of the hemorrhoids occur.

On inspection of the anus, advanced prolapsed hemorrhoids or strangulated, thrombosed hemorrhoids are immediately apparent. Uncomplicated prolapsed hemorrhoids are red or purple lesions covered with anal mucosa on their inner aspect and skin on their outer aspect. Longstanding prolapsed hemorrhoids may have a rather pale or white appearance due to squamous metaplasia in the anal mucosa. Internal hemorrhoids are not usually palpable on digital examination of the rectum, but longstanding hemorrhoids may become palpable if there is much fibrous tissue deposition within their substance.

At proctoscopy internal hemorrhoids become apparent when the instrument is withdrawn through the anal canal. The red mucosa of the hemorrhoids bulges into the lumen of the instrument when it is withdrawn beyond the anorectal ring; and it is usually apparent that there are essentially three major masses located in the left lateral, right posterior, and right anterior positions. The size of the hemorrhoids is appreciated if the patient is asked to bear down as the proctoscope is withdrawn, and in advanced cases this may result in complete prolapse of the hemorrhoids through the anus when the instrument is removed.

External   Hemorrhoids.   External hemorrhoids are found at or just outside the anal orifice, and they are diagnosed by simple inspection of the anus. The external hemorrhoid is a subcutaneous anal or perianal hematoma, but skin tags occurring in the perianal region are also often referred to as external hemorrhoids. Many of these skin tags are not associated with any obvious pathology, but in some cases a skin tag may be the remnant of a perianal hematoma, or it may be associated with an anal fissure.

Hypertrophic Anal Papilla.   The cutaneous serrations which give prominence to the pectinate line or mucocutaneous junction of the anal canal are referred to as anal papillae; and in some patients one or more of these papillae may become hypertrophic. The hypertrophic papilla is essentially a fibrous structure covered with skin, and it may attain significant size.

Symptoms arise because of prolapse of the papilla through the anus, and pain may be a feature of this condition. A prolapsed lesion is apparent on inspection of the anus, and the hypertrophic anal papilla is palpable on digital examination of the anal canal. Proctoscopy shows a white, polypoid, smooth lesion originating at the pectinate line, and it may be evident that several papillae are hypertrophic. Symptomatic lesions are removed under anesthesia with the aid of a bivalve speculum.

Anal Fissure. Anal fissure is a common complaint causing patients to seek proctologic advice. The fissure is a crack in the cutaneous lining of the lower part of the anal canal. It commonly occurs in the midline posteriorly, and occasionally in the midline anteriorly. The vast majority occur in otherwise healthy individuals, and the etiology is uncertain. A small proportion are associated with some underlying pathology such as Crohn's disease.

The cardinal symptom of an anal fissure is pain. This is usually related to defecation but it may persist for a variable time thereafter, and it may be aggravated by exercise or movement. Rectal bleeding is not uncommon, and pruritus ani may be a feature in chronic cases.

The diagnosis of an anal fissure is most readily made by simple inspection of the lower anal canal after separation of the buttocks. In most cases some degree of sphincter spasm is associated with this painful lesion, and an edematous skin tag may be present at the lower edge of the fissure. In acute cases it can be seen that the fissure is a superficial crack in the skin which bleeds readily when the skin is stretched. In chronic cases the base of the fissure consists of fibrous tissue, and in some cases the transverse fibers of the internal sphincter may be seen.

Digital examination of the anal canal may be painful, and it may achieve nothing apart from eliciting sphincter spasm. Some induration around the edges of the fissure may be apparent in chronic cases.

Proctoscopy is usually not possible owing to the painful nature of the lesion. If it is possible, it may be apparent that there is hypertrophy of an anal papilla at the upper border of the fissure.

In Crohn's disease anal fissures may be multiple. These fissures may have an indolent, edematous, unhealthy appearance; and they may be associated with ulceration of the anus or perianal skin.

Anal Infection. **Anorectal Abscesses.** Abscess formation in the anorectal region is relatively common. Most abscesses are pyogenic infections, and they are seldom associated with demonstrable pathology in the intestine. A minority of cases are associated with underlying diseases such as Crohn's disease or ulcerative colitis, and a few are caused by specific infections such as actinomycosis or tuberculosis.

The idiopathic or common type of anorectal abscess is thought to start out as an infection of the anal glands, which then extends through the anal musculature and results in abscess formation.[15,38] The abscess may be confined to the anal canal as an intersphincteric or submucous abscess, or it may present outside the anal canal as a perianal or ischiorectal abscess.

The clinical presentation of anorectal abscesses depends on the location. Pain, pyrexia, and a variable degree of systemic upset are characteristic features. Ischiorectal and perianal abscesses present as painful perineal swellings.

Proctoscopy in these patients should be deferred until the patient is anesthetized for surgical treatment of the abscess, and then a careful examination of the anal canal should be made with the bivalve speculum. In the case of perianal and ischiorectal abscesses, a careful search should be made for an internal communication within the anal canal. If such communication with the abscess cavity exists it is most likely to be found in the region of the anal crypt, and the anal crypts should be carefully examined with a malleable probe. In practice, however, an internal opening into the anal canal is often demonstrated more readily after the abscess cavity has been opened. A fistulous track may then be demonstrated by the passage of a probe or director from within the abscess cavity.

An intermuscular or submucous abscess has often burst into the lumen of the anal canal by the time the patient seeks attention, and the cavity is palpable on digital examination of the anal canal. In early cases a tender, brawny swelling is palpable below the anorectal ring. Proctoscopy reveals this swelling; or more commonly, when the abscess has already drained into the anal canal the orifice of the abscess cavity is apparent.

Anal Cryptitis. A limited infection of the anal glands may result in inflammation of an anal crypt. Acute infection of an anal crypt presents with clinical features similar to those of an early intersphincteric abscess, and some cases may progress to the formation of an anorectal abscess.

At proctoscopy acute cryptitis is apparent as swelling, reddening, and tenderness affecting one of the anal valves; and it may be possible to express pus from the affected crypt.

Low-grade, chronic anal cryptitis was described by Buie[8] and Bacon,[1] but it is not readily found at proctoscopy and its existence has been challenged.[19]

Syphilis. A primary syphilitic infection or chancre may resemble an anal fissure, but close inspection reveals that the syphilitic lesions are associated with considerable induration; there is often a symmetrical lesion in the opposite side of the anal canal, and enlargement of the inguinal lymph nodes occurs. The diagnosis of primary syphilis is made by bacteriologic examination of the discharge from the lesion, and the blood serology may be positive by the time the patient presents for examination.

Secondary-stage syphilitic lesions appear as warts or condylomas in the lower anal canal and perianal region, and they may be associated with lesions in the skin elsewhere and in the mouth. These anal lesions may be confused with nonsyphilitic venereal warts and condyloma acuminata, which also occur in the anal region. However, the blood serology tests for syphilis are always strongly positive in patients presenting with secondary stage lesions.

Tuberculosis. Tuberculous ulceration occurs rarely in the anal region, but it may resemble an ordinary anal fissure. However, as the lesion progresses it tends to resemble an ulcer with undermined edges more than a fissure. The diagnosis may be made by biopsy of the lesion and bacteriologic culture of a tissue specimen.

Anal Fistula. Anal fistulas may occur as a complication of such disorders as Crohn's disease or ulcerative colitis, in lymphogranuloma infection, and in association with actino-mycosis or tuberculous infections. Occasionally an anal fistula may be one of the presenting features of an anorectal carcinoma. However, in the vast majority of cases there is no demonstrable cause or pathology apart from the fistula, and these idiopathic fistulas probably result from previous pyogenic abscesses or anal gland infections.

The fistulous track may be subcutaneous, submucous, or transsphincteric; the fistulas are classified as high or low depending on whether the internal opening of the fistula is above or below the anorectal ring. The majority enter the anal canal below the anorectal ring at the level of the anal crypts.

Primary anal fistulas commonly present with a mucopurulent perianal discharge, anal irritation, and recurrent abscess formation. On inspection of the anus, one or more fistulous openings may be apparent. The indurated track of the fistula may be palpable in the perianal region, and digital examination of the anal canal may detect an area of induration or the internal opening of the fistula. It is important to establish the relationship of an internal opening to the anorectal ring. A low anal fistula entering the anal canal below the anorectal ring can be treated surgically with little risk of postoperative fecal incontinence, but fistulas communicating with the rectum present a much more difficult problem. This relationship of the internal opening to the anorectal ring is generally appreciated better in the conscious patient than in the anesthetized subject. Anesthesia causes relaxation of the anal muscles, and it may make interpretation of the anatomic features difficult. An attempt should be made to pass a malleable probe along the fistulous track from the external opening in the conscious patient, and in some cases the probe can be made to enter the anal canal.

Proctoscopy is of considerable value in the assessment of anal fistulas. When an internal opening is found with the Milligan-Morgan proctoscope, it is usually possible to establish the relationship of the opening to the anorectal ring. The bivalve speculum is used for examination of anal fistulas in the anesthetized patient prior to surgery. The fistulous track is explored with a probe or probe-pointed director; and when attempts to pass the probe through the external opening fail, it may prove possible to identify the internal opening on proctoscopy and pass the probe through the internal opening.

Anal Tumors. Tumors may arise in the mucosa of the anal canal or in the anal skin.

Mucosal Tumors. Benign tumors arising from the mucosal surface of the anal canal are rare, although in theory any of the benign tumors of the rectum could also occur in the glandular mucosa of the anal canal. The majority of tumors arising in the mucosa of the upper part of the anal canal are carcinomas. These are either tumors that have commenced primarily in the anal canal or are lesions which originated in the rectum and have extended downward into the anal canal. By the time the patient presents for examination it may be difficult to determine precisely the site of origin. The tumor may be annular and constricting, proliferative, or ulcerating, and the features are similar to those of a rectal carcinoma.

Tumors of Anal Skin. *Anal Warts or Papillomas.* Papillomas occurring in the skin of the anal canal and perianal region are quite common. Their appearance has some resemblance to that of papillomas or warts elsewhere in the skin, except that the anal lesions are quite friable, and they may bleed readily when traumatized. They are often associated with an anal discharge and maceration of the anal skin. Anal papillomas are probably caused by a virus transmitted by sexual contact, and they are found quite frequently in homosexuals.[44]

It is important to differentiate these tumors from syphilitic warts and squamous carcinoma of the anus. The question of syphilis is readily resolved by serologic tests, and a biopsy of the anal lesion is performed if serious doubt arises regarding the nature of the tumor.

Squamous Carcinoma. About half of the malignant tumors of the anus and anal canal are squamous carcinomas. The tumor may be an ulcerating lesion, and in its early stages it may be mistaken for a simple anal fissure. Alternatively, it may be an annular tumor causing stenosis of the anal canal, or it may be a proliferative growth. The vagina may be involved in female patients.

The symptoms associated with anal carcinoma include pain, swelling, bleeding, mucous discharge, and alteration of bowel habit. Fecal incontinence may occur when there is extensive destruction of the anal sphincters or when fistulation into the vagina occurs.

Generally there is little difficulty in establishing the diagnosis. Like malignant tumors of the rectum, an anal carcinoma has a characteristic induration. The diagnosis is confirmed by biopsy.

Other Malignant Tumors. Other malignant tumors rarely occur in the anal canal or perianal skin. The presenting features of these tumors may resemble those of carcinoma, but some tumors may be confused with such benign conditions as an anal fissure or a thrombosed external hemorrhoid.

A basal cell carcinoma may occur in the anus or perianal skin. On inspection of the anus or at proctoscopy an irregular ulcer is found with raised, everted edges. Marked induration of the tumor is apparent on digital examination.

A malignant melanoma is even less common than a basal cell carcinoma. It may present as a small polypoid tumor, and the blue or black pigmentation of the lesion may lead to confusion with a thrombosed hemorrhoid. Other tumors may have a more proliferative appearance or they may be ulcerative, and their appearance suggests a malignant process.

Very rarely a colloid-producing adenocarcinoma may occur low in the anal canal and perianal tissues. The origin of these tumors is uncertain, and it has been suggested that they arise from aberrant anal mucosa,[13] the intermuscular anal glands,[51] and the transitional epithelium at the mucocutaneous junction of the anal canal.[19]

The notable clinical feature of this tumor is that it may present outside the anal canal without producing a lesion in the epithelium of the anal canal. Occasionally the anal skin is affected, however, and an erythematous or eczematous lesion may be found. The diagnosis is made by biopsy.

REFERENCES

1. Bacon HE: The Anus, Rectum and Sigmoid Colon, 3rd ed. Philadelphia, Saunders, 1949
2. Barlow D: Simple ulcers of the caecum, colon and rectum. Br J Surg 28:575, 1941
3. Barron J: Office ligation of internal hemorrhoids. Am J Surg 105:563, 1963
4. Bensaude R, Bensaude A: Sur une forme particuliere d'angiome caverneux du rectum, l'angiome cutaneo-muquex ou genito-perineo-rectal. Presse Med 40:1739, 1932
5. Bensaude R, Lambling A: Discussion on the

aetiology and treatment of fibrous stricture of the rectum (including lymphogranuloma inguinale). Proc R Soc Med 29:1441, 1936

6. Billson FA, deDombal FT, Watkinson G, et al: Ocular complications of ulcerative colitis. Gut 8:102, 1967

7. Bochus HL, Staub WR, Finkelstein L, et al: Life history of nonspecific ulcerative colitis: relation of prognosis to anatomical and clinical varieties. Gastroenterologia 86:549, 1956

8. Buie LA: Practical Proctology. Philadelphia, Saunders, 1937

9. Crile G Jr, Turnbull RB Jr: The role of electrocoagulation in the treatment of carcinoma of the rectum. Surg Gynecol Obstet 135:391, 1972

10. Cynn WS, Rickert RR: Ischaemic proctosigmoiditis: report of a case. Dis Colon Rectum 16:537, 1973

11. deDombal FT, Burton I, Goligher JC: Recurrence of Crohn's disease after primary excisional surgery. Gut 12:519, 1971

12. Dukes CE, Bussey HJR: Sarcoma and melanoma of the rectum. Br J Cancer 1:30, 1947

13. Dukes CE, Galvin C: Colloid carcinoma arising within fistulae in the anorectal region. Ann R Coll Surg Engl 18:246, 1956

14. Edwards FC, Truelove SC: The course and prognosis of ulcerative colitis. Gut 5:1, 1964

15. Eisenhammer S: The anorectal and anovulval fistulous abscess. Surg Gynecol Obstet 113:519, 1961

16. Gabriel WB, Morson BC: Carcinoid of rectum with lymphatic and liver metastases. Proc R Soc Med 49:472, 1956

17. Galley HG: Combustible gases generated in the alimentary tract and other hollow viscera and their relationship to explosions occurring during anaesthesia. Br J Anaesth 26:189, 1954

18. Gardner EG: A genetic and clinical study of intestinal polyposis, a predisposing factor for carcinoma of the colon and rectum. Am J Hum Genet 3:167, 1951

19. Goligher JC: Surgery of the Anus, Rectum and Colon, 3rd ed. London, Bailliere Tindall, 1975

20. Goligher JC, deDombal FT, Burton I: Surgical treatment and its results. In Skandia Symposium on Regional Enteritis (Crohn's Disease). Stockholm, Nordiska Bokhandelns Forlag, 1971

21. Grinnell RS, Lane N: Benign and malignant adenomatous polyps and papillary adenomas of the colon and rectum. Int Abstr Surg 106:519, 1958

22. Hammer B, Ashurst P, Naish J: Diseases associated with ulcerative colitis and Crohn's disease. Gut 9:17, 1968

23. Jensen T: Rectal gonorrhoea in women. Br J Vener Dis 29:222, 1953

24. Knox WG, Miller RE, Begg CF, et al: Juvenile polyps of the colon; a clinicopathologic analysis of 75 polyps in 43 patients. Surgery 48:201, 1960

25. Lead Article: Beyond the examining finger. Lancet 2:1185, 1974

26. Lieberman W: Syphilis of the rectum. Rev Gastroenterol 18:67, 1951

27. Lockhart-Mummery HE, Morson BC: Crohn's disease of the large intestine. Gut 5:493, 1964

28. Madigan MR, Morson BC: Solitary ulcer of the rectum. Gut 10:871, 1969

29. Marston A: Patterns of intestinal ischaemia. Ann R Coll Surg Engl 35:151, 1964

30. McGovern VJ, Goulston SJM: Ischaemic enterocolitis. Gut 6:213, 1965

31. Minichan DP: Removing polyps through the sigmoidoscope: a method of removing adenomatous polyps with reduced risk of hemorrhage. Dis Colon Rectum 17:678, 1974

32. Morson BC: Precancerous lesions of the colon and rectum. JAMA 179:316, 1962

33. Morson BC: Precancerous lesions of the upper gastrointestinal tract. JAMA 179:311, 1962

34. Morson BC, Lockhart-Mummery HE: Anal lesions in Crohn's disease. Lancet 2:1122, 1959

35. Morson BC, Pang LSC: Rectal biopsy as an aid to cancer control in ulcerative colitis. Gut 8:423, 1967

36. Morton WA, Johnstone FRC: Rectal carcinoids. Br J Surg 52:391, 1965

37. Neuman HW, Bargen JA, Judd ES Jr: Clinical study of 201 cases of regional (segmental) colitis. Surg Gynecol Obstet 99:563, 1954

38. Parks AG: Pathogenesis and treatment of fistula-in-ano. Br Med J 1:463, 1961

39. Riddell RH: The extent of rectal premalignant change in ulcerative colitis. Gut 15:822, 1974

40. Salazar M, Jackman RJ: Reasons for incomplete proctoscopy. Dis Colon Rectum 12:19, 1969

41. Smiddy FG, Goligher JC: Results of surgery in treatment of cancer of the large intestine. Br Med J 1:793, 1957

42. Speare GS: Melanosis coli. Am J Surg 82:63, 1951

43. Stout AP: Tumors of the colon and rectum (excluding carcinoma and adenoma). In Turell R (ed): Diseases of the Colon and Anorectum, Vol 1. Philadelphia, Saunders, 1959, p 295

44. Swerdlow DB, Salvati EP: Condyloma acuminatum. Dis Colon Rectum 14:226, 1971

45. Swerdlow DB, Salvati EP, Rubin RJ, et al: Electrosurgery: principles and use. Dis Colon Rectum 17:482, 1974

46. Thayer WR: Crohn's disease (regional enteritis): A look at the last four years. Scand J Gastroenterol (Suppl)6:165, 1970

47. Watts JMcK, Thompson H, Goligher JC: Sigmoidoscopy and cytology in the detection of microscopic disease of the rectal mucosa in ulcerative colitis. Gut 7:288, 1966

48. Welin S: Modern trends in diagnostic roentgenology of the colon. Br J Radiol 31:453, 1958

49. Williams C, Teague R: Colonoscopy. Gut 14:990, 1973

50. Wright V, Watkinson G: Sacro-iliitis and ulcerative colitis. Br Med J 2:675, 1965

51. Zimberg YH, Kay S: Anorectal carcinomas of extramucosal origin. Ann Surg 145:344, 1957

33

Pancreoscopy

J. Meyer-Burg

The pancreas is unfortunately an organ for which reliable diagnostic procedures are not yet available. The various diagnostic tests, primarily endoscopic ones, with which various surrounding organs could be inspected were not utilized for the pancreas. However, diseases of the pancreas, primarily carcinoma and chronic pancreatitis, definitely seem to be on the increase. This organ has now become a consideration in the field of laparoscopy with direct vision and inspection.

TECHNIQUES FOR PANCREATIC ENDOSCOPY

Three endoscopic techniques of inspecting the pancreas are now available.

Supragastric Pancreoscopy

Supragastric pancreoscopy[4] permits inspection as well as palpation and biopsy of the body of the pancreas through the smaller omentum (Figs. 1 and 2). The patient is placed on his right side with the head of the table elevated (an electrically driven endoscopic table is desirable). A Lumina* laparoscope with a 130-degree optic is advanced under the left lobe of the liver. The backside of the scope is used to avoid damage to the liver, and the lobe is then elevated by the scope. All laparoscopies are

*Manufacturer: R. Wolf Endoscope Co., Knittlingen, West Germany. Distributor: R. Wolf Medical Instrument Corp., 7046 Lyndon Avenue, Rosemont, Ill. 60018.

carried out under local anesthesia with sedative and analgesic premedication. If the patient is not obese, the form, color, and consistency of the body of the pancreas can be evaluated (Figs. 3–9, Plate D).* In our opinion this technique gives the best results without great difficulties. In older, thin patients practically all parts of the pancreas between the left lobe of the liver and the anterior surface of the stomach can be inspected without further manipulations.

The laparoscope is usually introduced into the abdomen two fingerbreadths above and two to the left of the umbilicus. A biopsy is performed under vision if pathologic changes are seen. Additional instruments are introduced through a second trocar, inserted superiorly (above) the laparoscope. Biopsies can be obtained with thin needles (1.0 mm OD) for cytologic examination, and with a sharp biopsy forceps or a Menghini needle (1.4 mm OD) for histologic examination.

Inspection of the Head of the Pancreas

The head of the pancreas can be inspected[1] in thin patients at the duodenal curve without difficulty (Fig. 5, Plate D). If necessary, the greater omentum can be perforated to allow better visualization as well to obtain biopsies of the area. One can also gain an impression of the condition of the head of the pancreas by pushing aside the fat-containing omentum with a probe.

*All color plates appear at the front of the book.

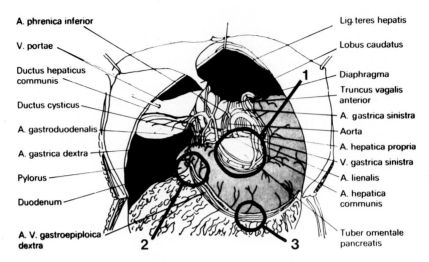

A. phrenica inferior

V. portae

Ductus hepaticus communis

Ductus cysticus

A. gastroduodenalis

A. gastrica dextra

Pylorus

Duodenum

A. V. gastroepiploica dextra

Lig. teres hepatis

Lobus caudatus

Diaphragma

Truncus vagalis anterior

A. gastrica sinistra

Aorta

A. hepatica propria

V. gastrica sinistra

A. lienalis

A. hepatica communis

Tuber omentale pancreatis

FIG. 1.   Topography after elevating the left lobe of the liver and removing the lesser omentum. The circles (1, 2, and 3) show the areas of the pancreas that can be inspected.[2]

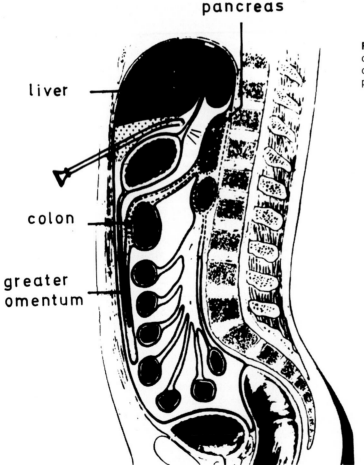

pancreas

liver

colon

greater omentum

FIG. 2.   Location of the pancreas on a lateral view. Representation of the technique of supragastric pancreoscopy.[3]

Infragastric Pancreoscopy

Infragastric pancreoscopy[5] is carried out with a prograde vision laparoscope; additional instruments are required to penetrate the greater omentum below the stomach. The laparoscope is introduced through this perforation, allowing inspection of the parts of the body as well as the tail of the pancreas.

Other Techniques

Further possibilities of inspecting the pancreas (e.g., retroperitoneoscopy as well as using flexible fiber instruments to permit entry through the foramen of Winslow) are currently of little value and are primarily of academic interest only.

RESULTS OF SUPRAGASTRIC PANCREOSCOPY

In 500 consecutive laparoscopies carried out between 1971 and 1972 (Table 1) we were able to examine directly parts of the body of the pancreas in 282 cases (56.4 percent). In 16 cases (3.4 percent) parts of the pancreas could not be seen but diagnostic evidence of a pancreatic involvement was nevertheless evident. In 202 cases (40.4 percent) the pancreas could not be inspected. The cause for failure in 124 cases (61.4 percent) was excessive fat or the lesser omentum. In 78 cases (38.6 percent) there were numerous adhesions in the upper abdomen from previous surgery. In one case a presumptive diagnosis of carcinoma was made on the basis of an indirect finding: pancreatic protrusion. This diagnosis was not confirmed at laparotomy, where no pathology was found. We have not experienced the reverse problem (i.e.,

as far as we know, we have not overlooked a carcinoma of the pancreas at laparoscopy). On one occasion a pseudocyst was misdiagnosed as a carcinoma.

The normal pancreas (Figs. 3, 4, 5, Plate D) is characterized by its fine nodular appearance and its pink to yellowish color. It can always be distinguished from the adjacent caudate lobe of the liver. The lesser omentum, normally a thin transparent peritoneal membrane, contains a small number of vessels and lymph channels, and can usually be lifted off the pancreas quite easily with a probe.

In resolving acute pancreatitis (Fig. 6, Plate D), the organ is erythematous and indurated. Usually one or more areas of calcification following fatty necrosis can be identified.

In chronic pancreatitis (Fig. 7, Plate D) the symmetrical nodularity of the surface disappears. One can see whitish-gray flat regions with adhesions between the lesser omentum and the pancreas as well as the undersurface of the liver. The consistency is markedly firm. Macroscopically it is difficult to differentiate from a pancreatic neoplasm, but the protrusion observed with a tumor is not present. The organ appears small. Our cytologic results are (as expected) unsatisfactory, as connective tissue material is frequently difficult to recognize cytologically.

Pancreatic carcinoma (Figs. 8, 9, Plate D), in contrast, is easy to diagnose: It is usually extensive because patients do not consult a physician until the lesion is at an advanced stage. At laparoscopy one often discovers liver metastases, a distended gallbladder, or cholestasis (Table 2). Usually the pancreatic neoplasm manifests as an increase in volume, with a grayish white mass, irregularly formed and stone hard, pushing the lesser omentum anteriorly. These findings allow identification without difficulty. At the border of the tumor there is often conspicuous vascularity. In 35 cases of laparoscopically diagnosed pancreatic carcinoma we had to revise the diagnosis twice. In one case a fist-sized tumor was identified under the antrum, but the omentum and the antrum itself prevented direct inspection. The head and the body of the pancreas were firm. We did not perform a biopsy for cytologic or histologic study because of the overlying omentum. Laparotomy was performed on the basis of clinical symptoms, high secretin-pancreozymin values, and angiographic changes suspicious for neoplasm. A fist-sized pseudocyst in the

TABLE 1.   Results of Supragastric Inspections of the Pancreas During 500 Laparoscopies

Finding	No. of Cases
Parts of the pancreas seen	282
Parts of the pancreas not seen	202
Normal pancreas	214
Carcinoma of the pancreas	33
Chronic pancreatitis	24
Resolving acute pancreatitis	2
Pancreatic pseudocyst	4
Cystic pancreas	1

head of the pancreas with accompanying chronic pancreatitis was found. In the second case the suspected diagnosis of pancreatic carcinoma was not confirmed, and the pancreas proved to be normal. Altogether laparoscopy was more successful in establishing a diagnosis than all other diagnostic methods available (Table 3).

RESULTS AND RISKS OF PANCREATIC BIOPSY

Pancreatic tissue for cytology was removed in 52 patients (Fig. 10). Each organ was punctured several times (up to five) in various places. In 16 cases a biopsy (usually more than one) was performed using a Menghini needle. In four cases a biopsy were used.

Based on our experience, we recommend fine needle aspiration under direct vision. Biopsy is indicated only if there is macroscopic or palpable evidence of a neoplasm. Results with the needle aspiration are good. Of 35 laparoscopically diagnosed pancreatic carcinomas, 28 were aspirated. In 25 cases (89 percent) a diagnosis

of a malignant pancreatic process could be cytologically established (Fig. 11).

We have not encountered any complications in our series of biopsies, although in one case there was moderate bleeding in the pancreatic capsule. Moreover, there has been no increase in the serum amylase, no fistula formation, and no symptoms of peritonitis.

On reviewing the literature (Table 4) it appears that the great reluctance to biopsy the pancreas should be carefully reconsidered. Of 896 biopsies carried out by various methods listed in the literature, there were six mortalities (0.67 percent) and 24 (2.68 percent) other complications reported.

DISCUSSION

The inspection and palpation of parts of the normal pancreas require critical interpretation. The diagnostic accuracy can undoubtedly be improved with increased experience. A biopsy is not always necessary, similar to the case of a macroscopically normal appearing liver. When the pancreas has a normal appear-

TABLE 2.   Laparoscopic Results in 20 Cases of Pancreatic Carcinoma

Case No.	Locali- zation*	Inspect. and Palpat.	Cytol. Findings	Histol. Findings	Metas- tases	Cour- voisier	Cholo- stasis
1	H-B	Pos.	Neg.	Neg.	Neg.	Pos.	Pos.
2	H	Pos.	Neg.	Neg.	Pos.	Neg.	Neg.
3	—	Pos.	Pos.	Neg.	Pos.	Pos.	Pos.
4	H-B	Pos.	—	—	Pos.	Pos.	Pos.
5	—	Pos.	Pos.	—	Pos.	Neg.	Neg.
6	H	Pos.	—	Pos.	Neg.	Pos.	Pos.
7	H	Pos.	Pos.	Pos.	Pos.	—	Pos.
8	H-B	Pos.	Pos.	Pos.	Pos.	Pos.	Pos.
9	H	Pos.	—	—	Neg.	Pos.	Pos.
10	H-B	Pos.	Pos.	?	Pos.	Pos.	Pos.
11	H-B	Pos.	Pos.	—	Pos.	Neg.	Pos.
12	H-B-T	Pos.	Pos.	—	Neg.	Neg.	Neg.
13	H-B-T	Pos.	Neg.	?	Neg.	Neg.	Neg.
14	H-B	Pos.	Pos.	Pos.	Pos.	Pos.	Pos.
15	B-T	Pos.	Pos.	?	Pos.	—	Pos.
16	—	Pos.	Pos.	Pos.	Pos.	Neg.	Neg.
17	H-B	Pos.	Pos.	?	Neg.	Pos.	Pos.
18	—	Pos.	Pos.	—	Pos.	Pos.	Neg.
19	—	Pos.	Pos.	Pos.	Pos.	Pos.	Pos.
20	H-B	Pos.	Neg.	—	Pos.	Pos.	Pos.
No. positive			13/17	6/4/13	14/20	12/18	14/20

H indicates the head, B the body, and T the tail of the pancreas. Pos. indicates positive findings; Neg. indicates negative findings; question mark (?) indicates questionable findings.
Data are from Meyer-Burg.[3]

TABLE 3. Comparison of the Laparoscopic Results with Other Diagnostic Modalities in the Pancreatic Carcinoma

Case No.	Op.	Autop.	Pancreoz. Secretin	Diabetes Mell.	Angiography	Alkal. Phos.
1	Pos.	—	—	Neg.	—	Neg.
2	—	Pos.	—	Neg.	—	Bord.
3	—	—	—	Neg.	Pos.	Bord.
4	—	Pos.	—	—	Pos.	Pos.
5	—	—	—	Pos.	—	Neg.
6	Pos.	—	Pos.	Pos.	—	—
7	Pos.	—	—	Neg.	Neg.	Neg.
8	—	Pos.	—	Neg.	—	Pos.
9	Pos.	—	Pos.	Neg.	Pos.	—
10	Pos.	—	—	Neg.	Pos.	Bord.
11	Pos.	—	Pos.	Pos.	—	Pos.
12	Pos.	—	Pos.	Pos.	Neg.	Bord.
13	Pos.	—	Pos.	—	—	—
14	Pos.	—	—	Pos.	Neg.	Bord.
15	Pos.	—	—	Neg.	—	Bord.
16	—	—	—	Neg.	—	Bord.
17	Pos.	—	Pos.	Pos.	—	Bord.
18	—	—	—	Pos.	—	Neg.
19	—	—	—	Neg.	—	Bord.
20	Pos.	—	—	Pos.	—	Bord.
No. positive			6/6	8/17	4/7	12/16

Pos. indicates positive findings; Neg. indicates negative values; Bord. indicates borderline values; Op. indicates laparoscopy; Autop. - Autopsy.

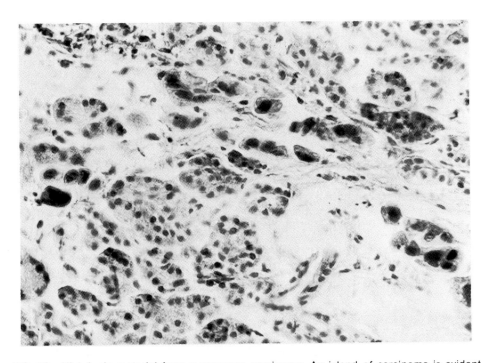

FIG. 10. Histologic material from a pancreas carcinoma. An island of carcinoma is evident (Menghini biopsy).

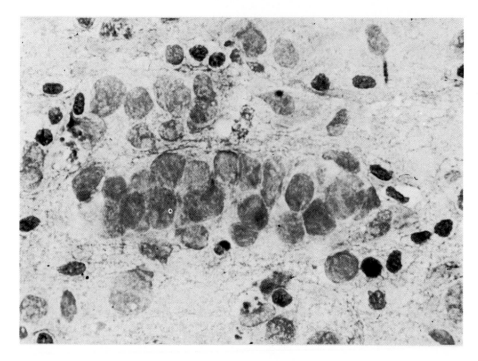

FIG. 11. Cytology specimen from a carcinoma of the pancreas Pappenheim stain. ×480.

TABLE 4. Risks of Various Biopsy Techniques in the Pancreas

Author	Method	No. of Cases	Complications (No.)	
			Fatal	Nonfatal
Probstein et al. (1949)	Wedge resection	28	—	—
Kirtland (1951)	Vim-Silverman	2	—	1
Crile et al. (1952)	Vim-Silverman	11	—	—
Belding (1954)	Sharp scoop	5	—	—
Elman et al. (1955)		41	—	—
Lukens et al. (1956)	Wedge resection	68	—	2
Spjut et al. (1957)	Wedge resection	68	—	3
Coté et al. (1959)	Vim-Silverman	99	—	2
	Wedge resection	110	—	—
Schultz et al. (1963)	Vim-Silverman	25	3	2
	Wedge resection	130	2	7
	Both	4	—	—
Loeschke (1966)	Vim-Silverman	2	—	1
	Menghini	1	—	—
Forsgren et al. (1968)	Vim-Silverman	32	1	1
	Wedge resection	18	—	—
Hess (1969)	Vim-Silverman, wedge resection	43	—	—
Lund (1969)	Vim-Silverman, wedge resection	55	—	5
Christoffersen et al. (1970)	Fine needle	28	—	—
Pantzar et al. (1972)	Fine needle aspiration	61	—	—
Meyer-Burg (1972)	Fine needle aspiration	45	—	—
	Menghini + forceps	20	—	—
Total		896	6 (0.67%)	24 (2.68%)

ance the study can rule out a pancreatic process as the cause of upper abdominal symptoms. We have been confronted with this question more frequently in recent years as the diagnostic techniques concerned with the surrounding organs have improved.

Biopsy of the pancreas for cytologic study has proved highly accurate. In contrast, biopsies using the Menghini needle and biopsy forceps gave positive results in only four of nine cases of carcinoma. In three further cases only chronic pancreatitis could be diagnosed histologically, and in two cases no pancreatic tissue was obtained.

It should be remembered that when taking a biopsy specimen from even an extensive carcinoma it is possible to remove only a chronically inflamed area. It must always be remembered that only a positive biopsy with evidence of malignancy permits a definitive diagnosis. At this time we feel that a fine needle for obtaining cytologic (aspiration) material carries a lesser risk and results in greater accuracy. Increasing experience and overcoming our initial reservations can improve the results.

It must be pointed out that parts of the pancreas and only the surface can be examined. However, that is relevant for all laparoscopically examined organs. If sufficient experience has been acquired one should be able to draw conclusions concerning the entire organ from the limited detail observed.

It is critical to remember that this method for inspecting the pancreas can scarcely be considered a valuable technique for the early diagnosis of carcinoma. Unfortunately the patients do not come to the physician with early symptoms. Furthermore, it can be assumed that a carcinoma does not arise in the periphery (i.e., on the surface) but rather in the center, usually in the head of the pancreas.

Nevertheless, direct pancreoscopy represents an extension of the laparoscopic possibilities. More than that, pancreoscopy can make a substantial contribution to pancreatic diagnosis and must be given its proper place along with other diagnostic tests available for determining pancreatic disease.

ACKNOWLEDGMENTS AND NOTES

The author is indebted to Dr. George Dechet for translating this paper into English.

The photos in Plate D were taken with instruments from Fa. Richard Wolf (Knittlingen, Germany) using Agfa CT 18 film.

REFERENCES

1. Look D, Henning H, Luders CJ: Darstellung und Biopsie des Pankreaskopfes bei der Laparoskopie. Z Gastroenterol 10:109, 1972
2. Meyer-Burg J: Moderne Pankreasdiagnostik internist. Praxix 14:37, 1974
3. Meyer-Burg J: Peritoneoscopy in carcinoma of the pancreas: report of 20 cases. Endoscopy 5:86, 1973
4. Meyer-Burg J: The inspection, palpation and biopsy of the pancreas by peritoneoscopy. Endoscopy 4:99, 1972
5. Strauch M, Lux G, Ottenhann R: Infragastric pancreoscopy. Endoscopy 5:30, 1973

EDITORIAL COMMENT

J. Meyer-Burg died during the prime of his life, leaving behind many projects reflecting his innovative mind. This chapter itself is a new approach to an old problem, throwing some light onto one of our greatest diagnostic difficulties—the pancreas. We hope that his colleagues will continue his work and ideas.

It is interesting to note that biopsy of the pancreas became taboo for surgeons because of the fear of complications. Gastroenterologists perhaps have more courage; they perform multiple suction biopsies using a fine needle and claim a high yield of positive cytology. However, these findings must be followed up and confirmed before we can advocate that the procedure be done on a more routine basis.

THE EDITOR

34

Endoscopy of the Small Bowel

Walter D. Gaisford

A new type of gastroscope called the fiberscope was introduced by Hirschowitz et al. in 1958,[8] and modifications appeared rapidly. Improved versions of the original fiberscope enabled the endoscopist to visualize the entire duodenum readily with a variety of end- and side-viewing instruments.

The development of instruments for colonoscopy was not begun until some 10 years later. Initial reports on colonoscopy were discouraging until Overholt[16] reported favorable experience with the use of a fiberscope to extend the range of sigmoidoscopy to the proximal sigmoid and descending colon. After early experience proved successful in fiberendoscopic examination of the left side of the colon, efforts were made to reach the cecum and ileocecal valve area. Even before the development of fiberoptics, a technique of retrograde intubation of the cecum with a colonic tube was described and demonstrated radiographically by Hoff in 1928.[9] Passage of a string or tube by mouth through the gastrointestinal tract in order to attach the tip of the colonoscope at the anus for easier retrograde guidance was proposed by Provenzale et al.,[18] Torsoli et al., [20] Hiratsuka,[7] and Provenzale and Revignas.[17] However, this technique soon appeared to be an unnecessary precaution as success in direct intubation of the colonfiberscope into the cecum was reported by Nagasako et al.[12] Wolff and Shinya,[22] Gaisford,[4] and Williams and Muto.[21]

The next logical step in endoscopic exploration of the alimentary canal was intubation of the ileocecal sphincter for examination of the terminal ileum and further direct insertion of longer upper gastrointestinal scopes into the jejunum. Direct intubation of the ileocecal sphincter and endoscopy of the terminal ileum was first reported from Japan by Nagasako et al.[11,13,14] More recently in the United States Gaisford[5] reported a similar successful experience in retrograde endoscopy of the terminal ileum.

The "blind area" for alimentary canal endoscopy—between the midjejunum and the lower ileum—quickly became illuminated by new instrumentation and techniques reported by Deyhle et al.,[3] Classen et al.,[2] and Wolff and Shinya.[23] With the aid of the transintestinal guide tube or string described by Blankenhorn et al.,[1] Deyhle et al.[3] and Classen et al.[2] were able to pass a fiberscope successfully through the entire small bowel for examination and biopsy. Recently Wolff and Shinya[23] utilized a special small-bowel fiberscope resembling a Miller-Abbott or Cantor tube for examination of the entire small bowel. The latter instrument does not allow for biopsy or obtaining cytology specimens.

INDICATIONS

The indications for consideration of small-bowel fiberendoscopy are as follows:

1. Unexplained gastrointestinal blood loss where esophagogastroduodenoscopy and colonfiberoscopy are negative
2. Small-bowel inflammatory disease
3. Malabsorption syndromes
4. During surgical exploratory celiotomy when a suspected small-bowel lesion cannot be found
5. Small-bowel tumors
6. Multiple polyposis of the gastrointestinal tract

These indications are listed in order of relative importance with respect to frequency and the value of endoscopic findings.

In the patient with gastrointestinal blood loss as manifested by one or more episodes of occult or chronic rectal bleeding that is neither black nor bright red but rather maroon, the small bowel must be considered as a possible site of bleeding. If esophagogastroduodenoscopy and colonfiberendoscopy to the cecum are negative and the appropriate x-ray contrast studies have failed to reveal an obvious site of chronic or recurrent bleeding, total small-bowel endoscopy is indicated.

In the patient with acute gastrointestinal hemorrhage, esophagogastroduodenoscopy with an appropriate end-viewing fiberscope (i.e., Olympus GIF-D 100 cm) is indicated early, as soon as the patient has been initially resuscitated. If the upper gastrointestinal tract is negative to the midduodenum and clinically the bleeding seems to be from the upper tract, a longer end-viewing fiberscope (i.e., Olympus CF-LB 186 cm, or Olympus JF-D 200 cm) can be intubated perorally through the entire duodenum and well into the lower jejunum. When the acute bleeding source is not identified by these endoscopic approaches or when the bleeding is bright red rectal hemorrhage, an emergency selective mesenteric arteriogram is the procedure of choice.

Intestinal malabsorption syndromes (e.g., sprue) and small-bowel inflammatory disease (e.g., regional enteritis) can be documented by small-bowel endoscopy and confirmed by biopsy in patients where the diagnosis was only suspected and not shown by other diagnostic approaches. The location and extent of the small-bowel pathology can be determined by endoscopy and biopsy. This may be helpful in deciding on the need for and extent of surgical treatment. Medical treatment of these conditions may be accurately followed by serial endoscopy and biopsy.

Operating room small-bowel fiberendoscopy during celiotomy with unopened bowel may be helpful in cases of gastrointestinal bleeding where the bleeding site is still obscure even after abdominal exploration.

Neoplasms of the small bowel are not common and in the past have been unexpectedly diagnosed by the surgeon during operation or the pathologist at autopsy. Small polyps and isolated small-bowel diverticula are difficult to isolate and evaluate at exploratory surgery.

Small-bowel fiberendoscopy should prove useful in the diagnosis of these conditions, and small-bowel polypectomy via the fiberendoscope will certainly become part of the armamentarium of skilled endoscopists.

PATIENT PREPARATION AND ANESTHESIA

Patient preparation varies according to the part of the small bowel to be examined and the technique used. For direct-insertion jejunofiberendoscopy, the preparation and premedication of the patient is the same as for esophagogastroduodenoscopy. The patient is fasted for 6 hours and mildly sedated with intravenous meperidine (Demerol) 50 mg titrated slowly with intravenous diazepam (Valium) 5 to 15 mg to a state of cooperative somnolence. Anticholinergic drugs such as atropine 0.4 to 0.6 mg maybe given intravenously or intramuscularly, but I prefer not to use atropine in most patients. Normal secretions and peristalsis have not interfered with endoscopy, and the peristalsis has usually aided insertion of the fiberscope.

For terminal ileofiberendoscopy the mechanical bowel preparation is similar to that for total colonoscopy. I prefer 2 days of low-residue diet, 36 hours of clear liquid diet, 2 ounces of castor oil 10 to 12 hours before the examination and high tap water enemas 2 hours before the procedure, repeated until the enema returns are clear. Mild sedation with intravenous meperidine and diazepam is produced as outlined above for jejunoscopy. Anticholinergic drugs are avoided so that normal peristalsis of the terminal ileum assists intubation of the fiberscope through the ileum. Both of the above techniques for direct examination and biopsy of the jejunum and terminal ileum are performed on an outpatient basis.

Peroral transintestinal tube intubation techniques require admission of the patient to the hospital, intravenous fluid supplements, and nursing care for several days. Both general anesthesia[3] and only mild parenteral sedation[2] have been used after the transintestinal tube reaches the anus, when the fiberscope is advanced through the entire small bowel.

With the prototype long small-bowel scope used by Wolff and Shinya[23] the examination is also done on inpatients with intravenous fluid supplements. However, this scope resembles a

Miller-Abbott or Cantor long intestinal tube and can be intubated without any special sedation or anesthesia.

INSTRUMENTATION AND TECHNIQUES

The current methods of small-bowel fiber-endoscopy include:

1. Direct insertion of the fiberscope perorally into the jejunum
2. Intraoperative peroral or peranal insertion of the fiberscope through the small bowel with passage of the scope assisted by the operating surgeon through the surgically opened abdomen
3. Direct insertion of the fiberscope per rectum into the ileum
4. Direct insertion of the fiberscope through an ileostomy stoma
5. Pulling the fiberscope through the gastrointestinal tract from above or below with the aid of a previously passed transintestinal mercury-weighted tube
6. Peroral intubation of the fiberscope through the small bowel by pushing the scope over a previously passed transintestinal tube, which is drawn through the forceps channel of the instrument and used as a guide
7. Peroral passage of a special long small-intestinal fiberscope which resembles a Miller-Abbott or Cantor tube and is introduced in the same manner

Direct-Insertion Jejunofiberendoscopy

The introduction of fiberscopes into the jejunum by direct insertion without using the transintestinal string or tube method has been reported to be unsuccessful in 70 percent of

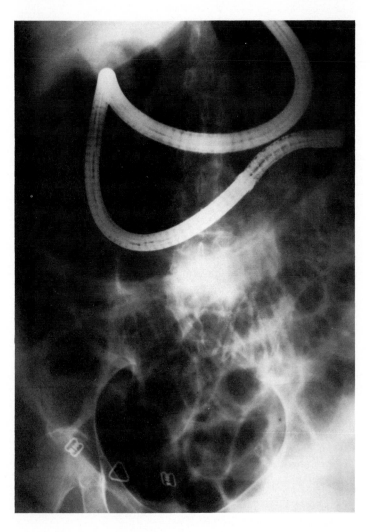

FIG. 1. Fiberendoscope (Olympus CF-LB 186 cm) inserted through the duodenum to the first part of the jejunum.

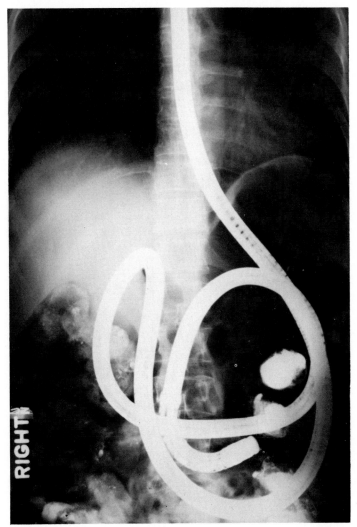
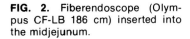

FIG. 2. Fiberendoscope (Olympus CF-LB 186 cm) inserted into the midjejunum.

cases according to Classen et al.[2] However, Gaisford,[6] using the Olympus CF-LB 186 cm end-viewing fiberscope, directly intubated the middle or lower jejunum successfully in all of six patients in whom it was attempted (Figs. 1 through 3). In three cases the examination was done for bleeding below the duodenum, and in three others for clinical suspicion of small-bowel enteropathy associated with malabsorption syndromes. The examination is done with the patient awake, lying on his left side after mild intravenous sedation.

Ogoshi et al.[15] reported the use of a new end-viewing small-caliber fiberoptic endoscope for peroral passage and visualization of the jejunum in 250 patients. The scope is 10 mm in diameter, 162 cm in effective length, and has four directional bending angles. The biopsy channel is 2.8 mm to accommodate a suction biopsy similar to but smaller than the Rubin tube. Target biopsy is also possible with a biopsy forceps passed through the channel. These authors also advanced the scope under direct visual control and concluded that this was more helpful in avoiding mucosal injury than fluoroscopic control.

Using a similar prototype Olympus duodeno-jejunoscope, Salmon et al.[19] reported peroral passage and jejunal examination in seven patients. Two other patients with ileostomies (following Crohn's disease) were examined through their stomas, and two additional examinations were performed during laparotomy with the instrument passed perorally through

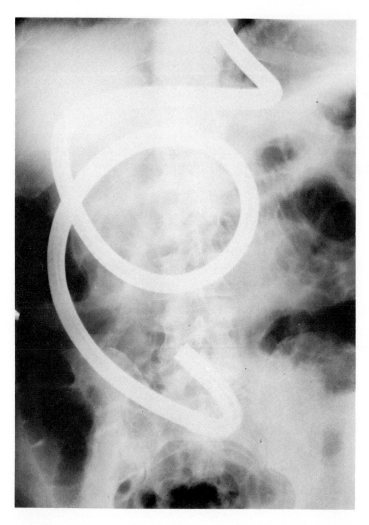

FIG. 3. Fiberendoscope (Olympus CF-LB 186 cm) inserted into the lower jejunum.

the unopened bowel to the ileocecal sphincter.

The advantages of this method are safety, simplicity, immediate examination, excellent visualization, photography, and direct forceps biopsy (Fig. 4A, B, Plate E; Fig. 4E).* The disadvantage is that usually only the jejunum can be visualized, and examination of the ileum requires a different approach.

Intraoperative Small-Bowel Endoscopy During Surgical Celiotomy with Unopened Bowel

There are occasions when, even after careful upper gastrointestinal and colon fiberendoscopy, the surgeon, with the patient's abdominal contents surgically exposed and palpated,

All color plates appear at the front of the book.

cannot identify the precise site of small-bowel bleeding or neoplasm. In this situation a long fiberendoscope can be inserted perorally or peranally by the endoscopist with the operating surgeon assisting the passage of the scope through the small bowel by manual palpation. Gaisford[6] has used this technique with the Olympus CF-LB 186 cm fiberscope on four patients in the operating room to help find the site of bleeding and specific lesions in the bowel which could not be isolated by other means.

Direct-Insertion Terminal Ileofiberendoscopy

It was demonstrated by Nagasako et al.[11,13,14] and more recently by Gaisford[5] that the ileocecal sphincter can be intubated with relative ease using standard colonfiberscopes.

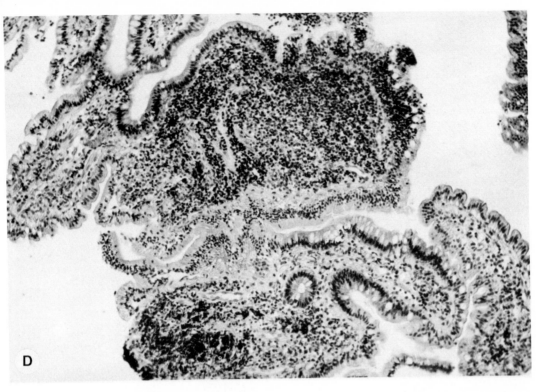

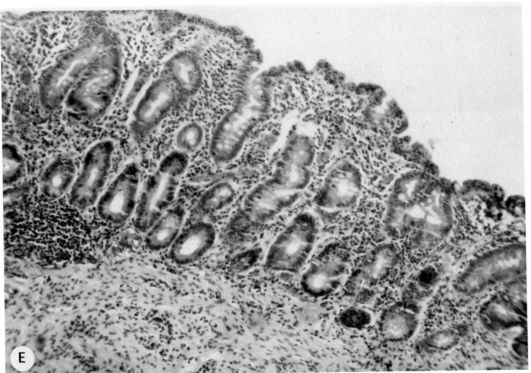

FIG. 4 D. Microphotograph of biopsy of nodule in terminal ileum showing lymphoid hyperplasia. **E.** Microphotograph of biopsy of midjejunum in patient with sprue. The villi are flattened and atrophic and there is chronic inflammatory reaction. (Parts **A, B,** and **C** appear in the color section at the front of the book, Plate E.)

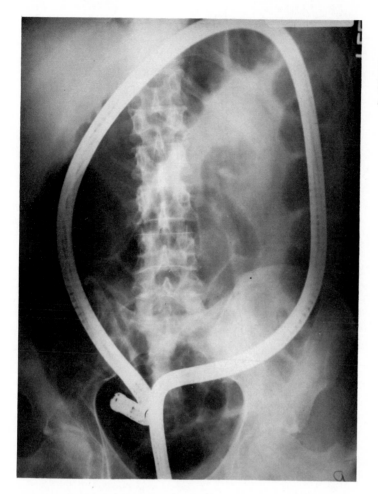

FIG. 5. Fiberendoscope (Olympus CF-MB 110 cm) intubated through the ileocecal sphincter and into the terminal ileum.

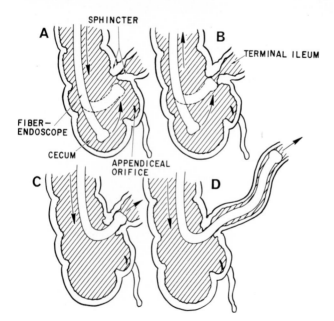

FIG. 6. Intubation of the ileocecal sphincter with the colon fiberscope and insertion into the terminal ileum. **A.** Flexion of the scope tip and positioning just proximal to the sphincter. **B.** Further flexion of the tip and gradual withdrawal of the scope to "pull" open the sphincter. **C.** Forward and medial insertion of the scope tip through the sphincter as its orifice comes into view. **D.** Further active insertion of the scope from the anus and directional control of scope tip in coordination with ileal peristalsis allows the ileum to advance over the scope distances up to 50 cm.

In most patients the distal terminal ileum can be intubated and visualized with a 110-cm colon fiberscope[5] (Fig. 5). The patient is examined as an outpatient after a mechanical bowel preparation (see above) and only light intravenous sedation. With the patient on the operator's left side the colonfiberscope is inserted into the cecum using abdominal palpation.[5] Fluoroscopy was used routinely by Nagasako et al.[11] but not at all by Gaisford,[5] although there are occasional patients with unusual flexure configurations in which

fluoroscopy might be helpful. With the patient on his left side the orifice of the ileocecal sphincter is not often directly visualized before intubation. Intubation of the sphincter is accomplished by: (1) flexion of the scope tip and positioning just proximal to the sphincter; (2) further flexion of the tip and gradual withdrawal of the scope to "pull" open the sphincter; (3) forward and medial insertion of the scope tip through the sphincter as its orifice comes into view; (4) further insertion of the scope from the anus and directional control of

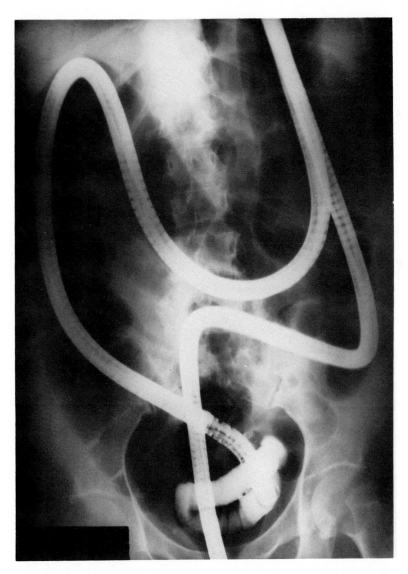

FIG. 7. Fiberendoscope (Olympus CF-LB 186 cm) intubated through the ileocecal sphincter and into the terminal ileum. Water-soluble radiopaque contrast medium (Renografin 60) is injected into the ileum via the biopsy channel.

the scope tip in coordination with ileal peristalsis, allowing the ileum to be advanced over the scope distances up to 50 cm[5] (Fig. 6). Manual palpation of the abdomen is sometimes helpful in guiding the fiberscope through the ileocecal sphincter and into the ileum. Cine and still photography and biopsy can be performed at any level of insertion (Fig. 4). With the fiberscope inserted into the terminal ileum, contrast segmental ileography can be performed as described by Gaisford[5] (Fig. 7). The latter technique may be helpful in identifying Meckel's diverticulum and enables radiographic contrast examination of ileum beyond the reach of the fiberscope. Injection of contrast material through the biopsy channel of the scope is best done under fluoroscopic control. A cuffed balloon may be placed near the tip of the scope and inflated during injection of contrast material in order to prevent reflux of dye back in the ileum and cecum distal to the scope tip.

Direct Insertion of the Fiberscope Through an Ileostomy Stoma

Gaisford[6] used the Olympus CF-MB 110 cm colonfiberscope in three patients with regional enteritis and permanent ileostomy stomas to perform retrograde ileofiberendoscopy and biopsy. Salmon et al.[19] also reported using a smaller-caliber prototype fiberscope (Olympus FIS IVa) for examining two patients with ileostomy stomas. The patient is fasted for only a few hours, and mild intravenous sedation is given. With the patient in the supine position the scope is easily inserted directly through the stoma. With gentle abdominal palpation and occasional rotation of the patient, the scope is advanced gently and carefully through the ileum under visual control, taking advantage of normal peristalsis to aid insertion. Extent and severity of recurrent or residual Crohn's disease can be evaluated by direct inspection and biopsy.

Pulling the Fiberscope Through the Gastrointestinal Tract

Transintestinal intubation of the entire gastrointestinal tract by means of a small plastic tube as described by Blankenhorn et al.[1] has been used to pull a variety of instruments through the gastrointestinal tract from above or below (Figs. 8 and 9). Deyhle et al.[3] used this method to introduce the Olympus colono-

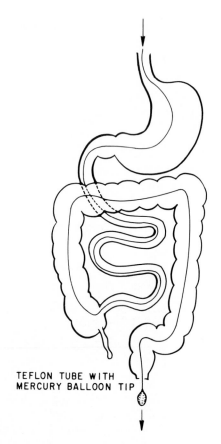

TEFLON TUBE WITH MERCURY BALLOON TIP

FIG. 8. Teflon tube with mercury balloon tip passed perorally and carried by peristalsis out the rectum.

scope CF-LB 186 cm into the small intestine in two patients with gastrointestinal bleeding of unknown origin. The 1.5-mm transintestinal tube with a mercury-weighted balloon tip is passed transnasally 1 or 2 days before the examination. After passage of the tube through the anus (Fig. 8), the fiberscope is attached at the oral end of the tube. By pulling at the anal end the fiberscope advances through the gastrointestinal tract (Fig. 9). Deyhle et al.[3] performed this technique under fluoroscopic control over 1 to 2 hours, and their two patients were given general anesthesia. This technique provides complete inspection of the entire small bowel and biopsies under direct vision.

Pushing the Fiberscope Perorally over a Transintestinal Tube Guide

Classen et al.[2] reported another technique of total small-bowel endoscopy with 2- and 3-meter fiberscopes (Olympus JF-D prototypes)

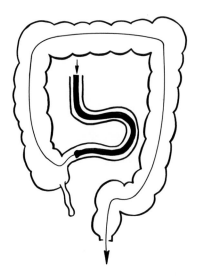

FIG. 9. Fiberendoscope intubated orally and guided or pulled through the gastrointestinal tract with previously passed transintestinal Teflon tube.

also utilizing prior transintestinal intubation as per Blankenhorn et al.[1] Two to 5 days before the examination the patient swallows the 1.6-mm Teflon tube with the mercury-weighted bag tip. After complete transintestinal passage (Fig. 8) the tube is drawn through the biopsy channel of the fiberscope and is used as a guide. Tension is applied to the oral and anal ends of the transintestinal Teflon tube, and by pushing the fiberscope over the tube the tip of the instrument is advanced through the small intestine under direct vision and/or fluoroscopic control. While direct inspection of the entire small bowel is afforded with this technique, no biopsy is possible since the Teflon guiding tube is through the biopsy channel of the fiberscope.

Peroral Transintestinal Intubation with Balloon-Tipped, Long, Small-Intestine Fiberscope

Wolff and Shinya[23] utilized a special small-intestine fiberscope for examining the entire small bowel (Fig. 10). The instrument resembles a Miller-Abbott or Cantor tube, and the balloon at the tip facilitates its advance. It is introduced in the same manner as the long intestinal tube and reaches the ileocecal valve within 48 hours. The examiner then withdraws it slowly, examining the small-intestinal mucosa as he does so. This instrument has no facilities for biopsy or obtaining cytology specimens.

RESULTS

The experience thus far with small-bowel endoscopy is relatively small, but the reported early results and lack of complications are very encouraging. These results are summarized in Table 1.

DISCUSSION

The small bowel is no longer the "blind spot" in endoscopic diagnosis. Partial upper small bowel, partial terminal small bowel, and total small bowel endoscopic examination have recently all proved feasible and safe, but each technique has some limitations and reservations. The techniques of direct intubation and examination of the proximal jejunum and terminal ileum with standard fiberscopes have been established as safe, successful, and useful. This extension of routine upper gastrointestinal and colonfiberendoscopy will become a standard technique in every major endoscopic laboratory. The main clinical usefulness of jejunal and terminal ileal examination and biopsy is in accurately determining the presence and extent of chronic or acute mucosal-submucosal inflammatory disease (i.e., Crohn's disease) and malabsorption diseases (i.e., nontropical sprue). Although radiologic contrast studies often show evidence of late changes in the small bowel in these conditions, direct endoscopy provides a more accurate diagnosis in earlier stages which can be confirmed by direct biopsies. These techniques have the advantages of: (1) outpatient performance of the examination; (2) mild or no patient discomfort with light sedation; (3) simple bowel preparation; (4) safety to the patient; and (5) no need for fluoroscopy. The major disadvantage of course is that the middle small bowel—lower jejunum and proximal ileum—are rarely visualized.

The several techniques of total small-bowel endoscopy as described previously by Deyhle et al., [3] Classen et al.,[2] and Wolff and Shinya[23] appear now to have only limited clinical usefulness. The major clinical application of total small-bowel endoscopy is probably in the patient with chronic or recurrent alimentary tract blood loss in whom careful upper gastrointestinal endoscopy and total colonfiberendoscopy and terminal ileoscopy have not revealed the source of bleeding. Lesions such as

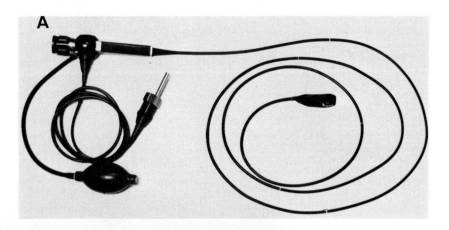

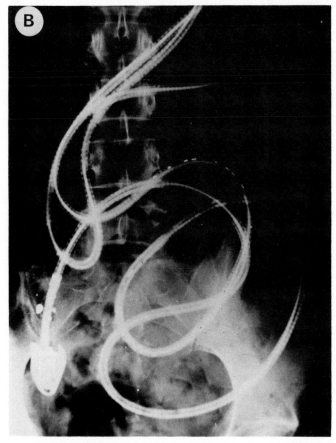

FIG. 10. **A.** Small-intestine endoscope, which is passed in similar fashion to a long intestinal (Miller-Abbott) tube. **B.** Position of instrument at 48 hours, prior to withdrawal.

small-bowel polyps, other small-bowel tumors, diverticula, telangiectasias, and localized regional small-bowel inflammatory disease should be diagnosed and localized by total small-bowel endoscopy. These particular lesions, although uncommon, are extremely difficult to diagnose by all other techniques and even on the operating table can be most exasperating to the surgeon trying to localize a source of unknown bleeding. Each of these techniques has the advantage of total small intestinal examination. The disadvantages are: (1) the need for patient

TABLE 1. Early Results of Small-Bowel Endoscopy

Author	Part or Amount of Small Bowel	Fiberscope	Technique	Indications	No. of Exams/Successes	Findings*
Deyhle et al.[3]	Total small bowel	Olympus CF-LB 186 cm	Peroral scope pull-through with transintestinal tube (biopsy)	GI blood loss	2/2	No bleeding site identified
Classen et al.[2]	Total small bowel	Olympus JF-D 200–300 cm	Peroral scope push-through over transintestinal tube guide (no biopsy)	GI blood loss (3); ?Crohn's disease (3); ?lymphocytic hyperplasia (2); diarrhea (7)	15/11 terminal ileum, 3 jejunal ileum, 1 jejunum	Crohn's disease (3); lambliasis (1); normal (9); incomplete exam (2)
Nagasako et al.[11,13,14]	Terminal ileum 10–50 cm	Machida FCS 188 cm	Colonoscopic intubation of ileocecal sphincter with fluoroscopy (biopsy)	Lower abdominal symptoms	100/66	Lymphoid hyperplasia
Gaisford[5]	Terminal ileum 10–15 cm	Olympus CF-LB 186 cm, CF-MB 110 cm	Colonoscopic intubation of ileocecal sphincter without fluoroscopy (biopsy)	Lower abdominal symptoms; GI blood loss	75/73	Lymphoid hyperplasia
Salmon et al.[19]	Upper jejunum	Olympus FIS IVa 162 cm	Peroral direct insertion (Rubin suction biopsy) during laparotomy to ileocecal valve	Suspected jejunal disease	7/7	Sprue; Crohn's disease
Ogoshi et al.[15]	Upper jejunum	Olympus 162 cm,	Peroral direct insertion (Rubin suction biopsy)	Survey examinations	2/2	Nonspecific jejunitis
Gaisford[5]	Jejunum	Olympus CF-LB 186 cm	Peroral direct insertion (direct biopsy)	GI bleeding; diarrhea	250/?	Sprue; Menetrier's disease
Wolff and Shinya[23]	Total small bowel	Olympus small intestine scope	During laparotomy to ileocecal valve Peroral as Miller-Abbott or Cantor tube (no biopsy)	Suspected small-bowel disease	6/6 / 2/2	Ruled out small-bowel source

*There were no complications reported.

hospitalization for 2 to 4 days; (2) greater patient discomfort requiring either heavy sedation or general anesthesia; (3) the need for fluoroscopic control in the methods of Deyhle et al.[3] and Classen et al.;[2] and (4) a probable complication risk although as yet unreported. The small-intestine scope being investigated by Shinya seems to be the simplest and easiest for the patient and the endoscopist; but until successful, practical experience is reported, its value remains hypothetical. Both the technique described by Classen et al.[2] with the guide tube through the biopsy channel and the long small-intestine scope approach of Wolff and Shinya[23] have the major disadvantage of having no biopsy facility. This seems to be a major deterrent to their practical use. As Classen et al.[2] pointed out, however, a future small-bowel scope could be provided with an additional (second) biopsy channel at the cost of increasing the diameter of the instrument or at sacrificing the glass fiber bundle size.

The use of standard and prototype fiberscopes for examining the small bowel in the operating room during celiotomy is still being investigated. Only a few cases have been reported: Salmon et al.[19] reported two and Gaisford[6] four patients. In two of my patients and in those two reported by Salmon et al. operating room small-bowel endoscopy to the ileocecal sphincter was used to rule out the small bowel as the source of alimentary tract blood loss. In another patient I was prepared to use intraoperative fiberendoscopy of the small bowel but did not require it since a small benign bleeding polyp was just palpable in the upper ileum. Preoperatively the patient had had multiple upper gastrointestinal contrast studies and barium enemas, upper gastrointestinal endoscopy, total colon fiberoscopy, and terminal ileoscopy and selective mesenteric arteriography—all of which were normal. The patient was an ideal candidate for total small endoscopy per the method of Deyhle et al., and if it had been performed it is likely that the small (1.5 cm) pedunculated bleeding polyp in the upper ileum could have been removed by the electrosurgical snare technique via the fiberscope. Instead it was excised by simple enterotomy, the excision being through its pedunculated base.

As Morrissey[10] noted, the current methods of examining the total small intestine are still in relatively primitive form, and further development of instruments is necessary which will allow improved techniques for propelling an endoscope through the small intestine.

REFERENCES

1. Blankenhorn DH, Hirsch J, Ahrens EH: Transintestinal intubation: technic for measurement of gut length and physiologic sampling at known loci. Proc Soc Exp Biol Med 88:356, 1955
2. Classen M, Firiihmorgan P, Koch H, et al: Peroral enteroscopy of the small and large intestine. Endoscopy 4:157, 1972
3. Deyhle P, Jenny S, Fumagalli J, et al: Endoscopy of the whole small intestine. Endoscopy 4:155, 1972
4. Gaisford WD: Gastrointestinal fiberendoscopy. Am J Surg 124:744, 1972
5. Gaisford WD: Fiberendoscopy of the cecum and terminal ileum. Gastrointest Endosc 21:13, 1974
6. Gaisford WD: Fiberendoscopy of the small bowel. In preparation.
7. Hiratsuka S: Technique for insertion of colon fiberscope by means of intestinal guide string. Gastroenterol Endosc 12:209, 1970
8. Hirschowitz BI, Curtiss LD, Peters CW, et al: Demonstration of a new gastroscope—the fiberscope. Gastroenterology 35:50, 1958
9. Hoff HC: Retrograde intubation of the cecum. Am J Roentgenol 20:226, 1928
10. Morrissey JF: Small intestinal fiberscope. Gastrointest Endosc 20:76, 1973
11. Nagasako K, Takemoto T: Endoscopy of the ileocecal area. Gastroenterology 65:403, 1973
12. Nagasako K, Endo M, Takemoto T, et al: The insertion of the fibercolonscope into the cecum and the direct observation of the ileocecal valve. Endoscopy 2:123, 1970
13. Nagasako K, Yazawa C, Takemoto T: Biopsy of the terminal ileum. Gastrointest Endosc 19:7, 1972
14. Nagasako K, Yazawa C, Takemoto T: Observation of the terminal ileum. Endoscopy 3:45, 1971
15. Ogoshi K, Hara Y, Ashizawa S: New technic for small intestinal fiberoscopy. Gastrointest Endosc 20:64, 1973
16. Overholt BF: Flexible fiberoptic sigmoidoscope. CA 19:81, 1969
17. Provenzale L, Revignas A: Colonic electrical activity recording and total fiberoptic colonoscopy: two new applications of transintestinal intubation. Am J Gastroenterol 56:137, 1971
18. Provenzale L, Camerada P, Revignas A: La coloscopia totale trans-anale mediante una metodica originale. Rassegna Med Sards 69:149, 1966
19. Salmon PR, Brown P, Burwood R, et al: Examination of the duodenum and jejunum employing a new fiberoptic enteroscope. Gut 14:823, 1973

20. Torsoli A, Arullani P, Casale C: An application of transintestinal intubation to the study of the colon. Gut 8:192, 1967
21. Williams C, Muto T: Examination of the whole colon with the fiberoptic colonoscope. Gut 13: 322, 1972; Br Med J 3:278, 1972
22. Wolff WI, Shinya H: Colonfiberoscopy. JAMA 217:1509, 1971
23. Wolff WI, Shinya H: Modern endoscopy of the alimentary tract in current problems in surgery. Yearbook Medical Publ Chicago, 1974, pp 50–51

35

Amnioscopy

Erich Saling
Joachim W. Dudenhausen

Amnioscopy, developed in 1961 and first reported in 1962,[19] is used to detect fetal danger during late pregnancy and the onset of labor before rupture of the membranes. The forewaters are inspected through the intact membranes after insertion of a conical tube (amnioscope) into the cervical canal. Clear (Fig. 1, Plate E)* or milky (by the emulsion of vernix) amniotic fluid is a sign of normal fetal conditions. Green (Fig. 2, Plate E) or yellow amniotic fluid, as well as a reduced volume or lack of amniotic fluid (positive amniotic findings), indicate impending danger.

TASK OF AMNIOSCOPY

Amnioscopy does not allow an exact diagnosis of the present state of the fetus, but it enables us to make a reliable selection of cases with increased hypoxic risk to the fetus, particularly during the last weeks of pregnancy. If during this time the examination of the mother or the case history have indicated intrauterine danger, amnioscopy helps either to exclude this suspicion or, in the presence of positive amnioscopic findings, to confirm it. Whenever amnioscopic findings indicate placental insufficiency or reduced oxygen supply due to other causes, the condition of the fetus should be further examined with more exact methods.

All color plates appear in the front of the book.

INDICATIONS FOR OPTICAL EVALUATION OF AMNIOTIC FLUID

Late Pregnancy

Optical evaluation of amniotic fluid is indicated during late pregnancy whenever placental insufficiency is suspected (Table 1). Gestosis (toxemia) and postmaturity are the most frequent causes of suspected placental insufficiency, although it is also found in other abnormalities or complications, e.g., late conception, diabetes mellitus, erythroblastosis. Placental insufficiency can also be suspected in dysmaturity, which is often the result of reduced nutritive partial function of the placenta.

Gestosis. To establish the severity of gestosis, Goecke and Schwabe[7] proposed a scoring system—the gestosis index (GI; Table 2)—which we have included in our list of indications for optical evaluation of amniotic fluid. The best type of supervision by optical evaluation of amniotic fluid of a fetus in danger due to gestosis is a combination of transabdominal amniocentesis between the 33rd and 36th week and amnioscopy after the 36th week. Therefore obstetric departments that have the facilities for transabdominal amniocentesis, in order to avoid major risk to mother and child (e.g., after placental localization), should prefer optical evaluation of amniotic fluid by amniocentesis before the 37th week. Departments without these facilities can carry out amnioscopy in

TABLE 1.   Indications for Optical Evaluation of Amniotic Fluid

Late Pregnancy

Amniocentesis as main supervision method
A. Gestosis
1. 33rd–36th week (GI >4): amniocentesis every 4th day (in addition to intermittent use of cardiotocography). Repeated amniocentesis allows simultaneous control of fetal lung maturity.

Amnioscopy as main supervisory method
2. After 36th week, weight >2500 g: amnioscopy every 2nd day.
a. GI <4: begin amnioscopic supervision when gestosis symptoms do not disappear after 3 days with therapy.
b. GI >4: immediately begin amnioscopic supervision.
B. Suspicion of postmaturity
1. From 7th day after calculated term, every 2nd day.
2. Young primipara (≤18 years), elderly primipara (≥30 years), elderly multipara (≥40 years): from calculated term, every 2nd day.
3. In additional risk (e.g., critical past history): from 14 days before calculated term, every 2nd day.
C. Other suspicion of placental insufficiency
1. Late conception: from 14 days before calculated term; every 2nd day.
2. Suspicion of dysmaturity (in addition to other methods of supervision).
a. Slight dysmaturity (weight between 3rd and 10th percentiles): after 36th week, every 2nd day.
b. Advanced dysmaturity (weight under 3rd percentile): after 36th week, daily.

Amnioscopy as additional supervision method
D. Diabetes mellitus
1. Manifest, not detected early enough, or not sufficiently treated latent diabetes: after 36th week, every 2nd day.
2. Detected early enough and sufficiently treated latent diabetes: from 14 days before calculated term, every 2nd day.
E. Rh erythroblastosis: after 36th week, every 2nd day.

Onset of Labor (After 36th Week)
A. Slow starter: daily as long as spontaneous contractions are present.
B. Admission amnioscopy.

Amnioscopy for Other Reasons (Not Supervision)
A. As a safe method for artificial rupturing of the membranes (high presenting part).
B. Differentiation of the type of premature rupture of the membranes (high or low rupture).
C. Antepartum uterine hemorrhage—differentiation between placenta previa and presence of membranes that can be ruptured.
D. Suspicion of intrauterine death.

GI is the gestosis index.

moderate gestosis during the last 6 weeks of pregnancy, and in severe cases even up to 8 weeks before term. The same applies to cases where amniocentesis is technically not feasible (e.g., anterior wall placenta).

The danger of premature labor is normally small if amniocentesis is carried out long before the due date. The frequency of accidental rupture of the membranes is 1 to 2 percent.

Amnioscopy should be continued every second day until

1. Gestosis symptoms disappear after treatment (we recommend continued amnioscopic evaluation for 1 week after the disappearance of gestosis symptoms, since meconium is sometimes evacuated shortly after symptoms have disappeared).
2. Meconium-stained amniotic fluid has been diagnosed.
3. Labor begins (admission amnioscopy).

Postmaturity.   Fetuses are in danger in cases of real postmaturity. Perinatal mortality increases after term, particularly after the end of the 41st week.[2] The cause of this intrauterine fetal danger is placental insufficiency. The risk for postmature fetuses is particularly great when there is an additional dysfunction of the placenta due to gestosis.

We recommend amnioscopy in women without other complications after the sixth day post term. For young and older primiparas and older multiparas we propose that amnioscopy be performed from the calculated term date onward. If there are additional risk factors (e.g., intrauterine death in past pregnancies) we recommend that supervision by amnioscopy be started 2 weeks before the calculated date.

If postmaturity is suspected amnioscopic control should be continued on alternating days until

1. Labor begins (admission amnioscopy).
2. Meconium stained amniotic fluid appears.
3. Reduced volume or complete lack of amniotic fluid has been diagnosed.

Reduced volume or complete lack of amniotic fluid is a pathologic finding, since this supports the suspicion of postmaturity. Amnioscopic supervision of the fetus, however, is no longer possible, because passed meconium cannot be carried to the forewaters for lack of a vehicle.

Late Conception.   If the first pregnancy occurs 3 to 5 years after a child has been desired, implantation failure and therefore placental insufficiency can be expected more fre-

TABLE 2.   Scoring Criteria for Classification of Gestosis (Gestosis Index)

Parameter	Scoring Criteria			
	0	1	2	3
Edema after bedrest	None	Tibial	Generalized	—
Weight gain/wk (g)	<500	500–750	>750	—
Proteinuria (g/100 ml)	<0.5	0.5–2	2–5	>5
BP (systolic)	<140	140–160	160–180	>180
BP (diastolic)	<90	90–100	100–110	>110

After Goecke and Schwabe.[7]

quently. In these cases we recommend starting amnioscopy 2 weeks before the calculated date.

Dysmaturity. If there is the suspicion of dysmaturity on the basis of ultrasonography, or estrogen or HPL levels, the reason should be sought primarily in nutritive placental insufficiency. In order to detect respiratory insufficiency early enough, we recommend amnioscopic supervision in cases with slight dysmaturity after the 36th week, performed every second day, and daily in cases with more severe dysmaturity.

For the indications described above, optical evaluation of amniotic fluid is used as the main method of supervision for the high-risk fetus during late pregnancy. Further control methods are normally not necessary to recognize hypoxic danger, since usually there is passage of meconium as an early sign of hypoxia.

For two further indications—diabetes mellitus and erythroblastosis—amnioscopy is an additional control method since meconium is not always discharged as in the other conditions, which are usually connected with hypoxia. Here we should use primarily other diagnostic methods: in diabetes, cardiotocography in spontaneous labor or the oxytocin load test, estrogen determination; in erythroblastosis, spectrophotometry of the liquor amnii. Nevertheless, we should not renounce amnioscopy. If meconium is discharged, clinical measures should take into account the additional hypoxic risk to the fetus.

Onset of Labor

Admission Amnioscopy. When a woman is admitted to the obstetric department with beginning labor at term and intact membranes, a correct diagnosis of the state of the fetus is important. We recommend that as a first measure amnioscopy be performed immediately after admission. This routine amnioscopy permits us to recognize those cases in which the fetus is in hypoxic danger because of the hemodynamic changes at the onset of labor which may be due to a latent placental insufficiency. When the amniotic fluid is clear, amnioscopy enables us to pass through the preparation period more safely. If the amniotic fluid is green or absent, however, other methods of intensive supervision must be employed immediately. Among 1,000 admission amnioscopies in 1972, we found that 10.8 percent revealed meconium-stained amniotic fluid.[10] Bollinger et al.[4] reported 18 percent pathologic findings in admission amnioscopy.

Slow Starters. Hypoxic danger to the fetus is high in women who at the beginning of labor have only slight contractions over a prolonged period. In these cases we frequently find discharge of meconium,[6] which can be detected by daily amnioscopy.

Other Clinical Indications for Amnioscopy

Artificial Rupture of the Membranes. If the membranes must be artificially ruptured, amnioscopy sometimes provides greater security for the fetus, e.g., to avoid cord prolapse when there is a high presenting part.[1,17,18]

Differentiation of Premature Rupture of the Membranes. After breaking of waters amnioscopy helps us to distinguish rupture of the membranes at the lower pole from high rupture. If the membranes at the lower pole are still intact, it can be either a high rupture or a misinterpretation. A high rupture is less dangerous than rupture at the lower pole (cord prolapse, ascending infection).

Antepartum Hemorrhage. If pregnancy must be terminated because of uterine hemorrhage, amnioscopy can serve to confirm or exclude placenta previa. Because of possible intensification of the hemorrhage the examination should generally be made with standby operation facilities. It is surprisingly often possible, particularly in cases with cephalic presentation, to see the membranes through the amnioscope and to rupture them, in spite of the hemorrhage, delivering the child vaginally.

Suspicion of Fetal Death During Late Pregnancy. With a recently dead fetus due to placental insufficiency, we normally find meconium. With absent fetal heart sounds and meconium-stained amniotic fluid we recommend rupturing the membranes and attempting fetal blood analysis. In a dead fetus it will either not be possible to obtain blood from the scalp in spite of repeated incisions or the pH values of the blood sample will be extremely low (under 6.8). There are, however, fetal deaths (e.g., due to premature separation of the placenta) without passage of meconium. When the fetus has been dead for more than 24 hours amniotic fluid is typically flesh colored.

TECHNIQUE OF AMNIOSCOPY

The patient is placed on an examination table or on the edge of the bed. The external genitalia are cleaned with a desinfectant solution. The degree of softening of the cervix and its position, the degree of cervical dilatation, and the relationship are determined. In most cases the cervical canal admits one finger during the last weeks of pregnancy. In about one of five patients this is not the case, and careful digital dilatation of the cervical canal must be carried out—or when labor is to be avoided, transabdominal amniocentesis. According to the width of the canal, an amnioscope of 12, 16, or 20 mm diameter is then introduced (Fig. 3). The larger amnioscopes are preferable because they provide better visualization and hence more reliable conclusions.

After some practice it becomes easy to replace the examining finger in the cervical canal with the endoscope tube, i.e., by "blind approach." The instrument has been successfully inserted when the posterior cervical lip can be palpated around the tubus. The inexperienced operator might find it easier to insert the instrument after visualization and fixation of the cervix by speculum. This "controlled approach" has two inherent disadvantages: (1) A placenta previa may be missed if the cervical canal was not examined digitally; and (2) more instruments are necessary (sterile speculum).

After passing the internal os of the cervix

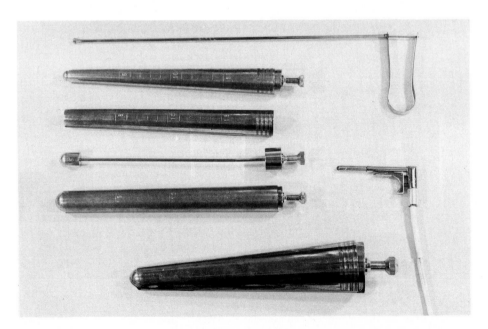

FIG. 3. The sizes of the amnioscope from top to bottom are 12, 16, and 20 mm in diameter at the tip of the conic-shaped tube. Obturator is seen in the middle. Top: Special applicator for small swabs. Bottom: Tubes for fetal blood sampling. At the right, flexible (white) fiberoptic cable connected to a rectangular fiberoptic light carrier for illumination; this can be clipped on each tube.

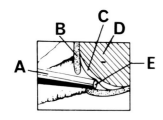

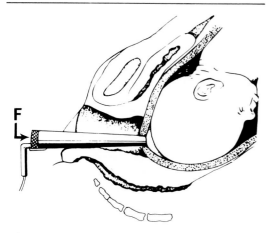

FIG. 4. Amnioscopy. Top: Insertion. A, Amnioscope. B, Cervix. C, Forewaters. D, Fetal head. E, Obturator. Bottom: Observation (F).

the instrument is advanced 1 cm into the uterus toward the sacral hollow in an approximate 30-degree angle. After removal of the obturator the lower pole of the amniotic sac can be visualized by somewhat retracting the instrument and by bringing it into a horizontal position. Later it may even be pointed upward. Vaginal secretion, mucus, or blood may be removed carefully with small swabs, which are inserted with a special applicator.

For reliable evaluation of the amniotic fluid, one must visualize a light-reflecting surface, which is behind the layer of fluid. The light skin of the presenting fetal part or large flakes of vernix serve this purpose. The amniotic fluid can then be examined as if it were contained in a cuvette consisting on one side of the transparent amnion and on the other of the light background (Fig. 4). It is essential to apply the eye as closely as possible to the instrument. It need not be said that experience is necessary to judge the color of the fluid.

By moving the instrument slowly along its longitudinal axis deeper layers of amniotic fluid can be inspected. Meconium flakes can be recognized when the fluid is put into motion by quickly moving the instrument back and forth a few millimeters.

When the membranes are tightly applied to the fetal head there is probably no amniotic fluid present. To rule out the possibility that only the lowermost portions of the membranes are adherent, or that they are pressed against the scalp by the instrument, the endoscope must be inserted more deeply, between the head and lateral uterine wall, until resistance is encountered. If the same findings are also present here, the diagnosis of oligohydramnios can be considered proved.

Accurate inspection of the amniotic fluid is of great importance because even slight discoloration must be taken as positive amnioscopic findings. For the inexperienced examiner it is often difficult to recognize this slight greenish discoloration.

PATHOPHYSIOLOGIC BASIS

Meconium-stained amniotic fluid indicates a slight hypoxic crisis in the fetus which took place a few hours or even days previously. The meconium passage is explained by the so-called oxygen-conserving adaption of the fetal circulation.[16-18] This means that the vessels in the organs which are not vital to intrauterine life (lung, spleen, thymus, adrenals, kidneys, pancreas, muscles, skin, intestinal tract) are constricted, reducing blood circulation and oxygen supply. The hyperperistalsis of the intestines which causes the passing of meconium is said to be the result of local hypoxia. The oxygen saved is now available to the vital organs (brain, heart, placenta). By the oxygen-saving mechanism of reduced blood flow in wide areas of the fetal circulation, total oxygen consumption of the fetus becomes lower with reduced oxygen supply.

We found that except for diabetes and erythroblastosis almost all hypoxic situations of the fetus during late pregnancy are accompanied by meconium passage. On the other hand, passage of meconium rarely occurs without symptoms of intercurrent fetal danger.[20]

Passage of meconium is an early warning sign of a hypoxic critical situation. If we measure the metabolic acidity briefly after the amnioscopic diagnosis of meconium-stained fluid, we find preacidotic values (pHqu40 7.24 to 7.20) in 6.5 percent and slightly acidotic values (pHqu40 7.19 to 7.15) in 1.7 percent. During the entire course of labor the acidity in fetal blood is frequently increased among women with meconium-stained amniotic fluid: 11 percent are preacidotic and a further 11 percent are acidotic values.[5] This result indicates that these were clearly high-risk cases requiring intensive supervision during labor (by cardiotocography and fetal blood analysis).

The lower antepartum mortality rate among amnioscopically supervised fetuses as compared to nonsupervised fetuses is clear proof that passage of meconium is an early warning symptom. If it were a late symptom, the antepartum mortality of amnioscopically supervised fetuses with passage of meconium should be higher than the antepartum mortality in the total group. The contrary is the case.

CLINICAL CONCLUSIONS AFTER PATHOLOGIC AMNIOSCOPIC FINDINGS

If an obstetric department has all the important and usual facilities for supervision of the fetus during late pregnancy, it should proceed according to Table 3. If the hospital uses amnioscopy only as a supervision method during late pregnancy, we recommend, in the presence of pathologic amnioscopic findings, rupturing the membranes and performing fetal blood analysis to determine the state of the fetus. We believe that if meconium is passed it is much more advantageous for all, even premature fetuses, to induce labor than to ignore this sign and wait. Otherwise hypoxic organ damages or even antepartum fetal death is risked. Danger for the child arising from accidental premature birth is slight in relation to the benefit for the group of fetuses with meconium passage.

SAFETY OF AMNIOSCOPIC SUPERVISION

The significance of amnioscopy for the supervision of high-risk fetuses is shown in the lower perinatal mortality of children supervised with this method. Perinatal mortality in our group does not correspond fully to the World Health Organization definition, since only children supervised amnioscopically and dead after the 34th week of pregnancy are covered—none after the 27th week—but all children who died during labor and after birth before the seventh day of life are contained in this group.

Between the introduction of amnioscopy in 1961 and 1973 we performed amnioscopy during late pregnancy in 11,379 women. In 62 cases the indication was suspicion of intrauterine death, and in 454 cases a suspected rupture of membranes. Therefore amnioscopy was used in only 10,863 pregnancies as a method of supervising high-risk fetuses. Out of this group 119 fetuses died. This means a mortality of 1.09 percent, the antepartum mortality being 0.11 percent. The mortality of 1.09 percent can be considered very low, especially when we take into account that the group of amnioscopically supervised fetuses is a selection of high-risk fetuses.

Among the 12 antepartum intrauterine deaths were two cases with premature separation of the placenta, two fetuses were a second twin, and in two other cases the cause was not established in spite of pathologic evaluation. The remaining six cases were, in our view, methodologic failure of amnioscopy. The term failure is applied if the last amnioscopy showed clear amniotic fluid and the fetus died within 48 hours or up to the onset of labor. In 10,863 amnioscopically supervised pregnancies six failures means a failure rate of 0.6/1000. During the first years of amnioscopy intrauterine fetal death occurred in one diabetic patient and one case of Rh erythroblastosis. Since in diabetes and erythroblastosis we no longer rely on amnioscopy alone, the failure rate would probably be even lower under present conditions.

DANGERS OF AMNIOSCOPY

The greatest danger of amnioscopy— ascending infection[8,9]—has not led to high maternal puerperal morbidity (subfebrile and febrile temperatures).[8,9,15] Some reports[11,12] have indicated that leukocytic infiltration in the membranes and the umbilical cord were more frequently observed in women after amnioscopy.

It is of clinical importance to know whether the fetus is at high risk. For this purpose studies in fetal morbidity are important. A morbidity comparison of fetuses of women with and without amnioscopy performed by Boenisch[3] did not show a higher rate in amnioscopically supervised infants. The rate of accidental rupture of the membranes is about 1 to 2 percent.[14,18]

It is also interesting to know how frequently

TABLE 3. Clinical Conclusions Drawn from Biochemical and Biophysical Findings in Late Pregnancy

Amniotic Fluid	Calculated Fetal Weight (g)	Prenatal Lung Maturity Tests	CTG During Spont. Contract. or Oxytocin Load Tests	HPL or Estrogens	Bishop Score	Clinical Conclusions
Clear or milky	>2,500	+	Path.	Normal	≥7 <7	Induction of labor Continued intensive supervision
Clear or milky	>2,500	+	Normal	Path.	≥7 <7	Induction of labor Continued intensive supervision
Clear or milky	>2,500	+	Path.	Path.	≥7 <7	Induction of labor Continued intensive supervision
Clear or milky	<2,500	−	Normal/ Path.	Normal/ Path.	≥7/<7	Continued intensive supervision*
Green	>2,500	+	Normal/ Path.	Normal/ Path.	≥7/<7	Induction of labor
Slightly meconium stained	<2,500	−	Normal/ Path.	Normal	≥7/<7	Continued intensive supervision*
Severely meconium stained	<2,500	−	Path. Normal	Path. Normal	≥7/<7 ≥7/<7	Induction of labor Continued intensive supervision
No fluid obtained	>2,500 <2,500 <2,500	? ? ?	Normal/ Path. Path. Normal	Normal/ Path. Path. Normal	≥7/<7 ≥7/<7 ≥7/<7	Induction of labor Induction of labor Continued intensive supervision*

*Promotion of lung maturity.

amnioscopy induces uterine contractions. Labor begins in about 25 percent of the women at term, and for these women induction of labor is not necessarily a disadvantage. It was a disadvantage in the past, however, when women with gestosis symptoms (if supervision during the 33rd to 36th weeks was necessary) had premature labor. We increasingly use amniocentesis during these weeks of pregnancy to avoid premature birth.

To answer a similar question—i.e., if amnioscopy leads to premature rupture of the membranes—our patients were checked for the rate of premature rupture of the membranes during the years before the introduction of amnioscopy (1958 to 1960) and after its introduction (1962 to 1967).[13] The rate of premature rupture of the membranes during both periods was about 25 percent.

AMNIOTIC FLUID EVALUATION IN COMBINED BIOCHEMICAL AND BIOPHYSICAL SUPERVISION OF THE FETUS IN LATE PREGNANCY

In addition to optical evaluation of the amniotic fluid for supervision of the high-risk fetus during late pregnancy, today we particularly use certain other measures:

1. Determination of fetal size with ultrasound (combined thoracocephalometry)
2. Cardiotocography during spontaneous contractions or after oxytocin load test
3. Prenatal lung maturity examinations
4. HPL determination in the maternal serum
5. Estrogen determination in the maternal plasma or urine
6. Spectrophotometry of liquor amnii

Among these methods amnioscopy is a very suitable broad screening technique because of its simplicity and high reliability. Nevertheless, in special high-risk cases we look for additional safety and so also employ the abovementioned diagnostic techniques.

Since several of these methods are relatively new we must expect that our clinical judgments may change as soon as new experience is gained. Therefore our lists of clinical indications (Table 1) and clinical measures (Table 3) cannot be seen as definitive.

REFERENCES

1. Barham K: Amnioscopy amniotomy: a look at surgical induction of labor. Am J Obstet Gynecol 116:35, 1973
2. Bickenbach W: Die Übersterblichkeit der Kinder bei übertragenen Schwangerschaften. Geburtshilfe Frauenheilkd 7:3, 1947
3. Boenisch H: Amnioskopie und Morbidität beim Neugeborenen. Dissertation, Berlin, 1973
4. Bollinger J, Hochuli E, Eberhard J, et al: Hat die Amnioskopie heute noch ihre Berechtigung? Fortschr Med 90:937, 1972
5. Bretscher J: Pränatale Diagnostik. In Schwalm H, Döderlein G (eds): Klinik der Frauenheilkunde und Geburtshilfe, Band III. Berlin, Urban & Schwarzenberg, 1970
6. Browne ADH: Discussion. Cited by Saling E: Comments on optical evaluation of the amniotic fluid by amnioscopy: summary of the chairman. In Huntingfort PJ, Hüter KA, Saling E (eds): Perinatal Medicine, 1st European Congress. Stuttgart, Thieme, 1969
7. Goecke C, Schwabe G: Vorschlag einer Stadien-Einteilung der Gestose. Zentralbl Gynaekol 42:1439, 1965
8. Hengst P, Budeck J: Untersuchungen zur Keim-Aszension durch Amnioskopie. Zentralbl Gynaekol 94:842, 1972
9. Hengst P, Budeck J: Zum Einfluss der Amnioskopie auf den Wochenbettverlauf. Zentralbl Gynaekol 94:835, 1972
10. Herzog W: Die Bedeutung der Aufnahme-Amnioskopie. Dissertation, Berlin, 1974
11. Horky Z, Amon K: Rundzelluläre Infiltrationen der Eihäute nach Amnioskopie. Geburtshilfe Frauenheilkd 27:1065, 1967
12. Imholz G: Erste Erfahrungen mit der Amnioskopie. Gynaecologia (Basel) 160:190, 1965
13. Klein H: Häufigkeit vorzeitiger Blasensprünge nach vorausgegangenen Amnioskopien. Dissertation, Berlin, 1972
14. Kubli F: The optical evaluation of amniotic fluid. In Huntingford PJ, Hüter KA, Saling E (eds): Perinatal Medicine, 1st European Congress. Stuttgart, Thieme, 1969
15. La Roche G: Vaginale Eingriffe bei Schwangeren und Fieber im Wochenbett. Dissertation, Berlin, 1967
16. Saling E: Oxygen-conserving adaptation of foetal circulation. In Apley J (ed): Modern Trends in Pediatrics, Vol. 3. Glasgow, Butterworths, 1970
17. Saling E: Das Kind im Bereich der Geburtshilfe. Stuttgart, Thieme, 1966. English edition: Foetal and Neonatal Hypoxia in Relation to Clinical Obstetrical Practice. London, Arnold, 1968
18. Saling E: Die O_2-Sparschaltung des fetalen Kreislaufes. Geburtshilfe Frauenheilkd 26:413, 1966
20. Vujic J: Amnioscopically determined meconic fluid without clear etiology at the start of delivery. In Horsky J, Stembera ZK (eds): Intrauterine Dangers to the Foetus. Amsterdam, Excerpta Medica Foundation, 1967

The authors requested significant changes in the text and the tables; unfortunately, the request was made after the text had been set and printing had proceeded. Because of possible changes in methodology or results, it is recommended that the interested reader contact the authors directly.

36

Colposcopy

Duane E. Townsend

The use of magnification to assist the physician to examine diseases of the human body in great detail encompasses the specialties of ophthalmology, otolaryngology, neurosurgery, and gynecology. Gynecologic uses of optical enlargement dates back to 1925 when Hans Hinselman[11] of Hamburg, Germany developed the colposcope for the early detection of cervical cancer.[2] At the time of his studies it was believed that cervical cancer began as miniature nodules. Hinselman believed that with magnification and improved illumination these small tumors should be detectable. Instead of miniature tumors an unexpected variety of fascinating normal and abnormal tissue patterns were encountered. Encumbered by the tumor nodule theory, and restricting most of his efforts to clinical interpretation, confusing concepts were developed which led to a terminology that was cumbersome, lengthy, occasionally contradictory, and difficult for English translation.

Ries[30] attempted to introduce colposcopy in the United States in 1931. Speaking before the Chicago Obstetrics and Gynecology Society, he reviewed the concepts upon which it was based and concluded that colposcopy provided an avenue for the reduction of deaths from cervical cancer. However, his advice was virtually ignored, and with the introduction of cytology during the 1940s[25] what little interest there was in colposcopy in North America waned.

Over the next two decades efforts were made to reintroduce the technique in the United States. Invariably it was placed in competition with cytology, and invariably it proved to be inferior for cervical cancer detection.[10,19,20,38]

Cytology was more economical, considerably easier to learn, and had a lower rate of false-negative results. As a result of this competitiveness numerous critics sprang up, and at one time colposcopy was called the greatest gynecologic hoax in this or any century; in a prominent author's book, the colposcope is indexed as "the uselessness of."[37]

However, colposcopy in North America did not die; on the contrary, interest in this technique has suddenly mushroomed. This increased interest is directly related to several significant developments: (1) A logical, scientifically based, simplified terminology based on new concepts was introduced.[2,3,14,15] (2) Improved reference materials, teaching aids, and instructional methods were developed. (3) Articles appeared in the English literature pointing out the value of colposcopy in avoiding the hazards and complications[36] of diagnostic conization in the patient with the abnormal Papanicolaou test, i.e., a test suggestive of dysplasia or worse (class III or worse).[1,4,5,8,12,13,18,21–24,31,32,34,35] (4) Colposcopy is recommended primarily as a technique to assist the physician in the examination of the visible portion of the female genital tract (i.e., vulva, vagina, and cervix) therefore not placing it in competition with but rather complementing cytology. In patients with preinvasive cervical neoplasia, cytology can suggest the presence of the neoplastic process; colposcopy can determine its location and extent.

Colposcopy should be differentiated from colpomicroscopy, another method to examine the cervix. Colpomicroscopy uses a magnification between 150× and 200×. Moreover, it is more difficult to master, requires an expert knowledge in cytology, and takes a considerably longer period of time to carry out.

COLPOSCOPIC EXAMINATION

Examination of the visible portion of the female genital tract by colposcopy takes no more than a few minutes. If the patient happens to have an abnormality the examination is longer, but it rarely exceeds 15 to 20 minutes in experienced hands. Initially the vulva is inspected in a systematic fashion. Any abnormal tissue is sampled. A nonlubricated speculum is then slipped into the vagina, and the cervix is exposed. All excess mucus and cellular debris are gently removed with dry cotton balls or gauze sponges. A cytologic sample is first taken with a saline-moistened cotton tip applicator from the cervical canal followed by a thorough scrape of the squamocolumnar junction. The vaginal pool should be avoided because of its high rate of false-negative results.[9,29] The squamocolumnar junction is recognized with the naked eye as that junction between the smooth pink squamous epithelium and the reddish granular columnar epithelium.

Three percent acetic acid delivered by soaked cotton balls is used to cleanse the cervix and the anterior and posterior vaginal fornices. The colposcope is then swung into view and focused on the cervix. The transformation zone and the squamocolumnar junction are viewed. The color tone and vascular architecture are carefully examined. It is recommended by some authors that the vascular architecture be viewed before acetic acid is applied, using saline to keep the tissue moist. However, should acetic acid be applied initially, the vascular changes reappear once the acetic acid effect has lessened, i.e., 3 to 4 minutes.

After the squamocolumnar junction and the transformation zone have been thoroughly inspected, any abnormal or suspect areas are biopsied. If the patient should have an abnormal Papanicolaou test and the entire limits of the squamocolumnar junction are not visible, she must undergo some type of canal sampling, preferably with an endocervical curette.

Once the cervix has been examined the vagina can be viewed in its entirety by gradually withdrawing and rotating the speculum. The vaginal epithelium folds down over the end of the speculum permitting an end-on view of this tissue. A bimanual examination completes the procedure.

Bleeding is seldom a problem after biopsies since the specimens are taken with special instruments (i.e., Kevorkian) which remove only a small piece of epithelium and stroma.[28] However, excessive bleeding is easily controlled with Monsel's solution (i.e., ferric subsulfate) and cotton balls.

Depending on the results of the Papanicolaou test and tissue sampling, logical and appropriate management may be initiated. Details of management are covered in the latter part of this chapter.

TRANSFORMATION ZONE

One of the major concepts on which contemporary colposcopy is based is the transformation zone. An understanding of this area is vital not only to colposcopy but also in comprehending the origin and development of the cervical neoplasia. The transformation zone is defined as that area of the cervix or cervix and vagina that was initially covered by columnar epithelium and which (through a process called metaplasia) has been replaced all or in part by squamous epithelium.

It has been generally believed for many years that the cervix is normally covered by squamous epithelium and that the presence of columnar tissue on the ectocervix is an abnormal location for this tissue. Studies in Australia[3] complemented by those in the United States have conclusively shown that columnar tissue normally exists on the ectocervix in at least 70 percent of females and extends onto the vagina in an additional 4 to 5 percent. Moreover, the location of columnar epithelium on the ectocervix is determined during embryologic development.

Embryologically the fallopian tubes, uterus, cervix, and vagina are derived from the paired müllerian ducts. Initially the vagina is lined by columnar epithelium; but early in fetal life a stratified cuboidal epithelium, which eventually differentiates into squamous epithelium, begins to displace (caudal to cranial) this müllerian-derived columnar tissue. All of the columnar epithelium in the vagina and a variable portion of the ectocervical columnar tissue is replaced in the balance of female fetuses.

Therefore the location of columnar tissue on the ectocervix, and in a few cases on the vagina, is not the result of outward growth as once believed but has been in residence since embryogenesis. The initial replacement of the columnar tissue by cuboidal epithelium apparently ceases around the fifth gestational month. Therefore any further replacement of the columnar tissue by squamous tissue is probably accomplished through the process referred to as metaplasia. It has been suggested that this normal physiologic transition from columnar to squamous epithelium is most active during three phases of an individual's lifetime,[3,14] i.e., fetal life, adolescence, and during the first pregnancy. The process is enhanced by an acidic environment and is no doubt influenced by steroids such as estrogen and progesterone. In the fetus metaplasia probably occurs as a response to maternal steroids. Following delivery metaplasia slows owing to a reduction in steroids and the neutral secretions of the vagina. With the onset of menstruation and establishment of a bacterial population, the vagina becomes more acidic. When ectocervical columnar tissue is exposed to the acidic environment, the transformation process is activated.

The replacement of columnar by squamous epithelium occurs both as a peripheral ingrowth from the original squamous tissue laid down early in fetal life as well as from multipotential cells that are adjacent to columnar epithelium. The greatest contribution from any one source probably occurs randomly. In instances where the peripheral ingrowth appears to be the major contribution, an irregular border of the metaplastic squamous epithelium is found at the periphery of the grapelike columnar epithelium. In cases where there is an equal or greater contribution from the multipotential cells, islands of squamous metaplasia are found within the area covered by columnar tissue.

The initial phase of transformation from metaplastically derived islands is a fusion of the grapelike columnar tissue forming ridges. On the surface of the ridges the glandular epithelium is lost and is replaced by immature metaplastic squamous epithelium. Accompanying this process is an infiltrate of inflammatorylike cells. The multiple foci of metaplastic epithelium broaden, coalesce, and eventually join the peripheral contribution from the original squamous epithelium. Gland openings become prominent and appear as white spots or rings from which mucus may be expressed. The openings permit the egress of mucus from the deeper secreting columnar cells which are afforded protection from the acidic environment by the buffering effect of the mucus. Whenever the gland openings become occluded and the buried columnar epithelium continues to secrete mucus, Nabothian cysts form. The complete transformation from columnar to squamous epithelium requires many years. Patients who are on oral contraceptives seem to have a slower transformation rate probably because of the buffering effect of increased mucus production as a response to the high concentration of steroids contained within the pills. As a patient ages the transformation zone matures, the Nabothian cysts and gland openings disappear, and the squamocolumnar junction is usually found at or just within the external os. The junction then gradually moves up the canal. The upward migration is extremely slow because of the neutral pH of the environment.

During the teenage years the transformation zone is characterized by areas of columnar epithelium intermingling with metaplastic squamous epithelium. As an individual matures the sheets of metaplastic squamous epithelium enlarge, and gland openings and Nabothian cysts are prominent. With advancing age the transformation zone becomes less apparent, and only its very fine vascular structure reveals its location. In some cases the metaplastic squamous epithelium appears slightly whiter than the original squamous epithelium. This is due to an increased number of relatively large nuclei in the intermediate and parabasal cell layers. It is of interest that when these immature cells exfoliate and are picked up on a Papanicolaou smear they are occasionally misinterpreted as mild dysplasia or atypia. Moreover, in some instances this immature metaplastic squamous epithelium lacks sufficient glycogen and only partially stains with iodine.

In most women a normal transformation zone develops and the cytology is normal. However, in a few instances, due to an as yet unknown cause or causes, a DNA change occurs in the immature metaplastic squamous epithelium, potentially malignant tissue develops, and an atypical transformation zone evolves. It is within the atypical transformation zone that the abnormal patterns that characterize the earliest forms of cervical neoplasia reside.

Atypical Transformation Zone

A transformation zone is classified as atypical when one or more of the following patterns are viewed: white epithelium, mosaic structure, punctation, leukoplakia, and abnormal vascular patterns. Although each pattern may exist as a separate and distinct entity, in most cases several patterns exist simultaneously. In fact the atypical vascular pattern associated with neoplasia is never found alone and always appears with either white epithelium, punctation, mosaic structure, or leukoplakia. Although each pattern of the atypical transformation zone is a separate entity, they are all primarily white epithelium which, when having certain vascular structures, take on specific appearances (i.e., punctation, mosaic structure, or atypical vessels). Leukoplakia is generally reserved for the raised white plaque that is due to hyperkeratosis. Leukoplakia is recognized with the naked eye, before the application of acetic acid; white epithelium, mosaic structure, and punctation are more apparent after the application of acetic acid. The abnormal patterns that make up the atypical transformation zone are invariably sharply demarcated from the surrounding areas. They are found within the boundaries of the original squamocolumnar junction, the junction that developed around the fifth month of fetal life, and the physiologic junction—that which is observed at the time the patient is examined. Except for leukoplakia and atypical vessels, one edge of the lesion is invariably located at the physiologic squamocolumnar junction.

White epithelium is due to an increased number of nuclei which also have an increase in DNA. When light from the colposcope illuminates an area with increased nuclear concentration the light does not completely penetrate the tissue and is reflected back to the instrument. As a consequence, these areas appear white. The optical density and therefore the degree of whiteness vary directly with the nuclear concentration. Normal epithelium, which has small pyknotic nuclei, is pinkish white. Dysplasia and carcinoma in situ, which have varying degrees of nuclear density, vary in degrees of whiteness.

White epithelium due to neoplastic tissue is usually unifocal, slightly raised, and sharply demarcated from surrounding normal tissue. An example of white epithelium is presented in Figure 1. Note that the lesion is unifocal.

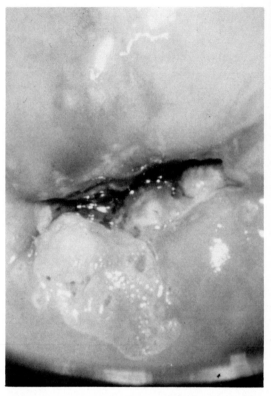

FIG. 1. Colpophotograph of cervix from a 19-year-old female with a Papanicolaou test suggestive of moderate dysplasia. There is an atypical transformation zone on the posterior lip characterized by white epithelium. The os is in the center of the photograph. The posterior border of the lesion is quite sharp. Directed biopsy showed moderate dysplasia. Entire limits of the lesion could be seen just at the external os, and the patient had cryosurgery avoiding the hazards of a major operative procedure.

In cases where the individual villous capillaries are retained, completely or partially, punctation and mosaic structures predominate. Punctation is the result of the retention of each individual villous capillary during the metaplastic process. Instead of fusing, the villi persist and the abnormal nuclei mutiply around the villi. As the abnormal epithelium expands, the villi are compressed so that only the individual capillary remains. When viewed on end the capillaries appear as red dots (Fig. 2).

Mosaic structure is likewise due to preservation of many of the villous capillaries, but in this case some villous capillaries are lost and those remaining link to one another to form a mosaic pattern (Fig. 3). Mosaic structure and punctation can be considered exact opposites of

FIG. 2. Colpophotograph of a 26-year-old female whose Papanicolaou test was suggestive of carcinoma in situ. On the anterior lip was extensive atypical transformation zone characterized primarily by punctation, which is quite diffuse, with a scattered area of early mosaic formation. Gland openings are apparent. The entire limits of this lesion could be seen; directed biopsy showed carcinoma in situ. Diagnostic conization was unnecessary, and the patient had primary hysterectomy because she had extensive pelvic relaxation.

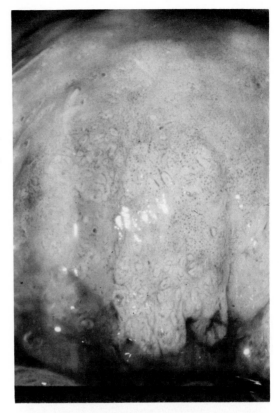

FIG. 3. Colpophotograph of a 23-year-old female whose Papanicolaou test was suggestive of carcinoma in situ. Colposcopically patient had a large atypical transformation zone characterized by mosaic structure. The mosaic pattern is quite regular and therefore not suggestive of an invasive lesion. The lesion extended well into the endocervical canal, and the patient required diagnostic conization because the curettage of the canal was positive.

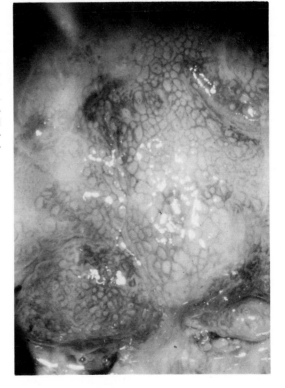

one another, although neither carries any greater or lesser degree of significance; they often coexist (Fig. 4).

Infrequently the abnormal epithelium produces an excess amount of keratin resulting in leukoplakia. Leukoplakia alone is usually not significant; however, each keratinized plaque must be thoroughly sampled since it is impossible to recognize any significant vascular pattern beneath the keratin crust (Fig. 5).

The last abnormal pattern viewed in the atypical transformation zone is atypical vessels. This is the most important entity since it may herald the site of early invasive carcinoma. It is an infrequent finding. An atypical vascular structure rarely if ever exists alone; occurring with it is either white epithelium, punctation, mosaic structure, or leukoplakia.

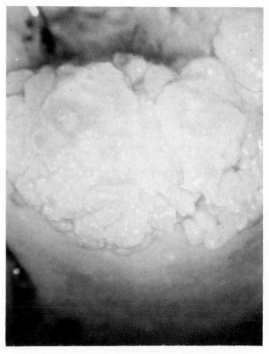

FIG. 5. Colpophotograph of leukoplakia in a 21-year-old female. In this case the heavy white keratinized plaque was due to condyloma; however, patterns identical to this have been seen overlying intraepithelial neoplasia. As a consequence, all leukoplakias must be thoroughly sampled because of the possibility of a neoplastic component.

The vascular patterns considered atypical are usually termed "commas," "spaghetti," "corkscrews," or "earthworms." They must be differentiated from the regular branching normal vessels often present over Nabothian cysts. Examples of atypical vessels are shown in Figure 6, which should be contrasted with the regular branching vessels over Nabothian cysts in Figure 7.

COLPOSCOPICALLY OVERT CARCINOMA

There are instances when to the naked eye there is no evidence of invasive carcinoma. However, when these patients are examined colposcopically, features consistent with invasive disease are apparent, i.e., raised irregular surface contour and markedly atypical vascular pattern. In these cases the colposcope is particularly valuable in pinpointing the exact area to sample for early diagnosis and prompt

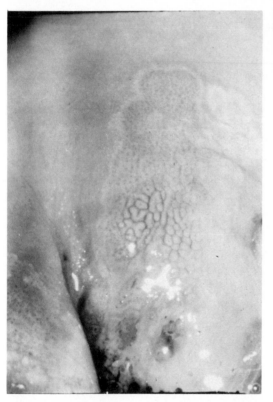

FIG. 4. Colpophotograph of a 32-year-old female whose Papanicolaou test was suggestive of carcinoma in situ. Colposcopically the patient had an atypical transformation zone characterized by punctation and mosaic structure. The limits of the lesion could be seen, and the borders of the lesion were fairly sharp. Directed biopsy shows severe dysplasia, and the patient had cryosurgery as definitive therapy.

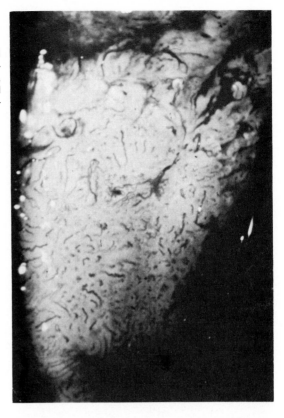

FIG. 6. Colpophotograph demonstrating atypical vascular structures in a patient with invasive carcinoma. The blood vessels are quite irregular. Terms such as "commas," "corkscrews," and "spaghetti" have been given to the irregular vascular patterns seen with invasive carcinoma.

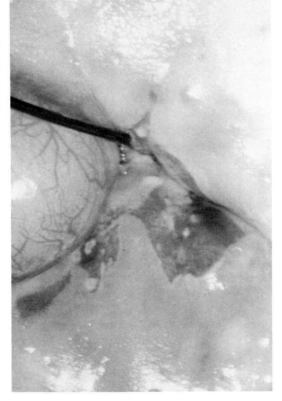

FIG. 7. Colpophotograph of a 40-year-old female with a large Nabothian cyst present on the left border of the photograph. The dark strings of the IUD are passing out of the anterior portion of the os. Note that the regular branching of vessels over the Nabothian cyst are quite dissimilar to those seen in Figure 6.

initiation of therapy. Examples of colposcopically overt carcinoma are shown in Figures 8 and 9.

SATISFACTORY OR UNSATISFACTORY EXAMINATION

Critical to every colposcopic evaluation in the patient with an abnormal Papanicolaou test or in routine colposcopic screening is the ability to view the entire limits of the active or physiologic squamocolumnar junction. If the entire limits of this important landmark cannot be seen, the examination must be judged

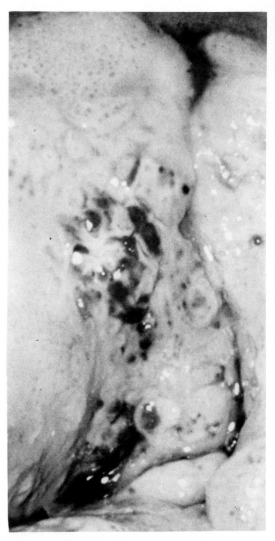

FIG. 9. Colpophotograph of a colposcopically overt carcinoma in a 54-year-old patient whose Papanicolaou test was class I. Colposcopy was done because of unusual discharge and postcoital bleeding. Note the extensive heavy white epithelium with an irregular surface contour. There are areas of coarse punctation high on the anterior portion of the lesion. In the center portion are areas of hemorrhage which overlie an atypical vascular pattern. Note that the border between normal and abnormal tissue is fairly sharp. Directed biopsy showed early invasive carcinoma.

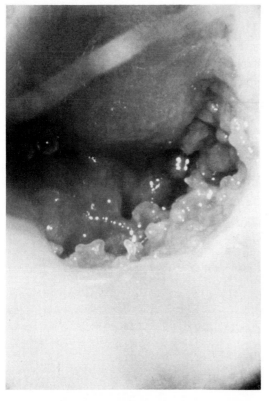

FIG. 8. Colpophotograph of a cervix in a 42-year-old female whose Papanicolaou test was suggestive of carcinoma in situ. Blind biopsies showed carcinoma in situ. Colposcopically on the posterior lip between 4 and 6 o'clock was an area of invasive carcinoma in the canal characterized primarily by an irregular surface contour. Irregular vessels and white epithelium were not the component in this particular case, but the surface contour, an important factor in colposcopic grading, was the predominant picture. Directed biopsy showed invasive squamous cell carcinoma.

unsatisfactory and invasive cancer in the patient with the abnormal Papanicolaou test cannot be excluded. However, if invasive cancer has been recognized and confirmed by biopsy, the patient has had appropriate evaluation. In those cases where preinvasive cervical

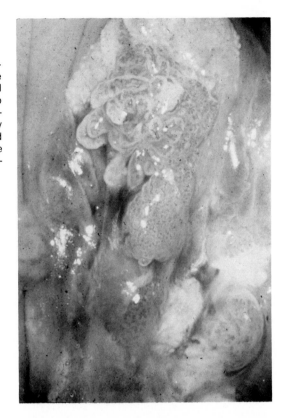

FIG. 10. Colpophotograph of cervix of a 19-year-old pregnant female who was referred to the institution for conization because of an abnormal Papanicolaou test. Grossly the cervix appeared to have a raised, irregular, friable lesion, which on colposcopy was consistent with papilloma. A biopsy was taken of the papilloma, which was confirmed histologically. Patient then proceeded with the pregnancy, delivered uneventfully, and the papilloma and condyloma disappeared spontaneously.

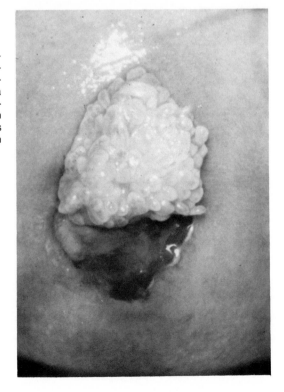

FIG. 11. Colpophotograph of cervix of a 17-year-old female with a raised, irregular lesion suspicious for invasive cancer. Colposcopically the classic irregular surface contour ascribed to condyloma acuminata is apparent. Directed excision biopsy revealed condyloma acuminata, and since the lesion was completely excised no further therapy was necessary. Patient also had a small condyloma on the vulva.

neoplasia is present or suspected and the entire junction cannot be seen, the examination must be followed by some type of canal sampling, i.e., endocervical curettage. Depending on the results of the curettings, further evaluation may be necessary, i.e., diagnostic conization.

OTHER COLPOSCOPIC FINDINGS

The largest subdivision of colposcopic findings is comprised of those which usually have minor significance. Most frequently encountered include condyloma, papilloma, cervical polyps, true erosions (which are usually traumatic due to speculum insertion), vaginocervicitis, and atrophic epithelium.

The most important of the miscellaneous patterns are papilloma and condyloma (Figs. 10 and 11) since they may give rise to abnormal Papanicolaou tests particularly during pregnancy when they are most frequently encountered. They are recognized by their striking surface contour and vascular pattern. Most are associated with vulvar and vaginal condyloma and are usually multifocal. They should always be biopsied because there have been instances where an inexperienced colposcopist mistook a keratinizing invasive cancer for condyloma.

With the recognition of the above colposcopic patterns it is possible to classify these changes according to a simplified and logical terminology (Table 1).

TABLE 1. Colposcopic Terminology

Normal colposcopic findings
1. Original squamous epithelium
2. Columnar epithelium
3. Typical transformation zone

Abnormal colposcopic findings
1. Atypical transformation zone
   a. White epithelium
   b. Punctation
   c. Mosaic structure
   d. Leukoplakia
   e. Abnormal blood vessels
2. Suspected invasive cancer

Unsatisfactory colposcopy

Other colposcopic findings
1. Vaginocervicitis
2. True erosion
3. Atrophic epithelium
4. Condyloma, papilloma

GRADING ABNORMAL PATTERNS

With experience, it is possible to grade the abnormal transformation zone and to make an extremely accurate prediction as to the histologic diagnosis. Factors considered in grading include the vascular structure (i.e., regular or irregular); surface contour (i.e., flat, depressed, smooth, or irregular); color and opacity or degree of whiteness; and line of demarcation of apparently normal epithelium. The green filter enhances the color tone differences and vascular changes; the latter are perhaps best viewed before acetic acid application. The most important factor in grading is the degree of whiteness, which is directly related to the nuclear density. The earlier forms of dysplasia are less white than carcinoma in situ and early invasive carcinoma. Immature metaplastic squamous epithelium may appear white owing to the increased number of immature nuclei. However, it is possible to differentiate it from dysplastic epithelium in that the border between the metaplastic and normal epithelium is usually irregular whereas the border between normal and potentially neoplastic tissue is invariably sharp.

Most of the abnormal patterns are unifocal, although in some instances multifocal appearances are seen. Multifocal disease is confined to the ectocervix and lies within the transformation zone. Cases of neoplastic disease high in the canal and low on the ectocervix without an intervening bridge of tissue have not been found in the nontraumatized cervix.

APPLICATION OF COLPOSCOPY

Abnormal Papanicolaou Test

The single greatest value of colposcopy is in the patient whose Papanicolaou test is abnormal (i.e., suggestive of dysplasia or worse, or class III or worse), be she pregnant, nonpregnant, postirradiation, or with an infection. With colposcopy it is possible to offer the patient a method of therapy based as much on the extent of the neoplastic epithelium as on the histologic diagnosis. In some cases the lesser forms of dysplasia are vast and are more dangerous than small focal areas of carcinoma in situ. Invariably the preinvasive lesion is found within the transformation zone and with one border at the physiologic squamocolumnar junction (PSC). The lesions stay superficial for many years but eventually develop into invasive cancer.[6,7,16,17,26,27] In over 90 percent of women with abnormal Papanicolaou tests, colposcopy coupled with appropriate biopsies can either confirm or exclude the presence of invasive cancer. When invasive cancer can be excluded without the need for conization, the patient can be treated in the manner most appropriate for her age, desire for childbearing, size of lesion, and histologic diagnosis.[4,13,14,33,35]

Depending on the ability to view the limits of the PSC, patients are triaged into several treatment categories (Fig. 12).

Entire Limits of Physiologic Squamocolumnar Junction (PSC) Seen

If the entire limits of the PSC and the lesion are viewed, it is only necessary to take one to three biopsy specimens from the most colposcopically abnormal appearing area. Endocervical curettage (ECC) is not necessary in these patients since they do not have disease beyond the upper limits of the lesion. However, ECC has been performed routinely in our program for several reasons. First, it permits an expeditious grouping of patients into two major categories based on the presence or absence of neoplastic disease in the curettings. Second, the multifocal concept of cervical neoplasia is an unproved entity and needs to be substantiated or refuted by experience. Third, the early asymptomatic cytologically negative adenocarcinoma may be revealed by routine curettage. Last, patients with a negative curettage are rarely found to have invasive cancer.

Several treatment techniques can be employed in those patients in whom noninvasive disease is present. Outpatient methods include excision biopsy, cryosurgery, and hot cautery. Excision biopsies are used when lesions are 1 cm or less. Once the lesion has been treated, patients are seen every 3 months for 1 year and then every 6 months thereafter with cytology and colposcopy.

Surgery is recommended in the minority of patients with preinvasive cervical neoplasia. Therapeutic conization is used in those patients who refuse outpatient therapy or in individuals who are considered poor follow-up risks. Hysterectomy is restricted to patients who desire sterilization by hysterectomy or who have some other gynecologic problem such as pelvic relaxation, uterine myoma, chronic salpingitis, adenomyosis, etc. A simple vaginal or abdominal hysterectomy is sufficient. A vaginal cuff excision is necessary only when neoplastic tissue extends onto the vagina (less than 5 percent of the time).

Entire Limits of the Lesion Not Seen

In about 10 percent of the patients with an abnormal Papanicolaou test the lesion extends well into the endocervical canal or is present solely within the canal. In these patients a firm and vigorous ECC should be carried out since invasive cancer may be diagnosed by canal sampling. Those patients in whom there is evidence only of dysplasia or carcinoma in situ must undergo diagnostic conization. Depending on the results of the conization further treatment may be necessary. If invasive cancer is found, radical surgery or irradiation is undertaken. When microinvasive cancer is present, a simple hysterectomy is sufficient.

If only preinvasive disease is present and the conization has cleared the lesion, treatment is complete. On the other hand if the cone biopsy has not cleared the lesion, either repeat conization or hysterectomy must be employed. In

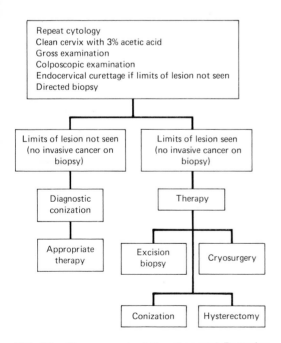

FIG. 12. Management of the abnormal Papanicolaou test.

properly performed conizations this should occur in no more than 5 percent of instances.

In the nonpregnant patient colposcopy has significantly reduced the need for diagnostic conization. In most cases during the reproductive years the entire limits of the lesion can be viewed. In those cases where the lesion does extend into the canal, its upper limits can often be viewed with an endocervical speculum. In patients with an abnormal Papanicolaou test during pregnancy, the most atypical area is seen and sampled. Colposcopy in pregnant patients is more difficult because the colposcopic patterns are exaggerated owing to the increased vascularity of the organ. An additional problem in these patients is an inflammatory component. When redundant vaginal folds prevent adequate visualization the blades of the speculum must be fully extended. Another speculum is placed at a 90-degree angle, and its blades are fully extended. Cervical mucus during pregnancy is quite tenacious and requires gentle teasing to avoid bleeding. Enzymatic powders containing papaya derivatives may be helpful in lysing the mucus. Those patients who have a diffuse punctation due to inflammation should have local therapy for at least 2 to 3 weeks before a final decision is made regarding the most atypical area for sampling. Biopsies during pregnancy are often associated with brisk bleeding, and for this reason we now restrict our biopsies to those patients in whom only carcinoma in situ or early invasive cancer is suspected. When biopsies are taken, a thick Monsel's solution (i.e. ferric subsulfate) is close at hand along with a generous supply of cotton balls. Biopsy sites are immediately cauterized followed promptly by a cotton ball pack, which is left in situ for 15 to 20 minutes.

Following radiotherapy the Papanicolaou test is occasionally abnormal. With colposcopy it is possible to locate the areas of white epithelium due to radiation-induced dysplasia. These areas may be subtle, and the intravaginal application of estrogen cream enhances the contrast between normal and abnormal tissue. Since minimal therapy is required for radiation-induced dysplasia the patients are spared the need for hospitalization and possible traumatic radical surgery. In other cases an early recurrence may be picked up, thereby permitting a more expedient route for further therapy.

Benign Changes

Physicians are often faced with a patient who has a red, "angry" appearing cervix. Colposcopic evaluation in these instances permits an accurate assessment of the red epithelium, assuring both the physician and the patient that a more serious problem is not present. The red, hypertrophied, granular appearance is invariably due to the single-cell columnar epithelium overlying the highly vascular stroma. This appearance is exaggerated in the patient taking birth control pills and may be accentuated when the patient has some type of vaginal infection. Patients with cervical polyps can be assessed by colposcopy. In most cases the base of the polyp can be viewed.

The vaginocervicitis of trichomoniasis often has a classic appearance and be diagnosed readily with colposcopy. Hepatic infections of the cervix have no characteristic appearances, although small vesicles may be seen. The later stages of ulceration may be small, although in some cases it may be so extensive the cervix is totally involved resulting in a picture not too dissimilar from invasive carcinoma.

Vulva

Vulvar disease amenable to colposcopic evaluation includes inflammatory, benign, premalignant, and malignant lesions. Papillomas and condylomas are particularly amenable to colposcopic evaluation. Several young patients were referred to our clinic diagnosed clinically as having condyloma but not biopsied; when viewed colposcopically abnormal epithelial foci were noted, which on biopsy proved to be Bowen's disease.

Vulvar neoplasia is frequently multifocal, and with the colposcope it is possible to locate all foci. In cases where only a single focus is present local therapy is used thereby avoiding disfiguring surgery. The most frequent pattern encountered is white epithelium, which may have a keratin crust. Total excision is necessary whenever the lesions are keratinized. Mosaic structure and punctation are infrequent since the vulva lacks columnar epithelium. Although herpes genitalis has no specific characteristics, evaluation may disclose vesicles, permitting an early initiation of therapy and possibly aborting the full-blown disease.

Vagina

The predominant patterns of the vagina are white epithelium and punctation; however, where there has been columnar tissue in the vagina (particularly at the apex) or in diethylstilbestrol (DES)-exposed offspring, then all the features seen in the transformation zone such as mosaic structure, punctation, leukoplakia, and atypical vessels may be present. It is important in evaluating vaginal intraepithelial lesions that Lugol's solution be used to assist in locating the foci, which may be hidden in vaginal folds.

Diethylstilbestrol-Exposed Offspring

The recent finding of clear cell adenocarcinoma as well as other abnormalities in DES-exposed offspring provide the colposcopist with a fertile field for investigation. To the naked eye it is almost impossible to know the extent of the changes on the vagina and cervix in the DES-exposed individual. With the colposcope it is possible to assess precisely the changes which usually preclude the necessity of multiple punch biopsies, which are mandatory when only a naked eye examination is carried out. Although clear cell adenocarcinoma is relatively rare in DES-exposed offspring, squamous cell lesions are beginning to be seen with alarming frequency. Since these abnormalities are occurring in very young individuals, a colposcopic evaluation becomes mandatory in any DES-exposed offspring who has an abnormal Papanicolaou test.

Invariably a large transformation zone is present since the normal embryologic replacement of columnar tissue by cuboidal epithelium is impaired. The transformation zone usually covers the entire ectocervix and extends on the vagina occasionally down to the introitus. Examples of colposcopic changes encountered in DES-exposed offspring are seen in Figures 13 through 15.

Research and Education

With the aid of the colposcope it is now possible to demonstrate in a logical manner the development of both benign and malignant disease of the cervix, vulva, and vagina. It is particularly satisfying to point out those areas

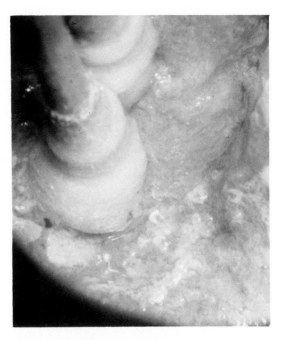

FIG. 13. Colpophotograph of the posterior fornix of a 17-year-old DES-exposed female. Cotton tip applicators are elevating the cervix to point out the irregular surface contour of adenosis. The areas of white epithelium present are metaplastic. Adenosis is found in about 35 to 40 percent of DES-exposed offspring.

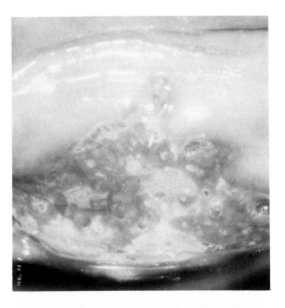

FIG. 14. Colpophotograph of the midvagina in a 23-year-old DES-exposed female showing the distal extent of the adenosis. Numerous gland openings and focal area of adenosis are present.

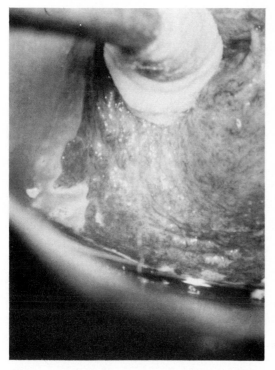

FIG. 15. Colpophotograph of the posterior fornix of a 21-year-old DES-exposed offspring. The cotton tip applicator is elevating the cervix, pointing out the irregular surface contour of adenosis on the posterior fornix. Adenosis and metaplastic squamous epithelium (the epithelium that replaces the adenosis) is found predominantly in the 12 and 6 o'clock positions in the DES-exposed offspring. In this case the very sharp border between metaplastic squamous epithelium and columnar epithelium is present along the left side of the photograph. The original squamous epithelium is seen on the extreme left border of the photograph.

where cervical neoplasia is most likely to occur so that Papanicolaou sampling is more accurate, thereby lowering the rate of false-negative results. In patients where specific tissue sampling is needed for research, one can precisely locate the area and take a small sample without significantly disturbing the cervical architecture or surface epithelium.

Infertility

In selected cases colposcopic inspection of the infertile patient is helpful in determining the cause of postcoital bleeding and has been of assistance in collecting cervical mucus. Whether the use of the instrument has been of significant value in enhancing the possibility of fertility remains to be determined, although it does provide a more thorough assessment of the cervix in the infertile individual.

COMMENT

Currently the availability of colposcopy is limited. Certainly every major teaching hospital and university should be employing this technique for patient care as well as providing a consultation service for the community. The Medical College of Wisconsin has developed an innovative program to make colposcopy available on a consultation basis for the entire state by organizing hospital-based colposcopy clinics in major communities. A similar program is being developed in southern California at several major community hospitals.

Colposcopy is eminently suited to office gynecology, and its utilization is particularly applicable to group practice. However, the interested solo practitioner may also find the instrument useful with sufficient frequency to warrant its acquisition. It is anticipated that the current interest in colposcopy will lead to its widespread use, and that it will finally take its place as an indispensable adjunct to the diagnostic armamentarium of the gynecologist.

REFERENCES

1. Beller FK, Khatamee M: Evaluation of punch biopsy of cervix under direct colposcopic observation (target punch biopsy). Obstet Gynecol 28:622, 1966
2. Coppleson M, Pixley E, Reid B: Colposcopy. Springfield, Ill, Charles C Thomas, 1971
3. Coppleson M, Reid B: Preclinical Carcinoma of the Cervix Uteri. New York, Pergamon Press, 1967
4. Creasman WT, Weed JC, Curry SL, et al: Efficacy of cryosurgical treatment of severe intraepithelial neoplasia. Obstet Gynecol 41:501, 1973
5. Donohue L, Meriwether D: Colposcopy as a diagnostic tool in the investigation of cervical neoplasias. Am J Obstet Gynecol 113:107, 1972
6. Fox CH: Time necessary for conversion of normal to dysplastic cervical epithelium. Obstet Gynecol 31:749, 1968
7. Fox CH: Biologic behavior of dysplasia and carcinoma in situ. Am J Obstet Gynecol 99:960, 1967
8. Gondos B, Townsend DE, Ostergard DR: Cytologic diagnosis of squamous dysplasia and carcinoma of the cervix. Am J Obstet Gynecol 110:107, 1971

9. Graham RM: The Cytologic Diagnosis of Cancer. Philadelphia, Saunders, 1964

10. Hill E: Preclinical cervical carcinoma, colposcopy and the "negative" smear. Am J Obstet Gynecol 95:308, 1966

11. Hinselman H: Verbesserung die inspektionsmöglichkeiten von vulva, vagina und portio. Munch Med Wochenschr 73, 1733. Cited by Coppleson et al.[2]

12. Hollyock VE, Chanen W: The use of the colposcope in the selection of patients for cervical cone biopsy. Am J Obstet Gynecol 114:185, 1972

13. Kaufman RH, Connor JS: Cryosurgical treatment of cervical dysplasia. Am J Obstet Gynecol 109:1167, 1971

14. Kolstad P: Carcinoma of the cervix, stage 0. Am J Obstet Gynecol 96:1098, 1966

15. Kolstad P, Stafl A: Atlas of Colposcopy. Baltimore, University Park Press, 1972

16. Koss LG: Significance of dysplasia. Clin Obstet Gynecol 13:873, 1970

17. Koss LG, Stewart FW, Foote FW, et al: Some histological aspect of behavior of epidermoid carcinoma in situ and related lesions of the uterine cervix—long term prospective study. Cancer 16:1160, 1963

18. Krumholz BA, Knapp RC: Colposcopic selection of biopsy sites. Obstet Gynecol 39:22, 1972

19. Limburg H: Comparison between cytology and colposcopy in the diagnosis of early cervical carcinoma. Am J Obstet Gynecol 75:1298, 1958

20. Navratil E, Burghardt E, Bajardi FWN: Simultaneous colposcopy and cytology used in screening for carcinoma of the cervix. Am J Obstet Gynecol 75:1292, 1958

21. Ortiz R, Newton M: Colposcopy in the management of abnormal cervical smear in pregnancy. JAMA 109:44, 1971

22. Ortiz R, Newton M, Langlois PL: Colposcopic biopsy in the diagnosis of carcinoma of the cervix. Obstet Gynecol 34:303, 1969

23. Ortiz R, Odell L: Observations on the use of the colposcope for cervical neoplasia: lying-in. J Reprod Med 4:97, 1970

24. Ostergard D, Gondos B: Outpatient therapy of preinvasive cervical neoplasia: selection of patients with the use of colposcopy. Am J Obstet Gynecol 115:783, 1973

25. Papanicolaou GN, Traut HF: Diagnosis of Uterine Cancer by the Vaginal Smear. New York, Commonwealth Fund, 1943

26. Richart RM: Influence of diagnostic and therapeutic procedures on the distribution of cervical intraepithelial neoplasia. Cancer 19:1635, 1969

27. Richart RM: Natural history of cervical intraepithelial neoplasia. Clin Obstet Gynecol 10:748, 1967

28. Richart RM: The handling of small tissue samples for pathologic examination. Bull Sloane Hosp 9:113, 1963

29. Richart RM, Vaillant HW: Influence of cell collection techniques upon cytological diagnosis. Cancer 18:1474, 1969

30. Ries E: Erosion, leukoplakia and the colposcope in relation to carcinoma of the cervix. Am J Obstet Gynecol 23:393, 1932

31. Stafl A, Mattingly RF: Colposcopic diagnosis of cervical neoplasia. Obstet Gynecol 41:168, 1973

32. Thompson BH, Woodruff JD, Julian CG, et al: Cytopathology, histopathology and colposcopy in the management of cervical neoplasia. Am J Obstet Gynecol 114:329, 1972

33. Townsend DE, Ostergard DR: Cryocauterization for preinvasive cervical neoplasia. Reprod Med 6:55, 1971

34. Townsend DE, Ostergard DR, Mishell DR Jr, et al: Abnormal Papanicolaou smears: evaluation by colposcopy, biopsies and endocervical curettage. Am J Obstet Gynecol 108:429, 1970

35. Tredway DR, Townsend DE, Hovland DN, et al: Colposcopy and cryosurgery in cervical intraepithelial neoplasia. Am J Obstet Gynecol 114:1020, 1972

36. Villasanta U, Durkan JP: Indications and complications of cold conization of the cervix. Obstet Gynecol 27:717, 1966

37. Way S: The Diagnosis of Early Carcinoma of the Cervix. Boston, Little Brown, 1963

38. Wilds PL: Is colposcopy practical? Obstet Gynecol 20:645, 1962

37

Experience with Fetoscopy and Fetal Blood Drawing

John C. Hobbins
Maurice J. Mahoney

Perhaps the most important contributing factor to recent progress in the field of prenatal genetic diagnosis has been the availability of amniotic fluid through amniocentesis. However, despite these advances the material analyzed reflects the fetal condition indirectly, and investigators in the field have recently sought more precise information by attempting to visualize the fetus and to obtain samples of fetal blood and skin.

In 1956 Mori[5] obtained an extramembranous view of the fetus by inserting a flexible endoscope inside the cervix. In 1971 Kadotani and his group[4] successfully obtained a biopsy of fetal skin with a Vim Silverman needle directed under radiologic image intensification. In 1973 Scrimgeour[7] reported 19 cases in which he visualized the intrauterine cavity via a fiberoptic endoscope 2.2 mm in diameter. An incision was made in the maternal abdomen and a portion of the uterus exposed. The instrument was then inserted into the intrauterine cavity, and a suture was placed in the uterus around the puncture site. After establishing in these patients that it was possible to view the fetus in utero, the procedure was then attempted in an additional six patients who had delivered previous babies with central nervous system abnormalities. The pregnancies were to be allowed to continue depending on the information obtained at endoscopy. In one of the six patients visualization was impossible and the pregnancy was terminated. In four of the women in which the procedure was

performed, three pregnancies were continuing and one patient delivered a normal baby at 38 weeks. In the last patient, although it was difficult to examine the fetus because of its size, spina bifida was not seen on fetoscopic examination. The pregnancy continued until the 34th week of gestation, at which time the patient delivered a baby with a small bifida. In 1972 Valenti[8] first reported his ability to view the fetus at the time of hysterotomy with an endoscope 6 mm in diameter, as well as to obtain a skin biopsy and withdraw fetal blood from a placental vessel and the umbilical cord.

In 1972 we designed a technique to visualize specific fetal areas and to obtain fetal skin biopsies. Because it would be desirable to accomplish this without subjecting the patient to general anesthesia, hospitalization, or major operation, we required an endoscope of extremely small diameter. The instrument we have been using* contains a solid optic lens surrounded by fiberoptic bundles which transmit light, all enclosed within a thin steel shell. The outer diameter is 1.7 mm, and the angle of visualization is 55 degrees in air. The endoscope is contained within an introducing cannula with an outer dimension of 2.2 mm, approximately the diameter of a 14-gauge needle. In our early experience with fetoscopy[3] we were surprised by the ease with which a blood vessel on the posterior placenta could be viewed; so a cannula was designed measuring

Needlescope, Dyonics, Woburn, Mass.

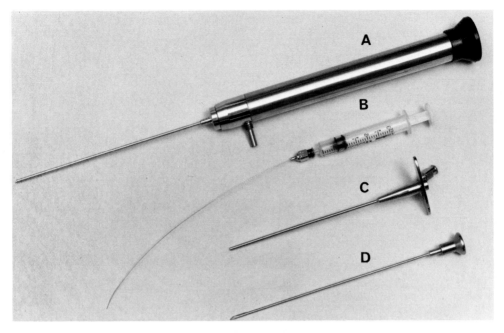

FIG. 1. Needlescope. A, Endoscope. B, Blood-drawing needle. C, Cannula. D, Trocar. (From Hobbins JC, Mahoney MJ: Fetoscopy and fetal blood sampling. The present state of the method. Clin Obstet Gynecol 19, 1976)

2.2 × 2.7 mm which would contain the endoscope and a 27-gauge blood-drawing needle[2] (Fig. 1).

Since our method is heavily dependent upon information obtained by ultrasound prior to and during fetoscopic examination, the procedure is performed in the ultrasound laboratory.

METHODS

The procedure to be described has been performed in patients about to undergo abortion between the 15th and 22nd weeks of gestation. The protocols utilized were approved by the Human Investigation Committee of Yale University School of Medicine, and informed consent was obtained from all volunteers in the study.

The exact positions of the intrauterine contents are determined by preliminary ultrasonic evaluation. The placenta is localized and the margins accurately identified; the fetal back, cranium, and small parts are identified, and a suitable abdominal insertion site is chosen. If the fetal back is to be viewed, an appropriate insertion site is selected over this area. If blood is to be drawn from a blood vessel on the placental surface of a posterior placenta, an abdominal insertion site is chosen over the area

of the fetal extremities. After the patient's skin is infiltrated with a local anesthetic, a cannula and sharp trocar are inserted through the central hole of an ultrasonic transducer,* which lies on the patient's abdomen. The instrument is then advanced into the amniotic cavity. The cannula tip emits an echo clearly perceived on an A-mode oscilloscope pattern; it is separate from other echos produced by the fetus, uterus, and placenta (Fig. 2). Therefore it is possible throughout the procedure to determine the exact position of the cannula tip within the uterus. The trocar is removed and clear fluid obtained if the cavity has been entered cleanly. The endoscope is inserted through the cannula and the contents of the intrauterine cavity then examined.

If a fetal biopsy is to be obtained, an area is chosen on the fetal scalp where scalp hair can be seen in all quadrants of the visual field. At the best optic distance the tip of the scope is no more than a few millimeters from the biopsy site. As the endoscope is removed, the operator is careful to maintain the position of the cannula in relation to the fetal scalp. Biopsy forceps is inserted through the cannula, and aided by the A-mode oscilloscope the forceps is di-

*Needle Aspiration Transducer, Picker Electronics, New Haven, Connecticut.

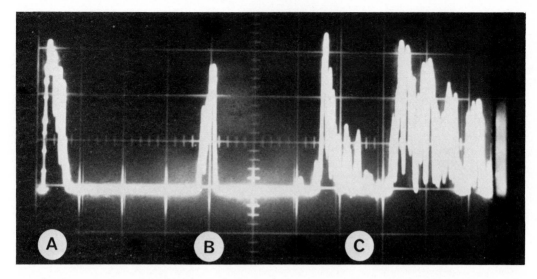

FIG. 2. A-mode display depicting endoscope in middle of amniotic cavity. A, Anterior uterine wall. B, Endoscope. C, Placenta.

rected the remaining few millimeters toward the fetal scalp. A very small scalp sample of fetal skin is obtained, and the sample is placed in cell culture.

If we wish to draw fetal blood from an accessible placenta, the specially designed cannula with a Y sidearm and a channel alongside the endoscope is used. A suitable vessel is selected which courses along the chorionic surface of the placenta; a 27-gauge needle is advanced alongside the endoscope, and under direct visualization the needle is inserted into the placental vessel (Fig. 3). Blood is aspirated

through the syringe attached to the hub of the needle. Another sample of amniotic fluid adjacent to the punctured vessel is obtained as the needle is withdrawn from the placenta. A small polyethylene catheter is placed through the cannula at the end of the procedure, and the cannula is withdrawn. Abortion is initiated by the injection of prostaglandin $f_{2\alpha}$ ($PGF_{2\alpha}$) through the catheter. In 13 patients the abortion was postponed for a period of 14 to 24 hours to observe the short-term effects of the procedure.

RESULTS

We have now successfully gained entry to the uterine cavity and visualized limited areas of the fetal anatomy in 65 of 74 cases (Table 1). The skin biopsies obtained grew well in cell culture, and karyotypes were available within 7 to 10 days.

Of the eight times we failed to gain access to the intraamniotic cavity, we were unable to

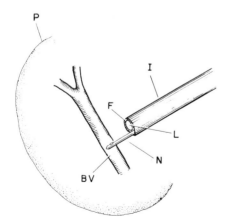

FIG. 3. Distal end of the endoscope with a 27-gauge blood-sampling needle. I, Introducer cannula. F, Fiber optics. L, Viewing lens. N, Needle. BV, Fetal blood vessel. P, Placenta. (From Hobbins and Mahoney[2])

TABLE 1.   Intrauterine Visualization

Procedure	No.
Successful intraamniotic entry	65
Extraovular placement (previous surgery in 4 of 8)	8
Extrauterine placement	1

penetrate the fetal membranes in all but one of the cases. It was clear that the cannula tip was in the intrauterine cavity, but the membranes were actually being advanced into the cavity by the instrument. It is noteworthy that in four of these instances the patients had had previous pelvic surgery with abdominal scarring. In the remaining case where intraamniotic entry was not accomplished there was a delay during the procedure. The patient's bladder filled more quickly than was anticipated, and an inadvertent cystotomy was performed. The fetoscopic procedure was canceled, and the patient had no other complications.

We obtained a suitable sample of fetal blood for hemoglobin synthesis studies in 22 of 25 patients. The only failure (1/20) in a posteriorly located placenta occurred when our needle tip passed alongside the vessel and we were able to sample only maternal blood from the underlying intravillous space. Withdrawal of fetal blood from an anterior placenta was attempted in five patients by inserting the endoscope through the placenta to visualize a vessel on a lateral or fundal extension of this placenta. In two cases we obtained a suitable sample for hemoglobin studies; in another we obtained a mixed sample with 1 percent fetal cells. We were thus successful in three of five cases.

The amniotic fluid specimen adjacent to the punctured vessel very often contains a higher percentage of fetal cells than the placental aspirate. The fetal vessel is quite mobile, and the needle often passes through both walls of the vessel; therefore the placental aspirate has a significant percentage of maternal blood drawn from the intravillous space.

No problems were encountered in the 13 patients in whom we postponed abortion. There was neither bleeding, rupture of membranes, nor unusual uterine activity. Fetal heart tones were present before initiation of abortion in all patients. One patient experienced abdominal discomfort immediately after the endoscopic procedure, but this abated after 20 minutes.

Fetal blood loss has been calculated in each of 16 patients by estimating the total amount of fetal blood (via a fetal red cell count) in a small sample of amniotic fluid and adding that volume to the amount aspirated into the syringe at the time of the procedure. The total fetal blood loss varied from 0.2 to 2.5 ml. As indicated in Table 2, most fetuses lost no more than 1 ml of blood. The percentage of fetal blood loss was calculated by a method based on fetal weight, which includes the volume of fetal blood in the placenta.[6] The percentage loss varied between 0.5 percent (a 0.2-ml blood loss in a 190-g fetus at 18 weeks' gestation) and 15 percent (representing a 1.6-ml blood loss in a 65-g fetus at 15 weeks' gestation). In the majority of cases the fetal blood volume was depleted by less than 5 percent.

DISCUSSION

Many problems have been encountered in the development and utilization of this method for intrauterine visualization. Perhaps the greatest difficulty to overcome are the limitations of the instrumentation. Because of the nature of the procedure it is essential to use an instrument of extremely small diameter, but with present instrumentation this limitation of endoscope thickness imposes significant magnification problems and thereby greatly reduces the field of vision. It is very difficult to examine completely specific areas of the fetus. We have been unable, for instance, to scan the entire spine visually. Therefore it would be impossible to exclude a diagnosis of spina bifida in a fetus at risk for this condition.

The fetal membranes are often difficult to penetrate. They are loosely attached to the underlying decidua; and if penetration cannot be accomplished with the first thrust of the trocar and cannula, it is often impossible to enter the intraamniotic cavity on that day. Sometimes the membranes close off whole areas from visualization. In the eight cases where it was impossible to gain intraamniotic entry, it was

TABLE 2. Fetal Blood Loss

No. of Fetuses	Calculated Volume Lost (ml)	No. of Fetuses	Percent of Fetal Blood Volume
Range of loss	0.2–2.5	Range of loss	0.5–15
10/16	<1.0	12/16	<5
4/16	1.0–1.5	3/16	5–10
2/16	>1.5	1/16	15

apparent ultrasonically that the cannula tip was in the middle of the intrauterine cavity, but the membranes were being pushed forward by the endoscope. This problem has been alleviated somewhat by making the trocar extremely sharp, but this phenomenon will always plague those attempting fetoscopy.

It has been extremely valuable to choose an abdominal insertion site from ultrasonic information in order to accomplish the desired aim of the procedure. For instance, if we wish to obtain fetal blood from a posterior placenta, we must direct the instrument to the desired area before the fetus moves and visualization is impaired by a portion of the fetal anatomy. The fetus is less mobile in a vertex presentation than in a breech position or a transverse lie.

It is often difficult to examine the genitalia, cord insertion, or facial structures because of the flexed position of the fetus, but this is more easily accomplished with the fetus in the transverse lie. It has been possible to move the fetus into a desirable position by utilizing gravity and a variety of positioning maneuvers with the mother.

In drawing fetal blood there is concern about the effect on fetal homeostasis and development by acute depletion of the fetal blood volume. It could be expected that any detrimental effect would depend on the amount of blood lost from the fetal circulation. As indicated, one 15-week fetus was deprived of 15 percent of its blood volume. This may well represent potential insult. In all but two cases the loss was below 10 percent. We have observed the blood to clot within seconds of the vessel puncture. This may be due to thromboplastic properties of amniotic fluid, histamine release from underlying tissue, or other factors. In any case, we are now performing the procedure at 18 weeks' gestation in continuing pregnancies. At this stage of pregnancy the amniotic fluid is very clear (the fluid later becomes more opaque), and 1 cc of fetal blood represents no more than a 4 percent deficit to the fetal blood volume. It has been possible, as reported,[1] to study globin chain synthesis with the fetal blood obtained. With this information it is potentially possible to identify a fetus with sickle cell disease and α- or β-thalassemia. The possibilities of diagnosing many other diseases will be even greater, however, once pure fetal blood can be obtained more consistently. In addition, the availability of a small volume of blood may become very important for monitoring the adequacy and safety of treating a fetus in utero.

It has been demonstrated by investigation in intrauterine visualization and sampling of fetal blood that it is technically feasible to obtain more direct information about the fetus during early pregnancy. Attention is now being directed to the dangers of these procedures to the fetus and to a continuing pregnancy. This work is already in progress. There is a strong indication that with increasing sophistication of ultrasonic instrumentation an invasive procedure to view the fetus may be unnecessary. The potential use of fetal blood in the diagnosis of hemoglobinopathies and other inherited and acquired diseases, however, certainly warrants further investigation.

REFERENCES

1.   Chang H, Hobbins JC, Cividalli G, et al: In utero diagnosis of hemoglobinopathies: hemoglobin synthesis in fetal red cells. N Engl J Med 290:1067, 1974
2.   Hobbins JC, Mahoney MJ: In utero diagnosis of hemoglobinopathies: technic for obtaining fetal blood. N Engl J Med 290:1065, 1974
3.   Hobbins JC, Mahoney MJ, Goldstein LA: New method of intrauterine evaluation by the combined use of fetoscopy and ultrasound. Am J Obstet Gynecol 118:1069, 1974
4.   Kadotani T, Sato H, Oama K, et al: A technical note on the antenatal chromosome analysis by transabdominal fetal skin biopsy. Jap J Hum Genet 16:42, 1971
5.   Mori C: A study on the intrauterine selfmovement of early human fetus by hysteroscopy and its recording on the film. Jap J Obstet Gynecol 3:4, 1956
6.   Morris JA, Hustead RF, Robinson RG, et al: Measurement of fetoplacental blood volume in the human previable fetus. Am J Obstet Gynecol 118:927, 1974
7.   Scrimgeour JB: Other techniques for antenatal diagnosis. In Emery AEH (ed): Antenatal Diagnosis of Genetic Disease. Edinburgh, Churchill Livingstone, 1973, pp 49–52
8.   Valenti C: Endoamnioscopy and fetal biopsy: a new technique. Am J Obstet Gynecol 114:561, 1973

38

Hysteroscopy

Hans Joachim Lindemann

Hysteroscopy, also called metroscopy or uteruscopy, was introduced to discover intrauterine pathology first by Pantaleoni in 1869.[36,37] His first patient was a 60-year-old woman with recurring bleeding in whom he discovered a mucous polyp. The instrument was an open tube with proximal illumination developed by Desorméaux in 1865[5] for inspecting the urinary bladder. Only after introduction of the cystoscope by Nitze[31] in 1877 did a larger interest in hysteroscopy develop. After invention of the electric globe and introduction of the telescope in conjunction with the examining instrument inside the cavity, as well as the installation of optical lenses into the apparatus, the endoscopic technique became possible as it is known to us today.

Reports from physicians from many countries about their work during the past 100 years have encouraged the development of the diagnostic technique—improving the instruments as well as increasing the number of fields to be examined. The outgrowth of hysteroscopy is reflected in the works of several authors.[2–4, 9–12,14,25,27, 32,35,40,41,43,50] They all utilized endoscopes similar to the cystoscope, and used water as the distention and visibility medium for the cavum uteri.

In 1957 Norment[33] reported a new method. He inserted a hysteroscope with a rubber balloon attached to its tip into the cavum uteri and consequently filled it with air. Silander[45,46] modified this technique in 1962 by filling the balloon with water instead of air. The annoying bleeding from the endometrium which impaired one's vision was eliminated because of the resultant pressure of the balloon against the cavity walls. Schmidt-Matthiesen[42] still spoke about this balloon technique in 1966. However, the method was once again abandoned in favor of liquid. In 1966 Agüero et al.[1] reported on the application of hysteroscopy during pregnancy in the 8th to 40th weeks in order to observe pathologic intrauterine situations. This indication, however, was then not pursued any further. The same year Maleschki[23] publicized a new method for hysteroscopy. He reported that using a flat mirror which, by means of an optical system reflects an image to the exterior, he was able to observe small segments of the womb and hence recognize the cycle phase. In 1968 Menken[24] reported using Luviskol, a polyphenylpyrrolidone solution instead of water as a distention and visibility medium. In 1970 Edström and Fernström[8] gave their first findings using a dextran solution. This method and those of Quinones[38] (who used a 5 percent glucose solution) and Lindemann[18,22] (i.e., the published hysteroscopic CO_2 method), being the most recent advances, are described in the subsequent sections of this chapter.

HYSTEROSCOPY

Endoscopic examination of the uterine cavity allows the gynecologist to observe the endometrium, ostium, and anatomic appearance (Figs. 1–6, Plate E*). One may examine both the normal and the bleeding uterus as well as recognize parts of the retained placenta after

All color plates appear at the front of the book.

493

abortion, polypous growth, submucous fibroids, carcinoma, and malformations. Probing the uterus to determine its size, shape, or pathologic and/or anatomic changes was the method of choice. In addition, hysterography and today hysteroscopy offer further information. Clarification of intrauterine pathology no longer depends on a blind technique or on a probe being introduced. The endoscopic examination permits, under visual control, target biopsy of suspicious tissues of the uterine cavity that would have been unnoticed by a probe, hysterography, and curettage. In the case of recurring metrorrhagia, curettage, even repeated several times, still does not provide a satisfactory histologic answer. Hysteroscopy provides additional valuable data. On many occasions the gynecologist unsuccessfully scrapes around the source of bleeding. Pathologic areas can be removed only after their location has been determined. Early carcinoma of the corpus can be discovered by visualization and can then be histologically confirmed.

Hysteroscopy is useful in the diagnosis and therapy of intrauterine infertility. Such changes as polypous growths of the endometrium (which may block the ostium), fibroids (which act like an intrauterine pessar), smoothly embedded submucous fibroids, and synechia (the cause for implantation difficulties) can be seen and diagnosed with ease. The endoscopic view enables treatment or, rather, removal of pathologic changes by means of target abrasions, biopsies, or electrosurgery.

It should be pointed out also that there is increased application of the hysteroscope for transuterine tubal sterilization. This minor procedure can be carried out in a few minutes under a local anesthesia as an outpatient procedure and will play a more dominant role in the future. It is a safe operation provided the surgeon has mastered the technique and will eventually replace other techniques like laparotomy or those done through the laparoculdoscope.

TECHNIQUE

A clear view into the uterus necessitates distending the cavity to achieve sufficient space between the endoscope and the endometrium. The oldest method consists of filling the cavity with water, a technique still practiced by Mohri[26,28] and Sugimoto and Nishimura.[47] Similar to cystoscopy, water is instilled into the uterus from a container located 95 cm above the patient. The result is distention of the uterus with a pressure of 35 mm Hg. When the cavity pressure exceeds 55 mm Hg, water flows through the tubes into the abdominal cavity. The distention facilitates endoscopic observation, but on the other hand the fluid can escape into the peritoneum causing irritation. The major disadvantage of this method lies in the fact that one's vision is impaired, sometimes totally, when there is bleeding from the endometrium. This is one of the reasons hysteroscopy has not become more popular.

Viscous solution replaced water later in the development of this technique. Quinones[38] utilized a 5 percent glucose solution to obtain sufficient distention as well as improved vision. This fluid is instilled into the uterus with an approximate pressure of 100 mm Hg. However, bleeding frequently still prevents a clear view. The glucose solution finds its way also into the abdominal cavity. Apparently no complications have been described when employing glucose.

In recent years a 32 percent dextran solution has been recommended by Edström and Fernström[8] and Joelsson et al.,[15,16] and was adopted by Neuwirth et al.[29,30] About 50 ml of dextran solution is necessary to instill into the cavum. The disadvantage of impaired vision occurs less frequently because dextran does not mix with blood in such highly concentrated solution. The blood, in the form of red drops, floats in the viscous, but the liquid remains clear. Although dextran provides better visibility, its viscosity has certain disadvantages. The solution does not run out of the cavum uteri easily, necessitating that the uterus be rinsed with glucose, saline, or water. In addition, unless the instruments are not immediately rinsed and cleaned, they could be damaged.

I have employed CO_2 pneumometra since 1970[18,19,21,22] as medium both for distention and to create visibility. The pneumometra, necessary for endoscopy of the uterus, is established by inflow of CO_2 gas, 40 to 80 ml/minute, with a cavity pressure of 40 to 100 mm Hg. The amount of gas necessary is individual, depending on the size of the uterine cavity, consistency of the myometrium, diameter of the tubes, as well as the gas escape into the peritoneum. A hysteroscope adaptor[22] should be used to prevent this escape of gas. By means of the guide sheath of the adaptor, the hystero-

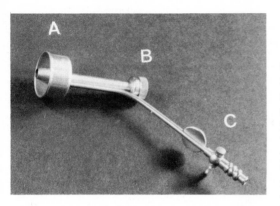

FIG. 7. Hysteroscope adapter. **A**, Vacuum suction cup. **B**, Valve of the channel for the hysteroscope sheath. **C**, Channel for use of negative pressure (vacuum).

scope can be inserted into the cavum uteri as deeply as required. A suction cup at the tip of the guide sheath is attached to suction and to the cervix to ensure a satisfactory seal (Fig. 7). The Hysteroflator* (Fig. 8) insufflates the gas under a constant pressure of 200 mm Hg. The volume can be varied individually, depending on the size of the uterus as well as the size and patency of the tubes. A permanent pneumometra for hysteroscopy is provided. An electronic device measures and records the amount of insufflated CO_2 constantly. Gas flow is limited to a maximum of 100 ml/minute. With this apparatus we avoid complications that occur with other types of insufflators, e.g., excessive pneumoperitoneum, cardiac arrhythmias. The excellent visibility is due to creation of a gas cushion instead of a water curtain mixed with blood.

ENDOSCOPES

The author believes that the forward-oblique Hopkins-Storz telescope† with a diameter of 4 mm is most suitable. The design of the hysteroscope sheath allows insufflation of CO_2, and an instrument channel allows the use of a probe, biopsy forceps, electrocoagulator, or dye injection under visual control (Fig. 9). The outside diameter of the hysteroscope including telescope is 7 mm.

PROCEDURE

Several hysteroscopic techniques were mentioned above. The only difference among them is the distending medium. All such agents must be introduced into the cavity under pressure in order to maintain the "bottle neck" pressure created by the narrowing at the ostium to retain the distention. This bottle neck pressure is created by the stagnation of flow of the distending medium inside the uterine cavity (the uterus is the bottle and the tubes are the neck). A certain distance should be kept between the working end of the telescope and the uterine wall in order to secure optimal vision. The patient is placed on the operating table in the lithotomy position. After the usual preparation of the vagina, a bimanual examination is carried out. The anesthesia may be general or local. We prefer the paracervical blockade with 7 ml of a 1 percent Scandicain* or 1 percent Xylonest solution† on each side. Dilatation of the cervical canal to Hegar 7 is the next step and should be carried out carefully. The dilator tip is inserted only over the internal os in order to prevent contact with the fundus of the uterus; otherwise artificial bleeding can occur.

The hysteroscope is inserted into the uterus with the hysteroscope adaptor. Be aware that the tip of the hysteroscope should not touch the lining of the cavity and should project just over the internal os. The suction cup of the hysteroscope adaptor is applied to the cervix with a suction of approximately 400 mm Hg, ensuring a tight seal to avoid escape of CO_2. The light source is connected via a fiberoptic cable to the hysteroscope, and the CO_2 insufflator linked with a tube to the sheath. Check that all locks and stopcocks of the hysteroscope sheath and the adaptor are closed. If the system is not fully sealed, it is difficult to achieve a pneumometra.

We start with a 40 ml/minute insufflation. Under observation it can be seen how the uterine cavity, normally a flat cleft, gradually unfolds. If the flow is not enough, it can be increased but should not exceed 100 ml/minute. Most examinations require a volume of 40 to 60 ml/minute. The bottle neck pressure varies from 40 to 80 mm Hg. If the tubes are closed,

F. M. Wiest KG, Reichpietschufer 20, 1 Berlin 30, West Germany.
†Manufacturer: K. Storz, Endoscopy Co., 7200 Tuttlingen, P.O. Box 400, West Germany.

M. Woelm Co., Max-Woelm-Strasse, 3440 Eschwege, P.O. Box 840, West Germany.
†AB Astra, Södertälje, Sweden.

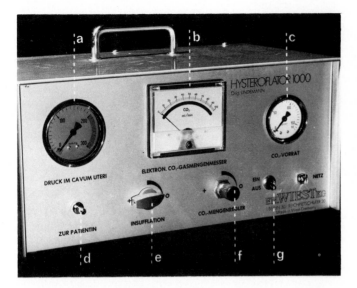

FIG. 8. CO_2 insufflation apparatus, Hysteroflator 1000. **a,** Manometer to measure intrauterine pressure. **b,** Electronic CO_2 volume gauge monitor. **c,** Manometer to control CO_2 cylinder. **d,** CO_2 connection to patient. **e,** Switch for gas insufflation. **f,** CO_2 gas regulator. **g,** Electric on-off switch.

intramurally or in the abdomen, the gas flow decreases. At this point the insufflation of gas is automatically stopped.

The most suitable time for this examination is during the early proliferation phase. During this period one encounters little if any secretions, and bleeding from the endometrium is minimal. If it is performed in another cycle time, bubbles originating from insufflation of the gas into the mucus or blood may impede visibility. With experience one can readily recognize that both mucus and blood are removed through the tubes by means of the gas inflow. A clear view of the inside of the uterus is obtained. Any pathologic anatomic changes are seen with ease, because the endometrium is not yet highly developed. Polyps, flat embedded submucous fibroids, and other anomalies can be differentiated. A 2- to 3-minute period of observation is sufficient to acquire enough information about the condition in the uterine cavity. The insufflated CO_2 in the abdominal cavity is well tolerated by the patient. If pain in the shoulders should occur, similar to those from symptoms after pertubations, it disappears within a short time.

TISSUE SAMPLING

Insufficient Information with Curettage

With the optical biopsy forceps a sample can be removed from any suspicious appearing tissue for histology under accurate visual control.

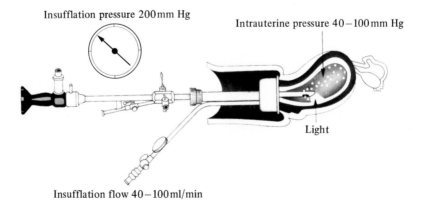

Insufflation pressure 200 mm Hg

Intrauterine pressure 40–100 mm Hg

Light

Insufflation flow 40–100 ml/min

FIG. 9. Hopkins-Storz hysteroscope. Telescope with sheath introduced in uterine cavity.

It is possible to discover small pathologic changes that would have been overlooked using the blind curettage technique.

Noninformative Hysterosalpingography

Small carcinomas, submucous fibroids, or small bleeders are not always detected by hysterosalpingography. During 980 random hysteroscopies, we discovered evidence of pathologic changes in 27.5 percent of an arbitrary sampling (Table 1).

TABLE 1. Hysteroscopic Results of 980 Patients

Diagnosis	No.
Corpus carcinoma	3
Uterus arcuatus	5
Uterus bicornis unicollis	3
Uterus subseptus	10
Synechiae	30
Fibromas	49
Polyps	81
Polypous endometrium	89
Total	270 (27.5%)

Infertility–Sterility

In searching for the causes of infertility and sterility, the hysteroscopic findings are of great help. Among 110 infertile patients, we were able to find intrauterine pathology in 60.4 percent. In most of these cases a pathologic cavity would not have been diagnosed by either curettage or hysterosalpingography (Table 2).

TABLE 2. Hysteroscopic Results of 110 Infertility Patients

Diagnosis	No.
Uterus arcuatus	3
Uterus subseptus	3
Uterus bicornis	3
Fibromas	4
Synechiae	13
Polypous endometrium	22
Polyps	23
Total	71 (60.4%)

Hysteroscopy plus Laparoscopy

The use of hysteroscopy in conjunction with laparoscopy is advantageous; both intrauterine and pelvic pathology can be discovered in one session. Generally we apply both methods simultaneously in infertility cases to examine the appearance of the ovaries, the condition of the tubes with reference to their motility, the effect of adhesions, and the patency using simultaneous chromopertubation. With a transuterine catheter probe introduced under laparoscopic control, an occlusion of the tubes in the intramural part may be recognized and/or excluded. The hysteroscope in this application is also used as a uterus elevator and for instillation of dye material.

Therapy

The removal of synechiae and pedunculated submucous fibroids can be effected.

Sterilization

Transuterine tubal coagulation in the intramural part can be performed by this technique. Sterilization is accomplished by inserting an electroprobe into the intramural part of the tube to a depth of 5 mm. The probe [17,20] has a 1 mm diameter and a coagulation surface 5 mm in length (Fig. 10). An insulation cap, 1.5 mm long, is attached at the tip to prevent overheating of the wall or adjacent organs. Coagulation is applied with a high-frequency current, and the temperature that reaches the tissue is 80 to 90 C. When the tissue surrounding the ostium has become white, sufficient damage of the endothelium and muscle layer of the tube has been achieved to ensure scarring and closure of the ostium. A separate coagulation probe is used for each tube; otherwise carbonized tissue accumulates on the surface of the probe and functions as an insulating cover. Possible failures in which only one tube has been successfully coagulated are prevented in this manner.

A scarred closure of the ostium develops approximately 12 weeks after this procedure. So far, results of all applied methods indicate a success rate of 92 percent during a follow-up period of 3 months to 2.5 years.

COMPLICATIONS

Complications have not been reported in the literature. However, through personal communication Sugimoto[48] mentioned one perfora-

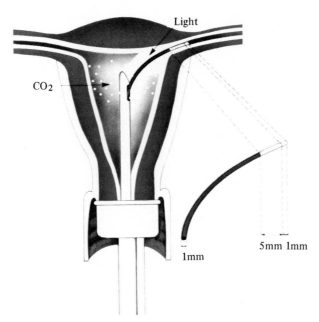

FIG. 10. Coagulation probe introduced under visual control for sterilization.

tion of the bowel. We have had two perforations of the uterus among 1,600 hysteroscopies. In one of these cases coagulation resulted in necrosis and perforation of the small intestine. In the other case the perforated tube was the only sequela of the procedure. These complications could have been prevented with proper precautions. In two cases clinical symptoms of pelvic peritonitis were observed but subsided with conservative treatment. The procedure should never be performed on one side only, followed by the other a few weeks later. Both sides should be done at the same time to avoid bacterial migration and pelvic peritonitis. The current survey indicates that hysteroscopy seems to result in fewer complications than hysterosalpingography.[44]

In a few cases CO_2 complications were observed (e.g., cardiac arrhythmias and even cardiac arrest) probably due to acidosis. In each case too much gas, up to 1,000 ml/minute had been insufflated and possibly entered the bloodstream. Inadequate insufflation apparatus was used. All these patients recovered without further consequence. To gather data about CO_2 administration we undertook blood gas measurements (pH, P_{CO_2}, P_{O_2}) during 55 hysteroscopies. We extended the observation time to 20 minutes and found no significant changes in the blood gases in these patients. There was

also no difference if the procedure was done under local or general anesthesia. The amount of CO_2 that can be absorbed depends on: (1) P_{CO_2}; (2) pH; (3) oxygen saturation of the hemoglobin; (4) temperature; and (5) blood flow per minute. According to the experiments of Hoeffken[13] we know that humans can tolerate additional CO_2—in a concentration up to 62 ml CO_2 per 100 ml blood.

In our animal experiments we tried to determine the relationship of varying concentrations of CO_2 and the ensuing complications. In a group of 20 German shepherds various amounts of CO_2 were injected for 15 minutes into the vena femoralis under a pressure of 200 mm Hg. The following measurements were made in all animals: (1) arterial blood pressure; (2) arterial blood pH, P_{CO_2}, P_{O_2}; (3) electrocardiographic (ECG) changes; (4) heart rate; and (5) respiratory rate. Clinical symptoms were also observed.

We noted that up to a flow rate of 200 ml/minute for 10 minutes there were no significant changes in the blood gases, blood pressure, or ECG and no other symptoms. After this time we observed changes in these values. A flow rate of 400 ml/minute or more caused an increase in the heart rate as well as deeper respirations. There were also changes in the ECG: extrasystoles and a depression of the ST

TABLE 3. Influence of I.V. CO_2 Insufflation in Dogs on pH, Pco_2, Po_2, Respiration, and Heart Rate

Time of Examination (minutes after beginning insufflation)	pH	Pco_2	Po_2	Respiration (breaths/min)	Heart Rate (beats/min)*
Dose: 100 ml/min					
Before	7.48	29.7	102.1	36	168
3	7.46	33.2	100.0	28	160
5	7.45	32.7	100.1	26	161
7	7.43	31.3	97.0	32	152
9	7.44	30.9	94.1	32	152
11	7.43	30.9	92.9	32	148
13	7.45	30.5	93.0	32	152
15	7.43	30.1	93.3	28	150
Dose: 120 ml/min					
Before	7.46	32.2	98.0	36	160
3	7.44	37.9	95.5	28	148
5	7.43	27.2	117.7	28	160
7	7.44	30.3	98.4	32	142
9	7.42	29.2	94.5	32	142
11	7.43	33.9	94.2	30	150
13	7.43	34.7	94.5	32	142
15	7.44	33.0	97.8	30	152

There were no electrocardiographic abnormalities in any of the dogs.

TABLE 4. Influence of I.V. CO_2 Insufflation in Dogs on pH, Pco_2, Po_2, Respiration, and Heart Rate

Time of Examination (minutes after beginning insufflation)	pH	Pco_2	Po_2	Respiration (breaths/min)	Heart Rate (beats/min)	ECG*
Dose: 200 ml/min						
Before	7.45	25.3	96.3	78	152	0
Before	7.46	27.2	103.2	78	152	0
3	7.42	33.4	107.8	78	152	0
5	7.42	33.1	102.2	92	156	0
7	7.42	31.7	100.7	76	160	0
9	7.42	32.2	96.9	72	168	0
11	7.42	31.0	100.8	76	160	0
13	7.42	32.3	96.9	60	172	0
15	7.43	32.5	98.8	60	172	0
Dose: 400 ml/min						
Before	7.45	30.5	100.3	94	200	†
3	7.44	33.9	103.2	54	250	†
5	7.44	28.1	100.2	52	192	†
7	7.45	32.2	96.2	56	262	†
Dose: 1,000 ml/min‡						
9	7.43	30.1	132.4	60	230	†
11	7.26	44.6	92.6	40	168	†
13	7.22	60.5	64.1	0	60	†
15	7.16	63.6	58.8	0	23	†
18	Exitus					

0, without pathologic results.
†See text.
‡A dose of 1,000 ml/min was insufflated during the 9- to 11-minute period.

segment. The P_{CO_2} level in arterial blood increased, the P_{O_2} decreased, and the pH changed to produce a slight acidosis. Clinical symptoms (tachycardia, tachypnea, and restlessness) were produced. The blood pressure and pupillary reflex remained nearly the same. Increasing the CO_2 injection up to 1,000 ml/minute for 2 minutes resulted in bradycardia, increased P_{CO_2}, sharply decreased P_{O_2}, and a pH change toward acidosis. Four minutes after CO_2 injection the reflexes were extremely diminished and apnea occurred. The blood pressure dropped from 100 mm Hg to 50 mm Hg and lower. The ECG showed arrhythmia and bundle branch block of the right heart (Tables 3 and 4).

At present we can say that the threshold dose of toxic reactions is about 400 ml/minute for dogs. The lethal dosage was 400 to 1,000 ml/minute. Death occurred after a latency period of about 60 seconds. Autopsy performed immediately after death showed no signs of a CO_2 embolus. The main reason for these symptoms is the acidosis created by the too-high gas flow rate (insufflated gas quantity per minute).

To prove the safety of any gas to be injected intravenously, it must be demonstrated that the entire amount could be tolerated if it were shunted from the right to the left heart through a septal defect. Therefore we injected CO_2 directly into the carotid artery of another group of German shepherds. The flow rate was 100 ml/minute under a pressure of 200 mm Hg. No significant clinical symptoms to indicate embolism were detected. We can confirm the experimental work of Oppenheimer et al.,[34] Durant et al.,[7] Stauffer et al.,[49] and Hoeffken et al.[13] who also did animal experiments to prove the safety of CO_2.

If we are to transfer these observations to humans we must take the smaller blood volume of the dogs and compare it with humans to determine the limits of comparability. The tolerated quantity of CO_2 is directly proportional to the cardiac output. Only when a greater volume of CO_2 gas per minute is used can complications be expected; problems can be avoided if appropriate volume and pressure are applied.

We must assume that a CO_2 hysteroscopy using the above-mentioned insufflation values is safe. Rubin,[39] reporting collective figures from 380 authors, noted that there were no CO_2 complications among 80,000 tubal pertubations.

CONTRAINDICATIONS

Hysteroscopy should not be carried out in the presence of purulent endometritis, infected pelvic inflammatory disease, heavy bleeding from the uterine cavity, or pregnancy.

SUMMARY

After a history of more than a hundred years, hysteroscopy has progressed so far as to gain an important place among the various examination techniques. Direct visual inspection of the uterine cavity enables the examiner to carry out diagnostic and therapeutic measures on this organ. In most cases it is superior to previous blind techniques like curettage. Our experience of 1,600 hysteroscopies resulted in only two complications and no mortality.

The technique also allows transuterine sterilization by means of coagulation of the tubes, which can be accomplished as an office procedure. The favorable comparison with laparoscopy and culdoscopy under identical indications are discussed.

REFERENCES

1. Agüero OMD, Aure M, Lopez R: Hysteroscopy in pregnant patients—a new diagnostic tool. Am J Obstet Gynecol 94:925, 1966
2. Bánk EB: Erfahrungen mit der Metroskopie. Zentralbl Gynaekol 82:23, 1960
3. Bumm E: Verh Dtsch Ges Gynaek 6:524, 1895
4. David Ch: L'endoscopic Uterine (Hysteroscopie) Applications au Diagnostic et au Traitement des Affections Intrauterines. Paris, G. Jaques, 1908
5. Desorméaux AJ: De l'Endoscope et des ses Applications au Diagnostic et au Traitement des Affections de l'Urethre et de la Vessie. Paris, Bailliére, 1865
6. Dickinson RJ: Simple sterilization of women by cautery stricture at the intrauterine tubal openings, compared with other methods. Surg Gynecol Obstet 23:204, 1916
7. Durant TM: Body position in relation to venous air embolism: roentgenologic study. Am J Med Sci 227:509, 1954
8. Edström K, Fernström J: The diagnostic possibilities of a modified hysteroscopic technique. Acta Obstet Gynecol Scand 49:327, 1970
9. Englund S, Ingelmann-Sundberg A, Westin B: Hysteroscopy in diagnosis and treatment of uterine bleeding. Gynaecologia 143:217, 1957
10. Gauss CJ: Hysteroskopie. Arch Gynaekol 133:18, 1928

11. Haselhorst L: Our experience with the hysteroscope. Zentralbl Gynaekol 59:2442, 1935
12. Heineberg A: Uterine endoscopy; an aid to precision in the diagnosis of intra-uterine disease, a preliminary report, with the presentation of a new uteroscope. Surg Gynecol Obstet 513, 1914
13. Hoeffken W: Fortschr Roentgenstr 86:292, 1957
14. Hyams MM: Sterilization of the female by coagulation of the uterine cornu. Trans Am Assoc Obstet Gynecol Abdom Surg 47:263, 1934
15. Joelsson I: Experience Using Dextran in Hysteroscopic Sterilization. Intercontinental Medical Book Corp, New York
16. Joelsson I, Levine RU, Moberger G, et al: Hysteroscopy as an adjunct in determining the extent of carcinoma of the endometrium. Am J Obstet Gynecol 111:696, 1971
17. Lindemann HJ: Hysteroscopic sterilization using carbon dioxide. In: Hysteroscopic Sterilization. Intercontinental Medical Book Corp, New York
18. Lindemann HJ: Historical aspects of hysteroscopy. Fertil Steril 24:230 1973
19. Lindemann HJ: Pneumometra für die Hysteroskopie. Geburtschilfe Frauenheilkd 33:18, 1973
20. Lindemann HJ: Transuterine Tubensterilisation per Hysteroskop. Geburtshilfe Frauenheilkd 33:709, 1973
21. Lindemann HJ: The use of CO_2 in the uterine cavity for hysteroscopy. Int J Fertil 17:221, 1972
22. Lindemann HJ: Eine neue Untersuchungsmethode für die Hysteroskopie. Endoscopy 4:3, 1971
23. Maleschki V: Die moderne Zervikoskopie und Hysteroskopie. Abl Gynaekol 88:20, 1966
24. Menken FC: Ein neues Verfahren mit Vorrichtung zur Hysteroskopie. Endoscopy 3:200, 1971
25. Mikulicz-Radecki F von, Freund A: Ein neues Hysteroskop und seine praktische Anwendung in der Gynäkologie. Z Geburtshilfe Gynaekol 92:13, 1927
26. Mohri T: V. Kongress der Deutschen Gessellschaft für Endoskopie in Erlangen, 10.–12. März 1972. In: Research of Tubaloscopy. Schattauer Verlag, Stuttgart
27. Mohri T, Mohri C (Japanese): World Gynecol Obstet 6:48, 1954
28. Mohri T, Mohri C (Japanese): Gynecol Obstet 20:26, 1953
29. Neuwirth RS: Results of a pilot program. In: Hysteroscopic Sterilization. New York, Intercontinental Medical Book Corp
30. Neuwirth RS, Levine RU, Richart RM, et al: Hysteroscopic tubal sterilization. Am J Obstet Gynecol 116:82, 1973
31. Nitze M: Beobachtungs und Untersuchungsmethode für Harnrohre Harnblase und Rectum. Wien Med Wochenschr 24:651, 1879 (Platin)
32. Norment WB: Improved instruments for diagnosis of lesions by hysterogram and water hysteroscope. NC Med J 10:646, 1949
33. Norment WB: Hysteroscope in diagnosis of pathologic conditions of uterine canal. JAMA 148:917, 1952
34. Oppenheimer MJ, Durant TM, Stauffer AM, et al: In vivo visualization of intracardiac structures with gaseous carbon dioxide; cardiovascular-respiratory effects and associated changes in blood chemistry. Am J Physiol 186:325, 1956
35. Palmer MR: Un Nouvel Hysteroscope. Presented at the Société de Gynécologie et Obstetrique de Paris meeting, June 1957
36. Pantaleoni D: Med Press (Lond) 8:26, 1869
37. Pantaleoni D: Cited by Silander[45]
38. Quinones R: Tubal catheterization: applications of a new technique. Am J Obstet Gynecol 114:5, 1972
39. Rubin JC: Utero-tubal Insufflation. St. Louis, Mosby, 1947
40. Rubin JC: Uterine endoscopy, endometroscopy with the aid of uterine insufflation. Am J Obstet Gynecol 10:313, 1925
41. Schack L: Unsere Erfahrungen mit der Hysteroskopie. Zentralbl Gynaekol 60:1810, 1936
42. Schmidt-Matthiesen H: Die Hysteroskopie als klinische Routinemethode. Geburtshilfe Frauenheilkd 26:1489, 1966
43. Schroder C: Über den Ausbau und die Leistungen der Hysteroskopie. Arch Gynaekol 156:407, 1934
44. Schultze GK, Erbslöh F: Gynäkologische Röntgendiagnostik. Stuttgart, Enke, 1954
45. Silander T: Hysteroscopy through a transparent rubber balloon in patients with carcinoma of the uterine endometrium. Surg Gynecol Obstet 114:125, 1962; Acta Obstet Gynecol Scand 42:284, 1963
46. Silander T: Hysteroscopy through a transparent rubber balloon. Surg Gynecol Obstet 114:125, 1962
47. Sugimoto O, Nishimura I: Hysteroscopic studies on female infertility due to intrauterine abnormalities. In: VII World Congress on Fertility and Sterility, Tokyo, October 1971. Amsterdam, Excerpta Medica, 1973
48. Sugimoto O: Personal communication, 1973
49. Stauffer HM, Durant TM, Oppenheimer MJ: Gas embolism: roentgenologic considerations, including experimental use of carbon dioxide as intracardiac contrast material. Radiology 66:686, 1956
50. Wulfsohn NL: A hysteroscope. J Obstet Gynaecol Br Emp 65:657, 1958

EDITORIAL COMMENT

At the Second European Congress of Endoscopy in 1975 two investigators (Semm and Beiler) reported 22 percent unilateral and 38 percent bilateral patent tubes and 32 percent unilateral and 9 percent bilateral open tubes after a follow-up of 3 months posthysteroscopic tubal sterilization with salpingography. These figures seemed to be a bit on the high side, and therefore the efficiency of the method must be carefully reevaluated. From the viewpoint of effectiveness, the late results of laparoscopic sterilization are much better.

It is possible that hysteroscopy is still a valuable procedure in certain cases of uterine pathology, biopsy under visual control, etc., but the sterilization aspects must be scrutinized before it is further urged for general use.

THE EDITOR

39

Laparoscopy in Diagnostic Gynecology

Hans Frangenheim

Gynecologic laparoscopy was preceded by gastroenterologic laparoscopy, and until 1944 their development was similar. It is amazing that the procedure was not adopted in gynecologic practice, since Kalk[44] in 1928 in Germany and Ruddock[42] in 1930 in the United States emphasized the value of laparoscopy for the diagnosis of unclear lower abdominal tumors. The development of culdoscopy by Te Linde[52] in 1939 and above all by Decker[6,7] in 1944 indicated that endoscopic methods might contribute to the diagnosis and therapy of gynecologic disorders. Palmer[36] in 1944 started to modify the gastroenterologic technique of laparoscopy for gynecologic demands, especially for diagnosis and therapy of sterility. He gave the final push for the integration of laparoscopy into gynecologic surgery.

The idea was taken up in Germany by Frangenheim[11,12,13] in 1954, in Italy by Albano and Cittadini[1] in 1962, and in England by Steptoe[50] in 1967. These educational centers started in loose cooperation to outline indications and contraindications. This experience was followed by the improvement of technique and instruments, and the development of additional equipment. Another area of progress during the late 1950s was the elaboration of operative laparoscopy, especially tubal sterilization, which first was mentioned by Anderson in 1937[2,39] and was finally made clinically practicable by Palmer and Frangenheim.

The final breakthrough of laparoscopy came with the introduction of cold-light endoscopy. The general interest for laparoscopy was manifested by numerous national and international

congresses,[40,44] beginning in 1964 and continuing to the present. These meetings showed the current standing of knowledge and development. In addition, the interested gynecologist was able to learn of recent developments in diagnostic and operative laparoscopy from various publications.

Because of linguistic barriers the basic publications comprising the development and progress of laparoscopy during the 1950s and 1960s did not cross the borders of the Old Continent. The monographs of Albano and Cittadini,[1] Cognat,[4] Frangenheim,[12] Gorga,[19] Menken,[29,30] Palmer,[33] Steptoe,[50] and Thoyer-Rozat;[53] Semm[45] the congress papers of the Palermo Symposium;[40] and recent publications of Cohen[5] and Clyman[3] may satisfy the interested reader. They outline the consequent development of a diagnostic method—laparoscopy—which to many gynecologists appears revolutionary.

INDICATIONS

No other discipline shows more possibilities for making use of laparoscopy than gynecology, and no other discipline has profited more from laparoscopy for its basic diagnostic procedures. During the past two decades critical evaluation of the method led to a variety of diagnostic and operative indications.[1,4,12,26,34,50,53] In many countries during these years the main application of laparoscopy steadily turned from the diagnostic to the operative field. Today in many parts of the world the major indication for laparoscopy is tubal sterilization (Fig. 1, Plate F).*

The indications for diagnostic laparoscopy include:

1. Evaluation of primary and secondary sterility; differential diagnosis of hormonal disturbances; suspected malformations of genital organs
2. Differential diagnosis of ectopic pregnancy
3. Differential diagnosis of adnexal tumors, particularly in menopause
4. Chronic pelvic neuralgic disease
5. Acute lower abdomen of unknown etiology
6. Suspected endometriosis
7. Suspected genital tuberculosis
8. Surgical indications
9. Pediatric indications

Indications for operative laparoscopy include:

1. Tubal sterilization (interval and post partum)
2. Aspiration of ovarian cysts
3. Biopsy or resection of ovarian tissue
4. Division of adhesions
5. Cauterization of endometriosis
6. Biopsy in suspected carcinoma or tuberculosis
7. Resection of sacrouterine ligaments
8. Ventrosuspension of the uterus
9. Liver biopsy

DIAGNOSTIC LAPAROSCOPY

Sterility

Steptoe's chapter in this volume is dedicated to the serious and extensive problems of sterility. There a number of fundamental publications concerning laparoscopy in ovarian dysfunction or endocrine disturbances (Fig. 2, Plate F) and particularly tubal sterility, many of which come from the French.[28,31,34,41,47,51]

Ectopic Pregnancy

In clinically obvious situations the diagnosis of an ectopic pregnancy generally is confirmed by puncture of the cul-de-sac. In rare cases of suspected intact ectopic pregnancy, early abortion with transuterine complications or large corpus luteum cysts with hemorrhage must be excluded. In these cases laparoscopy reveals about 40 percent of ectopic pregnancies with completely uncharacteristic history. As many authors emphasize, up to 60 percent of these are intact or old ectopic pregnancies. As a con-

*All color plates appear at the front of the book.

sequence, *since the introduction of laparoscopy the number of diagnosed and operated intact ectopic pregnancies is three times as high as before the laparoscopic era.* Under optimal conditions about 25 percent of ectopic pregnancies can be operated at an early stage, before they rupture and extensive blood loss increases the surgical risk (Fig. 3, Plate F).[12,21,23,31,53,54] In a review of the literature, 7 to 8 percent of intact ectopic pregnancies were found surgically (without laparoscopy) and 34 percent were found via laparoscopy.

Differential Diagnosis of Adnexal Tumors

The differential diagnosis of obscured adnexal tumors or masses is another important indication for laparoscopy. Even today too many patients undergo surgery. A considerable number of major operative procedures could be replaced by laparoscopy, with or without operative intervention. Preoperative laparoscopy should be done with the patient prepared for surgery in the case of a genital tumor, especially in the menopausal woman. In these women the differential diagnosis of myoma, ovarian tumor, or carcinoma of the sigmoid colon is sometimes difficult. We believe that laparotomy is indicated in obscured cases. Laparoscopy is preferable as a first measure since many of the patients present in a poor general condition, suffering from underlying diseases such as hypertension, cardiac failure, obesity, diabetes, etc. (Table 1).

TABLE 1. Differential Diagnosis for Operative Laparoscopy for Adnexal Tumors in 350 Menopausal Women

Diagnosis	%
No operation required	60.4
Operation suggested in two-thirds of cases: benign tumors	32.1
Transferred to surgery	7.5
Total	100

In more than half of the cases a benign tumor (e.g., myoma or ovarian fibroma) is found, and the patient avoids an unnecessary operation. One-third of the women have to be explored because of carcinoma or macroscopically unclear ovarian tumors. In cases where laparotomy is not advisable, evaluation of the dubious situation by ovarian puncture and aspiration is recommended. The material as well as the aspirate from the pouch of Douglas should be examined cytologically to exclude perforated carcinoma. Carcinoma of the colon is found in about 8 percent of the women, and they are then transferred to a surgeon's care.

Chronic Pelvic Neuralgia

Chronic lower abdominal pain that fails to respond to treatment or cases of chronic inflammatory processes without precise palpatory findings are major indications for laparoscopy. A careful psychiatric history is taken before laparoscopy to exclude psychologic factors. In 80 percent laparoscopy reveals nonpalpable pathology of the genital organs. Early endometriotic lesions or spastic, shortened, or fibrotic sacrouterine ligaments can explain the painful lifting of the portio as well as pain during intercourse. Often a hyperemia of the peritoneum shows the macroscopic appearance of "pelvic congestion."

In chronic constipation the sigmoid colon is fixed to the adnexal organs after old or chronic perisigmoiditis. Curtain or cordlike adhesions may cover large portions of the adnexal organs and eventually cause partial bowel obstruction. Other findings include hydatid cysts, hydrosalpinx, strangulated paraovarian cysts, or adhesions, which according to the filling stage of the colon with its peristaltic movements strangulate one organ or another.

Many findings can be treated definitively by operative laparoscopy. A considerable number of the patients have had lower abdominal discomfort for years. Sometimes when the information obtained after laparoscopy—that there is no etiology or that only minor changes were found—is explained to the patient a final cure is the result.

Acute Lower Abdomen

The differential diagnosis of acute or chronic lower abdominal disease is often difficult in light of the indication for explorative laparotomy. Performing a laparoscopy for the differential diagnosis of appendicitis, adnexitis, or ovarian abscess is easy. It helps also in suspected strangulation of ovarian tumors or suspected partial intestinal obstruction with an uncharacteristic course. In acute inflammatory disease such as pelvic or general peritonitis the diagnosis is rarely difficult, and therefore it is unnecessary to scope the patient. However, when a serious inflammation of the abdomen is unexpectedly found by laparoscopy, aggravation of the situation should not be anticipated. We recommend this examination in acute adnexitis because in case of a pyosalpinx surgical treatment might be preferable to prolonged conservative therapy. In acute ovarian abscess the treatment of choice is surgical revision immediately after laparoscopy, in the acute state. The postoperative course of an explored abscess shows considerably fewer complications than are seen with conservative treatment.[16,43,48]

Endometriosis

Laparoscopy is rarely required in cases of strongly suspected extended endometriosis. Smaller endometriotic lesions are frequently discovered as accidental findings in sterility diagnosis or when searching for the causes of chronic lower abdominal discomfort.

Genital Tuberculosis

The extent of genital tuberculosis varies considerably. It is discovered primarily as an accidental finding in sterility diagnosis. As long as there is an "inner tubal tuberculosis" (epitheloid cell tuberculosis), macroscopic diagnosis is doubtful. Miliary, peritoneal, or caseous adnexal tuberculosis is easy to diagnose.

To determine whether the process is cured, biopsies are required for histologic studies. The biopsy from smaller tuberculotic nodes is technically no problem. Biopsies from the fimbriated end of the tubes require careful manipulation because of the risk of excessive bleeding.[1,34]

Surgical Indications

The major surgical indication for laparoscopy is the differential diagnosis of appendicitis and adnexitis. This is also true for the numerous cases of so-called chronic adnexitis, which often manifests as neurovegetative pain.

A number of doubtful operations are performed because of suspected adhesions. About 40 percent of our sterility patients have had previous highly questionable operations.

Other entities where laparoscopy may help the surgeon are blunt abdominal trauma with suspected rupture of the liver or spleen, other intraabdominal hemorrhage, as well as suspected delayed posttraumatic hemorrhage.[8,14,16,17] Experienced laparoscopists can recognize inflammatory or malignant tumors involving the peritoneum or other intraabdominal organs.

The palpation rod introduced through an accessory trocar can be useful to inspect changes on the wall of the bowel, retraction or shrinking of tissue, or fixation of certain organs. The efficiency of laparoscopy in the diagnosis of acute pancreatitis is limited. On the other hand it can be valuable for staging a malignancy. If metastases are present unnecessary exploratory laparotomy can be avoided.

Pediatrics

Pediatric applications mainly consist of medical or surgical indications, and in gynecology for the evaluation of genital malformations (Figs. 4, 5, Plate F). This aspect is dealt with in detail in Chapter 31.

OPERATIVE LAPAROSCOPY

Tubal Sterilization

There are a great variety of possible operative interventions performed during laparoscopy. However, only a limited number of publications are available that report a large experience in this field.[3,4,9,34,55]

The only exception is tubal sterilization, which has become the major indication for operative laparoscopy. During the late 1950s this method was made available for clinical use by Palmer and ourselves. It was first recommended by Anderson[2] in the American literature.

Postpartum Sterilization

A large number of reports[9,34,39] concern experience with interval tubal sterilization. Postpartum sterilization is still debatable. The specific anatomic situation after delivery may render laparoscopy most difficult (e.g., a large, flabby uterus) makes it difficult to visualize the adnexal organs clearly, to manipulate at a safe distance from other organs, or to coagulate without a large risk. The tortuous, varicose, enlarged blood vessels of the mesosalpinx and the often extremely stretched and thin abdominal wall can cause technical difficulties (Fig. 6, Plate F).

Over a period of several years the following procedure proved efficient. It is performed on the fourth or fifth day after delivery. The patient receives an infusion containing uterus-contracting agents. The intrauterine probe is not always inserted, to avoid rupture of the episiotomy. If mobilization of the uterus is required a large curette is inserted into the uterus. All other probes disappear in the vast uterine cavity and may easily perforate the wall of the uterus.

Pneumoperitoneum should be performed with a moderate excess in pressure in order to accomplish a sufficient CO_2 cushion between the thin abdominal wall and the intraabdominal organs. Before inserting the trocar the abdominal wall should be lifted higher than usual. The trocar then safely reaches the space between the uterus and abdominal wall without injury to the uterine fundus. Insertion of the second trocar in the lower midline (borderline of pubic hair) must be done under careful visual control through the laparoscope. The patient is put in reverse (45-degree) Trendelenburg position, whereby the bowel falls backward toward the diaphragm.

During the postpartum period we prefer to perform only extended cauterization of the tubes, eventually on different sites. Division of the tubes is hazardous since there may be severe hemorrhage from the mesosalpinx. The incision is closed by sutures because of the thin skin and to prevent prolapse of the omentum.

Aspiration of Ovarian Cysts

Ovarian cysts are among the most common genital tumors, and a number of them are operated without proper indication. A better proposition is to puncture the capsule and aspirate it during laparoscopy. The aspirated fluid should be sent for cytologic study.[5a,31,32]

Most of the functional cysts do not refill. About 60 percent of the patients can avoid laparotomy. Exploration is necessary in cases of pseudomucinous cystoma, dermoid cyst, or suspected ovarian carcinoma. Depending on the arrangements with the patient in indicated cases, surgery can follow the endoscopic procedure.

During aspiration of cysts some serous content may be spilled into the peritoneal cavity. The question of spreading malignant cells then arises.[14·16·17·20·31] We never saw any detrimental consequences after aspiration of ovarian cysts. In some cases an early stage cancer was discovered by cytologic study while macroscopically the ovary seemed completely normal.

Biopsy and Resection of Ovarian Tissue

If ovarian cancer is suspected, sufficient tissue must be removed by means of the biopsy forceps. Sufficient tissue from both cortex and medulla must be recovered in cases of hormonal disturbances such as Stein-Leventhal syndrome or micromacropolycystic degeneration of the ovary. The recommended instrument for this purpose is the combined cauterization-biopsy forceps of Palmer. An incision of the capsule to a depth of 5 mm into the medulla with an electric knife in Stein-Leventhal syndrome produces the same outcome as a wedge resection. Incision of the capsule enhances the effect of those hormones soliciting ovulation. The effectiveness of the operation is limited to a period of 2 years.

Division of Adhesions

A division of adhesions should be performed only if a definite therapeutic success is expected. Curtainlike adhesions are most likely seen in sterility or in patients with chronic pelvic pain. Often a blunt dissection may be achieved by just moving the laparoscope. Other adhesions can be divided with the electric knife or forceps. After cauterization and transection, attention must be paid to bleeding. Division of adhesions also helps to avoid laparotomy—if we believe that adhesions can cause pain or discomfort at all.

Biopsy in Suspected Carcinoma or Tuberculosis

There is no difficulty in taking a biopsy from questionable tuberculotic nodes. Massive hemorrhage may arise, however, after biopsies from the fimbriated end of the tubes in cases of tubal tuberculosis. This bleeding can be arrested only by laparotomy, and so we do not recommend this procedure.

Large biopsies may be taken in the case of a suspected carcinoma for histologic study, differentiation of extended carcinoma, or evaluation of the effect of chemotherapy. In disseminated, inoperable ovarian cancer, laparoscopy should be performed rather than laparotomy. If in the case of inoperable carcinoma a perforation of adherent bowel can be anticipated due to laparoscopy, it can be avoided in the following ways.

A small circular incision is made around the distal part of the umbilicus through all layers. The palpating finger is inserted to determine if the intestine is adherent to the abdominal wall. If not, a purse-string suture is placed around the incised peritoneum, the trocar inserted, the suture tied around the instrument, and the abdomen closed in layers. The pneumoperitoneum is insufflated through the inserted trocar, and laparoscopy is performed as usual.[27]

Cauterization of Endometriotic Lesions

Cauterization of small endometriotic lesions produced better results than (hormonal) progestin therapy. Progestin only inactivates the lesions, which remain responsive to further hormonal stimulation. Only cauterization causes complete elimination of the lesion.

Resection of Sacrouterine Ligaments

So-called spastic-fibrotic sacrouterine ligaments may be divided with the electric knife in selected cases of chronic pelvic neuralgic pain, dysmenorrhea, or dyspareunia. This often causes long-lasting remissions. The procedure is recommended only if the patient is also prepared for immediate surgery. Because of the close proximity of large blood vessels there is a relatively high risk of severe hemorrhage. Large endometriotic foci situated on the sacrouterine ligaments can cause similar clinical symptoms. In this case extensive cauterization of the ligaments is preferable to resection.

Ventrosuspension

The clinical value of ventrosuspension is controversial. The supporters of laparoscopic ventrosuspension of the uterus claim that this is a lesser operation compared to other types of treatment and produces the same result. An accessory trocar is inserted in the right (or the left) midline of the abdomen. An advanced forceps grasps the middle portion of the round ligament, which is pulled through the abdominal fascia and sutured to it.

Liver Biopsy

Inspection of the liver surface should be routine. If pathologic changes are found, biopsy is recommended. This area should be dealt with only if the laparoscopist feels confident and is experienced.

Instruments for Operative Laparoscopy

Operative laparoscopy stimulated the development of a large variety of accessory instruments: cauterization forceps, cauterization-biopsy forceps, cauterization knife, scissors, probes, atraumatic forceps to grasp and mobilize organs, metallic loop for the cauterization and resection of the tubes, catgut and prolene loops for ligation of the tubes or to arrest bleeders, a scope that makes it possible to place tantalum clips around the tubes, etc. In addition, the use of electrosurgery requires perfect insulation of the additional instruments.

Technical Problems of Operative Laparoscopy

Operative laparoscopy has several problems that must be dealt with:

1. Choice of anesthesia.
2. Pneumoperitoneum. The insufflation set should have a built-in "quick flow" regulator to allow rapid insufflation.
3. Selecting a site for introducing a second trocar for additional instrumentation. There is no general rule. Transillumination of the abdominal walls helps to avoid large blood vessels. Insertion of the trocar in the midline at the border of the pubic hair (for cosmetic reasons) has proved practical and beneficial. In order to avoid bladder injury we insert the trocar cranially and obliquely through the abdominal wall. In the rare case of ventrosuspension or if another instrument is necessary, the incision can be made 4 cm laterally from the midline and 2 to 3 cm above the pubic hair (Fig. 7).
4. In operative laparoscopy there is a competition between interventions through a surgical laparoscope (single-puncture instrument) or through a second incision. Manipulation through a single-puncture laparoscope is more subtle and delicate and so are the instruments. Cauterization of

the tubes for sterilization is a more difficult task. Quite a number of pregnancies following sterilization performed through this single-puncture laparoscope have been reported. Another disadvantage is reduction of the visual field by the inserted additional instrument. Respiration can cause rhythmic movement of the entire instrument, making it difficult to reach the target organs. Manipulation of the accessory instruments is limited owing to the fact that they must move with the telescope, being inserted in one sheath. The single-puncture laparoscope is not recommended to the inexperienced laparoscopist. Manipulation of instruments inserted through a second incision is not restricted and is much easier and therefore less risky to the patient.

Contraindications

There is no defined absolute contraindication. This subject has been revised several times during the past years. There are, however, relative contraindications:

1. Intestinal obstruction with distention
2. Acute pancreatitis
3. Several scars due to previous explorations (adhesions)
4. Hernia (diaphragmatic, umbilical, large inguinal)
5. Late stage carcinomas, huge or extended abdominal tumors
6. Severe cardiac, circulatory, or respiratory insufficiency
7. Extreme obesity
8. Pregnancy after the 30th week

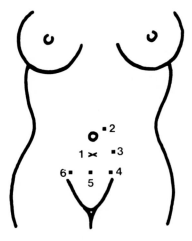

FIG. 7. Sites of incision for laparoscopy and for operative interventions through accessory (instrument) trocar. 1, Site of incision for the trocar 4 cm below the umbilicus. 2, Site of incision for the insufflation needle. 3, Another site of incision for insufflation or the trocar. 4, 5, and 6, Other sites for additional instruments in the midline, respectively, 4 to 5 cm lateral to the midline. 4 and 6, Sites selected by transillumination of the abdominal wall.

9. Limited technical ability and experience of the examiner

In my opinion there is only one absolute contraindication: if the condition of the patient is so poor that the anesthesiologist is hesitant or not willing to administer anesthesia. A situation in which only a neophyte is available to perform the laparoscopy without an anesthesiologist at hand and without the possibility of resorting to surgery if necessary should also be declared a relative contraindication.

Complications

Several complications are typical, and there are a number that are possible. They can be grouped as complications that arise with the preparation of the patient, with the technical performance, and with additional operative procedures (in the form of late complications).

Complications occur most frequently with insufflation of the pneumoperitoneum, insertion of the trocar, and operative interventions, especially when electrosurgery is used. Some complications (e.g., emphysema) are transitory, whereas others (e.g., persistent hemorrhage due to puncture of blood vessels or intestinal perforation because of some unexpected adhesions) can be treated only by laparotomy. This is also true for complications due to electrocauterization. Some of the complications may be fatal: perforation of the aorta, peritonitis after intestinal perforation, late hemorrhage, and cardiac or circulatory failure. In some countries such fatalities delayed acceptance of laparoscopy for a long time. So far no reliable data are available about type, number, and frequency of complications. We have tried repeatedly to deal with this complex question and have elaborated a list of proposals on how to prevent complications.

The Complications Committee of the American Association of Gynecological Laparoscopists (AAGL) compiled two series of elaborate questionnaires. These resulted in the first major statistics about complications and fatal incidents from this procedure (Table 2).[22,25,35,38,49]

There is no doubt that the reduction of mortality during the past 2 years (Table 2) is due to better education and more thorough training of the gynecologists. The frequency of minor complications remains the same since most are complications of the learning period.

TABLE 2. Type and Frequency of Complications

Parameter	1972		1973	
	No.	%	No.	%
Total laparoscopies	12,182	—	31,000	—
Diagnostic laparoscopies	5,000	—	10,000	—
Tubal sterilizations	7,182	—	21,000	—
Minor complications	130	10	?	—
Major complications	72	6	147	6
Mortality	3	0.3	8	0.15

Apart from the AAGL reports, we collected (personal information from different surgeons) 60 fatalities which occurred at laparoscopy during 1970-74:

Perforation of the iliac vein or artery, aorta, or vena cava	18
Intestinal perforation (necrosis post cauterization) with subsequent peritonitis	5
Anesthesia (death)	6
Gas embolism	3
Shock using electrosurgery (fibrillation?)	2
Postoperative or delayed hemorrhage	4
Not defined	3
Unknown etiology (Siegler, personal communication)	19

In comparison we compiled data of our clinic from 1954 until 1973. It includes the percentage of complications from 4,799 laparoscopies:

Mortality	0%
Transitional emphysema absorbed at the end of the procedure	4%
Minor hemorrhage from small blood vessels arrested and not requiring laparotomy	5%
Severe emphysema requiring termination of laparoscopy	0.2%
Perforation (bowel, stomach, cysts)	0.1%
Bleeding from puncture site with subsequent hematoma	1%
Cardiac and circulatory failure	1%
Exploration required	0.1%

The increasing number of operative laparoscopies did not increase the number of complications in our clinic. In the above statistics the number of fatalities show that the risk of laparoscopy almost approaches the risk of laparotomy or of major vaginal operations. In any case, most complications occurred during the physician's learning period.

Certain precautions help prevent them: appropriate training, limiting the performance of laparoscopy to qualified operators in large hospitals, proper choice of indications, attention paid to the safety rules.

It is true that laparoscopy, like any operation, is associated with certain risks. One aspect must be kept in mind: by performing laparoscopy, many laparotomies or vaginal operations can be avoided, and the indications for exploration confirmed in an earlier stage of the disease.

TECHNIQUE OF LAPAROSCOPY

It took us years of diligent work to rationalize and improve the technique of laparoscopy, and to reduce the necessary personnel and equipment to a minimum. We feel that the technique of gynecologic laparoscopy is not very much different from other laparoscopic procedures, but there are a few problems which should be discussed.

General Aspects

Laparoscopy should be performed only in an operating room that is also equipped to handle an emergency laparotomy. The set of instruments consists of various scopes and their trocars. Depending on the indication there are instruments with different diameters and directions of view (0 degrees or straightforward, 30 or 130 degrees forward oblique, 90 degrees or lateral, close-up, and photooptic), as well as a single-puncture surgical laparoscope. It is important to have an insufflation machine for the pneumoperitoneum.

The instrument set should be completed by additional tools for mobilizing the uterus (intrauterine probes, portioadapters, suction cannulas, etc.); instruments for operative interventions or mobilization of organs; those for the use of electrosurgery, coagulation, and cutting; low-voltage cauterization tools; pertubation apparatus to check tubal patency; and the anesthesia machine. The performance of all instruments should be tested prior to each operation.

Site of Insertion for Pneumoneedle and Laparoscope-Trocar

After long and extensive trials one transumbilical approach for insertion of both pneu-

moneedle and laparoscope-trocar proved to be the best and the easiest way. According to the situation, however, the laparoscopist must be aware of other sites as well. For example, he may be forced to choose another place of insertion for the pneumoperitoneum and the trocar—e.g., insertion of the insufflation needle 2 cm above the umbilicus to the left or in the lower third of Richter-Monro's line between the umbilicus and superior iliac spine (site for ascites puncture) in the case of space-occupying lesions or adhesions in or near the midline.

The gastroenterologist prefers to insert the laparoscope above the umbilicus to the right or left side. As a matter of fact the gynecologist may choose the same place or, even better, a site 4 cm below the umbilicus in the midline (Fig. 8). A Z-shaped (zigzag) penetration of the abdominal wall, layer by layer, is recommended by Semm.[46] This is meant to prevent abdominal herniation, which, however, was never described in the literature or seen in practice. In our opinion this is a needless safety measure based on purely theoretical grounds. It may even be dangerous (Fig. 9) because there is a high risk of damaging one of the great blood vessels.

Choice of Gas

Selection of the most suitable gas for pneumoperitoneum has been also the subject of

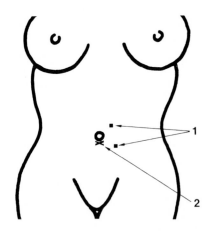

FIG. 8. Sites of incision for insufflation and insertion of the trocar. 1, Gastroenterology. Separate incisions. Two fingers below the umbilicus to the left: site for insufflation of the pneumoperitoneum. Two fingers above the umbilicus to the left: site for the laparoscope. 2, Gynecology. Combined site for the insertion needle and laparoscope through a sagittal incision at the distal part of the umbilicus.

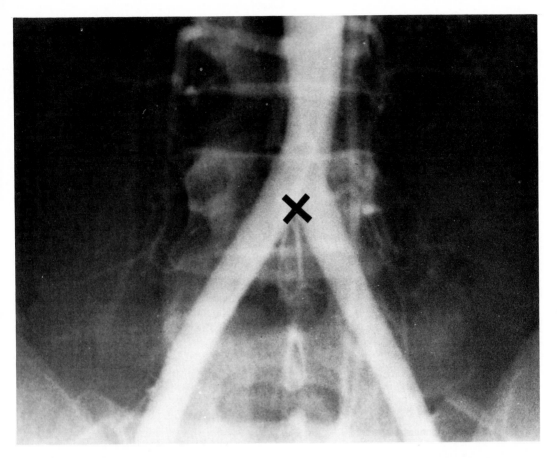

FIG. 9. Arteriography. The bifurcation of the aorta is seen below the umbilicus. It can be injured by a too-vertical insertion of the Verres needle or the laparoscopic trocar through the umbilicus. A Z-shape introduction of the trocar (a safety rule of the so-called pelviscopy) increases the risk of injuring blood vessels. For the less experienced operator a midline incision 3 to 4 cm below the umbilicus decreases the respective risks.

debates for several years. Available to us were room air, oxygen, nitrogen, nitrous oxide (N_2O), and carbon dioxide (CO_2). CO_2 is used most commonly. It has the fastest rate of absorption, causes no discomfort to the patient under general anesthesia, and offers the highest degree of safety with operative interventions where high-frequency electrosurgery is applied. Electric sparks might be the cause of explosions. The later point was deciding for CO_2. Instead of the unipolar procedure, however, there is now a tendency to substitute high-frequency electrosurgery to bipolar one with its much lower current requirement, or direct heat coagulation. Thus the main point for CO_2 is lost. It is generally known that the compatibility and the rate of absorption of N_2O is almost equal to that of CO_2. If laparoscopy is

done with local anesthesia, N_2O causes less discomfort to the patient. CO_2 is converted in the peritoneal fluid into H_2CO_3, which can cause some peritoneal irritation. As a consequence the patient becomes restless and starts to press. Other gases are less absorbant and could irritate the phrenic nerve and cause longer-lasting pain in the back.

The long experience of the gastroenterologists shows that in the days when no insufflation machine or gas for pneumoperitoneum were available, even room air was suitable for laparoscopy. This fact should be recognized, especially in countries which do not necessarily dispose of all technical equipment; it may also be considered in case of some defective equipment when there is a need to continue with older or more primitive methods.

Special gas insufflating machines have been constructed, almost all of which work on the same basic principle. It is recommended that machines with which the rate of insufflation is limited to a maximum of 1 liter/minute not be purchased. According to the changing needs of the operator a variable insufflation rate up to 3 liters/minute is desirable—not only to avoid wasting time during insufflation but also for use in difficult situations or complications and for varying the insufflation rate to achieve a slight excess in pressure, e.g., in postpartum sterilization. An automatic refilling system satisfies a certain demand for convenience without being able to guarantee absolute safety. Experienced surgeons prefer having the option of individual dosage. According to Semm, 10 to 12 mm Hg is the ideal intra-peritoneal pressure and should not be ex-ceeded. Of course clinical judgment, symmetri-cal distention of the abdomen, percussion, the patient's general condition (pulse rate, skin color, respiration, etc.) are of equal importance.

Steps of Performance

1. Preparation of the patient, adjustment of her po-sition on the operating table
2. Selection of anesthesia
3. Insufflation of the pneumoperitoneum
4. Procedure (laparoscopy)
5. Postoperative care

Preparation of the Patient. Prepa-ration consists of a gynecologic and physical examination. The latter is done by the anes-thesiologist. Generally but not always an enema is given before the premedication is administered. The patient is placed on the operating table, catheterized, and the anes-thesia started. Extreme elevation of the pelvis is necessary in a few situations, and only for short moments; longer times in this position result in cardiac and circulatory stress, fre-quently causing arrhythmia. A 15-degree Trendelenburg position is almost always sufficient.

Anesthesia. One of the most elemen-tary prerequisites for good diagnostic and operative laparoscopy, with minimal risk, is the appropriate selection of anesthesia. In gen-eral, there is no single exclusive anesthesia for different situations or for a different popu-lation. Principally there are two alternatives: local (or regional) and general anesthesia. Many pros and cons have been discussed in the same hospital where gynecologists perform laparoscopy using general anesthesia and gas-troenterologists local anesthesia, with the fol-lowing conclusion: All the above-mentioned anesthesia methods can be applied, but there are many factors influencing the choice. The individual sensitivity or threshold of the pa-tient to pain, the patient's age, and her general condition and/or underlying diseases—and therefore the resulting risks. Other factors are the particular indication, the personal skill and schedule of the operator, the length and kind of intervention (diagnostic or operative laparos-copy), the length of hospitalization, and finally the presence of an anesthesiologist.

If there is an anesthesiology department in the hospital the anesthesiologist should decide on the kind of anesthesia, according to his per-sonal experience, in consultation with the gy-necologist. It is the anesthesiologist who takes this responsibility, although it is partially shared by the gynecologist; of course the gynecologist is entirely responsible when no anesthesiologist is present or an anesthesiology technician performs the anesthesia. In practice, the following procedure has proved best. At-ropine and Thalamonal* are given for premedi-cation. For the induction of the anesthesia Brevimythal† is given, followed by fluothane inhalation anesthesia. Intubation is reserved for high-risk cases. Local or regional anes-thesia has not proved satisfactory for gyneco-logic laparoscopy. Even insertion of the intra-uterine probe is painful. Manipulation through accessory (operating) instruments causes peritoneal irritation, and the patient becomes restless.

Using the same technique the gastroen-terologist performs most laparoscopies under local anesthesia with good results. The main reasons for avoiding general anesthesia if pos-sible include the possibility of hepatic damage due to the anesthesia, high-risk patients, etc. These criteria are not rigid, and in certain types of patients intubation is still the method of choice. Depending on the differences among individuals and their reactions to pain, even gynecologic laparoscopy can be performed with local anesthesia as advocated by Wheeless.[55] The experience of our anesthesiologists who

---

*Dehydrobenzperidol plus fentanyl. Manufactured by Janssen Pharmaceutica I, Beerse I, Belgium.
†Manufactured by Eli Lilly, G.m.b.H 63 Giessen, Teichweg 3, West Germany.

surveyed all laparoscopies showed that the amount of narcotics for premedication, sedation, and local anesthesia was equal in terms of dosage to that used for general anesthesia. Each physician must decide on the type of anesthesia according to the local situation, the patient, the clinical picture, and the technical ability of the operator.

There is no doubt about the immense value of an anesthesiologist with good laparoscopic experience to both patient and surgeon. A well trained anesthesiologist recognizes many complications ahead of time. He can warn the operator and take immediate preventive measures. This is why we advocate and teach the use of a combined barbiturate-inhalation narcosis performed by an experienced anesthesiologist. It offers the best conditions for the technical performance of laparoscopy, provides more comfort for the patient, and finally fulfills all medicolegal aspects concerning safety rules.

Insufflation of the Pneumoperitoneum.
After the anesthesia is introduced a probe is inserted into the uterus for mobilization during the procedure. In 4,700 laparoscopies the Sellheim Tubus proved to be the instrument of choice.

This step is followed by disinfection of the abdomen. An incision of 0.5 to 0.8 cm is made, depending on the diameter of the scope, at the lower part of the umbilicus (Fig. 7). The abdominal wall is lifted with one hand and the insufflation needle inserted through the fascia and peritoneum (Fig. 7). The free position of the cannula is verified. Some authors recommend the aspiration test at this point; this is done by means of a saline-filled syringe and should indicate whether the cannula is inside a vessel, in the free peritoneal cavity, or inside an organ. The amount of gas depends on the size and structure of the body and the obesity of the patient, as well as the state of relaxation of the abdominal wall. Another factor is the different rates of gas resorption; the loss of gas beside the trocar or through a defective trocar gasket is not measurable, however. There is no general rule for the amount of gas necessary to accomplish a proper pneumoperitoneum.

A fatty abdominal wall makes it difficult to insert the trocar into the free abdominal cavity. If extensive preperitoneal emphysema is produced, laparoscopy cannot be performed with safety. Pneumoperitoneum can be attempted by inserting the pneumoneedle through the posterior vaginal fornix.

When enough gas has been insufflated into the peritoneal cavity, the Verres cannula is removed and the examination trocar inserted through the same incision by means of a drilling, pressing action. Trocars with triangular points are easier to insert than conical ones.

Great care is necessary at this point in the procedure, since a considerable number of complications, even fatal ones, occur here. The transumbilical technique especially demands great skill and instinct. Often there is no more than 2 cm between the abdominal wall and large blood vessels. In lean patients there is a high risk of injuring those blood vessels if the trocar is inserted too vertically or too vigorously.

If it is impossible to lift a fat abdominal wall with the hand in order to insert a trocar safely in the direction of the central pelvis, the wall can be elevated with a pair of sharp towel clips and held by the assistant.

With the trocar in place, the telescope can be introduced. While pushing the laparoscope forward it is necessary to verify that vision is not impeded by adhesions. In most cases it is impossible to go around adhesions between the omentum and the anterior abdominal wall. Insufficiently prewarmed telescopes become fogged; the optic can be cleared by rubbing it on the peritoneum of the anterior abdominal wall. When and if vision is secured the procedure may be started. The different organs are identified and if necessary brought into view by the accessory palpation rod or the atraumatic grasping forceps. Pertubation, hydropertubation, or operative interventions can follow the observation. The findings should be recorded by photography or cinematography. Once the gynecologic diagnosis is established, routine inspection of the middle and upper abdomen, including the liver, should follow. The laparoscope is then removed, the abdomen desufflated, and finally the shaft of the trocar removed. No special care is required for the incision. In most cases the elasticity of the skin approximates the wound edges sufficiently. Some antiseptic powder can be applied and a Band-Aid employed to cover the incision and hold the wound edges together.

A subcutaneous suture is advisable in older patients, in those with ascites, and in postpartum sterilizations. The incisions of additional instruments are covered with another Band-Aid.

The anesthesiologist should stand by until

the patient is fully awake. Depending on local conditions the patient may spend the night in the hospital, or she may be discharged the same day after being instructed about precautions and symptoms of late complications.

CLINICAL VALUE OF GYNECOLOGIC LAPAROSCOPY

Only a few gynecologists are fully aware of the clinical value of this examination. Over a 20-year period (1954 to 1974), 4,799 laparoscopies performed at our not particularly specialized clinic formed the basis of this evaluation (Table 3).

TABLE 3.   Indications for 4,799 Laparoscopies, 1954–74

Indication	No.	%
Sterility	1,638	34.1
Ectopic pregnancy	894	18.6
Adnexal tumor	776	16.2
Suspected carcinoma	140	2.9
Acute abdomen	245	5.0
Pelvic neuralgia	348	7.3
Endometriosis	137	2.9
Tuberculosis	67	1.4
Gastroenterologic problem	47	1.0
Tubal sterilization	477	9.9
Other operative interventions	20	0.4
Miscellaneous	10	0.2
Total	4,799	100.0

This list, compiled from the author's personal experience, shows the predominance of diagnostic indications. In many cases a great number of additional operative interventions were performed.

CONCLUSION

1. In many obscure situations laparoscopy allows diagnosis, even though all conventional diagnostic measures have failed.
2. The indications for gynecologic operations are greatly clarified, and in most cases surgery is found unnecessary.
3. In many cases operative laparoscopy can help to avoid laparotomy with its risks and prolonged hospitalization.

These advantages predominate in the field of diagnosis and treatment of sterility and infertility. The rate of successful sterility operations has increased because hopeless cases are distinguished beforehand. In our area about 75 percent of such women have severely damaged

tubes. Neither pertubation nor hysterosalpingography is of any reliable diagnostic value in these cases. Statistics concerning the results of sterility operations have proved that hopeless cases are excluded by laparoscopy, and only patients with a good chance are operated on. The 4 to 15 percent success rate without laparoscopy can now be compared with 21 to 26 percent successful sterility operations when preoperative laparoscopy is performed.[36] Laparoscopy is also valuable in the differential diagnosis of ectopic pregnancy and in undefined lower abdominal problems. It lowers the risk by clarifying the diagnosis at an early stage. The patients can be operated before massive hemorrhage or progressive peritonitis sequelae influence the general condition. In all high-risk patients with undefined adnexal masses, especially during menopause, it facilitates the decision of whether further surgery is necessary. The figures (Table 3) speak for themselves.

A great number of organic changes are revealed in patients with chronic or so-called neurovegetative disorders. Those patients form a large percentage of any gynecologic practice. Most of these lesions are not palpable or accessible by gynecologic examinations. Additional operative intervention at laparoscopy helps to avoid many operations, and proof that no organic changes are present often relieves the patient's pain.

Laparoscopic tubal sterilization as a means of modern birth control has received worldwide recognition. It has perhaps provided the greatest contribution to the wide acceptance of laparoscopy during recent years. Compared to this indication, all other interventions—such as for division of adhesions, aspiration of cysts, cauterization of endometriotic lesions, and the different biopsies—are small in number.

Problems of Training

The standard of laparoscopy depends largely on the teaching program and the teacher. The technique is relatively easy to learn for any skilled operator with dexterity. The real problem is in diagnosis, not technique. The best example is sterility diagnosis. Only a subtle knowledge of tubal morphology and pathology, as well as a long operative experience, allows a decision as to whether there is a good chance for surgically establishing fertility. Large hospitals often make the mistake of asking young, inexperienced surgeons to perform laparoscopy.

Furthermore, many older surgeons consider it a minor procedure, and this is definitely not the case. It is true that there is a small incision, short duration of performance, and brief hospitalization, but it must be emphasized that laparoscopy can carry all the risks of laparotomy if done by an inexperienced or careless operator. The high rate of complications (1.7 percent) and the great number of possible intraoperative accidents shows that laparoscopy requires a trained and experienced physician. The operator must be aware of all possible complications and should be able to cope immediately with any that arise. The increasing number of malpractice suits alone should warn against incompetence in the case of laparoscopy.

REFERENCES

1. Albano V, Cittadini E: La Celioscopia in Ginecologia. Palermo, Denaro, 1962
2. Anderson ET: Peritoneoscopy. Am J Surg 35:36, 1937
3. Clyman MJ: Operative culdoscopy. Obstet Gynecol 32:340, 1968
4. Cognat M: Coelioscopie Gynecologique. Villeurbanne (France), Simep, 1972
5. Cohen MR: Laparoscopy and Gynecography, Technique and Atlas. Philadelphia, Saunders, 1970
5a. De Brux ET, Palmer R, Mintz M: Cytology of para-uterine tumors punctured under coelioscopy. J Int Fed Gynaecol Obstet 5:247, 1967
6. Decker A: Culdoscopy. Philadelphia, Saunders, 1952
7. Decker A: Pelvic culdoscopy. In JV Meigs, SH Sturgis (eds): Progress in Gynecology. New York, Grune & Stratton, 1946
8. Fahrländer H: Die Laparoskopie bei abdominalen Notfallen. Dtsch Med Wochenschr 94:890, 1969
9. Frangenheim H: Coelioskopie und Douglaspunktion. In O Käser et al (eds): Gnyäkologie und Geburtshilfe, vol 1. Stuttgart, Thieme, 1964, pp 875–89
10. Frangenheim H: Complications of operative laparoscopy. In Proceedings: VIIth World Congress of Obstetrics and Gynecology, Moscow, 1973
11. Frangenheim H: Die Bedeutung der Laparoskopie für die gynekologische Diagnostik. Fortschr Med 76:451, 1958
12. Frangenheim H: Die Laparoskopie und Culdoscopie in der Gynekologie, 1st ed. Stuttgart, Thieme, 1959
13. Frangenheim H: Laparoscopy and Culdoscopy in Gynecology. London, Butterworth, 1972
14. Frangenheim H: Operative Eingriffe bei der Coelioskopie. Geburtschilfe Frauenheilkd 25: 1124, 1965
15. Frangenheim H: Sicherheitsmassnahmen zur Verhütung von Komplikationen bei der Laparoskopie. Endoscopy 3:10, 1971
16. Frangenheim H: Technical errors in peritoneoscopy. Ger Med Mon 80:705, 1965
17. Frangenheim H: Technische Fehler bei der Coelioskopie. Geburtshilfe Frauenheilkd 1:22, 1965
18. Frangenheim H: Über das Risiko bei der Laparoskopie. Presented at the Niederrheinische Gesellschaft für Geburtsheilkunde und Gynaekologie, Düsseldorf, 1971
19. Gorga RS: La Endoscopia Abdomino Pelviana. Sao Paulo, Ortiz, 1955
20. Graham JB, Graham R: Cul-de-sac puncture in the diagnosis of early ovarian carcinoma. J Obstet Gynaecol Br Commonw 74:371, 1967
21. Hope R: The differential diagnosis of ectopic gestation by peritoneoscopy. Surg Obstet Gynecol 64:229, 1937
22. Hulka JF, Söderstrom RM, Corson SL, et al: Complications Committee of the American Association of Gynecological Laparoscopists, 1972. J Reprod Med 10:301, 1973
23. Jamain B, Letessier A, Bonhomme J: Grossesse tubaire et coelioscopie. Rev Fr Gynecol 55:663, 1960
24. Kalk H, Bruhl W: Leitfaden der Laparoskopie und Gastroskopie. Stuttgart, Thieme, 1951
25. Keith L, Silver A, Becker M: Anesthesia for laparoscopy. Presented at the 1st International Congress of Gynecologic Laparoscopy, New Orleans, 1973
26. Kratochwil A: Laparoskopie bei unklaren gynaekologischen Befunden. In Proceedings: 1st International Symposium on Gynecologic Coelioscopy, Palermo, I.R.E.S., 1964
27. Loffer F, Pent D: An alternative technique of penetrating the abdomen for laparoscopy. Presented at the 1st International Congress of Gynecologic Laparoscopy, New Orleans, 1973
28. Lübke F: Die laparoskopie als diagnostisches Hilfsmittel in der Gynäkologie. Zentralbl Gynaekol 86:260, 1964
29. Menken F: Fortschritte der gynaekologischen Endoskopie. In L Demling, R Ottenjann (eds): Fortschritte der Endoskopie. Stuttgart, Schattauer, 1969
30. Menken F: Photokolposkopie und Photodouglasskopie: Indikation und Technik. Wuppertal (West Germany), Girardet, 1955
31. Mintz M, De Brux J: La biopsie per coelioscopie de l'ovaire dans les amenorrheés, spaniomenorrhees, et troubles ovulatoires. Soc Franc Gyn 40:1, 1971
32. Mintz M, Dupre-Froment J, De Brux J: Ponctions de 94 kystes parautérins sous coelioscopie et etude cytologique des liquides. Gynaecologia (Basel) 163:61, 1967
33. Palmer R: La Stérilité Involontaire. Paris, Masson, 1950
34. Palmer R: Les Exploratons Fonctionelles Gynécologiques. Paris, Masson, 1963
35. Palmer R: Security in Laparoscopy. Presented at the 1st International Congress of Gynecologic Laparoscopy, New Orleans, 1973
36. Palmer R: Technique et Instrumentation de la

Coelioscopie Transpariétale. Gynecol Obstet (Paris) 46:420, 1947

37. Philipps JM: The impact of laparoscopy in gynecological practice. J Reprod Med 9:4, 1972

38. Philipps JM, Keith DM, Keith L: Report of 1973: Survey on the state of the art of laparoscopy. Presented at the 1st International Congress of Gynecologic Laparoscopy, New Orleans, 1973

39. Power FH, Barnes AC: Sterilization by means of peritoneoscopic tubal fulguration: a preliminary report. Am J Obstet Gynecol 41:1038, 1941

40. Proceedings of the First International Symposium on Gynecological Celioscopy. Palermo, I.R.E.S., 1964

41. Pye A: Absence congénital d'uterus et aplasie vaginale: aspects endoscopiques. In Proceedings: 1st International Symposium on Gynecologic Laparoscopy, Palermo, I.R.E.S., 1964

42. Ruddock JC: Peritoneoscopy. Surg Gynecol Obstet 65:623, 1937

43. Samuelson S, Sjövall A: Complications of Gynecological Laparoscopy. Presented at the 7th Congress Scandinavian Association of Obstetrics and Gynecology, 1972

44. Schima ME, Lubell I, Davis JE, et al: Advances in Voluntary Sterilization. New York, American Elsevier, 1974

45. Semm K: Gynaekologische Laparoskopie. In H Schwalm, G Döderlein (eds): Handbuch der Klinik der Frauenheilkunde. 1:326 Munich, Urban and Schwarzenberg, 1970

46. Semm K: Prüfung der Tubendurchgängigkeit. In O Käser (ed): Gynaekologie und Geburtshilfe. Stuttgart, Thieme, 1969

47. Sharf M, Polishuk WZ, Peretz A: The value of endoscopy in the diagnosis of endocrine disorders. J Obstet Gynaecol Br Commonw 5:834, 1961

48. Sjövall A: Laparoscopy in the diagnosis of acute salpingitis. In Proceedings: 1st International Symposium on Gynecologic Celioscopy, Palermo, I.R.E.S., 1954

49. Söderstrom RM, Butler JC: A critical evaluation of complications in laparoscopy. J Reprod Med 10:245, 1973

50. Steptoe PC: Laparoscopy in Gynecology. Edinburgh, Livingstone, 1967

51. Swolin K: 50 Fertilitätsoperationen. Acta Obstet Gynecol Scand 46:234, 1967

52. Te Linde RW, Rutledge FN: Culdoscopy, a useful gynecological procedure. Am J Obstet Gynecol 55:102, 1948

53. Thoyer Rozat J: La Coelioscopie. Technique, Indications. Paris, Masson, 1962

54. Thoyer Rozat J, Dupay A: A propos d'unde série de 200 grossesses extrautérines. Sem Hop 632, 1960

55. Wheeless C: Laparoscopic sterilization: review of 3600 cases. Obstet Gynecol 42:751, 1973

EDITORIAL COMMENT

Hans Frangenheim is not only a master of the art of laparoscopy but a world authority of the topic and an excellent clinician with a sound judgment. His outstanding results and excellent teaching methods helped in achieving a wide acceptance of gynecologic laparoscopy in Europe and United States.

It is estimated that in the United States alone during the years 1971–75, 400,000 laparoscopies (diagnostic and sterilization) have been performed. Frangenheim's comments have to be taken seriously. A number of reported complications could have been avoided with better training. With the increase in experience the incidence is declining. Teaching programs established in the United States have already shown their favorable impact in the complication surveys. Because of the large amount of time and manpower required, these programs are chiefly carried out in university departments or in affiliated teaching institutions.

Diagnostic laparoscopy requires more know-how. The use of electrosurgical units, with their advantageous coagulation and cutting current for a variety of treatment procedures, such as sterilization, adhesiolysis, and endometriosis, drew attention to the potentials of bowel injuries. In certain cases lack of knowledge of the equipment and the peculiar behavior pattern (leakage) of radio frequencies can be blamed for injuries. But, in my experience, the proper training, e.g., learning when to activate and when to release the foot switch in the case of impaired vision, is needed to avoid excessive proximity to the bowel or a sudden obscuring peristaltic wave, which are factors that were more often responsible for complications. We have to acquire more data and information from the manufacturers about the electrosurgical units and accessories before using them. Rioux and Coutler (Reprod Med 13:6, 1974) and Corson (J Reprod Med 11:159, 1973) advocate the bipolar forceps that eliminates the necessity of the patient plate (another source of skin burns) and propagate the advantages of applying a lower voltage and lower current, using the bipolar instead of a unipolar technique.

Semm and Frangenheim employ a repeatedly heated grasping forceps with low voltage, eliminating the use of units operating with radio frequencies. I assume that the cooling period of a hot thermo element is slower than a bipolar forceps after the electrical circuit is interrupted.

In any event none of the improvements in employing coagulation produces heat below physiologic parameters. In the closed abdomen, modern endoscopic techniques cannot replace the judgment of the operator. Timing—knowing when to start or to stop coagulation, when not to apply current at all because of a peculiar or difficult anatomy, obscured vision, inadequate pneumoperitoneum, poor positioning of the accessory instrument, etc.—is the most important factor with which to be familiar. There is no procedure that does not carry, even in the best hands, at least a minimal calculated risk.

It is to Frangenheim's credit that during the years of his activities he has constantly focussed on the value of learning and teaching.

THE EDITOR

40

Laparoscopy for Infertility and Fertility

Patrick C. Steptoe

INFERTILITY

Introduction of modern techniques and instrumentation of gynecologic laparoscopy has permitted very detailed examination of the female pelvis. At the same time certain operative procedures such as adhesiolysis, biopsy, and aspiration of ovarian follicles can be carried out safely. As a result of these techniques there have been many advances in knowledge of the causes, management, and treatment of primary and secondary infertility in the female in recent years. Fortunately these advances coincided with a growth of biologic studies related to ova and spermatozoa, fertilization, and the early development of the embryo. The rewards of the combined clinical and scientific endeavors are remarkable.

Laparoscopy should be performed early in the investigation of infertility. Having established by means of the history and temperature charts the approximate timing of ovulation, laparoscopy is conveniently combined with a postcoital examination of the cervical mucus together with cytologic studies of the vaginal secretions. The endoscopic examination can also be done during the luteal phase of the cycle, thereby enabling the observer to diagnose the presence of one or more corpora lutea, and to carry out an endometrial biopsy at the same time. Naturally, disturbances of ovulation and menstruation may require more detailed preliminary investigation by hormone assays, and by examining hypothalamic, pituitary, and thyroid function. Although laparoscopy by comparison to tubal insufflation and hysterosalpingography (HSG) is a major pro-

cedure, the accurate, nonmisleading information obtained is so superior to these other investigations in relation to tubal function and pathology that it is more than justified—indeed is paramount. HSG, diagnostic curettage, and hysteroscopy are of more value for investigating uterine factors than problems of tubal and ovarian origin. HSG cannot accurately diagnose the causes of tubal kinking and misses altogether many cases of peritubal adhesions, ovarian adhesions, and early pelvic endometriosis. The timing of laparoscopy at midcycle allows one to assess the amount of follicular development in the ovaries, to assess the graafian follicle or follicles, and to judge the quality of ovulation and the formation of the corpora lutea. The laparoscope then is of great value in the diagnosis of three factors causing infertility: (1) uterine causes of infertility; (2) tubal and peritubal pathology; and (3) ovarian disorders causing infertility, including endometriosis, whether confined to the ovaries or affecting the surrounding peritoneum, uterus, and oviducts (Fig. 1).

Contraindications

Very few contraindications exist in the type of patient being investigated for infertility, as the majority are healthy women in their reproductive years. Patients who have compensated cardiac and circulatory disease may not be suitable for the induction of a pneumoperitoneum, which would increase abdominal pressure and disturb the balance of pressure between chest and abdomen. The risk of serious complications is reduced by the perfor-

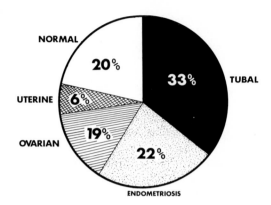

FIG. 1. Causes of 1,045 consecutive investigations of female infertility.

mance of laparoscopy under general anesthesia with controlled respiration through a cuffed endotracheal tube and marked relaxation of the abdominal wall by injected relaxants. A history of previous pelvic peritonitis, tubal infection, ovarian abscess, pelvic hematoperitoneum, and acute appendicitis does not preclude laparoscopy. Moreover, no contraindication exists after previous lower abdominal operations which may have produced adhesions, e.g., cesarean section, ventrosuspension of the uterus, operations on the oviducts or ovaries, and appendectomy. However, operations for previous generalized peritonitis or tuberculous peritonitis do increase the risks of laparoscopy in that adhesions may have fixed the bowel to the anterior abdominal wall. Perforation of the bowel might occur in introducing the instruments, or laparoscopy would be rendered valueless by the obstruction of vision caused by bowel and adhesions. Experienced laparoscopists are able to judge these risks by the ease or difficulty of obtaining a generalized pneumoperitoneum, and by probing of the abdomen with the induction needle.

Anesthesia

The advantages of *general anesthesia* were already mentioned, and indeed in the investigation of infertility general anesthesia is contraindicated only if the anesthetist finds the patient to be a poor anesthesia risk, which is unusual in this particular age group of patients. However, pregnancy would also probably be contraindicated in such poor-risk patients.

Epidural anesthesia is a good alternative to general anesthesia, since it can be controlled to effect complete relaxation of the abdominal wall. It has the disadvantage, however, of lowering the blood pressure; but if a moderate (30 degree) Trendenlenburg position is maintained and the intraabdominal pressure is not allowed to exceed 10 mm Hg, this does not constitute a problem. Epidural anesthesia allows introduction of all the necessary ancillary instruments.

Local anesthesia is not suitable for laparoscopy in the investigation of infertility because the operations which may be necessary at the time of the diagnostic procedure cannot be performed safely under such anesthesia. Even the diagnostic examination alone cannot be performed adequately under local anesthesia because of the necessity in most cases to introduce an ancillary probe or holding forceps (Fig. 2) so that the adnexae can be examined in every anatomic aspect. Although the examination is facilitated by using an angled (forward oblique) telescope, relevant details of isthmic and ovarian pathology often escape attention unless the organs are examined minutely and carefully by turning them over and from side to side under high-quality illumination. The safety of introduction of these ancillary instruments is increased when the angled laparoscope is used, illuminated by a light source of 300 watts that transmits light through the abdominal wall. Such a light source transilluminates even obese abdomens, and allows one to select a site about 6 to 8 cm from the midline, free from major epigastric vessels.

Alternative sites for the introduction of ancillary instruments are in the midline suprapubically and at various levels in and above the normal suprapubic hair line (Fig. 3). The fimbriae and abdominal ostium, for example, are best approached from a site relatively high, whereas the uterine cornu and tubal isthmus are readily reached lower down. All these approaches are facilitated by employment of a cannula locked in the uterus so that the uterus can be ante- or retroverted as desired, and moved from side to side.

Complications

If a vessel of the abdominal wall does bleed after introduction of ancillary instruments, it produces one of three results: (1) a hematoma forms on the abdominal wall; (2) the bleeding stops quickly with pressure; or (3) there is a persistent bleed into the abdomen. The first

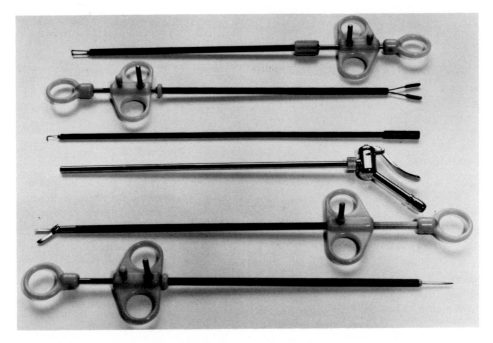

FIG. 2. Ancillary laparoscopic instruments. From top to bottom: Palmer biopsy-forceps drill. Steptoe atraumatic grasping forceps. Frangenheim diathermy knife. Steptoe suction probe. Diathermy scissors. Retractable coagulation knife or point.

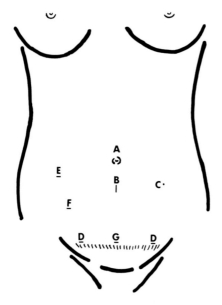

FIG. 3. Laparoscopic approach sites. A. Site most often used for both Verres needle and laparoscope. B. Alternate site for laparoscope in very fat women. C. Alternate site for Verres needle. D. Site for ventrosuspension. E. Approach to tubal fimbriae. F. Approach to ovary. G. Alternate approach to tubal isthmus.

can be treated by ice pack pressure and simple analgesics. The third is revealed by a constant drip of blood down the ancillary forceps; inspection of the peritoneal puncture site after removal of the ancillary instrument reveals a constant drip of blood; or there is a flowing trickle around the peritoneal surface of the abdomen. Inspection of the sites of introduction of these instruments by the laparoscope is an absolute necessity. If intraabdominal bleeding persists it is not usually necessary to open the abdomen or even explore the wound. In my experience bleeding can be controlled by passing a large half-circle cutting needle carrying a nylon thread through the abdominal wall to the peritoneum, observed by the laparoscope. A figure-of-eight suture is placed, which controls the bleeding, and the suture is removed the next day.

Uterine Factors in Infertility

Laparoscopy is of limited value in assessing uterine causes of infertility, although it may reveal endometriosis or uterine myomas causing obstruction of the oviducts at the cornu.

Minor congenital malformations of the uterus cannot be diagnosed by laparoscopy, but more serious ones ranging from incomplete union to complete nonunion of the müllerian ducts, and absence of part or all of the uterus, can be clarified by the laparoscope. It should be used after detailed endocrinologic and chromosome studies have been completed in cases of primary amenorrhea and genital malformations. If the vagina is absent the uterus may be represented by a peritoneal fold or a small nodule, or it may be hypoplastic. In Turner's syndrome a simple fold of peritoneum between bladder and rectum leads laterally to the infundibular pelvic ligaments. Very rudimentary oviducts may be present, and the ovaries are usually absent or markedly hypoplastic. In some cases the uterus is absent, but the ovaries are present in their normal sites. In such cases biopsy of the ovaries should be done by laparoscopy. Maturing follicles may be found. Even ovaries found in ectopic situations may also be found to be normal and not associated with testicular feminization syndrome. Such patients may not necessarily be permanently denied the possibility of pregnancy, since oocytes recovered from the woman may be fertilized in the future outside the body and subsequently implanted into a "surrogate" mother, particularly a blood relative.

Tubal Factors in Infertility

Carbon dioxide (CO_2) is the gas commonly used under general anesthesia for creating the pneumoperitoneum. This insufflated gas occasionally produces a hyperemia of the peritoneal vessels, and it is important to recognize this when examining the oviducts. True inflammatory conditions of the tubes are associated with a loss of mobility. CO_2 is preferred to nitrous oxide (N_2O), for the latter has certain disadvantages. With good general anesthesia the disturbance of P_{CO_2} is at a minimum when CO_2 is used, especially with automatic respiration. The absorption of N_2O from the peritoneum causes disturbance of both the anesthesia and the postanesthetic recovery, with the danger of precipitating anoxia. N_2O also may form explosive mixtures in the presence of small quantities of ether vapor or other gases, so that the use of high-frequency diathermy in the abdomen may well become dangerous. This latter disadvantage does not apply to CO_2.

Tubal Patency. It is well known that tubal patency can be tested by injecting CO_2 or colored solution through the tubes via the cervix. The latter is more efficient and accurate since CO_2 can readily escape along the insufflation cannula back through the cervix and vagina. Retrograde escape of dye solution is more readily prevented either by using cervical adaptors attached to the cervix, creating a vacuum, or using a cannula locked into the cervix by means of a spring. I have found the Cohen-Eder uterine cannula to be efficient and strong enough to withstand repeated use.

The blue solution should be a mixture of hydrocortisone sodium succinate with phosphate buffer 200 mg, streptomycin 250 mg, sodium methylene blue 1 percent 0.5 ml, normal saline to 50 ml, and then the pH adjusted to 7.3. Correctly adjusted this solution does not produce a chemical irritation of the oviducts and peritoneum. The flow of dye through the tubes can be observed by laparoscopy.

The flow should be free, without distention of individual parts of the tube. The presence of kinks in the tube or of internal adhesions due to old salpingitis is associated with irregular filling of the tubes and delay in escape through the fimbriated end. Before carrying out hydropertubation of the tubes, any pathologic condition should be carefully assessed. Marked damage, old inflammatory processes of such type that surgery is unlikely to assist, and suspicion of pyosalpinx are contraindications to attempted hydropertubation. Simple hydrosalpinges fill up with solution on testing and sometimes burst open through a very small opening even on moderate pressure of injection. Such perforations close again on ceasing the injection. Repeated attempts to open such tubes by perhydrotubations have no therapeutic value but may be of use in dispersing adhesions within the tubes.

Pathologic Tubal Lesions. Laparoscopy is of excellent value in discovering disturbances of fimbrial function as well as loss of tubal motility due to fine or heavy adhesions. *Obstruction of the intramural or isthmic portions* of the tube can be recognized during injection of blue solution; false results with this technique are unusual. In such suspected cases of cornual occlusion a hysterosalpingogram is of value to clarify the situation, but it can also be misleading. Before considering operative procedures on occluded tubes, detailed laparoscopic examination is of paramount importance, since this allows critical appraisal of the extent of the pathology and the chances of success. The selection of cases for surgery improves with the experience of the laparoscopist. Before the advent of laparoscopy selection of cases assessed only by gas pertubation and hysterosalpingogram gave a success rate no higher than 18 percent.[7] This has been improved to 25 to 30 percent[4] by the use of laparoscopy not only before but also after tubal surgery. The "second-look" laparoscopy allows one to deal with any recurrent fine adhesions and fimbrial stenosis by laparoscopic operative intervention.

Fine adhesions interfering with tubal function and ovum migration are best removed with the Frangenheim knife using unipolar diathermy current. Care must be taken not to damage the tube or any adherent bowel. It is best not to use diathermy scissors for adhesiolysis. Strictures of the abdominal ostium can often be dilated satisfactorily using a Palmer forceps to hold the fimbriae and an atraumatic Nordvall forceps to dilate the opening (Fig. 4).

Tubal biopsy of the ampullary area is occasionally indicated in suspected *tuberculous salpingitis.* The oviducts are swollen, thickened, and lack mobility. The fimbriae are edematous, blunted, and often rigid. If typical flat, whitish, tubercular nodules are present, the diagnosis is fairly simple; but in the absence of these, fimbrial biopsy can be diagnostic. This procedure, however, is fraught with the possibility of causing acute hemorrhage and should be carried out using two instruments: The Palmer biopsy forceps is used to steady the tube while a biopsy is performed with scissors. Any undue hemorrhage is stopped by passing the coagulating current through the Palmer forceps. In the case of tuberculosis there is therapeutic value in evacuating the CO_2 at the end of the procedure and replacing it with 2 to 3 liters of oxygen, which is not evacuated but left to absorb.

Pelvic and Ovarian Endometriosis

The incidence of pelvic and ovarian endometriosis as a factor in female infertility appears to be on the increase. It is often found when the sole complaint is that of infertility, particularly among women around 20 years of age in whom there is no associated dysmenorrhea or dyspareunia. The lesions may present as small, scattered, red, brown, or blackish cystic swellings 2 mm or so in diameter and affecting the ovarian fossae, uterosacral ligaments, pouch of Douglas, mesosalpinx, ovaries, oviducts, and even the peritoneum in front of the round ligaments and uterovesical folds. The cysts may be localized to any one of these sites remote from the usual area "polluted" by the retrograde menstrual flow through the oviducts. More extensive lesions provoke adhesions to other pelvic organs and may cause moderate to large ovarian cysts or tubal occlusion at any site along the tubes from cornu to abdominal ostium.

Treatment.   Small lesions should be destroyed by means of a diathermy coagulating point. The current is passed in very short bursts, 0.5 to 1 second usually being sufficient. The treatment can be applied to areas of the peritoneum and ovaries, with special care taken in the uterosacral region *not* to put the ureter at risk. Small surface ovarian endometriomas can be destroyed, and small or moderate cysts evacuated. It is important to remove any chocolate or tarry fluid by aspiration. Larger cysts may have to be removed by formal resection, but before doing so it may be expedient to adopt preliminary medical treatment.

When the uterus is retroverted, laparoscopic ventrosuspension is indicated to prevent fixation. Two small lateral incisions (right and left) are made in the hairline approximately 3 cm medial and below the anterior superior iliac spines. The actual site chosen on each side is dependent on transillumination to locate the epigastric vessels. Through these incisions the

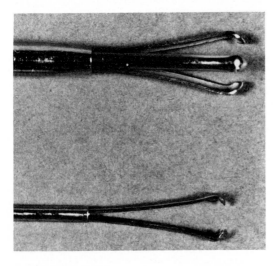

FIG. 4.   Nordvall dilating forceps (open).

round ligament on each side is grasped by means of the Palmer forceps approximately 3 cm from the cornu and is then pulled up and out through the incision. The loop of round ligament so formed is transfixed and ligated with nonabsorbable sutures, and stitched to the abdominal fascia, the redundant loop being excised. The incisions so formed are no more than 2 to 3 cm in length and are readily closed with a double Michel clip. This is removed the day after operation.

Medical treatment is indicated in nearly all cases by the exhibition of progestogens. Enovid 5 mg twice daily can be started and increased at 6-week intervals to 15, 20, and finally 30 mg/day, the whole course lasting 36 weeks. Suppression of menstruation and partial growth of the uterus are accompaniments of successful therapy, and the subsequent pregnancy rate in my series of 228 cases is 35 percent. Second-look laparoscopies in these cases at the conclusion of therapy reveals a high percentage of healing. The pseudopregnancy resulting from prolonged progestogen therapy reduces the amount of surgery necessary in the more severe cases; and because of this, primary excisional surgery should not be undertaken at the first laparoscopy. It should be delayed until the end of medical treatment.

Dysfunctional Ovaries

Hypoplasia of the ovaries is usually associated with primary amenorrhea, although occasionally a few ovulatory cycles may occur at about the time of puberty. Laparoscopy allows assessment of the size of the ovaries, which may vary from 1- to 3-cm streaks to almond-shaped ovaries one-half normal size. Biopsy at laparoscopy in such cases can establish the presence of rudimentary follicles in many cases, but the removal of even a small amount of ovarian tissue from hypoplastic ovaries is a disadvantage. The appearance of the ovary alone with deep bluish follicles up to 4 mm in diameter showing on the ovarian surface is of sufficient diagnostic value. Where such ovaries are associated with deficiencies of pituitary/hypothalamic function a good response to follicle-stimulating hormone (FSH) therapy combined with luteinizing hormone (LH) can be expected. The monitoring of response to such therapy is enhanced by second-look laparoscopy during the courses of treatment, as an adjunct to urinary or blood hormone assays. The developmental follicular response can be assessed numerically and by size estimation, and the imminence of possible ovulation can be judged. The indications for and timing of administration of LH, which is the trigger to ovulation, are facilitated. Superfolliculation and superovulation were successfully avoided in all patients treated in Oldham. Excessive follicular cyst formation giving rise to painful symptoms in patients can be treated at laparoscopy by aspiration of the cysts, and LH should not be given. Six pregnancies have been the successful outcome of cases treated in Oldham, and each has been a single pregnancy.

Disturbances of ovarian function are associated with *sclerosis of the ovarian surface*. The ovaries appear to be smooth, white, and porcelainlike. The condition may affect one or both ovaries. In the former cases ovulation takes place at irregular intervals, and in the latter ovulation does not occur. The ovaries may be of normal size (micropolycystic) or enlarged (macropolycystic). The author prefers the term "sclerocystic disease of the ovaries," and this nomenclature includes the typical Stein-Leventhal syndrome with its grossly enlarged sclerotic ovaries. Deficiency of follicular development and complete lack of luteinization is common to all these conditions.

The *macrosclerocystic ovaries* of the Stein-Leventhal syndrome can be treated at laparoscopy by (1) deep ovarian biopsy with the Palmer biopsy forceps; (2) splitting the ovarian capsule along the whole of the free border of the ovary; or (3) carrying out a laparoscopic wedge resection. The author performs the latter two techniques by employing the Palmer forceps introduced in the left side of the abdomen to hold the ovary steady, and the Steptoe diathermy point introduced on the right side of the abdomen to incise the ovary. The latter instrument has a protruding blade which can be adjusted from 0 to 2 cm in length. It cannot be overemphasized that such operative procedures require great technical experience on the part of the laparoscopist, as well as good instrumentation and lighting. Careful attention to safety factors must include maintenance of a clear gaseous space in the abdomen in which to work and constant surveillance of the whole of that space by means of an oblique distal lens (135 degrees). Constant attention to such detail avoids the danger of bowel burns.

Microsclerocystic ovaries are found at laparoscopy in cases of persistent secondary amenorrhea following administration of the contraceptive pill. Response to clomiphene and LH therapy can be expected in such cases, although occasionally more powerful follicle-stimulating therapy is required when pregnancy is desired by the patient. Four cases of premature menopause in women in their early thirties were diagnosed in Oldham by laparoscopy and ovarian biopsy. The tunica of the ovaries was typically "cerebellar" in appearance and sclerotic on histologic examination. There was complete absence of primordial follicles in the biopsy material, which was taken 1 cm deep in the ovary; and hyalinization of vessels was observed.

Microsclerocystic ovaries do not require immediate surgical treatment, but are best treated after laparoscopic diagnosis by clomiphene and human chorionic gonadotropin. This therapy is well known, but in Oldham we introduced modifications which have improved the results. Twenty-five patients were treated with clomiphene citrate 50 mg/day from day 3 of the menstrual cycle for 5 days; then the dose was increased to 150 mg/day. During 80 cycles of treatment the pregnancy rate was 28 percent with two abortions in nine pregnancies. Seventy-four patients were treated with clomiphene citrate as above with the addition of HCG 5,000 units on day 13 of the cycle. Coitus was timed at 32 to 36 hours after the HCG, based on the work of Steptoe and Edwards.[12] In 332 cycles of treatment the pregnancy rate was 48.6 percent with two abortions in 36 pregnancies. More recently the clomiphene citrate has been administered whenever possible from day 1 of the cycle, and the timing of the HCG has been based on the daily urinary output of estrogens from day 8 of the cycle onward. When the output reaches at least 50 μg, the result being available the following day, HCG is given at once and coitus timed for 32 to 36 hours later. The numbers of patients and cycles involved in this recent therapy are insufficient to report.

Disturbances of the Mechanism of Ovulation. Laparoscopic examinations of patients during various phases of the cycle allows assessment of the development of follicles, formation of the graafian follicles, actual rupture of the follicle, and formation of the corpus luteum. Ripening follicles, pink in color, which do not rupture may reach 1 cm in diameter and may number two or three in each ovary during a normal cycle. The graafian follicle reaches a larger size, becomes superficial, and the wall thins out. Vessels can be seen running over its surface. A thinner central area appears, the operculum. As ovulation approaches, the follicle becomes deeper pink and finally red. The wall of the follicle slowly gives way at the operculum, which expands to allow the ovum and the hemorrhagic jellylike mass of ripe follicular fluid to escape. Ovulation is not an explosion but a gentle oozing of the whole mass of follicular content. The fimbriae of the oviduct are usually in close juxtaposition to the ripe graafian follicle. The ovulatory mass is approximately 1 cm in diameter. After its expulsion a thin hemorrhagic fluid may leave the follicle, which rapidly heals to become the fresh corpus luteum. The stigma, measuring 1 to 2 mm across, can be recognized, but the follicle takes on a yellowish red tinge typical of the corpus luteum. The stigma disappears within a day or two, and the body becomes increasingly yellow. Such fresh corpora lutea can be identified during the luteal phase following ovulation, but their age cannot be estimated except in the fresh stage during the first days immediately after follicular rupture.

The mechanism of ovulation can be disturbed by the presence of ovarian adhesions, endometriosis of the ovaries, scars of ovarian operations, and old inflammatory scars particularly those following tuberculosis. It is also disturbed by cyst formation, whether of the retentive type or neoplastic.

Disturbances range from the complete cessation of visible follicular development to interference with the actual processes of rupture. The ovulatory mass may be fragmented and distorted so that the minute ovum may be lost to migration and reception by the oviductal fimbriae. In the diagnosis of infertility it is preferable to carry out the laparoscopic examination in combination with postcoital tests of the cervical mucus at the estimated time of ovulation so that disturbances of ovulation can be diagnosed. It must be remembered that such disturbances can occur in spite of the normality of all other parameters of ovulation.

Extended postcoital tests as described by Ahlgren[1] often reveal the presence of spermatozoa in the fluid aspirated from the oviduct. Oviductal fluid can be obtained readily from the tubes at laparoscopy by introducing a trocar and cannula through which a plastic cannula can be passed after removing the trocar. A long Tuohy needle is ideal for this

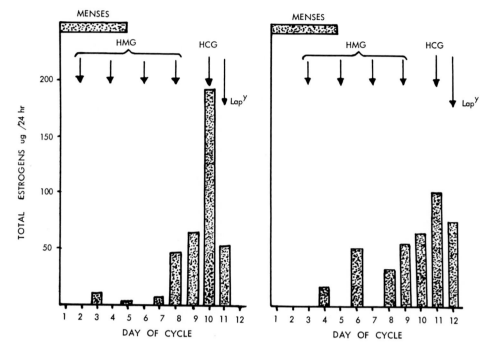

FIG. 6. Regimens of FSH and LH. The timing in the second regimen gives high recovery rates. HMG (12 ampuls) is given in divided doses. HCG (5,000 units) is given on day 11.

and allows a 1-mm polythene cannula to be introduced through the tubal ostium which is displayed when the fimbriae are grasped with an atraumatic forceps (Fig. 5, Plate G).*

The demonstration of spermatozoa in the tube or abdominal fluid has no real value in assessing an individual's infertility. Nevertheless Ahlgren showed that spermatozoa can migrate from the cervix to the tubal ampulla and abdominal cavity within 110 minutes. The migration time of 30 minutes reported by Rubenstein et al.[8] is questioned. Relatively few spermatozoa (estimated at not more than 200) were found by Ahlgren at the site of fertilization. These facts are valuable in that they indicate the value of adopting the technique of tubal aspiration to introduce spermatozoa directly into the oviducts in the case of oligospermic husbands. Such spermatozoa must first be cleaned, concentrated by slow centrifugation, placed with suitable culture media with controlled pH, and incubated for 2 to 3 hours at 37 C. The technique can also be used in cases of oligospermia that have failed to respond to all other therapeutic measures: An oocyte recovered from the female can be fertilized in vitro

All color plates appear at the front of the book.

with the male spermatozoa and placed, during the early stages of cleavage, into the oviduct of the ovum donor.

Collection of Oocytes by Laparoscopy. Preovulatory oocytes can be collected undamaged from the ovaries in three sets of circumstances:

1. After priming the ovaries with gonadotropins (FSH and LH) so as to cause maturation of several oocytes in vivo (Fig. 6)
2. After priming the ovaries with clomiphene and LH
3. After injecting LH alone in a natural cycle, a few hours before the anticipated LH surge

In all three methods the timing of laparoscopy is vital and is based on studies of oocyte maturation in vitro[2] (Table 1) and on the re-

TABLE 1. Maturation of Human Ovarian Oocytes in Vitro

Stage of meiosis	Interval from the beginning of culture (hours)
Diakinesis	25–28
Metaphase I	28–32
Metaphase II	ca 36

sults of a series of laparoscopies carried out at times varying from 29 to 40 hours after the LH injection[3,10] (Table 2).

TABLE 2. Timing of Ovulation by Laparoscopy at Various Intervals After Injection of HCG

After HCG (hours)	No. of patients	Evidence of ovulation
32–33	47	6 approaching ovulation?
36–36¾	4	0
37–38½	5	2 ovulating; 1 ovulated?
40–40½	2	1 with fresh corpus luteum
42	1	1 with fresh corpus luteum

Urinary estrogen assays are made in all cases to decide when the HCG (5,000 units) is to be given. Preovulatory oocytes are not recovered unless the output has reached 50 μg/day. Treatment with HCG can be withheld for a day or two until the ovarian response is satisfactory, or a boost of FSH can be given if the first method is in use. Good, large follicles are found with a high recovery rate of oocytes if the estrogen output has reached at least 100 μg on the day of laparoscopy.

Laparoscopy is best performed 32 hours after HCG administration. Even when the latter is used alone in an otherwise natural cycle, provided the estrogen output has reached 50 μg/day, at least one preovulatory oocyte and often two or three may be recovered.

The pneumoperitoneum, which is induced prior to passing the laparoscope, is achieved by using a modified gas mixture and not the conventional CO_2, NO_2, or O_2 gases. The mixture employed should be 5 percent O_2, 5 percent CO_2, and 90 percent N_2, which is also used as the gas phase during fertilization and subsequent cleavage of the embryo in vitro, for it maintains the pH of any culture added to the follicular aspirates during collection. The laparoscope is passed into the distended abdomen at the level of the umbilicus, and a holding forceps is introduced approximately 8 cm from the midline on one side of the lower abdomen through an avascular area pierced by the forceps trocar and cannula. The ovarian ligament is grasped to permit full examination of the ovaries and aspiration of the follicles. In a good response to gonadotropins, each ovary is moderately enlarged, by six to eight follicles varying in size from 1 to 3 cm in diameter; the follicles are thin-walled, blue pink, and on the ovarian surface (Fig. 7, Plate G). In a poor response the ovary is normal in size or only slightly enlarged, and follicles are less than 0.5 cm in diameter or lie deeper in the ovary.

Follicular contents are collected by means of an aspirator (Fig. 8). An 8-cm needle (1 mm diameter) introduced through the opposite side of the abdomen serves as a cannula so that the aspirating needle can be passed repeatedly into the abdomen during aspiration of individual follicles. The cannula is cleared by flushing with saline and heparin (1 IU/ml). The aspirating needle and its rigid transparent nylon tube are both 0.9 mm in diameter and lead to a small glass container with a capacity of approximately 8 ml. The point of the aspirating needle is inserted into an avascular area at the side of a follicle. Short-bevel needles are preferred, for all sizes of follicles can be pierced with minimal damage and little escape of follicular fluid, and the needle is changed if it becomes blocked. Each follicle is aspirated into

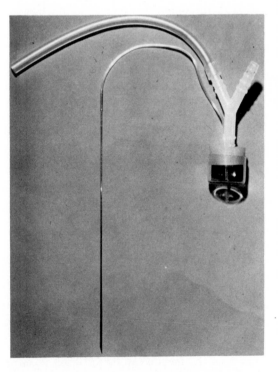

FIG. 8. Oocyte aspirator. Low-pressure suction is controlled by a finger on the Y-piece outlet.

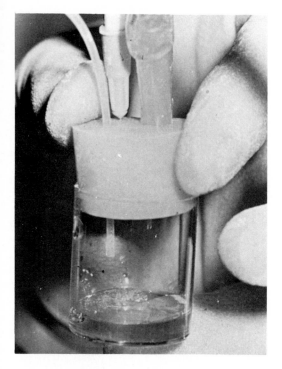

FIG. 9. Follicular aspirate.

a collecting chamber (Fig. 9) by means of gentle suction (approximately 12 cm Hg from a vacuum pump), and the remaining follicular aspirate is flushed out of the needle and tubing with heparinized (10 IU/ml) culture medium. The aspirate should flow into the chamber at about 2 drops/second; should the follicular fluid become contaminated with blood, the aspiration is stopped and the contaminated fluid collected separately into heparin. These washings are not discarded for oocytes may be found in them.

When aspiration is completed, the ovaries are inspected for any bleeding, which is usually very slight. Within 2 to 3 minutes the aspirated follicles fill with blood-stained fluid so that the ovaries appear unchanged in volume and with a number of dark blue follicles. The pelvis and puncture holes are carefully examined to ensure that there is no bleeding, and the cannulas are withdrawn. The gas mixture is evacuated from the abdomen, which is then filled with CO_2 to about 3 liters. This is then evacuated, and the procedure assists in washing out the nitrogen. The latter gas is absorbed slowly from the peritoneum, and if more than a small amount is left in the abdomen it gives rise to upper abdominal and shoulder pain. The laparoscope is then withdrawn and the patient returned to bed. The procedure takes about 20 minutes, and the patient makes a very rapid recovery.

One important modification is made in the general laparoscopic procedure. After emptying the bladder by catheter, the uterus is not disturbed by the usual cannula and vulsella forceps. The endometrium must not be invaded or damaged. Anteversion of the uterus is achieved by vaginal manipulation with the fingers and by abdominal holding forceps on the ovarian ligament.

Oocytes are collected from one-half to two-thirds of the follicles aspirated, a higher proportion being collected from larger follicles. Preovulatory oocytes are in diakinesis, metaphase I, or metaphase II when recovered. Their appearance is also typical, for they are surrounded by a thick, viscous mass of mucus-containing diffuse layers of cumulus cells; such oocytes are fertilized within a few hours. Classification of the oocyte enables the preovulatory follicles to be identified, and most are found to be the largest follicles in the ovary. Nonovulatory oocytes are surrounded by several layers of tightly adhering corona cells, and oocytes are considered to be atretic if there are no attendant corona cells.

Preovulatory ovarian oocytes collected by laparoscopy can be fertilized within a few hours. With recognition of certain needs in the culture media it is also possible to induce cleavage of such fertilized oocytes up to the blastocyst stage in vitro[11] (Figs. 10 and 11; Tables 3 and 4).

Indications for the use of in vitro systems of fertilization and cleavage of human oocytes are as follows:

1. In the treatment of infertility due to damaged, useless, or absent oviducts. This is achieved by reimplantation of the embryo into the uterus of the egg donor.
2. In the control of certain sex-linked diseases, e.g., hemophilia. Further studies are needed in the technique of sexing the embryos.
3. In the treatment of infertility due to oligospermia in the male partner which has failed to respond to other therapy. A pronucleate or cleaving ovum can be placed in the donor oviducts or uterus.
4. To test the fertilizing capacity of semen samples, in the development of contraceptive drug therapy for males.
5. For studying the causes of certain congenital deformities.

Some of the *contraindications* to laparoscopy

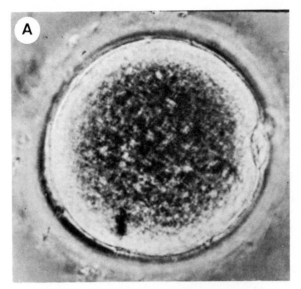

FIG. 10. Stages of in vitro fertilization of human oocyte. **A.** Human oocyte. **B.** Invasion of zona pellucida. **C.** Penetration of vitellum. (Continued)

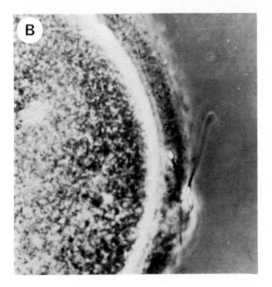

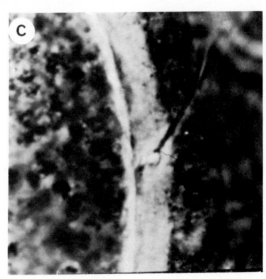

for oocyte recovery are based on observations showing a poor chance of recovery of preovulatory oocytes.

1. The urinary estrogen excretion of less than 40 to 50 μg/day on the day that HCG is given indicates that insufficient follicles have been stimulated, although some patients with much higher levels of urinary estrogens may have many small nonovulatory follicles. In general, levels higher than 100 μg/day are associated with the growth of several follicles. Hyperstimulation has been recorded on only one occasion and in a mild form. There were no serious clinical signs, and the patients returned to a normal menstrual cycle after a delay of some 20 days following oocyte recovery.

2. The second contraindication to laparoscopy is untreated ovarian endometriosis. These lesions may be small, but the distortion and fibrosis present in the ovary makes aspiration difficult and might interfere with subsequent luteinization. Treatment by gestagen therapy often improves the situation if endometriomas are small but usually must be applied for at least 9 months and must succeed in suppressing ovulation. The subsequent scars may increase the difficulty in recovering oocytes but do not prevent recovery of some preovulatory oocytes.

3. Many patients have had previous surgery such as salpingoplasty or salpingectomy, or they may have periovarian adhesions. For oocyte recovery the patient should have a healthy uterus and at least one accessible ovary. Periovarian adhesions may be removed during a preliminary op-

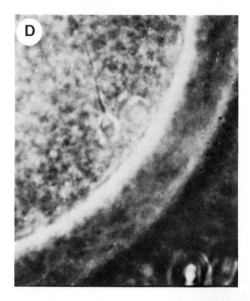

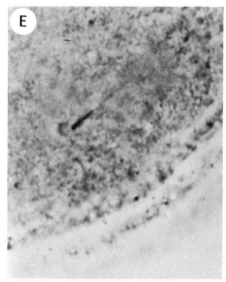

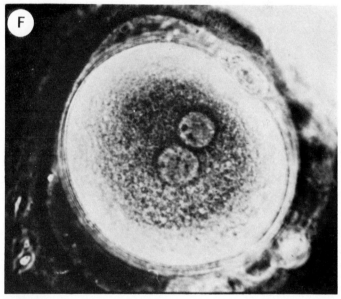

FIG 10. (cont.). **D.** Sperm in cytoplasm. **E.** Sperm head expanding. **F.** Pronucleate ovum.

eration, and the ovary placed into an accessible position. Such patients need at least one diagnostic laparoscopic survey to assess the necessity of any preliminary plastic surgery, and most will probably be suitable for oocyte recovery, even if the previous pelvic infections were extensive. The one reservation must concern tuberculosis infections, for the remaining severe thick adhesions may prevent laparoscopy or result in the failure of adhesiolysis designed to liberate the ovaries. It is essential that there be cornual occlusion on both sides; if it is suspected that an occluded tube or stump has a patent channel to the uterine cavity, coagulation should be applied to destroy such patency.

CONTROL OF FERTILITY

The role of laparoscopy in the control of fertility is now well established. It goes a long way toward the ideal form of female sterilization—which would be a procedure that is readily performed on an outpatient basis, immediately effective, yet readily reversible. It must not be forgotten, however, that the method of sterilization adopted must be efficient. To achieve permanent sterilization it is best to induce tubal occlusion so that sper-

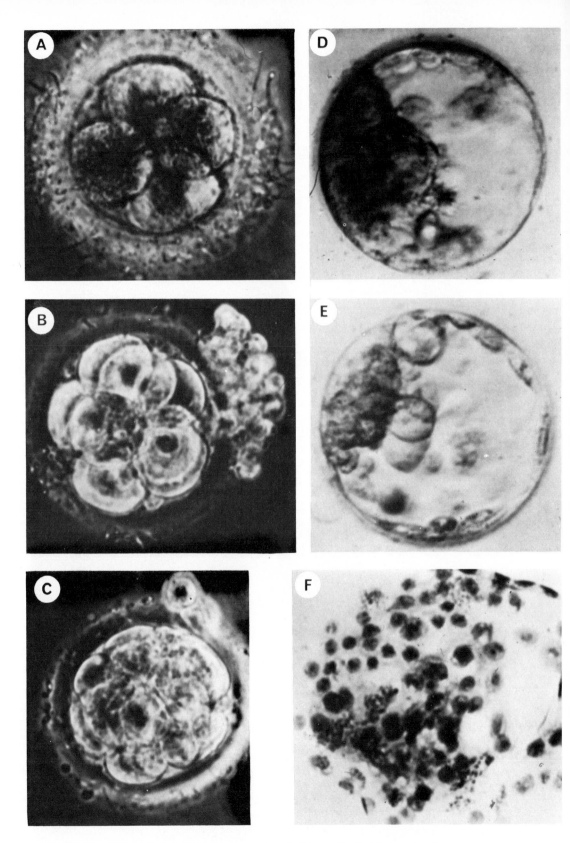

FIG. 11. Cleavage of fertilized human ova. **A.** Four-cell. **B.** Eight-cell. **C.** Morula. **D** and **E.** Early blastocysts. **F.** Dividing blastocyst cells.

TABLE 3. Bavister's Tyrode B Culture

Component	Concentration (mg/liter)
NaCl	7500
KCl	390
$CaCl_2$	200
$MgCl_2 \cdot 6H_2O$	100
$NaH_2PO_4 \cdot 2H_2O$	57
$NaHCO_3$	3,295
Na pyruvate	11
D. glucose	1,000
Bovine serum albumin	3,600
Phenol red	17
Penicillin	100 IU/ml

TABLE 4. Timing of Human Preimplantation Development in Vitro

Stage of Development	Time (hours)
2-celled	<38
4-celled	38–46
8-celled	51–62
16-celled	<85
Morula	111–135
Blastocyst	123–147

matozoa migration and ovum transport are effectively prevented. The failure rate of tubal ligation whether achieved by laparotomy or by the varied techniques of laparoscopy is high, four per thousand at best. In the interests of safety, however, these techniques and also that of tubal diathermy alone have been advocated.[4–6,9,12,13] However, it is this author's experience that diathermy and division of the tubal isthmus (Fig. 12; Fig. 13, Plate G) is the most effective method of procuring permanent sterilization, and it can be done with a high degree of safety. The adjacent mesosalpinx should be sealed by coagulation to achieve hemostasis.

Moreover, it is readily performed on an outpatient basis, a stay of about 8 hours being all that is necessary. The operation is performed under general anesthesia as described previously, utilizing the second puncture technique that is so necessary in the armamentarium of the diagnostic laparoscopist. It must be emphasized that the technique of diathermy/division is designed to bring about permanent sterilization. High-frequency diathermy is applied in short bursts of 1 to 2 seconds only. Bipolar diathermy may also be used with a reduction of the risks of diathermy injuries. Experience in diagnostic laparoscopy and supervised training in the operative technique is

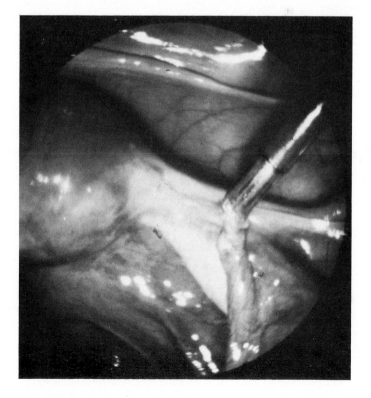

FIG. 12. Diathermy and division of right tubal isthmus.

essential before any such operations are undertaken independently by any surgeon.

"Reversible" Sterilization

Is it essential to secure tubal occlusion in order to prevent ovum and sperm migration? Intratubal plastic splints have been used for many years to assist in the maintenance of tubal patency during the healing phases following tubal surgery designed to restore the possibility of pregnancy. These devices appear to cause no significant damage to the oviducts. On occasion such splints have been left in the oviducts for long periods; no pregnancies have been observed when the splints are in place, but after removal of the devices pregnancy can and has occurred. It is probable that the introduction of intratubal devices into each oviduct *without* producing tubal occlusion is sufficient to prevent fertilization and ovum migration. The devices must be maintained in position as long as necessary. Tubal damage is reduced to a minimum if material of very low friction is used. Both Silastic and Teflon are very slippery and fulfill this criterion.

Flexible radiopaque rods of suitable material have been designed. The rods are 1 mm in diameter, but at intervals of 1 cm along the length there are protuberances of 1.5 mm in diameter (Fig. 14). The rods are 4 and 6 cm in length and are made by a molding process.

These devices are retained in position in the oviducts by means of a clip. At present the 1-cm Weck tantalum clip is used for this purpose, but instruments are being designed so that a spring clip of the Sundt-Kees type used in neurovascular surgery, which are readily removed, can be used. The clips are applied with moderate tension outside and across the oviducts into which the Silastic device has been inserted so that each clip lies between any pair of the rod's protuberances (Fig. 15). The Silastic rod is thus prevented from moving from its position because the diameter of the protuber-

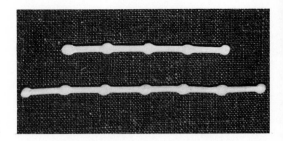

FIG. 14. Silastic intratubal devices.

ances plus the thickness of the tubal wall is too great to pass through the closed clip. The length of rod chosen depends on the width of the mesosalpinx between the tube and ovary. If this is short then the longer rod must be used so that the clip can be applied away from the narrow area, and so avoid occluding the vessels in that area. The intratubal devices and retaining clips can be delivered by three surgical methods.

Minilaparotomy. A small (3 cm) transverse suprapubic incision is made in the abdomen after first locking a uterine cannula into the cervix. An assistant elevates and directs the uterus into the small peritoneal incision by means of the cannula. The oviducts are readily elevated from the abdomen, facilitated by the use of two small retractors. A device is inserted into each tube and clipped in position and the oviducts are dropped back into the pelvis before closing the abdomen.

Culdotomy. The pelvis is entered through a small posterior fornix incision into the cul-de-sac. A Hegar dilator is used to retrovert the uterus strongly, so that the oviducts can be delivered readily one by one into the vagina for insertion of the devices. This route requires a normal, mobile uterus with no pelvic pathology. The risk of operative infection is increased by using this route. The operating culdoscope may also be used.

Laparoscopy. This method requires a general anesthetic of short duration and is

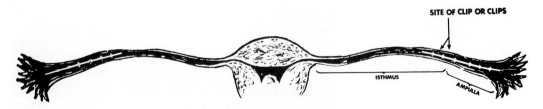

FIG. 15. Intratubal devices in position.

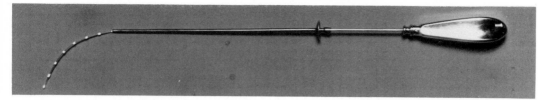

FIG. 16. Introducer for intratubal device.

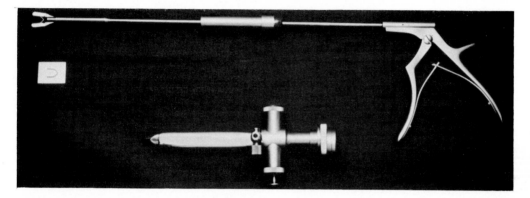

FIG. 17. Clip applicator with oval trocar and cannula. The 1-cm Weck tantalum clip is shown.

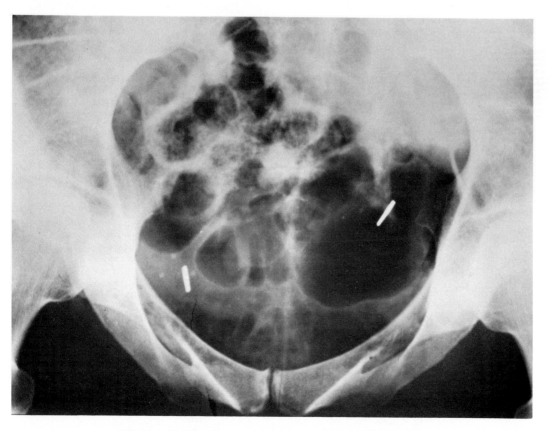

FIG. 18. Radiograph showing devices clipped into oviducts.

applicable to outpatients. The instrumentation consists of an angled laparoscope, an intrauterine cannula to raise the uterus to anteversion, atraumatic holding forceps introduced through a trocar and cannula to grasp the tubal fimbriae, a special trocar and cannula for carrying the devices into the abdomen and introducing them into the tubes, and a special clip applicator with its trocar and cannula (Figs. 16, 17).

The laparoscope is inserted at the umbilicus in the usual way after creating a pneumoperitoneum, and the clip applicator is inserted through a small medial transverse suprapubic incision in the hairline. The tubal grasping forceps is inserted to the left of the midline about 8 cm laterally and 3 cm below the umbilicus. The intratubal device applicator is introduced at a similar point on the right of the midline. Access to both tubes by the two insertions is readily achieved. The intratubal device is guided into the ampulla by means of the cannula and plunger, and the clip is applied as described above.

For laparoscopic technique the patient is admitted on the morning of operation. The procedure is carried out about 1.5 hours after premedication; the operating time is approximately 15 minutes; and the patient may go home in the evening—about a 10-hour admission. An x-ray film is obtained to check the position of the Silastic devices and clips after operation (Fig. 18). The patient returns on the third day to have three skin clips removed and to be reviewed clinically. Each patient is seen 1 month later when the radiologic examination is repeated. A second-look laparoscopy is now performed 3 to 9 months later.

Results

At the present time observations have been made in 14 women through some 110 cycles, with no pregnancies. No menstrual disturbances, bleeding, or pain have occurred. Second-look laparoscopy has been performed in six patients, and in each case the devices were in satisfactory position. In one the clip on one side was causing a small amount of tubal swelling. The clips are readily removed by a grasping forceps, and the devices can be removed easily at laparoscopy. The technique is still in its de-

velopmental phase—no attempts have yet been made to reverse the "sterilization."

While the author prefers laparoscopic diathermy/division of the tubes for permanent sterilization, this particular technique appears to be applicable in the younger age groups. Permanent sterilization performed in women in their twenties is a step to be taken with reluctance. In spite of the fact that the patient may be fully convinced at the time, her circumstances may change and the gynecologist will be faced with requests to undo the tubal damage. In spite of the improvements in such techniques including microsurgical methods, the results can never be certain. Intratubal devices of the kind described here may provide one answer and prove to be a step toward truly reversible sterilization.

REFERENCES

1. Ahlgren M: Migration of spermatozoa to the fallopian tubes and the abdominal cavity in women: student literature. University of Lund, 1969
2. Edwards RG: Maturation in vitro of human ovarian oocytes. Lancet 2:926, 1965
3. Edwards RG: Studies on human conception. Am J Obstet Gynecol 117:587, 1973
4. Frangenheim H: Proceedings, International Congress of the American Society of Gynecologic Laparoscopists, 1973 (in press)
5. Greene KR: Br Med J (correspondence) 2:54, 0000
6. Loeffler FE: Br Med J (correspondence) 2:444, 0000
7. Revaz C: Problemes chirurgeaux de la sterilite tubaire. Gynaecologia (Basel) 165:178, 1968
8. Rubenstein BB, Strauss H, Lazarus ML, et al: Sperm survival in women—motile sperm in the fundus and the tubes of surgical cases. Fertil Steril 2:15, 1951
9. Semm K: In Schima ME, Lubell I, Davis JE (eds): Advances in Voluntary Sterilization. New York, American Elsevier, p 253
10. Steptoe PC: Proceedings, International Congress of the American Society of Gynaecologic Laparoscopists, 1973 (in press)
11. Steptoe PC: The International Handbook of Medical Science. Oxford, Medical & Technical Publishing Co, 1972, p 45
12. Steptoe PC, Edwards RG: Laparoscopic recovery of preovulatory human oocytes after priming of ovaries with gonadotrophins. Lancet 1:683, 1970
13. Wheeless C: In Schima ME, Lubell I, Davis JE (eds): Advances in Voluntary Sterilization. New York, American Elsevier, p 252

EDITORIAL COMMENT

Patrick C. Steptoe, in addition to pioneering in the field of sterilization by means of the laparoscope, was among the first, in his early publications (see the references in Chapter 40), to draw attention to the fact that in the first series of patients, where the tubes were *coagulated only,* a larger-than-expected percentage of tube patency, leading to a greater incidence of pregnancies, was observed. This sequela necessitated the *coagulation* and the *division* of the tubes. After the first series of patients, his results on a long-term follow-up were excellent.

Investigators in the United States (Pent, Loffer, and Corson) and in Canada (Yuzpe and Rioux), who simply coagulate the tubes, claim for a large number of patients (approximately 4,000) results similar to those with coagulation and division. The complications resulting from transsection are also decreased by coagulation only.

The decision of the method that should be used will be based on follow-up reports in the next few years. During a recent complication survey (1974–75) of the American Association of Gynecological Laparoscopists (AAGL) amongst 924 gynecologists, it was found that 214 coagulate, 404 coagulate and divide, and 306 coagulate, divide, and obtain specimens for histology.

To decrease complications, such as tears in the mesosalpinx during transsection, followed by bleeding and bowel and skin burns, Hulka and Omran (Fertil and Steril 23:633, 1972) employed special clips, and recently Yoon and King (J Reprod Med 15:54, 1975) used silicone rubber rings to occlude the tubes.

More time is needed for evaluating the various pros and cons of these different techniques.

In the AAGL report 20,000 sterilizations had been performed in 1971, with a pregnancy rate two per 1,000 (0.2 percent); 40,000 sterilizations were completed in 1975, with a failure rate of 0.5 per 1,000 (0.05 percent). The last figure has to be interpreted with caution because of the short (six-month) follow-up period.

THE EDITOR

41

Gynecologic Urethroscopy

Jack R. Robertson

Viewing the interior of the bladder was first attempted by Phillip Bozzini of Frankfurt in 1804. He designed a long thin funnel, and light was reflected from a box containing a candle. Bozzini presented his instrument to the Faculty of Medicine of Vienna, but they were dismayed at such a contraption. There is no evidence it was ever used on a human.[2]

Pierre Ségalas simplified Bozzini's instrument and presented his version in 1826. It was a funnel with an interior that was highly polished to reflect light. It was intended to illuminate the bladder and ureteral orifices. Illumination was again by candles, and a concave mirror focused the light.[8]

Max Nitze, an instrument maker, is generally credited as the father of the modern cystoscope. He realized the problem was the external light source, and he felt a combination of lenses would enlarge the field of vision. He used a platinum wire as the source of illumination and filled the bladder with ice water to prevent thermal injury.[7]

In 1869 Nitze joined with Leiter, a skilled Viennese instrument maker, to produce a scope with a concave and a convex lens. It had a removable obturator which allowed the bladder to be filled with air or water for examination. A platinum wire was the light source, so water was still the preferred medium for examination.[2]

The invention of the incandescent lamp by Thomas Edison was a major step in making urology the exact science it is today. The heat of the bulb still required a water medium, however.

In 1893 Howard Kelly described a simple open speculum for examining the female bladder. The patient was placed in the knee-chest position, and the bladder distended with air when the scope was inserted. Kelly, a gynecologist, was the first to insert a ureteral catheter under direct vision.[4]

The American Surgical Society, a forerunner of the American College of Surgeons, met in Baltimore in 1900. A contest was held between Howard Kelly and Hugh Hampton Young, who is generally considered the father of modern urology in this country. Using his air cystoscope, Kelly inserted ureteral catheters in a female patient in just 3 minutes. Young equaled this time in a male patient using the catheterizing cystoscope developed by Leopold Casper of Berlin.[13]

In 1951 Ridley proposed indirect air cystoscopy. He placed a female patient in the knee-chest position and used the conventional cystoscope with air as the medium. The urethrovesical junction and urethra were difficult to visualize owing to heat from the light bulb and lack of a straightforward lens.[9]

Robertson put fiber optics into a Kelly-type female urethroscope. The instrument was excellent for examination of the urethrovesical junction and the urethra. A right-angled fiberoptic telescope could be inserted through the urethroscope for viewing the bladder.[10]

INTRODUCTION

Urinary continence is a blessing. Incontinence is one of life's miseries, and its cure remains a challenge. This is attested to by the numerous operative procedures that have been developed for the cure of stress incontinence.

The artificial isolation of the female urethra from the pelvis by the specialization of medicine has created a problem. The urologists use the female urethra (Fig. 1, Plate G)* as a resting place for their male telescope while they look around in the bladder. Gynecologists have developed innumerable operative procedures for stress incontinence, but they seldom do endoscopy.

Embryologically, anatomically, and functionally the lower urinary tract and the female genital tract are intimately related, and it is difficult to disassociate them despite the subspecialties of medicine. Congenital anomalies of the genital tract are frequently accompanied by anomalies of the urinary tract, showing the close embryologic relationship of these structures.

Urethroscopy with urethral and bladder pressure studies permit the gynecologist to do a comprehensive work-up of the female patient with both urinary and genital symptoms.

INDICATIONS

Pelvic pain, dyspareunia, and dysuria are common gynecologic complaints which may involve the lower urinary tract, the genital tract, or both. If genital disease of pathology is not found, then the urethra must be investigated as the source of these complaints.

Fifty percent of all women complain of urinary incontinence at some time during their lives. This may be secondary to chronic urethritis and cystitis or to some weakness of the urethra (e.g., a dysfunctional sphincter).

Stress incontinence as an isolated finding is uncommon. Most of these patients have superimposed urgency, and it is impossible to evaluate them adequately without the use of endoscopy. Other causes for incontinence which require endoscopic evaluation are the neurogenic bladder, urinary retention with overflow, urethral diverticulum, valvular vesicovaginal fistula, and ectopic ureter opening into the vagina or the urethra below the internal sphincter.

The patient with an asymptomatic cystocele and superimposed chronic urethritis is best managed by conservative measures such as urethral dilation and antibiotic and antispas-

All color plates appear at the front of the book.

modic therapy. This may cure her "stress incontinence" and thereby preclude the need for surgery.

The patient with stress incontinence, rectocele, enterocele, and uterine prolapse may have her incontinence cured by a Marshall-Marchetti-Krantz urethropexy, but procidentia often develops and she is required to go to a gynecologist for the remainder of her surgery. The compartmentalization of the female pelvis leads to the treatment of one problem while ignoring the other and is to the patient's disadvantage.

The absence of objective assessment of the patient with the symptom of stress incontinence is a handicap. Innumerable operations have been devised to strengthen the sphincter weakness. Chain cystograms[3] and cinécystography[6] demonstrate the anatomic configuration of the urethra and bladder, but they fail to show whether the loss of the posterior urethrovesical angle is due to sphincter weakness or a detrusor contraction. The patient with urinary incontinence from detrusor contraction may have. a history typical of true stress incontinence.

The conventional gynecologic work-up of the patient with urinary incontinence has been the chain cystogram. Jeffcoate and Roberts[5] felt that urinary continence depended on a posterior urethrovesical angle of 100 degrees. Their studies were done with a catheter.

The bead-chain technique was introduced by Hodgkinson.[3] The chain did not distort the urethra or limit its mobility. It also provided a good contrast for lateral views in the erect position. The anatomic changes which were felt to demonstrate stress incontinence were funneling of the bladder neck, undue descent of the bladder neck on straining, and loss of the posterior urethrovesical angle.

Green[1] believed that the angle of inclination of the urethra was part of the pathologic anatomy as demonstrated by cystograms. He classified patients as type I if loss of the posterior urethrovesical angle was present, and type II if there was also an abnormal inclination of the urethral axis. Chain cystogram is a complex procedure that never became popular.

CONTRAINDICATIONS

Acute infection is the only contraindication to instrumentation of the female urethra with

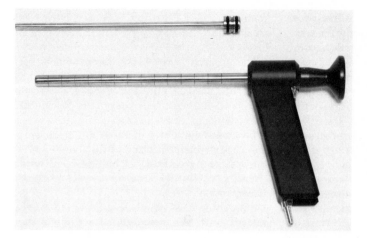

FIG. 2. Robertson CO_2 endoscopy telescope assembly. The instrument consists of a Hopkins endoscopic telescope, a handle with connections for the CO_2 gas supply, fiberoptic light bundle, and a plug-in gas obturating sheath enclosing the telescope shaft. A urethroscopy sheath is shown on the assembled instrument, and a diagnostic hysteroscopy sheath is shown above it.

concomitant urethral and bladder pressure studies. The procedure is preferably accomplished with a sterile lower urinary tract. Endoscopy of the urethra with gas obturation is a simple office procedure.

COMPLICATIONS

Whenever the lower urinary tract is instrumented there is a possibility of introducing infection. This occurs in a small percentage of patients. A short course of urinary antiseptic should be administered following endoscopy or an antiseptic solution injected into the bladder at the end of the procedure.

Endoscopic control allows the tip of the scope to be threaded into the bladder. It should never be forced to break up adhesions as these are best managed by dilation with an olive-tipped bougie. Meatal stricture occasionally prevents passage of the instrument with CO_2 acting as the obturator. This is best dilated with the bougie.

A small amount of bleeding may occur following instrumentation of a constricted urethra. In 10 years' experience using urethroscopy with CO_2 insufflation, the author has never seen a serious complication.

INSTRUMENTATION

The Robertson gas urethroscope consists of the Hopkins telescope with a straightforward view. The telescope fits into an airtight handle,

and the CO_2 is insufflated through the handle. The equipment* is easily assembled (Fig. 2).

Insufflation is accomplished with the Robertson CO_2 endoscopy monitor† (Fig. 3), which allows urethral and bladder pressure studies to be performed during endoscopy. The flow rate is variable from 30 to 120 cc/minute.

The endoscopy monitor has an X-Y recorder, which records the pressure in centimeters of water pressure and the volume of gas in cubic centimeters. The sensations experienced during bladder filling are recorded on the chart. The X-Y plotter makes a permanent record for the patient chart. The Robertson endoscopy monitor is a compact unit which has a dual-lamp, fiberoptic box, making the gas and light available from one source.

TECHNIQUE

The technique of urethroscopy and obtaining urethral and bladder pressure studies has been described by Robertson.[11] The patient is placed in the lithotomy position; a Sims speculum inserted into the vagina spreads the labia and makes the urethral meatus easily available. The CO_2 acts as an obturator and a urethral dilator. The urethral resistance is overcome by

*Manufacturer: Karl Storz K.G., PO Box 400, 7200 Tuttlingen, West Germany. Distributor: Karl Storz Endoscopy-America, Inc., 658 South San Vicente Boulevard, Los Angeles, Calif. 90048.
†Manufacturer and distributor: Browne Corporation, 203 Chapala Street, Santa Barbara, California 93101.

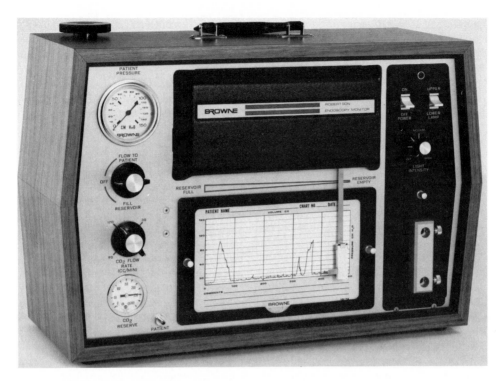

FIG. 3. Robertson CO_2 endoscopy monitor. The instrument includes a gas reservoir, gas flow controls and monitoring gauges, a pressure-volume X-Y recorder, and a dual-lamp fiberoptic light source. The instrument is portable and has been designed for both office and institutional CO_2 endoscopy procedures.

the force of the gas as the tip of the scope is passed into the bladder, and in this manner a urethral pressure profile is recorded. The average urethral pressure is 100 cm of water. In the patient with anatomic stress incontinence (Fig. 4, Plate G) it is 30 cm of water or less. The patient with infected periurethral glands or a urethral diverticulum (Fig. 5, Plate G) may extrude pus into the urethra.

On entering the bladder the normal intravesical pressure is 3 to 10 cm of water, and residual urine may be noted. The urine may be aspirated through the stopcock and measured; it is then sent for analysis and culture. Vesical pressure studies are made as the bladder fills. The sensations of bladder filling and fullness and of urge are all normally experienced with little or no increase in intravesical pressure. The patient with an unstable bladder (uninhibited neurogenic bladder) usually has an increased filling pressure, and undulations may be noted on the graph. Occasionally the bladder fills normally, but a cough or change in position precipitates an increase in filling pressure.

The bladder neck is evaluated as the tip of the scope is withdrawn from the bladder.[12] Normally the bladder neck closes, looking like a sphincter; and the urethra looks and functions like a sphincter. The patient who has true anatomic stress incontinence has a vesical neck which is lax and oval and closes sluggishly. The patient operated on unsuccessfully for urinary incontinence has a scarred, fixed bladder neck which closes looking like a drainpipe. When the scope is withdrawn to the external meatus, it is still not closed.

Another urethral pressure profile is recorded as the scope is pulled out through the urethra. The maximum urethral pressure is located about 2 cm from the vesical neck.

ANATOMY OF THE URETHRA

The urethra is a fibromuscular extension of the bladder. Its average length is 4 to 5 cm.

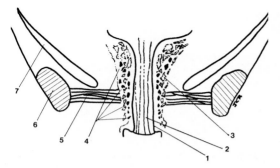

FIG. 6. Female urethra. 1, Mucous membrane. 2, Inner longitudinal layer of smooth muscle. 3, Outer circular oriented smooth muscle. 4, Lacunar vascular spaces. 5, Urogenital diaphragm. 6, Pubic bone. 7, Pubococcygeus muscle.

The lower two-thirds of the urethra is an integral part of the anterior wall of the vagina. The voluntary striated muscle which is part of the urogenital diaphragm inserts at midurethra (Fig. 6).

The female urethra is homologous to the prostatic portion of the male urethra. On the lateral aspect of the upper and middle thirds of the urethra are bands of connective tissue which insert into the pubic ramus, and in the female are called the pubovesical ligaments.

The urethral musculature is in two layers: an inner longitudinal and an outer circular layer. These muscular layers create an intraluminal urethral pressure. Although anatomists have never been able to identify a sphincter, the entire urethra functions like one.

URETHRAL PRESSURE PROFILE

The sphincteric action of the urethra may be assessed by obtaining a urethral pressure profile. This is measured as the scope passes through the urethra into the bladder and is then withdrawn through the urethra. The CO_2 acts as an obturator and a urethral dilator as the pressure is recorded on the Robertson endoscopy monitor.

The entering urethral pressure profile is low in patients with true anatomic stress incontinence (generally less than 30 cm of water). The sphincteric action of the urethra is assessed at the proximal urethra and at midurethra as the scope is withdrawn through the urethra. The scope is withdrawn until the vesical neck is

seen to close. The patient "bears down," which causes an increase in intraabdominal pressure that is transmitted, causing a rise in intravesical pressure. This increase is associated with partly transmitted and partly reflex activity, which raises the intraurethral pressure higher than the intravesical pressure, and continence is maintained. The urethra is observed to squeeze, and an increase in pressure is noted on the endoscopy monitor.

The same bearing down maneuver in the patient with stress incontinence causes a rise in intravesical pressure, which is not applied to the urethra owing to loss of support of the proximal urethra, and funneling occurs with opening of the vesical neck. Endoscopically the urethra is seen to open, and an increase in pressure is registered on the endoscopy monitor.

The bearing down maneuver in the patient with an uninhibited neurogenic bladder (unstable bladder) causes a detrusor contraction secondary to an increase in intraabdominal pressure. The bladder neck drops sharply and opens as an increase in pressure is registered on the graph (similar to an incompetent urethra). Those patients with true stress incontinence have a normal cystometrogram.

These maneuvers may be repeated at midurethra. The same findings are noted. However, patients with anatomic stress incontinence may be incontinent at the bladder neck but continent at midurethra.

Patients operated on unsuccessfully for stress incontinence may end up with the "battered bladder syndrome" and a "frozen urethra," which looks and functions like a drainpipe. These patients have no urethral pressure, and they are as incontinent as the patient with a vesicovaginal fistula (Fig. 7).

The graph in Figure 7 records from left to right. An entering urethral pressure profile is recorded as the scope is slowly inserted through the urethra. The CO_2 acts as an obturator and a urethral dilator. The urethral resistance is measured. The average urethral pressure is about 100 cm of water before the gas enters the bladder. The patient with urethral stricture may register a pressure of 150 cm of water. Patients with anatomic stress incontinence have a low urethral pressure profile.

Normally the bladder fills with little increase in intravesical pressure. The patient

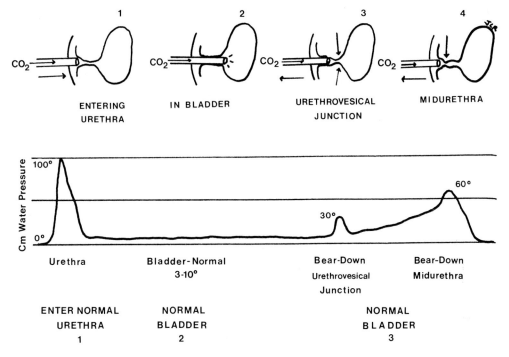

FIG. 7. Normal urethral pressure profile and normal cystometrogram. See text for details.

with an unstable bladder (uninhibited neurogenic bladder) has two different filling patterns. The first is an abnormal filling pressure (5 to 15 degrees) from the beginning with undulations on the graph (Fig. 7) representing small bladder contractions. The bladder fills normally in the second pattern until a cough or change in position causes abnormal detrusor contractions.

Competence at the vesical neck and at midurethra may be measured by instructing the patient to bear down. The tip of the scope is pulled back until the vesical neck closes. The patient is again instructed to bear down. Normally the urethra squeezes tight and a pressure is recorded on the graph.

The same maneuver in the patient with anatomic stress incontinence causes the bladder neck to drop and open with funneling, and a high pressure is registered on the graph. The bearing down maneuver in the patient with an unstable bladder precipitates a detrusor contraction, and the vesical neck opens.

The same maneuvers are repeated at midurethra. Some patients show incompetence at the vesical neck but have good tone and support at the midurethra and so remain continent.

DISCUSSION

Urinary continence may be viewed as a balance between the forces that retain urine in the bladder and the forces which expel it. Urinary incontinence is an imbalance of these forces—a sphincteric weakness, an abnormality of bladder action, or a combination of the two.

The factors involved in urinary incontinence as shown by endoscopy and urethral and bladder pressure studies are:

1. Unstable bladder (uninhibited neurogenic bladder) as determined by cystometrograms
2. Loss of support and function at the bladder neck and proximal urethra as determined by bearing down maneuvers
3. Malfunction of the voluntary sphincter at midurethra as determined by bearing down maneuvers

Removal of three-fourths of the terminal urethra by surgical incision does not produce incontinence providing the proximal urethra is competent. If the proximal urethra is incompetent, urine may enter the urethra with a sudden increase in intravesical pressure. However, it does not escape from the urethra if the voluntary sphincter is intact.

Endoscopy with urethral and bladder pressure studies are of particular advantage in the management of cystocele. It is generally believed that the surgical correction of a cystocele must be accompanied by repair of the urethra and bladder neck. It is believed that if this is not done a continent patient may be made incontinent. This is not always true. Occasionally a cystocele may develop behind a urethral stricture. Plication of the vesical neck in this patient may cause her to be unable to void for a month or 6 weeks. This problem is best treated by urethral dilation at surgery, and no sutures are placed at the vesical neck.

An unstable bladder is the most common cause for urinary incontinence in older women. This is secondary to cerebrovascular disease, which causes impairment of central inhibition. It is a common misconception that surgery prevents recurrent urinary tract infection in these patients, especially if they have a cystocele. Surgery may produce a good anatomic result, but the patient's incontinence may be worse.

The unstable bladder (uninhibited neurogenic bladder) may appear as one of two types on the cystometrogram. The first type shows an increase in intravesical pressure as soon as the bladder starts to fill. The second type is a low-capacity bladder in which a detrusor contraction is precipitated by a cough or sudden change in position. Treatment is by anticholinergic drugs combined with diazepam (Valium) to allow an increase in bladder capacity by preventing uninhibited contractions.

There are those who question the wisdom of the gynecologist doing urethroscopy—feeling that the urinary tract lies outside the gynecologist's domain. It seems logical that if the pelvic surgeon can place a large trocar in the abdomen and insert a telescope to visualize the pelvic contents, he should be able to perform endoscopy of a pelvic structure that is only 1 to 2 inches long.

Some instability of the female bladder is normal, as 50 percent of women have incontinence at some time during their lives. This is giggle incontinence and usually responds to perineal exercises. The reporting of cure rates for stress incontinence can be misleading. There is a difference in operating on a slender patient with giggle incontinence and on an obese diabetic with respiratory disease.

The female patient must be considered in toto. Too many women have become sexual and bladder cripples following operations for stress incontinence when their problem was actually bladder malfunction. Stress incontinence is uncommon as an isolated entity; these women frequently have superimposed urethritis and trigonitis. Associated anatomic defects such as uterine prolapse, rectocele, and enterocele may be present. It is a disservice to the patient to treat one problem and ignore the other. The compartmentalization of the female pelvis has led to poor results including unsuccessful or partial operations.

CONCLUSION

Most failures in the treatment of urinary incontinence are due to diagnostic and not operative failure. New instrumentation and endoscopic techniques make it possible to treat the urethra as a pelvic structure. The decompartmentalization of the female pelvis should lead to improved results and better patient care.

REFERENCES

1. Green TH Jr: Development of a plan for the diagnosis and treatment of urinary stress incontinence. Am J Obstet Gynecol 83:632, 1962
2. Herman JR: Urology: A View Through the Rectrospectroscope. New York, Harper & Row, 1973
3. Hodgkinson CP, Daub HP, Kelly NT: Urethrocystograms: metallic bead-chain technique. Clin Obstet Gynecol 1:668, 1958
4. Kelly HA, Burnam CF: Diseases of Kidneys, Ureters and Bladder, Vol I. New York, Appleton-Century-Crofts, 1922, Chap 9
5. Jeffcoate TNA, Roberts H: Observations on stress incontinence of urine. Am J Obstet Gynecol 64:721, 1952
6. Lund CJ, Benjamin JA, Tristin TA, et al: Cinefluorographic studies of the bladder and urethra in women. Am J Obstet Gynecol 74:896, 1957
7. Macalpine JB: Cystoscopy and Urography, 2nd ed. Baltimore, William Wood, 1936
8. Pousson A, Besnos E (eds): Encyclopédie Française d'Urologie. Paris, Doin et Fils, 1914–1923
9. Ridley JH: Indirect air cystoscopy. South Med J 44:114, 1951
10. Robertson JR: Air cystoscopy. Obstet Gynecol 32:328, 1968
11. Robertson JR: Gas cystometrogram with urethral pressure profile. Obstet Gynecol 44:72, No. 1, 1974
12. Robertson JR: Gynecologic urethroscopy. Am J Obstet Gynecol 115:986, 1973
13. Young HH: A Surgeon's Autobiography. New York, Harcourt, 1940

42

Pediatric Bronchoscopy

Dale Johnson
Stephen L. Gans

New instrumentation has increased the indications and safety of pediatric endoscopy and has caused alteration in many techniques. The breakthrough has come with development of miniature telescopes which provide a sharp and brilliant image, magnification, and a wide-angle view of hollow organ anatomy previously seen dimly or not at all. The small outside diameter of the optical telescope (2.7 mm) allows sufficient additional space within a bronchoscopic sheath for adequate airway plus an instrumentation channel. Ventilation can be controlled precisely in a closed system incorporated into the design of the instrument (Chapter 5). General anesthesia thus becomes the technique of choice for infants and children because of increased safety. Superb lighting, high-resolution optics, and safe control of ventilation and secretions facilitate more accurate inspection, complex endoscopic manipulations, photographic documentation, and careful teaching, all with added safety to the patient.

TECHNIQUE

Bronchoscopy in infants and children is most effectively and safely performed in the operating room. Advantages include the availability of accessory equipment, sterile technique, and most of all trained personnel in the event of difficulty. There is no way to avoid transfer of the patient's own oropharyngeal organisms into the lower airway during passage of the bronchoscope, but it is mandatory that outside organisms from the environment, the surgeon, or from unsterile instruments should be excluded. The desirability of general anesthesia for bronchoscopy in infants and children is an additional reason this procedure should be performed in the operating room.

The patient's head, along with the upper portion of his body is draped with sterile linen, and the surgeon should wear sterile gown and gloves to avoid contamination of the instruments. All instruments inserted into the airway should be sterile.

Proper position is obtained by flexion of the head and neck on the anterior chest, with subsequent moderate hyperextension of the head on the forward flexed neck. Introduction of the bronchoscope is facilitated by initial exposure of the cords with the larynogoscope. It is useful to place a moistened and partially opened gauze sponge over the upper lip and maxillary ridge on the right side for subsequent protection from trauma to the lip, gum line, or teeth (if present) by the bronchoscope.

The laryngoscope should be inserted from the right of the midline with the tip just at the base of the tongue and pointed toward the suprasternal notch. A forward, lifting motion against the base of the tongue exposes the cords by displacing the tongue to the left and elevating the epiglottis. A common error in infants involves *too-deep insertion* because the larynx is situated at a higher level than in the adult. Insertion of the blade too deeply or use of a blade too long for the infant results in airway obstruction from laryngeal occlusion or possible trauma to the epiglottis and upper larynx. The tip of the blade should be on the base of the tongue just at the tip of the epiglottis. As the tongue and epiglottis are lifted forward the blade should be advanced slightly into the vallecula to open and elevate the epiglottis further. Too-deep insertion has the reverse effect.

It is sometimes useful during initial insertion of the laryngoscope to stabilize the tongue and dental ridges with the thumb and first two fingers of the left hand while the laryngoscope is positioned gently with the right. Once the tongue is stabilized by the tip of the laryngoscope blade, the handle of the instrument is shifted to the left hand to leave the right hand free for manipulation of the bronchoscope.

The bronchoscope selected should be small enough to pass through the glottis and subglottic area without causing trauma. Conventional bronchoscopes of small size are difficult to use because vision through the small-diameter open pipe is so extremely limited. The new bronchoscopic telescopes eliminate this problem. The wide-angle view with the telescope inside even the smallest (2.5 mm) sheath gives excellent visualization (Fig, 1, Plate H).* The 2.5-mm sheath is used for most prematures, and the 3.0- or 3.5-mm sheaths are best for most full term infants. The larger sheaths have the advantage of a large air channel for control of respiration and simultaneous suctioning, as well as for the introduction and manipulation of instruments under telescopic vision.

With the glottis exposed by the laryngoscope, the bronchoscope is held like a pencil in the right hand and passed carefully through the cords under direct external vision, using the lip of the bronchoscope to separate the cords. An alternate and perhaps preferable method involves placing the lip of the bronchoscope just beneath the tip of the epiglottis and then passing it through the laryngeal vestibule and between the cords, utilizing the detailed and magnified view through the telescope. The point of greatest resistance is usually in the subglottic area at the lower rim of the cricoid. It is useful to visualize this passage as well. Once the bronchoscope is in the trachea the laryngoscope is removed from the pharynx. If the procedure is performed with visualization through the telescope the laryngoscope may not be necessary at all, or at least may be removed once the lip of the bronchoscope is beneath the tip of the epiglottis.

The bronchoscope with telescope permits continuous direct-vision suctioning through a

All color plates appear at the front of the book.

fine catheter inserted in the instrument channel. This saves time by maintaining a clear field during inspection. The capability for manipulating a soft suction tip while the telescope exposes the deep anatomy of the segmental bronchi permits great selectivity with the suctioning.

Fogging of the tip of the telescope is seldom a problem when the suction catheter is utilized throughout the viewing. Warming the telescope in water prior to insertion into the airway eliminates initial temporary fogging, as does a drop of sterile antifogging solution. The telescope is designed with an antifog sheath, and use of a small oil-free pump can deliver a fine stream of air over the tip of the lens to prevent fogging or fouling with secretions. In the smallest scope, however, the antifog sheath compromises the air channel, and it is preferable to use the telescope without the antifog sheath.

Biopsy and foreign body forceps have been miniaturized so that they pass through the instrument channel and can be used with the telescope in place. The small size of the jaws on the alligator forceps might appear initially to be a disadvantage, but this is not usually the case. The alligator teeth are used to grasp the edge of the object. The detailed view obtained through the telescope allows grasping of foreign objects with precision and security. Improved vision more than offsets any disadvantage from the small size of the forceps head. Occasionally, however, it is necessary to use a forceps of standard design through the open bronchoscopic sheath. In this circumstance the object is pinpointed and the bronchoscope positioned with telescopic viewing. The telescope is then removed, the proximal prism light inserted, and the manipulation performed through the open bronchoscope. Some foreign bodies such as marbles or glass beads defy grasping maneuvers because of their smooth surfaces. A Fogarty catheter passed under direct view beyond the foreign body and then inflated slightly can be withdrawn to move the foreign body out in front of it.

INDICATIONS

Airway Obstructive Problems

Management of airway obstruction in infants requires evaluation of the larynx and supraglottic structures as well as the tracheobronchial tree. The symptom of stridor is common to obstructive lesions above and below the cords, and proper diagnosis and management hinge on thorough evaluation of the entire airway. Except in obvious obstructive emergencies associated with foreign body aspiration, laryngeal trauma, birth asphyxia, or cardiac arrest, endoscopic maneuvers must be preceded by careful history, physical examination, and radiographic evaluation of the airway. Good-quality x-rays of the neck usually localize the problem and may even contraindicate further instrumentation, as in the case of acute infectious epiglottitis. Foreign bodies, tumors, stenosis, and extrinsic compression of the trachea, bronchi, and hypopharynx can usually be identified radiographically. Such prior localization adds safety and precision to any subsequent endoscopic procedures. *Bronchography,* however, is usually contraindicated in evaluation of the airway in small infants. Airway resistance varies inversely with the fourth power of the radius of the air passage. A thin layer of iodized oil on the surface of the small air passages can seriously compromise gas flow and exchange in a sick infant. Careful endoscopic evaluation using the new miniaturized ventilating bronchoscope with telescope is much safer and usually more rewarding.

Mass lesions of the hypopharynx and base of the tongue include hemangiomas, lymphangiomas, lingual thyroid, inflammatory abscesses, and rarely a rhabdomyosarcoma. Direct laryngoscopy usually provides the most satisfactory exposure of these lesions. Therapy of course depends on the nature of the lesion, but temporary tracheostomy is often required. The capillary hemangiomas usually involute spontaneously; the lymphangiomas often require excision; the abscesses require drainage; and the sarcomas require a combination of surgery, radiation, and combinations of antineoplastic drugs. A lingual thyroid sufficiently large to cause obstruction requires excision, but this is rare.

Acute inflammatory disease seldom requires endoscopic investigation, although they may cause serious obstruction. The clinical history of acute onset with stridor leaves a differential diagnosis of infection or foreign body. Acute infectious croup may be mimicked by a foreign body in the hypopharynx which produces irritation and secondary edema of the larynx, but the foreign body problems are usually associated with more acute onset plus a history of ingesting some object. X-rays may be very helpful in this differential diagnosis. Endoscopy is indicated only for foreign body removal. Acute epiglottitis should be diagnosed by the acute onset, systemic toxicity, extreme obstructive inspiratory stridor, and characteristic x-ray finding of the enlarged epiglottis on the lateral view. Endoscopic manipulation is contraindicated. Except in very specialized pediatric intensive care units, urgent tracheostomy in the operating room is the treatment for epiglottitis. Airway obstruction associated with diphtheria is rare nowadays. This formerly was recognized on inspection by the edema, exudate, and pseudomembrane formation in the pharynx.

Laryngomalacia is one of the more common congenital obstructive lesions of the upper airway. This lesion is characterized by an inspiratory stridor or croaking, often increasing during the first 6 to 12 months of life. Onset of symptoms may be during the first week of life, however. Progression in the degree of obstruction by instability and inspiratory prolapse of the supraglottic structures into the airway may require tracheostomy, but this is not common. Growth of the larynx brings stability to the arytenoids and false cords, and a spontaneous decrease and disappearance of symptoms.

Diagnosis can be made with the laryngoscope, but endoscopic evaluation of the larynx and trachea should be performed to rule out any lower lesions which might also be present with the common symptom of stridor. When the laryngoscope blade lifts the epiglottis there is some stabilization of the supraglottic structures and the stridor is decreased. The dynamics of the floppy supraglottic structures are therefore often better evaluated by the bronchoscopic telescope instead of the laryngoscope. The telescope placed just above the glottis reveals a more accurate picture of the "sucking inward" of the arytenoids, the false cords, and the omega-shaped epiglottis, which is often more curved than usual in this condition.

Cysts and laryngoceles may also cause inspiratory stridor. Internal laryngoceles may protrude between the true and false cords or bulge into the aryepiglottic fold. These usually have some connection with the interior of the larynx. Glottic cysts usually do not communicate with the internal larynx.[4] Therapy is by endoscopic aspiration or marsupialization.

Laryngeal webs may require urgent tracheostomy in affected infants. Most webs are incomplete posteriorly, but the opening may be too small to permit passage of an oral endotracheal tube. The webs may occur as a supraglottic fusion of the false cords, a glottic membrane between the true cords, a fusion of the anterior portion of the true cords, or as subglottic webs.[4] Infants with complete glottic obstruction rarely survive, but we have encountered an infant with a complete glottic membrane between the true cords plus a tracheoesophageal fistula at the cervical level, permitting survival until a tracheostomy could be performed. Therapy in incision or excision of the web may be facilitated by using the new bronchoscope with telescope, which can provide superior visualization and access to some subglottic and glottic problems. The same telescope can be used in conjunction with an infant urethral resectoscope instead of the bronchoscopic sheath for resection of some types of subglottic stenosis.

Vocal cord paralysis is an important cause of stridor in infants, and careful evaluation of cord movement by direct laryngoscopy should be performed with the infant essentially awake. Postoperative palsy may follow recurrent nerve injury associated with intrathoracic or cervical procedures, but congenital palsies (both uni- and bilateral) are seen. Extensive birth trauma or severe lesions of the central nervous system are usually associated with bilateral paralysis. Isolated right cord palsy may occur, but left cord paralysis is often associated with abnormalities of the heart and great vessels. Bilateral cord paralysis usually requires tracheostomy.

Obstructing neoplasms of the larynx in infants and children mostly take the form of benign, wartlike papillomatous growths. Recurrence has commonly accompanied excision and vaccine therapy.[8] There is current interest in cryosurgical or laser destruction of these lesions.

Foreign bodies in the upper airway are usually manifested by sudden choking, dyspnea, voice change, and occasionally death from asphyxia. Airway obstruction may also result from a large foreign body lodged in the upper esophagus. Buttons, pieces of plastic, pins, tacks, glass, egg shell, and all the various objects which infants and children place in their mouths have been recovered from the upper airway.

Laryngeal trauma may cause obstruction from edema and hematoma or actual cartilaginous fracture or disruption. The miniature bronchoscope with telescope has proved very useful in evaluating the extent of laryngeal injury. Tracheostomy is nearly always necessary as a temporary measure, but endoscopic evaluation may help to determine the need for an internal stent. Endoscopic reinspection of the airway prior to tracheal decannulation is also essential.

Acquired *subglottic stenosis* has increased in frequency with advances in management of respiratory problems in infants. Long-term intubations for assisted or controlled ventilation may be associated with chronic irritation in the subglottic cricoid region where the trachea is rigid and has its smallest diameter. The incidence is variable in newborn intensive care units, some claiming no incidence and others recognizing this as a significant complication of airway management. A loose fit of the endotracheal tube appears to be an important factor in prevention. Preexisting acute inflammatory disease of the upper airway, as in croup, has been associated with a high incidence of subglottic stenosis[9] following endotracheal intubation.

Stridor on inspiration and expiration is again a major symptom of this form of upper airway obstruction. Acutely, the subglottic reaction may be such that endotracheal extubation cannot be accomplished because of obstruction. Tracheostomy is necessary in this case, and therapeutic attack on the subglottic area is planned for a later time. In other situations the extubation is successful, but subsequent scarring and fibrosis result and cause subglottic narrowing with onset of stridor weeks or months later. Congenital subglottic narrowing also occurs, but the acquired postintubation variety is now more common.

The miniaturized infant bronchoscope with telescopes has greatly improved evaluation and management of acquired subglottic stenosis. Visualization of the narrowed area below the cords is more informative, and appropriate management can be planned. Thin, immature webs may require only a few dilatations using a laryngoscope and tapered dilators. More extensive involvement with a mature scar presents a complex problem in management. Injection of the stenotic ring with a steroid compound followed by dilatation has some experimental basis,[1] but the limited clinical experience with the technique is not conclusive.[10] Extensive scarring has been managed by excision and placement of a molded internal laryngeal stent.[2] One of the authors (D.J.) has managed subtotal occlusion of the subglottic airway by staged four-quadrant endoscopic excision of the subglottic scar, using the miniature telescope and the infant urethral resectoscope. Follow-up at 18 months on the first infant managed with this technique has revealed no recurrence of airway obstruction or stridor.

The therapeutic approach must be tailored to the degree of stenosis and to the extent and maturity of the scarring. Many of these problems improve greatly with time and growth of the trachea. The difficulties in managing an infant with a tracheostomy at home, however, justify approaches to relieve the obstruction and to remove the cannula from the trachea, providing that extreme risks are not involved by decannulation.

Post tracheostomy obstruction can be a problem. Decannulation difficulties in infants with tracheostomy are well known to those with experience on a large pediatric service.[3] Long and costly hospitalizations have resulted from the repeated failure to achieve extubation of an infant with a tracheostomy. Tracheal instability, inward deformity of a tracheal ring at the upper margin of the stoma, and an intraluminal granuloma either at the stoma or on the tracheal wall near the tube tip all may cause airway obstruction following tracheostomy tube removal.[6] Tracheal instability and deformity should be prevented by careful design of the initial tracheal incision (vertical through two or three tracheal rings). Cartilage should never be excised from an infant's trachea. Granulomas must be removed either by direct excision through the stoma or by endoscopic resection or fulguration.

Tracheoscopy for evaluation of the altered anatomy should be performed prior to decannulation. Instability of the anterior tracheal wall, inward encroachment on the lumen by cartilaginous deformity, or intraluminal granuloma can all be identified and corrective measures taken. The techniques involving trial occlusion of the tracheostomy tube or the use of progressively smaller tubes are not always practical decannulation techniques in small infants because the small airway may be filled by the smallest effective tube available. Endoscopic determination that intraluminal obstruction factors are absent allow sedation of the infant and decannulation in the intensive care unit. Occlusion of the stoma by a dressing to facilitate effective cough plus the administration of humid air, suctioning, and careful chest physiotherapy has permitted tracheal decannulation in every infant in our series, providing mechanical obstruction has been corrected first. Following spontaneous closure of the tracheostomy stoma within 5 to 7 days, endoscopic evaluation of the tracheal lumen should be repeated. An intraluminal granuloma may form during spontaneous closure of the stoma. One 3-month-old infant developed intraluminal obstruction and severe dyspnea 10 days following tracheal decannulation by one of the authors (D.J.). The initial endoscopic evaluation had revealed no obstruction. Subsequent excision of the granuloma at the stoma site, with direct tracheal closure, produced a normal airway.

An obstructing granuloma in the lower trachea or at the carina is more difficult to handle and is caused by pressure and irritation from the end of an indwelling tracheal tube. This may occur even with the newer soft plastic tubes if the length of the tube and its position are not properly adjusted. We have successfully resected a granuloma at the carina which was causing a valve-like obstruction of the right main bronchus. Excision was accomplished endoscopically with the miniature telescope and the infant urethral resectoscope.

Vascular rings, bronchogenic cysts, enteric duplication cysts, and mediastinal tumors all may cause tracheobronchial obstruction by extrinsic compression or deviation. Extrinsic pressure from vascular rings not uncommonly causes structural weakness in the compressed tracheal cartilage (tracheomalacia) so that instability of the tracheal wall and functional airway obstruction may persist following correction of the extrinsic pressure cause. Radiographic evaluation plays the major role in diagnosing these problems, but bronchoscopy is important in evaluating bronchogenic cysts and in postoperative management with tracheomalacia.

Congenital or postinflammatory stenosis of a bronchus may respond to endoscopic dilatation or limited fulguration or resection. Persistent stenosis with distal collapse or infection is more commonly handled by resection of the affected lung segment or lobe.

Foreign body obstruction of the airway is associated with significant mortality in infants and children 2 months to 7 years old.[11] Radiographic and endoscopic examination should be performed on the basis of a suspicious history. The characteristic story includes sudden choking, gagging, or coughing while chewing or sucking on particulate matter or food. Nut meats and bits of shell are common offenders, but raw carrot, bacon, pieces of plastic, chalk, beads, tacks, pins, beans, and many other objects have all been recovered from the airway.

The most severe and urgent obstructions occur at the laryngeal level. Tracheal obstruction is equally dangerous but less common. Once the foreign object slips into a bronchus the immediate threat to life is lessened.

Wheezing, cough, and audible clicking and air trapping may be apparent even to the parent, but more importantly physical findings may be completely absent even on careful examination. Early chest x-rays also may be completely normal if the object is not radiopaque and if it is situated in the airway without causing obstruction or air trapping. Inspiration-expiration films are more sensitive in suggesting air trapping and mediastinal shift. Lobar or segmental collapse and infiltration are late changes which should be prevented by early endoscopic examination and treatment. It cannot be overemphasized that a history suspicious of foreign body aspiration is indication for careful bronchoscopy.

Conditions Leading to Aspiration of Abnormal Tracheobronchial Secretions

Laryngotracheoesophageal cleft represents a failure of separation between the larynx and trachea anteriorly and the esophagus posteriorly. The extent of the cleft is variable. Mild clefts may involve only the larynx with a cleft between the arytenoids. Severe forms present with a common channel for food and respiration all the way to the thoracic inlet. The clinical picture of recurrent aspiration and cyanosis with feedings associated with abnormal voice or cry is suggestive, but the diagnosis must be confirmed by direct bronchoscopic visualization. Radiographic studies usually show massive aspiration. Precise definition of the lesion is difficult, and a swallowing study itself is hazardous for the infant. One patient from the literature had nine endoscopies over 46 months before the correct diagnosis was made.[5] The new infant bronchoscope with telescope allows precise evaluation of the laryngeal and tracheal anatomy, and with it the diagnosis appears obvious. Pettersson[7] is credited with the first successful surgical repair. Several cases

have been repaired since, including a case by one of the authors (D.J.).

Isolated "N-H" type tracheoesophageal fistula (TEF) presents a clinical picture similar to but less severe than the laryngotracheoesophageal cleft. Choking, coughing, and occasional cyanosis with feedings should raise the possibility of this diagnosis. Where investigation has been delayed in older infants, recurrent pulmonary infections are part of the symptom complex. Radiographic demonstration is usually achieved by flooding the upper esophagus with barium by catheter, but many small fistulas have been missed by x-ray studies. Other manipulative studies are not consistently accurate.

The isolated TEF can be identified precisely by direct visualization of the posterior tracheal wall with the infant telescopic bronchoscope. A fine catheter can be passed through the fistula under direct vision to aid subsequent localization during surgical repair. (Fig. 2, Plate H). In four of our cases the open fistula was demonstrated with the new bronchoscope after repeat radiographic studies of the esophagus failed to demonstrate any abnormality.

Congenital bronchobiliary fistula, with bile drainage from the right lobe of the liver into the right main stem bronchus, has been identified endoscopically as a cause of persistent pneumonia. Therapy of course involves transthoracic division of the fistula.

The *removal of viscid tracheobronchial secretions* and the management of atelectasis in infants following major surgical procedures or in pulmonary infections or fibrocystic disease usually do not require bronchoscopy. Prophylactic measures with humidification of inspired gas, systemic hydration, and skilled physiotherapy involving percussion, vibration, and postural drainage are usually effective. When mechanical suctioning is required it is best accomplished after passage of an endotracheal tube in the awake infant. Saline lavage via the tube with suctioning, artificial cough, and positive pressure inflation may be repeated several times. Bronchoscopy is occasionally necessary for selective therapy to specific lung segments.

ANESTHESIA

General anesthesia offers many advantages for bronchoscopy in infants and children, and it is the technique of choice under the following conditions:

1. An experienced pediatric anesthesiologist is available.
2. The bronchoscopic equipment is of modern design, which permits safe control of ventilation for indefinite periods even with respiratory paralysis.

In the small infant controlled ventilation in a semiclosed system using general anesthesia is much safer than heavy sedation and dependence upon spontaneous respirations. General anesthesia eliminates any movements which might cause injury during the instrumentation. Avoidance of psychic trauma and the unpleasant memory picture associated with examination is a very real benefit for the child. Finally, general anesthesia with complete control of the patient allows a careful, unhurried procedure that is pleasant and more advantageous for surgeon and patient alike.

RESULTS

The newly designed infant and child bronchoscopes with optical telescope have been available since 1971.* These instruments have improved our ability to visualize anatomic detail (Fig. 3, Plate H) and have lessened the possibility of complication. We have experienced few problems directly resulting from bronchoscopy performed with this equipment in 165 infants and children (Table 1). Six of the infants weighed less than 1800 g. One 10-month-old child had a croup following difficult instrumentation for removal of a glass bead in the left upper lobe. This procedure, though difficult, would have been impossible without the oblique view telescope and the flexible forceps. No infant or child has had major obstruction or required tracheoscopy as a result of bronchoscopic instrumentation, even though the small scope has been used to visualize or pass through significant stenotic areas.

Adequate visualization allows improved judgment regarding the safe limits of the procedure. One small infant did develop a tension pneumothorax following endoscopic dilatation of a congenital web occluding the bronchus intermedius on the right. This infant was origi-

Manufacturer: K. Storz, Endoscopy-America, Inc., 650 South San Vicente Boulevard, Los Angeles, California 90048.

TABLE 1.   Procedures Performed in 165 Infants and Children

Procedure	No. of Patients
Diagnostic	
Cord palsy: R/O lower airway obstruction	2
Congenital tracheal stenosis	4
Laryngotracheoesophageal cleft	3
Laryngeal cyst	2
Crush injury to airway	2
Lobar collapse	14
Lobar emphysema	3
Suspected TEF, natural or recurrent	48
Subglottic stenosis	4
Laryngomalacia	5
Tracheobronchomalacia	5
? Tracheal granuloma	4
Evaluation for tracheal extubation	7
Obstruction 2 degrees to neoplasm	1
Caustic burn of airway	3
Therapeutic	
Tracheal foreign body	3
Bronchial foreign body	13
Tracheobronchial lavage	3
Endoscopic resection of subglottic ring	7
Endoscopic resection of tracheal granuloma	11
Dilatation of tracheal stenosis	19
Dilatation of bronchial stenosis	2

nally treated for severe respiratory distress syndrome, had advanced pulmonary dysplasia, and had experienced two previous episodes of pneumothorax with positive pressure ventilation. We have not experienced failure in our series of foreign body removals using the new bronchoscopes. The smaller instruments provide a magnified and detailed view of both the foreign object and the grasping forceps during manipulation, and foreign body removal has become a safe and more efficient procedure.

COMPLICATIONS

The potential complications associated with instrumentation of the airway in small infants are all life-threatening. A significant possibility involves airway obstruction following mechanical trauma and subsequent edema of the epiglottis, true cords, or subglottic portion of the airway. Perforation of the trachea or a bronchus is possible, with resulting pneumothorax or pneumomediastinum. The introduction of infection through poor technique and contaminated instruments can also have serious consequences. Finally, inadequate control ventilation or partial mechanical obstruction of the airway during instrumentation can result in cerebral hypoxia and even cardiac arrest. The possibility that any of these complications will occur in the hands of an experienced surgeon has been measurably diminished by miniaturized equipment providing vastly improved visualization and secure control of ventilation.

REFERENCES

1. Ashcraft KW, Holder TM: The experimental treatment of esophageal strictures by intralesional steroid injections. J Thorac Cardiovasc Surg 58:685, 1969
2. Birck HG: Endoscopic repair of laryngeal stenosis. Trans Am Acad Ophthalmol Otolaryngol 74:140, 1970
3. Geenberg LM, Davenport HT, Shimo G, et al: Method for difficult decannulations in children. Arch Otolaryngol 81:72, 1965
4. Holinger PH: Clinical aspects of congenital anomalies of the larynx, trachea, bronchi and esophagus. J Laryngol Otolaryngol 75:1, 1961
5. Jahrsdoerfer RA, Kirchner JA, Thaler S, et al: Cleft larynx. Arch Otolaryngol 86:82, 1967
6. Lewis RS, Ludman H: Decannulation after tracheostomy in infants and young children. J Laryngol 79:435, 1965
7. Pettersson G: Inhibited separation of larynx and the upper part of trachea from oesophagus in a newborn: report of a case successfully operated upon. Acta Chir Scand 110:250, 1955
8. Shepkowitz NL, Worland M, Holinger P, et al: Evaluation of an autogenous laryngeal papilloma vaccine. Laryngoscope 77:993, 1967
9. Striker TW, Stool S, Downes J, et al: Prolonged nasotracheal intubation in infants and children. Arch Otolaryngol 85:210, 1967
10. Waggoner LG, Belenky WM, Clark C, et al: Treatment of acquired subglottic stenosis. Ann Otol Rhinol Laryngol 82:822, 1973
11. Weston JT: Airway foreign body fatalities in children. Ann Otol Rhinol Laryngol 74:144, 1965

43

Bronchoscopy with Rigid Instruments (Adults)

John E. Rayl

The word "bronchoscopy" was derived from the Greek words *bronkhos* and *skopein*. *Bronkhos* referred to the windpipe or trachea and possibly included both main bronchi. The interpretation of *skopein* was to see or to examine. Therefore the original definition of bronchoscopy was the act of examining the interior of the trachea and the two main bronchi with a lighted tubular instrument called the bronchoscope. Today bronchoscopy includes examination of the tracheobronchial tree as far peripherally as the fourth or fifth segmental division in each lung. This extent of examination is now possible through the combined use of the open bronchoscope with the 0-, 30-, and 90-degree telescopes and the flexible bronchofiberscope.

BRONCHOSCOPES

The Storz open bronchoscope with the Hopkins rod-lens telescopes (Fig. 1) and the Olympus bronchofiberscope used mainly as a flexible telescope (Fig. 2) are currently preferred for a complete diagnostic bronchoscopy. The Storz adult bronchoscope provides more room within its sheath (diameter 8.5 mm) than most other bronchoscopes and has a wide range of accessory endoscopic instruments including telescopic biopsy forceps. The Storz Hopkins rod-lens telescopes and accessory instruments are also available for infant-size bronchoscopes. The side arm of the Storz bronchoscope has connections for a respirator or anesthetic equipment when assisted respiration or general anesthesia is employed (Fig. 1C). The

magnified and wide-angle views through the Storz Hopkins rod-lens telescopes provide a brighter and more detailed image than the bronchofiberscope (Fig. 12, below). The forward (0-degree), forwardoblique (30-degree), and right angle (90-degree) telescopes permit inspection of the bronchi as far as the fourth or fifth subdivisions in the basal segmental bronchi of the lower lobes, the second subdivision of the medial and lateral segments of the middle lobe, and two subdivisions in the anterior, superior lingula, and inferior lingula of the left upper lobe. Visualization of additional subsegments of the right middle, left upper, and right upper lobes is obtained with the Olympus bronchofiberscope used as a flexible telescope through the Storz adult bronchoscope (Figs. 2A,D). *It should be emphasized that a conventional bronchofiberscope cannot be passed any further into the basal segmental bronchi of the lower lobes than a rigid telescope since their outer diameters are approximately the same.*

Contraindications to the use of the open (rigid) bronchoscope are the indications for the use of the flexible bronchofiberscope. Therefore use of the flexible bronchofiberscope is indicated where: (1) a tracheostomy tube has been present for a short duration; (2) a mechanical ventilator is necessary in a patient requiring a tracheostomy tube; (3) there is severe Marie Strumple arthritis or other orthopedic disability that prevents extension of the neck; (4) there is recent fracture of cervical vertebra(e); and (5) there is anklyosis of the mandibular joint causing inability to open the mouth.

A bronchoscopic examination with the flexible bronchofiberscope alone, whether through

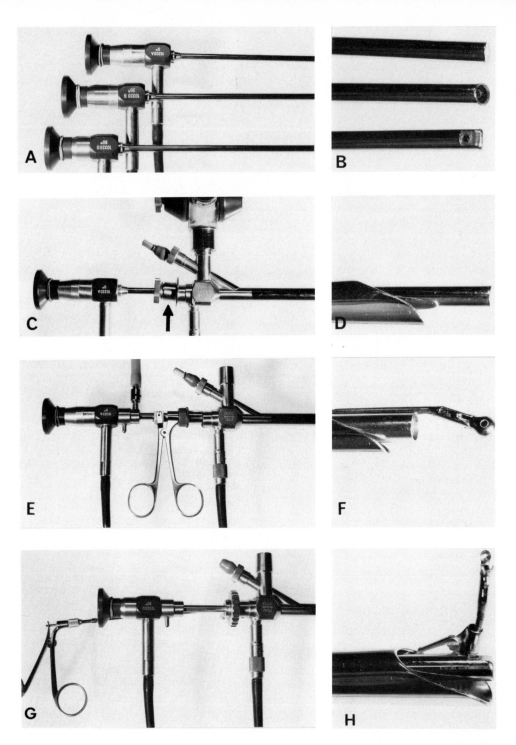

FIG. 1. Storz bronchoscopic equipment. **A.** Proximal ends of Hopkins rod-lens telescopes with fiberoptic light bundles. **B.** Distal ends of Hopkins rod-lens telescopes. **C.** Storz bronchoscope with ACMI adaptor (arrow) holding Hopkins 0-degree telescope. Connector for anesthetic gas machine is attached to side arm (top). **D.** Telescope (0 degrees) extended beyond distal end of bronchoscope for inspection of basal segments. **E.** Bronchoscope with telescopic biopsy forceps. **F.** Distal end of same assembly as in **E.** **G.** Bronchoscope with flexible cup biopsy forceps, 90-degree telescope, and deflecting device. **H.** Distal end, same asembly as in **G.**

FIG. 2. A. Olympus BF-B2 bronchofiberscope with flexible forceps in biopsy channel inserted into Storz bronchoscope. A Storz telescopic adaptor (not shown) can be used between bronchoscope and bronchofiberscope for air seal. **B.** Distal end of Olympus bronchofiberscope with extended cup biopsy forceps. **C.** Same as **B** with extended biopsy brush. **D.** Distal end of Storz bronchoscope showing the Olympus bronchofiberscope as used for examination of upper lobe bronchi. To obtain the 180-degree view shown here, pressure must be applied against the inferior wall of the upper lobe bronchi (arrow).

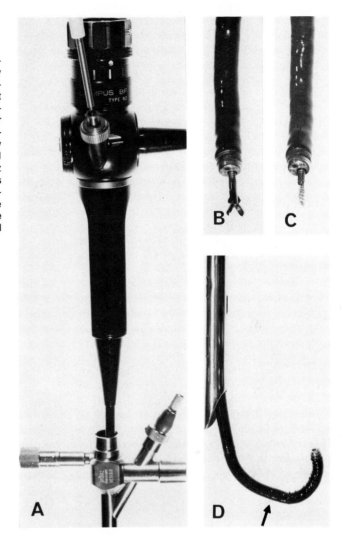

the nose, mouth, or endotracheal tube, is hampered by (1) impaired visual quality, a decrease in light transmission, and a narrower angle of view, which reduces the ease of orientation (Fig. 12, below); (2) inability to prevent spontaneous dislocation of the distal tip during cough; (3) difficulty in removing the instrument for cleaning the distal lens whenever necessary; (4) an extremely small orifice for removal of thick secretions or blood; (5) a biopsy forceps so small that the amount of tissue is often insufficient for diagnosis especially when the surface of an endobronchial tumor is covered by mucosa; and (6) a greater degree of hypoxemia than is incurred with the open bronchoscope. The bronchofiberscope cannot be used effectively for removal of most foreign bodies from the tracheobronchial tree.

In attempts to clean the flexible bronchofiberscope thoroughly there is danger that the cleaning fluid may enter and cause damage to the optical system. Solution sterilization is virtually ineffective since the optical end cannot be immersed. The only satisfactory method for sterilizing the flexible bronchoscope is with ethylene oxide. This method has the disadvantage of requiring an aeration period of 12 hours in an aerating machine or 72 hours in room air before it can be reused.

INDICATIONS FOR BROCHOSCOPY

The indications for diagnostic bronchoscopy include: suspected bronchogenic carcinoma; suspected benign endobronchial tumor; pulmonary bleeding of undetermined origin; obtaining bronchial secretions for bacteriologic studies; and preoperative evaluation prior to pulmonary resection.

The most frequent indication for diagnostic bronchoscopy is suspected bronchogenic carcinoma. This diagnosis should be considered when patients have: (1) nodular lesion(s) in their chest roentgenograms; (2) radiographic evidence of unresolved or slowly resolving pneumonia; (3) pulmonary hemoptysis or hemorrhage; (4) an increase in cough unrelated to acute respiratory infection; (5) recent onset of localized wheezing caused by partial airway obstruction, which may change with the patient's position; (6) absence of bronchovesicular breath sounds overlying a segment or lobe that indicates airway obstruction even though the chest roentgenogram may not reveal atelectasis; and (7) unexplained chest pain, polyarthritis, or symptoms of a metabolic disease beyond the fourth decade of life in a patient with a history of heavy cigarette smoking.

A benign endobronchial tumor may produce an insidious onset of airway obstruction. Wheezing may occur when obstruction of the airway is incomplete. When complete obstruction of a segmental bronchus occurs, atelectasis is not seen until secondary infection distal to the obstructing lesion interferes with cross ventilation through the pores of Köhn. Endoscopic differentiation between a benign and malignant endobronchial lesion requires a biopsy since the gross appearance may be misleading.

Bronchoscopy helps to localize the source of hemoptysis to a lobar or segmental bronchus so that a pulmonary resection can be done if bleeding should become life threatening. Attempts to localize the source of bleeding frequently lead to a diagnosis of bronchogenic carcinoma. Other causes of hemoptysis are acute bronchitis, bronchiectasis, tuberculosis, and severe mitral stenosis. Hemoptysis due to acute bronchitis typically occurs between the second and fourth weeks after the onset of acute respiratory infection when symptoms have almost subsided. Hemoptysis secondary to bronchogenic carcinoma is more frequently unassociated with an acute respiratory infection.

Occasionally a patient may have an inflammatory lesion that appears to be tuberculosis, although sputum smears and cultures have remained negative for acid-fast bacilli. Bronchial secretions collected at the time of bronchoscopy or during the first 24 hours following bronchoscopy may be the only specimen positive for these organisms.

Bronchoscopy done prior to a pulmonary resection should determine the precise location of the endobronchial tumor or other lesion to be resected, the presence of other unsuspected benign or malignant lesions, the existence of acute bronchitis, and unusual types of bronchial anatomy such as a tracheal bronchus leading to a pulmonary lesion in the right upper lobe. In patients with carcinoma a biopsy of the mucosa at the point of the intended pulmonary resection is advisable. Preferably the preoperative bronchoscopy should be performed early enough prior to thoracotomy to permit bacteriologic, cytologic, and histologic studies to be completed. Adequate time should also be planned for treatment of acute bronchopulmonary disease if it exists.

Therapeutic bronchoscopy may be performed to remove a foreign body and/or retained secretions, or in an emergency to establish an airway when an endobronchial or nasotracheal tube cannot be readily inserted for resuscitation. Therapeutic bronchoscopy should always be done when there is a history suggesting aspiration of a foreign body that may be radiographically nonopaque. Removal of the foreign body should be accomplished as early as possible since its continued presence often produces mucosal irritation, erythema, edema, large amounts of mucoid secretions, and subsequent atelectasis.

The goal to be achieved during therapeutic bronchoscopy in patients with retained secretions and impending atelectasis is to remove the secretions and determine if an obstructing organic lesion is present. Thick or tenacious bronchial secretions may require saline irrigation to reduce their viscosity sufficiently for removal through the suction cannula. Since acute bronchitis is frequently associated with atelectasis, gentleness during aspiration may reduce the degree of iatrogenic mucosal ecchymoses and thereby decrease the subsequent edema.

CONTRAINDICATIONS FOR BRONCHOSCOPY

Contraindications for bronchoscopy are relatively few in any patient who is psychologically prepared. If the endoscopic findings will not influence the future treatment of the patient regardless of what they may be, a diagnostic bronchoscopy should not be performed. A history of allergy to the anesthetic agent being employed is a contraindication to bronchoscopy unless another drug can be used. An acute bronchopulmonary infection, severe liver impairment, or kidney disease may contraindicate the use of general anesthesia. A large carcinoma of the tongue or larynx may obstruct the airway to such an extent that a bronchoscope cannot be safely passed without producing trauma and life-threatening postoperative edema.

CLINICAL EVALUATION OF PATIENT

The endoscopist should visit the patient prior to the bronchoscopy, telling him why the examination is being done and how it will be accomplished. The preoperative clinical evaluation of the patient should then lead the endoscopist to a tentative diagnosis.

The clinical evaluation should include the patient's history of cough, sputum, hemoptysis, dyspnea, wheezing, frequency of acute respiratory infections, pneumonia, tuberculosis and its chemotherapy, episodes of chest pain, weight loss, smoking habits, and alcoholic intake. The endoscopist should be aware of the medications the patient is receiving, especially bronchodilators, cardiac drugs, and antibiotics. Physical findings that should be carefully evaluated include temperature, pulse, masses in the neck found by palpation, heart and lung findings by auscultation, an enlarged nodular liver or other masses found by palpation of the abdomen, presence of clubbing of fingers or toes, and dependent edema. Pulmonary function studies and electrocardiographic (ECG) records should be studied in patients with respiratory or coronary insufficiency to determine if prophylactic oxygen therapy is indicated during bronchoscopy. A complete blood count, sputum bacteriology and cytology, and skin tests for tuberculosis and fungus diseases should be reviewed.

The above clinical evaluation can be accomplished effectively in a short time by utilizing a bronchoscopic worksheet that briefly outlines all of the important features of the clinical history, physical findings, and laboratory data. In the worksheet shown in Figure 3 only the

known portions of each date (month, day, year) are completed. Any symptom that has not occurred is indicated by a "0" on the line following the symptom title, and the remaining information is omitted.

Segmental Localization of the Roentgenographic Lesion

All chest roentgenograms should be reviewed, including recent upright posteroanterior (PA) and Bucky lateral chest views. The latter, with the side of the pulmonary lesion toward the film, provides more detail than a non-Bucky film. These roentgenograms are taken preferably in the upright position so that fluid, if present, tends to gravitate into a dependent position in the pleural space or pulmonary cavity. The upright position also allows the diaphragm to lower to the maximum degree during inspiration.

Roentgenographic localization of the pulmonary lesion to a segment or subsegement allows the endoscopist to pay particular attention to the bronchi leading to the lesion. If a positive diagnosis is not made during this special attention to the localized bronchopulmonary segment, a washing or brushing of the segmental or subsegmental bronchi may increase the probability of a diagnosis. Diagrams for localization of the bronchopulmonary segments according to the classification of Huber and Jackson[1] are helpful in determining the segmental localization of the pulmonary lesion (Fig. 4).

Right Upper Lobe. In the PA chest roentgenogram, the right upper lobe is generally above the transverse fissure, which should normally be found extending laterally from the right hilum (Fig. 4A). If the upper lobe is divided into thirds by lines radiating from the hilum to the chest wall, it is separated into the three segments. The apical segment (1) is the third that lies next to the upper mediastinum; the anterior segment (3) is located adjacent to the transverse fissure; and the posterior segment (2) is found between the apical and anterior segments.

In the right lateral Bucky chest roentgenogram, the upper lobe lies above the transverse fissure and anterior to the upper portion of the oblique fissure (Fig. 4B). The three segments in the right upper lobe can also be localized in the lateral view by dividing the lobe into thirds with lines extending from the hilum to the

A

Name ______ Social Security No. ______ Examination No.

Age Sex 1=Male 2=Female Race 1=Caucasian 2=Negro 3=Other Ward No. ______ Resident ______

Occupation ______ Last Employed MO. DAY YR. Cine Film No. ______

Admission Date Location of Patient 1=VAH Lake City 2=VAH Gainesville 3=Shands Date MO. DAY YR.

Code to be used below unless otherwise specified: 0=ABSENT OR NONE; 1=EQUIVOCAL OR OCCASIONAL; 2=PRESENT; 3=INCREASED

Chief Complaint ______

PULMONARY HISTORY

COUGH ______

Onset MO. DAY YR.

Present cough frequency

0=NO COUGH 1=OCCASIONALLY OR EQUIVOCAL 2=MORN. ONLY 3=DAYTIME 4=MORN & NIGHTS 5=DURING DAY & NT. 6=OTHER

Recent change in cough habit

Describe ______

SPUTUM ______

Onset MO. DAY YR.

Color 0=NONE 1=UNKNOWN 2=CLEAR 3=WHITE 4=GRAY OR BLACKISH 5=OCCASIONALLY YELLOW OR GREEN 6=USUALLY YEL. OR GRN.

Volume cc/24 hours

HEMOPTYSIS ______

No. Episodes

First Episode

Onset MO. DAY YR.

Last Episode

Onset MO. DAY YR.

Duration last episode days

Type 1=EQUIVOCAL 2=STREAKING ONLY 3=GROSS BLOOD

CHEST PAIN ______

No. episodes

First Episode

Onset MO. DAY YR.

Last Episode

Onset MO. DAY YR.

Duration last episode weeks.

Location 1=RIGHT 2=LEFT 3=BILATERAL 4=PRECORDIAL

OTHER PULMONARY FINDINGS ______

Asymptomatic X-ray lesion

Date ______ MO. DAY YR.

Metastatic lesion (clinically)

Location ______

Duration weeks.

CURRENT THERAPY ______ (during past week)

Bronchodilator Drugs:

List ______

Cardiac drugs

Digitalis

Other List ______

PHYSICAL FINDINGS

HEIGHT AND WEIGHT

Height inches

Present weight pounds

lbs. lost in mos

TEMPERATURE

Highest temperature in past week: °F

NECK

Masses 1=SUPRACLAVICULAR 2=ANTERIOR CERVICAL 3=POSTERIOR CERVICAL

Side 1=RIGHT 2=LEFT 3=BILATERAL

HEART

Murmur TYPE: 1=SYSTOLIC 2=DIASTOLIC 3=BOTH

Location 1=APICAL 2=AORTIC 3=BOTH 4=PULMONIC

EKG

Date ______ MO. DAY YR.

Findings:

Arrythmia

Coronary insufficiency

Myocardial infarction

LUNGS

Auscultatory Findings	RUL	RML	RLL	LUL Upr Div.	LUL Lingula	LLL
Bronchovesicular breath sounds						
Pleural Rub						

CHEST ROENTGENOGRAM

Rib lesions: RT LT

Pleural Effusion: RT LT

Mediastinal Widening:

Cardiomegaly: RV LV LA

Vascular enlargement (hilar): RT LT

Roentgenographic Lesions	RUL	RML	RLL	LUL Upr. Div.	LUL Lingula	LLL
Nodule						
Pneumonia						
Atelectasis						
Cavity, Abscess						
Fibrosis						
Pulmonary Vessels						

FIG. 3. **A.** Upper half of a computerized bronchoscopic worksheet for recording the pertinent pulmonary history, physical findings, and chest roentgenographic and laboratory data during the clinical evaluation of the patient. Symptoms that have not occurred are indicated by "O" on the line beside each symptom title. Only known portions of each date are recorded. (Continued)

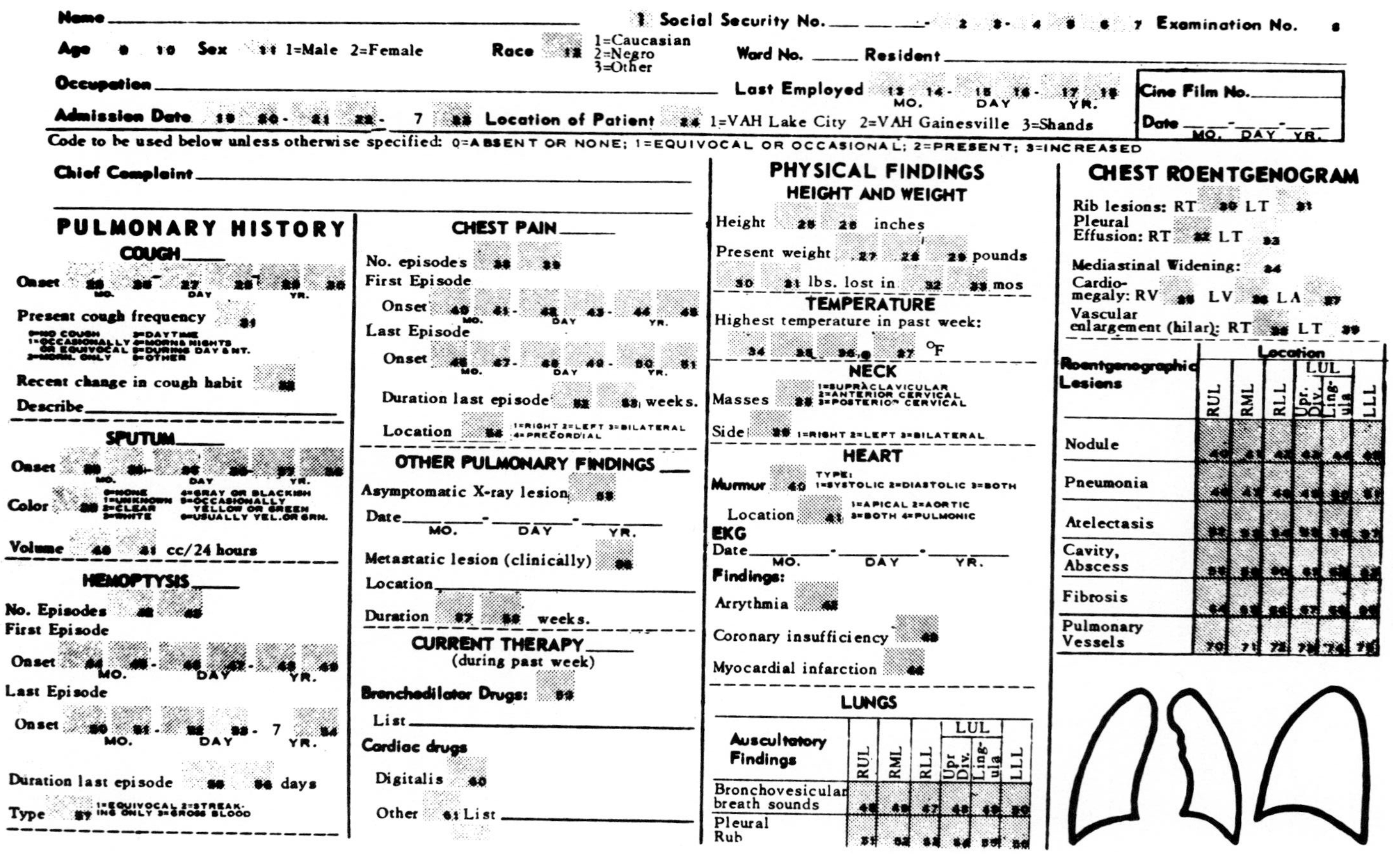

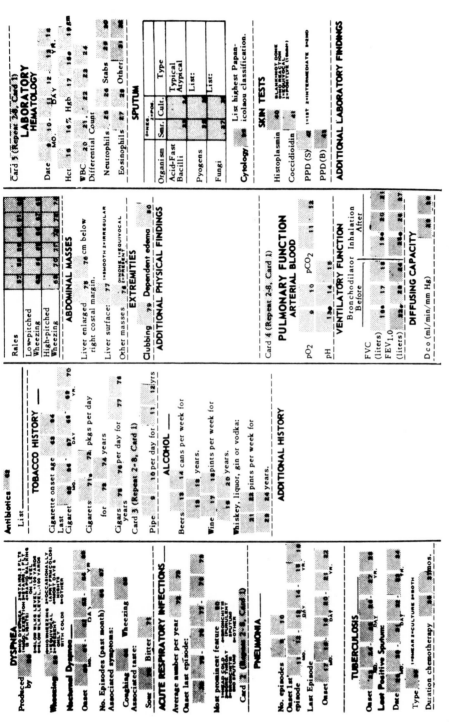

FIG. 3 (cont.). **B.** Lower half of a computerized bronchoscopic worksheet for recording the pertinent pulmonary history, physical findings, and chest roentgenographic and laboratory data during the clinical evaluation of the patient.

557

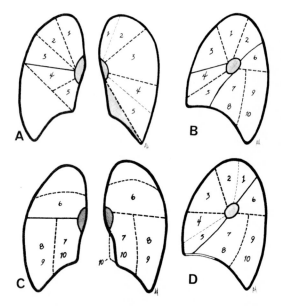

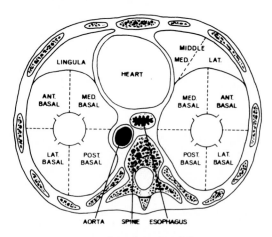

FIG. 4. A. Posteroanterior (PA) view showing roentgenographic localization of the bronchopulmonary segments in the right upper, right middle, and left upper lobes according to Huber and Jackson[1] classification. The transverse fissure separates the right upper and right middle lobes. The right upper lobe segments are apical (1), posterior (2), and anterior (3). The right middle lobe segments are lateral (4) and medial (5). The left upper lobe segments are apical subsegment (1), posterior subsegment (2), anterior (3), superior lingula (4), and inferior lingula (5). **B.** Lateral view showing roentgenographic localization of the bronchopulmonary segments of the right lung (anterior surface to the left). The transverse fissure and oblique fissure separate the right upper, right middle, and right lower lobes. **C.** PA view showing roentgenographic localization of the bronchopulmonary segments in the right and left lower lobes. The right lower lobe segments are superior (6), medial basal (7), anterior basal (8), lateral basal (9), and posterior basal (10). The left lower lobe segments are superior (6), medial basal subsegment (7), anterior basal subsegment (8), lateral basal (9), and posterior basal (10). The latter (10) extends behind the cardiac shadow, as indicated by the dotted line. **D.** Lateral view showing roentgenographic localization of the bronchopulmonary segments of the left lung (anterior surface to the left). The oblique fissure separates the left upper and left lower lobes.

upper rib cage. The posterior segment (2) is adjacent to the oblique fissure; the anterior segment (3) lies against the transverse fissure; and the apical segment (1) extends into the apex between the posterior and anterior segments.

Right Middle Lobe. In the PA chest roentgenogram the right middle lobe is located

within a triangle, formed superiorly by the transverse fissure, inferiorly by a line drawn from the lateral margin of the transverse fissure to the cardiophrenic angle, and medially by the cardiac shadow (Fig. 4A). A second line drawn inferiorly from the hilum, bisecting the middle lobe, separates it into lateral (4) and medial (5) segments.

In the right lateral Bucky chest roentgenogram, the middle lobe is located below the transverse fissure and anterior to the lower portion of the oblique fissure (Fig. 4B). It extends anteriorly to the chest wall immediately above the anterior costophrenic angle and inferiorly along the anterior surface of the diaphragm. A line drawn from the hilum to the chest wall just above the cardiophrenic angle divides the middle lobe into the lateral (4) and medial (5) segments.

Right Lower Lobe. In the PA chest roentgenogram, the lower lobe occupies the lower three-fourths of the right lung (Fig. 4C). The lower margin of the superior segment (6) is located near the level of the transverse fissure. Its upper margin lies approximately midway between the transverse fissure and the apex of the right lung. If the basal portion of the right lower lobe were divided into halves by a vertical line, the lateral half would contain the anterior (8) and lateral (9) basal segments, and the medial (7) and posterior (10) basal segments would occupy the medial half (Figs. 4C and 5).

In the right lateral Bucky chest roentgeno-

FIG. 5. Location of the basal and the supernumerary subsuperior segmental bronchi in the lower lobes are shown on transverse section through the lower thorax.

gram (Fig. 4B), the lower lobe lies inferior and posterior to the oblique fissure. The superior segment (6) occupies the portion of the lower lobe above a horizontal line drawn from the hilum to the posterior chest wall. Below this line the anterior (8) and medial (7) basal segments occupy the anterior half, and the lateral (9) and posterior (10) basal segments are found in the posterior half of the right lower lobe (Figs. 4B and 5).

Left Upper Lobe. In the PA chest roentgenogram, the left upper lobe occupies the apex and extends inferiorly to a line extending from the lower hilum to the costophrenic angle (Fig. 4A). When the upper lobe is divided into thirds, as indicated by the dark dotted lines, the upper third consists of the apical-posterior (1-2) segment, the anterior segment (3) is the fan-shaped middle third, and the lingula occupies the lower third. The apical-posterior segment can be further divided (as indicated by the lighter dotted line from the upper hilum to the chest wall) into the posterior subsegment (2), which lies adjacent to the mediastinal surface, and the apical subsegment (1), which occupies the apical portion. When the lingula is bisected by a line from the lower hilum to the chest wall, it separates the superior (4) and inferior (5) lingular segments.

In the left lateral Bucky chest roentgenogram, the left upper lobe is anterior and superior to the oblique fissure (Fig. 4D). The two dark dotted lines drawn from the hilum to the chest wall dividing the left upper lobe into three equal parts separate the apical-posterior (1-2), anterior (3), the lingular (4-5) segments, listed from the top downward. The additional light dotted line from the hilum bisecting the apical-posterior segment places the posterior subsegment (2) adjacent to the oblique fissure. A similar bisection of the lingula separates the superior (4) and inferior (5) lingular segments. The inferior lingular segment lies adjacent to the oblique fissure below the hilum.

Left Lower Lobe. In the PA chest roentgenogram, the lower lobe occupies the lower four-fifths of the left lung field (Fig. 4C). The superior segment (6) occupies the upper portion of the lower lobe. Its lower border is located on a horizontal line drawn from the midhilum to the lateral surface of the rib cage. The upper margin is approximately two-thirds the distance from this horizontal line to the apex. The basal segments extend from the lower margin of the superior segment inferiorly to the diaphragm. The medial basal subsegment (7) and the posterior basal segment (10) occupy the medial half of the basal portion of the lower lobe with the medial basal subsegment (7) extending to the heart shadow and the posterior basal segment (10) extending into the posterior sulcus (Figs. 4C and 5). The anterior-basal subsegment (8) and the lateral-basal segment (9) occupy the lateral half of the basal portion of the lower lobe.

In the left lateral Bucky chest roentgenogram, the lower lobe lies behind and inferior to the oblique fissure (Fig. 4D). The superior segment (7) occupies the upper portion and lies above a horizontal line drawn from the hilum posteriorly to the rib cage. The anteromedial basal segment (8-7) occupies the anterior half of the lower lobe below the superior segment (Figs. 4D and 5). The posterior basal (10) and lateral basal (9) segments lie in the posterior half of the basal portion of the lower lobe.

ANESTHESIA

Premedication

The most suitable premedication for bronchoscopy consists of adequate doses of a sedative, an analgesic, and a parasympatholytic drug. In the average patient these drugs are pentobarbital sodium 100 mg, morphine sulfate 10 mg, and atropine 0.4 mg given intramuscularly 30 minutes prior to examination. These dosages should be varied for the size, age, and degree of debilitation of the patient.

General Anesthesia

General anesthesia is rarely necessary for bronchoscopy; it has disadvantages and should not be a substitute for patient rapport and gentle endoscopic technique. Disadvantages to general anesthesia are cardiorespiratory problems secondary to periods of anoxia and absence of patient cooperation. Brief periods of anoxia during detailed telescopic visualization of the tracheobronchial tree in a patient under general anesthesia usually cannot be avoided. Patient cooperation is essential to ensure adequate ventilation and for performing certain maneuvers that are often helpful, e.g., breath holding, deep breathing, or coughing.

Topical Anesthesia

A 3 percent solution of freshly mixed cocaine provides good topical anesthesia and does not interfere with bacteriologic studies of the bronchial secretions. The cocaine solution is mixed just prior to use by placing 7 ml saline in a bottle containing 210 mg dry cocaine crystals. When administered transtracheally, this topical anesthesia is safe, rapid, effective, and well accepted by the patient. Since patient relaxation during the endoscopic examination is an important factor in ensuring his comfort, the topical anesthesia can be effectively supplemented by intravenous administration of either diazepam (Valium) or droperidol (Innovar). When droperidol is utilized, an anesthetist should always be available to ensure that the patient ventilates adequately and to assist in resuscitation if respiratory arrest should ensue.

Materials routinely used for transtracheal anesthesia are an alcohol sponge, syringe with needle, and cocaine solution. A 2-cc plastic Luer-Lok syringe allows rapid injection of cocaine solution through the 25-gauge needle without syringe breakage or loss of solution when the needle is forced off the adaptor of the syringe. The 0.75-inch needle is usually long enough to reach the airway without penetrating the posterior membrane of the trachea. A 1-inch 22-gauge needle may occasionally be required in an obese patient with a short, fat neck, but it should be used with care to prevent penetration of the posterior membrane.

The needle is inserted between the first and second tracheal rings or below this level. Laryngeal edema can occasionally be caused by inadvertent submucosal injection if the needle is placed above the first tracheal ring. When the needle is inadvertently passed through the tracheal cartilage, its lumen may become occluded with cartilage thereby preventing aspiration of air. During the first injection (2 cc), the patient is supine, the head lowered 15 to 20 degrees and the chin elevated. Anesthetic solution is injected only after it is unequivocally demonstrated that air can be readily aspirated. The hand is braced in such a way that displacement of the needle is prevented if the patient moves. The injection is then made as rapidly as possible. The patient should be encouraged to cough since the degree of supraglottal topical anesthesia depends, in part, on the volume of cocaine that is coughed into the patient's mouth with the first injection. He should then be instructed to spit out the cocaine from his mouth in order to decrease the total amount absorbed. In order to increase the peripheral distribution of the anesthetic solution during the second and third injections, the patient should be encouraged to withhold his cough. To help avoid coughing, the patient should be instructed to hold his breath momentarily until the tickling sensation disappears and then inhale slowly. The second injection of anesthesia solution (2 cc) is made with the patient sitting and leaning on his elbow toward the side opposite the principal pulmonary lesion. The third injection (2 cc) is made with the patient leaning in the same manner toward the side of the pulmonary lesion.

Adverse Reactions to Topical Cocaine Anesthesia. Before the administration of topical anesthesia, the endoscopist should always have the following items available in the event of a side reaction to the anesthetic agent: a mask for inhalation of oxygen, thiopental sodium (Pentothal) solution mixed in a syringe (25 mg/cc) for intravenous injection, a tourniquet, a battery-operated laryngoscope, an endotracheal tube of suitable diameter, and an anesthetic gas machine.

Cocaine anesthesia is a safe drug for topical anesthesia providing precautions are taken to prevent adverse reactions. Prior to its use the endoscopist should always inquire if there has been a previous cocaine drug reaction. The patient should be instructed to spit out any anesthetic solution coughed up from the airways prior to bronchoscopy in order to reduce the amount of cocaine absorbed. Persistent coughing during the bronchoscopic examination may be due to mucosal irritability secondary to acute bronchitis, and repeated administration of cocaine seldom reduces this coughing tendency. A total dose in excess of 210 mg should be given with extreme caution. Since the age of the solution increases the incidence of adverse reactions to cocaine, it is very important that the solution be mixed immediately prior to use.

Cocaine stimulates the central nervous system, and the most frequent side reaction is nausea and vomiting, which occurs within a period of 5 minutes. This adverse reaction readily responds to inhalation of oxygen by mask. Reflex retching that occurs only during intubation may not be related to the topical anesthesia since it is sometimes stimulated by the tip of the bronchoscope as it contacts the posterior pharyngeal wall.

A second type of adverse cocaine reaction, also secondary to central nervous system stimulation, is excessive talkativeness, restlessness, and excitement. Since this reaction may progress to tremors, clonic-tonic convulsions, and possibly death, immediate therapy is advisable. An intravenous injection of the thiopental sodium solution (25 mg/cc) should be given slowly until the patient shows visible evidence of improvement. A dose ranging from 50 to 125 mg (2 to 5 cc) is usually sufficient for this purpose.

The most severe adverse reaction to cocaine is acute cardiac failure due to the direct action of cocaine on the heart muscle. This reaction occasionally follows massive doses of cocaine, far in excess of the amount used for topical, transtracheal anesthesia. Treatment requires adequate ventilation of the patient through an endotracheal tube, appropriate intravenous fluids, stimulants, and cardiac massage.

Before topical anesthesia is supplemented with intravenous droperidol, an anesthetist should always be available and an intravenous infusion instituted. Adequate ventilation can usually be achieved by frequently reminding the patient to take a deep breath. Fewer than 1 percent of patients experience serious ventilatory difficulty after intravenous droperidol, and when it does occur the anesthetist can usually ventilate the patient satisfactorily until the examination is completed by attaching an anesthetic machine to the side arm of the Storz bronchoscope. Assisted ventilation can be continued following the bronchoscopy by inserting a cuffed endotracheal tube.

BRONCHOSCOPIC EXAMINATION

Position of the Patient

The patient is in a suitable location on the operating table when his head can be raised or lowered 45 degrees in each direction with the headpiece. One arm used for administration of intravenous fluids and for taking blood pressures may be conveniently placed under the draw sheet at the patient's side. The other arm is free, and the patient's hand is placed on his chest where it can be used to give predesignated signals in case of pressure or discomfort.

The height of the operating table should be adjusted for the convenience of the endoscopist. Excessive tilting of the table in the head-up or head-down position should be avoided as the flat supine position can help the patient to relax better during the bronchoscopic examination. The severe discomfort that some patients with arthritis have when they lie flat on their backs may be relieved by placing a folded sheet under the lumbar area. Occasionally a pillow under the knees gives the patient additional comfort.

Instructions to Patient Prior to Bronchoscopy

The patient should be instructed to lift his index finger under the sterile sheet and point toward his lips, teeth, or gums whenever he feels pressure or discomfort. The endoscopist should always remember that "vocal" anesthesia is just as important as "local" (or topical) anesthesia. That is, the endoscopist should talk repeatedly during the examination so the patient can anticipate every move before it is made.

Technique

Introduction of Bronchoscope. The headpiece of the operating table should be level and the patient's neck extended with the chin uppermost. The key to the introduction of the bronchoscope under local anesthesia is to encourage the patient to relax his tongue so that the endoscope can be kept in the midline or middle of the tongue, where it will be more comfortable during the examination. As the vocal cords are visualized, a great deal of pressure can be applied over the center of the tongue without discomfort to the patient. However, if the bronchoscopic tube inadvertently slips to the side of the tongue, lateral pressure produces periosteal pain and medial pressure gives the patient the sensation that his tongue is being avulsed from its lateral attachment.

The beveled tip of the bronchoscope should be directed upward and should not touch the posterior pharyngeal wall as the patient may experience reflex retching even though adequate anesthesia has been achieved. When the tip of the epiglottis is lying against the posterior pharyngeal wall, the bronchoscope may be slid beneath it from one side without stimulating the posterior pharyngeal wall. If the tip of the bronchoscope remains in the midline as the epiglottis is lifted, the arytenoids and the interarytenoid membrane should be the first structures visualized. In the event that the bronchoscope has been inserted too far beneath the epiglottis, the arytenoids and interarytenoid membrane may not be visualized. If this happens, the bronchoscope should be withdrawn slowly as the endoscopist looks from side to side until these structures are located. The inexperienced endoscopist must avoid passing the bronchoscope into the pyriform sinuses or esophagus, as instrumental perforation of the cervical esophagus may occur.

The arytenoids, interarytenoid membrane, and vocal cords are difficult to visualize in some patients with a relatively thick tongue and short neck. Pressure of the bronchoscope against the tongue is normally followed by counterpressure on the part of the patient. If the endoscopist lifts the tongue in stages and allows the patient to respond to the examiner's instructions to relax his tongue after each stage, this counterpressure may be lessened.

Vocal Cords. After the bronchoscope is used to lift the epiglottis, the false cords should be carefully observed for evidence of erythema, edema, asymmetry, or neoplasia. Direct inspection of the vocal cords during phonation (with the patient saying "E-E-E") will help to determine if they approximate symmetrically in the midline. A wide-angle view for detailed visualization of the vocal cords can be obtained with the forward-viewing telescope. If the anterior commissure is difficult to visualize in this manner, a 30-degree telescope will help to bring it into view. In the event that a large laryngeal tumor is discovered, the endoscopist should determine if the bronchoscope can be safely passed through the remaining opening in the larynx. Secondary inflammation and edema might result from trauma to neoplastic tissue and cause subsequent life-threatening airway obstruction.

As the bronchoscope approaches the vocal cords, they often tend to close reflexively. It is good practice to turn the beveled tip of the bronchoscope from the anterior position to the vertical position routinely as the vocal cords are approached. As the bronchoscope is passed between the vocal cords, the tip should be rotated into the posterior position. Rotated in this

manner, the tip separates the vocal cords without trauma and pushes the arytenoids and/or false cords away as the beveled tip is passed into the trachea. If the bronchoscope is not easily introduced in this manner, further anterior elevation and rotation of the tip of the bronchoscope in the same or opposite direction often frees an impinged arytenoid or false vocal cord.

If the endoscopist observes that the patient is having difficulty breathing due to reflex closure of the vocal cords during introduction of the bronchoscope, he should immediately advise the patient to hold his breath for a few seconds. As soon as the patient takes a breath, the vocal cords usually reopen spontaneously so that the bronchoscope can be passed between the vocal cords into the trachea. However, if the patient cannot breathe after this interval and the vocal cords do not separate, the bronchoscope should be immediately removed from the pharynx to prevent undue apprehension by the patient. If laryngospasm continues after the bronchoscope is removed, the endoscopist should reassure the patient and instruct him to inhale slowly and deeply with each breath until his lungs are full.

Trachea. The trachea should be inspected throughout its entire length. The entrance points of the transtracheal anesthetic needle, seen anteriorly between the first and second tracheal rings, provides a good landmark to begin this examination. The wide-angle view provided by the forward telescope is essential for a panorama of the entire tracheal lumen as the bronchoscope is passed downward. Such findings as a tracheal bronchus or invagination of the posterior membrane or tracheal cartilages by an extraluminal mass are seldom missed when inspection is routinely made in this manner.

The lateral and anteroposterior diameters of the tracheal lumen should be approximately equal, and the tracheal cartilages should have a symmetrical appearance. The normal degree of anterior bulging of the posterior membrane in the cervical trachea may sometimes be mistaken for a retrotracheal mass, but this membrane is usually soft and should be easily displaced posteriorly. Below the thoracic inlet the posterior membrane should normally bulge inwardly only during forced expiration or cough.

The distal tip of the bronchoscope should remain in the center of the airway lumen as the tracheobronchial tree is inspected. The thoracic inlet is the pivot point for all changes in the direction of the bronchoscope. Pressure should never be applied against the bronchoscope to change direction, but all movements of the distal end are made by moving the patient's head in the opposite direction. The position of the patient's head is changed by the endoscopist using his right hand placed on the occiput and two fingers of the left hand on the teeth or gums and hard palate. As the head position is changed, the endoscope is lifted off the gums or teeth with the left thumb as it is moved in or out of the airways. Since sudden violent forward movements that accompany cough could conceivably cause the tip of the bronchoscope to perforate the posterior tracheal membrane, the endoscopist must hold the head rigidly enough to prevent these movements.

Carina.   Normally the middle third of the carina should not exceed 2 mm in thickness. Since mucosal edema and expiratory shortening may seemingly increase the width of the carina in some patients, it is best to observe it during a maximum inspiration. During inspection of the carina, it is also important to observe the angle between the main bronchi to rule out the presence of a subcarinal mass.

Side of Preference for First Examination.   Initial examination of the lung on the side opposite the lesion in the chest roentgenogram is preferred unless the endoscopist feels that the patient will not tolerate a complete bronchoscopy. If there are bilateral lesions on the chest roentgenogram, initial examination of the right side is preferred before rotating the patient's head into the more uncomfortable position for examination of the left bronchial tree. In a patient who has hemoptysis and a negative chest roentgenogram, it is best to inspect initially the side in which the greater amount of blood is seen. If active bleeding cannot be located following removal of all blood, the endoscopist can return to the same side later to detect new evidence of bleeding.

Right Main and Intermedium Bronchi. The right main bronchus (RMB) is the portion of the right bronchial tree extending from the level of the carina to the inferior margin of the right upper lobe orifice (Figs. 6 and 7). The bronchus intermedius (BI) extends from the inferior margin of the right upper lobe (RUL) orifice distally to the bifurcation into the middle (RML) and lower lobe (RLL) bronchi. Horseshoe-shaped cartilages similar to but smaller than those in the trachea are found in the right main and intermedius bronchi.

Right Upper Lobe Bronchus.   The RUL bronchus arises at approximately right angles from the right main bronchus (Fig. 6). The RUL takeoff is usually located in the 3 o'clock position (Fig. 7). The upper lobe bronchus divides by a trifurcation (65 percent) or a bifurcation (35 percent) into three segmental bron-

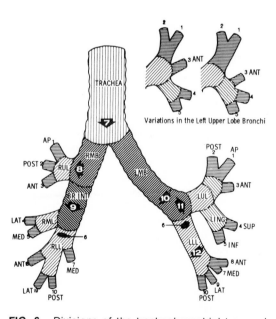

FIG. 6. Divisions of the tracheobronchial tree and common variations in the left upper lobe bronchus. Segmental bronchi and their corresponding numbers are shown. Black arrows with white numbers indicate position of the views seen in Figures 7 through 12.

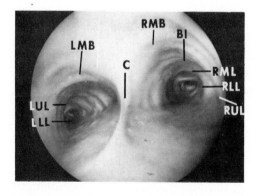

FIG. 7. Endoscopic view (0-degrees) from lower trachea showing carina (C) that separates the left main (LMB) from the right main (RMB) bronchus and the bronchus intermedius (BI). On the left is the left upper (LUL) and lower (LLL) lobe bronchi. On the right are the orifices of the upper lobe (RUL), the middle lobe (RML), and the lower lobe (RLL) bronchi.

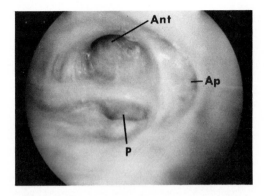

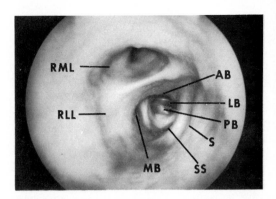

FIG. 8. Endoscopic view from right main bronchus with the 90-degree telescope showing trifurcation of right upper lobe bronchus into anterior (Ant), apical (Ap), and posterior (P) segments. Transverse mucosal ridges are seen along the inferior margin inside the anterior segmental bronchus.

FIG. 9. Endoscopic view (0-degrees) from the bronchus intermedius shows the transverse spur that separates the right middle (RML) from the right lower (RLL) lobe bronchus. The orifices of superior segmental bronchus (S) at 5 o'clock and the medial basal segmental orifice (MB) at 9 o'clock are seen just inside the RLL bronchus. At a more distal level are the anterior basal (AB), lateral basal (LB), and posterior basal (PB) segmental bronchi. A supernumerary, subsuperior posterior basal bronchus (SS) is seen between the medial and anterior basal bronchi.

chi. As visualized with a right angle telescope, the most frequent positions of the three segmental orifices in a trifurcated upper lobe bronchus are: posterior (2) between 5 and 9 o'clock, anterior (3) between 9 and 1 o'clock, and apical (1) between 1 and 5 o'clock (Fig. 8). Infrequently subdivisions of the segmental bronchi can be visualized with the 90-degree telescope. Up to the third and occasionally the fourth segmental branches in each of the three upper lobe segments can be visualized with a bronchofiberscope used as a flexible telescope.

Right Middle Lobe Bronchus. The RML bronchus arises anterior to the horizontal spur, which separates it from the lower lobe bronchus (Figs. 7 and 9). This bronchus can usually be visualized as far as its segmental divisions with a forwardoblique telescope (30 degrees) or with a forward telescope (0 degrees) if the head is lowered 30 degrees and the chin elevated and rotated to the left. The RML bronchus extends anteriorly and laterally for a distance of 2 to 3 cm where it bifurcates into medial and lateral segments (Fig. 6). The medial segment (4) is usually located medially and anteriorly, and the lateral segment (5) is located laterally and posteriorly. The primary subsegmental branches can frequently be seen with the 0- or 30-degree telescopes when they are passed into the middle lobe bronchus. The third or fourth subdivisions can usually be visualized in the same manner with the flexible bronchofiberscope.

Right Lower Lobe Bronchus. The RLL bronchus arises at the distal end of the bronchus intermedius posterior to the horizontal

spur that separates it from the middle lobe bronchus (Figs. 7 and 9). The first RLL branch is the superior segment, which arises between 4 and 6 o'clock just inside the lower lobe bronchus (Fig. 9). An anatomic landmark in the right bronchial tree is the location of the superior segmental orifice opposite and immediately below the inferior spur of the middle lobe bronchus. This landmark can be used for reorientation whenever necessary. The inferior spur of the middle lobe can be used for locating the level of the superior segmental bronchus with the 90-degree telescope. With a right angle (90-degree) or forwardoblique (30-degree) telescope, the second or third branches of the superior segmental bronchus can frequently be visualized.

The second branch of the lower lobe bronchus is the medial basal (MB) segment, which is usually located between 8 and 10 o'clock approximately 15 mm below the superior segmental orifice (Figs. 6, 7, and 9). Primary and occasionally secondary branches of this segment can be visualized with a forward or forwardoblique (30-degree) telescope.

The third branch of the lower lobe bronchus is usually the anterior basal (AB) segment, which is found between the 1 and 3 o'clock position approximately 5 to 10 mm below the medial basal orifice (Figs. 6 and 9). With the forward-viewing telescope extended beyond the

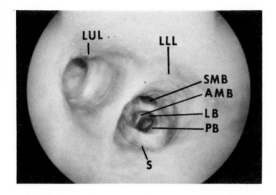

FIG. 10. Endoscopic view from the left main bronchus with the 0-degree telescope showing the inferior spur of the left upper lobe (LUL) that separates it from the lower lobe (LLL) bronchus. Fine transverse mucosal ridges are seen along the inferior margin of the LUL bronchus. The characteristic position of the orifice of the superior segmental bronchus (S) in the lower lobe is at 7 o'clock. Midway between the superior segmental orifice and the orifices of the anteromedial (AMB), lateral (LB), and posterior (PB) basal segments is a supernumerary subsuperior medial basal bronchus (SMB), which is seen in only 2 percent of patients.

bronchoscopic sheath (Fig. 1D), the third or fourth subsegmental branches can usually be seen. Approximately 2 percent of patients have no separate medial and anterior basal bronchi, but instead have a combined anteromedial basal bronchus located between 11 and 2 o'clock.

The orifices of the lateral basal and posterior basal segmental bronchi are separated by an almost vertical spur which lies 0.5 to 2.0 cm below the anterior basal bronchus (Fig. 9). The lateral basal segmental bronchus originates to the right of this spur and the posterior basal segmental bronchus to the left. Up to the fifth or sixth subdivisions of these two basal bronchi can often be visualized with the forward telescope.

Supernumerary bronchi are frequently found in addition to the four basal bronchi named above. These extra lower lobe bronchi are called subsuperior basal segmental bronchi, and are named for the basal segment they supplement (Figs. 5 and 9). They supply the lungs between the superior segment and the remaining portion of the corresponding basal segment. A method for naming the supernumerary subsuperior basal bronchi in the right lower lobe is to divide the basal bronchial lumen into four quarters (Fig. 5). Beginning with the quarter located between 9 and 12

o'clock and proceeding clockwise, the subsuperior bronchi are named subsuperior medial basal, subsuperior anterior basal, subsuperior lateral basal, and subsuperior posterior basal.

Left Main Bronchus. The left main bronchus (LMB) arises to the left side of the carina, is approximately 6 cm in length, and ends at the bifurcation into the left upper (LUL) and lower (LLL) lobes (Figs. 6, 7, and 10). It is slightly curved, with its concave surface located medially and inferiorly, and it is surrounded on three sides with horseshoe-shaped cartilages similar to those in the main and intermedius bronchi on the right. The left main bronchus may assume a more transverse position when there is upward traction secondary to apical fibrosis or atelectasis of the left upper lobe.

Left Upper Lobe Bronchus. The LUL bronchus is seen endoscopically arising from the left main bronchus between 9 and 12 o'clock, and its length varies from 2 to 15 mm (Fig. 10). In 65 percent it divides by bifurcation into upper (UD) and lower or lingular (LD) divisions (Figs. 11 and 12), and in 35 percent by trifurcation. Whether the left upper lobe divides into two or three branches usually depends on the position of the anterior segment (Fig. 6). When a bifurcation is present, the anterior segment may arise from either the upper or lower division, or it may arise between the upper and lower divisions to form a trifurcation. Visualization of the upper lobe bronchus with a right angle telescope usually reveals a

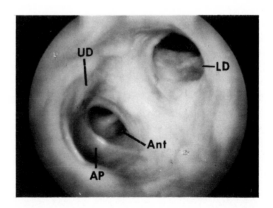

FIG. 11. Endoscopic view (90 degrees) inside the left upper lobe bronchus from the left main bronchus, showing a bifurcation into an upper (UD) and a lower or lingular (LD) division. In the upper division the orifice of the apical-posterior segment (AP) and a subdivision of the anterior segment (Ant) is seen.

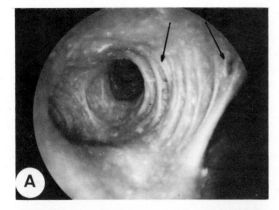

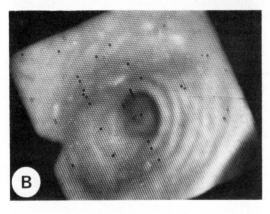

FIG. 12. Left upper lobe bronchus showing small light particles of inflammatory exudate on mucosal surface, transverse mucosal ridges, and dilated ducts of mucous glands (arrows) characteristic of chronic bronchitis. **A.** Hopkins rod-lens telescopic view. **B.** Olympus flexible bronchofiberscopic view.

Additional visualization of the subsegmental bronchi in all of the left upper lobe segments requires the use of the bronchofiberscope as a flexible telescope.

Left Lower Lobe Bronchus. The LLL bronchus arises medially and posterior to the upper lobe bronchial orifice at the bifurcation of the left main bronchus (Fig. 10). The first branch is the superior segmental bronchus, which arises in the 7 o'clock position just below the inferior spur of the left upper lobe bronchus. After the left upper lobe bronchus has been inspected with the right angle telescope, the superior segment of the lower lobe can be visualized by rotating the telescope 90 degrees in counterclockwise direction and sliding the tip downward 1 cm into the lower lobe bronchus.

Approximately 3.0 cm below the superior segment the lower lobe bronchus usually divides into three basal segmental bronchi (Fig. 6). The first basal segmental bronchus is the anteromedial basal (AMB), which is located to the left and anteriorly (Fig. 10). Its characteristic appearance is the division within a short distance into anterior (AB) and medial (MB) basal subsegments by a spur that lies almost perpendicular to its inferior spur (Fig. 13).

Occasionally (in fewer than 2 percent of instances) the anterior and medial basal subsegments arise separately. In this event the me-

centrally placed spur if a bifurcation is present (Figs. 11 and 12) or a centrally placed orifice if division is by trifurcation. Secondary branches of the anterior segment and the orifices of the superior and inferior lingular segments can usually be visualized with the 30- and 90-degree telescopes. Secondary branches in the superior and inferior lingular segments can frequently be seen with a 0- or 30-degree telescope passed directly into the lingular bronchus. In some patients the tip of the 90-degree telescope can be passed into the lingular bronchus, and secondary branches of the apical posterior segments can frequently be seen. When an anterior segmental bronchus arises from the lower division, a 90-degree telescope may be passed up to 1.5 cm inside the lingular bronchus to visualize its secondary branches.

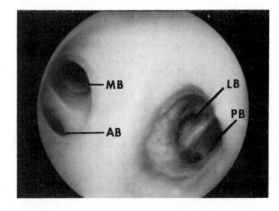

FIG. 13. Endoscopic view (0 degrees) in left lower lobe showing the three basal segmental bronchi. The characteristic vertical spur inside the anteromedial basal bronchus separates the anterior (AB) from the medial (MB) subsegments. The lower lobe bronchus continues until it divides into the lateral (LB) and posterior (PB) basal bronchi.

dial basal bronchus arises midway between the superior and anterior basal segmental bronchi. If this occurs the characteristic symmetrically placed vertical spur inside the anterior basal bronchus is absent.

If there is a typical perpendicular spur in the anteromedial basal bronchus in addition to a bronchus arising between 12 and 3 o'clock, it is considered to be a subsuperior medial basal bronchus (Figs. 10 and 13). The first or second branches of the anterior and medial subsegments can usually be visualized with the 0- or 30-degree telescopes.

The spur between the lateral (LB) and posterior (PB) basal segmental bronchi is usually found 0.2 to 1.0 cm more distally (Figs. 6 and 13). The lateral basal segmental bronchus lies between the anteromedial and the posterior basal segmental bronchi, and it can frequently be visualized with the forward telescope as far as its fifth subdivision. Visualization of the fifth subdivision of the posterior basal segmental bronchus usually requires forward movement of the head to obtain the required posterior direction of the 0-degree telescope. When the basal segmental bronchi are not arranged in the positions described above, it is necessary to name the basal bronchi by the area of lung they supply—the medial basal leads toward the left cardiac border, the anterior basal toward the left anterior axillary line, the lateral basal to the left posterior axillary line, and the posterior basal toward the left posterior sulcus (Fig. 5).

Supenumerary or extra bronchi arising from the left lower lobe bronchus are called subsuperior basal bronchi, and as in the right lower lobe these bronchi are named for the basal segment they supplement (Fig. 5). All of the subsuperior segmental bronchi in the left lower lobe arise only a short distance above the orifices of the basal segmental bronchi except the subsuperior medial basal bronchus (Fig. 10).

ENDOSCOPIC FINDINGS

In addition to the variations in anatomy of the tracheobronchial tree described above, diagnostic bronchoscopy reveals endoscopic findings characteristic of chronic bronchitis, acute bronchitis, and/or bronchogenic carcinoma.

Chronic Bronchitis

Marked variations in the lateral and vertical diameters of the trachea and main bronchi are sometimes seen in patients with longstanding chronic bronchitis, e.g., increase in width of the trachea due to flattening of the cartilaginous arch and stretching of the posterior membrane, or a "high-dome" type with marked narrowing in the width of the tracheal lumen. In patients with the former variation, narrowing or collapse of the airway may be observed during forced expiration or cough due to invagination of an attenuated posterior membrane. The lumen of the "high-dome" tracheal deformity, which is exclusively observed in patients who began regular cigarette smoking before adolescence, may collapse from side to side during cough.

In patients with severe chronic bronchitis and emphysema who have a flattening of the cartilaginous arches in the trachea, the carina may initially appear thickened since the posterior membrane may be invaginated so far anteriorly that only the normally blunted anterior third of the carina is visible. In these patients the thin middle third of the carina is not seen until a maximum inspiratory effort is made.

The endoscopic features of chronic bronchitis are dilated ducts of mucous glands, transverse mucosal ridges, and longitudinal light-colored bands beneath the mucosal surface. Dilated ducts are seen endoscopically as small holes or depressions in the mucosal surface, which are best visualized with the magnified views of the rigid bronchoscopic telescopes (Fig. 12A). Although chronic bronchitis is generalized, dilated ducts are more easily observed in the upper-lobe bronchi, the right middle lobe bronchus, and near the ends of the cartilaginous arches in both main and intermedius bronchi. The duct openings are sometimes obscured by mucosal edema when acute bronchitis is present.

Transverse mucosal ridges are usually seen more prominently during bronchoscopy in the right middle, left upper, and the basal segmental bronchi of the lower lobes (Figs. 8 and 12). The development of transverse mucosal ridges appears to be secondary to degeneration of the smooth muscle bundles in the lamina propria. Light and electron microscopic studies of bronchial mucosal biopsy specimens in our laboratory have revealed evidence suggesting smooth muscle degeneration in patients with longstanding chronic bronchitis. The degenerative process is sporadic; and when the normal muscle bundles alternate with the degenerated bundles, transverse mucosal ridges are formed. Therefore on longitudinal microscopic section of the mucosa, the transverse ridges contain bundles of smooth muscle, and the depressions have little or no smooth muscle.

Longitudinal light-colored bonds are due to linear collections of collagen fibers in the submucosa of patients with longstanding chronic bronchitis. These bands are seen most frequently in the lower trachea and can often be seen extending into both main bronchi, the right upper lobe bronchus, and the bronchus intermedius. The presence of these light bands appears to denote a degree of bronchial irritability in these patients since bronchospasm is frequently seen to develop in the lower lobe bronchi during the course of the bronchoscopic examination.

An endoscopic diagnosis of mild chronic bronchitis is made when two or more of the features described above are present in two or more areas of the tracheobronchial tree. Chronic bronchitis is considered moderate in severity when a few of these features are prominent in several areas, and is severe when several are seen in many areas of the tracheobronchial tree.

Acute Bronchitis

The endoscopic features of acute bronchitis may be seen alone or in combination with the findings of chronic bronchitis. Four features of acute bronchitis are the presence of mucosal erythema, mucosal edema, bronchospasm, and purulent exudate.

Mild mucosal erythema may be detected by irregular mottled areas of redness. Moderate erythema is present when the mucosal redness is uniformly increased and ecchymosis appears after the mucosa has been gently rubbed with one of the bronchoscopic instruments. Marked erythema is present when there is a further increase in redness of the mucosa, and bleeding often occurs after the same mild degree of trauma.

Mucosal edema causing thickening of the mucosa may be associated with erythema in acute pyogenic bronchitis or with mucosal pallor in allergic bronchitis. Blunting of normally thin spurs between bronchial divisions is usually the first detectable evidence of mucosal edema. As the edema increases there is progressive loss of the normal bronchial mucosal pattern, and the endoscopic findings of chronic bronchitis are progressively obscured. Indentations between the cartilaginous rings of the trachea, the main bronchi, or the bronchus intermedius are partially or completely obliterated by mucosal edema; and if the edema is severe, separate cartilaginous rings may not be identified. Mucosal edema also produces narrowing of the bronchial lumen, which is more apparent in the smaller bronchi.

Bronchospasm is frequently associated with acute bronchitis and is characterized by the presence of longitudinal mucosal ridges and a concentric decrease in the bronchial diameter. When the longitudinal mucosal ridges are seen on tangential view, their width and height are approximately equal. In the lower lobe bronchi longitudinal ridges produced by bronchospasm may extend around the circumference of the lumen, but they are more prominently seen along the posterior surface. Longitudinal mucosal folds always appear more prominent when small amounts of blood collect in the depressions between the ridges; they are less prominent or may not be seen at all when significant mucosal edema is present.

The longitudinal mucosal ridges of bronchospasm must be differentiated from the longitudinal light-colored bands of chronic bronchitis described above. The mucosa over the light bands is usually flat, although the edges may be slightly raised. Differentiation may be difficult in the lower lobes since the light bands appear to be continuous with the top surface of the longitudinal mucosal ridges caused by bronchospasm.

The longitudinal mucosal ridges of bronchospasm must also be differentiated from the widened or thickened longitudinal mucosal folds associated with mucosal lymphatic obstruction by carcinoma. The width of the lymphatic obstructive type of longitudinal mucosal folds is three or four times the height, whereas in bronchospasm the width and height of the ridges are almost equal.

Purulent exudate seen endoscopically in the tracheobronchial tree may be associated with acute bronchitis; however, it may originate from inflammation in the smaller bronchi, bronchioles, or a parenchymal lesion, e.g., pneumonia or acute lung abscess. Purulent exudate may vary from thin cloudy mucus, or mucopus, to exudate so thick it tends to occlude the aspirating tube or solidify in the bottom of the Luken's tube after it has been aspirated. A layer of pus may also coat the mucosal surface so thinly and uniformly that it is not detected until it rolls up in front of the bronchoscope or the forward telescope that has been slid along the mucosal surface. The presence of the pus on the surface can be verified by washing the bronchial mucosa with a small amount of saline and then inspecting the aspirate. It is always good practice to examine the Luken's tube after bronchoscopic examination since the purulent content of the bronchial secretions may not be adequately appreciated during bronchoscopy.

A diagnosis of mild acute bronchitis in any portion of the tracheobronchial tree is made when there are three or more endoscopic findings of minimal severity. Moderate and severe acute bronchitis is indicated by corresponding increases in the number and severity of the endoscopic findings.

Bronchogenic Carcinoma

From the endoscopic viewpoint, neoplasms may be classified as extrabronchial or intraluminal. An extrabronchial mass may be detected by noting the presence of localized protrusions of two or three cartilaginous rings into the lumen of the trachea or main bronchi. An extrabronchial mass should also be suspected if there is a localized anterior bulge in the posterior membrane during deep inspiration and the mucosa can be seen sliding up and down over the bulge during respiratory movements. Normally a maximum inspiratory effort should completely flatten the posterior membrane during examination of the trachea and main bronchi.

Widening of the carina by mucosal carcinoma usually produces irregular changes in the mucosal pattern which can easily be seen with the magnified view of the forward or 30-degree telescope. Subcarinal masses may tend to flatten the angle of the carina and may also produce a convex deformity of the medial and/or posterior walls of the main bronchi.

An intraluminal neoplasm may involve only the mucosal surface or may protrude into the lumen and produce varying degrees of airway obstruction. A malignant neoplasm that is confined mostly to the mucosal surface is usually more anaplastic than one that is predominantly intraluminal. The more anaplastic neoplasms may resemble a severe acute inflammation since the mucosa appears to have a thickened, irregular, dark, erythematous surface. The surface of the less malignant tumor may be devoid of mucosa and have a smooth, irregular, or ulcerated surface. The better differentiated malignant neoplasm is often covered by mucosa.

In evaluating a neoplasm the endoscopist should make the following observations: (1) location of its upper limits; (2) degree of fixation of the involved bronchi; (3) extent of airway obstruction; (4) evidence of mucosal lymphatic obstruction; and (5) the most suitable location for biopsy. As the upper limits of a neoplasm are localized, it is important to determine the extent of resection that would be required to transect the bronchus a satisfactory distance above the tumor. A mucosal biopsy specimen should be taken at this point to determine if the area is free of carcinoma.

Complete fixation of a bronchus suggests a nonresectable lesion and usually denotes direct continuity between the bronchial lesion and the mediastinal structures, vertebrae, and/or ribs. Fixation of the right upper lobe bronchus should be suspected when its orifice is inspected with the 90-degree telescope and it does not move inferiorly or superiorly with a maximum inspiratory and expiratory effort. Fixation of the intermedius or lower lobe bronchi can be detected by the absence of movement with respiration and a sensation felt through the bronchoscopic instruments suggesting that the mass is solidly fixed. This sensation is similar to that felt when a suction cannula is tapped against a solid concrete surface.

Estimation of the location and extent of airway obstruction is helpful in determining if atelectasis is impending after accumulation of secretions. Evaluation of the degree of acute bronchitis and/or purulent exudate below a bronchial obstruction is helpful in determining the need for aggressive medical management prior to the initiation of pulmonary resection or radiation therapy.

Involvement of the mucosal lymphatics by carcinoma is frequently associated with edematous thickening of the mucosa and the presence of wide longitudinal mucosal ridges that often extend downward to the neoplastic lesion. The width of these longitudinal folds may vary to such an extent that they mimic the longitudinal mucosal folds of bronchospasm. This differentiation is enhanced when carcinoma has produced an eccentric bronchial lumen. Biopsy of the bronchial mucosa in a thickened longitudinal fold may reveal carcinoma within distended lymphatics.

The most suitable location for a biopsy of a bronchial neoplasm is along its superior margin, where direct pressure with a bronchial sponge can be subsequently applied in the event of excessive bleeding. This location is especially important if the neoplasm is found to have prominent blood vessels over its surface. Most bleeding subsequent to a biopsy subsides within 5 minutes, during which time the endoscopist must keep the airway free of blood. Therefore when bleeding appears to be excessive, the endoscopist should immediately place the patient in the Trendelenburg position so that the proximal end of the bronchoscopic tube tilts downward. Blood can then drain freely to the outside rather than be aspirated into the airways. If bleeding continues beyond a period of 5 minutes, pressure on the biopsy site with a bronchial sponge sparsely moistened with a 1:2000 solution of Adrenalin is helpful in bringing the bleeding under control. The endoscopist should be very cautious in the use of Adrenalin in hypertensive patients.

Benign Neoplasms

Benign lesions in the tracheobronchial tree are relatively rare. Benign intraluminal or extrabronchial lesions may sometimes be suspected, but their differentiation must await the biopsy findings. Therefore all endoscopic tumors must be considered to be malignant until a biopsy and histologic diagnosis can be established.

REFERENCE

1. Huber JF, Jackson C: Correlated applied anatomy of the bronchial tree and lungs with a system on nomenclature. Dis Chest 9:319, 1943

44

Flexible Fiberoptic Bronchoscopy

L. Penfield Faber

The flexible fiberoptic bronchoscope described by Ikeda et al.[14] has become estabished as an important tool in the assessment and management of pulmonary disease. Clinicians and investigators have described the many advantages of this versatile instrument,[9,23,31] and its extended diagnostic capabilities make it mandatory that all physicians performing tracheobronchial endoscopy be familiar with its use. For those familiar with tracheobronchial anatomy, the technique of fiberoptic bronchoscopy is readily acquired. Direct visualization of pathology at the segmental and subsegmental level has become an increased benefit to physicians dealing with pulmonary problems.

INSTRUMENTATION

Several instruments are commercially available and all features must be assessed prior to purchase. The external diameter of the instrument is important to those who are performing fiberoptic bronchoscopy to establish a diagnosis of malignancy. In this instance the bronchoscope is preferably passed through an endotracheal tube, which permits rapid removal and reinsertion of the scope to obtain bronchial brush and biopsy specimens. If the brush or biopsy forceps is pulled back through the channel of the instrument, some of the specimen may be lost, and the rate of positive results decreases. A fiberoptic bronchoscope with an external diameter of 5.7 mm is readily inserted through an 8-mm (32 Fr) endotracheal tube, which is easily passed in adults and adolescents. If bronchial brushing and biopsy are rarely carried out, the external diameter of the scope is not critical.

The larger the internal diameter of the aspirating channel, the more versatile is the instrument. Brushes and flexible biopsy forceps are easily passed through the standard 1.8- or 2.0-mm channels, and thick secretions can be aspirated. Bronchoscopes under 4 mm external diameter do not have an aspirating channel. Although visualization of sixth and seventh order bronchi is beneficial, the inability to brush a lesion or aspirate secretions is a significant disadvantage. Most physicians have only one or two instruments, and so these should provide maximum all-round utilization.

Various degrees of flexion and in some instances rotation are available on the different instruments. The ability to flex the tip of the instrument over 100 degrees in two directions (one plane) allows for easy manipulation of the tip of the scope into all segmental orifices. Scopes with a larger external diameter at the tip cannot be passed as far peripherally, which is a disadvantage when subsegmental visualization is attempted.

It is not difficult to become adept at passing the instrument into any segmental orifice, and only a short period of practice is required with either cadavers or commercially available models of the tracheobronchial tree.

The clarity of the visual field should be carefully assessed prior to purchase of any instrument. The visibility is usually of good quality, but there are some differences among instruments.

The cold light supply is an added cost, and varying amounts of illumination are available.

Increased illumination is needed for photographic and television purposes only. The standard available light source for each instrument is adequate for routine visualization of the tracheobronchial tree and 35-mm photography. A camera can be purchased which fits on the eyepiece of each instrument. The photographs obtained are of good quality, and no professional training is required. A camera is an accessory that provides limitless educational value to both students and other physicians.

Teaching adapters are available which allow a second viewer to see the anatomy as the operator carries out the procedure (Fig. 1). These adaptors are attached to the eyepiece and are an invaluable teaching aid. They are a mandatory part of the instrumentation in any teaching hospital.

The instruments are fragile, and all personnel handling them must be trained in their use. It is recommended that in-service educational sessions be held for all physicians, house officers, and nursing personnel who use and clean the instruments. Carelessness can result in serious damage. Any time the instrument is removed from the operating room to be used elsewhere in the hospital it should be signed out by the physician, who then becomes responsible for the care of the instrument.

ANESTHESIA

Topical anesthesia is the preferred method for performing routine flexible fiberoptic bronchoscopy. General anesthesia[32] is usually required only for prolonged examinations in a search for in situ carcinoma.

Commonly used topical agents are cocaine (5 and 10 percent), lidocaine, tetracaine, and benzocaine. The incidence of adverse affects with any of these agents is directly proportional to the dose administered, and the minimal amount that provides effective anesthesia is always recommended. Lidocaine 4 percent is a very satisfactory topical anesthetic, and toxic or sensitivity reactions rarely occur at recommended adult dosages of 200 mg or 1.5 mg/pound body weight. Adolescent and childhood dosages should vary as a function of age and weight. Equipment and drugs to coun-

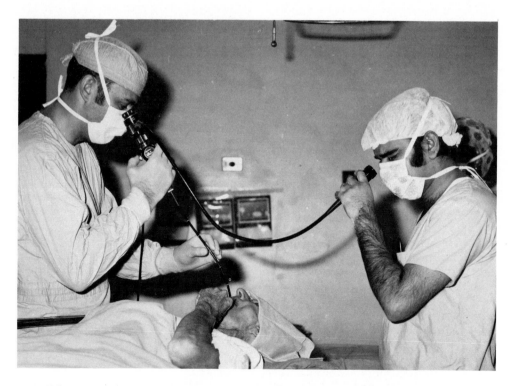

FIG. 1. Tracheobronchial anatomy can be easily viewed through a teaching adapter.

teract any systemic reaction must be readily available. Reactions are usually central nervous system excitation or cardiovascular depression. Precise placement of the anesthetic agent is mandatory for complete assessment of the tracheobronchial tree so that coughing and patient discomfort do not occur. Laryngospasm rarely occurs if topical anesthesia is properly carried out.

Topical anesthesia can be applied by many methods. Our technique is to spray the pharynx and epiglottis with 2 percent lidocaine and then instill 3 to 4 ml of 4 percent lidocaine into the tracheobronchial tree, utilizing a curved cannula with indirect mirror laryngoscopy.

A common method of topical anesthesia is to instill the agent as the scope is introduced.[29] The nasopharynx or oropharynx is sprayed with the topical solution to provide comfortable passage of the nasopharyngeal airway or the instrument itself. The epiglottis and vocal cords are directly visualized through the scope, and the topical agent is then instilled on them. Satisfactory anesthesia of the larynx is achieved after a brief waiting period, and the instrument is passed into the upper trachea. The topical solution is injected in succeeding amounts as the scope is advanced into the trachea and main stem bronchi. Care must be taken that as the anesthetic is aspirated to clear the tracheobronchial tree for further visualization it is not mixed with secretions for bacteriologic study as these agents are known to inhibit bacterial growth. It also may have some effect on cytologic assessment of malignant cells, and for this reason we make every effort not to aspirate the topical agent into either our bacteriologic or cytologic specimens. This method of anesthesia is ideal for bedside aspiration of secretions.

Another method of instilling the topical anesthetic agent is by ultrasonic nebulization or with various types of air- or oxygen-driven aerosols. Usually 4 percent lidocaine is utilized with this technique. The method requires 5 to 7 minutes of inhalation, and if it is necessary to examine several patients during an operative session this can be somewhat slow. In our experience ultrasonic nebulization is unsatisfactory in providing adequate anesthesia of the larynx, and so we routinely utilize direct or indirect visualization to apply the topical anesthetic.

Topical anesthesia can also be achieved by instilling the agent through a needle inserted into the trachea through the cricoid cartilage. Effective anesthesia of the vocal cords may not be accomplished by this method, and bleeding may be a minor complication.

If a general anesthetic is to be utilized, it can be carried out through an endotracheal tube with a side adapter. There are several commercially available adapters that permit insertion of the instrument while ventilation is maintained.[27] An air seal around the flexible fiberoptic bronchoscope at the adapter opening is required so that the anesthetic gas is not lost and an adequate tidal volume is maintained.

Premedication is administered to both inpatients and outpatients. Morphine or meperidine (Demerol) along with hydroxyzine and 0.6 mg atropine are used routinely in appropriate dosages. Atropine decreases saliva and excessive secretion. Diazepam is reserved for the very apprehensive patient and is used intravenously when needed.

FACILITIES

It is not recommended that flexible fiberoptic bronchoscopy be an office procedure. It should be carried out in the operating room or in properly equipped endoscopy rooms. Adverse reactions to anesthetic agents or complications may occur during the procedure, and it is mandatory that appropriate equipment and personnel be immediately available.

Bedside examination can be readily performed by physicians familiar with the instrumentation and those able to handle any complications that might ensue. It is not recommended that routine diagnostic evaluation be done at the bedside. This technique is reserved for aspiration of secretions in an extremely ill pulmonary or postoperative patient and for the assessment of tracheal mucosa in patients on long-term ventilatory support.

Outpatient bronchoscopy can be readily accomplished. Premedication is given to the patient in a waiting area where he can recline on a cart and be appropriately gowned. The same space is used for postendoscopy recovery. Patients return home accompanied by an adult, as the effect of the premedication and anesthetic agent does not permit them to travel alone. Outpatients should be examined in the endoscopy suite in the same manner as hospitalized patients are.

INSERTION

A commonly accepted method of inserting the flexible fiberoptic bronchoscope is through the nasopharynx and into the trachea.[22] The advantage of this method is that after the instrument is passed through the nasopharynx, the epiglottis and larynx readily come into view and the scope is virtually dropped into the trachea. Nasopharyngeal airways facilitate passage of the scope.[36] The scope can also be passed through the oropharynx in a similar manner (Fig. 2).[3] The instrument does not pass as readily into the larynx with this technique, and somewhat more expertise is required. A protective bite block should be used if the patient is uncooperative as he may bite the instrument and damage some of the fibers.

A significant disadvantage with the nasal technique is that if a brushing or biopsy is done it is inconvenient to both the operator and the patient to remove and reinsert the scope several times to obtain an adequate number of specimens. When a brush specimen is obtained, the brush should not be pulled back through the instrument as a portion of the specimen may be lost in the channel. The use of a long thin plastic tube to act as a sheath for the brush partially obviates this disadvantage. This method of insertion is most satisfactory when only visualization or aspiration is required.

The flexible scope may also be easily introduced through the rigid bronchoscope. The latter must have a lumen large enough to accommodate the flexible scope, and ease of passage should be tested before the procedure is begun. Despite almost filling the lumen of the rigid scope, ventilation is usually adequate.

Our preferred method of inserting the flexible bronchoscope is through an oral endo-

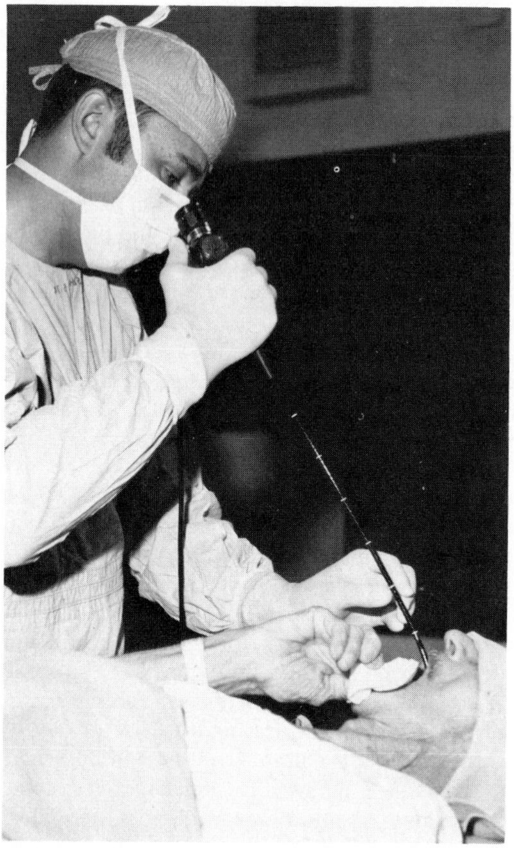

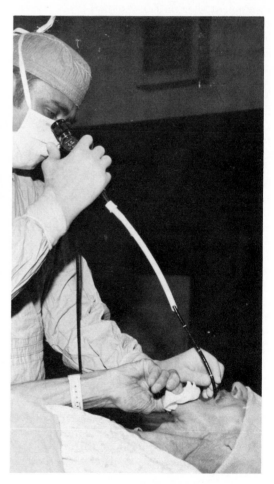

FIG. 2. Flexible bronchoscope has been inserted through the oropharynx and into the trachea.

FIG. 3. Endotracheal tube has been threaded to the proximal portion of the bronchoscope.

tracheal tube, *which provides constant airway control.* Supplemental oxygen or ventilation can be given quickly if indicated. This is a significant advantage when dealing with hypoxic patients.[15,38] An 8-mm (32 Fr) or 8.5-mm (34 Fr) uncuffed endotracheal tube is lubricated and threaded back over the length of the flexible fiberoptic bronchoscope to the proximal end (Fig. 3). With the patient in a supine position, the neck slightly extended, and the patient holding his own tongue, the flexible bronchoscope is passed through the oropharynx and into the trachea. Unsuspected pathology can be detected by careful assessment of the epiglottis, pyriform sinuses, arytenoids, and vocal cords. The tip of the flexible scope is then passed 2 to 3 cm above the carina. With the scope acting as a stylet, the endotracheal tube is guided over the flexible fiberoptic bronchoscope through the larynx and into the trachea (Fig. 4). This method requires satisfactory anesthesia of the larynx and upper trachea, as the patient coughs forcibly and develops laryngospasm if the anesthetic is not properly placed. We have not failed to pass an endotracheal tube utilizing this method in more than 800 procedures. The endotracheal tube is then taped in place or held by an assistant who also views the procedure through the teaching adapter. The endotracheal tube is easily tolerated by the patient during the course of the entire examination (Fig. 5). The tube is a sheath and permits rapid withdrawal and reinsertion of the scope for brushing, biopsy, and lens cleaning. Immediate airway control is always provided.

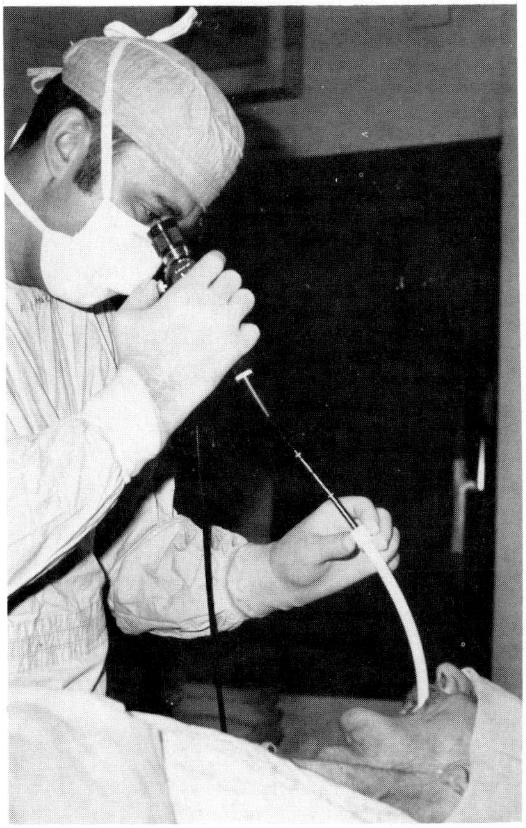

The endotracheal tube can be inserted by direct visualization, but this method is time-consuming and more traumatic to the patient. Supplemental oxygen can be delivered directly through the tube itself or by attaching a side arm adapter. The flexible fiberoptic bronchoscope can be passed through tracheostomy tubes, tracheostomy stomas, and side arm attachments of tracheostomy tubes while the patient is on controlled mechanical ventilation.

The operator should wear a cap and mask and be in appropriate surgical attire. Although not a sterile procedure, bronchoscopy should be carried out in as clean an atmosphere as possible. Handling the instrument with the bare hands and being attired in a laboratory coat

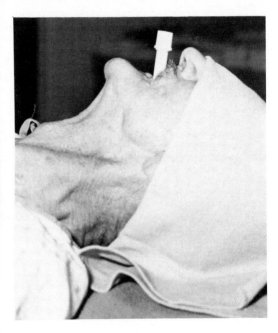

FIG. 4. Endotracheal tube is passed through the larynx and into the trachea. The fiberoptic bronchoscope acts as a stylet to direct the endotracheal tube.

FIG. 5. Endotracheal tube in satisfactory position.

TABLE 1. Clinical Experience with Flexible Fiberoptic Bronchoscopy

Indication	No. of Patients
Suspected lung cancer	555
Retained secretions	266
Inflammatory disease	181
Chronic pulmonary disease	160
Cough and normal x-ray	78
Hemoptysis and normal x-ray	32
Esophageal lesions	28
During and after thoracotomy	15
Difficult intubation	8
Total	1,323

over street clothes is not recommended. Contamination of the airway of a debilitated or sick patient can occur and is to be prevented if at all possible.

CLINICAL INDICATIONS

We have utilized the flexible fiberoptic bronchoscope in 1,323 patients (Table 1). The flexible bronchoscope has proved so advantageous it has now become the primary instrument for performing diagnostic and therapeutic bronchoscopy. Approximately one-half of the patients undergoing flexible bronchoscopy were examined for the possibility of pulmonary malignancy. Another large group underwent aspiration bronchoscopy following thoracotomy

and other surgical procedures. These were carried out in the intensive care units of the hospital and at the bedside. The opportunity to visualize pathology at the segmental and subsegmental level has made the instrument indispensable in assessing many other types of pulmonary problems.

Pulmonary Malignancy

The flexible bronchoscope permits the endoscopist to visualize mucosal changes of pulmonary malignancy at the segmental and subsegmental level. Prior to the development of this instrument, bronchogenic and metastatic carcinoma could be seen directly only in the major bronchi, and indirectly in lobar orifices with telescopes. Direct visualization and biopsy of tumors at the segmental and subsegmental level has increased the preoperative diagnosis of pulmonary malignancy in many series.[9,13,16] Coupled with fluoroscopic image intensification the more peripheral lesions can be brushed or curetted, and a diagnostic accuracy of 80 to 85 percent can be achieved.[38]

Flexible biopsy forceps (Fig. 6) are available for biopsy of hilar and more peripheral lesions. These forceps have also been utilized to obtain specimens of peripheral lung tissue for histologic and bacteriologic study (Fig. 7). The flexible biopsy forceps do not obtain a large specimen, and it is difficult to biopsy small lesions on the side of a major bronchus. The

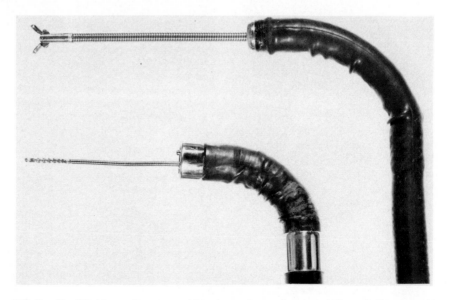

FIG. 6. Flexible biopsy forceps and brush can be easily passed through the channel.

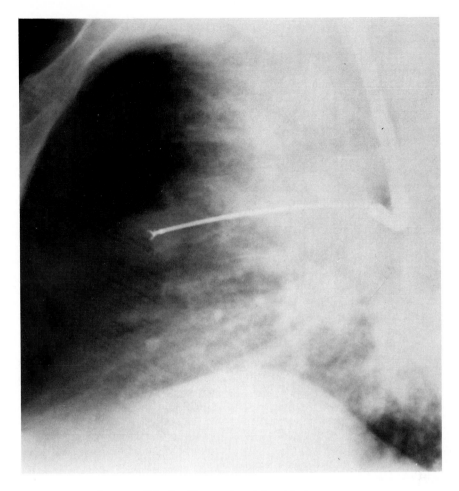

FIG. 7. Biopsy of peripheral lesion.

bronchial spur can be safely biopsied with flexible instruments as a large specimen is difficult to obtain and complications of bleeding are negligible. A larger 3-mm biopsy cup forceps was recently described by Marsh,[16] and as instrumentation is improved more efficient and larger biopsy forceps will become available.

The brush (Fig. 6) has become an indispensable part of flexible fiberoptic bronchoscopic evaluation for pulmonary malignancy. Brushing of hilar, lobar, segmental, subsegmental, and peripheral lesions is readily carried out. Bronchial brushing can identify the histology of a pulmonary malignancy, and at the present time approximately 75 percent of our positive bronchial brushings have been correctly classified as to histologic type. Bronchial brush specimens can establish the diagnosis of metastatic pulmonary malignancy, lymphomas, adenomas, and rare neoplasms of the respiratory tract. As our confidence has increased with histologic confirmation of cell type by bronchial brushing we have tended to rely less on biopsy specimens, although if the pulmonary lesion is readily accessible, biopsy is always carried out. However, there is no concern if a positive brush is obtained but the biopsy fails to yield a positive result.

These techniques have encouraged cooperation between the clinical and pathology services and provide significant material for diagnostic study. Continued communication between endoscopist and pathologist is important. Discussion of the clinical findings in the patient assists a competent cytopathologist in making an accurate histologic interpretation.

The flexible instrument has proved advantageous in bypassing significant distortion or obstruction of major bronchi caused by inflammation or pulmonary malignancy.[19] A tumor compressing a left main bronchus does not permit passage of a rigid instrument to the left upper lobe. A flexible scope can usually bypass the angulation, and direct visualization of the involved lobe or segmental orifice is accomplished. When preoperative irradiation is used, this can be beneficial as histologic confirmation of carcinoma could be obtained only by utilizing the flexible instrument. Visualization of distal, partially obstructed main bronchi is most helpful when contemplating pulmonary sleeve resection.

Cytologic diagnosis of pulmonary malignancy is occasionally made on a cough specimen, and radiographic assessment reveals no discernible lesion. Utilizing the flexible fiberoptic bronchoscope under general anesthesia, careful inspection, aspiration, and biopsy of all segmental orifices may be carried out. Recent studies[24] described the location of these small or in situ pulmonary malignancies by careful segmental evaluation and biopsy. Without this instrument these patients would have remained untreated until the x-ray showed a positive shadow which indicated the site for pulmonary resection.

Increased confidence in results obtained with the flexible bronchoscope in the assessment of pulmonary malignancy has permitted us to observe some pulmonary densities that once would have been resected. Most thoracic surgical services have had the experience of resecting suspicious lesions that turned out to be benign. As diagnostic accuracy with the flexible scope and bronchial brushing increases, one can more confidently observe a lesion that is thought not to be pulmonary carcinoma. However, a negative study for a highly suspicious pulmonary lesion does not negate thoracotomy if the clinician still feels that cancer exists.

We have performed flexible bronchoscopy in 555 patients with suspected pulmonary malignancy (Table 2). Pulmonary malignancy was confirmed in 364 patients by either diagnostic studies, subsequent thoracotomy, or autopsy

information. The diagnosis of primary bronchogenic carcinoma was made in 307 patients, and the remaining 57 had metastatic lesions. Utilizing the flexible scope with accurate placement of the brush or biopsy forceps we were able to establish the diagnosis of malignancy in 264 patients for a diagnostic accuracy of 73 percent. Direct visualization of a definite mucosal pathologic alteration was seen in 219 of these patients (60 percent). Many of these lesions were at the segmental and subsegmental position and could not have been detected by rigid endoscopy. Routine utilization of fluoroscopic control increases diagnostic accuracy in the peripheral lesions and should be utilized whenever possible.

Our initial brushing procedures were carried out by selective catheterization of the bronchus with a premolded catheter. The diagnostic accuracy was only 49 percent (23 of 47) in patients subsequently proved to have a pulmonary malignancy. The flexible fiberoptic bronchoscope has permitted more accurate placement of the brush in patients with bronchogenic carcinoma, and we have achieved a positive diagnostic accuracy of 78 percent (238 of 307). Our overall accuracy in both primary and metastatic lesions in 73 percent, which represents a 50 percent increase over our previously utilized fixed-catheter method (Table 3).

TABLE 3. Diagnostic Accuracy in Pulmonary Malignancy

Malignancy	No. of Patients	Positive Brush Biopsy	
		No.	%
Proved pulmonary malignancy	364	264	73
Primary bronchogenic carcinoma	307	238	78
Metastatic pulmonary lesions	57	26	46

Positive results in 57 patients with metastatic pulmonary malignancy have not been as satisfactory. We made a correct diagnosis in 26 of 57 patients for a diagnostic accuracy of 46 percent (Table 4). It is well known that metastatic pulmonary lesions do not involve bronchial mucosa as often as the primary malignancies do, and this may account for the decreased accuracy. Cytopathologic examination of brushing material has established the diag-

TABLE 2. Flexible Fiberoptic Bronchoscopy in Patients with Pulmonary Malignancy

Malignancy	No. of Patients
Suspected pulmonary malignancy	555
Proved pulmonary malignancy	364
Primary bronchogenic carcinoma	307
Metastatic pulmonary malignancy	57

TABLE 4. Metastatic Pulmonary Malignancy

Type	Pos	Neg
Adenocarcinoma	12	9
Lymphoma	7	5
Renal	1	4
Sarcoma	2	3
Other	4	10
Total	26 (46%)	31

nosis of lymphoma, Hodgkin's disease of the lung, and metastatic sarcoma.

Atelectasis, Aspiration, and Lung Abscess

The flexible fiberoptic bronchoscope has provided a safe and nontraumatic method for aspirating tracheobronchial secretions at the bedside[35] (Fig. 8). We have used the flexible instrument in 266 patients without serious morbidity or mortality. The great majority of these procedures were carried out at the bedside using topical anesthesia. The ease and expediency with which this procedure can be done at the bedside negates the need to transport a patient to another area of the hospital or to an endoscopy suite. Selective lobar and segmental aspiration is accomplished under direct vision. The flexible bronchoscope is less traumatic than rigid instruments, and the already inflamed tracheobronchial mucosa is minimally traumatized.

The 2-mm channel provides an adequate

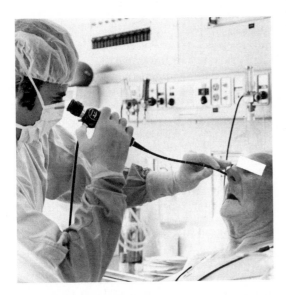

FIG. 8. Bedside aspiration of secretions.

lumen for irrigation and aspiration of even thick secretions. In our series of 266 cases we have had to resort to rigid endoscopy to remove thick, tenacious material on only three occasions. Continued saline irrigation and aspiration loosens and removes almost all secretions. Suction traps are routinely used to collect material for immediate bacteriologic study. Repetitive procedures are more readily accepted by the patient, and there is less reluctance on the part of the physician to bronchoscope patients for retained secretions.

Hypoxia does occur during the aspiration, and the physician must be careful that suction is not administered for prolonged periods.[1] Matsumoto and DeLaurentis[17] demonstrated a fall in arterial oxygen tension during suctioning of the airway. Oxygen should be administered to the patient prior to the procedure. Supplemental oxygen can be delivered through the nares, the mouth, or available channels on some of the fiberscopes. Cardiac monitoring should be utilized when available and particularly on postoperative patients in the intensive care unit.

Immediate bronchoscopy can be carried out when aspiration of gastric contents is suspected.[10] Often these patients are hypoxic and in severe respiratory distress. In these instances an endotracheal tube must be utilized to establish an adequate airway so that assisted ventilation can be implemented. The tracheobronchial tree is irrigated with saline to remove all aspirated material. The endotracheal tube may be left in place at the completion of the procedure for continued assisted ventilation.

Early assessment of a lung abscess is readily accomplished with the flexible scope.[35] Bronchial obstruction distal to a normal lobar orifice can be visualized, and a brushing or biopsy specimen obtained at the segmental level if malignancy is suspected. Aspiration of the obstructed bronchus can promote bronchial drainage and expedite healing of the abscess. Application of epinephrine to swollen mucosa may promote shrinkage and allow drainage. Patient comfort, segmental and subsegmental visualization, and segmental aspiration for cytologic and bacteriologic study are significant reasons for early fiberoptic bronchoscopy in all patients with lung abscess.

We have performed flexible bronchoscopy on 22 patients with asthma, none of whom were in status asthmaticus. Mucous plugs were removed with saline irrigation, and there were no associated complications. Goodman[12] reported significant improvement in a small series of cases using a lavage solution of 250 cc saline with 30 cc 20 percent acetyl cysteine, 250 mg prednisone, and 0.5 cc isoproterenol (Isuprel). Blood gases should be monitored in the severe asthmatic, and hypoxia treated with supplemental oxygen. Patient comfort and nontraumatic aspiration provide a safe and reliable method for treating the asthmatic patient.[7]

Hemoptysis

The great majority of patients experiencing hemoptysis should have early bronchoscopic evaluation. It is important for the clinician to locate the bleeding site and assess segmental and subsegmental mucosal alterations. This permits confidence in appropriate therapy, and the ease of fiberoptic bronchoscopy allows repetitive examination to evaluate therapeutic improvement and to be certain that the diagnosis remains firmly established.

On many occasions coughing spreads blood throughout the entire tracheobronchial tree, making it difficult to localize a bleeding site at the segmental and subsegmental level with any type of bronchoscope. Major bronchial abnormalities are readily detected with all bronchoscopes. Selective lobar and segmental saline lavage can be carried out with only the flexible bronchoscope, and the site of active bleeding identified in a significant number of patients.[28] With the tip of the instrument in the lobar or segmental orifice, blood from the remainder of the tracheobronchial tree does not obscure the field, and continued aspiration and lavage permit direct visualization of each orifice. Mucosal changes can be brushed or biopsied when indicated.

Massive hemoptysis (life-threatening) can present a significant viewing problem. When active bleeding occurs during flexible bronchoscopy, airway control is mandatory. An endotracheal tube should be inserted to deliver supplemental oxygen, permit the bronchoscope to be rapidly removed and reinserted for cleaning of the lens, and provide for more expeditious aspiration of the trachea. Vigorous bleeding during the procedure often obscures the viewing lens, and despite copious lavage it can be difficult to visualize the pathology. In our experience on three occasions it was necessary to remove the fiberscope and insert a rigid instrument to allow faster and more efficient suctioning through a large channel. This provided the opportunity to biopsy lesions not clearly seen through the fiberscope. Life-threatening hemoptysis is best evaluated by open tube bronchoscopy.[39] This type of bleeding requires airway control, rapid and efficient aspiration of blood, and larger instruments to compress or biopsy a bleeding site quickly.

Packing an active bleeding source requires the use of a rigid bronchoscope. Epinephrine pledgets have also been used successfully to control bleeding. On one occasion large clots could not be removed with the flexible scope and the rigid instrument had to be inserted to remove the clots and permit visualization of the bleeding site.

In most cases the flexible bronchoscope is an excellent instrument to evaluate hemoptysis. Bleeding obscures the lens, but irrigation usually clears it. The rigid bronchoscope should always be available for severe active bleeding and is the instrument of choice in massive hemorrhage.

Our experience with hemoptysis includes 32 patients who presented with a normal chest x-ray. The site of bleeding was identified in 22 of these patients, and with bronchograms a diagnosis was established in 24 of the 32 patients. The bronchogram is performed following completion of the bronchoscopic examination through a catheter placed through the nasopharynx into the trachea.

Use During Surgery

The fiberscope can provide valuable assistance during pulmonary resection. A bronchial anastomosis can be inspected to determine that the lumen is adequate and that there are no discrepancies in approximation.[18] We have utilized the instrument immediately after a pulmonary resection when excessive secretions were still present or the dependent lung had been contaminated during the procedure. The bronchoscope is inserted through any two-channel adapter while continued ventilation is maintained by the anesthesiologist.

Sleeve or bronchoplastic resections require early and often repetitive bronchial aspiration. The fiberoptic bronchoscope permits direct magnified visualization of the suture line,[26] and secretions are aspirated with minimal trauma to the anastomosis. When this type of aspiration is done with a rigid scope there is always concern about anatomic disruption. The flexible scope can be safely passed through the anastomosis for selective lobar and segmental aspiration. Patient acceptance permits repetitive aspirations when indicated. All sleeve and bronchoplastic procedures undergo routine bronchial aspiration during the first 48 hours, and the flexible bronchoscope has made the procedure more efficient.

Endoscopy During Mechanical Ventilation

Patients on a mechanical ventilator are readily examined and aspirated with the flexible scope.[27] Two-way adapters permit continuous ventilation during the bronchoscopy.[2,20]

Prior to the procedure the expired minute ventilation or tidal volume should be measured. As most side arm adapters for bronchoscopy do not provide an air-tight seal at the point the bronchoscope enters the adapter, the ventilator volume must be increased during the bronchoscopy so that the same prebronchoscopic expired ventilation is maintained. When bronchoscopy is done through an endotracheal tube of 8.5 mm (34 Fr) or larger, resistance to air flow is minimal.[27,32] Patients with Po_2 below 60 mm Hg should have the Fio_2 (fractional inspired oxygen) increased during the procedure to prevent arrhythmias and possible cardiac arrest. Coughing is controlled with 2 percent lidocaine injected into the trachea prior to bronchoscopy. The opportunity to inspect and aspirate segmental bronchi while adequate continued ventilation is maintained is a significant advantage of the flexible scope. Mucous plugs removed from segmental bronchi must be missed by more conventional catheter aspiration and rigid bronchoscopy.

Intubation over 48 hours is often associated with tracheal mucosal damage, and these changes can be readily assessed by frequent bronchoscopy.[2] The necessity for repositioning the endotracheal tube and altering the cuff site is readily detected. The position of the tip of the endotracheal tube can be noted, and if it impinges on the carina or penetrates the wall of the trachea the position can be changed.

Some patients require mechanical ventilation for many days or weeks. Bronchoscopy can identify tracheal damage or stricture and appropriate therapy be instituted. Secretions are readily removed from a narrowed trachea, but strictures cannot be dilated with the flexible instrument.

We have bronchoscoped 96 patients during continuous mechanical ventilation. There has been no significant morbidity or mortality associated with any of these procedures. The opportunity to aspirate the tracheobronchial tree selectively in an unhurried fashion is a significant advantage.

Gas Sampling

Patients with chronic parenchymal disease are ideal candidates for selective lobar gas sampling. These values can assist in determining the physiologic function of a diseased lobe by measuring the contribution of each lobe to total gas exchange.

This determination can assist the surgeon in deciding whether resection or decortication is indicated when a surgical procedure is carried out. A balloon on the tip of the scope facilitates these collections.[11]

Difficult Intubation

Patients with cervical arthritis, foreshortened mandibles, and prominent incisor teeth may present difficult intubation problems. A similar problem occurs in the group of patients with craniofacial anomalies. A patient with cervical spinal cord trauma may require a general anesthetic for other associated injuries, and with the flexible fiberscope intubation can be performed while cervical traction is maintained. This entire group of patients can be easily intubated with the aid of the flexible bronchoscope.[5,33] Topical lidocaine anesthesia is used on the larynx and in the trachea as for routine fiberoptic bronchoscopy. For an average adult patient an 8.5-mm (34 Fr) endotracheal tube is threaded over the scope back to the proximal end of the instrument. The scope is then introduced into the trachea, and the tube is passed over the scope through the vocal cords and into the trachea. We have intubated patients for a general anesthetic on eight occasions by this method.

Other Uses

In 1973 Crispen and Van Baarle[8] described the use of the flexible scope in visualizing the internal anatomy of peripheral arteries. Blood can be flushed from an isolated segment of vessel, and a clear view of atheromatous intima can be noted. Following endarterectomy the surgical result can be directly visualized and even modified through use of the flexible biopsy forceps. This technique requires gas sterilization of the instrument prior to its use.

Thoracoscopy was accomplished with the flexible scope by Senno et al. in 1974.[25] The bronchoscope is passed through a previously inserted 32 Fr chest tube. A T-shaped connector is used to attach the chest tube to a water seal system so that the amount of pneumothorax can be controlled. Biopsy or curettings of abnormal pleural surfaces can be easily obtained. The chest tube is left in place to expand the lung following the procedure.

Bronchograms are readily performed after completion of fiberoptic bronchoscopy. Supplemental anesthesia in dilute solution can be administered if the cough reflex has returned. When the bronchogram is done immediately following bronchoscopy a second procedure is unnecessary and hospitalization time is shortened. We prefer to insert a curved 16 Fr Stitt catheter through the nasopharynx and into the trachea for the bronchogram. The large catheter allows rapid injection of contrast material for screening bronchograms. The quality of the bronchogram is not altered by doing it immediately after the bronchoscopy.

We do not use the flexible scope as a conduit for instillation of contrast material as the instrument might be damaged. It is also difficult to clear bronchographic contrast material entirely from the channel of the fiberscope. Selective bronchograms can be done using a long plastic catheter inserted into the appropriate lobe or segment by direct visualization.

Utilizing the flexible scope, catheters have been placed in selected lobes for lobar lavage in the treatment of alveolar proteinosis. Sackner et al.[23] described this technique in 1972 in treating the respiratory distress syndrome; and if further reports document the efficacy of this procedure it could have significant therapeutic results. Utilization of a balloon cuff on the tip of the scope as described by Goldberg "would provide occlusion of the lobar orifice preventing spill of the lavage solution into other portions of the lung."[11]

DISADVANTAGES

As yet there is no satisfactory method for examining the tracheobronchial tree of infants with a flexible scope. Flexible fiberscopes with a 2 or 3 mm external diameter are available, but they do not have an aspirating channel, which is a significant limiting factor. It is often desirable to obtain bronchial washings for bacteriologic study and to clear the airway of retained secretions following a protracted illness or surgical procedure. The larger flexible fiberoptic scope cannot assist ventilation and obstructs the larynx of the infant. We have had no experience with the small 2-mm flexible scope, and until one is developed with an aspirating channel we do not contemplate utilizing it. It is still necessary to perform endoscopy in infants with the standard rigid bronchoscope.

Adolescents can be successfully examined with the flexible bronchoscope following appropriate premedication and topical anesthesia. If the procedure is carefully explained, the patient is usually most cooperative. In critically ill children when topical anesthesia is mandatory, we have bronchoscoped and aspirated secretions in younger age groups. Children can be intubated under general anesthesia and examined through the endotracheal tube if laryngeal size permits the passage of a 32 Fr endotracheal tube.

Foreign body removal requires a variety of forceps as a forceps that can grasp a peanut may be ineffectual for retrieving a pin. Flexible biopsy forceps are small, and the grasping pressure exerted is not adequate for the dislodgment of many foreign bodies. Foreign body forceps for use with the flexible scope are currently being developed, and those with a large cup must be inserted retrogradely into the channel. This technique is somewhat cumbersome, and at the present time foreign bodies are not easily removed by flexible fiberoptic bronchoscopy. It is our practice that when a foreign body is identified we convert to rigid instrumentation and effect removal with standard foreign body forceps.

Following bronchoplasty or sleeve resection of the tracheobronchial tree, suture material often produces granulation tissue which partially obstructs the lumen. It then becomes necessary to remove the granulation tissue and offending suture. Since a strong forward grasping forceps is needed for this operation, we have rarely been successful in removing bronchial sutures with the flexible biopsy forceps.

Dilatation of tracheobronchial strictures cannot be accomplished with the flexible instrument. Removal of granulation tissue at a stricture often initiates brisk bleeding, and a large aspirator for rapid removal of the granulation tissue is required. Forceful dilatation of a stricture requires an instrument with a large lumen which provides an adequate airway, and one that is firm enough to bypass the scar tissue. It is doubtful that any type of flexible instrument will ever be developed to permit this therapeutic procedure.

Thoracic surgeons feel that the inability to assess carina or main bronchial fixation is a significant disadvantage of the flexible instrument. As we have become more experienced with the instrument this has not proved to be the case. Carina widening is easily detected, and submucosal pathology is more clearly visible with the flexible visualization.

Biopsy specimens are small and on occasion may not be diagnostic.[37] Several bites of the lesion should always be obtained. Our excellent results with cytologic examination of bronchial brushing has partially negated this disadvantage. The operator should not be discouraged by failure to obtain diagnostic specimens on his initial attempts as continued practice will improve his results. It is difficult to obtain an adequate submucosal biopsy specimen with the flexible forceps when sarcoid or submucosal invasion of malignancy is suspected. Our results have been unsatisfactory in this regard.

COMPLICATIONS

Credle and co-workers in 1974 reported a major complication rate of 0.08 percent and a mortality of 0.1 percent in a survey of 24,521 fiberoptic bronchoscopies.[6] Premedication and topical anesthesia were related to 11 major complications, and 11 others were directly associated with the procedure.

One of the most frequent causes of complication with any endoscopic procedure is the inappropriate use of topical anesthesia. Inappropriate use includes excessive amounts and inaccurate placement. Toxic reactions can be avoided if the safe (milligram per kilogram) dose is known for each agent along with its other pharmacologic actions. Reactions often occur when the patient coughs excessively and supplemental anesthesia is administered. This problem can be avoided if the anesthetic agent is given in carefully measured amounts, and known safe levels are not exceeded.

Patients with excessive secretions and chronic bronchitis can present particular problems in achieving satisfactory topical anesthesia. Atropine should be used as a premedication, and dilute solutions of the topical anesthetic agent provide a wider margin of safety.

Laryngospasm as a complication can be avoided if the topical anesthetic is placed directly onto the vocal cords and the bronchoscope is not passed until satisfactory anesthesia is achieved. When laryngospasm does occur it is most likely a direct result of the anesthesia not being accurately placed on the larynx and cords. The operator must always visualize the cords for effective anesthesia.

Premedication in excessive amounts may cause respiratory depression and a fall in blood pressure. Drug dosage should be selected on the basis of age, weight, and general clinical condition. Premedication can be eliminated in the severely debilitated or hypoxic patient.

Complications directly associated with the procedure are usually cardiac arrhythmias or respiratory compromise. Supplemental oxygen must always be given to the hypoxic patient. Use of an endotracheal tube provides airway control, and assisted ventilation can be implemented if needed. The internal diameter of the tube must be large enough to permit passage of the bronchoscope and allow adequate ventilation.

Bronchospasm is a result of direct irritation of the tracheobronchial tree and usually responds to bronchodilators. Known asthmatic patients should be bronchoscoped with caution, and facilities and medication should always be available to treat hypoxia and severe bronchospasm.

Debilitated patients and those with severe chronic obstructive pulmonary disease must be carefully assessed prior to the procedure and bronchoscoped with care. Premedication and topical anesthesia are administered in minimal amounts, and supplemental oxygen is always given. The procedure should not be prolonged, and cardiac monitoring is used as indicated.

Laryngospasm has not occurred in our series, and bronchospasm has responded to bronchodilators on three occasions. There was one fatality in our group of patients—a direct result of mycoardial infarction that occurred 30 minutes after an uncomplicated procedure.

Complications from fiberoptic bronchoscopy

are minimal if premedication and topical anesthesia are administered in safe amounts, patients are carefully evaluated prior to the procedure, and supplemental oxygen is administered when indicated.

CLEANING AND STERILIZATION

Complete sterilization of the instrument can be accomplished only by gas sterilization. This method requires a period of time for airing to permit release of the toxic gas from the plastic material of the scope. If the bronchoscope is used almost daily, gas sterilization cannot be performed very often.

Methods of cleaning the flexible fiberoptic bronchoscope are related to the frequency of its use. On a busy endoscopic service where five to eight patients may be examined during a limited operative time, cleaning the scope between each use cannot be as lengthy as when only one procedure a day or every other day is performed.

Sackner et al. described "wet sterilization" of the instrument, accomplished by inserting the flexible portion into a tube filled with 0.5 percent povidone-iodine (Betadine).[21·23] The scope is immersed for 20 minutes and then irrigated with sterile saline, dried, and repackaged. This technique permits only one patient to be examined daily. A more rapid turnover of patients requires that two or even three bronchofiberscopes be available.

The flexible portion of the scope can be immersed in glutaraldehyde. Ten minutes of soaking almost completely sterilizes this portion of the instrument. The proximal control portion of the flexible fiberscope cannot be submerged as the solution enters the instrument and destroys the fiber bundles.

Frequent use of the scope may cause a small defect to appear in the rubber covering at the tip of the instrument. If such a defect is detected it should be repaired as solutions leaking through this defect damage the fibers.

At the present time there is no universal method of cleaning or sterilizing the instrument. Fiberscopes have been damaged by glutaraldehyde, povidone-iodine, and occasionally alcohol. Accidental leakage of cleaning solution or water into the control mechanism at the head of the instrument results in distortion of the visual field or destruction of the fiber bundles. All methods require competent, highly trained nursing personnel who can carefully and expeditiously cleanse the instrument and prepare it for the next patient.

It is our practice to clean the scopes after each use by the following method. The inner channel is brushed to clear all debris. It is then vigorously flushed in both directions with a solution of 30 percent alcohol followed by sterile saline. The external covering of the flexible portion of the scope is cleansed with soap and water followed by wiping with 30 percent alcohol and sterile saline. The proximal end of the scope is wiped with 30 percent alcohol, and the instrument is then placed on a sterile drape ready for its next trip. Occasional bacteriologic cultures following this cleaning method have failed to reveal any pathologic organisms. However, extensive control analysis has not been carried out.

When a patient with tuberculosis is bronchoscoped, the instrument should be gas sterilized. Tuberculosis organisms have been reported to be obtained from the inner channel of the instrument after standard cleaning procedures. We use the rigid bronchoscope when tuberculosis is a possibility.

The American Cystoscope Company* recently developed a flexible fiberoptic bronchoscope that can be totally submerged in any sterilizing solution desired. A separate Luer-Lok opening has been constructed into the proximal control head. A pressurized air source is connected to this opening, and air at 2 pounds per square inch is forced through the control mechanism of the scope. When the instrument is totally immersed, the air passes out through any nonwater-tight connections and prevents seepage of the cleansing agent into the inner workings of the scope. We have totally immersed this instrument in glutaraldehyde for 30 minutes with no resulting damage. Thorough flushing and cleaning of the scope must be done after the use of glutaraldehyde. The trials and bacteriologic studies with this instrument will be continued.

TRAINING

The amount of training necessary for the performance of flexible fiberoptic bronchoscopy remains undefined. The reported large number

American Cystoscope Makers Incorporated, Pelham Manor, New York.

of flexible bronchoscopies with rare complications attest to the relative ease and safety of the procedure. If it were as difficult as rigid endoscopy, the internist would have abandoned the flexible scope. His continued enthusiasm with a limited training background in topical anesthesia, rigid endoscopy, and oral intubation further signifies the relative ease and safety of the procedure.

Training endoscopists to perform only flexible endoscopy will eventually leave a void when rigid techniques are required.[4] This void may be obviated by improved instrumentation that permits removal of foreign bodies, infant bronchoscopy, and the removal of bronchial sutures. However, it is doubtful that the flexible scope can be developed to such proficiency that all of these procedures can be carried out. The rigid endoscope will undoubtedly always have a place in the care of the tracheobronchial tree.[30]

Hospitals permitting the performance of these procedures must establish guidelines and criteria as to who can perform the procedure and what training background is required.[34] The Joint Commission on Hospital Accreditation already requires delineation of privileges for all staff members. National specialty societies must combine their efforts and establish training guidelines for hospital accreditation committees to follow.

At many institutions bronchoscopes are done only by the bronchoesophagologist, but at others they are done by the otolaryngologist, the thoracic or general surgeon, and the internist. It is the responsibility of each interested group of physicians to combine their efforts and patient material to provide broad based and well supervised training programs. They must define the time needed for endoscopy training in order to be qualified to do flexible bronchoscopy, as well as, most importantly, how many procedures should be done by the trainee. It is difficult to select rigid bronchoscopy as a procedure of choice if you have never seen it performed or attempted it yourself. A trainee should spend the minimum of 3 months on a busy endoscopy service. He should participate in a minimum of 100 endoscopic procedures and learn the fundamentals of rigid bronchoscope insertion. These criteria can be easily met on a combined or active endoscopy service. If they are not met, the credentials committee of the hospital should not permit the physician to perform endoscopy of any type. Certificates can be given to attest to the completion of a required training program.

A small cadre of supertrained endoscopists must be maintained at major teaching institutions. They must have received extensive experience in all aspects of endoscopy and will be the referral center for any complicated endoscopic problem. Establishment of this type of program requires the utmost cooperation of all interested specialties.

Postgraduate programs are given annually or semiannually in many teaching centers, and trainees in pulmonary disease, medical or surgical, should be encouraged to attend these sessions. Practical experience is gained and newer techniques are discussed. The flexible fiberoptic bronchoscope is a "superscope" but the problem of training and certification must be answered.

CONCLUSION

The flexible fiberoptic bronchoscope represents a significant advancement in bronchoscopic instrumentation. Endoscopic, therapeutic, and diagnostic capabilities have been significantly increased by the use of this instrument. For any endoscopic physician to remain versatile and "flexible" he should be familiar with the use and advantages of the flexible fiberoptic bronchoscope.

REFERENCES

1. Albertini R, Harrel JH, Moser KM: Hypoxemia during fiberoptic bronchoscopy. Chest 65:1, 1974
2. Amikam B, Landa J, West J, et al: Bronchofiberscopic observations of the tracheobronchial tree during intubation. Am Rev Resp Dis 105:747, 1972
3. Atocha J: Tracheobronchial fiberoscopy. Conn Med 37:107, 1973
4. Benfield J: About flexible fiberoptic bronchoscopy. Ann Thorac Surg 16:538, 1973
5. Conyers A, Sallace D, Mulder D: Use of the fiber optic bronchoscope for nasotracheal intubation: case report. Can Anaesth Soc J 19:654, 1972
6. Credle W, Smiddy J, Elliott R: Complications of fiberoptic bronchoscopy. Am Rev Resp Dis 109:67, 1974
7. Credle W, Smiddy J, Shea D, et al: Fiberoptic bronchoscopy in acute respiratory failure in the adult. N Engl J Med 288:49, 1973
8. Crispin H, Van Baarle A: Intravascular observation and surgery using the flexible fiberscope. Lancet 1:750, 1973
9. Faber LP, Monson DO, Amato J, et al: Flexible

fiberoptic bronchoscopy. Ann Thorac Surg 16: 163, 1973

10. Fleming WH, Bowen JC: Early complications of long-term respiratory support. J Thorac Cardiovasc Surg 64:729, 1972

11. Goldberg E: Personal communication, 1974

12. Goodman AH: Conference on Flexible Fiberoptic Bronchoscopy. La Jolla, California, 1973

13. Ikeda S: Flexible bronchofiberscope. Ann Otol Rhinol Laryngol 79:916, 1970

14. Ikeda S, Yanai N, Ishikawa S: Flexible bronchofiberscope. Keio J Med 17:1, 1968

15. King E: Expanding diagnostic and therapeutic horizons—fiberoptic bronchoscopy. Chest 63: 301, 1973

16. Marsh B, Frost JK, Erozan YS, et al: Flexible fiberoptic bronchoscopy its place in the search for lung cancer. Ann Otol Rhinol Laryngol 82:757, 1973

17. Matsumoto T, DeLaurentis D: Tracheal aspiration and fiber optic bronchoscopy. JAMA 221:1163, 1972

18. Payne W, Leonard P, Miller D, et al: Physiologically based assessment and management of tracheal strictures. Surg Clin North Am 53:875, 1973

19. Rath G, Schaff J, Sninder G: Flexible fiberoptic bronchoscopy techniques and review of 100 bronchoscopies. Chest 63:689, 1973

20. Renz L, Smiddy J, Rauscher C, et al: Bronchoscopy in respiratory failure. JAMA 219:619, 1972

21. Sackner M: Use of betadine in bronchofiberscopy. Chest 64:280, 1973

22. Sackner M, Landa J: Bronchofiberscopy: to intubate or not to intubate! Chest 63:302, 1973

23. Sackner MA, Wanner A, Landa J: Applications of bronchofiberscopy. Chest 62(Suppl):705, 1972

24. Sanderson DR, Fontana RS, Woolner LB, et al: Bronchoscopic localization of radiographically occult lung cancer. Chest 65:608, 1974

25. Senno A, Moallem S, Quijano ER, et al: Thoracoscopy with the fiberoptic bronchoscope. J Thorac Cardiovasc Surg 67:606, 1974

26. Shimada K, Gondos B, Benfield J: Photofiberoptic bronchoscopic findings during lung transplant rejection. Arch Surg 106:774, 1973

27. Shinnick JP, Johnston RF, Oslick T: Bronchoscopy during mechanical ventilation using the fiberscope. Chest 65:613, 1974

28. Smiddy J, Elliott R: The evaluation of hemoptysis with fiberoptic bronchoscopy. Chest 64: 158, 1973

29. Smiddy J, Ruth W, Kerby G, et al: Flexible fiberoptic bronchoscope. Ann Intern Med 75: 971, 1971

30. Spence W: Fiberoptic endoscopy and bronchoscopy. JAMA 226:353, 1973

31. Stubbs S, Rosenow EC III: Flexible fiberoptic bronchoscopy. Minn Med 56:831, 1973

32. Tahir A: General anesthesia for bronchofiberscopy. Anesthesiology 37:564, 1972

33. Taylor PA, Towey RM: The broncho-fiberscope as an aid to endotracheal intubation. Br J Anaesth 44:611, 1972

34. Tucker G Jr, Olsen A, Andrews A Jr, et al: The flexible fiberscope in bronchoscopic perspective. Chest 64:149, 1973

35. Wanner A, Landa J, Nieman R Jr, et al: Bedside bronchofiberscopy for atelectasis and lung abscess. JAMA 224:1281, 1973

36. Wanner A, Zighelboim A, Sackner M: Nasopharyngeal airway: a facilitated access to the trachea: for nasotracheal suction, bedside bronchofiberscopy, and selective bronchography. Ann Intern Med 75:593, 1971

37. Wilson JA: The flexible fiberoptic bronchoscope. Ann Thorac Surg 14:686, 1972

38. Zavala D, Richardson R, Mukerjee P, et al: Use of bronchofiberscope for bronchial brush biopsy. Chest 63:889, 1973

39. Zavala DC, Rhodes ML, Richardson RH, et al: Fiberoptic and rigid bronchoscopy, the state of the art. Chest 65:605, 1974

45

Indirect Endoscopic Examination of the Larynx and Nasopharynx

Paul H. Ward
George Berci
Thomas C. Calcaterra

Indirect examination of the larynx began during the early nineteenth century when Bozzini[4] in 1807 used a candle and mirror to visualize the pharynx and vocal cords. Garcia[5] improved on the technique and examined the vocal cords of many of the prominent singers of his time. The first head mirrors were held in the examiner's teeth and only later were they attached to a headband. The technique underwent gradual improvement, and with the addition of the incandescent light developed by Edison at the turn of the century mirror examination was further facilitated and has become an increasingly popular standard office procedure.

In 1879 Nitze developed the first endoscopic telescope, which was almost immediately introduced into urology, gastroenterology, bronchoesophagology, and laryngology. Laryngologists readily recognized the potential application of the telescope for the indirect examination of the larynx and nasopharynx. Its small size relative to the mirror, increased viewing field, and magnification of the objective without beam glare significantly improved the quality of the examination.

The telescope endoscopic systems have undergone continual improvement with replacement of the distal light bulb by quartz rods and fiberoptic transillumination. In general, however, they have failed to replace mirror techniques for routine use in spite of the superiority of the examination. Undoubtedly

responsible for this failure has been the increased mechanical complexity, expense of the equipment, cumbersomeness in sterilization, and the necessity of retraining the examiners. The recent invention of a new rod-lens system by Hopkins and its application to endoscopy telescopic equipment by Karl Storz* has promised a revolution in quality of examination and photography.

The new lens system is compared with the conventional lens system in Figure 1. In essence, the air-containing spaces between the conventional series of lenses have been replaced by glass rods with polished ends separated by small "air lenses." The optics of this new invention are such that light transmission and magnification are significantly increased, thereby providing a brighter and more easily perceived image. The improved resolution of depth and breadth of field facilitate observation of details. These attributes enabled miniaturization of the instruments while maintaining fiberoptic illumination and adding an "antifog" airflow system (Fig. 2). Perhaps the most attractive feature is the ease with which still or movie cameras and teaching attachments can be coupled to the new telescopes. This adds a new dimension to the examination and docu-

*Manufacturer: Karl Storz Endoscopy, KG. Tuttlingen, West Germany. Distributor: Karl Storz Endoscopy America, Inc., 658 So. San Vicente Boulevard, Los Angeles, Calif. 90048.

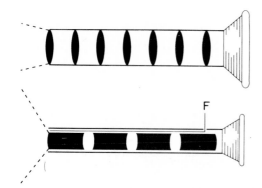

FIG. 1. Top, Conventional endoscopic telescope with assessories of glass lenses (in black) separated by air interspaces. Bottom, In the Hopkins rod-lens system the air interspaces have been replaced with glass rods with polished ends separated by small "air lenses." Noncoherent fibroptics (F) surround the image-transmission lenses and transmit the light.

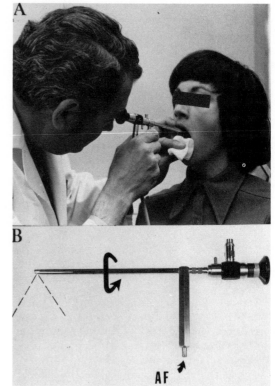

FIG. 2. **A.** New Hopkins rod 90-degree (right angle) telescope being used in a patient. The larynx and nasopharynx can be examined by rotating the telescope 180 degrees. **B.** The telescope is ensheathed in a thin 5.5-mm tube with a handle that facilitates manipulations and is attached to a low-pressure air flow system (AF) that prevents fogging by continual delivery of air over the instrument.

mentation, particularly where accurate assessment of the pathology and the maintenance of accurate follow-up records of the patient's treatment and progress are of paramount importance.

INDICATIONS

Examination of the relatively inaccessible larynx, pharynx, and nasopharynx is usually performed during the routine otolaryngology examination. At present relatively few other physicians have developed the capability of efficiently using head mirrors and the various-sized nasopharyngeal and laryngeal mirrors. The technical capability of visualizing these areas is one of the reasons for the existence of the specialty of otorhinolaryngology.

It is common practice for physicians to treat patients with complaints referable to these areas of the body symptomatically for a week or two and then refer them to the specialist if the symptoms persist. For example, sore throats, dysphagia, and hoarseness are treated as inflammatory disease with antibiotics, and only on failure of the symptoms to subside are the patients eventually referred to a specialist who may visualize with mirrors a tumor of the pharynx, larynx, or base of the tongue. There are many tragic delays in making a definitive diagnosis of malignancy and other diseases of

these difficult to visualize areas of the body. Even the specialist may experience difficulty in determining the pathology in young patients, those with hyperactive gag reflexes who are difficult to examine, and in cases where there are abnormalities of the physiologic mechanisms. The use of right-angle telescopes in these instances may provide a markedly improved examination. The new telescope described in this chapter greatly facilitates examination of these areas and requires only moderate initial expenditure and minimal training experience for its use. It is anticipated that it will become standard examining equipment in the offices of all physicians who manage diseases of these areas and the body as a whole. The radiotherapists in our institution, for example, now have these instruments and are thus able to examine and follow the lesions during radiotherapy treatment of patients with lesions in the nasopharynx, larynx, and pharynx.

Because of the rapidity of the otolaryngology examination and the cleansing and sterilization time requirements, most otolaryngologists continue to use the mirrors for conventional examination of nonsymptomatic areas. Based on the experience in our clinic, the improved features of the examination, potential for still and moving picture photography, and videotape documentation make the new Hopkins rod telescopes essential for evaluation of symptomatic or pathologic cases. In view of the markedly improved resolution of the system, enabling detection of preclinically symptomatic lesions, it is likely that as sterilization problems are solved this instrument will be more widely used for routine examinations.

CONTRAINDICATIONS

There are no contraindications to indirect examination of the larynx, pharynx, and nasopharynx with either mirror or telescope except in unusual situations. In those patients too ill to be examined sitting upright in a chair, the telescope often proves of great value, giving better visualization than mirror examination. In patients with extremely severe gag reflexes who have a history of reactions to topical and local anesthesia and in whom per-

sistent symptomatology demands examination, resort to direct laryngoscopy may be required.

ANESTHESIA

The larynx, pharynx, and nasopharynx of 80 to 90 percent of patients can be examined adequately either with mirrors or the telescope without anesthesia. A similar number of patients require a topical anesthetic (i.e., 10 percent cocaine, 5 percent Xylocaine, etc.) in the form of a spray to reduce the gag reflex for both mirror and telescopic examination. When photography is performed all patients are anesthetized topically because of the 5 to 10 minutes of discomfort and gag reflex stimulation initiated by the repeated introduction of the larger instruments. If the examinations cannot be conducted without anesthesia or with topical anesthesia, and symptoms are not rapidly responsive to therapy, direct examination under general anesthesia is indicated. Indirect examination is not conducted under general anesthesia.

TECHNIQUE

The use of the head mirror and various-sized laryngeal and pharyngeal mirrors requires considerable practice and skill with personal instruction and extensive practice. The posi-

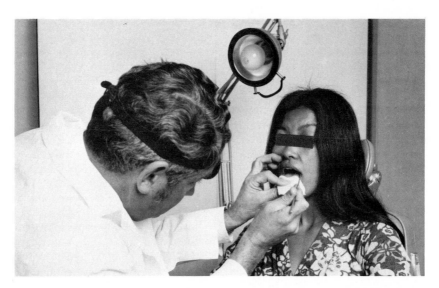

FIG. 3.   Conventional head mirror is used for laryngeal mirror examination of the larynx of a patient.

tioning and technique of performing indirect mirror examination of the larynx and pharynx is illustrated in Figure 3. Important considerations are the focal length of the head mirror and the positioning of the patient's head and the light to be reflected. The tongue is gently grasped with gauze and pulled outward and downward. An effort is made not to touch the base of the tongue while introducing the mirror since this is the strongest stimulus to the gag reflex. The mirror is gently placed against the soft palate and uvula, which are pushed upward and posteriorly thereby placing the mirror in line with the larynx and pharynx.

A smaller mirror is used for the nasopharyngeal examination, and a metal tongue depressor is placed on the tongue as far back and to one side as the patient will tolerate. The tongue is depressed strongly, and the mirror is introduced between the lower margin of the palate and the depressed tongue. Again, these maneuvers are performed as gently as possible, and effort is made not to touch any of the surrounding structures more than is absolutely necessary. The disadvantages of limited mirror-objective size, reversal of the object, lack of magnification, fogging, beam reflection, and difficulty in obtaining photographic documentation have long been recognized and tolerated. The mirror examination continues to be practical for routine examinations of the larynx, pharynx, and nasopharynx primarily because of the low cost of the equipment and the ease of sterilization. Telescopic examination eliminates many of the drawbacks of the mirror examination. The technique of introducing the new Hopkins rod telescope for indirect examination of the larynx is demonstrated in Figure 2A.

The examination instrument consists of a telescope with a 90-degree direction of view and a 50-degree viewing angle, incorporating in the sheath (total outside diameter 6 mm) the antifog arrangements and the fiberoptic light guide for the illumination. The instrument is connected via a 6-foot fiberoptic flexible bundle to an external light source and a small aquarium pump to provide positive air pressure in the front of the objective. This antifog apparatus if not connected can be substituted for with ease by warming the tip of the telescope in a bowl of warm water. The antifog device has the great advantage that in case of prolonged examination the instrument does not have to be withdrawn for prewarming. In case of forced phonation and coughing, the working end does not become covered by moisture or secretions. The patient is seated in an examining chair with the head comfortable, rested on the head rest. The patient's tongue is grasped and pulled forward, and the telescope inserted. After introduction the axis of the telescope or the eyepiece can be elevated or lowered according to the patient's anatomy (short neck, overhanging epiglottis, short distance between the back of the tongue and the posterior wall of the pharynx). Under visual control the telescope can thus be optimally positioned. The image is a direct view (rather than a mirror image) and the quality is remarkable. The enlarged panoramic view of the larynx and pharynx is presented in one field. The image is much brighter than the reflected beam through the mirror, and glare from reflecting surfaces is eliminated. The larger image field makes orientation for the expert as well as the novice much easier.

In some patients with active gag reflexes who are difficult to examine and in others where there are abnormalities of the physiologic mechanisms the brief glimpses provided by the mirror or the telescope may be inadequate for formulation of a sound diagnosis. Le Jeune,[7] Holinger,[6] and Berci and co-workers[1-3] stressed the value of moving pictures for analysis of abnormalities involving motions of the larynx. They further emphasized that the fleeting glimpse or observation lasting only a fraction of a second may provide an inadequate and inaccurate diagnostic impression. Telescopes have provided markedly improved examination but previously have been impractical for routine photography because of the bulky and unwieldy equipment and the inadequate transmission of light. The improved optics and magnification produced by this new invention allows incorporation of a surrounding fibroptic light bundle that provides better visualization and adequate light for photography, which is achieved by simple coupling of the still and motion picture camera to the telescope (Fig. 4).

The new rod-lens system and its development gave impetus to and made possible the redesign of new telescopic instruments and accessory equipment. For teaching institutions and for conferences where it is desirable for a number of students, residents, and other physicians to visualize lesions of these areas the newly developed side arm offers significant advantages (Fig. 5).

This side arm consists of a beam splitter with

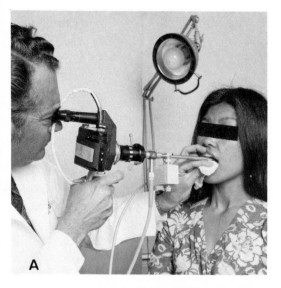

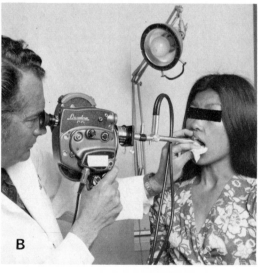

FIG. 4. Demonstration of the simplicity of the camera-telescope coupling and the technique of photographing the patient's larynx with a still (**A**) and a moving picture (**B**) camera.

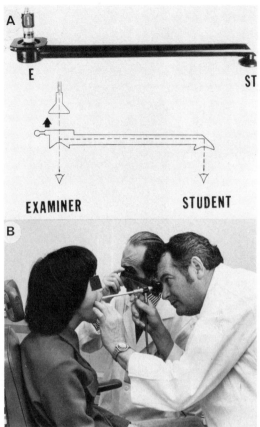

FIG. 5. **A.** Student teaching attachment (ST) coupled to the telescope eyepiece (E). The line illustration shows that the optical system does not cause any significant light loss to the examiner's eye. **B.** Teaching side arm in use, enabling simultaneous observation of the examination by two observers.

a newly designed optical transmission system. The teaching arm attachment is easily coupled to the telescope, and as the examiner advances or moves the instrument the student or observer can follow exactly the technique and the view through the teaching side arm eyepiece, which displays the same image. The student or observer is placed a convenient distance from the examiner. The side arm is lightweight and does not affect or restrict the examiner's position or view. This new observation system has improved light transmission and image fidelity that far surpass the coherent fiberoptic bun-

dle viewing systems where distortion and light loss are inherent properties. The side arm is more durable and less expensive than the coherent fiberoptic bundle teaching attachments. This equipment is now used routinely in our weekly head and neck tumor conference. The side arm attachment makes it possible for a number of observers to visualize the laryngeal, pharyngeal, or nasopharyngeal pathology with minimal discomfort whenever patients with lesions in these areas are presented.

Photographs and movie strips stimulate increased interest when patients are presented in absentia and provide excellent follow-up assessment. The advantage to the patients, students, and conference participants when the lesion can be seen before diagnosis and management are discussed is self-evident. Study of postoperative and posttherapy movies of the

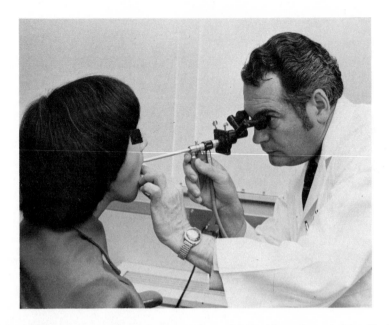

FIG. 6.   Telescope in use examining the patient with the binocular eyepiece attached.

laryngeal motions may be of significant value in determining why some patients aspirate, do not aspirate, and have an excellent or conversely a poor voice following conservation surgery. It is anticipated that teaching movies now in progress, the use of film strips for case presentations to panels, and the application of videotape recordings will contribute significantly to future educational endeavors. A binocular eyepiece system that can be attached to the telescope is under development; and just as the monocular microscope has almost totally been replaced with binocular lenses, the same appears likely for this instrument in the future (Fig. 6).

RESULTS

The new Hopkins rod telescopes have been used to examine several thousand patients and have been put into routine use in the UCLA Hospital clinic for the examination of any patients having symptoms or lesions referable to the larynx, pharynx, or nasopharynx.

Examples of routine photographs taken from patients are shown in Figure 7 (Plate H).* Currently under evaluation is the instant Polaroid reproduction of transparent slides into permanent color photographs that can be placed in

*All color plates appear at the front of the book.

the patient's chart and sent to the referring physician. Permanent moving pictures are easily obtained in those instances where detection of minimal pathologic abnormalities and impairment of movements are of paramount importance (Fig. 8). Permanent records of this type facilitate treatment follow-up of progression or regression of the pathology.

The same instrument is employed to examine the nasopharynx by rotating the telescope 180 degrees. The breadth and depth of field provide a comprehensive view of the entire nasopharynx (Fig. 7, Plate). The superior magnified view includes in one field eustachian tubes, choanae, fossa of Rosenmüller, vault and base of the septum, posterior turbinates, and dorsal surface of the palate. Photography of lesions of the larynx, pharynx, and nasopharynx allows objective measurement and assessment of the effectiveness of the various treatment modalities. The telescope provides visualization for accurate biopsy of lesions in this area with either curved or transnasally passed straight forceps. New information on velopharyngeal closure was obtained by studying photographs and movies of the nasopharynx of normal subjects and of patients with velopharyngeal insufficiency, before and after Teflon injection.[10]

Otolaryngologists, neurosurgeons, and others in recent years have experienced the transition periods during which they used the naked eye,

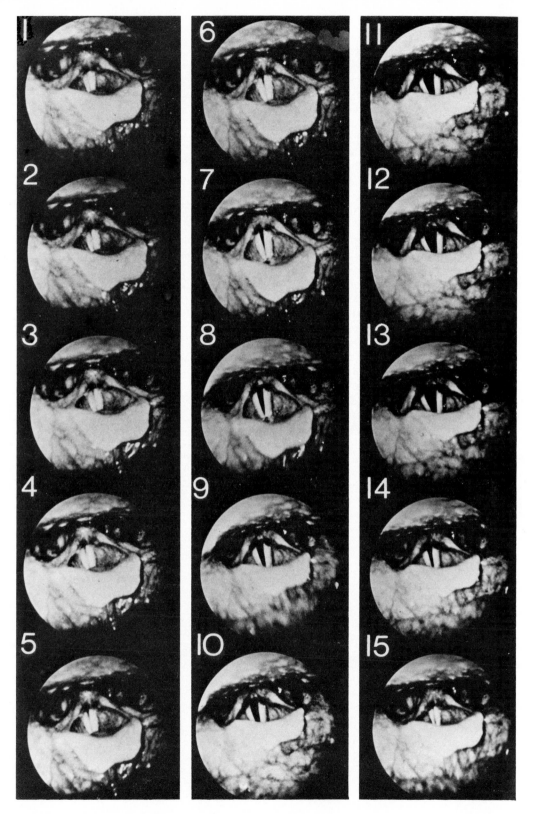

FIG. 8. Enlargement of a 16-mm movie film strip taken through the Hopkins rod telescope. Frames 1 through 15 clearly demonstrate the stationary midline position of the paralyzed left vocal cord. The epiglottis is at the bottom since the telescope gives a direct image rather than the customary reversed mirror image.

loop magnification, and then became dependent on the microscope. The improvement in diagnostic and surgical technical performance for them is no longer in question. Few modern otologists neglect to examine a pathologic ear or to complete any ear operation without using the microscope at some time during the procedure. The same is now applicable to our technical state of the art in examination of the larynx and nasopharynx. New instruments are now available that provide such improved and superior evaluation potential that the superior specialist can no longer "get by" without them. Retraining the examiner is simple but requires effort and some initial increase in examination time. The enthusiasm which the residents and staff have shown and their literal demand for the opportunity to use this instrument during its clinical trial state is indicative of their recognition of its value. They repeatedly inquire of the availability of a similar examination setup for their future offices. These new instruments offer perhaps even more to the family physician and his patients. The technical ability needed to visualize the larynx, pharynx, and nasopharynx with the new telescopes is far less than that required to learn to use mirrors.[9] It is anticipated that by including the Hopkins rod telescope in his examining armamentarium the family physician will be able to examine the pharynx, larynx, and nasopharynx, and arrive at an accurate early diagnosis without having to treat diseases of these areas symptomatically. Early diagnosis and appropriate referral for treatment should improve survival statistics for patients with life-threatening disease.

REFERENCES

1. Berci G, Caldwell FH: A device to facilitate photography during indirect laryngoscopy. Med Biol Illus 13:169, 1963
2. Berci G, Fleming WB, Dunlop EE, et al: New endoscopic technique for the examination and cinematography of the nasopharynx. Cancer 20:2013, 1967
3. Berci G, Kont LA: A new optical system in endoscopy. Br J Urol 41:564, 1969
4. Bozzini: Cited by Mettler CC, Mettler FA: History of Medicine. Toronto, Blakiston, 1947
5. Garcia: Cited by Mettler CC, Mettler FA: History of Medicine. Toronto, Blakiston, 1947
6. Holinger PH: Photography of the larynx, trachea, bronchi and esophagus. Trans Am Acad Ophthalmol 46:153, 156, 1942
7. LeJeune FE: Motion picture study of laryngeal lesions. Surg Gynecol Obstet 62:492, 1936
8. Nitze M: Eine neue Beobachtungs und Untersuchungsmethode fur Harnrehre und Harnblase. Wien Med Wochenschr 24:650, 1879
9. Ward PH, Berci G, Calcaterra TC: Advances in endoscopic examination of the respiratory system. Ann Otol Rhinol Laryngol 83:754, 1974
10. Zwitman DH, Ward PH, Sonderman JC: Variations in velopharyngeal closure assessed by endoscopy. J Speech Hear Disord (in press)

46

Direct Endoscopic Examination of the Larynx

Paul H. Ward

Almost a century passed between the first reported indirect candle-lighted mirror examination of the larynx by Bozzini[2] in 1807 and the first direct laryngoscopy examinations reported by Kirstein[10] in 1895. Using an L-shaped tongue depressor laryngoscope, the vocal cords and the tracheal bifurcation were visualized—and direct laryngoscopy was born. One of the primary problems (which still persists) was the difficulty in visualizing the anterior commissure. Early clinicians also found mastery of the technique difficult, the equipment expensive, and the necessity of illumination by the primitive electrical systems cumbersome.

The development of laryngoscopes evolved in several directions with many modifications within each group. The conventional tube handle type was associated with Brunings,[3] Jackson,[8] Mosher,[14] Ingals,[7] and Clerif.[5] Modifications by adding leverage arms that attach to the scopes or handles and provide self-retaining support are associated with Roberts,[15] Somers,[16] and Lewy.[11] The original suspension laryngoscope blade is an L-shaped tongue depressor with tapered ends, a mouth gag, and a complicated suspension apparatus that moves up and down, and forward and backward. This instrument was introduced by Killian[9] and modified by Albrecht,[1] Lynch,[13] Holinger,[6] and others.

The suspension laryngoscope provides an excellent view of the larynx but has failed to gain widespread use. The necessity for the use of general anesthesia, the complexity and cumbersomeness of the apparatus, and the propensity to induce lacerations of the tissues of the oropharynx in the hands of the inexperienced operators probably explain its lack of popularity.

Recent modifications and advances have been made which facilitate visualization of the anterior commissure, provide a wider translaryngoscopic working distance, and provide additional light via fibroptics, allowing microscopic visualization and photography.[12] The slotted laryngoscope with a 3- to 4-mm opening on the side facilitates working simultaneously with two instruments. It also provides better visualization and placement of the needle for Teflon injection.

The incorporation of self-contained battery-supplied light sources within the handle that connect directly with the fibroptic bundle transmitting light to the end of the laryngoscope have decreased the size and awkwardness of the instrumentation but have yet to receive wide usage.

INDICATIONS

Unlike indirect laryngoscopy, which can be performed with relative ease and minimal equipment in almost any physical setting, direct laryngoscopy is a surgical procedure performed in a specially equipped operating or endoscopy room. Furthermore, when indirect visualization with mirrors and telescopes is possible the overall view and examination are superior to those usually possible on direct examination. There are therefore specific indications for direct laryngoscopy, and indiscriminate use of the procedure should be discouraged.

Examination of the larynx of infants and young children generally requires direct laryngoscopy for adequate visualization. Any patient with hoarseness, stridor, hemoptysis, or other signs and symptoms of laryngeal and/or pharyngeal disease in which the area cannot be visualized because of a strong gag reflex or because of abnormal anatomic relationships, and who does not respond to short-term symptomatic treatment (1 to 2 weeks), has a strong indication for direct laryngoscopy.

Whenever there is difficulty interpreting the pathologic findings of indirect laryngoscopy, with the diagnosis requiring biopsy and removal of pieces of tissue, and when delicate endolaryngeal surgical operative procedures are contemplated, direct laryngoscopy is indicated. Partial visualization of the larynx by indirect means in symptomatic patients is unacceptable, and direct laryngoscopy in most cases allows visualization, inspection, and biopsy of the anterior commissure, ventricles, epiglottic tubercle, and subglottic region as indicated. In summary, the direct view, normal outer posterior and lateral plane relationships, more natural depth and color perception, and the opportunity to assess mobility and tissue texture by instrumental palpation as well as to explore and biopsy obscure inaccessible areas are the advantages of direct laryngoscopy over indirect laryngoscopy.

Following direct trauma to the larynx with possible fractures of the cartilage in which lacerations, edema, and bleeding prevent assessment of the degree of damage, direct laryngoscopy can contribute greatly to the evaluation of, determination of necessity for, and planning of exploratory surgery. The prolonged persistence of excessive postirradiation edema (beyond 6 months) for carcinoma of the larynx requires direct laryngoscopy and multiple biopsies because of the high probability of recurrence.

CONTRAINDICATIONS

The contraindications to direct laryngoscopy are relative, and each situation and case must be individually assessed. Special care must be taken when introducing the laryngoscope into the laryngeal lumen in patients with impending upper airway obstruction since the additional trauma could add to the obstruction and require emergency tracheotomy.

In these instances an appropriately sized bronchoscope should be available. If the decision is made to pass through the partially obstructed area, the bronchoscope can be introduced and the tracheostomy performed with the bronchoscope in place. This provides an adequate airway and increases the safety during the performance of tracheostomy. Early diagnosis and treatment of the underlying laryngeal pathology, with the saving of many lives, has resulted from adherence to these precautions.

The disadvantages of hospitalization, preparation, and expense of the operative team and equipment, and the risks of trauma, sedation, and anesthesia must be accepted when the indications for direct laryngoscopy are present.

ANESTHESIA

Direct laryngoscopy can be performed on most patients using either topical, local, and/or general anesthesia. Selection of the specific type of anesthesia for each patient requires experience and good judgment. Except for specific instances, the choice is left up to the patient after informing him of the hazards of general anesthesia and the slight discomfort that may accompany local anesthesia. In tense, anxious, nervous, and highly emotionally labile patients general anesthesia is preferred and may be mandatory. Patients with short stocky necks, receding chins, or markedly protruding upper incisors are candidates for general anesthesia. Topical and local anesthesia are indicated whenever evaluation of cord mobility is desirable, as in laryngeal paralysis and cricoarytenoid fixation or for testing phonation after injection of a paralyzed vocal cord with polytetrafluoroethylene (Teflon). The stomach should be empty if possible before laryngoscopy regardless of the anesthesia selected.

TOPICAL ANESTHESIA

The success of topical anesthesia is dependent on a relaxed patient. Adequate explanation of the proposed examination does much to help the patient relax. This attitude must be enhanced with sedation sufficient to produce drowsiness and yet still leave the patient awake enough to cooperate. The combination of sedative drugs and dosages used are tailored to the individual patient, eliminating any drugs to which there is a history of allergic reaction. Usually morphine or meperidine is the basic drug and is combined with atropine and a short-acting barbiturate or hydroxyzine (Visterol) or diazepam (Valium) administered in dosages based on the individual's weight, sex, age, and general health. If the patient can tolerate morphine it is the drug of choice because of its superior pain-relieving and euphoria-producing qualities.

The topical anesthetic usually depends on the preference and experience of the laryngologist. Whether cocaine, lidocaine, or tetracine is used, it is imperative that the physician be aware of the toxic dosages of each drug and accordingly limit the amount used.

The patient is most easily anesthetized by having him sit up with his legs dangling over the edge of the examining table. The palate, oropharynx, and throat are sprayed several times with the solution. The mist is sprayed as the patient inspires so that some is carried into the larynx and trachea. Applicators with cotton are dipped in the anesthetic solution, and the excess liquid is squeezed out. The applicators are gently passed over the tongue into the pyriform sinuses where they are held for 30 to 60 seconds. With the tongue held out the applicator can be used to paint the anesthetic solution over the epiglottis and aryepiglottic folds. The larynx is visualized with a mirror, and several drops of the solution are then dropped over the surface of the cords into the laryngeal lumen. The patient is allowed to assume the supine position and is ready for draping and laryngoscopy.

Currently popular among some of the younger laryngologists is the addition of blocking the superior laryngeal nerve by injecting 1 or 2 cc of local anesthetic (i.e., 1 percent lidocaine). This is accomplished by palpating the hyoid bone near its lateral margin. The needle penetrates the skin, a small amount of anesthetic is injected, and then the lateral lip of the hyoid is palpated with the needle, which is allowed to roll caudally over the hyoid, at which point the anesthetic is injected into the area. The author feels after considerable experience that the injection of local anesthesia is·

probably not necessary if adequate time has been spent in meticulously administering a good topical anesthetic.

GENERAL ANESTHESIA

The trend in recent years has been to perform more procedures under general anesthesia probably because of the increased comfort to the patient. The newer, rapidly acting anesthetic drugs and the increase in superiorly trained anesthesiologists has also influenced the trend toward general anesthesia.

An increase in the use of suspension microlaryngoscopy, which is very difficult to perform and uncomfortable to the patient under topical anesthesia, has also contributed to the shift in the use of general anesthesia. While performing suspension laryngoscopy, and in most instances of conventional laryngoscopy, a small cuffed tube (16 Fr.) is introduced into the larynx after adequate sedation and induction. The laryngoscope is then passed anterior to the tube, which nestles in the posterior commissure. The tube can be manipulated so that this area can be inspected before or at the completion of the procedure. The tube, even though small, is frequently in the way, and a new technique using a segment of cuffed tube placed below the glottis with insufflation of jets of anesthetic under pressure through a small-lumen tube (utilizing the Venturi effect) provides adequate respiratory exchange and greatly facilitates performance of the procedure.[4]

When only a very short working period is required and an experienced anesthesiologist is available, the apneic technique can be used. The cuirass or body respirator is extremely awkward and marginally effective. It is rarely used now. Particularly important to the success of laryngoscopic examination is good communication between the surgeon and anesthesiologist so that a clear understanding of what is to be accomplished is understood by both specialists.

TECHNIQUE

The technique, posturing, and instruments utilized for direct laryngoscopy are the same for either local or general anesthesia. In the past elaborate gowning and sterile precautions

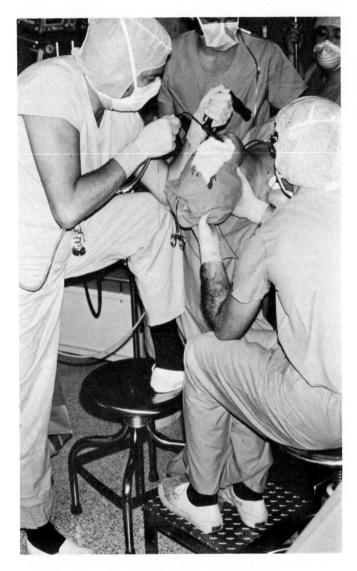

FIG. 1. Properly positioned patient, laryngoscopist, assistant, and anesthesiologist. The head of the patient, who is lying supine, is flexed on the chest and then extended at the occipitoatloid articulation. This positioning tilts the epiglottis and larynx anteriorly, facilitating entrance into the laryngeal lumen.

were routine. This has proved unnecessary, and the procedure is now treated as a surgically clean operation with sterilization of the instruments and the wearing of sterile gloves. No infections or untoward effects have been encountered from this more realistic approach, and the excess expense to the patient is avoided. The variety of laryngoscopes—Jackson, Holinger, or other modifications—come in several sizes (i.e., child, adolescent, and adult). Special beveled-tip anterior commissure scopes are selected whenever the lesion is located anteriorly and better exposure of the area is indicated. A slotted laryngoscope is usually selected if microlaryngoscopy, Teflon injection,

or other single and multiple instrument manipulations are to be performed.

After selecting the appropriate laryngoscope the patient is placed in a dorsal recumbent position. Positioning the head is crucial and is best performed by an assistant holding the head (Fig. 1). The neck is first flexed so that the chin touches the manubrium; then the cranium is extended at the occiput, thrusting the chin into the air. Similar positioning can be achieved by placing a roll of folded sheets under the patient's shoulders and also by utilizing a mechanical headrest. Proper positioning is necessary, for it serves to lift the epiglottis away from the posterior pharyngeal wall and open up the laryngeal lumen. A moistened sponge is placed over the upper teeth to form a protective cushion. The laryngoscope is introduced gently over the surface of the tongue and then is angulated at about 45 degrees to the patient's body axis. The epiglottis is identified, and the laryngoscope tip is dipped posteriorly to slide past the epiglottis and lift it forward. The arytenoids and posterior commissure are visualized, and the laryngoscope is passed into the laryngeal lumen. Sometimes mild external pressure over the thyroid cartilage facilitates penetration of the laryngeal lumen.

The endoscopist should develop a routine pattern of examining the vallecula, pyriform sinuses, epiglottis, aryepiglottic folds, posterior commissure, false cords, ventricles, true cords, and subglottic areas. The observations made and the biopsies performed can then be entered in a uniform way in the operative report.

RESULTS

The addition of direct laryngoscopy to indirect laryngoscopy, and the correlation of the findings with the radiologic (tomographic and laryngographic) results has added greatly to our understanding of the pathologic and physiologic mechanisms of the larynx. The direct inspection of the larynx of infants and newborns with respiratory distress, stridor, or abnormal cry has resulted in early diagnosis and has saved many lives. Rational, appropriate management of congenital lesions, cord paralysis, papillomas, and other lesions of the larynx has resulted from the development of direct laryngoscopy.

Biopsy of suspicious lesions in adults has provided early diagnosis of carcinoma, enabling immediate treatment and improved survival rates. Direct laryngoscopy has also facilitated the surgical removal of many benign lesions of the larynx. Translaryngoscopic surgery has expanded to include excision of webs with keel insertion, injection of paralyzed vocal cords with Teflon, arytenoidectomy, and local resection of low-grade, superficial glottic carcinomas.

The laryngoscope has perhaps received its greatest use in the newly developing field of anesthesiology where it is used in almost every patient for direct inspection and intubation of the larynx and trachea. Little did its inventor realize the widespread use this valuable tool would receive.

REFERENCES

1. Albrecht W: Die Bedeutung der Schwebelaryngoskope fur das Kindersalter. Arch Laryngol Rhinol 28:1, 1913
2. Bozzini PH: Der Lichleiter Oder Beschreibung einer einfachen Vorrichtung und ihrer Anwendung zur Erleuchtung innerer Hohlen und Zwischenraume des lebenden animalischen Korpers. Weimar, 1807
3. Brunings W: Die Direkte Laryngoskopie, Bronchoskopie und Oesophagoskopie. Wiesbaden, Carl Ritter, 1909. Cited in Mettler CC, Mettler FA: History of Medicine. Toronto, Blakiston, 1947
4. Carden E, Ferguson G, Crutchfield WM: A new silicone elastome tube for use during microsurgery on the larynx. Ann Otol 83:360, 1974
5. Clerif LH: In Jackson C, Coates GM (eds): Photography of the Larynx in the Nose, Throat, Ear and Their Diseases. Philadelphia, Saunders, 1929, p 748
6. Holinger PH: An hour-glass anterior commissure laryngoscope. Laryngoscope 70:1510, 1960
7. Ingals EF: Direct laryngoscopy. In Transactions of the American Laryngology, Rhinology, and Otolaryngology Society. 1911, p 26
8. Jackson CL: Indications for direct laryngoscopy. Ann Otol 48:926, 1939
9. Killian G: Suspension laryngoscopy. In Transactions of the 3rd International Congress on Laryngology and Rhinology, Berlin. Part 2, 1911, p 112
10. Kirstein A: Autoskopie der Larynx und der Trachea (Besichtigung ohne Spiegel). Arch Laryngol Rhinol 3:156, 1895
11. Lewy RB: Gear-power detachable laryngoscope holder and simplified position for direct laryngoscopy. Arch Otolaryngol 58:444, 1953
12. Lewy RB: Depth perception in laryngoscopy. Arch Otolaryngol 72:383, 1960
13. Lynch RC: Technic of suspension laryngoscopy. Laryngoscope 25:840, 1915
14. Mosher HP: Direct examination of the larynx and of the upper end of the esophagus by the lateral route. Boston Med Soc J 48:189, 1908
15. Roberts SE: A self-retaining dual distal lighted laryngoscope with screw-driven fulcrum lift. Trans Am Acad Ophthalmol Otolaryngol 56:91, 1952
16. Somers K: Direct laryngoscopy and description of self-retaining attachment for the laryngoscope. Arch Otolaryngol 55:484, 1952

47

Pediatric Laryngology

Eugene G. Flaum

The operative procedure to evaluate or treat laryngeal disease or in gaining exposure for passage of an endotracheal tube or a broncho-scope is called direct laryngoscopy. This may be performed either when a patient is awake or when he is under a general anesthetic. What-ever the reason may be for the passage of a laryngoscope, one should always examine the oral cavity, oro- and hypopharynx, and the lar-ynx. The procedure should always follow direct guidelines. One must be acutely aware of the normal anatomy and the abnormalities which might be present. Whether a surgeon is intro-ducing a rigid bronchoscope or a nonsurgeon is inserting an endotracheal tube, the glottic chink (the area between the true vocal cords) should be well visualized. Injuries to the glottis and the surrounding hypopharynx are much more common when the procedure is performed by a physician who is not completely aware of his inadequacies. The blade of the laryngoscope can be a dangerous weapon. Fractured teeth and tears of the palate, tonsillar pillars, walls of the hypopharynx, or vocal cords are not un-common.

Inspiratory stridor, change in the voice or cry, or the necessity for assisted ventilation are the main indications for performing a direct laryngoscopy. Inspiratory stridor is the hall-mark of upper airway distress. Quite often there is also an expiratory phase (i.e., laryn-gotracheobronchitis, tracheal stenosis, or a foreign body of the tracheobronchial tree). Ex-piratory stridor alone is never an upper airway phenomenon.

Direct laryngoscopy should always be per-formed in a completely controlled situation, al-though often it is not. During resuscitation in a hospital room or ward, chaos may prevail. There usually are more personnel than are necessary, and a team approach to the intuba-tive procedures is lacking. Another area where complications occur is in the delivery room. Here the obstetrician is involved with two pa-tients instead of one.

The general principle of a laryngoscope is that it has a handle and a viewing portion. There are numerous sizes and shapes. The Flagg laryngoscope is used during intubation. This is a battery-operated scope with a light bulb attached near the tip of the blade. The batteries are located in the handle, making the instrument too bulky to perform operative laryngoscopy adequately. The blades might be curved or straight. I can see no use for the curved blade in the pediatric age group.

The Jackson laryngoscope (Fig. 1) is used primarily by a laryngologist. The handle is parallel with the blade, with a perpendicular bar at the proximal end of the scope. The view-ing portion, which is completely enclosed, may be opened with the removal of the inferior half in a sliding fashion. This scope, because of the slightly flattened tip, is ideal for evaluating virtually the entire larynx and hypopharynx. Also following passage of a bronchoscope, the laryngoscope can be easily removed following displacement of the sliding piece. The sizes best suited for pediatric work are those scopes 9 to 12 cm. The light source can easily be converted from the old battery box-powered light source to the newer fiberoptic system.

The Holinger anterior commissure laryngo-scope (Fig. 2) is used for those cases where vis-

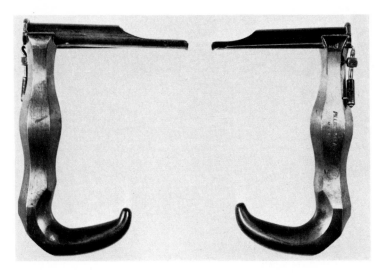

FIG. 1. Jackson laryngoscope.

ibility in the anterior one-third of the cords might be difficult. The scope is similar to the Jackson type, only the tip is more acute and the viewing area is complete without a sliding portion.

At Cedars-Sinai Medical Center in Los Angeles, we are using the Storz pediatric laryngoscope (Fig. 3). The barrel of the blade is approximately a three-fourths arc and open on the side. This opening facilitates introduction of a suction tip or a bronchoscope. The prismatic light deflector is built in the handle and connected via a flexible fiber light-carrying bundle to an external light source.

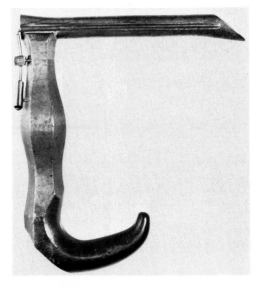

FIG. 2. Holinger laryngoscope.

ANATOMY

It is extremely important to be fully acquainted with the topographic anatomy from the oral cavity to the hypopharynx and larynx. The oral cavity extends from the lips anteriorly to the anterior tonsillar pillars or palatoglossus muscle posteriorly. It contains the alveolar ridge, gingivae, teeth, floor of the mouth, palate (hard and soft), and the anterior two-thirds of the tongue. While performing direct laryngoscopy, the patient is in an inverted position, with the tongue and floor of the mouth superiorly and the palate inferiorly. The posterior or free margin of the soft palate has a redundant fleshy mass—the uvula—extending from its midportion. In the upright individual this is easily seen since it is vertically placed when one is examining the oropharynx. In the endoscopic position it frequently is lying on the posterior pharyngeal wall.

The entrance to the oropharynx is bound by the palatine tonsils (located just posterior to the palatoglossus) and the posterior tonsillar pillars (palatopharyngeus muscle) laterally, the posterior one-third of the tongue inferiorly, and the posterior portion of the uvula superiorly. The oropharynx extends from the soft palate superiorly to the tip of the epiglottis inferiorly. The walls of the oropharynx are bound by the lateral and posterior walls and the oral cavity and base of the tongue anteriorly.

The most critical anatomy to the endoscopist lies in the hypopharynx. This area extends

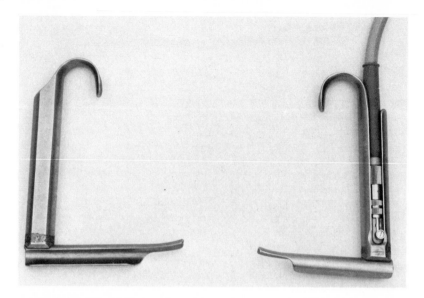

FIG. 3. Storz pediatric laryngoscope (available in three sizes). A prismatic light deflector is inserted into the handle and connected to a fiberoptic light cord to an external source. The blade is approximately three-quarters of an arc and open on one side. (Manufacturer: Storz Endoscopy Co., Tuttlingen, West Germany)

from the tip of the epiglottis superiorly to the cricopharyngeus or the introitus of the cervical esophagus inferiorly. The laryngeal surface of the epiglottis, the arytenoid cartilages, and the cricoid cartilage lie anteriorly, and the pharyngeal walls laterally and posteriorly. During relaxation the arytenoids and cricoid might lie directly against the posterior pharyngeal wall. The larynx lies at the level of the third to the sixth cervical vertebrae. It is composed of multiple paired and unpaired cartilagenous structures connected by membranous and ligamentous attachments. When one examines the larynx from its superior surface, the paired arytenoids and central epiglottis are noted. The tip of the epiglottis is usually sharp and almost leaflike in appearance. At times it might be omega-shaped—i.e., it might be curled in a posterior direction so that its lateral edges almost touch each other (as is seen in laryngomalacia). The width of the epiglottis is greater toward the base. The aryepiglottic folds are membranous bands which attach the base of the epiglottis to the arytenoids. These folds are usually noted in an anterolateral direction because of the more laterally placed arythenoid cartilages. The glottic chink or opening lies in a midline position, medial to the aryepiglottic folds, posterior to the epiglottis, and anterior to the interarytenoid region. This will be de-

scribed further later. Just anterior to the epiglottis and posterior to the base of the tongue lie the paired valleculae. These are shallow pouches and constitute an area of prime importance to the endoscopist. The tip of the laryngoscope should be introduced into it and against the base of the tongue in order to obtain a nondistorted view of the larynx when the scope is elevated in a superior direction. Two other pouches, the piriform sinuses, are located just lateral to the glottis. Their medial walls are formed by the lateral edges of the aryepiglottic folds. They extend inferiorly, being formed anterolaterally by the thyroid cartilage ala, and laterally and posteriorly by the pharyngeal walls. This is a common place for a traumatic intubation. It should also be noted that bronchoscopes and endotracheal tubes are frequently introduced to the postcricoid region.

The false and true vocal folds, with the central glottic chink or space, are located in a central position. The false or ventricular bands are formed by the mucous membrane and submucosal tissue, along with the lateral portion of the internal thyroarytenoid muscle. They are actually medially extending shelflike projections from the aryepiglottic folds. The true cords are formed by the vocal ligaments, internal thyroarytenoid or vocalis muscles, and the surface mucosa. Since they extend more medially than the false folds, they are easier to examine. A portion of the true cords, however, is hidden by the overlapping of the false cords. The intervening space is called the ventricle. The glottic chink is the actual area between the true cords and therefore leads to the subglottic airway and trachea (Figs. 4, 5).

TECHNIQUE

It is imperative to understand the anatomy prior to passing a laryngoscope, whether it be for intubation purposes or operative laryngoscopy. One should always follow a general procedure. Be sure the light source is in working condition (for the laryngoscope and bronchoscope if it is to be used). Check the suction apparatus. Is the tubing of proper length, and is the pressure adequate? The instruments should be within close reach. This includes the laryngoscope, endotracheal tube, or bonchoscope, and suction catheter or suction tube.

Positioning the patient is probably the most important step in direct laryngoscopy. With adequate extension of the neck—whether the head is rotated on a slightly elevated head rest, or a rubber ring or bolster is placed under it—the trachea and larynx are brought into a position parallel with the cervical spine. *A curved laryngoscopic blade should never be used in pediatric patients.* Following the introduction of a straight blade into the proper position (Figs. 6, 7), a direct view of the larynx, subglottic airway, and upper trachea is noted.

The infant has no teeth to worry about. In older children the teeth might be loose or easily displaced if the scope is passed in a midline position. Always check the teeth to make sure all are firm and if any are loose; try to avoid them, rather than finding a missing one following the procedure. The central portion of the posterior one-third of the tongue is higher than the lateral aspects. If one passes the scope from

FIG. 4. Xeroradiograph of the upper airway. h, hypopharynx. e, epiglottis. v, vallecula. fvc, false vocal cord. tvc, true vocal cord. s, subglottic airway. t, trachea.

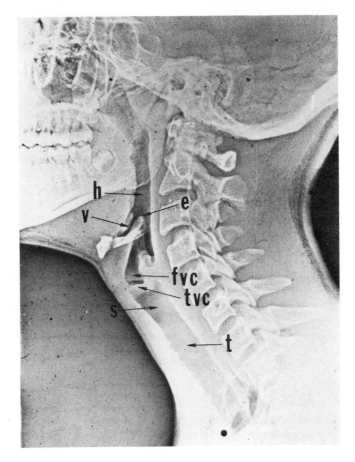

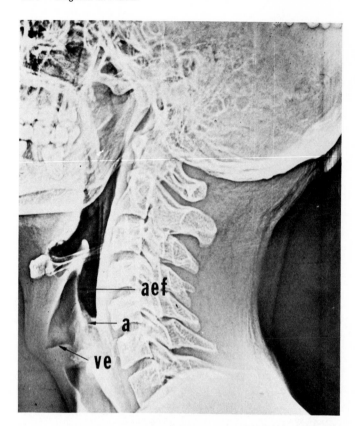

FIG. 5. Xeroradiograph of the upper airway. aef, aryepiglottic fold. a, arytenoid. ve, ventricle.

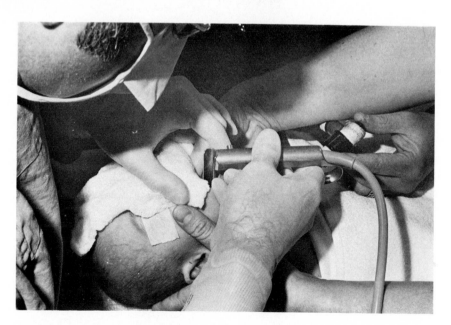

FIG. 6. Passage of laryngoscope with the right hand, the head being held in an extended position in a rubber ring.

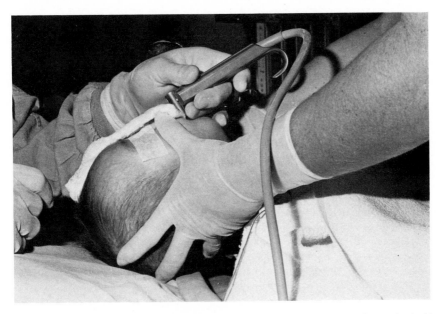

FIG. 7. Following passage of the laryngoscope to the level of the larynx, it can be held with the left hand, leaving the right hand free for instrumentation or passage of a bronchoscope.

a position slightly to the right of the midportion of the oral cavity, it is easier to get a view of the vallecula and the epiglottis (which may be placed slightly anteriorly). If a scope is passed over the midportion of the tongue, it may fall or be forced to one side or the other with the thrust of the tongue. The tip of the blade of the scope can then be advanced, carefully noting the surrounding anatomic structures. Following a quick but adequate evaluation of the supraglottic structures and the base of the tongue, the blade may be placed against

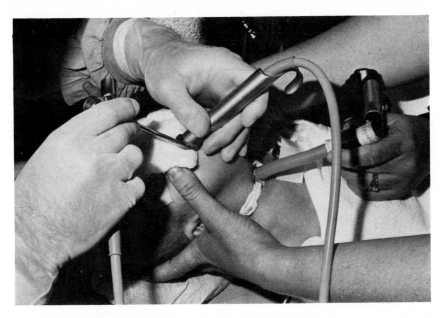

FIG. 8. With the laryngoscope in place, a bronchoscope is positioned with the right hand. Anesthesia is applied via tracheostomy.

one of two objects. If the larynx is being examined during operative laryngoscopy, it is advisable to place the blade against the base of the tongue, anterior to the lingual surface of the epiglottis. With elevation of the tip of the blade, the laryngeal structures are usually easily brought into direct view without abnormal stretching of the aryepiglottic folds or true or false vocal cords. If this still does not allow visibility of the glottis, the blade tip may be inserted under the glottic surface of the epiglottis and elevated once again. This second position is advised for the times when the procedure is done to pass an endotracheal tube. It is quite frequently easier to pass a bronchoscope (Fig. 8) with the blade of the laryngoscope against the base of the tongue, thus displacing the epiglottis forward with the tip of the bronchoscope. I feel that it is much safer and easier to pass a bronchoscope through a well placed laryngoscope in the pediatric age group.

Laryngoscopy should never be performed alone. A team approach should be used in all instances. In operative laryngoscopy the team should include, in addition to the surgeon, an anesthesiologist, scrub nurse, head-holder, and circulating nurse. *There should be no compromise in this arrangement.*

Whether a case is done under anesthesia or without, an anesthesiologist should be present in the operating room with the apparatus at the opposite side of the patient from where the scope is to be passed. It would be helpful if all endoscopists would work from the right side. This would be beneficial for a smoothly working team. The anesthesiologist should have an appropriately sized mask and mouthpiece handy. He should also have a laryngoscope, endotracheal tubes, and proper attachments for possible assisted ventilation.

The head-holder should be fully acquainted with positioning the child, and if the procedure is done awake he should know how to immobilize the patient. This member of the team should be positioned on the right with his arms and body straddling the child. The hands should be held on either side of the face, keeping the thumbs just under the malar eminences and the fingers over the ears toward the occiput. Be sure the hands are not over the mandible, as this obviously would restrict the surgeon's access to the oral cavity.

The scrub nurse, with the endoscopic equipment, should be located off to the right, in position to be able to hand the instruments between the head-holder and surgeon. Even though a laryngoscopy might be the only procedure planned, a bronchoscope should be on hand to assist with ventilation if severe respiratory distress develops.

The surgeon should be in a completely relaxed position. It is advisable that the table be set at the proper height so that the surgeon feels comfortable while performing the procedure in a sitting position. The handle of the scope should be held in the right hand and guided with the left. When the proper depth is reached he may hold it with both hands or switch it to the left if an instrument, suction tip, or bronchoscope has to be used during the procedure. The upper anterior or anterolateral alveolar ridge or teeth may be used as a fulcrum, provided precaution is taken to minimize any possible injury to this area. This might consist of a small surgical sponge placed between the scope and the instrument.

It is advisable to have a cardiac monitor during all endoscopic procedures. Displacement of the hypopharynx or larynx frequently causes vagal reflexes and subsequent arrythmias. The same is also noted with various anesthetic agents or with relaxants such as succinylcholine. Whenever the surgery is performed under a general anesthetic, a good functioning intravenous line should be available. Whether hypnotics, relaxants, or emergency medications during resuscitation are to be used, the intravenous route is the quickest and most reliable.

COMPLICATIONS

The blade of the laryngoscope can be a dangerous weapon, despite having a blunted tip. It is most important to be aware of the complications because their consequences can be life-threatening. This section is designed to describe the complications in a systematic or anatomic approach, rather than by severity.

A parent can easily see a swollen, bleeding lip or tongue, or a fractured or lost tooth. At times this is of greater concern than the content of the surgical findings. It is extremely important to make sure the lips are not compressed between the gingivae or teeth and the scope. Contusions, abrasions, or lacerations are not uncommon. It is advisable to check the teeth prior to passing a scope. Try to avoid loose ones and be aware of missing teeth prior to surgery; and if a tooth is extremely loose, it may have to be removed.

The tongue frequently is caught between the teeth or gingivae and the scope. Abrasions and contusions are uncomfortable to the bottle-fed infant. Swelling of the tongue might follow prolonged laryngoscopic procedures. This condition is usually of minimal importance. As the scope is progressing toward the oropharynx, the tonsils and soft palate might become easy targets. Swelling of the uvula or hemorrhage from the tonsils is seen occasionally.

The major complications are noted with hypopharyngeal and laryngeal injuries. Tears in the lateral and posterior pharyngeal walls or in the pyriform sinuses might lead to bacterial seeding into the retro- or parapharyngeal spaces with subsequent local abscesses or mediastinitis. Occasionally one sees massive hemorrhage from mucosal tears in the hypopharynx. This can lead to a quick demise unless intubation and subsequent control of the hemorrhage, in that order, are carried out. More common than that are the glottic injuries, where dislocation of the arytenoids or tears of the true or false cords might occur. This can happen with the tip of the scope or with an endotracheal tube or bronchoscope during an improper passage.

PATHOLOGIC CONDITIONS

As noted by Ferguson[12] the quality and type of stridor might give a clue to the position and type of pathologic conditions present. He noted that high-pitched noises during inspiration usually indicate trouble within the larynx, whereas low-pitched stridor is usually located deeper in the tracheobronchial tree or in the pharynx. Wheezing or expiratory stridor is usually due to obstruction of the secondary bronchi and bronchioles. To and fro stridor suggests main airway obstruction below the larynx (i.e., extrinsic compression of the trachea or tracheal stenosis).

Infants with airway obstruction usually eat poorly and display slow growth. They might have problems controlling their own secretions (i.e., saliva) and might even have increasing obstructive symptoms during feedings.

The disorders which cause inspiratory stridor or voice changes in the pediatric age group cover a wide range of categories. These may be outlined as follows:

- Infectious disorders: epiglottitis, laryngotracheobronchitis, diphtheria, tonsillopharyngitis, tuberculosis
- Neuromuscular disorders: recurrent laryngeal nerve paralysis, myasthenia gravis, Mobius' syndrome, supranuclear lesions, poliomyelitis, Guillain-Barré syndrome
- Metabolic disorders: hypocalcemia, hypothyroidism
- Benign tumors: cysts, laryngocele, papilloma, hemangioma, screamer's nodes, aberrant thyroid, fibroma
- Malignancies: rhabdomyosarcoma, chondrosarcoma, fibrosarcoma, lymphoma
- Congenital anomalies: webs, atresia, stenosis, laryngeal cleft, laryngomalacia, craniofacial abnormalities
- Foreign body
- Allergy
- Trauma: blunt, prolonged intubation (faulty instrumentation)

Infectious Disorders

This section includes some of the most critical of all etiologic factors for airway distress. Some infections have a quick onset and cause severe stridor (i.e., acute epiglottitis and laryngotracheobronchitis), and in others the airway problem is of gradual onset during the progression of the disease (i.e., tonsillopharyngitis, tuberculosis, and diphtheria).

Acute Epiglottitis. Acute epiglottitis, which also includes acute supraglottitis[8] and acute supraglottic laryngitis,[22] is an inflammatory disorder which causes severe cellulitis and edema of the supraglottic structures (i.e., epiglottis, aryepiglottic folds, arytenoids, and false vocal folds). The organism most often cultured is *Haemophilus influenzae* type B. Other organisms less often found are *Pneumococcus, Streptococcus,* and *Staphylococcus.*

Clinically one sees a child, usually 3 to 6 years of age, sitting forward, drooling, and presenting with a muffled voice. He is usually pale, tired, and extremely stridorous. Temperatures often reach the 104 F range. Miller[21] in 1949 noted that the child sits with his head in a forward position in order to increase the greatly narrowed supraglottic airway. The onset is usually insidious, and the obstruction may rapidly worsen. The diagnosis is usually made by noting the clinical appearance of the child. Attempting to visualize the erythematous epiglottis with a tongue blade could, in some instances, cause increased respiratory distress because of aspiration and laryngospasm. Radiologic evidence of an increased supraglottic mass might be of assistance; however, x-rays are contraindicated if the child is in severe respiratory distress. Whenever epiglottitis is contemplated as a diagnosis, the safest approach is to have an experienced endoscopist view the larynx via direct laryngoscopy and be prepared to intubate the child (rigid bronchoscope or endotracheal tube) if the disease is present. My experience and training stresses the use of a bronchoscope followed by tracheostomy. It is generally felt in our community that a tracheostomy affords the safest form of management. As noted by Ballenger[2] "in many early cases, with vigorous conservative therapy and constant observation, tracheostomy may be avoided." Over the past few years articles have appeared in the literature advising endo- or nasotracheal intubation as the treatment of choice. It is the general opinion among otolaryngologists in Los Angeles that unless an experienced endoscopist can sit with the patient until the edema has subsided this form of treatment is more hazardous than considering the complications associated with tracheostomy.

The average time until decannulation is approximately 5 days, and the general length of hospitalization is 6 or 7 days. It has been noted by the authors who advocate the more conservative approach that the period of intubation is 1 to 2 days less, thus shortening the length of hospitalization. The tracheotomized child is able to take oral fluids at least by the next day and is generally a more cheerful patient.

Along with establishment of an airway, it is advisable to use a broad-spectrum antibiotic such as ampicillin for controlling the infection. The tracheal secretions are generally inspissated. Frequent suctioning, instillation of saline into the trachea, and increased humidification (by croupette or tracheostomy collar) are also recommended.

Laryngotracheobronchitis. Also called croup or acute subglottic laryngitis, this refers to an infection in which the immediate subglottic airway becomes narrowed by submucosal edema. It is generally considered to be caused by a virus and is most prevalent during the winter months. Various viruses have been isolated, and it is thought that bacterial growths are probably due to secondary infections. Among the bacteria cultured, streptococci, staphylococci, pneumococci, and *H. influenzae* are the most common.

Acute laryngotracheobronchitis is an inflammation which probably begins in the subglottic region (conus elasticus) and later extends to the trachea and bronchi, and may also cause a pneumonitis. The mucosa in the region of the conus elasticus becomes edematous, and the subsequent thick, viscous transudation causes crusting and increasing obstruction. The use of decongestants frequently makes this situation worse. The lack of moisture in the air might also predispose to a life-threatening status.

The disorder is manifested by a barklike cough and inspiratory stridor. Unlike the child with epiglottitis, this patient is able to swallow easily, but because of prolonged air hunger and lethargy might not want to. The severity of this disease is quite varied, but the majority of cases are mild with little or no fever and stridor. Most of the patients are 1 to 3 years of age. The characteristic cough usually starts abruptly during the evening hours. Most of children have a self-limited course following treatment with mist and a mild cough mixture. Their illness might pass during the night. Mills[23] noted that the plasma cortisol level is at its lowest during the period from midnight to 4 AM. He labeled this disorder allergic croup.

In the more severe cases the stridor becomes worse and the child becomes more restless because of the severe hypoxia. The length of the inspiratory phase is much greater than during expiration. Frequently a biphasic stridor develops. The heart rate increases along with a rise in the respiratory rate. Chest retractions deepen, and alar flaring becomes prominent. Treatment in this patient should be started rapidly as respiratory failure could develop at any time.

Treatment can be medical and surgical. Surgical intervention (i.e., tracheostomy or intubation) enters the picture if medical management fails. Antibiotics, steroids, and humidification constitute the recommended medical regimen. Ampicillin, because of its broad spectrum, is the antibiotic of choice. We frequently use intermittent doses of dexamethasone (Decadron) intramuscularly over the first 12 to 24 hours, and then if good progress is made the use of oral corticosteroids is considered. Administration of racemic epinephrine has been proposed by many, and the cure rate is high. The one problem with local application of epinephrine and other sympathomimetic drugs is that the rebound phenomenon sometimes causes an increase in stridor. Regarding the question of intubation versus tracheostomy, refer back to the section on epiglottitis. The length of time until decannulation is much more variable than with supraglottic infections because the subglottic area is the narrowest portion of the upper respiratory tract.

Diphtheria. This disease is caused by a gram-positive bacillus *(Corynebacterium diphtheriae)*. The incubation period is 3 to 10 days, with a relatively slow onset of malaise, fever, and sore throat. Respiratory distress follows quickly because of the continued formation of a membrane over the mucosal linings of the palatine tonsils, nasopharynx, larynx, and occasionally the tracheobronchial tree. Neurologic problems occur 2 to 6 weeks later from release of the toxin.

Although this disease is extremely rare in the United States, sporadic outbreaks in the states bordering Mexico still occur. Immunization programs have generally been very successful. Because of the severity of the disease and the fact that sporadic cases still occur, we should remain aware of this disorder.

Diagnosis is made by discovering the firmly adhering grayish membrane, which when removed causes a moderate amount of bleeding. The membrane has a musty odor. Cultures should be placed on a Klebs-Loeffler medium; smears often show the characteristic organism.

Treatment consists of penicillin and diphtheria antitoxin (following appropriate skin tests to rule out allergy). The child might develop increasing stridor because of the obstructing membrane. Occasionally the membrane has to be removed via direct laryngoscopy and bronchoscopy, and there may be a strong consideration for tracheostomy.

Occasionally postdiphtheritic paralysis of the soft palate, pharynx, and larynx develops. The child should be watched closely following resolution of the membranous period of the disease, as this can occur weeks later.

Tonsillopharyngitis. This infection should be considered a possible cause for upper airway distress in a child. Waldeyer's ring is a mass of lymphatic tissue encompassing the base of the tongue, palatine area, and nasopharynx. Chronic benign hypertrophy and a subsequent severe infectious state can cause severe respiratory distress. Many different organisms have been noted to cause edema, cellulitis, and exudate formation over the tonsillar and adenoid tissue. Among these are group A β-hemolytic streptococcus, *C. diphtheriae*, adenoviruses, infectious mononucleosis, and the Coxsacki viruses. Occasionally exudates are associated with acute leukemia. Treatment is medical, with the appropriate antibiotics. In the very rare patient with severe respiratory distress, emergency measures are instituted to establish an improved airway (i.e., tracheostomy). Tonsillectomy and adenoidectomy are recommended following resolution of the infectious state.

Tuberculosis. This occasionally causes the formation of somewhat friable granulomatous masses over the vocal cords. Usually it is seen in an older child or adult with hoarseness and no previous diagnosis of pulmonary tuberculosis. The actual number of patients with tuberculous granulomas in the upper airway who are under active treatment for pulmonary tuberculosis is greater than might be suspected. The reason for this is that these patients are frequently never examined by direct or indirect laryngoscopic examinations, and furthermore their symptoms of hoarseness and mild respiratory distress are relieved following adequate therapy.

Neuromuscular Disorders

This section includes a discussion regarding the etiologic factors which cause recurrent laryngeal nerve paralysis as well as other factors leading to laryngeal neuromuscular imbalance.

Recurrent Laryngeal Nerve Paralysis. Sensation to the larynx is carried via the superior laryngeal nerve, which is a branch of the vagus and is not a part of the recurrent nerve system. Paralysis of this nerve is usually secondary to an abnormality within the central nervous system (CNS).

The major innervation of the larynx is carried via the recurrent laryngeal nerves. The left one has a longer course as it passes under the arch of the aorta and is therefore more vulnerable by compression by intrathoracic lesions. The right recurrent nerve passes under the subclavian artery. The only laryngeal muscle not supplied by the recurrent nerves is the cricothyroid, and this innervation is via the external branch of the superior laryngeal nerve.

Unilateral motor paralysis is usually due to involvement of the peripheral nerve itself, as there is a bilateral cortical innervation to each side of the larynx. Bilateral paralysis secondary to a CNS disorder would have to be caused by a mass lesion, which is generally symmetrical and covering a large area. The only exception to that rule is if a lesion is located in the area of the decussation of the fibers, at or just above the nucleus ambiguus.

Bilateral vocal cord paralysis (abductor or midline) is often secondary to a severe CNS disorder but might also be present in an otherwise normal child. It occurs almost as often as unilateral paralysis during the newborn period. Some of the CNS disorders which cause this abnormality are: brainstem hemorrhage, Arnold-Chiari malformations, cerebral meningocele, or extensive cardiovascular malformations. Jackson[19] stated that posterior paralysis is due to pinching of the posterior branch of each recurrent nerve in the cricothyroid joint during delivery. He also noted that recovery of the nerve might take place within 10 days. The neck stretched during delivery and the umbilical cord wrapped around the neck are probably the leading peripheral causes for bilateral paralysis.

Fearon[10] stated that "bilateral abductor paralysis results in almost complete apposition of the vocal cords in the midline, creating a severe airway problem. The breathing in these patients was a very high pitched, stridulous character." Usually the voice is absent, and aspiration is common. Adductor paralysis is very rare, as this usually is of functional or hysterical causes. The patient is aphonic and has no stridor.

Unilateral paralysis (abductor or midline) is a peripheral phenomenon. Causes include: mediastinal cysts, cystic hygromas, cardiomegaly, thyromegaly, mediastinal adenopathy, lead poisoning, viral infections, or diphtheria. Another common cause of unilateral paralysis is stretching of the nerve during delivery. It is more likely to be left-sided and most often is secondary to a cardiovascular abnormality. Right-sided lesions are rare and are sometimes due to CNS disorders. An abnormal voice or cry is the major symptom. Occasionally stridor is evident, and it can be severe enough to cause cyanosis.

Diagnosis for laryngeal nerve paralyses is made by direct laryngoscopic examination. If the stridor and respiratory distress is severe, tracheostomy is advised. Paralysis caused by stretching of the nerves during delivery usually recovers early but might last as long as 9 months to a year. Repair of the cardiovascular malformation or removal of the mediastinal cyst or mass usually leads to rapid recovery of the paralyzed nerve. Arytenoidectomy via laryngofissure is occasionally done if the problem is not resolved.

Myasthenia Gravis. This is a disorder affecting the myoneural junction. Whether there is a block inhibiting acetylcholine from acting on the muscle receptor sites or it is tied up by a relative abundance of cholinesterase, the result is the same. Muscle weakness is the major symptom, and during the neonatal period this is manifested by excessive drooling, aspiration, and a weak or absent cry. Stridor is not a common finding. Farmer[7] described two groups of myasthenics: the neonatal transient group, who are born to myasthenic mothers and have a short, severe course of generalized weakness and dysphagia, and the neonatal persistent group, who have milder symptoms but a much longer course. These children are usually born to nonmyasthenic mothers. The edrophonium chloride (Tensilon) test is not recommended during the newborn period as its duration of action is too short to be useful. Neostigmine (Prostigmin) has a longer activity. A muscle biopsy discloses the presence of lymphorrhages, and antibodies may be found attached to the A-band on the muscle fibers. Endoscopic evaluation would reveal only the flaccidity and pooling of saliva. Treatment consists of prolonged use of cholinesterase inhibitors (i.e., pyridostigmine, neostigmine). Thymectomy has not proved advantageous in the pediatric age group.

Moebius' Syndrome. This disorder is described as a bilateral congenital facial paralysis occasionally coupled with other cranial nerve abnormalities. Weakness of voice, dysphagia, and stridor have been noted.

Supranuclear Lesions. These may also cause stridor and aspiration problems.

Poliomyelitis. Poliomyelitis is seldom seen anymore as immunization programs have controlled this once dreaded disease. Along with paralysis of the major muscle groups, bulbar involvement might ensue, causing paralysis of various cranial nerves. Respiratory distress, usually following weakness of intercostal muscles and the diaphragm is worsened with laryngeal nerve involvement. In these cases a tracheostomy is a necessity, despite using an apparatus such as the almost forgotten Drinker respirator. The prognosis is guarded with bulbar involvement.

Guillain-Barré Syndrome. Also called Guillain-Barré disease, infectious polyneuritis, or acute polyradiculoneuritis, this syndrome is usually described as an ascending paralysis which is self-limiting inasmuch as resolution usually occurs within less than 1 year from the onset. Permanent weakness is not characteristic as it is with poliomyelitis.

This syndrome often follows many other infectious diseases (i.e., infectious mononucleosis, typhoid fever, streptococcal infections, etc.). Changes in the CNS have been described and include chromatolysis of anterior horn cells and motor cranial nerve nuclei.[7] Wallerian degeneration, extending peripherally into the nerves, may occur in severe cases.

The disease usually affects, in centripetal fashion,[7] the extremities, then ascending to include the cranial nerves (VII and XI most commonly, and occasionally V, IX, and X). The paresis is occasionally asymmetrical at first but becomes symmetrical as the disease progresses.

The reason for mentioning this disorder is that there are variants which might attack the cranial nerves first. The ensuing laryngeal paralysis might necessitate a tracheostomy because of paralysis of the laryngeal musculature.

Diagnosis is made by the neurologic examination and by a cerebrospinal fluid (CSF) protein-cell dissociation. The cell count is usually normal, whereas the protein level is markedly elevated reaching a maximum within 10 to 25 days.

Metabolic Disorders

Hypocalcemia. Laryngospasm secondary to hypocalcemia might occur within the first week of life. Associated with rarer laryngeal problems are irritability, muscular twitchings, convulsions, and possible carpopedal spasms.

Hypothyroidism. In the older child hypothyroidism can lead to laryngeal polyps or polypoid thickening along the free margins of the vocal cords. This leads to hoarseness and usually no noticeable stridor. Treatment is directed at control of the thyroid problem and possible laryngoscopic removal of the polypoid tissue.

Benign Tumors

Cysts and Laryngoceles. Laryngeal cysts and laryngoceles should be discussed together as they sometimes have the same appearance during a laryngoscopic examination. Cysts, which represent remnants of the fourth branchial cleft,[2] are usually found in the lateral wall of the supraglottic area although they may protrude into the glottis or up into the aryepiglottic fold.[13] They also are periodically found arising in the vallecula, decreasing the movement of the epiglottis. True cysts are filled with thin, yellow-tinged fluid, although some are filled with thicker material making a diagnostic aspiration impossible.

Laryngoceles are noted to emanate from the laryngeal ventricle, and they might herniate anteriorly through the thyrohyoid membrane or laterally, appearing as a mass in the neck. An important differentiation is that these are air-filled sacs and they increase in size with crying or coughing. Radiologic assistance might be helpful, as occasionally the air-filled space can be noted anterior or lateral to the air passages.

Both cysts and laryngoceles can cause severe obstruction. If the laryngocele is of the internal variety (one which protrudes internally into the glottic lumen and not laterally), stridor can increase markedly with crying or straining. Treatment of cysts and internal laryngoceles are similar as endoscopic aspiration and marsupialization can be curative. The externally appearing laryngoceles should be treated via a lateral neck approach in order to remove as much of the cystic sac as possible. In the differential diagnosis of cystic masses in the neck adjacent to the larynx, one should consider the thyroglossal duct cyst and cystic hygroma.

Papillomas. These growths are benign tumors that constitute the most common neoplasm in children. In this age group they are almost always multiple, occurring in clumps. Most frequently they are found in the region of the anterior commissure, extending over the anterior one-third of the true and false vocal cords. They may be found in any position throughout the tracheobronchial tree, and if a tracheostomy is performed to relieve severe respiratory distress, the stoma may also be filled with papillomas.

These tumors are found in individuals anywhere from the newborn period throughout the preteen and adolescent years, into adulthood.[15] Papillomas are usually solitary in adults, in contrast to those seen in the pediatric age group, where they clump.

The symptoms range from simple hoarseness on one end of the spectrum to airway obstruction of the other. The history is one of gradual progression. The most common mode of therapy is intermittent laryngoscopic procedures with removal of the tumorous tissue using a biting forceps. The general plan for this therapy is that the airway is protected by intermittent surgical procedures until the growth of the papilloma ceases. The reason for cessation of the growth of these tumors is not understood. This usually occurs some time during early puberty. Approximately 50 percent of all laryngeal papillomas occur in children 3 to 16 years of age.

There have been numerous therapeutic programs undertaken, including the use of cryotherapy, laser, alkylating agents, heavy metals, and autogenous vaccines. Despite success in many instances, the safest form of therapy still appears to be surgical removal by an able endoscopist. Microsurgical procedures via suspension laryngoscopy is considered by many to be superior to standard laryngoscopic techniques. There is a feeling that the underlying tissues are cleaner following surgery. It should be noted, however, that since suspension procedures are done with an endotracheal tube in place, the tube should be removed prior to ending the procedure so as to ensure complete removal of the tissue. Standard procedures are done either with an endotracheal tube in place or by the apneic technique.

Hemangiomas. These lesions may be located in the subglottic area, causing moderate to severe obstructive symptoms. They often are firm and might range from white to blue. A clue to the presence of a subglottic hemangioma in a stridorous child is the finding of a similar lesion on the skin. The hemangioma is the most common tumor in children.

They may be present in the airway from the first or second week of life, but it may take 2 to 6 weeks more before symptoms appear. Lateral radiologic views of the neck often show a subglottic narrowing such as is seen with subglottic stenosis, laryngotracheitis (rarely seen in infants under 6 months of age), and other rare tumors, e.g., aberrant thyroid.

Katz and Askin[20] noted that steroid therapy dramatically reduced the size of hemangiomas of the skin during treatment for thrombocytopenia. This study prompted Cohen and Wang[4] to develop a study to evaluate the use of steroids on the head and neck. They used prednisone orally at a dose of 60 mg/sq meter/day, and following resolution of the symptoms (airway distress for laryngeal lesions) the dose was lowered to two-thirds and then one-half every other day.

I successfully treated one child with this disorder, without performing a tracheostomy. The child was 2 months of age when she arrived at the hospital retracting, cyanotic, and aphonic. Intramuscular dexamethasone was given prior to her arrival in the operating room. Her retractions ceased and a slightly hoarse cry was noted. There was no further cyanosis. Direct laryngoscopy without anesthesia was performed, during which a very dense subglottic mass was noted. It was blue and would not permit passage of a 3-mm bronchoscope. Since the respiratory status was stable, I elected to terminate the procedure and continue steroid therapy. The child had no further bouts of respiratory distress, and an endoscopic procedure done 1 week later disclosed an eccentric subglottic airway with no respiratory distress. She remained on intermittent oral therapy (every other day) for 6 months until she was asymptomatic while off the medications. Her chest wall hemangioma showed rapid regression during this period. Her growth rate has remained normal (1 year post therapy).

The most common method of treatment is to perform a tracheostomy and wait for resolution (usually about 2 years). Other forms of therapy include cryotherapy, irradiation,[8] and injection of sclerosing agents. The complications from these methods have led to the wait-and-see attitude (tracheostomy) and the use of steroids.

Screamer's Nodes. Also known as vocal nodules, screamer's nodes are benign elevations of inflammatory tissue occurring in the junction of the anterior and middle one-third of the true or membranous vocal cord. The formation of these lesions is usually from voice abuse. The hyperkinetic child who is always striving to be noticed frequently presents with chronic hoarseness. As voice abuse continues, the nodules may change from their softened erythematous state to a whitish, firm, fibrous mass. Rarely does a child need removal of the nodules, as when the voice abuse lessens there frequently is resolution of the nodules as well as their symptoms. The same is not always true in adults.

The nodules meet in the midline and as noted above are located between the anterior and middle thirds of the vocal cords. They are most easily removed via suspension microlaryngoscopy, where they are dissected free from the underlying submucosal tissue. The classic manner is to strip the mucosal lining along with the nodules from the underlying vocalis muscle along the free margins of the vocal cords. Voice rest for approximately 2 weeks is recommended following surgery.

Aberrant Thyroid Tissue. Such tissue within the subglottic airway or tracheal lumen is extremely rare but must be considered whenever a mass or narrowing is noted. Waggoner[33] grouped masses in this area into two categories: those arising during the pre- or neonatal period that violate the cricotracheal wall and are in continuity with the thyroid gland proper (false aberrant thyroid), and those developing in the embryo from an isolated, misplaced thyroid deposit (true aberrant thyroid). Treatment for each type differs; with the false type the defect through the wall of the airway must be cleared of thyroid tissue and closed, whereas the true type can be removed via endoscopic removal.

Fibromas. Intraluminal fibromas are extremely rare and are removed endoscopically. Neurofibromas may occur in the larynx, as well as elsewhere in Recklinghausen's disease. Treatment is laryngoscopic evaluation and removal.

Malignancies

Rhabdomyosarcomas. These lesions (Fig. 9) occasionally are noted in the region of the base of the tongue or within the glottic area, leading to respiratory distress. Fortunately they are rare. Other tumors that can cause respiratory embarrassment are *chondrosarcoma, fibrosarcoma, and lymphoma.*

Congenital Anomalies

Congenital Webs. According to Ferguson[13] congenital webs are caused by an arrest of development of the larynx at about the tenth week of fetal life. The mechanism is similar to that which produces atresia or subglottic stenosis in that there is a failure of dissolution of the fused lateral masses. Seventy-five percent are at the level of the cords, 12.5 percent are supraglottic, and 12.5 percent are subglottic. Holinger[16] reported these figures from 32 patients with congenital webs.

Webs may range from being thin and almost transparent to thick, fibrous masses. Webs are located anteriorly with a concavity posteriorly. The superior surface of the web is covered by squamous epithelium, and the undersurface with tracheal respiratory mucosa.

Webs might be small enough to be asymptomatic early in life, or they might cause severe stridor if a large enough area within the glottic chink is blocked. The cry may be weak or occasionally hoarse.

Treatment is varied. The thinner webs may be incised and dilatation carried out intermittently every 2 to 3 days until the raw edges are healed. Thicker webs may be able to be incised, dilated, or both. Stenting is used occasionally.

Atresia of the Airway. This refers to complete obstruction and is incompatible with life unless it is immediately recognized. The infant attempts to breathe, but the total obstruction causes deepening cyanosis and finally death. Although the cases are extremely rare, there have been reports of infants with true atresia being saved when early, lifesaving measures were undertaken. Holinger[16] noted one infant who was brought to his attention following an emergency tracheostomy performed a few minutes after delivery. This child was later found to have a total laryngeal occlusion. Fortunately a newborn has enough oxygen from the placental blood supply to maintain cerebral oxygenation for 4 to 5 minutes. Either breaking through a membranous atresia with a blade or bronchoscope or performing a tracheostomy are the only measures for saving a child with this malady.

Congenital and Acquired Subglottic Stenosis. The extent of the narrowing determines the severity of the symptoms. The stenosis is either cartilagenous or membran-

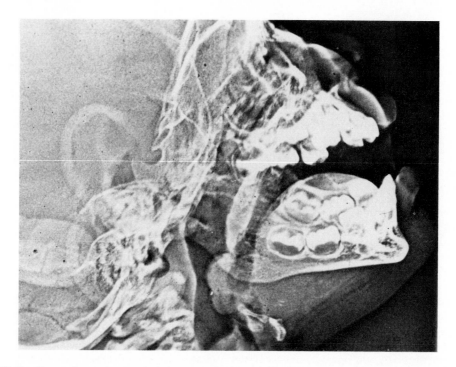

FIG. 9. Xeroradiograph of a rhabdomyosarcoma of the base of the tongue. The patient was noted to have audible inspiratory stridor and drooling.

ous, but one should be aware that other forms of soft-tissue masses might also be present (i.e., aberrant thyroid, hemangioma, fibroma).

The congenital stenoses usually are secondary to maldevelopment of the cricoid cartilage or of the conus elasticus. The conus is usually widest in the immediate subglottic area, but with abnormal development of this structure the narrowing might be evident as close as 2 mm from the undersurface of the true vocal cords. Occasionally a deformed cricoid cartilage is noted projecting into the subglottic lumen.[12] One case is brought to mind where a bronchoscope was passed through an extremely narrow subglottic airway, at which time a crescent wedge of cartilage was noted within the scope as it was passed into the upper trachea. Subsequent dilatations were much easier following that incident.

These children usually have stridor from birth, although at times it is not loud enough to be worrisome to the parent or the pediatrician. A history of recurrent bouts of croup in a child less than 6 to 9 months of age is common in this disorder. The stridor might be present only after or during an upper respiratory infection. As the repeated bouts of "croup" continue,

the severity of stridor increases. The voice is usually normal and strong.

Other laryngeal anomalies have been noted in children with this disorder, including complete absence of the epiglottitis or a congenitally small larynx. A subglottic area of 4 mm or less is abnormal and consequently dangerous.

Approximately one-half of the cases can be treated by intermittent endoscopic dilatations without a tracheostomy tube in place. The dilatations are gently done with several sizes of bronchoscopes or metal dilators at varying intervals of time. The other half have severe enough stridor to necessitate tracheostomy. Fearon[8] noted a high mortality rate (25 percent) in children with tracheostomies cared for at home. This has not been the experience among otolaryngologists associated with the University of Southern California. Fearon recommends an open operation with interposition of a portion of the thyroid cartilage to augment the cricoid ring. His results are reported as excellent. Some laryngologists advocate the use of a stent, which is in actuality a T-tube with the vertical limb through the tracheostome.

Acquired subglottic and tracheal stenosis following prolonged intubation (Fig. 10) leads me to believe that stenting be used in only carefully selected cases which have been refractive to other forms of treatment. Stenoses have been noted after as few as 5 to 7 days of intubation, despite the use of the newer softer plastic endotracheal tubes. The severity of the acquired stenoses in general is more severe in the infant than in the older child.

Laryngeal Cleft. This laryngotracheoesophageal cleft is caused by a failure of the dorsal fusion of the cricoid lamina so that the cleft can extend downward for quite some distance. As noted by Atkins[1] the cleft might run as far as the carina or just above. This has been called an esophagotrachea by many authors.

The extent of the cleft determines the severity of the symptoms. At times clefts have been noted to extend just through the interarytenoid area or also through the posterior portion of the cricoid. This child would of course be much less symptomatic than a child with the complete or common esophagotrachea. Cyanosis and aspiration of secretions or with feeding is common for all these infants. Of course it would be much more evident in the child with a common channel. The cry is usually weak or possibly absent.

The evaluation cannot be made adequately without endoscopy. X-rays might appear as an H-type tracheoesophageal fistula. Direct laryngoscopy may not determine the true defect if it is done in the hands of an inexperienced endoscopist. A laryngeal cleft can be missed if it is incomplete. Observation of the posterior commissure is mandatory during the procedure.

Shapiro and Falla[30] reported an 8-month-old infant with a cleft in whom the diagnosis was made by retrograde esophagoscopy via a gastrostomy. Numerous laryngoscopic examinations failed to describe the defect. Surgical repair was successfully performed through a lateral pharyngotomy incision.

Laryngomalacia. This is a term coined by Jackson[19] to describe a condition in which there is retardation of the normal development of cartilage. It does not describe a pathologic disorder. It is a self-limiting condition, which with further growth and increasing rigidity of the laryngeal framework becomes resolved.

Atkins[1] and other authors call this phenomenon congenital laryngeal stridor; Atkins notes that it is actually a symptom complex characterized by noisy breathing associated with greater or lesser degrees of respiratory

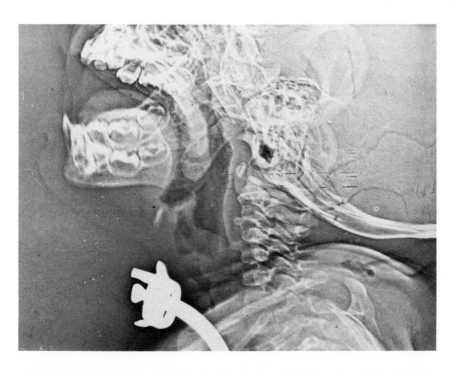

FIG. 10. Subglottic and upper tracheal stenosis following prolonged intubation.

obstruction. Occasionally, because of the generalized sternal retractions and intermittent respiratory distress, the infant fails to thrive.

The symptoms and signs are those of inspiratory stridor and a fluttering, crowlike cry. True respiratory embarrassment such as cyanosis is usually absent. The child can feed normally, although he might be stridorous. Frequently the sounds disappear while in a prone position and may be louder while lying supine.

The symptoms are caused by excessive folding of the omega-shaped epiglottis with shortening of the aryepiglottic folds. There is also some degree of flabbiness of the mesenchymal tissue of the larynx—thus the term laryngomalacia. The treatment consists of watchful waiting; only rarely is a tracheostomy needed. Fearon recently eliminated the need for a tracheostomy in one patient by suturing the epiglottis to the base of the tongue after removing the adjacent mucosa.[10]

Craniofacial Abnormalities. This constitutes a large group of varied congenital disorders. *Pierre Robin syndrome* most commonly is associated with respiratory distress. These children have micrognathia, a cleft palate, and glossoptosis. The third finding is one in which there is posterior displacement of the tongue and subsequent blockage of the pharyngeal airway. These patients present with episodic respiratory distress with cyanosis and then recovery. The child might be stable between attacks until a subsequent episode perhaps causes death. Treatment consists of attempts at careful oral feedings and close observation. Rickham and Johnston[28] described a special cradle in which the child can be placed face down, allowing the tongue to fall forward. They note that within 2 to 3 months there is sufficient growth of the mandible and training of the infant to breathe and feed properly to allow the child to pass out of the danger period. Occasionally a tracheostomy or possibly suturing of the tongue to the lower lip are recommended.

The only other abnormality which should be discussed in some detail is choanal atresia. There is a strong familial tendency with this disorder. Ferguson[13] notes that about 50 percent of the infants with choanal atresia have other, often more serious anomalies. The most important point is that the physician should entertain a high index of suspicion. A newborn who is struggling to breathe should be examined carefully to rule out bilateral obstruction of the posterior nasal choanae. It should be noted that infants are obligatory nasal breathers. They learn mouth breathing weeks or months later. If improvement of the respiratory status following opening of the mouth is noted, a presumptive diagnosis can be made. One should be aware that elevation of the mandible can improve the respirations in a child with severe laryngomalacia. The examiner should carefully attempt to pass plastic or rubber catheters through the nasal cavity into the naso- and then the oropharynx. Beinfield[3] noted that if a metal probe cannot be passed beyond 32 mm from the edge of the nostril, atresia is present. If it is passed 44 mm or more, patency is apparent. Other methods of diagnosis are x-rays with instillation of Lipiodol into the nasal cavity, or clinically by just dripping a small amount of methylene blue into the nose and observing for possible passage into the pharynx. It is advisable to obtain roentgenograms prior to attempting surgery. There are numerous procedures for opening the posterior choanae. It should be noted whether the atresia is membranous (10 percent) or bony (90 percent). An attempt at perforation with the placement of a catheter might be all that is necessary at first, following placement of an adequate oral airway. Emergency surgery is not necessary in this disorder. Intranasal or transpalatine procedures can be done following improvement in the infant's overall status.

Other conditions such as *complete nasal absence, partial absence,* and *duplication of the nasal septum* can also cause severe respiratory distress.

Foreign Bodies

An extremely important point to remember is that stridor need not be associated with an infectious state or anomaly. Foreign bodies of the larynx and hypopharynx may cause severe respiratory embarrassment. The material might be organic or inert. X-rays might be helpful (Figs. 11 and 12), although if a child is in severe respiratory distress the most logical approach would be to perform emergency endoscopy, rather than risking his life awaiting the taking and processing of films.

Suspicion of a foreign body being present

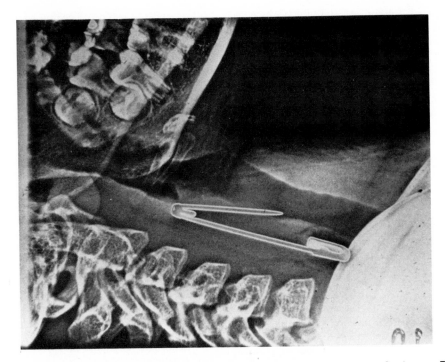

FIG. 11. Lateral view of an open safety pin in the hypopharynx and upper esophagus. This retarded child had dysphagia, mild stridor, and an elevated temperature.

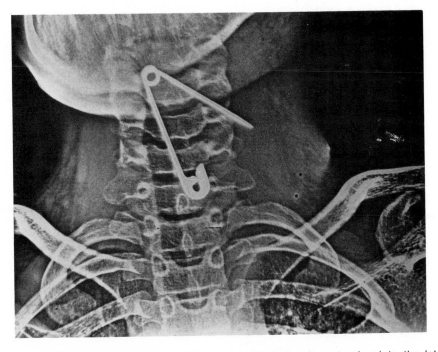

FIG. 12. Anteroposterior view of a foreign body, disclosing its extension into the lateral pharyngeal wall. There is an associated abscess.

would be most helpful, but frequently the child is already on the operating table when the foreign material is noted during the course of a diagnostic endoscopic procedure. Therefore varied sizes of grasping forceps should be readily available at the time the larynx is being examined. Fortunately most of the larger foreign bodies become lodged in the region of the cricopharyngeus or the upper esophagus.

Case Report. *A 5-month-old child was brought to the emergency room with a short history of severe respiratory distress. No infectious history was obtained, and the child was afebrile. He was retracting severely and was tired and pale. The stridor was noted to be to and fro in nature. X-rays were obtained by a pediatrician and disclosed a subglottic narrowing. The child was given 4 mg dexamethasone (Decadron) intramuscularly and one minum of 1:1000 epinephrine subcutaneously. The results were negligible. The child's breathing was still rapid, shallow, and noisy; and he continued to look very tired. Otolaryngologic consultation was obtained, and the child was immediately taken to the operating room. He was positioned on the operating table with an anesthesiologist standing by, giving oxygen by mask. A laryngoscope was then passed into the oropharynx, when the entire hypopharynx became black. The light was checked and was working. Then a tip of the epiglottis was noted. The black area was actually a large plastic refrigerator knob; because available instruments were too small and the "finger" too large, a tonsil snare was used to remove it. The upper portion of the knob measured 1.25 inches with a narrower portion beneath. The child made an uneventful recovery.*

Allergy

Pang[26] stated that "allergy of the larynx occurs in two forms, the acute or anaphylactic and the chronic." Angioneurotic edema is the disorder caused by the acute form. This phenomenon can occur anywhere from the lips to the larynx. It develops in tissue which has a loose areolar base, and the subsequent swelling occurs at a rather rapid rate. It is easy to diagnose swelling of the tongue, lips, or uvula. When the condition involves the larynx, however, the developing symptoms are of extreme importance in making the diagnosis. Because of the propensity for the tissues of the epiglottis, arytenoids, aryepiglottic folds, and the true and false vocal cords to become edematous following any insult (i.e., infections, local trauma, allergy), the airway can quickly become obstructed.

The allergic reaction can be caused by a myriad of allergens, e.g., foods, insect stings, inhalants, antibiotics. Treatment is aimed at rapid recognition of the problem and institution of medical therapy, which consists of subcutaneous injections of Adrenalin, intramuscular or intravenous corticosteroids (i.e., Solu-Cortef or Decadron), and antihistamines. Occasional the use of IPPB treatments with a bronchodilator in the nebulizer is helpful.

I have never witnessed a severe reaction in a child, although I have treated adults with this condition. These cases represent a spectrum from mild to moderate laryngitis, to severe laryngeal obstruction.

Case Report. *A 66-year-old female was brought to the hospital because of an acute onset of wheezing. She had no history of asthma or emphysema. Despite institution of a subcutaneous Adrenalin series, to-and-fro stridor appeared, and she then developed severe respiratory distress. Indirect laryngoscopy was attempted following a request for otolaryngologic assistance. She became very agitated and collapsed. A direct laryngoscopic examination disclosed massive hypopharyngeal and laryngeal edema. A bronchoscope was inserted just as she became apneic. A tracheostomy followed successful resuscitative measures. The patient began to show gradual resolution over a period of 48 to 72 hours following institution of a corticosteroid program. The etiology of this allergic reaction remained unknown.*

The chronic type refers to repeated bouts of laryngeal edema in an allergic individual. It should also be noted that hypothyroidism can cause a low-grade edematous state. Treatment for the chronic type is the same as the acute form except that a concentrated effort to search for the allergen (i.e., skin testing) should be carried out. A curative desensitization program should follow.

Trauma

Trauma can be grouped into three categories: blunt trauma, that which occurs after prolonged intubation, and that caused by faulty instrumentation. The latter was discussed under complications.

Blunt Trauma. This refers to any force which when applied to the anterior neck causes damage of varying degrees. Shumrick reported that "after intracranial injuries, obstructive damage of the airway is the second most common cause of death associated with trauma of the head and neck."[31] He also noted that the three most common symptoms are subcutaneous emphysema, aphonia, and persistent pain. The emphysema is noted by feeling crepitus while palpating the skin. Frequently there is swelling of the face, neck, and chest. If the air dissects into the mediastinum and pericardial tissues, cardiac tamponade might occur. With flattening of the thyroid cartilage following a fracture, the vocal cords may be drawn laterally, thus causing aphonia. Pennington[27] noted that in his series a vertical midline fracture of the thyroid cartilage was the most common site of injury in the larynx. Next were posterior displacement of the base of the epiglottis and rupture of the thyroepiglottic ligament, and tears and abrasions of the true and false cords. The resulting hematoma might cause respiratory embarrassment. Shumrick[31] noted that pain without the other symptoms should be evaluated further, as it might be a subtle sign of a fracture.

Other diagnostic aids include roentgenograms (plain views of the neck, xeroradio-graphs, or laryngograms) and indirect and direct laryngoscopy. Treatment might include an ironing-out of the fracture segments with a bronchoscope, performing an open reduction and possibly insertion of a stent. Strong consideration must be made regarding extremely close observation versus tracheostomy.

Prolonged Intubation. The complications secondary to prolonged intubation or intubation with an oversized tube are not uncommon. Inflammatory changes have been noted in the laryngeal and tracheal mucosa within as little as 18 to 24 hours. There are reports of 3 to 6 months of intubation in newborns with no respiratory difficulty noted at or following the time of extubation. There are also reports and personal observations which show definite subglottic and tracheal narrowing following 4 to 5 days of intubation with the same type of soft, "nonreactive" tube and under the same conditions. Because of these varying findings we feel that there is no rule of thumb concerning when to extubate an infant in favor of a tracheostomy. I do feel, however, that if a child must be intubated over 1 to 2 weeks and a long period of intubation is anticipated, and if he is over 1,500 g, a tracheostomy should be performed.

Scott[29] at Childrens Hospital of Los Angeles recently compared the external diameter of the

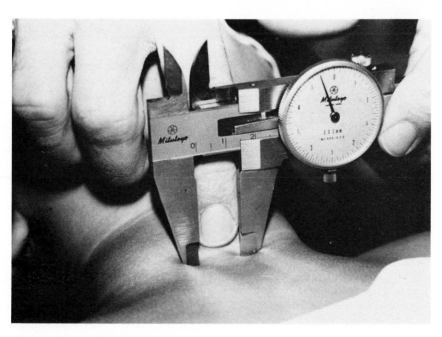

FIG. 13. Measuring the external diameter of the lower border of the cricoid cartilage. (Courtesy of E. Scott)

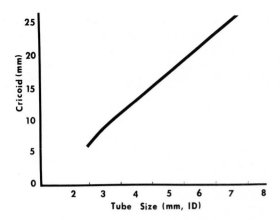

FIG. 14. Comparison between the external diameter of the cricoid and the internal diameter of the selected endotracheal tube, based on 100 patients. (Courtesy of E. Scott)

lower border of the cricoid cartilage (Fig. 13) with the recommended size of endotracheal tube. Figure 14 is a graph presented as a possible guide to selecting the proper sized endotracheal tube. Also included are formulas used at the same institution, which were also developed as aids for estimating sizes of endotracheal tubes as compared to the age of the patient (Tables 1 and 2).

TABLE 1. Comparative Diameter of Endotracheal Tubes

Metric, ID (mm)	French, OD
2.5	12
3.0	14
3.5	16
4.0	18
4.5	20
5.0	22
5.5	24
6.0	26

The type of injury from prolonged intubation can be quite varied. Laryngeal webs or granulomas are occasionally noted. The cry is often somewhat lower-pitched or at times almost nonexistent. Subglottic stenosis with or without a tracheal narrowing is probably more common than might be expected. Often a child is stridorous while crying, and normal at rest.

TABLE 2. Formulas for Estimating Sizes of Pediatric Endotracheal Tubes According to Patient's Age

Age	Metric, ID (mm)	French, OD
Premature	2.5–3.0	12–14
Newborn	3.0–3.5	14–16
One year and older	$\dfrac{16 + \text{age in years}}{4}$	18 + age in years

There might also be a change in the character of the voice.

In our hands the treatment is endoscopic. The stenosis is usually mild in nature, but because of the small size of the infant's airway it might take 6 months or longer until the problem is safely resolved. If the child's condition was severe enough for him to be tracheotomized, the course might be slightly longer because of the severity of the problem and because there might be a slight depression of the tracheal ring just above the tracheostomy. This might cause continuing stridor following removal of the tracheostomy tube if the size of the trachea has not increased sufficiently during the normal growth process.

Inability to move a vocal cord following injury to the arytenoid might present a different type of problem. Arytenoidectomy following a laryngofissure might be the procedure of choice.

REFERENCES

1. Atkins JP: Laryngeal problems of infancy and childhood. Pediatr Clin North Am 9:1125, 1962
2. Ballenger JJ: Diseases of the Nose, Throat and Ear. Philadelphia, Lea & Febiger, 1969
3. Beinfield HH: Bilateral choanal atresia in the newborn. Arch Otolaryngol 73:659, 1961
4. Cohen SR, Wang C: Steroid treatment of hemangioma of the head and neck in children. Ann Otol Rhinol Laryngol 81:584, 1972
5. Davison FW: Acute laryngotracheal infections in children. Otolaryngol Clin North Am June:69, 1968
6. Downs JJ, Striker TW, Stool S: Complications of nasotracheal intubation in children (letter to the editor). N Engl J Med 274:226, 1966
7. Farmer TW: Pediatric Neurology. New York, Harper & Row, 1964
8. Fearon B: Acute airway obstruction. In Disorders of the Respiratory Tract in Children.

Vol 2: Pediatric Otolaryngology, Philadelphia, Saunders, 1972, p 1213

9. Fearon B: Acute laryngotracheobronchitis in infancy and childhood. Pediatr Clin North Am 9:1095, 1962

10. Fearon B: Respiratory distress in the newborn. Otolaryngol Clin North Am June:147, 1968

11. Fearon B, Cotton R: Surgical correction of subglottic stenosis of the larynx. Ann Otolaryngol Rhinol Laryngol 81:508, 1972

12. Ferguson CF: Congenital abnormalities of the infant larynx. Otolaryngol Clin North Am 3:185, 1970

13. Ferguson GF: Congenital choanal atresia. In Disorders of the Respiratory Tract in Children. Vol 2: Pediatric Otolaryngology, Philadelphia, Saunders, 1972, pp 1002, 1213, 1169

14. Fitz-Hugh GS, Powel JB II: Acute traumatic injuries of the oropharynx, laryngopharynx, and cervical trachea in children. Otolaryngol Clin North Am 3:375, 1970

15. Holinger PH: Benign tumors of the trachea and bronchi. Otolaryngol Clin North Am June:219, 1968

16. Holinger PH, Brown WT: Congenital webs, cysts, laryngoceles and other anomalies of the larynx. Ann Otol Rhinol Laryngol 76:744, 1967

17. Holinger PH, Schild JA, Weprin L: Pediatric laryngology. Otolaryngol Clin North Am 3: 625, 1970

18. Hollingshead WH: Anatomy for Surgeons. Vol I: The Head and Neck. New York, Harper & Row, 1966

19. Jackson C, Jackson CL: Bronchoesophagology. New York, Saunders, 1950

20. Katz HP, Askin J: Multiple hemangiomata with thrombopenia. Am J Dis Child 115:351, 1968

21. Miller AH: Acute epiglottitis. Trans Am Acad Ophthalmol Otolaryngol 53:519, 1949

22. Miller AH: Hemophilus influenzae type B epiglottitis or supraglottic laryngitis in children. Laryngoscope 58:514, 1948

23. Mills IC: Clinical Aspects of Adrenal Function. Philadelphia, Davis, 1964

24. Moffitt OP Jr: Treatment of laryngeal papillomatosis with bovine wart vaccine. Laryngoscope 69:1421, 1959

25. Ogura JH, Biller HF: Reconstruction of the larynx following blunt trauma. Ann Otol 80: 492, 1971

26. Pang LQ: Allergy of the larynx, trachea and bronchial tree. Otolaryngol Clin North Am 7:719, 1974

27. Pennington CL: External trauma of the larynx and trachea: immediate treatment and management. Ann Otol Rhinol Laryngol 81:546, 1972

28. Rickham PP, Johnston JH: Neonatal Surgery. New York, Appleton-Century-Crofts, 1969, p 137

29. Scott E: Unpublished data, personal communication, 1975

30. Shapiro JJ, Falla A: Congenital posterior cleft of larynx. Ann Otol Rhinol Laryngol 75:961, 1966

31. Shumrick DA: Traumatic injuries of the upper respiratory tract. Otolaryngol Clin North Am June:403, 1969

32. Snow JB Jr, Rogers KA: Bilateral abductor paralysis of vocal cords secondary to Arnold-Chiari malformations and its management. Laryngoscope 25:316, 1965

33. Waggoner L: Intralaryngeal intratracheal thyroid. Ann Otol Rhinol Laryngol 67:61, 1958

34. Zobell DH: Massive neurofibroma of the larynx. Laryngoscope 74:233, 1964

48

Maxillary Sinoscopy

Peter Illum

Despite the fact that endoscopic examination of the maxillary sinus has been carried out since the beginning of the present century, there were only sporadic reports regarding the method until approximately 1950. In 1902 Reichert[18] and Hirschmann[10] used the newly discovered Nitze cystoscope for sinoscopy, introducing the endoscope through a dental alveolus. The method was later simplified by using a straight trocar introduced under local anesthesia into the maxillary sinus via the canine fossa[4] or via the inferior meatus of the nose in the same manner as is used for ordinary antral puncture.[15,21,22]

During the last 20 years the method has been reintroduced and the technique refined by many authors in Germany and Austria.[3,7,8,11,17,19,20,24] The sinoscopic picture in various diseases has been shown in colored drawings[3,5,10] and color photographs.[12,25]

Knowledge of the usefulness of the endoscopic examination in the maxillary sinus (sinoscopy) has never been widely disseminated. Since it is a simple examination and permits a direct view of the antral mucosa, it is a valuable supplement to the conventional methods of examination in paranasal sinus disease. Sinoscopy gives fairly exact information on the type and degree of pathologic changes in the sinus, thus permitting the correct method of treatment to be chosen with greater certainty than when relying on examination of the nasal cavity, x-rays, and antral puncture alone.

slightly more inconvenient for the patient than an ordinary antral puncture. During routine treatment of maxillary sinusitis with intubation using a short, split polyethylene tube we normally use a thick cannula, and it has been quite natural in all cases to inspect the mucosa. In this way considerable skill in the technique can be obtained. Sinoscopy, however, is somewhat more time-consuming in comparison to antral puncture, and it cannot be said to be indicated in all cases of maxillary sinus disease.

The indications for sinoscopy were discussed in particular by Pihrt,[17] Timm,[25] and Hütten.[11] A number of other situations in which sinoscopy is useful can be added to their lists:

1. No clinical symptoms but a positive x-ray examination
2. Clinical symptoms and negative x-ray examination
3. Roentgenologic, circumscribed changes in the maxillary sinus
4. Complete blurring of the maxillary sinus on the x-ray pictures
5. Sinus involvement in dentogenic infections
6. Malignant tumors of the palate, nose, or paranasal sinuses
7. Fresh fractures of the maxilla, especially the "blow-out fracture" of the floor of the orbit
8. For postoperative control after Caldwell-Luc operation
9. Patients previously subjected to maxillary sinus resection who are still having symptoms
10. Uncharacteristic facial pain, particularly in the second branch of the trigeminal nerve
11. Foreign bodies in the maxillary sinus

INDICATIONS FOR SINOSCOPY

There are no actual contraindications to sinoscopy in patients over 5 years of age, and the examination, at least in adults, is only

EQUIPMENT

The Storz equipment used (Fig. 1) includes a cannula (diameter 4.6 mm) and a trocar; we also use a Hopkins optic with a diameter of 4.4

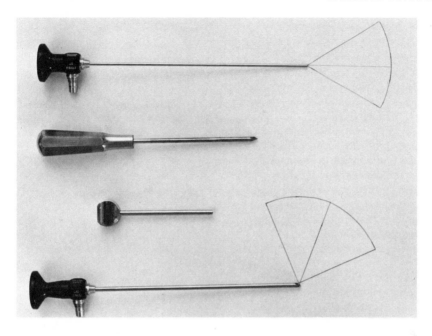

FIG. 1. The 70-degree (lateral) and 0-degree (straightforward) Hopkins telescope and trocar with cannula.

mm with a 70-degree (lateral) direction of view, the wide angle facilitating orientation. The equipment can be supplemented with a Hopkins miniature optic with a 2.7 mm diameter and a field of vision around the axis of 60 degrees. In addition, there is an external light source with a fiberoptic cable and photographic equipment, including an electronic flash generator (Fig. 2). The development of fiberoptic light and not least the Hopkins rod-

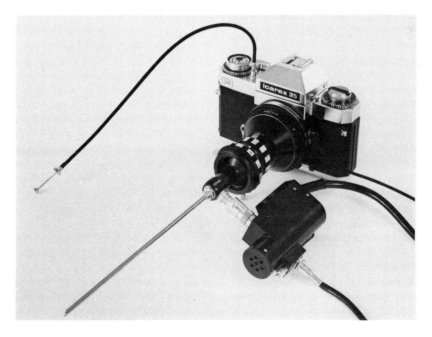

FIG. 2. Hopkins lateral telescope attached to a flash tube (in plastic cover) and a 35-mm still camera.

lens optics have been of vital importance in making the method simple, also permitting good color pictures to be taken for documentation and teaching.

TECHNIQUE

In adults sinoscopy can be performed under local anesthesia and applied in the usual manner below the inferior turbinate, as with the normal antral puncture. In order to ensure a clear view of the sinus, it is important to apply a local anesthetic containing a vasoconstrictor, going in below the middle turbinate near the ostium of the sinus; this reduces bleeding into the sinus after the puncture.

Premedication can be helpful in nervous adults, and general anesthesia may be necessary in cases of severe septal deformity or abnormal thickness of the medial wall of the sinus; it is always necessary in children. Sinoscopy should not be performed on small children owing to the small size of the sinus in relation to the diameter of the cannula.

The sinus is punctured with the cannula in the same manner as with a normal antral puncture. It is important that the cannula be introduced as far forward as possible into the inferior meatus, as the point of the optic is then situated in the middle of the sinus. Any secretion present can be removed by suction for bacteriologic examination without contamination from the nasal flora following removal of the trocar.

The sinoscope can now be introduced and the sinus inspected, while the optic is rotated and at the same time moved around in order to obtain the best possible view. It has been demonstrated in model studies that it is possible to obtain a view of all parts of the sinus with the exception of a small circular area of the lateral wall opposite the site of puncture.[12] This area (Fig. 3), which is the only site from which a biopsy can be obtained with the existing equipment, can be easily seen with the straightforward optic.

The photographic equipment can thereafter be attached to the optic. The mucosa can be seen through the reflex camera while the photograph is taken. Hellmich and Herberhold[8] recommend that the camera be mounted on a flexible teaching attachment, which simplifies manipulation of the equipment. However, this

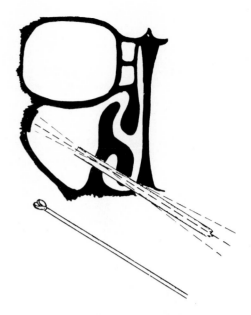

FIG. 3. The limited area on the lateral wall of the sinus from which a biopsy can be taken is the only place that cannot be inspected with the 70-degree optic. The straight optic can more than compensate for this, however.

considerably reduces the quality of the pictures.

If desired it is then possible to remove a tissue sample from the lateral wall of the sinus by means of a fine cup biopsy forceps. The value of histologic examination of this sample is discussed later.

In cases where there is secretion in the sinus we insert a small, split, polyethylene tube (Fig. 4). This is cut within the vestibule and is used for daily lavage of the sinus.

TECHNICAL DIFFICULTIES

Introduction of the rather thick cannula into the sinus seldom entails much more inconvenience to the patient than an ordinary antral puncture. As the examination takes somewhat more time than antral puncture, however, it is sometimes necessary to use general anesthesia in extremely nervous or senile patients. General anesthesia is also preferred in children. (Adenotomy, tonsillectomy, and/or paracentesis are frequently indicated at the same time.) In approximately 3 percent of the cases it is impossible to carry out the procedure owing to pronounced deviation of the septum or a

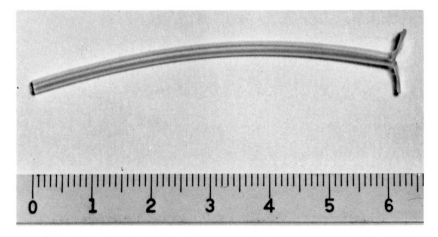

FIG. 4. A split polyethylene tube is used for insertion through the cannula for daily lavage in cases of sinusitis.

very thick osseous wall between the sinus and inferior turbinates. In such cases the introduction might be effected through the canine fossa.

A clear view of the sinus is frequently difficult to obtain owing to the presence of hemorrhage from the site of the puncture. As mentioned, application of a vasoconstrictor around the ostium of the medial turbinate considerably reduces this impediment, and with repeated suction or lavage using physiologic saline a clear view can usually be obtained. However, in approximately 5 percent of the cases it is impossible to obtain a good view. Similarly a clear view is also prevented by secretions or fluid from a cyst; these, however, can be removed by suction or lavage in nearly all the cases.

In 3 to 4 percent of the cases a view of the maxillary mucous membrane is obscured owing to the fact that the lens is positioned in close contact to the tissue. Perforation of the wall as far forward as possible in the inferior meatus ensures that the point of the optic is situated in the middle of the sinus lumen. Introduction further back can result in the point ending up under the mucosa of the medial wall. A very pronounced hyperplasia of the mucosa which fills the lumen similarly spoils the view. Palpation using the point of the endoscope permits an impression to be gained concerning the thickness of the mucosa, and by means of repeated suction it is usually possible to decide whether it is thickening of the mucosa or hemorrhage that is obscuring the view. In a few patients the point of the endoscope lies in

tumor tissue, and a biopsy should always be taken if a clear view cannot be obtained.

In a single case where the maxillary sinus was unusually flat, the author perforated the posterior wall of the sinus into the parapharyngeal space, but this did not produce any inconvenience to the patient. No other authors have mentioned such a complication.

ENDOSCOPIC APPEARANCE OF THE MAXILLARY SINUS

Normal Maxillary Sinus

The mucosa of the normal maxillary sinus (Fig. 5, Plate I)* is very thin and pellucid, and the yellow of the underlying bone can be clearly recognized. The fine blood vessels are easily seen. Upward and medially the ostium of the sinus can frequently be observed, and in some cases the accessory ostium as well. This region is more easily seen when the percanine puncture is used.[7,25] Posteriorly in the sinus is a depressed bluish area. This is the thin wall between the maxillary sinus and one of the posterior ethmoidal cellulae.

Sinusitis

In cases of acute maxillary sinusitis the mucosa is bright red and moderately swollen, with indistinct and dilated blood vessels and larger

All color plates appear at the front of the book.

or smaller amounts of mucopus. A special form is sinusitis maxillaris sicca,[24,25] which can be distinguished from the other forms by the bright red mucosa that is quite dry with no fresh secretion. This condition cannot be demonstrated by x-ray examination or antral puncture. The appearance is often marked by diffuse edema and slightly reddish mucosa. The larger blood vessels are dilated and dark. This picture is found with a catarrhal infection of the sinus;[2] however, it is presumed to be seen also in cases of acute sinusitis during healing.[25]

Chronic maxillary sinusitis usually gives a very mixed sinoscopic picture (Fig. 6, Plate I). The mucosa is swollen; in some areas it is edematous or polypoid and in others fibrotic. Small cysts are often seen, and large amounts of mucopus are frequently present. Special attention should be drawn to the region of the ostium, which is only seldom open (Fig. 7).

Other Diffuse Changes

In cases of hay fever or vasomotor rhinitis the mucosa is moderately swollen and covered with small pale, edematous papules with a "peachlike" appearance (Fig. 8, Plate I). The blood vessels cannot be seen.

In some cases the sinus can be more or less completely filled by large pale polyps having an appearance similar to that of nasal polyps

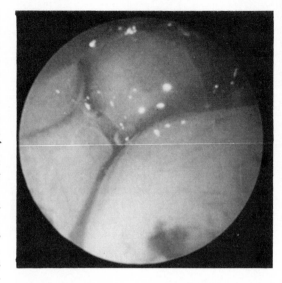

FIG. 9. Marked polyposis in the right sinus caused by prolonged nonseasonal allergy.

(Fig. 9). If infection has taken place also, the color is more or less reddish and mucopus is present. However, an allergic genesis should also be suspected.

Circumscribed Changes

A localized swelling on the x-rays of the maxillary sinus, often in the bottom of the sinus, is a frequent finding. The differential diagnosis can be established only by sinoscopy or exploration of the sinus.

A mucosal cyst apears yellowish, pellucid, and with smooth walls (Fig. 10, Plate I). The remaining mucosa is normal. These cysts are often of considerable size, and it is sometimes found that the sinoscope is positioned within the cyst. After evacuation by suction the membrane of the cyst collapses and a clear view of the sinus can be obtained. In other cases the cyst can be torn apart with the biopsy forceps, causing it to disappear. Occasionally quite small white or yellow cysts are present, which are called "intramural abscesses" in the literature. However, on histologic examination they are found to contain crystals of cholesterol.[12,19]

A solitary simple polyp is easily distinguished from a cyst as it appears similar to a nasal polyp, being grayish and semipellucid. A periapical dental infection, early in its course, frequently causes considerable localized edema in the bottom of the sinus (Fig. 11, Plate I).

Solid benign tumours are sometimes seen

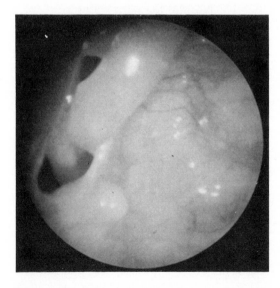

FIG. 7. The ostial region in a mild case of chronic left-sided sinusitis. Mucopus is passing through the open ostium. The lower border of the middle turbinate can be seen.

through the sinoscope. They are not semipellucid and are covered by normal mucosa (Fig. 12, Plate I). They are frequently so large that the cannula enters the tumor, thus preventing inspection. However, the biopsy obtained by endoscopy provides the histologic diagnosis.

Malignant Tumors

The sinoscopic appearance varies considerably in cases of malignancy, and the tumor is usually so large before the patient is referred to the specialist that the diagnosis can easily be made by x-ray examination; the histologic type can often be confirmed from a biopsy taken from a more accessible site than the maxillary sinus. The possibility of diagnosing a small tumor confined to the maxillary sinus, however, must be emphasized.

In cases of widespread tumor in the palate, nose, or paranasal sinuses sinoscopy can also be helpful as a supplement to clinical examination and tomography in establishing the extent of the tumor; this is useful information when planning the operation or deciding on the size of the field to be irradiated. During follow-up sinoscopy can be useful in disclosing early relapse. There is, however, a limitation to the usefulness of the method as biopsies can be obtained only from the posterior and lateral walls of the sinus. Development of an optical flexible biopsy forceps would greatly increase the value of sinoscopy in these cases.

Various Rare Conditions

Herpes zoster in the second branch of the trigeminal nerve gives typical elements in the maxillary sinus. Manifestations of diphtheritis and various types of tuberculous manifestations have been described in the older literature. Ectopic teeth can be found in the sinus (Fig. 13). The presence of foreign bodies, which can be teeth dislocated through the alveoli, glass splinters arising from a traffic accident, or forgotten tampons from an earlier operation, have also been described in the maxillary sinuses.

SINOSCOPY IN FRACTURES OF THE MAXILLA

In cases of fractures of the maxilla an exact picture of the fracture line is rarely possible

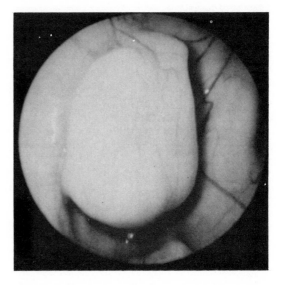

FIG. 13. An ectopic tooth covered by a thin mucous membrane situated in the lower part of the sinus.

from conventional x-ray films, and as there is often massive blurring of the sinuses tomography is rarely of any aid. In such cases sinoscopy can be helpful in finding the exact course of the fracture lines after removal of the blood by suction, thus making the choice of the method for fixation far easier. In those rare cases of a blowout fracture of the bottom of the orbital cavity the diagnosis is extremely important and without the help of sinoscopy very difficult.[23]

Sequelae after an earlier maxillary fracture can be observed sinoscopically as sharp projections of bony spicules covered by a normal mucosal membrane (Fig. 14). These patients may complain of facial pain in the second branch of the trigeminal nerve.

SINOSCOPY AND X-RAY EXAMINATION OF THE PARANASAL SINUSES

The results of sinoscopy and x-ray examination of the maxillary sinuses were compared by Illum et al.[13] In the majority of cases sinoscopy gave better differential diagnostic information than x-rays on the type and degree of changes in the sinus; in fact, quite often the x-ray diagnosis was either incorrect or insufficient. In a few cases sinoscopy showed completely normal conditions in the sinus despite distinct blurring of the x-ray film. The presence or absence

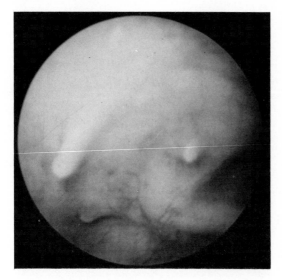

FIG. 14. Left sinus; sequelae after a previous fracture of the maxilla in a patient with facial pain. Several small bony spicules are seen.

of secretion was more precisely diagnosed by sinoscopy. However, in cases where a very slight diffuse swelling of the mucosa was present, the x-ray examination is more precise than sinoscopy, as this condition is very difficult to diagnose sinoscopically.

One often must treat patients who show a radiologic blurring of the sinus but whose clinical symptoms are absent or atypical. Following x-ray examination of 400 healthy subjects, Fascenelli[6] found radiologic abnormalities in 26 percent. It is doubtful if these changes can be taken as an expression of disease in all cases. Sinoscopy is of infinite help in the differential diagnosis, and especially in this type of patient there is the possibility of "catching" a maxillary sinus cancer in the very early stages.

Another distressing condition is to find normal x-ray pictures in a patient with clinical symptoms definitely suggesting maxillary sinus disease. However, it is well known that in these cases it is possible to find pronounced changes in the maxillary sinus, both circumscribed or diffuse, in the form of secretion and thickening of the mucosa.[2,13,19] Less comprehensive changes in the lower part of the maxillary sinus can be difficult to evaluate roentgenologically, especially in patients with teeth and particularly in children. In addition sinusitis acuta sicca, which can be demonstrated neither roentgenologically nor by an-

tral puncture, should be borne in mind.[25] Likewise, an otherwise asymptomatic sinusitis might be the cause of atypical facial pain.

In many cases one finds a circumscribed swelling in the sinus on the x-ray pictures. In this group (mucosal cysts, solitary polyps, localized edema, tumors) it is possible after sinoscopic evaluation to avoid a number of exploratory procedures on the sinus or repeated control examinations. In cases where the sinoscopic finding is uncertain or where a tumor is suspected, an exact diagnosis can readily be obtained histologically from an endoscopic biopsy or an explorative operation. The sinus is explored without delay when sinoscopy reveals a localized change, the nature of which is not familiar, even though malignancy is not obviously suggested.

When a total blurring of the maxillary sinus is present there are a number of diagnostic possibilities: (1) empyema with acute, subacute, or chronic maxillary sinus inflammation; (2) pronounced thickening of the mucosa of allergic or infectious genesis; (3) a cyst or tumor of benign or malignant character; (4) hematosinus. The radiologic examination offers no help in the differential diagnosis, and it is possible only to distinguish partially between them using antral puncture. Sinoscopy is usually conclusive; and even in cases where a clear view is not obtained because of contact between the lens and tissue, the endoscopic biopsy can help.

Thus it must be considered whether sinoscopy can replace x-ray examination in many cases as a normal method for examining the maxillary sinuses, especially when sufficient experience has been acquired. In cases where a tumor is suspected, x-ray examination is indispensible often supplemented by tomographic examination.

VALUE OF THE ENDOSCOPIC BIOPSY

During sinoscopy it is possible to obtain a tissue sample from the posterior wall of the sinus (Fig. 3) for histologic examination using a fine cup forceps. The normal mucosa is extremely thin, and the removal of tissue is difficult. With a pathologic membrane, the thicker the mucosa, the easier it is to remove a sample; a biopsy is successfully obtained in approximately 80 percent of all cases. Bauer[1] stated that there is good agreement between the sinoscopic examination and the microscopic appearance of a biopsy in cases of allergic and infectious diseases. In contrast Moesner et al.[16] found that there is no characteristic histologic finding corresponding to each type of sinoscopic picture, and so biopsy is of limited value in the differential diagnosis of the type of disease. It should be noted in particular that no difference was found in the occurrence of neutrophils, lymphocytes, edema, or fibrosis. However, there was a significant correlation between, on the one hand, basal membrane thickening, eosinophilia, epithelial and ciliary loss, and an increase in the number of goblet cells, and on the other hand the groups of polypous and fibrous types of sinusitis dominated by allergy. The problem of whether a single biopsy was representative with regard to the histology of the whole sinus was evaluated by comparison between two fortuituously chosen sites in the section removed at operation. A considerable difference was found from one site to another in the same sample, and it was concluded that a single biopsy was not representative of the whole sinus. Kashiwado et al.[14] state that a single biopsy was found to be representative in 80 percent of their cases.

It must therefore be concluded that histologic examination of mucosal biopsies using current techniques is of no great help in evaluating sinusitis. However, it can be of some use in the diagnosis of allergic conditions.

On the other hand, if malignancy is suspected or difficulty is encountered in obtaining a view of the mucosa during endoscopic examination, histologic evaluation is then of considerable value and it is often possible in such cases to ensure a far greater degree of certainty in the differential diagnosis than with x-ray examination or antral puncture alone.

The development of a flexible biopsy forceps guided by the telescopic view will increase the value of mucosal biopsy. It should be mentioned, however, that Hellmich[7] using the bimeatal sinoscopy technique (the optic is introduced through a cannula in the canine fossa and the biopsy forceps through another cannula, puncturing the sinus below the inferior turbinate) suggested a technique with which removal of a biopsy specimen (as well as minor therapeutic excisions) can be carried out under direct vision. The disadvantage with regard to this technique, as stated by Timm,[25] is that following puncture of the canine fossa small bone

splinters can be introduced into the maxillary sinus; moreover, in cases where the mucosa is thickened the end of the sinoscope is caught more easily in folds of the mucosa thus preventing a clear view of the interior of the sinus.

SINOSCOPY AND RESECTION OF THE MAXILLARY SINUS

In connection with the above-mentioned belief that histologic examination of a biopsy from the mucosa removed during sinoscopy could determine the type of sinusitis, several authors have presumed that the need for operative treatment of cases of sinusitis could be determined with reasonable certainty on the basis of sinoscopy and histologic examination.[1,2,17] In our studies it has been impossible, however, to demonstrate that the time of recovery following daily lavage through the polyethylene tube could be predicted with any certainty by sinoscopic evaluation; furthermore, the histologic evaluation is not conclusive with regard to the type or degree of sinusitis, and similarly the individual biopsy is not representative of the whole sinus.[16]

It must therefore be maintained that only the clinical evaluation of the course of conservative treatment can show whether a Caldwell-Luc operation is necessary. Sinoscopy can be of some value, however, when determining the time after which further conservative treatment must be considered useless.

Sinoscopy is useful in the postoperative control following Caldwell-Luc operation. Introduction of the cannula is easily accomplished through the fenestra formed below the inferior turbinate. The healing process, which is usually completed after approximately 2 months, can be followed by inspection (Fig. 15, Plate I) and biopsy removal.[1,17] In a very unfortunate case there was, after 3 weeks, reformation of a severely polypous mucosa, which on histologic examination contained ciliary epithelium and numerous mucous glands.

If the maxillary sinus is examined in a patient subjected to Caldwell-Luc operation some considerable time previously, it is frequently seen that the mucosa is slightly thickened, fibrous, but otherwise reactionless. Occasionally a viscous, gelatinous secretion is found despite the open fenestra. The mucosa often has sail-shaped scars with sharp edges (Fig. 16). Corresponding mucosal scars have been formed

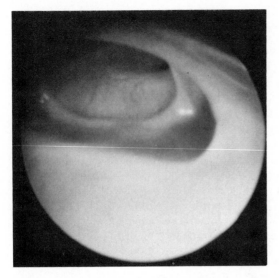

FIG. 16. Right sinus: Caldwell-Luc operation previously performed. There is a thin, slightly fibrous lining with sail-shaped mucosal scars.

experimentally in studies on dogs.[9] However, one-third of the patients, often those with severe symptoms, have a completely different sinoscopic picture. In these cases the mucosa is very swollen and polypous, and there are drops of purulent secretion scattered over the surface. In these patients the x-ray pictures are sometimes rather difficult to interpret owing to the considerable reaction in the surrounding bone, which produces greater or lesser blurring; in these cases sinoscopy is very helpful.

CONCLUSION

The technical improvements during the last years have simplified endoscopic examination of the maxillary sinus and have made it possible to produce excellent color photographs for documentation and educational purposes. However, sinoscopy has been used only to a limited extent, mainly in Germany and Austria. The examination is carried out under local anesthesia and usually does not entail much more inconvenience to the patient than an ordinary antral puncture. Sinoscopy is indicated in a great variety of maxillary sinus diseases, where it gives valuable information for the differential diagnosis and as a rule is superior to x-ray examination.

In addition to the obvious advantages obtained by direct inspection of the mucous membrane, the sinoscopic method permits removal of tissue samples from the mucous membrane; in cases of sinusitis the secretion can be removed for bacterial examination without contamination from the nasal bacteria, and a polyethylene tube can be inserted for daily lavage of the sinus.

Thus it is essential to disseminate the knowledge of this method, as many diagnostic operations on the sinus can be avoided in this manner, and the correct treatment of maxillary sinus disease can be readily chosen with greater certainty.

REFERENCES

1. Bauer E: Die normale und pathologische Histologie der Kieferhöhlenschleimhaut. Monatsschr Ohrenheilk 94:43, 1960
2. Bauer E, Wodak E: Die Kieferhöhle und ihre Krankheiten im endoskopischen Bild. Wien Med Wochenschr 109:404, 1959
3. Bauer E, Wodak E: Neuerungen in der Diagnostik und Therapie der Nasen-Nebenhöhlen. Arch Ohren Nasen Kehlkopfheilkd 171:325, 1957
4. Baum HL: A new method and a new instrument for endoscopic examination of the maxillary antrum. Laryngoscope 31:965, 1921
5. Bethmann W: Endoskopische Bilder aus gesunden und erkrankten Kieferhöhlen. Zahnaerztl Welt 8:606, 1953
6. Fascenelli FW: Maxillary sinus abnormalities. Arch Otolaryngol 90:190, 1969
7. Hellmich S: Bimeatal sinuscopy, technical and diagnostic improvements. Int Rhinol (Leiden) 10:37, 1972
8. Hellmich S, Herberhold C: Technische Verbesserungen der Kieferhöhlen-Endoskopie. Arch Klin Exp Ohren Nasen Kehlkopfheilkd 199:678, 1971
9. Hilding AC, Banovetz J: Occluding scars in the sinuses: relation to bone growth. Laryngoscope 73:1201, 1963
10. Hirschmann A: Ueber Endoskopie der Nase und deren Nebenhöhlen. Arch Laryngol Rhinol Otol 14:195, 1903
11. Hütten R: Kritische Betrachtungen zur Sinuskopie. Laryngol Rhinol Otol 49:118, 1970
12. Illum P, Jeppesen F: Sinoscopy: endoscopy of the maxillary sinus: technique, common and rare findings. Acta Otolaryngol (Stockh) 73:506, 1972
13. Illum P, Jeppesen F, Langebaek E: X-ray examination and sinoscopy in maxillary sinus disease. Acta Otolaryngol (Stockh) 74:287, 1972
14. Kashiwado T, Ohashi I, Suzuki T, et al: The mucocis membrane biopsy of the maxillary sinus for the window operation. Int Rhinol (Leiden) 4:67, 1966
15. Maltz M: New instrument: the sinuscope. Laryngoscope 35:805, 1925
16. Moesner J, Illum P, Jeppesen F: Sinoscopical

biopsy in maxillary sinus disease. Acta Oto-laryngol (Stockh) (in press)

17. Pihrt J: Bilan des examens de la cavité max-illaire par la sinoscopie. Rev Laryngol Otol Rhinol (Bord) 85:781, 1963

18. Reichert M: Ueber eine neue Untersuch-ungsmethode der Oberkieferhöhle mittelst des Antroskops. Berl Klin Wochenschr 39:401, 1902

19. Riccabona Av: Erfahrungen mit der Kiefer-höhlenendoskopie. Arch Ohren Nasen Kehl-kopfheilkd 167:359, 1955

20. Rosemann G: Zur endoskopischen Kieferhöhl-endiagnostik. Z Laryngol Rhinol Otol 40:935, 1961

21. Slobodnik M: Die direkte Untersuchung der Kieferhöhle dursch Endoskopie. Z Laryngol Rhinol 19:437, 1930

22. Spielberg W: Antroscopy of the maxillary sinus. Laryngoscope 32:441, 1922

23. Strupler W: Diagnose und Therapie der isolier-ten Berstungsbrüche des Augenhöhlenbodens. Arch Klin Exp Ohren Nasen Kehlkopfheilkd 201:57, 1972

24. Timm C: Die Endoskopie der Kieferhöhlen. Fortschr Med 74:421, 1956

25. Timm C: Die Wichtigsten Befunde bei der sinu-skopischen Untersuchung. Z Laryngol Rhinol Otol 44:606, 1965

EDITORIAL COMMENT

Recently a lateral-view telescope was developed with a guided biopsy forcep. Both can be introduced through a 5-mm trocar. During advancement the biopsy forceps is

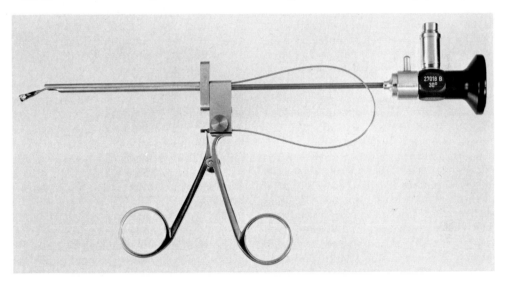

New design of a miniature biopsy forceps with a forward oblique telescope that can be intro-duced through the 5-mm trocar. By advancing the flexible biopsy forceps the jaws appear in the viewing field in a bent position. This addition facilitates biopsies from those areas which are difficult to see or to approach with a straight, rigid forceps and scope.
(Manufacturer: K. Storz Endoscopy K.G. 7200 Tuttlingen, P.O. Box: 400, W. Germany).

bent "around the corner" and brought into the visual field. Biopsies can now be obtained from those areas where Dr. Illum described difficulties.

THE EDITOR

49

Mediastinoscopy

Paul H. Ward

Diseases involving the mediastinum and thorax are often difficult diagnostic problems that in the past have often required exploratory thoracotomy to obtain a tissue diagnosis. In 1959 Carlens introduced mediastinoscopy as a promising, new, simple, and safe method for exploring, palpating, and biopsying lesions of the mediastinum under direct endoscopic vision.

Originally the procedure was used to determine the operability of bronchogenic carcinoma without resort to thoracotomy. Experience from a number of centers has now shown that it often can be helpful in the diagnosis of other diseases involving the mediastinum and particularly the paratracheal and carinal lymphatic system.[9] Diseases diagnosed by mediastinoscopy included metastatic tumors from other areas of the body, tuberculosis, histoplasmosis, sarcoidosis, mediastinal cysts, thymoma, Hodgkin's disease, lymphosarcoma and other lymphomas, liposarcoma, lipoma, silicosis, and vascular anomalies. Recently we even removed a foreign body by this technique.[19]

Mediastinoscopy received rapid acceptance throughout Europe. The procedure has been accepted for popular use more slowly in the United States and Canada perhaps in part because the name "mediastinoscopy which to some surgeons may," according to Pearson,[14] "suggest rather formidable and frightening possibilities and may conjure up visions of blind instrumental probing in among the great vessels and vital structures of the mediastinum." Widespread use of the procedure, however, has demonstrated it to be safe and to provide valuable diagnostic information,

often alleviating the necessity for more traumatic and risky thoracotomy. Over 26,000 cases have been accumulated in the European literature and more than 4,000 in the American literature.

The degree of mediastinal involvement in cases of bronchogenic carcinoma has always been difficult to evaluate. Laminography, esophagography, tracheobronchography, angiography, phlebography, lymphadenography, and gas mediastinography have proved helpful in attempts to assess this area. Often, however, additional information would have been beneficial.

Earlier efforts to acquire histopathologic proof of the metastasis of lung tumors to lymph nodes were made by Daniels[6] in 1949. He described the technique of removing the scalene fat pad and its contained lymph nodes, which in advanced cases sometimes contained metastatic tumor. Harken and co-workers[7] in 1954 were able to reach nodes in the primary drainage area by elaborating on the scalene node biopsy technique, and they approached the superior mediastinum by blunt dissection through the cervical fascia, passing either anterior or posterior to the subclavian vein. A laryngoscope was inserted, and biopsy of the homolateral paratracheal nodes was obtained with a laryngeal forceps. Radner[15] in 1955 pointed out the unnecessary hazards of the lateral approach and described five cases of paratracheal lymph node biopsy performed via a midline approach through a suprasternal incision. In 1959 Carlens introduced the technique of endoscopic midline approach to the mediastinum. He presented 100 cases of mediastinoscopy performed without complication. The midline approach under direct vision decreased the hazards of damage to the major vessels and pleura, and in addition allowed bilateral exploration, palpation, visualization, and biopsy of the paratracheal nodes. This approach also facilitated exploration of the region of the carina with biopsy of any nodes or other mediastinal masses encountered. A distinct advantage of the latter procedure is the increased probability of finding metastases in the primary drainage nodes rather than in the more distant secondary nodes of the scalene fat pad. The superiority of this logical extension of obtaining lymph nodes closer to the primary tumor lymphatic drainage area was documented by Johner et al.[10]

The recent literature on the surgical results in bronchogenic carcinoma leaves no doubt of the need for additional preoperative information concerning the extent of spread of the tumor. Harken et al.[7] expressed the opinion that "a technique that spares needless suffering for the hopelessly involved patient is as important as the extension of excisional therapy in an attempt to cure more people." We have entered an era of almost unlimited technical ability and are able to perform extensive lung and mediastinal resections. A number of thoracic surgeons can cite the example of an occasional survivor who has undergone pneumonectomy with mediastinal dissection for bronchogenic carcinoma. These same surgeons, however, usually fail to recall the high mortality and morbidity that accompanied the extended resections. Even with the advances in surgical technique, the 5-year survival rate of all patients with bronchogenic carcinoma remains at 9 to 10 percent.[2] About half of these tumors were nonresectible when the patient first consulted the surgeon. Among the resected cases, the 5-year survival rate has been reported at 19 to 28 percent.[5,11] Of the cases explored, an average of about 40 percent were found to be nonresectable, and the exploration provided no more than a tissue diagnosis. If the diagnosis and nonresectablility could have been determined by other means, these unfortunate victims could have been spared unnecessary thoracotomy with its accompanying risk of morbidity and mortality. For this large group of patients with such limited life expectancy, the mortality—which averages 10 percent or higher for thoracotomy and resection, and 3.5 to 9 percent for simple

exploration and biopsy—could have been avoided.

Mediastinoscopy offers promise as a method of determining the operability of patients with lung cancer. Reynders[16] initiated the use of mediastinoscopy in all patients with suspected bronchogenic carcinoma seen in their clinic. He found that the use of the information obtained from mediastinoscopy resulted in a drop in the incidence of unnecessary exploratory thoracotomies from 40 percent to less than 10 percent, decreased the number of surgical complications and deaths, and decreased the number of curative pneumonectomies while increasing the number of curative lobectomies.

The ever-increasing, more widespread experience with mediastinoscopy has demonstrated it to be a safe and relatively easy procedure to perform that can yield valuable information about the diseases of the chest and mediastinum.

INDICATIONS

As experience with mediastinoscopy has increased, the indications have become more sharply defined, although by no means static. The routine clinical tests such as blood and culture studies, bronchoscopy, cytology, etc. should not be neglected. Where palpable masses or enlarged supraclavicular or neck nodes are readily accessible, they should be biopsied prior to resorting to mediastinoscopy. In those cases in which all routine clinical studies are normal and mediastinal or hilar masses exist, mediastinoscopy frequently may provide the tissue diagnosis without resort to thoracotomy and its accompanying morbidity and mortality. The merit of mediastinoscopy in determining the spread of carcinoma of the lung to the primary regional lymph nodes has been well documented.[17] In some clinics all patients with pulmonary carcinoma undergo mediastinoscopy in an effort to determine the extent of spread of the tumor. The information obtained has often spared patients unnecessary thoracotomy. These persons have only a limited survival time and need neither the expense nor the morbidity and mortality risks that accompany thoracotomy. It is not the purpose of the procedure to determine the operability of the tumor, but rather to obtain information concerning the histologic type and the extent of tumor spread. For those surgeons who consider extended resection to be worthwhile, mediastinoscopy may yield information on the extent of mediastinal involvement to be encountered at surgery. For the others who consider unilateral, contralateral, bilateral, carinal, or any other combination of positive mediastinal lymph node biopsies as indications of nonresectability, this procedure has much to offer in the selection of patients. For those obviously non-resectable cases in which all efforts have failed to yield a tissue diagnosis, mediastinoscopy often provides a tissue diagnosis without resort to thoracotomy.

The rather typical exemplary inoperable case of bronchogenic carcinoma in which clinical laboratory tests were normal and bronchoscopy was negative is seen in Figure 1A. Mediastinoscopy under local anesthesia provided a tis-

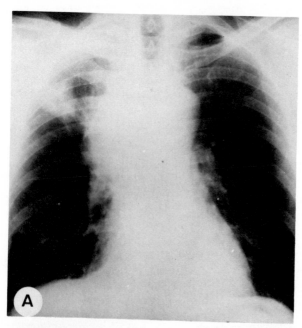

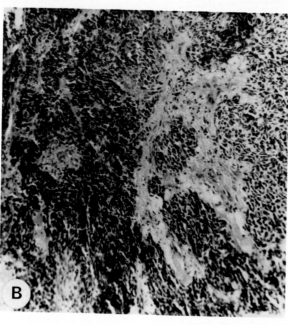

FIG. 1. **A.** Chest x-ray (PA) of right upper lobe infiltrate, right hilar mass, and mediastinal widening. **B.** Photomicrograph showing anaplastic carcinoma destroying the architecture of the mediastinal node.

sue diagnosis without resorting to thoracotomy and its accompanying morbidity and mortality (Fig. 1B). The patient was treated palliatively with radiation therapy. Without a tissue diagnosis many physicians would hesitate to administer radiotherapy.

Mediastinoscopy is invaluable in obtaining a tissue diagnosis of sarcoid. The positive his-

tologic diagnosis is obtained when sarcoid is suspected in 10 to 30 percent of cases by bronchoscopy, 50 to 70 percent of cases by scalene fat pad biopsy, and 95 to 100 percent of cases undergoing mediastinoscopy.[4]

The typical example of a patient with sarcoid diagnosed by mediastinoscopy (under local anesthesia) is seen in Figure 2A. This asymp-

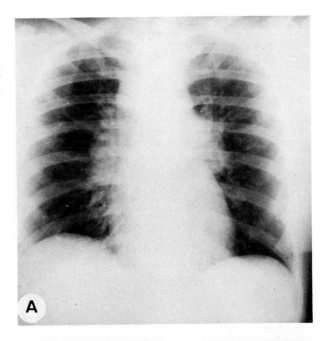

FIG. 2. **A.** Chest x-ray (PA) demonstrating hilar adenopathy. **B.** Photomicrograph of noncaseating granuloma in a mediastinal lymph node compatible with sarcoid.

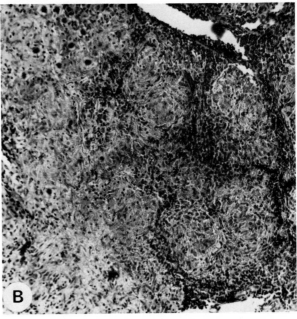

tomatic 33-year-old female with a normal physical examination demonstrated hilar adenopathy on chest x-ray. Bronchoscopy with washings for cytology was negative. The differential diagnosis included sarcoid, tuberculosis, fungus infection, and lymphoma. The latter were easily ruled out when histologic examination revealed the classic-appearing noncaseating granuloma (Fig. 2B).

Metastatic carcinoma of the breast was easily diagnosed in a 50-year-old white female who complained of shortness of breath and hoarseness of 3 months' duration. A left radical mastectomy had been performed 8 years previously for adenocarcinoma of the breast. X-rays of the chest revealed no hilar adenopathy (Fig. 3A). A tracheostomy was performed because there was bilateral recurrent nerve paralysis.

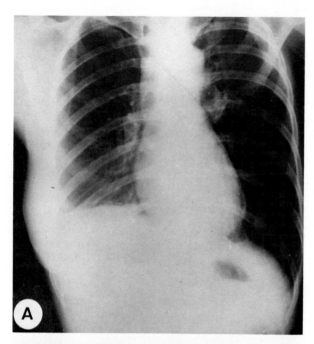

FIG. 3.   **A.** Chest x-ray (PA) of elevated right diaphragm and a small amount of atelectasis of the right lower lobe. The mediastinal width appears normal. **B.** Photomicrograph of adenocarcinoma in a mediastinal lymph node.

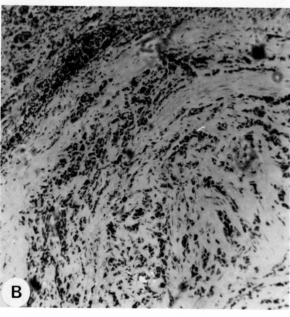

The dissection was extended into the mediastinum. The mediastinoscope was inserted and biopsy specimens were obtained (Fig. 3B), which contained adenocarcinoma similar histologically to the breast tumor removed 8 years previously. The absence of hilar enlargement on x-ray films made consideration of other causes for recurrent nerve paralysis essential. Mediastinoscopy permitted early diagnosis and confirmation of recurrent tumor; palliative radiotherapy was administered.

The diagnosis of probable malignant thymoma was confirmed in a 44-year-old woman who had pain in the right side of the chest and the sternal area for 3 weeks. X-ray films showed a rounded mass in the anterior mediastinum causing some indentation of the trachea just above the carina (Fig. 4A). Bronchoscopy,

FIG. 4. **A.** Chest x-ray (PA) of anterior superior mediastinal mass and widened upper mediastinum on the right. **B.** Photomicrograph of biopsies of mediastinal mass showing many dark-staining nuclei in the islands of small pleomorphic cells. This is compatible with a malignant thymoma.

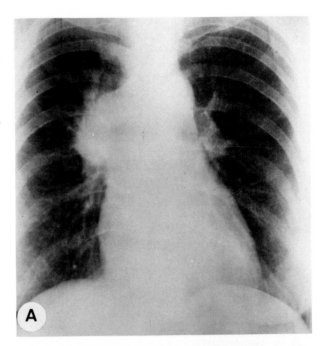

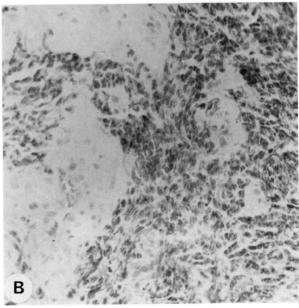

cytology cultures, and other conventional clinical tests were normal. Mediastinoscopy under local anesthesia permitted easy excision of biopsy material under direct vision of the mass, which was located anterior to the trachea. Following histologic study the pathologist reported the tumor to be a malignant thymoma (Fig. 4B). This patient was spared the thoracotomy that otherwise would have been necessary to obtain the tissue biopsy considered essential before radiation therapy. Her response to irradiation was excellent, and at last report, 2 years after diagnosis, she was symptom-free.

Lymphosarcoma was diagnosed in a 38-year-old man who complained of malaise, fever, cough, and hoarseness of 6 weeks' duration. On physical examination he appeared acutely ill, and his left vocal cord was paralyzed. An x-ray film showed a large, bilobed anterior mediastinal mass (Fig. 5A). A routine clinical examina-

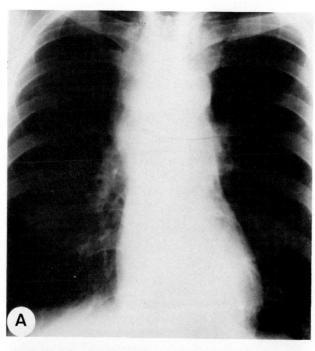

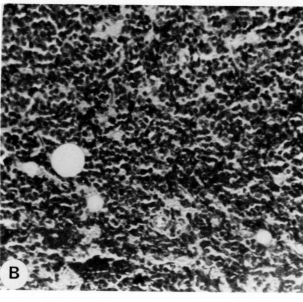

FIG. 5.   A. Chest x-ray (PA) of large bilobed anterior mediastinal mass.   **B.** Photomicrograph of mediastinal lymph node containing lymphosarcoma. The architectural structure of the lymph node has been replaced by immature lymphocytes.

tion and tests including bronchoscopy were normal. At mediastinoscopy done under local anesthesia, many enlarged paratracheal nodes were seen. A fixed mass of matted nodes was palpated in the arch of the aorta. A large lymph node was dissected free, and a frozen section of it showed lymphosarcoma (Fig. 5B). Radiotherapy was given, and the patient had an excellent response.

A most unusual application of mediastinoscopy was the removal of a bullet from the mediastinum of a 62-year-old man shot in the chest during a fight. The bullet entered the right side of the sternum and lodged in the superior mediastinum (Fig. 6). The wound became infected, and pus drained from it. On the seventh day after the injury the bullet was removed by mediastinoscopy under local anesthesia.

These are examples of the value and indications for mediastinoscopy. As mentioned previously, mediastinoscopy is indicated to determine if there is extension of pulmonary disease (inflammatory or malignant) to the mediastinum, as well as for obtaining a tissue diagnosis of any primary mediastinal pathology (i.e., bronchogenic cysts, benign and malignant tumors, infections, etc.).

The successful use of mediastinoscopy for implanting cardiac pacemakers has been reported.[4] We removed parathyroid adenoma by mediastinoscopy under local anesthesia in a patient too ill for general anesthesia,[20] and Carlens and Jepsen[4] found mediastinoscopy useful in performing thymectomy for patients with myasthenia gravis. There thus appears to be an ever-expanding group of indications for this valuable endoscopic technique.

CONTRAINDICATIONS

There are no absolute contraindications to the performance of mediastinoscopy. The utilization of local anesthesia makes it feasible to obtain a tissue diagnosis even in the extremely moribund high-risk patient. Relative contraindications are the presence of bleeding abnormalities and clotting defects. Most experienced mediastinoscopists who have attempted mediastinoscopy in the presence of the superior vena caval syndrome consider the excessive

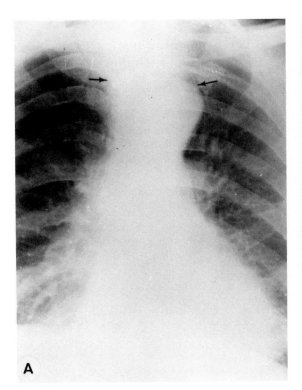

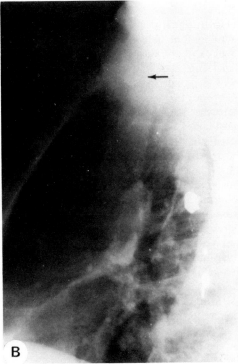

A **B**

FIG. 6. PA (**A**) and lateral (**B**) chest x-rays of a bullet (arrows) in the anterior mediastinum. The other metallic objects (from a previous fight) were in the soft tissues of the left axilla.

bleeding from the markedly dilated vessels a reason for withholding the procedure.

GENERAL ANESTHESIA

The majority of mediastinoscopies are performed under general endotracheal anesthesia. The belief that a general anesthesia is essential has been another detracting factor as far as the popularity of mediastinoscopy is concerned. Many thoracic surgeons argue that if a general anesthesia is to be given then thoracotomy followed by biopsy, frozen section, and definitive surgical extirpation is more reasonable than administration of two anesthetics—one for the diagnostic procedure and another for the definitive resection if indicated. General anesthesia facilitates the management of young patients (children) and patients who are emotionally labile. Furthermore, in the event of complications such as pneumothorax or injury to major vessels, the appropriate correction is better managed under general anesthesia.

LOCAL ANESTHESIA

Palva[12] stated, "The operation is always made in general anesthesia; local anesthesia would not be feasible when working as low down as at the bifurcation and main bronchi." Experience has demonstrated the latter statement to be incorrect. Having withheld mediastinoscopy for moribund patients on several occasions because of the hazards of general anesthesia, we decided to perform the procedure under local anesthesia. So superior were the results that we now reserve general anesthesia for those patients who refuse local anesthesia and for extremely nervous patients and children. In addition to eliminating the hazards of a general anesthesia, we have found many other advantages to the performance of mediastinoscopy under local anesthesia. The almost bloodless field allows better visualization and definition of the mediastinal structures with resulting increased safety. The operating room time is shortened, and the discomfort to the patient during and after the procedure is minimal. Throughout the procedure the patient can describe any discomfort or shortness of breath, which assists in the early detection and correction of pneumothorax,

bilateral recurrent nerve paralysis, and other complications. Never has the cliché, "If you haven't tried it, don't knock it," applied more aptly. Almost uniformly those who have the courage to try mediastinoscopy under local anesthesia readily recognize the significant advantages and increased safety. Most patients who have undergone both bronchoscopy and mediastinoscopy under local anesthesia feel that the discomfort experienced during mediastinoscopy is less than during bronchoscopy. Local anesthesia has attained a definite place in the performance of mediastinoscopy.[19-21]

RESULTS

Tucker, Ward, and Duvall collaborated in combining their series, which were presented to the AMA as an award-winning exhibit.[18] Table 1 summarizes the results of the 826 cases reviewed from their series of 1,076 mediastinoscopies.

The value of prethoracotomy mediastinoscopy as a screening procedure is obvious. Of all the patients who have thoracotomy for carcinoma of the lung, 40 percent undergo "futile" operations that actually decrease their survival time.

The most rewarding aspect of mediastinoscopy is the rapid acquisition of a definitive diagnosis when there is hilar adenopathy. It also helps to determine the presence of lym-

TABLE 1. Summary of Results of Mediastinoscopy Series

Mediastinoscopy	No.
Total mediastinoscopies performed[18]	1,076
Tucker	400
Ward	300
Duval and Koop	376
Total mediastinoscopies reviewed	826
Carcinoma of the lung	446
Positive	190 (42%)
Sarcoidosis	157
Positive	152 (97%)
Miscellaneous malignancies	
Miscellaneous metastatic	5
Head and neck	5
Breast	3
Hodgkin's disease	17
Lymphoma	10
Miscellaneous nonmalignant	29
Histoplasmosis	6
Tuberculosis	13

phoma, Hodgkin's disease, and infections, and assists in differentiating them from sarcoidosis. Appropriate treatment can be initiated without delay, additional morbidity and mortality are decreased, and the overall expense of hospitalization is diminished.

TECHNIQUE

It is essential that mediastinoscopy be performed in a general operating room with meticulous sterile technique. It is a sterile procedure and should not be considered comparable to other endoscopic procedures which are not sterile but surgically clean procedures. While complications in the hands of the careful operator are rare, the possibilities of pneumothorax and damage to the great vessels do exist and are much better managed in the general operating room.

The patient is placed supine on the operating table with the shoulders elevated by a shoulder roll or a sandbag. This extends the neck while leaving the head in the midline free to be turned to either the right or left. The neck, chin, and upper thorax are prepared and draped in a fashion similar to that required for a tracheotomy or thyroidectomy. When the procedure is performed under local anesthesia, the skin and suprasternal notch area are infiltrated with 1 percent Xylocaine with Adrenalin. The sympathomimetic drug is omitted in patients with hypertension or heart disease. A transverse 3- to 4-cm skin crease incision is made about 2 cm above the manubrium (Fig. 7). Midline dissection is carried down to the ventral surface of the trachea. Particularly important is the division of the pretracheal fascia since the plane of dissection is against the trachea posterior to this fascia. If this is not done the dissection may be in an improper plane, with the possibility of damage to the great vessels.

About 2 cc of 1 percent Xylocaine is injected into the lumen of the trachea to diminish the cough reflex. The index finger is then used to perform a major portion of the dissection. The finger gently dissects down the anterior surface of the trachea. It is usually possible to palpate the tracheobronchial angles and carina. Should the patient experience discomfort, 1 percent Xylocaine (several cubic centimeters) is placed in the wound and massaged into the mediasti-

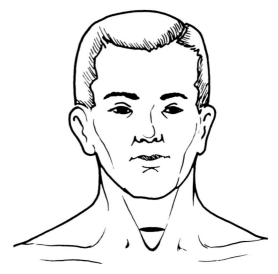

FIG. 7. Small suprasternal incision area used to approach the trachea and through which the mediastinoscope is introduced.

nal tissues. A remarkable evaluation of the upper mediastinum can be performed with the palpating finger. The aortic arch, innominate artery, and left common carotid artery are easily identified. Any enlarged paratracheal lymph nodes or tumor infiltrates in the mediastinum or against the mediastinal pleural walls can be felt and their adherence and mobility ascertained. Bleeding, particularly when the procedure is performed under local anesthesia, is negligible up to this point.

The mediastinoscope (which is like a modified child's esophagoscope) is introduced into the pretracheal space that has been prepared by finger dissection (Fig. 8). As the instrument is passed down the tract, care is taken always to keep the anterior tracheal wall in the field of vision. Further paratracheal and carinal dissection can be performed using a specially designed spreader or by a forceps modified to hold a small dissecting sponge. Delicate, blunt-tipped laryngeal scissors are used to divide small fibrous bands. Prior to dissection or division, possible blood-filled structures can be identified by means of a long hypodermic needle and aspiration. Sometimes exposed and to be protected are the superior vena cava and azygos veins on the right, and on the left the pulmonary artery as it crosses the left main bronchus anteriorly and the descending aorta as it passes behind the left main bronchus and

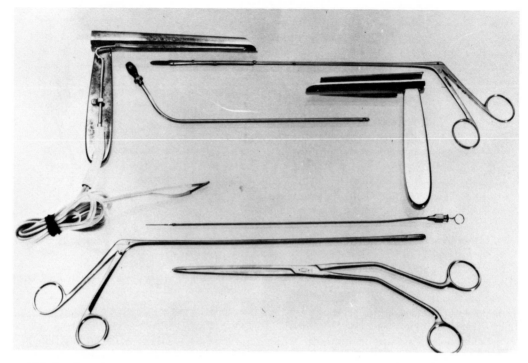

FIG. 8. Special instruments used in the performance of mediastinoscopy: mediastinoscopes, light carriers, suction tubes, long aspirating needle, cup biopsy forceps, laryngeal scissors, and dissecting instrument (spreader).

to the left of the esophagus. Care must also be taken not to injure the left recurrent nerve, which is much more ventrally located in the lower tracheal area near the bifurcation. Large pigment (carbon particles) containing lymph nodes literally bulge before the orifice of the mediastinoscope as the dissection progresses. Often masses of matted nodes can be freed and removed in toto. The anterior, superior, and inferior surfaces of the bronchial walls can be explored out to the pleural reflections. Biopsies are routinely taken of any tumor masses, the paratracheal hilar nodes on both sides, and the subcarinal nodes (Fig. 9). Cup or basket-type laryngeal forceps are used to obtain these biopsies. In the event of more profuse bleeding, Gelfoam and packing may be used. The packing can be removed and the Gelfoam left in place upon closing. On completion of the exploration the mediastinoscope is removed, allowing the mediastinal tissues to fall back against the trachea, which provides additional hemostasis. The wound is then closed in layers without drainage, and a gentle pressure dressing is applied over the neck incision. The operating time required for performing mediastinoscopy under local anesthesia is usually around 30 to 45 minutes. A significant portion of this time is required for frozen section preparation and analysis.

Discomfort is minimal postoperatively and is far less than that encountered after tracheostomy. The patients are ambulated the same day and may go home 1 to 2 days after mediastinoscopy.

COMPLICATIONS

The safety of mediastinoscopy in competent hands has been well documented.[8,13,17] There were no deaths in the combined series of 826 mediastinoscopies reviewed from the total 1,076 cases presented by Tucker et al.[18] (Table 2). None of the complications were life-threatening, even though many of the procedures in these combined series were performed by relatively inexperienced residents under close supervision. There were four patients in whom pneumothorax developed; in two of these

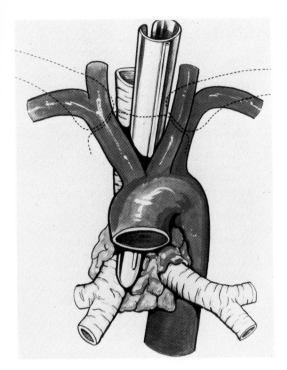

FIG. 9. Mediastinoscope in position to explore and obtain biopsies of paratracheal and carinal lymph nodes.

patients local anesthesia was used. Their complications were immediately recognized since they were awake and able to describe their chest pain. Chest tubes were inserted and placed under a water seal. The tubes were removed after 48 hours without sequelae. In five patients excessive bleeding required Gelfoam to be placed in the area and the wound was packed for 5 minutes. When the packing was removed there was no bleeding and the procedure was terminated. On completion of the pro-

TABLE 2. Complications in a Series of 1,076 Mediastinoscopies

Complication	No.
Subcutaneous emphysema	2
Pneumothorax	4
Wound infection	2
Esophageal injury	0
Recurrent nerve injury	5
Hemorrhage	5
Hypotension	0
Wound hematoma	1
Deaths	0
Complications in total series	1.7%

cedure in one patient, he was observed to be in respiratory distress, although he stated in a hoarse voice that he had no pain. In the sitting position mirror examination of the larynx revealed a bilateral vocal cord paralysis. Because there was potential easy access to the trachea through the mediastinoscopy incision, it was elected to maintain him in the sitting position and observe his course. Within 1.5 hours the effects of the local anesthetic had passed, and both vocal cords had regained normal movement. Five patients experienced permanent unilateral recurrent nerve injury and its accompanying hoarseness and voice changes.

In another patient efforts to dissect with the spreading forceps in a plane at right angles to the slit in the mediastinoscope broke the light bulb from its carrier. Fortunately the intact bulb stuck in the mediastinoscope and was discovered while preparations were being made for irrigating the mediastinum. Similar accidents can be prevented by always dissecting, with the spreading forceps, in the same plane as the mediastinoscope slit. If another plane of dissection is required, the mediastinoscope is rotated 45 to 90 degrees.

The morbidity and serious complications reported to date are no greater than for scalene node biopsy. The nonfatal complications reported in the literature have included pneumothorax, recurrent nerve paralysis, and bleeding from the superior vena cava, axygos vein, and bronchial artery. Carlens[3] reviewed some 60 publications on more than 4,000 patients and found astonishingly few serious complications. Palva[12] was able to find only two reported deaths. One was a 67-year-old man in severe respiratory distress with extensive mediastinal metastasis who never awakened from the anesthesia and died 1 hour after the procedure. The other was a 40-year-old woman with lymphosarcoma who died of cardiac arrest immediately after the operation. Bergh and his colleagues[1] subsequently reported two deaths in their series of 300 mediastinoscopies. One patient was a 67-year-old man with advanced carcinoma metastatic to the mediastinum who progressively deteriorated and died on the sixth day following mediastinoscopy. The other was a 75-year-old male who had oat cell carcinoma and did well until the tenth day when he developed a pneumothorax. In spite of correction of this problem, he continued to deteriorate mentally and physically, and died on the thirteenth day after mediastinoscopy. The authors felt it improbable that mediastinoscopy was directly responsible for either death.

The overall complication rate in our combined series was only 1.7 percent in spite of the often moribund condition of many of the patients. Minimization of complications can be achieved by better knowledge of the anatomy of the mediastinum, which can be acquired via autopsy room and cadaver dissections.

Palpation and aspiration of all structures prior to biopsy should serve to identify vascular anomalies and aneurysms, and to prevent injudicious biopsy. Most important is the initial step of beginning the mediastinal dissection in the midline beneath the pretracheal fascia and against the cleaned tracheal rings. This prevents entering an incorrect, more anterior compartment that is occupied by major vessels.

Our experiences, the illustrative cases presented here, and those reported by others substantiate the merit of mediastinoscopy as a diagnostic method for diseases of the superior mediastinum and thorax. The success and increased safety achieved by performing mediastinoscopy under local anesthesia should contribute to its increased acceptance in this country as a standard diagnostic procedure.

REFERENCES

1. Bergh NP, Rydberg B, Schersten T: Mediastinal exploration by the technique of Carlens. Dis Chest 46:399, 1964
2. Burford TH, Center S, Ferguson TB, et al: Results in the treatment of bronchogenic carcinoma. J Thorac Surg 36:316, 1958
3. Carlens E: Mediastinoscopy. Ann Otol 74:1102, 1965
4. Carlens E, Jepsen O: Mediastinoscopy. Otolaryngol Clin North Am June:171, 1968
5. Chamberlain JM, McNeil TM, Parnassa P, et al: Bronchogenic carcinoma: an aggressive surgical attitude. J Thorac Cardiovasc Surg 38:727, 1959
6. Daniels AC: Method of biopsy useful in diagnosing certain intrathoracic diseases. Dis Chest 16:360, 1949
7. Harken DE, Black H, Clauss R, et al: A simple cervicomediastinal exploration for tissue diagnosis of intrathoracic disease. N Engl J Med 251:1041, 1954
8. Jepsen O: Mediastinoscopy. Copenhagen, Einar Munksgaard Forlag, 1966
9. Jepsen O, Sorenson HR (eds): Mediastinoscopy: Proceedings of an International Symposium. Odense University Press, Denmark, 1971
10. Johner C, Conner G, Prochnow J: A comparison of mediastinoscopy and scalene node biopsy. Ann Otol Rhinol Laryngol 76:935, 1967
11. Johnson J, Kirby CK, Blakemore WS: Should we insist on "radical pneumonectomy" as a routine procedure in the treatment of carcinoma of the lung? J Thorac Surg 36:309, 1958
12. Palva T: Mediastinoscopy. Verlag S. Karger, A.G., Basel/New York, 1964
13. Palva T, Viikari S: Mediastinoscopy. J Thorac Cardiovasc Surg 41:206, 1961
14. Pearson FG: Value of Mediastinoscopy. Can J Surg 6:423, 1963
15. Radner S: Suprasternal node biopsy in lymph spreading intrathoracic disease. Acta Med Scand 152:413, 1955
16. Reynders H: Mediastinoscopy in bronchogenic cancer. Dis Chest 47:606, 1964
17. Tucker JA: Mediastinoscopy: 300 cases reported and literature reviewed. Laryngoscope 82:2226, 1972
18. Tucker JA, Ward P, Duvall A, et al: Exhibit presented at AMA convention, San Francisco, June 1972
19. Ward PH: Mediastinoscopy under local anesthesia. Calif Med 112:15, 1970
20. Ward PH, Stephenson S Jr, Harris PF: Exploration of the mediastinum under local anesthesic. Ann Otol 75:368, 1966
21. Ward PH, Stephenson S Jr, Harris PF: Mediastinoscopy, a valuable diagnostic procedure for evaluation of lesions of the mediastinum. South Med J 60:51, 1967

50

Otoscopy

Horst R. Konrad

Otoscopy is the visual examination of the ear canal and tympanic membrane. Middle ear structures can be seen through the tympanic membrane or through a perforation. This procedure requires light, a speculum which straightens out the ear canal and dilates the cartilaginous portion of the canal, and magnification to improve the visual detail.

In addition to the visual examination, otoscopy is also used to clean ear canals, remove foreign bodies, and culture secretions; and it serves as a first step in surgical procedures on the tympanic membrane, the middle ear, attic, and mastoid. After ear and mastoid surgery otoscopy is used to clean the ear canal and surgical cavity.

SPECULUM

The origin of the speculum is credited to Guy De Chauliac who lived during the fourteenth century.[5] This instrument was like the present-day expanding ear speculum. It was at first advocated for removal of foreign bodies and for ear surgery. The expanding speculum was later largely replaced by the closed speculum described by Gruber in 1838.[6]

The external auditory canal has a cartilaginous portion and a bony portion. In the adult the ear canal is rarely a straight tube. The tragus overhangs the anterior portion of the ear canal laterally, and the concha border of the ear canal overlaps the bony ear canal posteriorly.[3] In order to get a direct look at the tympanic membrane the tragus has to be pushed anteriorly and the concha posteriorly. An additional angulation of the medial ear canal superiorly requires tilting the upper part of the head away from the observer for good visualization of the tympanic membrane. A speculum is inserted into the external auditory canal to straighten it and to dilate the cartilaginous canal. Metal and plastic speculums of various sizes are available for this purpose. Some are oval, but most are round. The speculums are either hand-held or attached to a speculum holder or light source.

The adult ear canal is rarely round. In most cases the bony portion is oval or like an inverted trapezoid (Fig. 1). The greatest and least diameters were measured in 31 consecutive adult temporal bones, with these results: greatest diameter 6.8 ± 1.0 mm (standard deviation), least diameter 4.13 ± 0.7 mm. The measurements were performed at the bony cartilaginous junction. The speculum should have an oval shape in order to take advantage of the greatest amount of usable space in most ear canals (Fig. 2).

LIGHT SOURCE

Direct sunlight was the first light source described that was used to view the ear canal and tympanic membrane. It had already been recommended by Razes (AD 850–932)[5] and was very likely used by even earlier observers. Almost 1,000 years later various forms of simple and concave mirrors were described to direct light into the ear canal. Some of these were

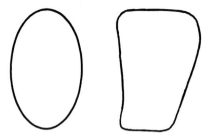

FIG. 1. The most common shape for the external auditory canal is oval or trapezoidal in the adult.

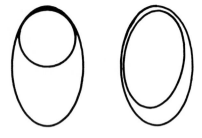

FIG. 2. An oval speculum uses more of the available space in the ear canal.

held in the teeth, others by hand.[6] The concave head mirror with its central hole as it is known today was developed from a mirror described by Hoffman in 1841.[7]

The recent development of small incandescent light sources has resulted in the development of light headlights which can be directed along the path of vision. This is somewhat easier to learn to use than the head mirror (Fig. 3).

The hand-held otoscope usually combines the speculum, the light source, and often the power supply. This is lighted by a small incandescent bulb with a lens to focus the light beam. Fiberoptic or other light conduit materials have been used to bring the light into the speculum without having a bulb obstruct part of the visual field. Flexible fiberoptic systems permit the use of high-intensity light sources,

including arc lamps to produce the light, which is then brought to the object from a distance (Fig. 4).

MAGNIFICATION

The $2\times$ to $4\times$ (magnification) optic loop has been in use for many years. It serves to give some magnification while leaving the hands free. Early mastoid surgery including fenestration and early middle ear operations were accomplished with the loop as the only source of magnification. This method was preferred by Lempert.[2] The Siegel speculum uses a magnifying lens, and in the Storz modification half the lens is left open to permit the use of instruments through the otoscope. In the pneumatic otoscope the lens also creates an airtight seal so that positive and negative pressure can be applied to move the tympanic membrane.

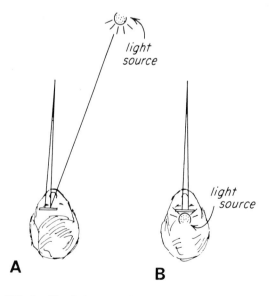

FIG. 3. The light path of the head light (**A**) is simpler than the light path of the head mirror (**B**).

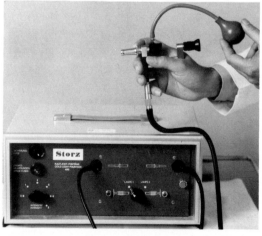

FIG. 4. A fiberoptic light source gives sufficient illumination for moderate magnification.

OPERATING MICROSCOPE

Nylén first described the use of the monocular microscope for ear operations in 1922. The lighted binocular microscope was first used by Holmgren in 1922.[2] This instrument (Zeiss binocular microscope) combined a light source with high magnification and added binocular vision, which is very important when manipulating small instruments near vulnerable structures. The binocular microscope not only revolutionized ear surgery, but when used in the clinic it greatly improved visual examination of the ear. With binocular vision, good lighting, and magnification it is possible to clean the ear canal and, through perforations, the middle ear and attic.

The short depth of field of the microscope presents a problem in examination, particularly at high magnifications. When this is coupled with limited mobility the clinical evaluation becomes difficult unless the patient is lying on a table or has his head supported. This is particularly apparent in children where a careful examination sometimes necessitates general anesthesia.

OTOSCOPE WITH HIGH MAGNIFICATION

In order to overcome some of these problems a new hand-held otoscope is being developed by Storz. This otoscope uses a flexible fiberoptic light carrier which brings the light to each side of the speculum. A 2× lens can be used to give a tight seal for pneumatic otoscopy and slight magnification. If higher magnification is desired, a second lens is moved into the field. This increases the magnification to 5×, which is sufficient for most clinical evaluation (Fig. 5). This instrument is hand-held and highly mobile, and has an even distribution of light and moderately high magnification. Work with the prototype suggests that modifications of the speculum could improve visualization.

PEDIATRIC OTOSCOPY

Several problems still remain in pediatric otoscopy. The ear canal in the newborn is shorter than in the adult. It is more circular, and the cartilaginous portion is smaller in circumference. In addition to this the infant usu-

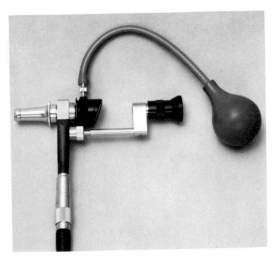

FIG. 5. Prototype of a high-magnification otoscope currently under development.

ally presents a moving target, which makes the use of a fixed instrument difficult. There is a need to develop an otoscope which takes advantage of the not yet developed tympanic ring, is hand-held, permits high magnification, has good mobility, and can move the tympanic membrane with positive and negative pressure.

Otologic disease is common in young children. The diagnosis of serous otitis media in infants is difficult. If the child is crying, the increased venous pressure makes it difficult to judge the color of the tympanic membrane. Fluid lines and bubbles are not a common finding in serous otitis, and the more subtle finding of mild retraction, a more prominent malleus, a darkening of the tympanic membrane, and decreased mobility must be observed to make the diagnosis. The subtle changes in early bacterial otitis media are also difficult to evaluate with currently available equipment. This is an area of otoscopy where new developments are needed.

OTOSCOPIC PHOTOGRAPHY

The difficulties which hamper otoscopy are compounded in otoscopic photography. Sufficient light must be brought in through the ear canal to expose the film properly. The image of the tympanic membrane must be enlarged sufficiently to cover the negative area. There has to be a minimum amount of movement between the tympanic membrane and the camera.

The first reported photographs of the tympanic membrane in a living person were by Stein in 1873. By 1922 Hegener reported a lighting system and camera capable of producing detailed stereoscopic photographs of the tympanic membrane.[1] Paul Hollinger has produced motion pictures with endoscopy including otoscopy. J. Brown Farrior and Richard Buckingham are recent contributors to otoscopic photography.

The attachment of a camera to an operating microscope facilitates photography during examination or operation. A motor drive to rewind the camera and a foot cable release as in the Robot camera or in the House Urban camera facilitates photography during sterile procedures. To get sufficient light to the film plane it is necessary to put an additional power surge through the light filament of the microscope light or to add the output from a flash unit to the light source. The power boost to the light source also gives sufficient light for the use of motion picture photography. The development of more sensitive emulsions has greatly helped in this area of photography.

REFERENCES

1. Denker A, Kahler O (eds): Handbuch der Hals-Nasen-Ohrenheilkunde. Berlin, Springer, 1926, pp 944–949
2. Dohlman GF: Carl Olof Nylen and the birth of the otomicroscope and microsurgery. Arch Otolaryngol 90:813, 1969
3. Hollingshed WH: Anatomy for Surgeons, Vol I. New York, Harper & Row, 1968, pp 184, 186
4. Mettler C: History of Medicine. Philadelphia, Blakiston, 1947
5. Politzer A (ed): Geschichte der Ohrenheilkunde, Vol I. Stuttgart, Verlag von Ferdinand Enke, 1913, pp 41, 153
6. Politzer A (ed): Geschichte der Ohrenheilkunde, Vol II. Stuttgart, Verlag von Ferdinand Enke, 1913, pp 71, 72
7. Roggenkamp W: Aus der Geschichte der Hals-Nasen-Ohren-Heilkunde: Der Ohrenspiegel. Z Laryngol Rhinol Otol 47:647, 1968

51

Anterior Rhinoscopy

W. Messerklinger

Anterior rhinoscopy refers to the examination done through the orifice of the nose with a nasal speculum, or endoscopy of the meatus of the nose with telescopes with various directions of view.

STANDARD EXAMINATION WITH A SPECULUM AND MIRROR

The cleft-shaped sinuses of the nose can be well illuminated and examined only when the light and the visual axis run coaxially. This is possible by applying indirect illumination: A paraboloid mirror in front of the eye collects and reflects the beam while a hole in its middle permits observation. The instruments must meet certain specifications:

- Illumination: 100 watts, opaque globe.
- Paraboloid mirror: Diameter 10 cm with a 1-cm hole in the center. It is affixed on the head by a strip and a ball joint (Fig. 1).
- Speculum: Among the various models we prefer the Hartmann-Killian type. According to the patient's age, the speculums are different in size and length (Fig. 2).
- Mirror: For examination of the apex of the vestibulum a postrhinoscopic mirror is employed (diameter 8 to 10 mm).

EXAMINATION TECHNIQUE

The patient sits in a chair. There is an adjustable light source on the right side next to the head, and the examiner sits on the right. With the reflector in front of his left eye, the examiner focuses the light by looking through the central hole so that the visual axis and the reflected light are parellel. Using this technique the right eye is protected against dazzling by the dorsum of the nose, and the left eye by the mirror.

For looking into the vestibulum, the tip of the nose is lifted and pressed toward the side to be examined, or the wing of the nose is pulled to the side. A small mirror held at an oblique angle under the nostril enables the operator to see into the apex of the vestibulum.

It is possible to look into the nasal cavity only by spreading the soft parts of the orifice of the nose. A nasal speculum is held in the left hand and the patient's head is held tight with the right hand; the closed instrument is then inserted 15 to 20 mm into the nose. The tip of the speculum must always point slightly laterally in order to avoid injury to the septal mucosa (Fig. 3). Thereafter the instrument is spread, and the sheath is lifted simultaneously (Fig. 4).

All sections of the anatomy are examined. While slightly bending the head forward the beginning of the inferior concha can be seen laterally; parts of the convex middle region of the inferior concha can be observed beneath the nasal fundus; and the septal base is located medially. If this part of the joint nasal meatus is large enough, a small part of the posterior epipharyngeal wall is also visible, as is the portion in front of it; by forming palatine sounds, the levator torus can be seen as a projecting wedge from below and laterally.

By slightly lifting the head, the agger nasi and the middle concha can be seen laterally. Between the middle concha and the lateral

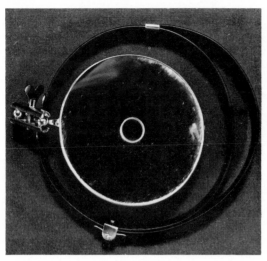

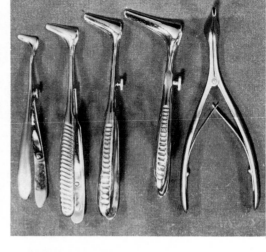

FIG. 1. Head mirror.

FIG. 2. Nasal speculums of different sizes.

nasal wall it is possible to look into the anterior part of the middle nasal meatus. Inspection of this region is of particular significance because it provides important indications concerning the condition of the nose, the paranasal sinuses of the first series (i.e., the frontal sinus, frontal ethmoid cells, and maxillary sinus), which is important in such entities as diffuse and circumscribed inflammation, edematous swelling, hyperplastic changes, polyps, and discharge from secretory ducts and tumor tissue. It was therefore attempted to improve this approach using Killian's speculum by inserting a

long blade into the middle nasal meatus and then spreading it. This "median rhinoscopy" yielded no further results and so was not used for diagnostic purposes.[3,4]

Medially the septum forms the boundary of the middle joint nasal meatus, which may show various deviations, ridges, and (approximately on the same level with the agger nasi) a tuberculum septi; in front of this, as well as beneath it, the locus Kiesselbach and a small fistulous opening as a rudiment of an organum vomeronasale can be seen.

When the head is bent backward it is impos-

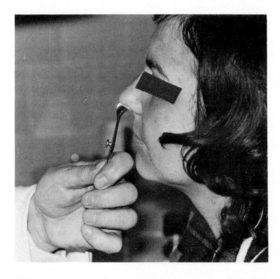

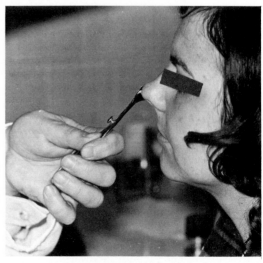

FIG. 3. The tip of the speculum is pointed slightly laterally in order to avoid injuries of the septal mucosa.

FIG. 4. The speculum is spread, and the shaft is lifted at the same time.

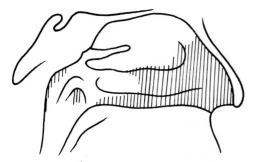

FIG. 5. Lateral wall of the nose. The shaded areas are visible by standard anterior and posterior rhinoscopy.

and the swollen region anemic by applying topical vasoconstrictors. Even with a reflector and speculum it is not possible to obtain a subtile exploration of the superior ethmoid region, the recessus sphenoethmoidalis, or even the meatuses of the nose with their ostia, sinuses, and fissures. Such a procedure is possible only with instruments that permit good illumination of even the remote areas, facilitating an atraumatic insertion into the nasal meatuses and clefts, with various directions of view. Special telescopes were developed to meet all these requirements.[5,6,7]

sible to look through a fine cleft between the middle concha and septum in the direction of the rima olfactoria. Rarely a small part of the superior concha can be seen. Polyps, a secretory duct, or other findings in this cleft indicate a disease of the paranasal sinuses of the second series (i.e., the inferior ethmoid cells or the sphenoid sinus).

The view into the nose from the front depends of course on the anatomic condition. The sections of the lateral nasal wall in the joint nasal meatus are thus visible (Fig. 5, shaded area), as is a small part of the anterior half of the middle meatus. A further improvement in inspection is provided by making the mucosa

RHINOSCOPY WITH A TELESCOPE

Many attempts have been reported to extend the frontal view into the nose to the meatuses by employing various instruments by Czermak,[1] Wertheim,[15] Voltolini,[14] and Rethi.[13] The first to succeed was Hirschmann,[2] who in 1901 inserted a cystoscope into the middle nasal meatus following a surgical intervention on the concha media or the ethmoid. Unfortunately this method was not employed until some years later. Reasons for this could be the discovery of the effects caused by cocaine and the possibilities offered by x-ray examinations. Most physicians believed there was no need for

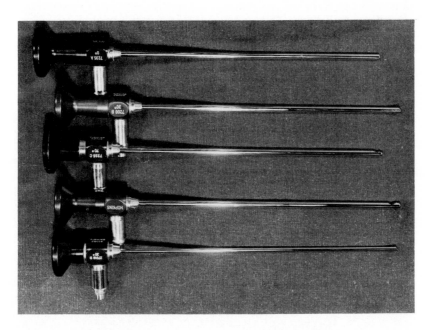

FIG. 6. From top to bottom (first four instruments): Hopkins telescopes with 0, 30, 70, and 120-degree directions of view. At the bottom is a small 30-degree telescope (2.8 mm OD). (Manufacturer: Storz Endoscopy Co., Tuttlingen, West Germany)

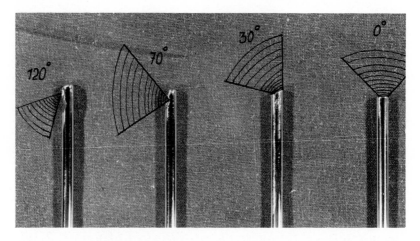

FIG. 7. Visual fields of the different endoscopes (120, 70, 30, and 0 degrees).

further improvements in rhinoscopy.[16] Probably the main reason for the lack of progress was the difficulties of anatomy—the bony boundaries and the narrow meatuses.

ENDOSCOPES

The Hopkins telescope with 30-, 70-, and 120-degree directions of view, 18 cm length, and 4 mm diameter are most suitable. Smaller optics are available for narrow regions (2.8 mm in diameter only with a forward oblique view of 30 degrees). The visual field of this instrument, however, is considerably restricted compared to those which are 4 mm in diameter (Figs. 6 and 7).

Polyethylene tubes (3 mm OD) with round tips are used for suction. A cannula with a guide for the soft suction tube is attached to the telescope (Fig. 8).

TECHNIQUE

The patient lies on the operating table facing the examiner, who sits on his left. The instrument table (Fig. 9) is on the examiner's left, and the light is positioned at the head of the operating table (Fig. 10).

Anesthesia of the mucosa is obtained with topical anesthetics. If a vasoconstrictor is added it should not influence the color of the mucosa. The procedure can be started 1 to 2 minutes later.

The 30-degree telescope is inserted, under vi-

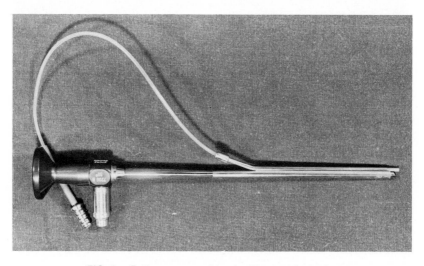

FIG. 8. Endoscope combined with a suction tube.

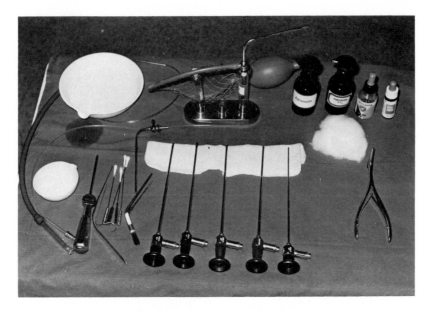

FIG. 9. Table with instruments for anterior rhinoscopy.

sion, into the joint meatus of the nose up to the choana. When the endoscope is too close to the mucous membrane, secretion on the objective disturbs the view. By using the forward oblique telescope the metal sheath is slightly longer. If secretion adheres, it is helpful to pull the instrument back into this tube in order to remove the secretion and regain free vision. The endoscope is reintroduced by changing the direction slightly to eliminate further contact with mucosa or secretion.

Following inspection of the epipharynx, the rhinoscope is slightly withdrawn and at the same time directed laterally or lateral-cranially to the nasal meatus, which is to be examined. Thereafter it is guided to the broadest part of the meatus. Sometimes it is easy to advance, but often slight pressure is necessary, perhaps in combination with slight withdrawal, to overcome a certain resistance and to reach the meatus. Very seldom a part of the concha is fractured. Bleeding creates difficulties for the examination but fortunately occurs rarely. Inserting the instrument and inspecting the meatus only from back to front means that the mucosa or the concha is pushed aside tangentially by the smooth sheath of the rhinoscope. Once the meatus is reached it is inspected from back to front. In some cases it is necessary to exchange the optic, which is possible during the procedure without difficulty.

This examination also achieves satisfactory visualization in cases of considerable deviation of the septum or in narrow noses of other eti-

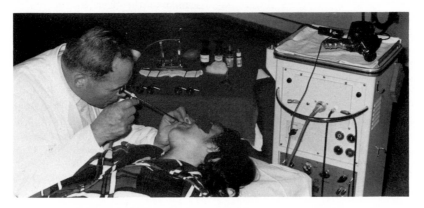

FIG. 10. Position of the patient during the procedure.

ology. Sometimes the impression is gained, mainly during the operator's learning period, that the nose is too narrow for introduction of an endoscope. When it is tried nevertheless, it may happen that one or the other mucosal area can be suddenly displaced and the nose may be easily scoped. The endoscope can also slide tangentially over a septal thorn that looked to be impassable. In case of a mechanical obstruction (e.g., a septal thorn reaching far back into the middle meatus) not permitting insertion into the sphenoethmoidal recess, it is possible to inspect this region. The 70-degree rhinoscope is inserted into the joint meatus and passed under the obstruction; one can then look up into the posterior region of ethmoid. If this method fails, a 120-degree endoscope is introduced into the epipharynx through the other nasal part, and this region is then inspected from behind, through the choana.

A certain amount of experience is required to be able to take full advantage of all the possibilities offered by endoscopy. Endoscopy enables recognition of a wide range of anatomic variations and pathologic changes.

The inferior meatus of the nose is a hall-like space open to the bottom, which is formed by the concave conchal area, the conchal sinus. Normally the lateral nasal wall protrudes into it. Apart from circumscribed or diffuse inflammation of the mucosa, all protrusions of the lateral upper wall into the lumen of the meatus caused by a pathologic process of the adjoining paranasal sinus are of interest. A lateral and cranial protrusion can fill the inferior meatus. It can be caused by a mucocele of the anterior ethmoid or a malignant tumor in the maxillary sinus of the anterior ethmoid. In this region malignant lesions often detach the mucosa from the bone without obvious infiltration or perforation. The ductus nasolacrimalis can open into the anterior lower meatus in various ways. The opening is funnel-shaped, and the duct can be visualized by means of a steeply angled optic. Sometimes branching of a small diverticulum can be seen. Diseases of the nasal mucosa or of the paranasal sinuses may involve the duct; narrowing the duct can cause epiphora.

The posterior part of the middle meatus, behind the bulla ethmoidalis, is also a hall-shaped space. Its medial wall is formed by a conchal sinus,[17] which is covered by mucosa that can easily become swollen. In the presence of disease there is a fine fissure at the margin of the concha.

The lateral wall behind and beneath the ostium of the maxillary sinus is only partially membranous; these parts are known as the nasal fontanelle.[17] Often an accessory maxillary ostium is found here. The mucosa of the fontanelle is highly susceptible to any kind of irritation—the nasal part as well as the maxillary part—but it also can be affected by itself. In a case a maxillary sinusitis the fontanelle is often swollen and bulges to such an extent that it blocks the middle meatus (inferior fontanelle) (Fig. 11, Plate J)* or fills the conchal sinus (posterior fontanelle). If the fontanelles are well developed they almost reach the maxillary ostium or can partly form its boundaries. Under such circumstances a swelling of the fontanelle, in the course of a case of maxillary sinusitis, can extremely narrow the ostium and cause a valve occlusion, creating difficulties in irrigating the maxillary sinus. The maxillary ostium is normally situated at the end of the hiatus semilunaris (Fig. 12, Plate J), sometimes, however, it is situated more toward the front, underneath the bulla ethmoidalis. It can vary in size, and its position can be anything from horizontal to vertical.

The anterior part of the middle meatus is an irregular and curved cleft that can be endoscoped in spite of its narrow shape, in most cases from back to front. Medially, this part is also surrounded in the back by the conchal sinus into which the bulla ethmoidalis often deeply projects (Fig. 13, Plate J); it is limited in the front by the head of the middle concha. In the head of the concha may be an osseous cell which normally opens in the conchal sinus and only seldom in the superior meatus, and sometimes they communicate with the anterior ethmoid sinus. The lateral wall of this region is formed in the back by the bulla ethmoidalis, which can vary in size. Normally the ostium is at the top, but sometimes it appears also in the front or in the back. The anterior ethmoid cells open in front of and behind the bulla, which is surrounded below by the hiatus semilunaris, which leads into the infundibulum (Fig. 14, Plate J). The ductus frontalis opens in various ways at the anterior end of the hiatus. The medial boundaries of the hiatus semilunaris or the infundibulum are formed by the processus

All color plates appear at the front of the book.

uncinatus. Its free margin is often bent medially, turning in the front into the agger nasi.

The anterior portion of the middle meatus of the nose can have many anatomic variations. For example, the head of the concha can appear to be normal. Just behind it, at the margin of the concha, however, a sagittal congenital fissure appears, separating the concha far to the back. Medially, in the front, the fissure continues upward (cranially) and forms a second head. The anterior head of the concha can be large, and the posterior medial head embodies a large turbinal cell. The concha can also be divided into two parts at the bottom by a delicate sagittal congenital fissure. It appears as if something is protruding laterally from the middle nasal meatus that looks like a concha in the middle meatus of the nose. However, it is only an enlarged processus uncinatus curved medially.

The difficulty in interpreting pathologic changes are thus demonstrated. For instance, a latent inflammation of infundibular cells which reach far to the front or anterior ethmoid cells can be concealed behind the protrusion of the agger nasi, but the disorder can also be a malignant tumor originating from there or perforating from the region of the lacrimal sac. Pathologic infundibular cells may be responsible for an infiltration of the processus uncinatus. The inflammation may be, for instance, the result of a spontaneous formation of concrements in the maxillary sinus which has spread through the ostium to the middle of the nasal meatus; on the other hand, it may be a mycotic infection of the maxillary sinus. Tissue projecting from the anterior middle meatus might be, among other things, a mucosal hyperplasia originating from the margin of the processus uncinatus or a bulla ethmoidalis which is enlarged toward the front. Polyps—if isolated, small, and squeezed into the upper part of the meatus—usually originate in the bulla ethmoidalis. Polypous tissue at the lower circumference of the bulla ethmoidalis can be a carcinoma which, still circumscribed, started at the ethmoidal cells. The mucosa of the head of the middle concha can develop an isolated hyperplasia; but solitary polyps can also arise from the neck or head of the concha. If the head of the concha seems to be elongated to the front, and the mucosa is studded with small starlike vascular markings, it may indicate a defined empyema of the frontal sinus or the anterior ethmoid. The same disease, however, may also enlarge the agger nasi to such an extent that the head of the concha disappears. When a bony cell in the conchal head is involved, the inflammation spreads to the external mucosa. Although this inflammation is often not very obvious, in most cases it causes a frontal fissure which clearly separates the conchal head from the conchal body at the free margin. The same disease, however, can also cause a diffuse hyperplasia of the mucous membrane of the conchal head or changes in a large polyp. In the case of perforation of an affected conchal cell it is possible that, apart from a permanent suppuration, a solitary polyp may evert from the perforation; or in the case of spontaneous healing, an ostium can remain in the conchal head.

When inserting a 30-degree telescope just in front of the choana between the septum and the posterior end of the middle concha toward the recessus sphenoethmoidalis, the plicae septi repeatedly appear at the upper margin of the choana. Going back toward the cranium, the ostium of the sphenoid bone, normally round or oval (Fig. 15, Plate J), is visible. Sometimes it is also possible to insert a small endoscope into the sphenoid sinus. In the case of acute sinusitis sphenoidalis the ostium is swollen, slit-like, and discharging pulsating secretion; however, after recurrent inflammations, it is narrowed by scarring or even divided by a synechia. A mucocele of the sphenoid sinus is recognizable by a nipple-shaped protrusion into the region of the ostium. If an epipharyngeal carcinoma grows into the bone, the whole anterior wall of the sphenoid bulges out and the mucous membrane shows typical small varicosities.

When directing the endoscope cranially and laterally, the superior and highest ethmoidal conchae appear with their ducts. Here we can also find a wide range of anatomic variations due to formation of partial conchae, conchal rudiments, etc. When after a short inspection the 30-degree endoscope is changed to one with a 70-degree angle it is often possible to look deeply into one or both nasal meatuses. Figure 16 (Plate J) shows the superior and highest concha. In the highest concha one cell has developed into an operculum, narrowing the posterior part of the rima olfactoria. At the bottom, between operculum and septum, the ostium sphenoidale is still recognizable; whereas in the highest nasal meatus the ostium of the operculum is well visible. By slowly reintroducing the rhinoscope between septum and middle concha, it is also possible to examine this region completely with its various origins and forms of the superior ethmoid conchae. There are possible variations. For instance, the superior concha can arise just behind the head of the concha media regularly from the medial space of the middle concha. The inflammatory changes of the superior meatuses and conchae are very similar to those of the concha media—i.e., there is a tumefaction of the conchal head when developed, fissures at the free conchal margin indicating a disease of the conchal sinus, etc. A chronic increase in intracranial pressure can cause slight symptoms in the environment of the recessus sphenoethmoidalis: Either the mucosa of this area pulsates (which is clearly visible through the endoscope by the light reflection), or there is marked swelling of the mucous membrane (without inflammation blocking the view into the sphenoid ostium) and a sagittal fissure develops at the free margin of the superior concha—probably as a sign of congestion.

Apart from the advantage of being able to examine all sections of the nose—which until now could not be seen without surgical intervention—rhinoscopy with the telescope offers further possibilities.[8,9,10,11,12]

SUMMARY

1. Introducing the Hopkins telescope into the deeper parts of the nose, near the mucous membrane, magnifies the area to such an extent that in the illuminated portions the ciliary movements are easily visible if there are no pathologic changes in the secretion.
2. By tagging the secretion with an insoluble powder that is easily seen, it is possible to observe movement of the secretion.
3. By staining cerebrospinal fluid with fluorescein, a nasal liquorrhea can be diagnosed and localized for appropriate operative management.
4. Finally, it is possible to perform various intranasal operations under the excellent visibility provided by endoscopy.

REFERENCES

1. Czermak JN: Uber die Inspektion des Cavum pharyngo-nasale und der Nasenhohle vermittels kleiner Spiegel (Rhinoskopie). Wien Med Wochenschr 17, 1860
2. Hirschmann A: Endoskopie der Nase und ihrer Nebenhohlen. Arch Laryngol Rhinol (Berl) 14: 195, 1903
3. Killian G: Uber Rhinoskopia media. Munch Med Wochenschr 33, 1896
4. Messerklinger W: Die Endoskopie der Nase. Monatsschr Ohrenheilkunde Rhinol Laryngol (Wien) 104:451, 1970
5. Messerklinger W: Endoskopie des unteren Nasenganges. Monatsschr Ohren Laryngol Rhinol (Wien) 106:569, 1972
6. Messerklinger W: Nasenendoskopie: Der mittlere Nasengang und seine unspezifischen Entzundungen. HNO 20:212, 1972
7. Messerklinger W: Nasenendoskopie: Nachweis, Lokalisation und Differentialdiagnose der nasalen Liquorrhoe. HNO 20:268, 1972
8. Messerklinger W: Technik und Moglichkeiten der Nasenendoskopie. HNO 20:133, 1972
9. Messerklinger W: Uber die Kieferhohlenfontanelle. Acta Otolaryngol (Stockh) 73:290, 1972
10. Messerklinger W: Uber pathologische Veranderungen der Kieferhohlenfontanelle. Arch Klin Exp Ohren Nasen Kehlkopfheilkunde 199:675, 1971
11. Messerklinger W: Zur endoskopischen Anatomie der menschlichen Siebbeinmuscheln. Acta Otolaryngol (Stockh) 75:243, 1973
12. Messerklinger W, Eggemann G: Uber die spontane Konkrementbildung in der Kieferhohle. (Ein Symptom der Kieferhohlen-Mykose?) Monatsschr Ohren Laryngol Rhinol (Wien) 107: 456, 1973
13. Rethi L: Ein Spiegel zur endonasalen Besichtigung. Prager Med Wochenschr 42, 1893
14. Voltolini R: Die Rhinoskopie und die Pharyngoskopie. 2. Auflage. Breslau, Verlag E. Morgenstern, 1879
15. Wertheim: Uber ein Verfahren zum Zwecke der Besichtigung des vorderen und mittleren Drittels der Nasenhohle. Wien Med Wochenschr 18–20, 1879
16. Zarniko C: Diagnostik der Nasenkrankheiten. Denker-Kahler: Handbuch der Hals-, Nasen-, Ohrenheilkunde. Berlin, Springer, Band 1, 1925
17. Zuckerkandl E: Normale und pathologische Anatomie der Nasenhohle und ihrer pneumatischen Anhange. Vienna, Verlag W. Braumuller, 1893

52

Thoracoscopy

Jacob Swierenga

Thoracoscopy is a diagnostic and therapeutic procedure that has been known for many years. It was first practiced by Jacobeus[2] in 1925 in Sweden to cauterize adhesions between the visceral and parietal pleura in the production of an artificial pneumothorax.

At that time artificial pneumothorax was commonly used in connection with the collapse therapy of tuberculosis. After this form of therapy was discontinued, thoracoscopy fell into disuse, only to be rediscovered much later. We first rediscovered it around 1950 in the diagnosis of spontaneous pneumothorax, and since that time the technique has proved to be of great value in a variety of diseases involving the pleura, thorax wall, mediastinum, and lung. The increasing importance of this examination is also attributable to the consistent improvement in the equipment. Distinct from the appliances used in former days, we now invariably employ what are called cold-light sources, the sources being localized outside the patient's body. We believe that thoracoscopy can be performed under local anesthesia at all times. Without question, the presence of a pneumothorax is imperative—i.e., if it does not exist it should be induced. Adhesions between the visceral and parietal pleura prevent the performance of a thoracoscopy in the majority of cases.

TECHNIQUE

The patient is premedicated with 200 mg Luminal and a small amount of morphine or a derivative thereof. Before thoracoscopy is undertaken, an x-ray picture is made to ascertain that a proper pneumothorax has been induced. The insertion site is determined according to the expected location of the anomaly. At this point (local) anesthesia is infiltrated by injecting a 0.5 percent Novocain solution. It is most important to ensure that the anesthesia infiltrates the intercostal space and the parietal pleura. Once the local anesthesia is given, a small skin incision is made with a knife, and a trocar is introduced. The thoracoscope is then passed through the trocar, and the examination can be started.

The thoracoscope, with its various optical systems, permits the inspection of almost the entire lung surface, the thorax wall, diaphragm, pericardium, and mediastinum. This modus operandi also allows the collection of further information about a possible diagnosis of lesions localized in one of these sites. During thoracoscopy a tissue sample of the parietal or visceral pleura may be taken. Similarly, a biopsy may be obtained from suspicious tissue of the mediastinum, pericardium, or diaphragm. In dubious cases it is also possible to perform a biopsy of an inspected anomaly by a specially designed biopsy needle.

Interpretation of the picture, however, is always important, and in fact is the most significant aspect of the examination. This calls for a wealth of experience. It is also possible to take a small specimen from the periphery of the lung if anomalies are seen. Once the thoracoscopy has been completed, the air of the pneumothorax can be aspirated by means of a temporarily inserted drain; or the pneumothorax may be maintained, for example, in those cases where an operation is to be considered.

Color figures for this chapter appear at the front of the book (Plate K).

INDICATIONS FOR THORACOSCOPY

Pneumothroax

The clinical picture of idiopathic spontaneous pneumothorax[4] has been recognized for many years. In former times it was argued that tuberculosis was an important condition in the genesis of this anomaly. It subsequently became evident that tuberculosis hardly played a role. Following the introduction of thoracotomy in the treatment of specific types of pneumothorax, blebs or bullae were found on the surface of the lung on several occasions. Since 1952 we have examined by thoracoscopy about 1,000 cases of spontaneous pneumothorax, with the following findings:

No abnormalities found	35%
Local adhesions between the visceral and parietal pleura	12%
Local, predominantly small blebs localized on a small portion of the lung, particularly on the apex	35%
Anomalies localized on the surface of the upper lobe	18%

A noticeable feature is that fewer anomalies were found during the early years than subsequently. In our view this is undoubtedly due to the refinement in the investigation technique. Depending on the anomaly detected by thoracoscopic examination, we make the decision as to the treatment. We feel that in spontaneous pneumothorax thoracotomy removal of the blebs and partial pleurectomy are necessary to avoid relapse. Pleurectomy and removal of the bullae may likewise be performed for moderately extensive small bullae. If the anomalies or adhesions occur to a minor extent we think that spraying with iodated talc (1:1,000) and drainage comprise sufficient treatment. In all instances continuous aspiration is applied at a pressure of approximately 30 mm Hg for 24 to 48 hours. If proper reexpansion is achieved after 48 hours there is nearly always splendid recovery. Relapse following such treatment is very rare. In our series of pleurectomies we did not observe relapses after spraying with 2 percent talc. They always occurred, however, if blebs or bullae were still present.[5]

Exudative Pleurisy

In many cases of exudative pleurisy a diagnosis can be established on the basis of clinical findings, e.g., by culturing pleural fluid containing bacteria or by cytologic examination of the pleural fluid in which carcinoma cells may be found.[1] In a number of instances, however, it is impossible to establish the cause of the pleurisy with any certainty. In our opinion a thoracoscopic examination is particularly useful in these cases. A prerequisite is the presence of fluid in the pleura. The fluid is aspirated and air instantly injected, inducing a pneumothorax. Thoracoscopy is performed, permitting exploration of the entire visceral and parietal pleura and the detection of any pathology that may be present. If anomalies are seen a tissue sample can be readily taken from the parietal pleura in particular, after which a pathologic and anatomic examination can be performed. This procedure has enabled us to make much progress in the diagnosis of patients with pleurisy. In 400 cases we have studied to date we could rapidly and adequately make the following diagnoses:

Tuberculosis	11.5%
Empyema	15.4%
Nonbacterial pleurisy	18.0%
Rheumatism and lupus erythematosus	3.0%
Primary pleural tumor	9.0%
Carcinomatous pleurisy	15.5%
Pleural fibrosis or pleural thickening of unknown genesis	19.0%
Hemothorax	3.3%
Transudate	3.0%
Miscellaneous	2.3%

Extreme importance is attached to the thoracoscopic examination in tuberculous pleurisy, which in contrast to previous means is a rapid method of forming a definitive diagnosis. The same is true for carcinomatous pleurisy where the cytologic examination of the pleural fluid is negative. This is so in 35 percent of our subjects. The cytology of the pleural fluid is negative in many cases (approximately 50 percent) of primary malignant pleurisy tumors (e.g., mesothelioma). If thoracoscopy can be performed, this procedure enables us to arrive at a diagnosis in 90 percent and nearly 100 percent, respectively, of the cases of mesothelioma and carcinomatous pleurisy. Thoracoscopy is not so important in other cases of pleurisy but nevertheless constitutes a welcome diagnostic adjunct.[3]

Thorax Wall and Mediastinal Tumors

In many cases of tumors of the thorax wall and the mediastinum, a very fine picture of the tumor can be obtained after induction of a pneumothorax and thoracoscopy. This procedure permits a splended direct-vision inspection of the tumor; if required, a biopsy can be performed at all times. In cases where a vascularized tumor might be present, or where, for example, the tumor has a cystic appearance, the desirability of a biopsy must be considered. Under these circumstances we think that it is advisable to probe the lesion before a biopsy is taken. When a very thin-walled cyst is found, for instance, all that can be said is that it is a cyst. Pneumothorax plus thoracoscopy has enabled us to make great progress in diagnosing cystic tumors as well. In fact, it is for this reason that we regularly proceed to thoracoscopy when mediastinal and thorax wall tumors are involved if the diagnosis cannot be established by other means. To date we have performed 200 thoracoscopies on the basis of this indication, and positive diagnoses were made in a high percentage of subjects. This applies to thorax wall and mediastinal tumors as well as to anomalies of the diaphragm.

Anomalies in the Lung Periphery

In recent years an increasing number of reports have appeared in the literature which describe the thoracoscopic diagnosis of anomalies in the periphery of the lung. Such anomalies comprise:

1. Diffusely scattered pulmonary anomalies for which no diagnosis could be established by means of conventional methods and for which the possibility of an open lung biopsy was considered. In these cases it is possible to produce a pneumothorax and subsequently to perform thoracoscopy. During thoracoscopy biopsies can be taken from different points of the lung. We have used this method only occasionally, and we do not recommend it because it does not ensure proper hemostasis; moreover, it involves the possibility of dealing with hypervascular lesions so that, for example, a pulmonary hemorrhage or air embolus may develop. Investigators who employed this technique, however, have not observed many complications.
2. Small, subpleural tumors in close proximity to the periphery. In these cases a diagnosis is sometimes made only with great difficulty, and the diagnosis is of paramount importance for therapy. In instances where it has been impossible to make a diagnosis by other means because of a closed thorax, pneumothorax plus thoracoscopy is the method of choice. A biopsy can be taken from the local focus if the anomaly is distinctly visible. We think that this is a great step forward, and for this reason we shall certainly continue to recommend this examination technique.

COMPLICATIONS

Complications are extremely rare after this procedure. Among 1,500 thoracoscopies only two patients developed an empyema, and both had uneventful recoveries. Hemorrhage resulting from excisions or biopsies was never observed. So far we have seen no complications resulting from lung biopsies or excisions, but we have not had a long experience with these procedures.

In carcinomatous pleurisy there is a possibility of spread of the carcinoma along the tract of the trocar insertion (implantation of tumor cells). We believe that this complication can be taken into account or accepted because of the advantages gained by this method of examination.

CONCLUSION

Thoracoscopic examination has been a valuable adjuvant in the diagnosis and treatment of:

1. Idiopathic spontaneous pneumothorax
2. Pleurisy
3. Disease and tumors of the thorax wall, mediastinum, pericardium, and diaphragm
4. Anomalies localized in the periphery of the lung or anomalies diffusely scattered throughout the lung

We have found that the percentage of positive diagnoses in a variety of diseases has distinctly increased since we have used this diagnostic examination procedure We also feel that the improved diagnosis has resulted in more efficient therapy, especially of spontaneous pneumothorax and various mediastinal thorax wall anomalies.

We believe that in the future thoracoscopy can find an even wider range of indications, and that the diagnostic capability can be further developed—e.g., by constructing a flexible thoracoscope. Such an instrument would afford a still better view of the areas of the lung situated on the mediastinal or the dorsomedial side. This is important since in some instances (e.g., in the case of a pneumothorax) a bleb or bulla is occasionally overlooked.

REFERENCES

1. Berquist S, Nordenstam H: Thoracoscopy and pleural biopsy in the diagnosis of pleurisy. Scand J Resp Dis 47:64, 1966

2. Jacobaeus HC: Die Thorakoskopie und ihre praktische Bedeutung. Ergeb Ges Med 7:112, 1925

3. Lloyd MS: Thoracoscopy and biopsy in the diagnosis of pleurisy with effusion. Q Bull Sea View Hosp 14:128, 1953

4. Sattler A: Zur Behandlung des Spontanpneumothorax mit besonderer Berücksichtigung der Thorakoskopie. Beitr Klin Tbk 89:395, 1937

5. Wagenaar JPM: De zogenaamde idiopathische spontane pneumothorax. Academisch Proefschrift Leiden 36, 1970

53

Transconioscopy

Henning Sørensen

Percutaneous puncture of the tracheal wall with introduction of a telescope for inspection of the subglottic space was first performed by Euler[4] in 1954. In 1967 Mårtensson[7] introduced transconioscopy in a large clinical study. Puncture of the cricothyroid membrane had previously been performed for bronchography,[3] tracheal anesthesia,[2] and physiologic studies of the trachea.[5]

Transconioscopy is a method for examination of the larynx and the subglottic space. It implies that the cricothyroid membrane is punctured percutaneously under local anesthesia and a telescope is introduced into the subglottic space, thus permitting retrograde inspection of the larynx.

The laryngeal lumen can be visualized by the following methods available for evaluating the nature and extent of pathologic processes:

1. *Indirect laryngoscopy* is the most important method in the detection of any disease in the larynx.
2. *Direct laryngoscopy* under general anesthesia should be performed in every case of laryngeal carcinoma if possible with the operating microscope. However, the fact that the visual axis coincides with the longitudinal axis of the larynx limits the possibility of inspecting the sinus Morgagni and subglottic space. Furthermore the laryngoscope often cannot be advanced beyond lumen-constricting tumors, which means that their caudal part cannot be inspected. Thus it may be impossible to determine the margins, especially the lower border of the tumor. Moreover, valuable information on the mobility of the vocal cords cannot be obtained during general anesthesia.
3. *Endoscopic inspection.* A telescope with a lateral view is introduced via the laryngoscope. This permits inspection in other than the longitudinal direction. The field of vision is limited, however, because of the rather small lumen of the larynx, and it may be difficult to avoid contact with the mucosa. Furthermore it is often impossible to advance a telescope beyond parts of an exophytic tumor.
4. *Roentgenologic examination* of the larynx may permit a more accurate determination of the tumor's extent than does laryngoscopy—especially when supplemented by tomography or laryngography. However, the x-rays cannot determine the nature of the pathologic contours—whether these are due to a malignant lesion, edema, or anatomic variations.

The most reliable determination of the true nature of the pathologic process is obtained by visualizing the surface structure and color of the lesion. The shortcomings of the above-mentioned methods of examination have led to the introduction of transconioscopy as a supplementary procedure.

TECHNIQUE

The patient is premedicated with morphine and scopolamine for sedation and to reduce secretions in the upper airways. The patient is placed in a supine position with the larynx presenting and easily palpable, with as much distance between the cricoid and the thyroid cartilage as possible.

After skin preparation, the site of puncture over the cricothyroid membrane is anesthetized with 1 percent lidocaine and the needle is inserted through the membrane. When the needle is in the subglottic space—which position-

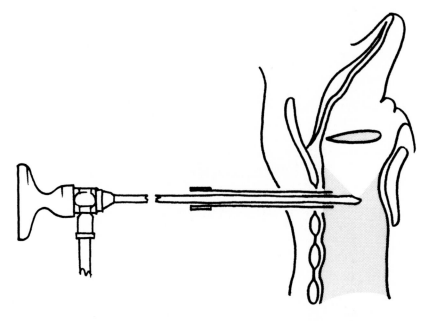

FIG. 1. Telescope in position in the subglottic larynx, introduced through the trocar.

ing can be assured by the withdrawal of air into the syringe—0.5 to 1.0 ml lidocaine is injected as a surface anesthesia. A horizontal incision 5 mm long is made in the skin, and a trocar (6 mm OD) is introduced through the membrane by even pressure while the larynx is fixed with the left hand. After removal of the stylet, a telescope (Hopkin's 70-degree telescope, 4 mm OD*) with fiber light is introduced through the trocar at a right angle to the longitudinal axis of the larynx (Fig. 1). The telescope has a wide range of mobility in the subglottic space. It may be rotated, moved in and out, and the angle of the telescope axis in relation to the larynx changed. By these movements the greater part of the larynx and the subglottic space can be inspected. The field of vision is 10 times as large as that which can be obtained by a telescope introduced via a laryngoscope.

The distance from the site of puncture to the border of the vocal cords is 1 to 1.5 cm. The border and undersurface of the vocal cords, as well as the anterior and posterior commissures, can be inspected; and the upper part of the trachea can be seen by rotating the scope. During inspiration the vocal cords are maximally abducted, thus permitting a view of the entire

posterior aspect of the epiglottis and the lower surface of the ventricular band. At phonation the picture is dominated by the arytenoid regions, which project into the view considerably and usually permit inspection only of the anterior half of the vocal cords. The movements of the larynx are clearly seen. In particular, it is easy to note differences in the mobility of the two sides. The Morgagni sinus and the upper surface of the vocal cords are not visible. Transconioscopy offers optimal illumination of the slanting mucosal wall just below the vocal cords, which is hidden in the shadow and outside the axis of vision at indirect and direct laryngoscopy. Even small anomalies such as hyperemia, patches of leukoplakia, or minute ulcerations are clearly visible, as well as slight impairments in the functional appearance.

INDICATIONS

The procedure is indicated in the evaluation of malignant tumors (Figs. 2–7, Plate L).*

Supraglottic Tumors

The caudal border of the supraglottic tumor can be seen, and the relation of the tumor to

Manufactured by K. Storz, Endoscopy Co., 72 Tuttlingen, PO Box 400, West Germany.

All color plates appear at the front of the book.

the vocal cords can be determined. Invasion of the vocal cord, which may be overlooked by direct laryngoscopy, can be demonstrated by transconioscopy. In large supraglottic lesions the growth of the tumor often impedes evaluation of the vocal cord at direct laryngoscopy, as it may be completely hidden by tumor. Also deeper infiltration in the tissue may be disclosed at transconioscopy by which information of the mobility is obtained. Thus with this technique a more accurate diagnosis of the mucosal changes of supraglottic tumors can be made, which may be important in the choice of therapy and ultimately in the prognosis of the disease.

Glottic Tumors

In glottic tumors accurate knowledge of the site and extent of the tumor is of paramount therapeutic and prognostic significance; even a small supraglottic or subglottic extension can change the outlook for the patient. A subglottic extension of a vocal cord lesion may be overlooked by direct laryngoscopy and x-ray tomography, but transconioscopy enables the subglottic extension to be definitely diagnosed in every case, and even observed by repeated examinations during or after a course of radiation therapy. An undiagnosed subglottic extension of a small vocal cord tumor may be the reason for therapeutic failure. It may be assumed that a number of glottic lesions not responding to irradiation had an extension that was not recognized at the beginning of therapy because of inadequate methods of investigation.

Subglottic Tumors

A primary malignant tumor in the mucous membrane in the subglottic space occurs very seldom but can be detected by transconioscopy. Most subglottic tumors occur as extensions of vocal cord lesions. Such extension of a carcinoma involves the lateral wall more often than the ventral wall.[1] The infrequent subglottic invasion to the ventral wall is very often visible at laryngoscopy, in which case the puncture for transconioscopy should not be performed. It is only by subglottic extension of larger glottic tumors that inspection of the anterior part of the subglottic space by laryngoscopy may be obscured. In such a case the

risk of puncture through malignant tissue is present.

The choice of therapeutic measures in malignant laryngeal diseases must be based on an exact determination of the site and size of the lesion. The margins of the tumor must be exactly assessed and the infiltration in the submucous tissue evaluated. Consideration of the possible submucosal modes of extension of a lesion may affect not only the lines of surgical excision but also the area of planned radiation.

As shown by Tucker,[10] submucosal extension also occurs in the subglottic larynx on the posterior wall. The difficulties in diagnosing a submucosal tumor infiltration are great, but transconioscopy may be of value in solving the problems in many cases.

Transconioscopy has been shown to be a valuable aid in improving on the diagnostic success rate for superficial malignant laryngeal disease compared with other available methods of examination.[7,8]

COMPLICATIONS

Transconioscopy is a simple procedure easily done under local anesthesia in outpatients. The patient can leave the hospital immediately after the examination without any discomfort.

Small hemorrhages within the larynx can occur, but rarely to such a degree that the examination is impeded, nor is it so profuse as to be manifested as hemoptysis. Among more than 100 cases examined by transconioscopy we have had only one in which the examination could not be carried out because of bleeding.

A small subcutaneous emphysema in the neck develops in about one-third of the cases and persists for a few hours. The coughing that provokes this emphysema may be avoided by proper application of local anesthesia before the puncture. Infection of the puncture canal is rarely seen.

The risk of perforation of the posterior wall of the subglottic space is minimal thanks to the thick cricoid cartilage, which offers effective protection, and was never seen in our clinic. Puncture through carcinomatous tissue may result in the cancer cells spreading through the puncture canal; it must be regarded as the most dangerous risk and the only real objection to this method of examination.[9,11] As mentioned, however, subglottic extension of a tumor is very seldom found in the ventral wall of the subglottis. In this site it is possible to recognize the lesion at laryngoscopy, except in a case in which inspection of the ventral wall is prevented by a large supraglottic tumor. However, subglottic extension of such a tumor occurs only at a very late stage, and therefore the risk may be regarded as slight. The evident value of transconioscopy in the topical diagnosis justifies the rather slight risk that this method of examination presents. Until now we have not observed a single case in which local recurrence could be proved to be due to transconioscopy. In cases where perforation of the cancerous tissue occurs, due regard to this must be taken in the therapeutic measures.

CONCLUSION

As transconioscopy has proved to be a highly reliable method for evaluating subglottic lesions, it is indicated in every case of carcinoma of the larynx in which subglottic extension cannot be excluded with certainty.

In large *supraglottic* tumors transconioscopy may be valuable in determining the lower margins, which may not be visible in direct laryngoscopy and which may prevent introduction of a telescope via the laryngoscope. Exact localization of the lower border of a supraglottic lesion is necessary for the evaluation of a partial laryngectomy.

A *glottic* tumor may project so much from the margin of the vocal cord that determination of its extent toward the caudal surface of the cord or to the mucous membrane of the subglottic space cannot be obtained by other methods of examination. Limitation of the lesion to the vocal cord is decisive for the performance of a partial saggital laryngectomy (cordectomy or hemilaryngectomy). When there is invasion of the subglottic space, other therapeutic measures should be taken (irradiation or total laryngectomy).

Small *subglottic* lesions may escape detection by other methods of examination but can be clearly seen during transconioscopy. Last but not least, the *mobility of the vocal cords,* which is of paramount importance in the evaluation of a deep infiltration of carcinomatous lesions, can always be seen at transconioscopy.

REFERENCES

1. Baclasse F: Radiographic diagnosis of tumours of the pharynx and larynx. In Modern Trends in Diagnostic Radiology. London, Butterworth, 1948
2. Bonica JJ: Transtracheal anaesthesia for endotracheal intubation. Anaesthesiology 10:736, 1949
3. Dietzel K: Endoskopiche Untersuchungsmöglichkeiten im Kehlkopf. Hals Nasen Ohrenheilkd 4:53, 1953/1954
4. Euler HE: Pertracheales tracheo-laryngoscopi. J Laryngol Rhinol 33:57, 1954
5. Ingelstedt S: Studies on the conditioning of air in the respiratory tract. Acta Otolaryngol (Stockh) [Suppl] 131, 1956
6. Mårtensson B: Transconioscopy in topical diagnosis of carcinoma of the larynx. Pract Otorhinolaryngol (Basel) 29:233, 1967
7. Mårtensson M, Fluur E, Jacobsson F: Aspects of treatment of cancer of the larynx. Ann Otolaryngol (Paris) 76:313, 1967
8. Sørensen H: Transconioscopy in laryngeal carcinoma. Arch Otolaryngol 92:28, 1970
9. Stell PM: Transconioscopy (correspondence). Arch Otolaryngol 93:338, 1971
10. Tucker G: Some clinical inferences from the study of serial laryngeal sections. Laryngoscope 73:728, 1963
11. Tucker G: Transconioscopy (correspondence). Arch Otolaryngol 93:540, 1971

Section IV: Special Subjects

54

Nephroscopy

Ruben F. Gittes
J. L. Williams

Early urologists endoscoped the kidney via a nephrotomy, usually in cases with an established nephrostomy tube tract, which permitted introduction of a urethroscope and removal of stones with Lowsley or Bumpus forceps.[7]

Operative pyeloscopy was developed over 25 years ago by Trattner and discussed in detail at the American Urological Association's meeting in 1948.[10] Trattner made a pyelotomy and sutured a metal valve into the opening. The sheath of his nephroscope was straight and 24 French (Fr.) in caliber. It was passed through the valve into the pelvis for a watertight connection (Fig. 1) and used standard optical telescopes. Because it was straight, the instrument demanded excessive manipulation of the kidney and contortions by the endoscopist who had to wear a sterile hood (Fig. 2).

It was the genius of the late Dr. W. F. Leadbetter that made him the father of the operative nephroscope we use today. In 1949 he reported[5] on the design, development, and clinical use of a nephroscope as a right-angled, one-piece instrument (Fig. 3). He described its

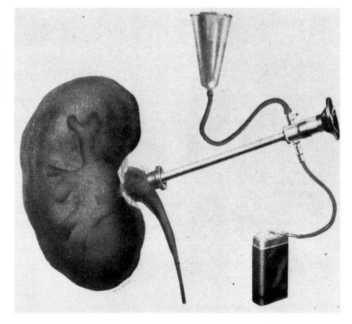

FIG. 1. Trattner's pyeloscope described in 1948. A metal flange was sewn into the renal pelvis for a watertight connection. (From Trattner: J Urol 60:817, 1948. Courtesy of the Journal of Urology.)

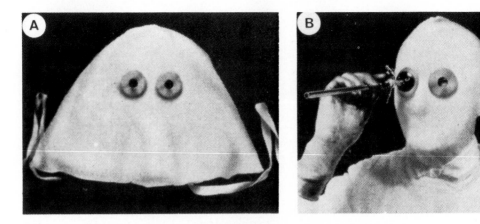

FIG. 2. Appearance of early nephroscopist in an attempt to prevent contamination of the wound while using Trattner's straight pyeloscope. (From Trattner: J Urol 60:817, 1948. Courtesy of the Journal of Urology.)

size as 22 Fr., "which allows it to enter infundibula and most calyces with comparative ease,"[5] and described its use through a simple pyelotomy to explore the renal collecting system systematically (Fig. 4). He was the first to report localization of hematuria to one diseased papilla via the nephroscope, permitting selective open surgery of that papilla.

Improvement of the optical transmission with a Hopkins lens system and fiberoptic light input have given us the current operating nephroscope with a 15 Fr. caliber and a 90-degree viewing angle.[11] It is made by Storz Instrument Company. As shown in Figures 5

and 6 it is similar to Leadbetter's design, but the exploring or horizontal portion of the shaft is shortened to 40 or 60 mm; furthermore the piece has only three built-in channels (optic, light, and water) with the option to clip on an instrumentation channel (Fig. 6) or a rigid forceps for biopsy or stone removal (Fig. 7). A notable and most useful development is the atraumatic stone forceps designed by Hertel,[3] shown in action in Figures 7 and 8.

Another and very different instrument is available for nonoperative, transurethral nephroscopy. Developed by the Japanese and called a pyelonephroscope,[8,9] it is designed to

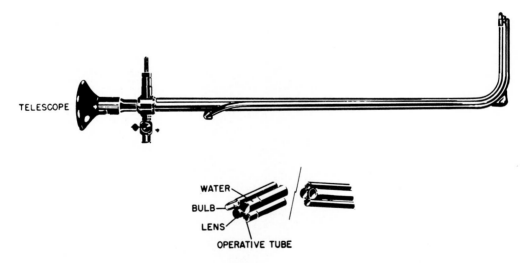

FIG. 3. Right-angled nephroscope introduced by Leadbetter in 1949. The operative tube was incorporated into the shaft as a fourth channel.

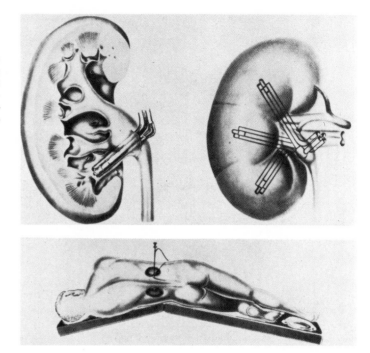

FIG. 4. Leadbetter's nephroscope in use. This technique led to the first reported surgical excision of a renal papilla for hematuria localized by nephroscopy. (From Leadbetter: J Urol 63:1006, 1950. Courtesy of the Journal of Urology.)

be passed through a cystoscope much like a large ureteral catheter. However, the currently available units represent, at best, a compromise between the limits of miniaturization of flexible fiberoptics and the specifications required for clinical usefulness. The individual fibers are 10 μ thick and cannot be reduced further without an unacceptable loss of optical resolution. The light-gathering compound lens at the tip of the bundle is the smallest ever made. As a result, the current limits of miniaturization of the optics have achieved an outside diameter of 2.7 mm (8 Fr.). This is close to the maximum caliber able to be threaded into the normal ureter from the bladder. The instrument thus has no room for an irrigation

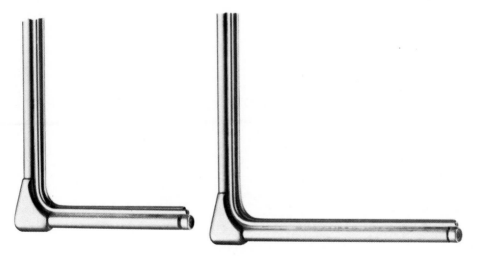

FIG. 5. Tips of Storz nephroscopes, with a 40 and 60 mm side area, incorporating the three channels needed for observation: rod-lens telescope, fiberoptic light input, and irrigation duct. Actual size is depicted.

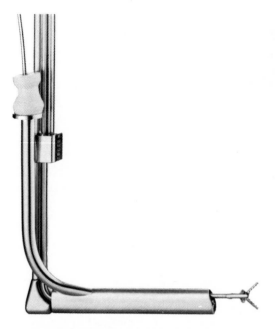

FIG. 6. Instrumentation channel shown attached to 60-mm tip Storz nephroscope, with alligator forceps in place.

channel. Certainly the inclusion of a channel for irrigation/manipulation will be necessary before any pyeloureteroscope becomes generally useful, since the urine is so often turbid with blood or debris in cases in which the upper urinary tract presents a diagnostic problem.

Current research in optics has achieved prototype instruments with 5-μ fibers and 0.5-mm lenses which will inevitably lead to the development of a pyeloureteroscope permitting directional manipulation into calyces, fluid irrigation, direct-vision biopsy, and fulguration.

INDICATIONS

The applications of the nephroscope have remained the same as envisioned by Leadbetter.[5]

Calculi

The operative nephroscope has rapidly become a valuable adjunct in all operations for renal calculi. About 90 percent of calyces may

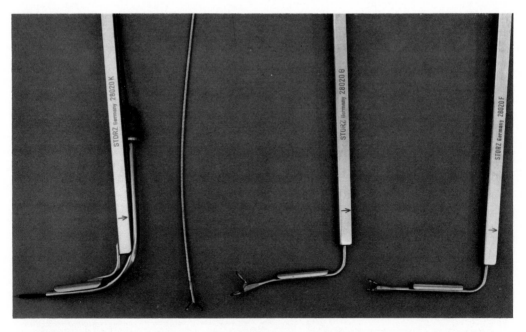

FIG. 7. Attachments for nephroscopic instrumentation. On the left is the hollow instrumentation channel with a Bugbee fulguration electrode in place and a flexible alligator forceps alongside, as in Figure 6. On the right is the Hertel stone forceps and a rigid biopsy forceps, both of which attach to the nephroscope shaft.

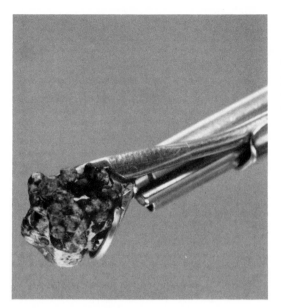

FIG. 8. Hertel forceps in action, with calyceal calculus grasped in its nontraumatizing round jaws.

be visualized with the Storz nephroscope according to published data,[3-11] and so calyceal calculi are prime targets for localization and removal with the nephroscope. We believe that the availability of the nephroscope has greatly increased the indications for surgery on small renal calculi. It used to be true that such a surgical attack ran a high risk of being in vain, with blind probing and manipulation that only further harmed the kidney and forced the frustrated urologist to leave behind both the stone and some of the patient's confidence in him. That possibility no longer colors our decision as to whether any given patient with calyceal calculi should have open surgery. In fact, we had one case in which a kidney had hydroureteronephrosis from ureterovesical obstruction, as well as a 1.5-cm calculus in the lower calyx, with infected urine. It was possible at the time of ureteroneocystoscopy to reach up to the large renal pelvis with blunt dissection and introduce the nephroscope with its stone forceps to remove the loose calculus in the kidney, sparing the patient an extended or even separate incision.

In staghorn calculi nephroscopy is indicated to achieve more complete removal of residual fragments following extraction of the pelvic portion of the calculus.

Renal Hematuria

Direct nephroscopy adds a new dimension to the diagnostic and therapeutic management of persistent unilateral renal hematuria. The uncommon cases of such "essential" hematuria can now be investigated with arteriography, retrograde studies, and careful cytologic washings of the renal pelvis. When these are negative, an open nephroscopic exploration during a persistent bleeding episode provides the opportunity to determine the source of the bleeding and to treat it with partial nephrectomy or fulguration.[2]

Renal Papillary Tumors

Carefully selected patients may be candidates for biopsy, fulguration, and resection of intrarenal papillary tumors with the nephroscope. Thus patients with recurrent papillary tumors with a low-grade cytology or brush biopsy of an intrarenal lesion, especially those with a solitary kidney, are candidates for nephroscopic visualization of the lesion and treatment by local resection.

Clearly lesions with a high-grade malignant cytology and large lesions in an expendable kidney are not to be treated with the nephroscope. Standard surgical therapy is indicated instead.

CONTRAINDICATIONS

The only contraindication considered an absolute one is the presence of a known transitional cell carcinoma of the renal collecting system, which could be better treated by total nephrectomy. The obvious danger in such a case is that opening the pelvis and flushing out malignant cells can cause local tumor spread. We have not had such a complication. Any fixed radiolucent defect in the collecting system should have urinary cytology and, if possible, transureteral brushings taken before considering open nephroscopy. Yet in exceptional cases with a solitary kidney, nephroscopic resection or fulguration of the lesion may be indicated, particularly if it is small and of low-grade malignancy.

The presence of acute infection, often associated with calculi, is not a contraindication if antibiotic coverage is being provided and if tissue infiltration is avoided by use of low irrigation fluid pressures and a generous pyelotomy. It may be noted here that, by contrast, ureteropyeloscopy could be very dangerous in a similar situation since the instrument necessarily obstructs the infected kidney.

Another contraindication to be considered is the presence of active tuberculosis, which would necessitate a period of prior treatment. It is difficult to imagine an indication for nephroscopy in such a case anyway. Also, a relative contraindication is the presence of a very delicate intrarenal pelvis, particularly with surrounding scar tissue in the renal hilus and perinephric scarring.

TECHNIQUES

Simple Calculi

In simple renal calculi, whether lodged in a distant calyx or floating in a large renal pelvis, we have invariably been able to visualize the calculus with the nephroscope. In about two-thirds of such cases the Hertel forceps can be used to grasp the stone under direct vision and retrieve it with the nephroscope. Depending on the size of the infundibulum, this can be accomplished with a stone up to 1 cm or even more in diameter. In the rest, either the infundibulum is too delicate to allow reinsertion of the nephroscope with forceps attached or the calculus is too large to pass through the infundibulum safely.

In cases where we cannot bring the calculus safely out with the nephroscope, we resort to making a nephrotomy over the point of light transmitted through the renal parenchyma by the tip of the nephroscope; then while watching through the nephroscope, we grasp the stone with forceps introduced through the nephrotomy and extract it with minimal damage to the collecting system.

Staghorn Calculi

We have continued to use a Gil-Vernet exposure of the pelvis and a large pyelotomy, transverse and arcuate under the overhanging renal parenchyma. Then with gentle manipu-

lation the pelvic portion of the stone is delivered, grasped with a right-angle or a Randall's clamp using a gentle, rocking motion. We intentionally fracture the branches of the calculus which are anchored by their flared bulbous tips inside the calyces, rather than risk tearing infundibula with forceful traction. The nephroscope is then introduced. All residual pieces visualized are removed—either through a nephrotomy, with nephroscopic monitoring (as described earlier) or with the Hertel forceps.

It must be stressed that the mucosal edema and the fluttering epithelial shreds raised inside the kidney by the stone manipulation impair the vision, and it is possible to overlook the entrance to the calyx and thus fail to see a stone fragment. Therefore x-rays must be taken of the kidney while the patient is still on the table at the end of the nephroscopic extractions. It is not uncommon to find a missed fragment on the first x-ray. The nephroscope is then reinserted and that area searched for the overlooked calyx, which in our experience is usually in the posterior midportion of the kidney, i.e., in the substance of the kidney closest to the surgeon working through a posterior pyelotomy. The entrance to such a calyx is missed in the stone-damaged pelvis unless the surgeon rolls the kidney away from himself and tips the foot of the nephroscope toward him.

The irrigation duct is often used to complete the evacuation of small stone fragments or organic debris which could become the nidus for recurrent stones if left behind. These fragments and debris are not usually seen in the operative x-rays. However, with the nephroscope they can be seen and irrigated out under vision, using intermittent hand pressure spurts on a syringe attached to the input irrigation line. Although other nephroscopists[4] have used a Fenwal pressure irrigation system similar to those used to speed the infusion of blood packs, we feel that such pressure may rupture fornices and extravasate fluid when the infundibulum is narrow and prevents an easy runoff of fluid around the nephroscope. A very recent report describes modification of the irrigation system using a Water Pik, which has a pulsatile fluid delivered under pressure that can be controlled with a dial and seems to be safer. We have not tried it, but it looks promising.[1]

Low-Grade Tumors

A tumor of the collecting system requires special attention to walling off the kidney after its full mobilization, using linen packs. A suction nozzle is to be kept continuously adjacent to the pyelotomy to aspirate all effluent and avoid potential seeding of tumor. The tumor or suspicious mucosa is visualized; then the rigid biopsy forceps is attached to the nephroscope (Fig. 7) and a cold biopsy taken for frozen section. If indicated, resection can be accomplished either with repeated bites of the rigid forceps or with the alligator forceps (Fig. 7). The base and bleeding points are fulgurated with the insulated Bugbee forceps (Fig. 7) and electrocautery.

RESULTS

Our experience with the use of the nephroscope reviewed for a 24-month period (3/72 to 2/74) included 58 cases, of which 49 were patients with calculi (Table 1). Our overall experience now exceeds 75 cases.

TABLE 1.   Cases Involving Operative Nephroscopy at University of California Medical Center, San Diego, March 1972–February 1974

Pathology	No.	%
Calculi	49	84
Intrarenal hematuria	8	14
Intrarenal tumor	1	2
Total	58	100

Review of the cases with calculi reveals that 16 of the 49 cases were staghorn calculi (Table 2). The failure rate (i.e., the persistence of opaque fragments of calculi not visualized or removed completely) was a sobering 31 percent among the staghorn calculi, but it occurred in only one case (3 percent) of the nonstaghorn cases. Whenever the final operative x-rays showed residual fragments in the kidney and we could not visualize them and wash them out with the nephroscope, we have left a nephrostomy tube for later chemical dissolution of the fragments. This procedure required the use of Renacidin solution with a strict adherence to

TABLE 2.   Review of Nephroscopy in Patients with Calculi, March 1972–February 1974

Type	No.	No. with Residual Stone Fragments Postop	%
Solitary calyceal calculus	8	0	0
Multiple calculi, separate	25	1	4
Staghorn calculi	16	5	31

the precautions set forth by Nemoy and Stamey.[6] While we have had no recurrences of calculi as yet, longer follow-up will be needed to confirm our current enthusiasm for this technique.

Photographic documentation of the appearance of the renal calculi and their nephroscopic removal has been practiced in selected cases, with both still photography and movies. Examples are illustrated in Figures 9–11 (Plate L)* and Figure 12.

In renal hematuria we have had 100 percent success in narrowing the possible source of bleeding to at least the calyx involved. In five cases we proceeded to excise a full-thickness wedge from the midportion of the kidney containing the bleeding calyx.[2] The other three were treated with lower-pole partial nephrectomy. All were cured of the hematuria. We have not yet settled for a simple fulguration of the bleeding source through the nephroscope because we feared a recurrence if the vascular lesion was not completely extirpated. However, the histology of several of the cases[2] does indicate that Bugbee fulguration could have been effective for the mucosal or submucosal microvascular malformations involved in half of the cases.

The one patient whose tumor was explored and treated with the nephroscope did well, but the peculiarities of the case preclude generalizations. A papillary lesion (Fig. 13) had grown to discernible size in the upper calyx of a solitary kidney. Previously the entire ureter and part of the renal pelvis of that kidney had been resected and replaced with an ileal ureter connected to the bladder because of coincident multiple grade II transitional cell tumors. Although the patient was a 50-year-old severe

*All color plates appear at the front of the book.

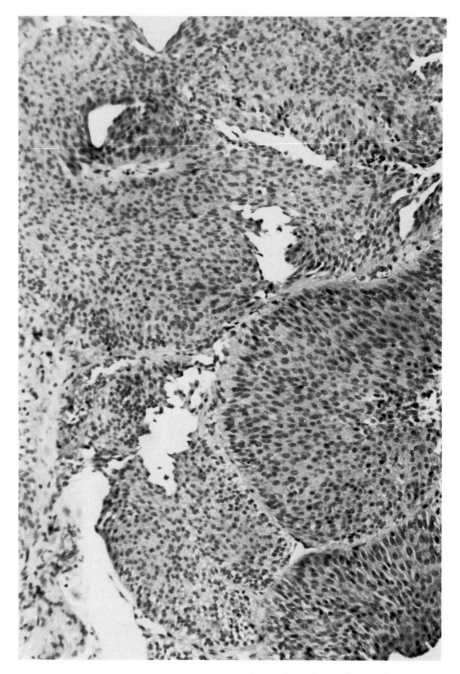

FIG. 12.   Low-power view of a histologic section of a fragment of calyceal tumor taken via the nephroscope in the case shown in Figure 13.

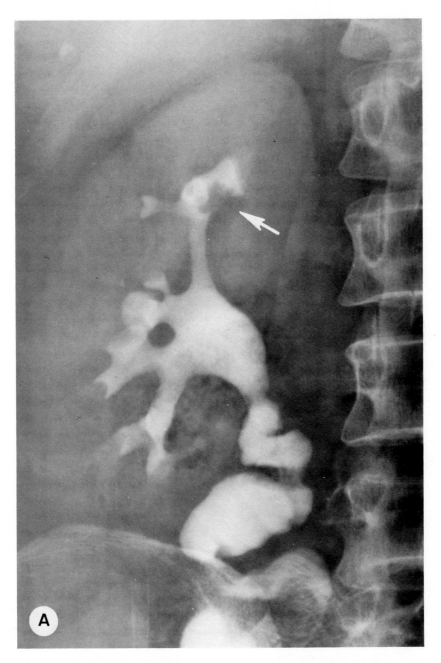

FIG. 13. Sequential x-ray views of a tumor in a solitary kidney biopsied, partially resected, and fulgurated through the nephroscope.   **A.** Urogram of 2/2/73, showing a sessile papilloma of the upper calyx (arrow). The pelvis was drained by an ileal ureter some 3 years earlier to replace a ureter afflicted with multiple low-grade tumors. (Continued on pp. 674–75)

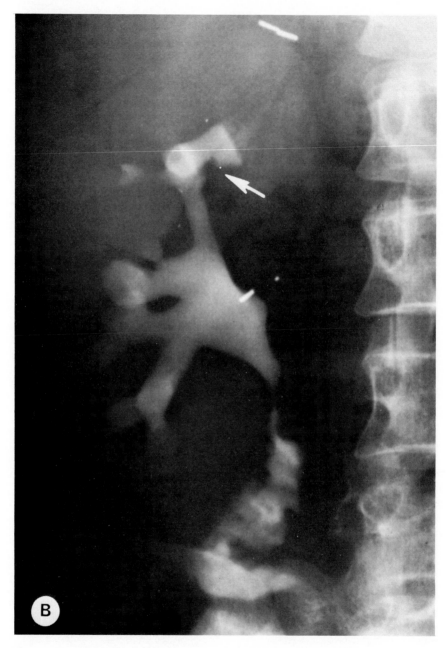

FIG. 13 (cont.).   **B.** Urogram of 3/5/73, one month after nephroscope resection and fulguration. Surgical clips are evident. The outline of the tumor is reduced to a small truncated stump (arrow). (Continued)

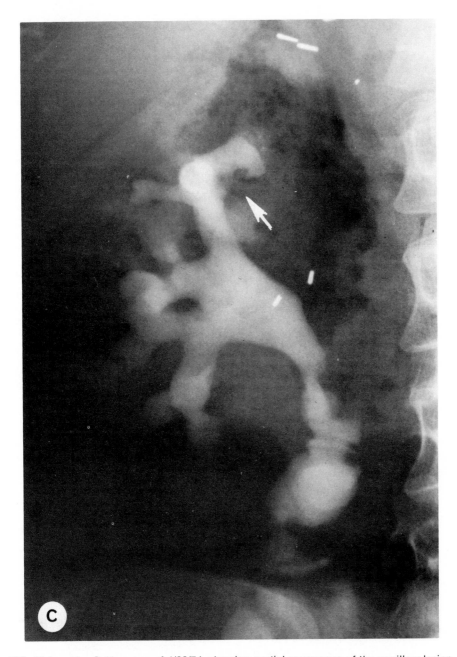

FIG. 13 (cont.).   **C.** Urogram of 4/22/74, showing partial recurrence of the papillary lesion.

diabetic, he had avoided urinary infection and his serum creatinine was normal.

Repeated cytologic studies of his urine failed to reveal clearly malignant cells (class III). It was decided to explore him nephroscopically: A biopsy submitted for frozen section showed a low-grade tumor, and morcellation of the papillary lesion was carried out with the biopsy forceps, alternating bites of the alligator forceps with fulguration with the Bugbee electrode. The papillary lesion was reduced to a square stump, solidly fulgurated. The integrity of the collecting system was maintained. The endoscopic photos were lost owing to technical failure of the camera. The histology of one of the fragments of the tumor is illustrated in Figure 12, and the follow-up x-rays of the kidney in Figures 13B and C. It is clear that if the lesion had proved to be of higher grade we would probably have removed the upper pole of the kidney with the tumor—and the regrowth of the stump now evident may yet require such a procedure. We proved to ourselves, however, that biopsy and surface fulguration of a low-grade intrarenal lesion is feasible and potentially curable without sacrifice of functional kidney tissue.

COMPLICATIONS

Wound infection was documented in only one case of nephroscopy, a remarkable rate of under 2 percent. This was a man with a solitary kidney with large calyceal calculi in whom a movie was made of the endoscopic use of the Hertel forceps.

Intraoperative bleeding was not increased during stone surgery with nephroscopy. On the contrary, avoidance of blind grasping with Randall forceps and elimination of the forceful dragging of large stone fragments through narrow infundibula reduced both the trauma to the mucosa and the degree of intrarenal bleeding.

There was one case of severe postoperative bleeding in a woman with polycystic kidney disease whose right lower pole was removed after nephroscopy showed it to be the source of her chronic bleeding. The postoperative bleeding was extrarenal and was ascribed to an unexpected clotting defect, not to intrarenal trauma. She is well 2 years after surgery, with no further hematuria. One patient had a pulmonary embolus after nephroscopy and seg-

mental excision of the midportion of the right kidney. There were no surgical deaths in the entire series.

CONCLUSION

Renal endoscopy has been made possible, practical, and safe by technical advances in instrumentation. Operative nephroscopy has become an indispensable adjunct to stone surgery in many centers, including our own. It has extended our horizons in the management of both intrarenal hematuria and low-grade tumors of the renal collecting system.

Further technical developments are expected to improve transureteral, nonoperative renal endoscopy to the point that it may be used diagnostically even in renal hematuria and infected kidneys. For the present, such ureteropyeloscopy is not usually practicable or safe. Improvement of the instrumentation is a high priority goal for current research.

REFERENCES

1. Gibbons RP, Correa RJ, Cummings KB, et al: Use of Water-Pik and nephroscope. Urology 5:605, 1974
2. Gittes RF, Elliott ML: Renal cortical rest and chronic hematuria: a syndrome treated by mid-kidney partial nephrectomy. J Urol 109:14, 1973
3. Hertel E: Entwicklung der operativen Pyeloskopie. Urologe [A] 12:116, 1973
4. Hertel E: Intraoperative nephroscopy. Urology 4:13, 1974
5. Leadbetter WF: Instrumental visualization of the renal pelvis at operation as an aid to diagnosis: presentation of a new instrument. J Urol 63:1006, 1950
6. Nemoy NJ, Stamey TA: Surgical, bacteriological, and biochemical management of "infection stones." JAMA 215:1470, 1971
7. Rupel E, Brown R: Nephroscopy with removal of stone following nephrotomy for obstructive calculus anuria. J Urol 46:177, 1941
8. Takagi T, Go T, Takayasu H, et al: Small caliber fiberscope for visualization of the urinary tract, biliary duct and spinal canal. Surgery 64:1033, 1968
9. Takayasu H, Aso I, Takagi T, et al: Our new pyelonephroscope for observation of the upper urinary tract. Endoscopy 4:105, 1972
10. Trattner HR: Instrumental visualization of the renal pelvis and its communications: proposal of a new method; preliminary report. J Urol 60:817, 1948
11. Vatz A, Berci G, Shore JM, et al: Operative nephroscopy. J Urol 107:355, 1972

55

Arthroscopy

Jan Gillquist
Sten-Otto Liljedahl

Arthroscopy was introduced in Japan by Takagi 50 years ago.[13] The early instruments allowed a fairly clear view of the interior of the knee joint, but the technique was difficult and not generally accepted. Several instruments have been developed since then, the instruments of today having a diameter of about 5 mm. Arthroscopy was initially employed mostly in Japan. Trials in Europe and the United States did not result in more frequent use.

Basic information about arthroscopy of the knee joint is compiled in the excellent volume by Watanabe et al.[14] During the last few years there has been an increasing interest in arthroscopy, and many authors[5,6,8] have reported their experience with the Japanese arthroscopes.[14] These instruments were equipped with a conventional lightbulb, and were available in diameters of 4.0 to 6.0 mm. The telescopes were made with an oblique, lateral, and straightforward view, the viewing angle ranging from 35 to 100 degrees. The telescope and accessory instrument (e.g., that used to take a biopsy specimen) were introduced through a separate incision.

The need for diagnostic improvement in certain disorders of the knee joint makes arthroscopy an attractive approach. Diagnostic efforts have previously been performed by exploratory arthrotomy. As arthrotomy is not without risk, arthroscopy is a reasonable alternative.

METHOD

For some years we have used an arthroscope manufactured by Storz.* Unfortunately we have no experience with the Watanabe arthroscope, and therefore a comparison is impossible.

The Storz arthroscope consists of two trocars with telescopes, one 4 mm and the other one 5 mm in diameter (Fig. 1). The small telescope is used together with a biopsy instrument (Fig. 2) and the slightly larger one to inspect the knee joint. This telescope is equipped with a fiberoptic light transmission system using an external source (in contrast to the Watanabe arthroscope). The viewing angle in the joint is 70 degrees for the larger and 45 degrees for the smaller telescope. Included in the set of instruments is a pair of hooks[7] specially designed for testing the menisci, cartilage, or cruciate ligaments (Fig. 3). The telescopes have only a straightforward view. Together with the arthroscope, a flash light source (Storz) and a camera can be used. Our pictures were taken with a Nikon F 35 m/m camera with a 200-mm lens and Kodak High Speed Ekta-

*Manufacturer: K. Storz Endoscopy Co., 72 Tuttlingen, PO Box 400, West Germany. United States distributor: K. Storz Endoscopy of America Inc., 658 S. San Vincente Boulevard, Los Angeles, California 90048.

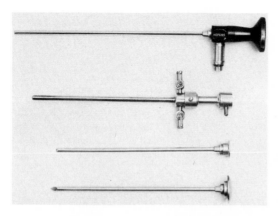

FIG. 1. Larger Hopkins telescope (4.0 mm) and trocar with obturators.

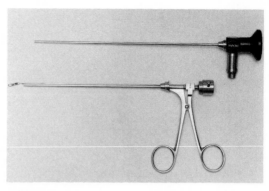

FIG. 2. Smaller Hopkins telescope (2.7 mm) and biopsy forceps.

chrome (ASA 160) 35-mm color film. We have also used a Paillard 16-mm movie camera with Kodachrome II film to record some investigations. During the filming a special light source made by ACMI* was used.

TECHNIQUE

Arthroscopy is performed with the same precautions as arthrotomy. The patient is prepared as for an operation of the knee joint. The surgeon and assisting nurse wear sterile gowns, caps, masks, and gloves. The patient should be placed on the operating table with a folding foot plate, as the knee must be flexed to 90 degrees during the examination.

A tourniquet may be used, although we consider this step unnecessary. Furthermore, the normal appearance of the synovia and the vascularization of the structures are lost under bloodless conditions. Thus in our opinion the examination should be made without obstruction of the blood supply to the leg. Bleeding in the joint seldom interferes with the procedure.

Any type of anesthesia may be used. We have tried both spinal and local anesthesia, and at present prefer spinal or general anesthesia, which produces at least partial muscle relaxation. This enables the surgeon to force the joint into various positions, making the examination easier. If local anesthesia is used there is also a risk that the patient may suddenly move the leg, which can damage the telescope.

Before insertion of the arthroscope, the joint is filled with 100 ml sterile isotonic, isothermic saline. The pressure in the joint cavity, after complete filling, is about 60 cm of water. Higher pressures are reached in normal knee joints.

To fill the joint, a 1.5-mm plastic catheter with an internal needle* is inserted in the suprapatellar pouch; the needle is withdrawn and the joint filled by means of a 20-ml syringe (Fig. 4). A piece of plastic tubing is connected to the catheter through a stopcock, which enables the joint to be emptied when needed. Continuous irrigation of the joint is not necessary.

The arthroscope may be inserted according to Watanabe et al.,[14] either medial or lateral to the patellar tendon or medially or laterally above the patella. These are the approaches most often used by other authors. However, for some time we have found it more convenient to use a single approach in most cases.[7] Accordingly, in the majority of our cases introduction of the arthroscope centrally through the patellar tendon gives a very satisfactory view of the knee joint. In a few cases, where the patella is the center of interest, the superior approach is necessary for a complete examination.

The knee is bent to 90 degrees. A small stab wound is made transversally about 1 cm below the apex of the patella (Fig. 5). The trocar with the sharply pointed obturator is then introduced through the skin and the subcutaneous fascia (Fig. 6). The sharp obturator is exchanged for a blunt one, and the trocar is advanced into the joint cavity and up under the patella. During this maneuver the leg is suc-

*American Cystoscope Makers Inc., 8 Pelham Parkway, Pelham Manor, New York 10803.

*Manufacturer: AB Stille Werner, Box 4051, S-102 61 Stockholm, Sweden.

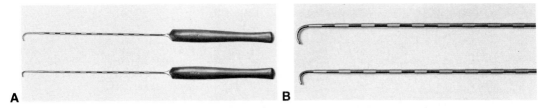

FIG. 3. **A.** Hooks used during arthroscopy. Note the markings on the shafts indicating 5-mm intervals. The hook with the short end is used to test the menisci and the cartilage, and the one with the long end the cruciate ligaments. **B.** Close-up view of the hooks.

FIG. 4. The joint is filled with isotonic, isothermic saline through a plastic catheter inserted in the suprapatellar pouch from the lateral side.

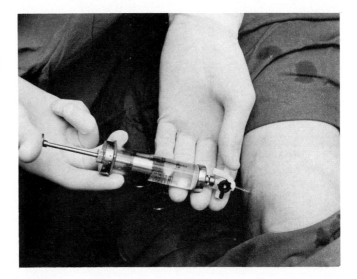

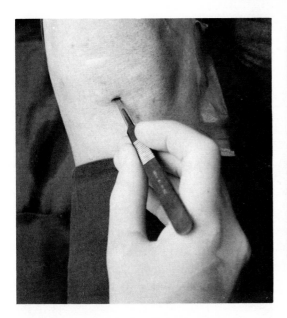

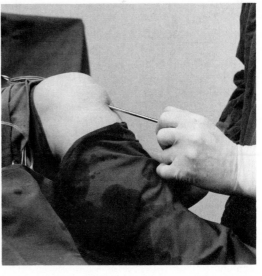

FIG. 5. A small stab incision is made through the skin about 1 cm below the apex of the patella. The patellar tendon should not be incised.

FIG. 6. The trocar and sharp obturator are introduced through the stab wound and the patellar tendon. Before the trocar is inserted into the joint through the synovia, the sharply pointed obturator is exchanged for a blunt one.

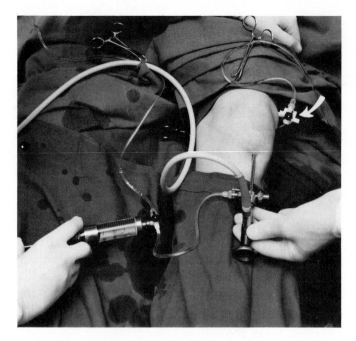

FIG. 7. System used for irrigating the joint with saline. The fluid leaves the joint through the catheter on the lateral side *(arrow)*.

cessively straightened out, the obturator withdrawn, and the telescope introduced through the trocar.

The light carrier and irrigating system are connected. The latter consists of three pieces of plastic tubing connected with a three-way stopcock. One part is connected to a bottle of isotonic saline, one to the arthroscope, and one to a 20-ml syringe. This allows the assisting nurse to flush the joint on request (Fig. 7).

The hook is introduced by a separate incision when the joint has been inspected. It should be introduced from either the medial or the lateral side of the joint line (Fig. 8).

The knee is flexed to 160 degrees, and inspection of the joint starts in the femoropatellar compartment. The appearance of the synovia in the suprapatellar bursa and cartilage of the patella is noted. If the knee joint is flexed during inspection of the femoropatellar joint the congruency of the joint surfaces can be estimated. The knee is now flexed to 90 degrees again. The instrument is slowly withdrawn, until the tip can be introduced into the femorotibial joint. The cartilage of the femur and tibia condyles is inspected as are the two cruciate ligaments. The anterior cruciate ligament is easily identified as a well defined ligament structure with somewhat twisted fibers (Fig. 9, Plate M).*

All color plates appear at the front of the book.

The normal vessels in the synovia, as well as the arteries deeper in the ligament, can be seen if the fluid pressure in the joint is not too high. Usually a double vessel can be identified crossing transversally over the midportion of the ligament. The arthroscope might also be ad-

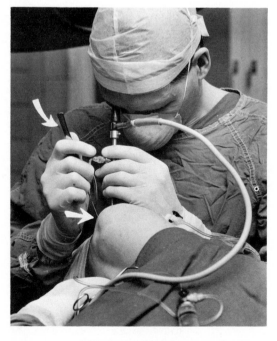

FIG. 8. Hook inserted from the medial side (arrow).

vanced along the ligament up to the posterior femoral attachment (Fig. 10). The posterior cruciate ligament is usually covered by a rather thick synovia, and no ligamentous substance is normally seen at the superior (femoral) attachment. However, if the ligament is followed downward and backward, the synovia becomes thinner, and normal ligament fibers can be seen through the synovia. As a rule the vessels of the posterior cruciate ligament are hidden by the synovia. Much more experience is required to identify the posterior cruciate ligament than the anterior one.

The inspection continues with the *medial meniscus*. When the knee joint is flexed to 90 degrees the anterior part of the meniscus may be seen. One can inspect the meniscus from the edge of the synovial attachment as far as the middle of the meniscus. The medial compartment, from the medial collateral ligament and backward, is rather narrow in a normal joint, and inspection is usually impossible. However, if the deep portion of the medial collateral ligament (the medial capsular ligament) is ruptured, the medial recess is wider, which makes it possible to advance the arthroscope further, about 1 cm backward along the attachment of the medial meniscus. A much better view of the posterior part of the meniscus is obtained, however, if the knee is extended under the arm of the investigator (Fig. 10). During manipulation with extension and slight flexion, alterna-

tively, the arthroscope might be advanced under visual control to the posterior horn of the medial meniscus. This is possible with the 5-mm telescope in about half the examined knees, and the whole medial meniscus can be visualized. Care must be taken not to damage the cartilage with the tip of the arthroscope. In some knees the posterior horn might be seen at some distance, but a closer view is impossible. In these instances the meniscus might be tested with the hook, and any rupture will be revealed (Fig. 11, Plate M). If there is a linear rupture of the capsular attachment of the posterior horn, the meniscus can be drawn into the joint with the hook and the diagnosis made. The diagnosis of small tears at the edge can also be made by using the hook.

The *lateral meniscus* is examined mainly in the same way as the medial one, but on this side the investigation is much easier. The posterior horn of the lateral meniscus often has a more anterior position in the joint than the medial one. Inspection of the posterior horn of the lateral meniscus can be accomplished in every knee. Usually the arthroscope can be advanced over and under the attachment of the meniscus. The rather deep recess at the lateral attachment of the lateral meniscus can also be inspected. The meniscus is also tested with the hook to demonstrate any small ruptures that may be there. By doing so, we have seen small holes in the attachment of the meniscus and

FIG. 10. With the patient's leg extended under the arm of the surgeon, the arthroscope can be manipulated into the posterior compartments of the joint.

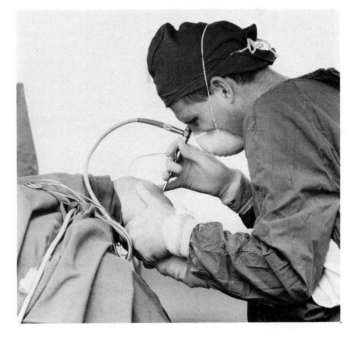

tiny horizontal tears on the edge of the meniscus, inserting just the end of the hook.

The cartilage of the condyles is examined with the knee joint in various positions, thus revealing any lesions of the weight-bearing surfaces. Biopsy may be taken after exchanging the larger telescope for the smaller one. Any pathologic lesions are photographed. After the examination the joint is emptied, the arthroscope withdrawn, and the small stab wound covered with a surgical tape (Fig. 12). Bacteriologic cultures are taken from the irrigating fluid before and after arthroscopy in every case.

The majority of our patients are examined as outpatients and are thus allowed to return home after 3 to 4 hours. The knee is supported by an elastic bandage. Walking and ordinary physical activities are allowed immediately and sports activities after 3 days. A follow-up is routinely arranged after 10 days and then according to the demands of the disease.

ARTHROSCOPY AS A DIAGNOSTIC AID

Synovitis

Watanabe et al.[14] have given a rather complete description of the various forms of villi

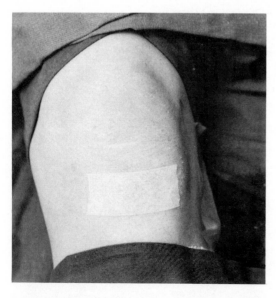

FIG. 12. The examination is completed, and the small stab wound is covered with a surgical tape.

seen in different kinds of synovitis. In our limited experience, however, the diagnostic value of arthroscopy in various cases of synovitis has been minimal. Biopsy specimens from the synovial membrane are always taken in cases of undetermined synovitis. So far, the microscopic examination has resulted in a diagnosis of "nonspecific synovitis." The difference between our experience and that of Watanabe et al. might be explained by the fact that purulent, syphilitic, and tuberculous arthritis are very rare in our country. The diagnosis of rheumatoid arthritis is usually made from other, more reliable signs than the arthroscopic picture. O'Connor[11] recently demonstrated that the diagnosis of crystal-induced synovitis made by arthroscopy is more reliable than that made by roentgenograms. Therefore in cases of recurrent swelling of the knee joint of uncertain etiology, we consider arthroscopy well worth a trial.

Lesions of the Meniscus

Medial Meniscus. The anterior part of the medial meniscus is easily examined, and the posterior parts may be examined with sufficient accuracy by using a hook. In a typical case of rupture of the medial meniscus, after a rotational trauma with locking symptoms and typical pain, arthroscopy is superfluous. However, when it is difficult to distinguish the pain of a partial rupture of the medial collateral ligament from that caused by a linear rupture of the capsular attachment of the meniscus, arthroscopy is of definite value. With the hook, examination of the medial meniscus by arthroscopy is more reliable than that by exploratory arthrotomy. In a study in which the diagnostic accuracy of physical examination (by an experienced physician), arthrography, arthroscopy, and arthrotomy was compared, it was found that rupture of the medial meniscus was diagnosed as accurately by arthroscopy as by the other methods (Fig. 13).[2]

Lateral Meniscus. The lateral meniscus can be more completely examined by arthroscopy than the medial one. When the hook is employed, practically no rupture of the lateral meniscus escapes the examiner. On the other hand, the physical diagnosis as well as arthrography are often difficult in the case of a torn lateral meniscus. Thus when suspicion of a rupture of the lateral meniscus is not verified

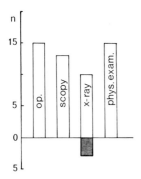

FIG. 13. Diagnostic results in cases of a torn medial meniscus. Open columns, Correct diagnoses. Black columns, False diagnoses. The hook was not used in this investigation.

by arthrography, arthroscopy should be performed. If arthrography raises suspicion of a rupture of the lateral meniscus, arthroscopy is helpful, as arthrography sometimes gives a false-positive result. We found that the diagnostic accuracy of arthroscopy is superior compared with all the other procedures in cases of rupture of the lateral meniscus.[2]

Lesions of Ligaments

Anterior Cruciate Ligament. The anterior cruciate ligament is easily examined. In the case of a recent rupture, the tear and the ends of the ligament are usually identified without difficulty. The ends of the ligament usually appear thick and swollen, and sometimes even bleeding vessels are seen. If the joint is continuously irrigated during the examination, this bleeding is not disturbing. The ligament is usually torn in the middle of the substance, with the shorter end in the upper part. The hook may be used to identify any ligament fibers left in place. Occasionally a few thin threads of ligamentous tissue can be seen in the posterior part of the ligament, and in others the major part of the ligament is intact with only a synovial rupture. A forward drawer test may be made to obtain information about the continuity of the ligament. Often in cases with an old rupture of the anterior cruciate ligament, no remnants of ligament can be seen. Only a small part covered with synovial tissue at the lower attachment, or adherent to the posterior cruciate ligament, is observed (Fig. 14, Plate M). In these cases identification of the ligament remnant is difficult. However, the

place occupied by the anterior cruciate ligament in a normal joint is empty, and the arthroscope can easily be advanced far back toward the posterior capsule, lateral to the posterior cruciate ligament. Small strands of tissue are usually found at the normal superior attachment of the anterior cruciate ligament.

A rupture of the distal (tibial) attachment of the anterior cruciate ligament is also easily diagnosed by endoscopy. Usually there is a bony fragment torn loose with the ligament. This fragment is easily identified by means of the hook. In some cases plain radiographs show a fracture of the intercondylar notch of the tibia. This is often interpreted as a rupture of the distal end of the anterior cruciate ligament. In some cases, however, we have been able to identify a fragment of the bone lateral and posterior to the attachment of the anterior cruciate ligament, with the main part of the ligament intact. When traction is placed on the ligament by the hook in these cases, the bone fragment is not dislocated at all. The fracture in these cases is unimportant and immediate quadriceps exercises can be instituted. Therefore we consider a fracture in the vicinity of the attachments of the cruciate ligaments as an indication for arthroscopy. The result of the examination indicates if arthrotomy is necessary.

Posterior Cruciate Ligament. Identification of the posterior cruciate ligament may be difficult for an unexperienced examiner. With the aid of the hook, however, the posterior cruciate ligament can always be tested. A rupture of the ligament usually occurs in the lower, posterior attachment, mostly with a piece of bone attached to the ligament. In these cases the diagnosis is easy to make on plain x-ray films, and arthroscopy is not considered of any value. If, however, a rupture of the posterior cruciate ligament is suspected because of the presence of a "backward drawer" sign, and the roentgenogram is normal, arthroscopy is necessary. In these cases arthrography is practically never of any help, as it is very difficult to visualize a rupture of the posterior cruciate ligament in the substance, even if the examination is made with lateral views during the "backward drawer" test.

The experienced arthroscopist can determine whether the rupture is in the superior or the inferior attachment. This must be known in order to position the patient on the operating table properly; a rupture in the posterior end must be approached from the popliteal fossa, and a rupture in the superior end from the anterior side of the knee. In these cases the hook is very helpful in determining the site and completeness of a rupture. If the rupture is in the posterior part of the substance of the ligament, the free end may be drawn into the joint and the diagnosis established. If a bone fragment is attached to the ligament, the interior of the joint is mostly normal. A rupture of the anterior-superior attachment is seldom complete, although almost invariably two-thirds of the ligament is torn loose. The free ends may be caught with the hook and drawn forward (Fig. 15, Plate M). During a "backward drawer" the tension in the ligament may also be felt with the hook. An early diagnosis using arthroscopy in these cases is very important as ruptures eventually lead to atrophy. At present there is no way of replacing a posterior cruciate ligament undergoing atrophy.

Rupture of the Collateral Ligaments. A rupture of the medial collateral ligament can be diagnosed by arthroscopy. During the acute phase the accompanying rupture of the capsule above or below the medial meniscus can often be identified using the hook. In cases with an old lesion of the deep portion of the medial collateral ligament, the diagnosis is more difficult. However, a wide recess may be found at the superior or inferior attachment of the ligament.

Nevertheless, a *single* rupture of the medial collateral ligament is not an indication for arthroscopy, as the diagnosis is made with satisfying accuracy by physical examination. A rupture of the lateral collateral ligament is extraarticular, and arthroscopy in these cases is used only to exclude intraarticular injury (e.g., a rupture of the anterior cruciate ligament).

Combined Injuries

As a rule traumatic injuries to the knee joint result in combinations of lesions.[1,10,12] The most common combination is rupture of the medial meniscus, medial collateral ligament, and anterior cruciate ligament. This combination has been called "the unhappy triad."[12] In our investigation of the diagnostic accuracy of arthroscopy, we found that parts of this triad were often overlooked at physical examination as well as at arthrography. Arthroscopy, on the other hand, revealed the whole combination in most cases (Fig. 16).

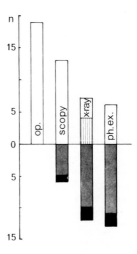

FIG. 16. Diagnostic results in 19 cases with various combinations of lesions in the knee joint. Open columns, Correct diagnoses. Striped columns, Uncertain diagnoses. Shaded columns, One item of the combination misses. Black columns, False diagnoses.

Cartilage of the Joints

Femoropatellar Joint. Inspection starts with the suprapatellar bursa and the cartilage of the femoropatellar joint. The congruency of the joint surfaces is tested, as a deviation of the patellar surface is usually seen in cases with recurrent patellar luxation or subluxation. Small injuries to the cartilage on both surfaces of the patella in its lower part can easily be seen in most cases from the described central infrapatellar approach. However, if a complete view of the patella is important a suprapatellar approach should be used too. During examination of the joint in various degrees of flexion, the correspondence of lesions on the patella with lesions on the femoral condyles may be seen. In patients who complain of diffuse pain around the patella after a fall to the ground, we have seen fractures in the cartilage of the patella often occupying an area about 1 cm in diameter. Corresponding lesions in the femoral condyles have also been noted. In patients with complaints commonly diagnosed as "chondromalacia of the patella" the cartilage of the patella has been shown to be fragmented. In this way the diagnosis of chondromalacia of the patella is based on the observation of a pathologic lesion and not on nonspecific complaints. We consider arthroscopy to be of diagnostic value especially in these cases with complaints that are difficult to classify. Often an early osteoarthrosis that is impossible to diagnose on roentgenogram can be detected. In fact, there may be surprisingly large damage to the cartilage without the roentgenograms showing an abnormality.

Femorotibial Joint. The weight-bearing surfaces are readily inspected during arthroscopy. Injuries to the cartilage as well as early changes of degeneration (fragmentation, slight yellow color, matt appearance, diminished elasticity) are easily identified by inspection and by testing the cartilage with the hook. Early arthrosis is an easy diagnosis, which cannot be made with certainty by any other means. In this way arthroscopy helps to diagnose cases with an unspecific clinical picture.

Osteochondritis Dissecans. Even though the diagnosis of this condition is usually made with great accuracy by x-ray, arthroscopy is of definite value as it can show whether the fragment is firmly or loosely attached in the bed and therefore if operation is necessary. The integrity of the cartilage over the fragment may be readily shown by arthroscopy, and the attachment of the fragment tested by the hook.

Loose Bodies. Loose bodies are easily found by endoscopy, even when they contain only cartilage and thus cannot be seen on roentgenogram. In some cases the loose bodies may be caught with the biopsy instrument or by the hook, and removed. However, large loose bodies must be taken care of in the usual manner, by exploration.

ARTHROSCOPY IN ACUTE CONDITIONS

Some authors consider arthroscopy to be contraindicated during acute conditions.[5] The reason is that a hemarthrosis obscures the view. We have tried arthroscopy in 25 acute cases with bleeding into the joint and succeeded in obtaining a clear view by irrigation. In fact, arthroscopy has been very helpful in our acute cases, allowing us to make therapeutic decisions much earlier than we would have without arthroscopy. In cases of a recent rupture of the anterior or posterior cruciate ligament, the diagnosis may be made immediately after the accident by arthroscopy, whereas by arthrography and physical examination the diagnosis is difficult during the first week.[9] We consider arthroscopy to be diagnostically helpful in acute cases.

ARTHROSCOPY DURING THE FOLLOW-UP PERIOD

We have also used arthroscopy in 20 patients subjected to reconstruction of the cruciate ligaments. At first the indication was suspected injury after a new trauma, but over the years the list of indications has expanded to include cases with nonspecific complaints after operation, e.g., pain or persistent swelling. The wider indication was possible because arthroscopy in our hands was free from complications.

In this way it has been possible to follow, visually and by biopsy, vascularization of a part of the patellar tendon transposed into the joint to replace the anterior cruciate ligament (Fig. 17, Plate M).[4] The results of this investigation are published elsewhere.[3] In some cases with the complaint of persistent swelling, the cause was found to be a piece of suture material that had become loose in the joint (Fig. 18, Plate M). In other cases in which instability returned after the operation, a degenerated tendon strip was found. In yet others the symptoms were due to a ruptured meniscus (injured during a new accident), and the transposed tendon strip looked like a normal cruciate ligament, the joint being quite stable. In patients complaining of pain or persistent locking symptoms after meniscectomy, arthroscopy revealed a rupture of a remaining part of the meniscus, usually the posterior horn. These patients became symptom-free after a total meniscectomy.

THERAPEUTIC EFFECT OF ARTHROSCOPY

We regard arthroscopy as a diagnostic method, although in limited cases, as described above, loose bodies might be extracted through the arthroscope. Watanabe et al.[14] and O'Connor,[11] however, described a therapeutic effect of arthroscopy, especially in patients with synovitis or osteoarthrosis. We have noted also in these cases that the examination is often followed by a symptom-free interval, sometimes lasting several weeks. This unspecific effect is ascribed to the irrigation of the joint during arthroscopy. Especially in cases with osteoarthrosis, a large amount of detritus is washed out of the joint during the investigation. We regard this "therapeutic" effect entirely as a side phenomenon and do not include it as an indication for the procedure. However, it should be remembered that other therapy instituted immediately after arthroscopy can be followed by subjective improvement, mainly due to the arthroscopy alone.

COMPLICATIONS

There have been no complications in our 280 arthroscopies during the last few years. Not a single infection has been observed; and the bacteriologic cultures from the joint fluid before and after arthroscopy in the last 150 cases have never produced any growth. This means that the precautions taken are adequate. With the same principles, Watanabe et al.[14] report no infection in more than a thousand cases. If the rules are strictly followed, the risk of infection is probably overestimated. However, one should avoid arthroscopy in patients inoculated with virus hepatitis, as this disease may be transmitted to another patient by the instrument, in spite of sterilization by gas, fluids, or autoclaving.

We have not seen any other complications after arthroscopy either. The patients sometimes complain of a slight stiffness of the knee for 2 to 3 days, but physical activity is practically never limited. There has never been an exudate necessitating aspiration of the joint.

The anesthesia used in our cases has not been followed by complications. There is of course a theoretical risk when general anesthesia is given, but arthroscopy is performed mostly in otherwise healthy people, and so the anesthesia risk can be regarded as minimal. If a condition is present which would increase this risk, the determination to perform arthroscopy should be considered more carefully. In such a case arthroscopy is carried out only if knee surgery seems necessary, should endoscopy reveal any pathology. In such a case arthroscopy and operation should be done during the same anesthesia session.

INSTRUMENTAL FAILURES

In the early part of our series we had two failures with the small telescope. Once it broke during cleaning before it was sterilized, and another time the lens became foggy. On one occasion the objective lens of the larger telescope was damaged by the hook during ar-

throscopy; the hook was accidentally rubbed against the front of the telescope inside the joint. No harm was done to the patient. However, when the hook is used, care should be taken that contact with the telescope is avoided.

The small telescope (2.7 mm) was used to inspect the joint in the early part of our series. As this results in a rather limited field of vision, the diagnostic accuracy is lower than when the larger telescope (4.0 mm) was employed. It is recommended therefore that the smaller telescope be used only for taking biopsy specimens in the knee joint.

ARTHROSCOPY OF
THE ANKLE JOINT

We have tried the smaller telescope in 15 ankle joints. The indication has been to find out if there was damage to the cartilage of the talus or the tibia in patients complaining of posttraumatic pain a long time after the initial injury (fracture or ligament rupture) was healed.

The ankle joint is filled with about 10 ml isotonic isothermic saline, and the telescope is introduced from the lateral side of the joint. In all cases it has been possible to inspect the talus and the anterior part of the joint surfaces of the tibia. Different parts of the joint surface of the talus are brought into view by moving the foot. Defects and injuries to the joint cartilage have been diagnosed in cases where no injury was seen on x-ray films. It is probably possible to obtain information using the arthroscope in the ankle joint, although in our opinion the indications for it are less frequent than for arthroscopy of the knee joint.

INTERPRETATION OF
THE ARTHROSCOPIC PICTURE

Even if a clear view of the interior of the joint is obtained by today's arthroscopes, interpretation of the appearance is difficult. All authors in this field have reported the same difficulties at the beginning. According to our experience, about 50 examinations are necessary before any diagnostic accuracy is attained. In the first part of our series almost every other arthroscopy result gave an inaccurate diagnosis. With an increasing number of cases false diagnoses become rare. These difficulties are the same as encountered in all other types of endoscopy, and the demands are the same: Arthroscopy should be performed only by an experienced endoscopist, and the examinations should be done frequently. The best results are obtained when only one or two surgeons in each institution are performing arthroscopy.

When a young surgeon wishes to become familiar with arthroscopy, exercises at autopsy in the pathology department are recommended. In this way the anatomy of the knee joint as seen through the arthroscope can be studied thoroughly and at leisure.

SUMMARY

Our experience of arthroscopy in 280 cases has convinced us that this procedure is of definite value in diagnosing various conditions of the knee joint. The main indications are the following:

1. Diagnosis of early damage to the joint cartilage
2. Diagnosis of injuries to the cruciate ligaments, especially in the acute phase and when there is uncertainty as to the location of a rupture of the posterior cruciate ligament
3. Diagnosis of a rupture of the lateral meniscus in uncertain cases
4. Diagnosis of small ruptures of the medial meniscus
5. Diagnosis and removal of loose bodies
6. In follow-up examinations after intraarticular surgery, e.g., reconstruction of the cruciate ligaments
7. To take biopsy specimens in cases of synovitis of unknown origin

It is possible that new and improved instruments will increase the use of arthroscopy. Furthermore, other joints may be examined with arthroscopes of a smaller caliber.

REFERENCES

1. Alm A: Old injuries of the ligaments of the knee joint. Acta Chir Scand 140:283, 1974
2. Alm A, Gillquist J, Liljedahl SO: The diagnostic value of arthroscopy of the knee joint. Injury 5:319, 1974
3. Alm A, Gillquist J, Strömberg B: The medial third of the patellar ligament in reconstruction of the anterior cruciate ligament: a clinical and histologic study by means of arthroscopy or arthrotomy. Acta Chir Scand [Suppl] In press
4. Broström L, Gillquist J, Liljedahl SO, et al: Behandling av invetererad ruptur av främre korsbandet. Lakartidningen 65:4479, 1968
5. Casscells SW: Arthroscopy of the knee joint. J Bone Joint Surg 53-A:287, 1971
6. Gallannaugh S: Arthroscopy of the knee joint. Br Med J 3:285, 1973
7. Gillquist J, Hagberg G: The technique of arthroscopy of the knee joint. In preparation
8. Jackson RW, Abe J: The role of arthroscopy in the management of disorders of the knee. J Bone Joint Surg 54-B:310, 1972
9. Liljedahl SO, Gillquist J: Innere Verletzungen des Kniegelenkes bei Sportlern. Munch Med Wochenschr 114:1371, 1972
10. Liljedahl SO, Nordstrand A: Injuries to the ligaments of the knee. Injury 1:17, 1969
11. O'Connor RL: The arthroscope in the management of crystal induced synovitis of the knee. J Bone Joint Surg 55-A:1443, 1973
12. O'Donoghue DH: Treatment of Injuries to Athletes. Philadelphia, Saunders, 1970, p 512
13. Takagi K: Practical experiences using Takagis arthroscope. J Jap Orthoped Assoc 8:132, 1933
14. Watanabe M, Takeda S, Ikeuchi H: Atlas of Arthroscopy. Tokyo, Ikagu Shoin Ltd, 1968

56

Cystoscopy and Transurethral Endoscopic Surgery

Robert B. Smith
Joseph J. Kaufman

Although effective transurethral endoscopic surgery has been developed largely during the twentieth century, the possibility of utilizing the urethra as a route for internal surgery fascinated physicians for centuries. Blind procedures per urethram were certainly used in the millenium before the Christian era. Galen in 150 AD is given credit for the first attempt to destroy urethral strictures by forceful urethral catheterization with a rigid tube. The extent to which this technique was used during subsequent centuries is difficult to determine from the fragmentary reports available in medical historical literature. A significant advance was made by Ambrose Paré in 1575, when he employed a sound with a sharp fin to ream an opening in the urethra and bladder neck area (the forerunner of our contemporary internal urethrotomy).

Little progress was made during the next two and a half centuries until James Guthrie in 1834 reported cutting the bladder neck with a knife concealed in a catheter. Mercier perfected the procedure 2 years later by devising a urethrotomy blade for incision of the vesical neck. He gave no mortality statistics, although he reportedly used this method in over 300 cases. First to use electrical coagulation in transurethral surgery, Bottini in 1874 employed galvanocautery for blind coagulation of the bladder neck.

After Nitze developed the first practical cystoscope in 1877, transurethral surgery began to progress rapidly. Edison's invention of the in-candescent lamp in 1879 resulted in the disposal of the cumbersome cooling system necessary for Nitze's hot platinum wire. Pioneer urologic surgeons could now visualize disease processes that had been treated blindly for centuries.

D'Arsonvall first performed transurethral fulguration of various lesions using a low-frequency current in 1882, but the invention of the vacuum tube by De Forest in 1908 gave impetus to the utilization of electrosurgical currents for endoscopic surgery. Beer of New York was the first surgeon to use a high-frequency current in clinical urology. In 1910 he successfully coagulated a bladder tumor under direct vision. One year earlier Hugh Young introduced the cold-punch procedure for prostatectomy, but lack of hemostasis was a serious disadvantage in this blind approach.

Stevens and Bugbee performed successful coagulation of the bladder neck using a steel wire, and in 1914 Luys described massive electrical coagulation of the bladder neck and prostate employing an air cystoscope. Successful results with this procedure depended on sloughing of necrotic tissue.

In 1918 Braasch modified Hugh Young's cold-punch technique, and for the first time "resection" of prostatic tissue under direct vision was possible. Caulk adapted a low-frequency electrocautery unit to the cold-punch procedure in 1920, and 3 years later transurethral surgery as we know it today began, with the development of a high-frequency cutting current by Collings and Wappler. The following year Bovie and Liebel perfected a highly damped coagulation current and undamped cutting current that allowed the first "true" electroresection of tissues. The discovery in 1925 of the nonconducting Bakelite sheath by Walker further improved transurethral electroresection. Collings successfully incised the bladder neck under direct vision that same year, and in 1926 Stern invented the first modern resectoscope. Although he removed tissue with an undamped current, he did not control bleeding in this archetypal procedure. A momentous advance was made by Bumpus in 1926 when he combined the Braasch cold-punch procedure with high-frequency coagulation of the prostatic fossa, thereby markedly reducing the morbidity and mortality rates. In 1931 D. M. Davis became the first to adapt effectively a unified cutting and coagulation current to Stern's resectoscope, and the same year McCarthy modified Stern's design to allow the instrument to cut toward rather than away from the operator, thus giving the endoscopic surgeon increased control. McCarthy incorporated the fore-oblique telescope from his panendoscope into the resectoscope. In 1939 Nesbit devised the first one-handed instrument, utilizing a spring device, thus freeing the other hand for rectal examination and manipulation during a procedure; and in 1940 Iglesias developed his resectoscope, one of those most commonly used today.

The greatest advances in endoscopic surgery during the past 30 years have been improvements in the illumination and optics of viewing telescopes (see discussion of the fiberoptic light source and the Hopkins solid lens system telescope, below). With the availability of better light sources and optics, it has been possible to develop a teaching attachment to enable the fledgling urologist to view transurethral procedures while in progress. The addition of the direct vision 0-degree lens is also gaining an important place in various phases of transurethral surgery.

SURGICAL ARMAMENTARIUM

When the surgeon embarks on an endoscopic procedure, it is essential that an array of instruments be immediately available to him. Certainly many complications encountered in transurethral surgery have been attributable to shortcuts employed because the appropriate instruments were not readily available.

The armamentarium for standard adult endoscopic procedures should include a full set of *Van Buren sounds* (Nos. 18 Fr through 30 Fr). No size should be missing since overly rapid dilation of a stricture is a major cause of false passage. Likewise, *bougies* should be available for urethral calibration, as should *filiforms* with woven silk followers or *Le Forte sounds*. An *urethrotome* should also be handy.

A full selection of *resectoscope sheaths* insulated with Bakelite, Fiberglass, or Teflon in sizes 24, 26, 27, or 28 Fr is mandatory, although we rarely use the larger sheaths. Sheaths with short beaks are preferable, as the likelihood of injury to the urethra or trigone is less than when long-beaked sheaths are used. For similar reasons the beak should be inspected for smoothness. Appropriate *obturators* are necessary for each sheath size. It is sometimes helpful to have available an obturator with a screw tip which can accommodate a filiform thread. Copious amounts of water-soluble jelly and 1 percent hydrocortisone ointment for proper lubrication of sounds and sheaths are de rigueur.

The Hopkins lens has improved visualization during transurethral procedures and certainly has helped to decrease operating time. Lenses with 30- and 70-degree viewing angles are essential, and a 0-degree (direct vision) lens, though not mandatory, is often helpful. With the wide-angle 70-degree lens, a retrospective lens is rarely necessary. A *fiberoptic light source* is obviously part of a modern suite, and extra bulbs for this light source or an alternate unit should be available.

Two *resectoscopes* should be available, the design of which may be the choice of the individual surgeon. We prefer a one-handed instrument of the Iglesias or Nesbit design in order to liberate the opposite hand for rectal or suprapubic manipulation, but other endoscopic surgeons are at ease with two-handed instruments.

A full selection of appropriate *resectoscope loops* should be available, both in regard to loop size and wire caliber. The thinner the wire, the better is the cutting and the poorer the coagulating capacity of the loop. Therefore the thin-wired loop is particularly useful in the resection of fibrous prostates. In resecting the succulent adenomatous gland, a loop with a larger-caliber wire is preferable to effect hemostasis. Several loops of each size should be available in case of loop breakage. The color coding of the loops according to size should be familiar to the surgeon. A firm *brush* should be included in the setup to facilitate cleaning the resectoscope loops during the procedure.

If a one-handed instrument is employed, an *O'Conor rectal shield* should be used to allow periodic rectal manipulation without contamination. The rectal portion of the shield should be well lubricated to prevent irritation and possible injury.

If unsuspected vesical or urethral calculi are encountered, a *lithotrite* of the surgeon's choice should be available. Similarly, *flexible* and *rigid grasping forceps* are useful in the event that material cannot be removed from the bladder by manipulation of the resectoscope loop. Although frequent levering of the resectoscope sheath successfully evacuates fragments of tissue from the bladder, the *Toomey syringe* or *Ellik evacuator* is helpful for rapid extraction of vesical debris. To facilitate filling of the Ellik evacuator, a deep pan of sterile irrigating fluid should be prepared. The Ellik evacuator should be checked for bulb strength and for sites of possible leakage. The connecting hose should be of large caliber, rigid, and short, with an airtight seal between the glass phalange and the nozzle that adapts to the resectoscope sheath.

Generous stores of suitable *irrigating fluid* are imperative. Distilled water is safe for brief procedures, such as bladder tumor resection, cystolitholapaxy, and resection of fibrous bladder necks. Because of the possible risk of hemolysis, many urologists feel that it is contraindicated in standard transurethral prostatic surgery, despite its advantages of low cost and superior optical properties. There is a growing body of evidence indicating that this danger has been overstated, and many urologists use distilled water for all transurethral surgery. The "ideal" solution should be nonelectrolytic and isosmotic. Solutions composed of 5 percent mannitol, 1.8 percent urea, 4 percent glucose, or 1.1 percent glycine readily satisfy these criteria, and with improved optical and illumination systems good visualization is not a problem in any case. Because of the ismotic diuretic effect of mannitol, this is our preferred solution. Commercially prepared sterile bottles or plastic bags with appropriate tubing are vastly superior to the old bell jar fluid storage with its inherent risks of contamination.

Surgical instruments for performing vasectomy, meatotomy, or perineal urethrotomy should be available. A minimum set should include two towel clips, four straight hemostats, one Adson thumb forcep, scalpel, and needle holder. The type of suture material depends on the preference of the surgeon.

Two *electrosurgical units* should be available in case of malfunction of the primary one. The type of such units, again, is the individual surgeon's choice. Desirable features include a weighted foot pedal that remains relatively stationary during the procedure. A sound mechanism with which cutting and coagulation current can be differentiated by ear is helpful in preventing the wrong pedal from being pressed inadvertently. Imperative is a warning light or buzzer to detect short circuits or improper patient grounding. The new solid state electrosurgical units are superior instruments in our experience.

The *operating table* should be freely adjustable by the surgeon. The tray should be large in order to facilitate collection of irrigating fluid and resected tissue. The ideal table should have radiologic capabilities should emergencies arise in which cystography or urethrography are necessary. Occasionally an extra anesthetic may be avoided if retrograde pyelograms are performed in conjunction with contemplated endoscopic surgical procedures. *Adjustable chairs* that are semi- or completely automatic are an added luxury for the endoscopic surgeon. Operating time may be decreased by minutes if the surgeon can easily adjust the patient's or his own relative position.

A modern *endoscopic surgical room* should be equipped with a floor drain and overhead surgical light. The walls should be leaded, and permanent x-ray equipment provided if possible. The cystoscopy room ideally is not only clean but sterile, so that if a complication arises it can be managed in the same room. Transportation of an anesthetized patient to another operating suite is sometimes necessary because of this, and occasionally other operating suites may not be immediately available for open procedures.

Extra "luxury" features include installation of a built-in electrosurgical unit, permanent xenon or halogen light sources for endophotography or endocinephotography of interesting pathologic lesions, and fluoroscopy with image intensification. The endoscopic operating room of the future will undoubtedly include closed circuit television equipment as an educational aid.

PATIENT PREPARATION AND EVALUATION

Patients undergoing major endoscopic urologic procedures should have evaluations identical to those for major open surgery. The cardiac status is especially important, as he may be challenged by massive shifts in fluid volume and serum electrolyte composition, especially during transurethral resection of the prostate. It is important to know the renal reserve of the patient to ensure his ability to handle extra fluid volume. Serum creatinine, PSP determination, and creatinine clearance are adequate tests for this purpose. If compromised renal reserve is detected, attempts should be made to identify its etiology and to correct it prior to operation if possible (i.e., catheter drainage in cases of longstanding obstructive uropathy). If renal function impairment is not reversible, modification of the operative plan (e.g., staged resection of the prostate) may be necessary.

Urine culture and sensitivity determinations are mandatory in preparation for transurethral procedures. Patients with significant urinary bacterial growth should be given an appropriate parenteral antibiotic agent pre-, intra-, and postoperatively to decrease the risk of bacteremia. Prophylactic coverage with antibiotics in patients with sterile urine preoperatively is optional.

Since hemostasis in transurethral surgery is a problem not infrequently, a coagulation profile should be obtained prior to any major transurethral procedure and specific deficiencies corrected. When a coagulopathy exists that is difficult or unreasonably costly to correct, alternative surgical plans may be necessary (e.g., total prostatectomy rather than a transurethral prostatectomy in hemophiliac subjects).

It is our practice to obtain preoperative intravenous pyelograms on all patients undergoing major transurethral surgery to serve as baseline studies as well as to detect pathology that may influence the operative approach. If vesical diverticula are found, cystograms with postvoid films should be obtained to determine if they empty. Uroflowmetric and cystometric determinations are helpful in differentiating confusing neurogenic and obstructive lesions.

ANESTHESIA

The choice of anesthetic agents may be left to the discretion of the anesthesiologist and the patient. *Spinal anesthesia* is our personal preference, since during the postoperative period the patient is less restless and coughs less, thus reducing the risk of postoperative hemorrhage. Spinal anesthesia allows the patient to respond to pain in the event that an untoward complication such as intraperitoneal extravasation should occur. Spinal anesthesia should be of sufficient duration to cover possible inadvertent occurrences, and it should be given to a level of at least T9—otherwise the patient may feel discomfort from vesical distention.

Blood loss should be monitored by both the surgeon and the anesthetist; if excessive, the volume and hemoglobin of irrigating fluid should be measured to determine its extent. The anesthetist must be alert to the signs and symptoms and be prepared to treat water intoxication syndrome of transurethral prostatic resection. Parenteral steroids and antibiotics should be readily accessible in case of intraoperative sepsis. When hemostasis is being secured at the end of the procedure, the anesthetist should ensure that the patient has at least normal preoperative blood pressure. Hypotension may mask significant arterial bleeding, which may be the source of troublesome hemorrhage during the postoperative period.

When positioning the patient for an endoscopic procedure, the legs should be well padded to protect against nerve injury from the knee braces. For more extensive procedures the legs should be wrapped to guard against venous stasis and possible subsequent embolic events. The electrosurgical grounding plate must have adequate patient contact covering a large area without causing pressure on bony prominences.

TROUBLESHOOTING IN TRANSURETHRAL SURGERY

Mechanical Difficulties

It is beyond the scope of this chapter to describe all the possible mechanical malfunctions that may occur during transurethral surgery. The best means of preventing such problems is to require that technical personnel who care for the instruments routinely check all equipment after each case. If the surgeon closely inspects his instruments while assembling them, he may also uncover potential sources of difficulty.

If a loop does not cut through tissue satisfactorily, the machine should be checked for proper setting. The resectoscope loop should also be checked to ensure that it is well secured in the resectoscope and not broken. The attendant should be responsible for seeing that the patient is properly grounded; if a problem still exists, the power cord should be changed. An ionic solution such as saline can cause dissipation of the electric current. A simple taste test prevents this from causing faulty tissue cutting. Finally, if the problem is still not corrected, an alternate electrosurgical unit should be used.

Troublesome air bubbles which obscure the operator's view are usually due to insufficient fluid in the drip chamber or to air in the water tubing. Interrupting the procedure to fill the drip chamber and to irrigate the water line solves this problem. If tissue tends to stick to the loop during resection, it is usually because of an unclean loop or a blended cutting current, with too great a coagulation component. One of the most annoying problems is when resected tissue remains attached to the bladder wall or prostatic fossa. This is generally due to faulty positioning of the resectoscope loop within the sheath. The same problem occurs when the surgeon releases the cutting pedal prematurely, before the loop is withdrawn into the sheath. On the other hand, a "heavy" foot causes damage to the sheath.

Problems Encountered in Instrument Introduction

Phimosis may be severe enough to cause difficulty in passing instruments. If this is so, a circumcision should be performed to facilitate instrument introduction and to allow better antiseptic preparation. During the postoperative period phimosis may trap secretions and cause poor urethral drainage around the catheter, possibly leading to severe urethritis, stricture formation, and even sepsis. The standard instruments in an endoscopic armamentarium for a vasectomy or a meatotomy should include those used for circumcision.

Meatal stenosis of congenital, inflammatory, traumatic, or iatrogenic origin may be present.

Not only can it prevent passage of a resectoscope, it may also cause "instrument drag," which hampers the surgeon's maneuverability. Meatal stenosis during the postoperative period is also a cause of poor urethral drainage with all its potential sequelae.

Meatotomy should be adequate. Incomplete incision may fail to prevent subsequent damage and possibly lead to postoperative meatal stenosis, which may often be more symptomatic than the original condition. Bougie-à-boule calibration of the meatal area determines the proximal extent of a stenosis. If the stenotic area is long, it may be wise to perform an *internal urethrotomy* or a *perineal urethrostomy*.

Opinion is divided as to whether the meatotomy should be made dorsally or ventrally. Dorsal meatotomy causes less subsequent spraying of the urinary stream but limits the extent of the incision; hemorrhage is often a subsequent problem. We are more satisfied with the ventral meatotomy. If it becomes necessary to perform a "radical" meatotomy to ensure proper instrument mobility, reconstruction of the meatus utilizing a frenular flap may be performed.

Urethral strictures or *false passages* often represent problems for the surgeon. Mild strictures may be dilated with Van Buren sounds, but false passages are a common hazard in the anesthetized patient. Sounds should never be forcibly introduced. The free hand in the rectum is often helpful in obviating false passage formation.

Should a false passage be encountered, urethroscopy with a 0-degree lens is helpful in guiding a filiform through the urethra. Dilation with woven silk followers is then performed. Timberlake obturators with a screw tip to accomodate the filiform threads are helpful in ensuring proper passage of the resectoscope sheath. If one cannot satisfactorily negotiate the true urethral passage, the procedure is then best terminated and attempted at a later date.

Ninety percent or more of male patients can accept a 26 Fr resectoscope without difficulty. In the small percentage who cannot, urethral strictures are not uncommon, usually occurring at the fossa navicularis, penoscrotal junction, or membranous portions. The liberal use of 1 percent hydrocortisone ointment as a lubricant and employment of the smallest sheath possible minimize this complication. If, after apparently satisfactory dilation and lubrication, the resectoscope does not move freely in and out of the urethra, an internal urethrotomy or perineal urethrostomy should be considered.

When *internal urethrotomy* is performed, the urethrotome needs only to be set at 36 Fr; and only one "cut" should be made at the 12 o'clock position. As the fibrous septum between the corpus cavernosa is relatively avascular, hemorrhage is rarely a problem. If the penis is held perpendicular to the pubis during internal urethrotomy, injury to the membranous urethra is avoided. When "prophylactic" internal urethrotomy is performed, a catheter is necessary for only 48 to 72 hours postoperatively. Surgeons who favor internal urethrotomy point out its technical ease and speed, and the fact that there are no external wounds to heal. However, complications of internal urethrotomy include sepsis, hemorrhage, subsequent stricture formation, and severe chordee formation (in 0.9 percent of patients).

Perineal urethrostomy is advocated by many urologists to bypass distal urethral strictures. In patients with a short suspensory ligament of the penis or a long phallus, it is invaluable in facilitating maneuverability of the resectoscope. Valk[30a] and others advocate its routine use in transurethral prostatic resection when resectable tissue is expected to exceed 40 g in weight. Perineal urethrostomy is considered by many surgeons, however, to be a cumbersome, difficult, and often time-consuming procedure. If the incision is not kept in the midline, brisk hemorrhage can result.

A simple and successful method uses resectoscope sheaths of different sizes. In order to employ this technique, the distal urethral must be dilated to a sufficient caliber to accommodate a 24 Fr resectoscope sheath. The 24 Fr sheath is passed into the bulbous urethra to the point where the urethra turns upward toward the urogenital diaphragm. The fenestra of the resectoscope beak is then readily palpable in the perineum. After ensuring that the fenestra is in the midline, a small incision is made, just large enough to allow the small sheath to be passed through the urethral wall, exiting via the perineum. Then, using a 26 Fr or 28 Fr sheath with the 24 Fr Timberlake obturator, which fits snugly into the proximal end of the 24 Fr sheath, the larger sheath is passed into the distal urethra as the smaller sheath is withdrawn. The 24 Fr obturator is replaced in the larger sheath by an appropriate obturator. The larger sheath is then passed into the proximal urethra and bladder, taking care to "hug" the anterior wall of the bulbous urethra as the turn toward the urogenital diaphragm is negotiated.

Sutures are not necessary with this technique. The larger sheath tamponades the perineal urethrostomy site, and hemorrhage is rarely a problem. If during the course of the procedure the resectoscope is inadvertently extracted from the perineal urethrostomy site, the entire maneuver should be repeated. One should never attempt simply to push the sheath back through the perineal urethrostomy, as severe urethral injury and hemorrhage may result. During the postoperative period the catheter should not exit via the perineal urethrostomy site unless absolutely necessary, as delayed wound healing and prolonged urinary leakage can occur from this site. If a Foley catheter is left indwelling for the customary 72 hours following transurethral prostatis resection, coursing the entire urethra, perineal leakage is rare when the catheter is removed. Urethral strictures at the site of perineal urethrostomy are extremely rare.

Erections during transurethral surgery are another possible annoyance. They may occur with any mode of anesthesia and often persist stubbornly, despite all therapeutic measures. A trial of hypotensive anesthesia is of occasional benefit. If a patient is under spinal anesthesia, a judicious trial of amyl nitrate inhalation may be attempted. If the erection persists, perineal urethrostomy can bypass the problem, but hemorrhage may occur if the incision veers from the midline. Temporary cessation of manipulation may allow the phallus to detumesce. Under no circumstances should the procedure simply continue, since forcing the instrument through the erected penis may result in meatal and urethral injuries. Occasionally procedures must be terminated.

Obturator nerve stimulation during transurethral resection of a bladder tumor or prostate is occasionally bothersome. A strong adductor contraction causes sudden movement of the thigh, which may lead to perforation of the bladder or prostatic capsule. If the patient is under general anesthesia, the administration of muscle relaxants circumvents this problem. Muscle relaxants obviously cannot be given to the patient under spinal anesthesia. Usually by resecting "sensitive" areas at the initiation of bladder filling, the magnitude of this problem is decreased. Instillation of local anesthesia around the obturator nerve is of occasional benefit. If an obturator reflex does occur, the surgeon must immediately release his foot from the pedal to prevent serious injury. Perforation may lead to premature termination of the procedure and necessitate a second anesthesia at a later time.

TRANSURETHRAL URETHRAL SURGERY

Urethral Strictures

The treatment of urethral strictures which impede the passage of instruments for other transurethral procedures has already been discussed. These strictures are usually asymptomatic and are an incidental finding. Most symptomatic urethral strictures may be managed by periodic dilations, using either Van Buren sounds or filiforms and followers, as discussed previously. The institution of a more aggressive approach in treating symptomatic urethral strictures depends on the ease and frequency of dilation, the degree of patient discomfort, and the incidence of septic complications following such instrumentation. If infected urine is present, the patient should be given an appropriate antibiotic agent 24 to 48 hours before undergoing dilation. If a stricture is easily dilated, with little chance of causing a false passage, and dilations are required at greater than 3-month intervals, we favor conservative therapy. If dilations are technically difficult or must be performed at more frequent intervals, consideration of a more aggressive approach is warranted.

Injection of local steroids (e.g., dexamethasone) into the area of stricture at the time of dilation may retard the re-formation of strictures. This injection may be given percutaneously, using direct vision urethroscopy to observe the accuracy of the injection site. Malleable needles (6 Fr) are available for direct transurethral instillation under vision. Injection of a solution of six parts dexamethasone and four parts lidocaine (1 percent) may decrease patient discomfort; 2 cc or less of this solution is usually sufficient. Reports regarding the efficacy of the treatment, however, show conflicting results.

If this approach is not successful, the surgeon should opt for therapeutic internal urethrotomy or open surgical urethroplasty. The indications and techniques of urethroplasty are beyond the purview of this chapter.

Only slight modifications are necessary in the aforementioned technique of internal urethrotomy when this procedure is performed to remedy stubborn symptomatic strictures. The incision is still made in the fibrous intercavernous septum at the 12 o'clock position; the relatively dull blade of the urethrotome —set at 38 Fr—should sever only the rigid unyielding strictured areas. The penis should also be held perpendicular to the pubis to eliminate the possibility of sphincter injury.

A straight Otis urethrotome is the preferred instrument. Employment of a urethrotome with a screw tip that can be attached to a filiform guards against extension of a false passage. Because it is often difficult to pass a urethral catheter following an internal urethrotomy, the use of this filiform in combination with a *Council catheter and guide* often aids in subsequent catheter passage. The catheter should be left indwelling for 6 to 8 weeks, depending on the severity of the stricture. The use of Silastic catheters has decreased the frequency of urethral reactions and improved the success rate of internal urethrotomy. Small fenestra cut into the urethral portion of the catheter allow drainage of purulent urethral material into the catheter, further decreasing the likelihood of urethritis and subsequent stricture formation. For the patient the main disadvantage of this procedure is the inconvenience of long-term catheter drainage. If failure should result, repeat internal urethrotomy or open urethroplasty may be performed. In our experience internal urethrotomy has not compromised the success rate of subsequent urethroplasty.

Some endoscopic surgeons indicate the use of a Collings knife to incise a strictured area electrically. Its use should be restricted to short, dense strictures. Often the stricture is replaced by severe, dense scar tissue, however, resulting in a tighter or longer stricture than originally encountered. Therefore for the dense, short stricture, we advocate excision with primary reanastomosis.

Urethral Polyps and Condylomas

Urethral polyps and condylomas, though rare, may be difficult to manage. Poorly planned attempts at transurethral resection may lead to widespread dissemination of the lesions to areas of denuded, traumatized mucosa. Use of a *flexible cup biopsy forceps* to remove the bulk of the lesion followed by chemical or electrofulguration of the base is often successful. Resection with an electrosurgical loop is rarely indicated because of the high incidence of subsequent brisk hemorrhage and stricture formation. Only localized lesions should be treated transurethrally.

If multiple lesions exist they are best treated chemically with topical urethral installation of 5 percent 5-fluorouracil cream[10] or 0.5 percent colchicine;[13] both medications have proved effective. If these measures are not successful, marsupialization of the involved segment of the urethra with open excision of the lesions may be necessary. After a minimum 6-month period of observation for recurrence, the urethra may be closed employing standard second-stage urethroplasty techniques.

Urethral Foreign Bodies and Stones

Urethral foreign bodies and calculi in most instances can be removed with gentle transurethral manipulation and the use of rigid grasping forceps, e.g., Lowsley's forceps. Proximal periurethral pressure, applied either manually or with a tourniquet at the base of the penis if the object is distal enough, is employed to prevent retrograde movement of the object. Forcible injection of a water-soluble lubricant against this proximal pressure usually dilates the distal urethra and simultaneously lubricates the object, facilitating removal. When extracting an object, care must be taken not to include urethral mucosa in the jaws of the grasping forceps. However, after dilation of the urethra with a lubricating jelly, external manual manipulation alone may be successful. If antegrade manipulation is not possible, attempts to move the object in a retrograde fashion into the bladder usually allows the object to be snared. Occasionally external urethrotomy or suprapubic cystostomy become necessary to extract such objects.

Transurethral Sphincterotomy

Occasionally in patients with *neurogenic dysfunction of the detrusor* significant residual urine remains despite all attempts to correct outflow obstruction and to increase the tone of the detrusor by either medical or surgical means. *Spasm of the external urinary sphincter* often causes such imbalance of micturition. External sphincter spasm may be suspected if the patient describes a hesitant, interrupted urinary stream. The diagnosis may be confirmed either by measurement of intraluminal urethral pressure or by electromyographic studies of the pelvic floor musculature.

Staged transurethral sphincterotomy is often successful in correcting this problem. The therapeutic range between success, continued retention, or incontinence is small indeed. It is better to have the patient return on another day if residual urine is still present than to err on the side of incontinence—although often the latter is preferable in patients with large amounts of residual urine and partially decompensated upper tracts. Many patients favor the use of an external condom type of urinal, rather than a stomal appliance. Sphincterotomy obviously holds less operative risk than its alternative—ileal loop diversion. If penile complications ensue secondary to external collecting devices, supravesical diversion may be performed subsequently.

Transurethral sphincterotomy is performed with an Otis urethrotome or by electroresection of the sphincter with a Collings knife. We favor the latter method. A pure cutting current is used, incising the sphincter initially at the 12 o'clock area. The incision should extend into the corpus spongiosum. Brisk hemorrhage is an expected sequela, and although bothersome it rarely represents a significant complication. Coagulation of bleeding points should not be performed since stricture formation occurs. If significant residual urine still remains, additional incisions are made judiciously at a later time. If incontinence or a membranous urethral stricture should result, supravesical urinary diversion may then be performed as a last resort. We have, however, observed several dramatic successes from transurethral sphinc-terotomy in patients who were facing possible supravesical diversions.

TRANSURETHRAL RESECTION OF THE BLADDER NECK

Great care should be exercised when making the diagnosis of *primary bladder neck contracture,* especially in the female patient. In years past this was a greatly overdiagnosed lesion; recent data have shown it to be a rare lesion indeed. Primary bladder neck contracture in the male is usually secondary to adenomatous hypertrophy of the posterior commissural lobe, rather than to a true fibrous median bar. The former is part of a more generalized process involving other prostatic lobes. Resection of this isolated area therefore rarely corrects the obstructive problem. Although primary bladder neck contracture secondary to a median bar does exist, its incidence is much lower than previously cited.

Bladder neck contracture may also occur secondary to *generalized detrusor hypertrophy,* as in cases of distal urinary obstruction (i.e., posterior urethral valves) or of hypertonic neurogenic dysfunction of the bladder. The functional degree of contracture in selected cases may be quite significant and occasionally causes continued obstruction despite correction of the primary etiologic factor. In our view this lesion is best treated by open YV-plasty of the bladder neck, rather than by transurethral resection.

Iatrogenic fibrous contracture of the bladder neck is the most frequently encountered form of bladder neck contracture, resulting from either transurethral or open prostatectomy, or from previous bladder neck resections. Circumferential resection of the bladder neck with indiscriminate fulguration may lead to this complication. Occasionally it is a sequela to radical prostatectomy. This type of contracture frequently causes a high-grade obstructive lesion, and the bladder neck orifice may be of only pinpoint size.

Neurogenic dysfunction of the bladder neck is another important cause of bladder neck obstruction. This *functional obstruction* should be distinguished from anatomic obstruction seen in neurologic dysfunction with generalized detrusor hypertrophy. Obstruction from spas-ticity of the external urinary sphincter should also be differentiated from this entity by the use of urethral pressure studies or by electromyography of the pelvic floor musculature. Recent experience with phenoxybenzamine (Dibenzyline) in cases of bladder neck obstruction secondary to neurogenic dysfunction has been encouraging, and such patients may be spared bladder neck resection.

Transurethral Bladder Neck Resection in the Female

Diagnostic Evaluation. Detection and quantitation of the degree of bladder neck obstruction in the female is difficult, and the diagnosis should be made with circumspection. The cystoscopic appearance of the bladder neck in female subjects is often misleading. In our experience *voiding ciné studies of the bladder neck* are most important in documenting the functional significance of this lesion. *Bougie-à-boule calibration* of the bladder neck may be of benefit, especially in fibrous contractures. These findings must also be present to support a cystoscopic impression of bladder neck contracture. Bladder trabeculation and residual urine are helpful indicators, but care must be taken to rule out distal obstructive lesions of neurogenic disease as a cause of apparent bladder neck contracture. If with overdistention of the bladder the outlet still appears obstructive as viewed from the distal urethra and has a blanched appearance, a significant bladder neck contracture is probably present.

Technique. Scrupulous attention to technique is imperative in performing trans-urethral bladder neck resection in the female. The distal extent of the resection must be carefully monitored. As the resection is carried distally, the urethra may appear obstructive, luring the resectionist into cutting too far distally, resulting in incontinence. Resection should be restricted to the proximal one-fourth to one-third of the urethra. It is helpful to mark the distal extent of the proposed resection with light fulguration prior to commencing resection. Whenever possible, resection should preserve the muscle fibers in the anterior and posterior portions of the bladder neck, since these fibers which aid in vesical neck opening during micturition extend into the distal urethra. A deep incision with the Collings blade at 5 and at 7 o'clock is the preferred method. As mentioned earlier, circumferential resection with a loop invites subsequent fibrous contracture. Use of a pure unblended cutting current with precise and minimal fulguration of bleeding points further decreases this likelihood. A finger in the vagina for palpation is helpful in determining the completeness of the resection. A catheter should be left indwelling for a minimum of 48 hours postoperatively.

Fibrotic bladder neck contracture in the female may respond well to "overdilation" with a *Kollman dilator* opened to 40 Fr. Similarly bladder neck obstruction secondary to neurogenic dysfunction may also occasionally be benefited. In this instance the entire urethra should be dilated.

Complications. *Hemorrhage* and *recurrent bladder neck contracture* are not altogether uncommon, and *incontinence, perforation,* and *fistula formation* are serious complications of bladder neck resection in the female.

Careful attention to technical detail will guard against incontinence. Postoperative hemorrhage rarely requires repeat fulguration; prolonged catheter drainage usually suffices. Perforation into the vagina heals spontaneously with prolonged catheter drainage in most instances. Open surgical repair is occasionally necessary if the perforation persists. Delayed fistula formation usually results from widespread tissue necrosis, which causes the tissue to spread during the healing process. Surgical repair in this instance is usually necessary.

Transurethral Bladder Neck Resection in the Male

On only rare occasions in cases of primary bladder neck contracture in the male does resection of the apparent obstruction of the bladder neck suffice. It is usually necessary to resect adenomatous tissue involving other prostatic lobes. In performing bladder neck resection in cases of neurogenic dysfunction, a full resection of the entire prostatic fossa should be performed, resecting all adenomatous tissue to favor a successful result. The prostatic fossa and bladder neck are converted into a conical funnel. Continence is maintained by the external striated urinary sphincter. Care should be exercised to avoid perforating the bladder neck; it is preferable to repeat the resection at a later date if residual urine persists, rather than to overresect the bladder neck. A therapeutic trial

of phenoxybenzamine should precede any bladder neck resection for neurogenic disease.

Fibrous contractures of the bladder neck in males are best treated with a Collings knife. An initial incision at 6 o'clock is usually adequate and should extend to transect all circular fibers. If this does not spring the bladder neck open, incisions in additional quadrants (10 and 2 o'clock) may be made until the desired effect is obtained. Resectoscope loops may also be used for this purpose. Concomitant circumferential local injection of triamcinolone transurethrally may decrease the incidence of subsequent recurrent contractures.[8] Occasionally open YV-plasty of the bladder neck is necessary if subsequent contracture occurs.

Retrograde ejaculation is a common sequela to any surgical procedure involving the bladder neck. The patient should be informed of this possibility.

TRANSURETHRAL RESECTION OF THE PROSTATE

Electroresection of the Prostate

Indications for Surgery. The decision to perform prostatectomy by any method should be made on the basis of subjective and objective signs of obstruction. Residual urine signifying vesical decompensation is a usual prerequisite. Occasionally, however, patients may suffer severe obstructive symptoms and still void to completion. In such selected cases where micturition is an ordeal, prostatectomy may be indicated. Patients undergoing prostatectomy for irritative symptoms only may find their symptoms no better—and possibly worse—after an ill-advised prostatectomy. In borderline candidates uroflowmetry indicating urine flow rate well below normal is of importance; trabeculation is another important finding. In patients with possible neurogenic disease a cystometrogram is essential. Cystoscopy is necessary to confirm the preoperative impression, but rarely should a decision to operate be made on cystoscopic findings alone. The primary value of cystoscopy is to exclude other obstructive lesions and to help select the operative approach.

The latter decision is largely one of individual preference. The size of the prostate is an important consideration, although there is no absolute size limit for *transurethral prostatec-tomy*. Rather than institute such a size limit, a time limit of about 1 hour for resection should be the surgeon's guide. Transurethral resections lasting longer than an hour are associated with a high incidence of complications, e.g., water intoxication, urethral strictures, sepsis, and excessive blood loss. If completion of the resection within 1 hour cannot be anticipated, open prostatectomy should be selected. Some surgeons prefer to resect in two stages if the gland is too large to manage during an initial 1-hour period. While this is appropriate if the prostate is larger than anticipated, we question the judgment in performing a *planned* two-stage resection. The necessary second anesthesia and possible septic sequelae in such cases favor one-stage open prostatectomy. On the other hand, in poor-risk or very old patients it is possible to resect one lateral lobe or the middle and one lateral lobe only and still obtain an excellent functional result. This is preferable to an incomplete resection of all lobes, since the incidence of poor operative slough and hemorrhage is increased in the latter but not in the former case.

Small fibrotic glands should almost invariably be removed by the transurethral route. Carcinoma of the prostate causing lower tract obstruction should also be managed transurethrally.

Associated pathology such as vesicoureteral reflux, vesical calculi, diverticula, and vesical neoplasm may alter the decision in regard to the route of prostatectomy.

Patient preparation and evaluation have been discussed previously.

Vasectomy.   Controversy still exists in regard to the efficacy of prophylactic vasectomy in preventing epididymitis in patients undergoing transurethral resection of the prostate. Evidence exists both for[6,26,27] and against[17,21] vasectomy. In a well controlled study by Rinker and associates[26] consisting of 1,029 patients in whom unilateral vasectomy was performed, the incidence of epididymitis in nonvasectomized patients was 4.2 percent, compared to 0.39 percent in the vasectomized patients. Schmidt and Hinman[27] noted a threefold difference in the incidence between the vasectomized and nonvasectomized groups. Lynn and Nesbitt[21] and Haralambidis and Spinelli,[17] however, noted no significant difference. Since 1963 when Kendall[18] demonstrated a 30 per-

cent incidence of bacterial growth when excised vas segments were cultured from patients who had had an indwelling catheter for more than 3 days, it was felt that vasectomy in this group would be hazardous for fear of trapping infection within the epididymis. A more recent study by Brooks and associates,[6] however, demonstrated a reduction in the incidence of epididymitis after vasectomy in patients with prior catheter drainage (20.5 percent versus 0 percent). Although the series is small, it shows that in certain instances vasectomy may be beneficial in this group. We feel that the reason for these diverse conclusions, all from seemingly well conceived studies, must be the result of individual surgical variations.

If vasectomy is to be performed, the percutaneous method or the standard exposure, excision, and ligation method are superior to a simple "vas crush." In our personal experience vasectomy is not performed routinely.

Surgical Technique for Benign Prostatic Hypertrophy.   Prior to commencing resection of obstructing adenomatous prostatic tissue, it is mandatory that thorough *cystoscopic evaluation* be made. The bladder should be the first area examined, as cystoscopic manipulation in the prostatic urethra may cause troublesome and obscuring hemorrhage. The 0- or 30-degree lens is employed for the resection, but a 70-degree lens allows more complete inspection of the bladder wall. The presence of coexisting *bladder tumors, diverticula,* or *vesical calculi* must be excluded. If found they should be dealt with prior to the initiation of prostatic resection.

It has been taught that if *transitional cell carcinoma* of the bladder coexists with obstructive benign prostatic hypertrophy, the bladder tumor should be excised immediately and the prostatic resection deferred until a later time. Seeding of the prostatic fossa with transitional cell carcinoma was a feared sequela if the tumor was not excised first. In an important communication by Green and Yalowitz[15] this fear was found to be unwarranted. The incidence of tumor recurrence in the areas of the vesical neck and prostatic urethra was identical in both the one- and two-stage procedures.

Bladder diverticula of small capacity with an open neck need no therapy if the preoperative cystogram reveals complete emptying of the diverticulum. By contrast, if the neck is small and residual urine is present in the diverticulum, transurethral incision of the diverticular neck is advisable to decrease the possibility of development of transitional cell carcinoma in the diverticulum. Diverticula of larger size are generally best treated by open excision.

Vesical calculi when present should be handled by litholapaxy prior to resection.

After associated vesical pathology has been excluded or properly treated, careful evaluation of the obstructing *adenoma* should be made in regard to its anatomic relationship to the trigone, bladder neck, verumontanum, and external urinary sphincter. These relationships must be indelibly fixed in the surgeon's mind before resection is begun.

The distance from the adenoma to the trigone is an important determination. As the trigone hypertrophies and the length of the prostatic fossa increases, this distance decreases, making trigonal injury more likely. After the bladder neck and trigone are inspected to determine the amount of middle lobe tissue present, the appropriate resection is planned. The length of the prostatic urethra proximal to the verumontanum should be measured with respect to the length of the loop excursion. If the fossa is shorter than a loop excursion, care must be taken during the resection to avoid encroaching on the trigone and ureteral orifices. The extent of the prostatic tissue distal to the verumontanum should also be determined to help protect against injury to the external sphincter. The bulk of the adenoma should be judged by palpation of the cystoscope with a finger placed in the rectum. It is especially important to gauge the thickness of the adenoma at the posterior vesical neck, one of the common potential sites of perforation. The external sphincter should then be visualized in relation to the verumontanum and the apex of the prostate; during resection it is imperative that the surgeon be able to differentiate between the cut surface of adenoma and that of muscle tissue, as the spatial relationships of the external sphincter, verumontanum, and adenoma are constantly changing.

The sheath of the resectoscope should be well lubricated with a water-soluble jelly or 1 percent hydrocortisone ointment and inserted with an appropriate Timberlake obturator. Under no circumstances should the sheath be advanced without the obturator in place. A 24 Fr sheath suffices for most resections and should

be used in preference to larger sheaths except when massive adenomas exist. As mentioned previously, a 26 Fr or 27 Fr resectoscope loop can be accommodated in a 24 Fr sheath, and a 28 Fr loop in a 26 Fr sheath; it is rarely necessary to use a 27 Fr or 28 Fr sheath. If after satisfactory dilation and lubrication the sheath "drags," an *internal urethrotomy* or *perineal urethrostomy* should be performed. If instrument drag occurs in midprocedure, a smaller sheath should be substituted wherever possible. If a 24 Fr sheath is already in use, an internal urethrotomy or perineal urethrostomy may be necessary.

The order in which lobes are resected is done largely by individual choice; it is not the purpose of this chapter to promote one method in preference to another. Ideally, a neophyte resectionist employs various methods during the initial phases of his training so that he may determine which method best suits his talents. Variant adenomatous configurations may induce a surgeon to deviate from his routine pattern, but whenever possible a uniform method should be followed. A detailed anatomic discussion of all techniques is beyond the scope of this chapter.

It is our practice to begin resection of the *posterior bladder neck area* and *middle lobe* as an initial step. The flow of irrigating fluid from the prostatic fossa into the bladder is improved by this maneuver, and resected chips of adenomatous tissue flow more readily into the bladder. Another advantage of beginning in this area is that resection of the middle lobe and posterior bladder neck can be completed early in the procedure, when the surgeon is fresh and visualization is still optimal. This reduces the risk of trigonal injury or perforation of the posterior bladder neck. When circular muscle fibers of the posterior bladder neck are seen, resection in this area is terminated. One should be especially careful not to use widespread coagulation in the area of the bladder neck lest a bladder neck contracture ensue. Only "pinpoint" fulguration should be employed.

The anterior portion of the neck is next resected. Again, by performing this part of the resection early, better visualization is afforded the surgeon while he is still fresh, decreasing the likelihood of perforation at the anterior bladder neck, another high-risk area. The resection then proceeds to the 11 o'clock to the 1 o'clock position. In order to facilitate the resection, the patient should be elevated in relation to the surgeon. The resectoscope beak should be set at the level of the verumontanum. When resecting the length of the prostatic adenoma, the sheath of the resectoscope is depressed as the loop is swept back in order to resect deeper at the midpoint of the prostatic fossa; this makes the fossa into the shape of a barrel, the bladder neck and prostatic apex forming the top and bottom of the barrel, respectively. The adenoma is thinnest in the anterior portion of the prostatic fossa, and care must be taken not to perforate this area. Once this portion of the resection is completed, the anterior attachments to the lateral lobes are then freed, allowing both lateral lobes to fall posteriorly, making subsequent lateral lobe resection easier. The surgeon no longer needs to operate with the lens upside down. Resection in the extreme 12 o'clock position is the last resected, to decrease the possibility of early entry into venous sinuses. After hemostasis is obtained, attention is then turned to lateral lobe resection.

The order of resection of the lateral lobes is generally determined by the left- or right-handedness of the surgeon. Most right-handed surgeons feel that resection of the right lateral lobe is easier, and so they may elect to begin with the more awkward left side while there is only minimal distortion of the prostatic fossa. Resection is performed beginning at the upper medial portion of the lobe, progressing laterally at each level until true prostate and the surgical capsule are seen. Resection is continued in the next lower layer, in a medial-to-lateral direction. The resectoscope beak should be positioned so that the verumontanum is often in view; this is to protect the external sphincter from injury. Whenever possible, full use of the loop's sweep should be made, resecting the entire length of the prostatic adenoma with each excursion. In small prostates where a loop excursion may exceed the length of the prostatic fossa, special care must be taken not to encroach on the trigone. If the prostatic fossa is markedly enlongated, two loop excursions may be necessary, or the sheath should be moved to the apex while the loop is still extended. This latter method is quicker and facilitates a smoother resection. If the lateral lobes appear so bulky that three loop widths do not complete resection laterally into the area of the surgical capsule, it is preferable to employ an *encirclement technique,* rather than the side-to-side, step-down technique. With a large prostate resection time may be significantly reduced if a suprapubic punch cystostomy is placed prior to the resection. One then does not have to stop resection periodically to empty the bladder, as the suprapubic cystostomy tube allows continual runoff of irrigating fluid. Iglesias has developed a new modified sheath with continual inflow and outflow channels with suction.

In the encirclement technique the anterior portion of the resection is performed as with small adenomas. After the anterior portion has been resected to gain sufficient space for the sheath to maneuver, the encirclement technique is begun. A deep groove is created between the adenoma and the surgical capsule; care must be taken near the bladder neck and apex in regard to the lateral extent of the resection. This groove is carried posteriorly on each side to the 5 and 7 o'clock positions, where the main vascular supply to the prostate is located. The bulk of the lateral lobes is then devascularized, facilitating their subsequent rapid removal. By manipulation of the adenoma with a rectally placed finger (if a one-handed instrument is used), more rapid resection is possible.

During the final stage of the procedure the *apical adenomatous tissue* lying distal to the verumontanum is resected. The external urinary sphincter should be visualized to guard against injury; the beak of the resectoscope should be placed just proximal to the sphincter. Any apical tissue that protrudes into the lumen of the prostatic fossa as viewed from the area of the membranous urethra should be resected. We do not routinely incise the posterior bladder neck or interureteric ridge with a Collings blade.

Following resection the bladder is evacuated of prostatic chips with an Ellik evacuator or Toomey syringe, and final hemostasis is achieved. If open venous sinuses cause excessive bleeding, catheter traction should be employed during the initial postoperative period. The surgeon should ensure that the blood pressure level at the final stage of the procedure is at a normal level prior to removing the resectoscope. Hypotension may mask significant arteriolar bleeders.

A 22 Fr or 24 Fr Foley catheter should then be inserted and connected to straight drainage. If clots form and obstruct the catheter lumen, intermittent hand irrigation usually suffices to remove them. We prefer this type of catheter drainage to the three-way Foley under continuous irrigation, feeling that the latter may cause continued bleeding.

If catheter traction is employed, at least 30 cc of fluid should be placed in the balloon to ensure that the balloon remains outside the prostatic fossa. This allows contraction of the prostatic capsule, a major hemostatic mechanism. When large adenomas are resected, a correspondingly large volume should be placed in the balloon. Traction may be applied with meatal pressure, using a moist sponge tied around the catheter or weighted traction (<1 pound) over the foot of the bed. Traction should be terminated at 1 hour. If bleeding persists, traction should be intermittently released to prevent pressure necrosis of the meatus or bladder neck.

Surgical Technique for Carcinoma of the Prostate. The indications for operative intervention in carcinoma of the prostate are the same as those for hyperplasia. Since almost all carcinomatous glands causing obstruction are extensive stage C lesions, *total prostatectomy* in most cases has no place in their management. In early stage C lesions, however, total prostatectomy may be an appropriate palliative procedure to obviate recurrent episodes of lower tract obstruction. Extensive stage C lesions causing obstruction must be treated by *transurethral resection,* as the infiltrative nature of the carcinoma does not allow for *open enucleative prostatectomy.*

When there is massive neoplastic involvement of the prostate producing obstruction, many urologists favor perineal needle biopsy to confirm the diagnosis, followed by *orchiectomy* and *estrogen therapy.* Controversy exists whether in fact *hormonal therapy* is justified for obstructive disease, or if its use should be held in abeyance until the patient becomes symptomatic from metastatic disease. We do not intend to advocate one approach over the other; when benign adenomatous hyperplasia exists in conjunction with carcinoma and is the prime lesion responsible for outlet obstruction, however, transurethral prostatectomy should be performed. Cystoscopic evaluation is helpful in differentiating between obstruction caused by adenomatous hyperplasia and massive infiltrative carcinoma.

Recent enthusiasm for *radiation therapy* for stage C carcinoma of the prostate has also modified the traditional role of transurethral resection of prostate (TURP) in its management. In fact, many patients with complete or near-complete retention may be managed well by catheter drainage and radiation therapy, with or without adjunctive hormonal treatment. Six or seven weeks, however, are often required for sufficient shrinkage of the prostate (and subsidence of radiation reaction) before the catheter can be removed and the patient is able to void. Although it is thus possible to obtain significant shrinkage of neoplastic glands with radiation therapy, we prefer transurethral resection for this group of patients. If transurethral resection of a prostatic carcinoma has been performed and subsequent radiation therapy is contemplated, it is probably best to defer the initiation of irradiation for 6 to 8 weeks following the resection to allow reepithelialization of the prostatic fossa. Fewer irritative symptoms seem to result. If the patient has already received a full course of irradiation and later develops lower tract obstruction, transurethral resection may be performed without major problems. Delayed healing of the prostatic fossa sometimes occurs but rarely is bothersome. There is, however, a higher incidence of urethral stricture in patients who have had prior irradiation.

Special care must be taken in cases of carcinoma of the prostate, since the incidence of *postoperative bleeding* is more common in these patients than in those who have benign disease. A *prothrombin time, platelet count,* and examination of the urine for *fibrinolysins* should be part of the preoperative evaluation. If troublesome postoperative hemorrhage ensues, *primary fibrinolysis* and *primary intravascular coagulation* must be ruled out. Fibrinolysis may also occur in conjunction with disseminated intravascular coagulation.[5] Fibrinolysis secondary to *urokinase* is easily detected by incubating a blood clot in a urine sample. If clot lysis occurs, *epsilon aminocaproic acid* (EACA) should be administered immediately by the intravenous route, and later converted to oral therapy.

The administration of EACA to patients who have both fibrinolysis and disseminated intravascular coagulation (DIC), however, is hazardous. Primary intravascular coagulation must be ruled out prior to instituting EACA therapy. A diagnosis of DIC is made when the patient is found to be thrombocytopenic and hypofibrinogenemic, with an associated increase in the prothrombin time (secondary to a decrease in the concentration of accelerator globulin). Decreased levels of prothrombin and factor VIII (antihemophilic factor) further substantiate the diagnosis. DIC is managed with intravenous heparin in a dose of 150 to 400 mg per 24-hour period. Continuous intravenous infusion is preferable to the intermittent intravenous or subcutaneous methods. If associated urokinase activity is present, EACA may be added to heparin after the clotting factors (platelet count, fibrinogen, and prothrombin) have begun to return to normal. Transfusion with fresh blood is an important adjuvant in that it replaces depleted coagulation components.

If carcinoma exists in conjunction with hyperplasia, the surgical technique remains essentially the same as with benign adenomatous obstruction. If the prostate is extensively involved with carcinoma, however, some modification in technique may be necessary. A cross-step resection such as that used in small adenomatous hyperplasia (i.e., medial-to-lateral) is preferable to the encirclement technique. Often there is anatomic distortion; the bladder neck and membranous urethra may be the only remaining landmarks. With extensive carcinoma the urethra is often so rigid that maneuverability of the sheath is limited; resection may initially have to be performed in the rigid areas to facilitate maneuverability of the sheath. In prostatic obstruction secondary to scirrhous carcinoma, a "channel cut" often suffices for relief of obstruction, as tissue will not fall into the fossa as with adenomatous tissue. Care must be taken in the region of the apex.

Surgical Technique for Prostatic Abscess. Modern antibiotic treatment has made prostatic abscess a rare lesion. In the course of a transurethral resection, however, it is not uncommon to encounter small pockets of contaminating purulent material which persist following acute or chronic episodes of infection. Fortunately these pockets are usually sterile.

Occasionally a patient presents with acute obstructive symptoms secondary to a prostatic abscess. The abscess areas are often fluctuant but occasionally may be so firm as to resemble carcinoma. Prior to the days of modern antibacterial chemotherapy, *incision and drainage* by the perineal exposure was the procedure of choice. Today the transurethral route is preferred, but resection of the abscess should be deferred until the patient has been placed on appropriate parenteral wide-spectrum antibiotic coverage. If the patient presents with acute retention, however, a small urethral catheter or punch suprapubic cystostomy may be necessary until antibiotic therapy has been instituted. Transurethral resection may then be performed.

The abscess is commonly seen bulging into the lumen of the prostatic urethra. Simple unroofing of the most prominent portion of the bulge is usually all that is necessary. If significant hyperplasia is also present, this can be resected at the same time or at a second sitting, depending on the general status of the patient.

Surgical Technique for Prostatitis. Transurethral resection should be employed only rarely in patients with prostatitis (and patients should be properly forewarned of the possible failure of transurethral resection to relieve their symptoms). Obstructive urinary symptoms must not be confused with irritative symptoms; the latter are often worsened by an ill-advised resection. When prostatitis is associated with adenomatous obstruction or with *prostatic calculi,* and if the patient has severe debilitating symptoms, a properly performed resection may be of benefit. A "radical" transurethral resection offers the best chance for symptomatic relief in these patients. All tissue surrounding the prostatic calculi should be resected. Since prostatic calculi reside between the adenoma and the surgical capsule, resection should extend well into the surgical capsule in an attempt to resect most of the inflamed tissue. Coagulation should be used sparingly to decrease subsequent fibrosis in the prostatic fossa. If severe symptoms persist, *total prostatectomy* may be the only means of benefiting such patients.

Surgical Technique for Prostatic Urethral Valves. A detailed discussion of the technique for proper resection of prostatic urethral valves is found in Chapter 57.

Complications of Transurethral Electroresection of the Prostate. *Hemorrhage* is the most common complication following transurethral prostatic surgery. Complete preoperative evaluation of the coagulation profile of the patient is a valuable prophylactic measure. Careful electrofulguration of arterial bleeders decreases the chances of delayed hemorrhage resulting from sloughing of necrotic tissue secondary to massive fulguration of the prostatic fossa. Blood pressure must be at normal levels near the termination of the procedure to ensure that significant bleeding points are not masked by hypotension. Bleeding venous sinuses respond to catheter traction; indiscriminate fulguration of venous sinuses does not control this type of bleeding and may even result in additional hemorrhage. Catheter irrigation should be instituted only when the catheter is obstructed, as irrigation may displace clots from venous sinuses, causing renewed hemorrhage. For this reason the use of routine three-way continuous catheter irrigation is discouraged.

It is only rarely necessary to return a patient to the cystoscopy suite for control of hemorrhage. After thoroughly evacuating the bladder and prostatic fossa of clots, examination for bleeding sites should be performed, using the irrigating fluid under low pressure. Appropriate fulguration may then be accomplished. Occasionally open surgical exploration may become necessary, with direct fulguration or suture ligation of bleeding sites; a circumferential bladder neck suture may be of benefit in stubborn cases. Only under rare circumstances should it be necessary to leave a pack in the prostatic fossa.

Undermining of the trigone with associated ureteral injury is a result of careless technique. If this does occur, a cystogram should be performed to exclude *intraperitoneal perforation*. If perforation has not occurred, nothing further need be done. If present to a significant degree, intraperitoneal perforation can be managed with open cystotomy and closure of the defect. Fulguration near the injured ureteral orifice should be avoided, as it increases the risk of subsequent obstruction. An intravenous pyelogram should be performed in these patients postoperatively to rule out obstruction.

Water intoxication may occur when venous sinuses are opened early in the course of a resection, or when resection time is prolonged. Hypertension and mental confusion are the predominant symptoms. Fluid restriction and administration of a potent diuretic agent should be instituted. In patients with severe hyponatremia, judicious administration of hypertonic saline (3 percent) may be necessary. The use of a 5 percent mannitol solution as an irrigating medium helps to obviate this complication because of its osmotic diuretic effect.

Hemolysis should not occur if an isosmotic irrigating fluid is used.

Urethral strictures occur in approximately 5 percent of patients following transurethral resection of the prostate. The membranous urethra, penoscrotal junction, and fossa navicularis are common sites for such strictures. Gentle technique with proper preliminary urethral dilatation and instrument lubrication is an important prophylactic measure. By using the smallest available instrument and by limiting the resection time to less than 1 hour, the incidence of stricture formation can be further decreased. If a preexisting stricture is found, or if the urethra is simply too small to accept the smallest resectoscope sheath comfortably, *internal urethrotomy* or *perineal urethrostomy* should be performed to bypass the stricture. Use of a small-caliber Silastic catheter during the postoperative period also reduces the incidence of stricture. The prophylactic passage of a 22 Fr sound 8 weeks postoperatively allows a stricture to be detected before it becomes severe enough to cause a management problem. Periodic dilation usually takes care of this complication.

Symptomatic *perforation* of the bladder neck and prostatic capsule should occur only rarely. With perforation early during the resection, large amounts of fluid may be extravasated into the retroperitoneal space, causing significant discomfort. Spinal anesthesia allows the extravasation to be discovered while the patient is still in the cystoscopy room where appropriate therapeutic measures may be undertaken without delay. General anesthesia often delays the diagnosis, requiring the patient to be returned to the operating suite for treatment. Additional general anesthesia is usually required, whereas spinal anesthesia usually persists for a sufficient duration to take care of this complication.

If abdominal distention is noted and the patient complains of abdominal discomfort a cystogram should be performed. If an intraperitoneal perforation has occurred, the patient should be explored and the site of the perforation closed through a cystotomy incision. Expectant therapy with catheter drainage and diuretics may often suffice if a small perforation has occurred; close observation of the patient is imperative. Only *small retroperitoneal perforations* are managed with catheter drainage. These perforations occur quite commonly and usually remain undiagnosed. *Large retroperitoneal perforations* are often associated with severe discomfort. A small suprapubic incision should be made in such cases and a Penrose drain placed in the retropubic space. If the urine was infected preoperatively, appropriate parenteral antibiotic coverage should be initiated at once, if it has not already been administered. Prophylactic antibacterial coverage is not necessary in patients with sterile urine preoperatively.

Incontinence is a feared complication of any form of prostatectomy. The patient must be forewarned of this possibility. The incidence of permanent urinary incontinence following transurethral resection of the prostate should be less than 0.5 percent. Temporary incontinence is more common but usually resolves within a few days or weeks. Improvement in the degree of incontinence can be seen up to 1 year postoperatively. Rarely is an antiincontinence procedure indicated without having observed the patient for signs of improvement for a minimum of several months.

Infected urine during the postoperative period is common and is difficult to remedy completely until the prostatic capsule has reepithelialized. If infected, the patient should be given appropriate antibacterial coverage followed by antibiotic suppression for 8 to 12 weeks postoperatively. During the healing phase the presence of pyuria is expected and does not necessarily indicate infection. Cultures should be taken to justify the administration of antibiotic agents—and even then, antimicrobal therapy may lead only to drug resistance or superinfection.

Postoperative Management of Transurethral Prostatectomy. It is imperative that the catheter drain well during the postoperative period. An obstructed catheter causes distention of the prostatic capsule with resultant hemorrhage. Intra- and postoperative parenteral furosemide (20 to 40 mg) facilitates postoperative diuresis and helps to keep the catheter patent. Intravenous fluids should be given in adequate volumes (150 to 175 cc/hour), unless they are contraindicated because of congestive heart failure or water intoxication syndrome. *Bladder spasms* may indicate an obstructed catheter. If clots in the bladder are ruled out as a cause of the spasms, appropriate anticholinergic agents may be administered. The average period of catheter drainage is 3 days.

The patient should be kept at bed rest during the initial 24-hour period following prostatectomy. Full ambulation is allowed on the first postoperative day, but the patient should be discouraged from sitting for prolonged periods of time. Bowel movements should be kept soft to prevent excessive straining during this period. If an enema is necessary, it should be given with extreme caution because of possible rectal perforation. Heavy lifting should be avoided during the first 4 to 6 weeks after surgery.

Cryosurgery of the Prostate

Indications. In 1964 Gonder and associates[14] reported on experimental prostatic cryosurgery. Since this time several communications regarding the procedure have been presented in the urologic literature, with varying degrees of success reported. Initially cryosurgery was advocated as an alternative to transurethral electrosurgical prostatic resection, but the disadvantage of prolonged catheter drainage and the associated high incidence of postoperative urinary retention (15 to 20 percent) secondary to obstruction by necrotic tissue fragments have dampened enthusiasm for this procedure. That final results are unpredictable is also cause for concern; as the amount of tissue destruction depends on the amount of blood flow to the prostate, differences in prostatic vascularity can cause variable results. The histologic type of obstructing prostatic tissue may cause further variance in results. A fibrous muscular hypertrophy of the prostate is much more resistant to cryogenic destruction than is an adenomatous gland. However, since this procedure may be performed using only topical anesthesia, it may have a place in the treatment of hyperplasia in the extremely poor-risk patient.

Renewed interest in prostatic cryosurgery occurred with reports by Soanes and associates[28] demonstrating regression of metastatic lesions of carcinoma of the prostate following cryodestruction of the primary lesion. Three patients were noted to respond in this preliminary report. Gursel et al.[16] noted subjective responses in regard to relief of pain in 8 of 11 patients undergoing this form of therapy, but objective remission of metastatic lesions was noted in only one patient. Repeat cryosurgical procedures were used to boost the immune response. Albin and associates[1] reported antiprostatic antibodies detected by elution techniques in patients with prostatic carcinoma who had undergone sequential cryotherapy. Drylie and Hahn,[11] however, failed to detect antiprostatic antibodies when canine prostates were similarly treated. Since most patients with metastatic disease are immunologically depressed,[7] it is difficult to evaluate this method of immunotherapy. Whether immunostimulation with specific antiprostatic tumor antibodies actually occurs in prostatic carcinoma patients undergoing sequential cryotherapy remains to be proved.

Technique. Cryogenic destruction of the prostate may be performed under topical or low spinal anesthesia. A thermocouple is placed in the posterior prostatic capsule near the apex, transperineally. A rectal probe should also be inserted. The bladder is filled with air (250 to 300 cc) to keep the trigone and bladder wall away from the cryosurgical probe; an air leak can cause trigonal and bladder injury. The cryoprobe is then inserted into the prostatic mass, monitoring its position with a finger placed in the rectum. When properly positioned, the reference knob on the probe should be 0.8 cm distal to the apex of the prostate for small glands, 0.4 cm distal for moderately enlarged glands, and at the apex for markedly enlarged glands.[9]

Liquid nitrogen is then allowed to flow into the probe. The flow is continued until the temperature in the posterior capsule is −20 C. This usually takes 10 to 20 minutes depending on the size and vascularity of the prostate or if the rectal thermocouple approaches 0 C, the procedure is abruptly terminated to avoid rectal injury.

A Foley catheter is inserted soon after the cryosurgical probe is removed, as the gland becomes markedly edematous during the immediate postoperative period, making subsequent passage of a catheter difficult. Sloughing of necrotic tissue begins 2 to 3 days later. Recurrent catheter obstruction may be a problem. The catheter should be left indwelling for 10 days. Most necrotic debris is passed during the first 2 to 3 weeks postoperatively. Subsequent acute obstruction from debris is a common occurrence, often necessitating secondary electroresection. Rectal or bladder injuries are potential problems if technical details are not strictly adhered to. The precise role of prostatic cryosurgery in clinical urology is still to be determined.

TRANSURETHRAL BLADDER SURGERY

Transurethral Resection of Bladder Tumors

This section does not purport to discuss in detail which malignant vesical neoplasms should be managed by transurethral resection. Most low-grade, noninvasive bladder tumors may be managed satisfactorily by the transurethral route. The extent to which higher-grade invasive carcinomas should be managed transurethrally depends on the patient in question and on the skill of the endoscopist.

Endoscopic Evaluation and Biopsy of Vesical Neoplasms. Accurate clinical staging and histologic grading are essential before a rational therapeutic plan can be formulated for a particular patient. Bimanual examination under anesthesia should be done prior to transurethral biopsy. After a thorough cystoscopic examination to exclude other lesions, resection is begun. The base of the lesions should be biopsied, exposing muscle fibers. Another specimen which includes deep muscle fibers is then taken from this base and submitted separately. Tumor in this specimen indicates a stage B2 lesion. Completeness of the resection is confirmed by the pathologic examination. Random biopsies should also be taken in normal-appearing areas to rule out in situ lesions. Each random area specimen should be labeled as to location and submitted in a separate pathology container.

Surgical Technique of Therapeutic Resection. After determining that resection of the lesion is feasible, resection proceeds from the top to the bottom of the lesion. Distilled water is our preferred irrigating medium because of its superior optical properties and its cytotoxic osmotic effect on free-floating tumor cells. The bladder should be filled with sufficient fluid to carry the normal bladder wall away from the lesion. Hemostasis should be maintained throughout the procedure to allow optimal visualization. After the lesion has been completely resected, further tissue below the obvious lesion should be resected and submitted as a separate pathologic specimen. Tissue around the entire circumference of the lesion must also be resected to ensure the completeness of the resection. The border of the lesion should be fulgurated. If resection is complete it is unnecessary to fulgurate widely the base of the lesion, as this merely delays wound healing.

In the late stages of the resection, the bladder should not be overdistended as perforation of thin areas may result. Lesions near ureteral orifices should be resected as if they were in any other area of the bladder, but fulguration should be limited to prevent subsequent ureteral obstruction. Lesions in the anterior portion of the bladder are often inaccessible to the resectoscope. Suprapubic pressure by the surgeon or by an assistant, with the bladder partially filled, often aids in resecting these difficult areas. The new right angle microlens is also useful in this procedure. Occasionally in cases of inaccessible or massive lesions, cystotomy with open loop resection becomes necessary. In selected cases of multiple low-grade neoplasms, lesions less than 0.5 cm in diameter may be safely fulgurated without resection, but generally most tumors should be resected so that they may be examined pathologically.

If a lesion less than 1 cm is resected, it is rarely necessary to employ postoperative catheter drainage. Large lesions require catheter drainage for 1 to 5 days, depending on both the size of the tumor and the depth of resection.

Complications. Hemorrhage following endoscopic resection of bladder tumors may be troublesome. It is imperative to keep the catheter clot-free, as overdistention of the bladder may lead to perforation. If repeated clot retention occurs, it is best to return the patient immediately to the cystoscopy suite for clot evacuation and fulguration.

Stimulation of the obturator nerve is a major cause of vesical perforation. To avoid this problem, bladder resection in the area of the obturator nerves should be performed with the bladder only partially filled.

Extraperitoneal perforation is not a serious complication unless extensive extravasation has occurred. In this instance suprapubic drainage should be instituted, as well as prolonged catheter drainage (for 5 to 7 days). Small extraperitoneal perforations need only catheter drainage.

Intraperitoneal perforation requires immediate exploration to repair the perforation and drain the extravasated fluid. Catheter drainage should be employed for 5 to 7 days postoperatively.

Transurethral Resection of Vesical Diverticula

The indications for transurethral resection of diverticular orifices are controversial. Small diverticula without residual urine need no treatment, whereas large diverticula should be managed by open surgical excision. Many urologists doubt that incision into the neck of a small diverticulum can be made in a manner that improves drainage without producing a vesical perforation and subsequent urinary extravasation. In selected cases, however, careful incision into the muscular rim around the diverticular orifice can be successfully accomplished using a Collings knife, and often improved drainage of the diverticulum is noted subsequently.

Transurethral Resection of Ureteroceles

Indications. Transurethral resection has only limited application in the management of intravesical ureteroceles. Obstruction caused by a ureterocele frequently is replaced by vesicoureteral reflux; therefore large ureteroceles with high-grade obstruction should be excised by open surgery so that the involved renal segment can be managed concomitantly. In this situation the base of the ureterocele also must be reinforced, as a hernialike defect is often present behind the ureterocele which would interfere with subsequent bladder emptying. Small ureteroceles rarely cause significant obstructive symptoms.

Occasionally small ureteroceles are associated with significant obstruction or stones and may benefit from transurethral "unroofing." Careful follow-up investigation for reflux is mandatory. If reflux occurs causing progressive upper tract changes or recurrent infections, an open surgical antireflux procedure must be performed.

Large ureteroceles with associated high-grade obstruction and pyonephrosis may be handled on an emergency basis, using transurethral resection as a means of rapid drainage in this acute situation. When the condition of the patient stabilizes, open repair can then be accomplished on an elective basis.

Technique. A variety of instruments may be employed in performing transurethral resection of a ureterocele. Meatotomy scissors are useful if they can penetrate the wall of the ureterocele; if not, a Collings knife or loop electrode may be used. The inferior portion of the ureterocele should be incised transversely, creating a flap-valve mechanism which may prevent subsequent reflux. If an associated stone is found, it can be extracted with grasping forceps if small enough, or crushed by a lithotrite if larger. During the postoperative period these patients must be followed closely with intravenous pyelograms and cystograms to monitor the status of the upper urinary tract.

Transurethral Ureteral Meatotomy

Indications. Transurethral ureteral meatotomy should be performed in very few instances because vesicoureteral reflux is a common sequela of this procedure. Occasionally meatotomy is indicated following ureteral reimplantation if obstruction appears to result from an excessively long submucosal tunnel. When carefully performed, meatotomy may benefit these patients, relieving the obstruction without causing reflux. Meatotomy is also occasionally justified if a ureteral calculus is lodged in the intramural ureter. The combined use of a stone basket often facilitates stone passage.

Technique. Flexible cystoscopic scissors offer precise control. If the incision is performed at the 6 o'clock position in the orifice, there is a low incidence of reflux, as compared to the reflux seen after incision at the 12 o'clock position. Fulguration should not be performed following meatotomy.

A ureteral catheter with a wire stylet protruding from the end may also be used to perform transurethral meatotomy. An electrosurgical unit is connected to the stylet and a pure cutting current employed for the meatotomy. This method facilitates a ventral (6 o'clock) incision, which is often technically difficult using meatotomy scissors.

Cystolitholapaxy

Indications. Vesical calculi may accompany bladder outlet obstruction. A bladder stone small enough to fit into a lithotrite may be crushed and removed transurethrally. Con-

traindications to cystolitholapaxy include a contracted or inflamed bladder and severe vesicoureteral reflux with infected urine. The presence of vesical diverticula, where crushed stone fragments may lodge, represents another contraindication to litholapaxy, as do severe urethral strictures or a large intravesical prostatic adenoma.

Technique. Many types of lithotrites are commercially available. We favor the use of a lithotrite with an incorporated lens system, rather than the blind model such as the Bigelow. Blind lithotrites are more powerful in stone-crushing capability, but they also cause more complications. Many urologists, however, are adept with "blind" instruments and see few complications.

Prior to performing cystolitholapaxy, the instrument should be checked for proper function. Occasionally lithotrites become fixed in an open position in the bladder because of mechanical malfunction; this requires cystotomy for removal. Surgeons should be well acquainted with the mechanics of any lithotrite to be used.

Preliminary progressive urethral dilation is important so that the lithotrite may be passed atraumatically into the bladder. Cystoscopy should precede litholapaxy to exclude any concomitant vesical pathology that might contraindicate litholapaxy. The configuration and size of the calculus is then also confirmed.

If a blind lithotrite is to be used, the bladder should be only one-third to one-half full to facilitate engagement of the stone in the lithotrite. When the lithotrite is in the bladder, the handle is raised 40 to 50 degrees to allow engagement. If the stone cannot be engaged at first, manipulation of the stone via the rectum is often helpful. After securing the stone, the lithotrite should be moved from side to side to be sure that the bladder wall has not been caught between the jaws of the lithotrite. The jaws are then closed and the entire process repeated until no further fragments can be engaged. An adequate volume of fluid must remain in the bladder to lessen the risk of damage to the bladder wall. Too much fluid, however, makes the calculus more difficult to engage.

When using a lithotrite with a lens system, it is best to have the bladder well filled as the calculus may be easily manipulated into the lithotrite under direct vision. With this visual control, the possibility of vesical perforation is decreased. Completeness of the litholapaxy is also ensured prior to removing the lithotrite. In summary, the main advantage of blind lithotrites is their capacity to manage slightly larger stones.

After completion of litholapaxy, a large resectoscope sheath is inserted and stone fragments are removed with an Ellik evacuator or Toomey syringe. Completeness of crushing and extraction should be confirmed cystoscopically.

Complications. Major complications include vesical perforation and hemorrhage. Catheter drainage with intermittent irrigation usually controls hemorrhage. Only rarely is severe hemorrhage seen, unless there has been trauma to an intravesical prostatic middle lobe. Vesical perforation should be confirmed by cystogram and managed as any other vesical perforation.

New Horizons in Lithotripsy. Fragmentation of vesical calculi using ultrasound or electrohydraulic lithotripsy appears promising.[2,12] The Russians pioneered the development of an electrohydraulic lithotriptor (Urat-1) about 12 years ago. This device produces an electrohydraulic shock wave in a liquid medium, which has been quite effective in fragmenting bladder calculi. A 10 Fr probe is inserted via a 24 Fr or 28 Fr sheath. Damage to the bladder wall does not occur unless there is direct contact with the probe on the bladder wall at the time of discharge. Pulse waves are controlled with the use of a foot pedal.

The ease with which fragmentation is accomplished is quite variable, depending on the composition of the stone. Soft stones (e.g., phosphate stones and some urate stones) are often completely fragmented with the first contact of the probe. Hard stones (e.g., oxalate stones) may require exploration with the probe until a disruption point is found. Since the instrument can be adapted to standard resectoscope sheaths, simultaneous fragmentation and extraction is possible.

Research into methods of lithotripsy of ureteral calculi is also in progress. As yet, no satisfactory commercial units are available.

Transurethral Ureteral Calculus Manipulation

Indications. When a ureteral calculus is lodged in the lower third of the ureter and is less than 1 cm in diameter, consideration may be given to transurethral stone manipulation; this should be preceded, however, by an attempt at expectant therapy. The presence of associated infection contraindicates manipulation, although an emergency open surgical procedure may be averted if a ureteral catheter can be negotiated above the obstructing calculus.

Technique. Endoscopic stone manipulation should be performed under x-ray control. A preliminary kidney-ureter-bladder (KUB) film confirms that the stone has not migrated during transportation of the patient to the endoscopy unit and the induction of anesthesia. Preliminary dilation of the distal ureter is of benefit, but one must take care not to elevate a mucosal flap which might preclude subsequent passage of a stone basket or loop. The safest method of transurethral stone manipulation is with the use of multiple ureteral catheters. After successfully passing two or three catheters above the calculus, the procedure is terminated. The catheters are left indwelling for 1 to 3 days; they are then twisted to engage the calculus and are slowly withdrawn. Although this extraction maneuver is not often successful, the ureter may be dilated sufficiently to allow spontaneous passage of the calculus during the next 24 to 72 hours.

If the multiple-catheter method is not successful, or if it is impossible to place multiple catheters above the stone, manipulation with a stone basket is indicated. Many endoscopists favor stone basketing as their primary procedure in preference to the multiple-catheter method. New baskets such as the Dormia are extremely useful but must be used cautiously. Ureteral perforation and avulsion as well as subsequent ureteral stricture are dangers even in the most experienced hands. Calculi with sharp irregularities may impale the ureter, causing injury on removal.

Only gentle traction should be placed on a basket. A delicate sense of touch is an invaluable asset in the successful manipulation of a ureteral stone. X-ray control confirms what the sense of touch suspects. The use of a basket with a long filiform tip facilitates reintroduction of the basket should the initial attempt at manipulation fail. Repeated passes of the basket in the event of failure, however, should be discouraged; if the stone has not been recovered after three or four attempts, the procedure is best terminated. A solitary ureteral catheter left indwelling after unsuccessful manipulation guards against pyelonephrosis and may dilate the ureter to allow subsequent spontaneous passage.

Many urologists favor the passage of an *Ellik* or *Zeiss loop catheter*. The renal pelvis should be sufficiently large to allow formation of the loop in the pelvis prior to withdrawing the loop down the ureter to engage the stone. If the attempt is successful, the loop should be left indwelling for 1 to 3 days after engagement without further manipulation, so that the stone may adhere to the loop.

Occasionally a basket or loop may become impacted in the ureter. If impaction is secondary to a tight ureteral orifice, meatotomy may be successful in releasing the instrument and the stone. If the site of impaction is not at the meatus, open surgery becomes necessary. The basket or loop should never simply be pulled out transurethrally in this instance, as ureteral avulsion may result from this practice.

Complications. If ureteral integrity is questionable following a manipulation, retrograde pyelograms should be performed immediately. Ureteral perforation or avulsion should be treated on an individual basis, employing the simplest method possible to reestablish urinary continuity.

An intravenous pyelogram should be routinely obtained 6 to 8 weeks following stone manipulation to rule out development of a delayed ureteral stricture. The latter occasionally responds to progressive ureteral dilation, which should be the initial therapy. Failure of this step may necessitate open surgical repair.

ADVANCES IN UROLOGIC ENDOSCOPY

Urologic endoscopy had its true beginning with the development of a direct-light cystoscope by Max Nitze in 1877. Prior to this, reflected light transmitted through a large-caliber hollow tube or transilluminated rectal light allowed only the briefest glimpse of the interior of the bladder or urethra. In fact until Nitze's invention, urologic endoscopy was merely a curiosity and had no real therapeutic applications despite the fact that such primitive urologic procedures as catheterization and "cutting for a stone" had been employed since the beginning of medical history.

In 1877 Nitze, along with the help of instrument maker Wilhelm Deicke, developed the first direct-light cystoscope. He presented it on October 2, 1877 to the Royal Medical Society in Dresden. Nitze[23,24] conceived his cystoscope by employing the simple principle summarized in his truism: "In order to light up a room, one must carry a lamp into it." He also thought of using a lens *system* to enlarge the visual image: Along with poor illumination, inadequate image size had been a major problem in the past. Prior to Nitze's development of a lens system, the visual field through a "cystoscope" was only 3 mm. In 1878 Nitze, working with Joseph Leiter, included a prism in his optical system, which further enlarged the visual field.

Yet this modified cystoscope, as well as the first instrument devised by Nitze and Deicke, was encumbered by a bulky water-cooling system. These first instruments consisted of a long metallic tube about 21 Fr in caliber. A "hot" platinum wire was placed at the tip for direct internal illumination. The design of this instrument was complicated by the fact that it was necessary to cool the platinum wire with a circulating current of water in order to avoid damage to the bladder from the incandescent platinum loop.

When Edison invented the incandescent light bulb in 1879, Nitze at once recognized the importance of this invention and quickly incorporated it into his cystoscopic design, finally enabling the awkward water-cooling system to be discarded. During the same year Nitze began work on endophotography, but it took him more than 10 years of experimental work to obtain a satisfactory photograph. Initially exposure times in excess of 1 minute were necessary; this in addition to the extremely coarse grain of the photographic emulsion resulted in insufficient detail for visualizing blood vessels: One shudders to imagine the patient's discomfort during these early attempts. By 1877 with improved light from an incandescent lamp and improved film, the first satisfactory pictures were obtained using exposure times ranging from 10 to 30 seconds. All of these pictures were of course black and white. It was therefore necessary to tint the pictures by hand with yellow and red; this coloring was especially helpful to the student's comprehension of actual endoscopic appearances. In 1894, Nitze published the first atlas in this field.[22]

Although there have been many dramatic improvements in illumination and in the optics of instruments available for urologic procedures, there have been few truly innovative techniques developed during the past 30 years in the field of urologic endoscopy. This is not to minimize the benefits afforded the urologist by the aforementioned advances—as with the better visualization provided by improved optics —with which the urologist is now able to perform procedures more expeditiously and more accurately than ever before. These improvements are reflected most dramatically in the field of pediatric endoscopy: whereas in the past inadequate illumination and restricted field size severely hampered our diagnostic acumen and therapeutic accuracy, we now have optimal visualization to perform pediatric procedures (Chapter 57).

Cystoscopy

Hopkins Rod-Lens System. The development of the Hopkins rod-lens system has been the greatest advance in urologic endoscopy since Nitze's invention of a direct light cystoscope in 1877. In a study performed by Berci and Kont[3] the Hopkins forward-oblique lens transmitted four times the light of the standard forward-oblique lens, and the Hopkins lateral lens was found to transmit twice the light of standard lateral lenses. Accordingly the Hopkins lens system yields brighter images of viewed objects and an overall increase in perception, consequently causing less viewer fatigue. Hopkins' wide-angle lens also allows faster orientation. With the smaller visual field yielded by a standard lens system, the viewer had to compile in his memory a "mosaic" of what he has seen, thereby decreasing his observational accuracy, in addition to lengthening the cystoscopic procedure. The Hopkins lens system with either a forward-oblique or lateral lens system has a viewing angle of 70 degrees, compared to the standard forward-oblique lens with a viewing angle of 30 degrees and the lateral lens with an angle of 52 degrees. Although it is true that the wider the viewing angle, the less magnification of objects, with the faster orientation afforded by the Hopkins lens system this is easily compensated for by moving the cystoscope closer to the object. The further addition of a 0-degree (direct vision) lens has been of great aid in visualizing urethral lesions and in performing transurethral operative procedures.

The improved light transmission of the Hop-

kins lens systems has permitted a decrease in the diameter of the telescope incorporating fibers for light transmission to 4.0 mm (Hopkins adult telescopes) and 2.7 mm (pediatric instruments).* This in turn has enabled the diameter of an adult sheath to be decreased to 15.5 Fr. An obvious result of these improvements is that for every given sheath size there is more room for working elements than ever before, especially in the pediatric units. A 10 Fr pediatric cystoscope can now accomodate a 3 Fr ureteral catheter, and an 11 Fr cystoscope a 4 Fr ureteral catheter. Pediatric resectoscopes as small as 10 and 11 Fr are now available. The Hopkins lens system provides superior optical resolution compared to conventional lens systems.

Fiberoptic Light Source. The invention of the fiber bundle principle of light transmission has been another major development in the field of urologic endoscopy. For the first time the light source and the endoscope are now physically divorced from each other. No longer does the sheath or telescope have to be removed as a result of bulb burn-out. The fiberoptic light source also has a higher intensity, as the fibers may be arranged around the lens.

A disadvantage of the fiberoptic light source is the slight yellow hue which the fiber bundle light imparts to the visual field. This problem has been a minor one, however, and becomes insignificant when compared to the benefits of fiber optics.

Binocular Endoscopy. Binocular eyepieces, readily detachable from the monocular eyepiece, are now available for standard cystoscopes. No loss of detail but some light loss is encountered within this system. Some viewers favor the binocular eyepiece, stating that faster perception and better visualization are possible with this lens system and that it causes less viewer fatigue.

Teaching Attachments. The improved illumination and better visualization afforded by the Hopkins lens system and the fiber bundle have revolutionized teaching attachments. It is now possible for both the endoscopist and the observer to have sufficient illumination for good visualization. With continuous observation by a student during endoscopic surgical

Manufacturer: Karl Storz Endoscopy, Tuttlingen, West Germany. Distributor: Karl Storz Endoscopy of America, Inc., 658 South San Vicente Boulevard, Los Angeles, California 90048.

procedures, the surgeon was previously hampered by the awkward standard fixed teaching attachment. The fiber coherent image bundle has made the connection between the cystoscope and the teaching attachment flexible, improving the maneuverability of the endoscope. With the flexible fiber teaching attachment, however, there is some loss of light and visual detail, as well as some up and down orientation (Chapter 4). With proper narration of the procedure by the surgeon to the observer, these problems are minor.

The primary importance of teaching attachments are in teaching students and house staff in regard to cystoscopic findings. The decreased maneuverability of the new rigid teaching attachments influences us to continue using a flexible system in the latter instance; however, the better detail afforded by the rigid system along with better light and easier orientation make it an attractive aid in the teaching of endoscopic vesical and urethral pathology.

Female Cystoscope. At the suggestion of Willard E. Goodwin, a new "female" cystoscope has been developed. Its large caliber accomodates all diagnostic endoscopic procedures, so only one sheath is needed per setup for any contemplated procedure. Its short length allows for easy maneuverability in the female patient compared to cystoscopes of conventional lengths.

Air Endoscopy. Air endoscopy has been used since the early days of cystoscopy. This technique, however, has important current applications. Because of the large caliber of the air endoscope, its use is almost exclusively limted to female urology. The patient is placed in the knee-chest or lithotomy position. Air cystoscopy is especially useful in the identification of sphincter functions, urethral diverticula, or urethral or vesical fistulas. Detailed discussion of this diagnostic modality (Chapter 41), however, is beyond the scope of this chapter.

Flexible Fiber Cystoscopes. The need for surgeons and diagnosticians to be able to explore all orifices and body cavities has led to the development of a flexible fiber cystoscope.[29,30] This new instrument has a viewing angle of 64 degrees and can be manipulated with a knob to adjust the bend of the distal end of the scope; the latter has a maximum range of 90 degrees in either direction. The cystoscope has a fixed focus and a depth of vision ranging from 5 to 60 mm. Illumination is via a fiber bundle; the light source is a halogen or xenon lamp. This flexible tube is 7 mm outside diameter. Its proximal half is semirigid to aid passage of the fiberscope into the bladder. The problems of an image less clear than that obtained with the Hopkins rod system have been partially circumvented by using coherent glass fibers in a scope. There is no doubt that the instrument allows improved visualization of the bladder neck compared to a standard retrospective lens systems, but at present it is not a mandatory inclusion in our standard urologic armamentarium.

Ultraviolet Cystoscopy. Whitmore and Bush[31,32] described the cystoscopic use of an ultraviolet light to demonstrate tumor fluorescence following the administration of tetracycline. While their study established an undeniable association between ultraviolet tetracycline fluorescence and carcinoma of the bladder, there is some question regarding its reliability in detecting *all* neoplastic lesions.

A fiberoptic bundle with ultraviolet-transmitting capacity is utilized in their study to carry the light source from a 200-watt mercury arc lamp. This produces a spectrum of visible and ultraviolet light with energy peaks at 366 nm (ultraviolet), 403 nm (violet), 430 nm (blue), 543 nm (yellow), and 577 nm (yellow). From prior studies by Bottiger[4] and Rall and associates,[25] light energy in the range of 366 to 430 nm excites tetracycline to fluoresce at a wavelength of 520 nm, causing a yellow gold color to be visualized. Cystoscopic observations are made in patients with suspected carcinoma of the bladder after they have been premedicated orally four times a day for 4 days with tetracycline hydrochloride. The ultraviolet cystoscopy should be performed 24 to 36 hours after the final dose of tetracycline.

Acridine orange has recently been used as a preferred source of fluorescence,[19] as its maximum excitation spectrum is brighter than that of the tetracycline fluorescence utilized by Whitmore and Bush.[31,32] More acridine orange concentrates in the tumor because it is directly applied, rather than taken orally. Acridine orange 0.1 percent (100 cc) is placed intravesically for 10 minutes prior to cystoscopy, then rinsed 20 times with water. A 300-watt xenon lamp is used as the light source, with a special fluorescein isothiocyanate interference filter (passes light between 380 and 505 nm), to obtain the excitation spectrum of acridine orange (490 nm).

The clinical experience of Whitmore and Bush[31,32] clearly establishes the presence of tetracycline fluorescence, but more data are needed before the clinical relevance of this diagnostic tool is determined. Seventy of 86 patients with obvious neoplasms fluoresced and 16 did not, yielding a false-negative rate of 18.6 percent. In their study it is difficult to determine how many lesions not visualized with standard cystoscopic or ultraviolet fluorescent means were positive, as random biopsies of nonfluorescent areas were not taken. In 175 patients with a strong past history of bladder tumors, however, 41 areas of cancer were confirmed by biopsy of fluorescent areas that had appeared to be either normal or merely inflamed in the standard cystoscopic examinations. All these patients, incidentally, had positive urinary cytologic findings. It is disturbingly evident that not all in situ carcinomas fluoresce; thus ultraviolet cystoscopy is not reliable in detecting sites of occult cancer in patients who have positive urinary cytologic studies. Moreover, in 28 of 175 patients previously mentioned, biopsies of fluorescent areas revealed nonmalignant changes, varying from normal tissue to atypia short of carcinoma in situ—a false-positive rate of 41 percent. The fact that Whitmore and Bush[31,32] did not have an interchangeable lens system may have caused a sampling error: When biopsies were performed it was necessary for the investigators to remove the ultraviolet cystoscope and replace it with one using a standard conventional light source, thus introducing the possibility that incorrect areas were biopsied.

Kioke[20] recently described an apparatus with interchangeable lens groups for fluorescent cystoscopy, photography, and biopsy purposes. In addition to a 300-watt xenon lamp source and a fluorescein interference filter for the ultraviolet light source, a special transformer supplies a small electric bulb with energy. The latter has a tungsten filament; for observation, 9 volts is passed through the filament, and for intravesical photography 30 volts. Thus photographs and biopsy procedures may be carried out without changing cystoscopes. This innovation should reduce sampling error and better reflect the true false-positive rate. Its use in high-risk patients in conjunction with standard periodic cystoscopy and urinary cytology is justified. Its incorporation into the standard battery of instruments for urology is questionable at this time; as yet, ultraviolet fluores-

cence has not detected a clinically unsuspected tumor (i.e., when cytologic examination and standard cystoscopic examination were both negative).

Endophotography

The superior resolution and wide viewing angle afforded by the Hopkins rod-lens system, along with the improvements in light sources and modalities of light transmission discussed above, have markedly improved the quality of endoscopic photographs. It is now possible to document cystoscopic findings in a practical, concise manner. These can then become a part of the patient's record, rather than the customary written cystoscopic report. The value of this documentation in both teaching and comparative patient follow-up is obvious.

Photographic Equipment. Any good single-lens reflex camera may be utilized. A special attachment is necessary to secure the camera to the cystoscopic eyepiece. Excellent visualization of the object through the camera is then possible, ensuring that the visualized object is the object photographed (Fig. 1).

Photographic Light Source. Three methods of illumination have been employed for endoscopic urologic photography. The first method utilizes a light source outside the patient's body—either a halogen or xenon lamp or an electronic flash. Light is conducted into the interior of the bladder via the fiber bundle. The advantage of the method is that the flash is divorced from the cystoscope, thus eliminating the possibility of bulb burn-out. Fibers may be arranged around the lens, allowing for more uniform illumination of the obejct to be photographed. A standard light source may be transmitted through the same fiber bundle for standard endoscopic viewing. Disadvantages of this method include a slight yellow hue imparted by the fiber bundle and the loss of some intensity with transmission of the light via the fiber bundle (10 percent loss per foot). In our experience, however, satisfactory photographs are easily obtained utilizing this type of light source, with minimal technical problems (Figs. 2–4, Plate M).*

In the second method a small electronic flash bulb at the tip of the cystoscope serves as the light source. Aside from the possibility of burn-out, there is a recharging period neces-

All color plates appear in the front of the book.

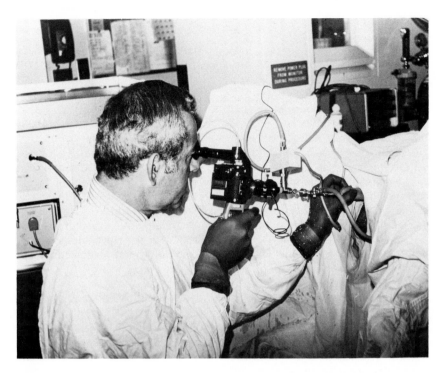

FIG. 1. Still photograph being taken through Hopkins telescope (external flash and Robot 352 camera).

sary for the flash bulb—several seconds, depending on the mechanism used—which makes rapid sequence photography impossible. This method of illumination is not recommended.

In the third method described and advocated by Kioke[20] a small electronic bulb is attached to the tip of the cystoscope, and high voltage is applied only at the instant of photography. Two filaments are placed within the small electric bulb. A 5-volt tungsten filament is used for observation, and a 12-volt filament for photography. Improvement in the quality of tungsten filaments now allows passage of up to 30 volts in the 12-volt filament without breakage, whereas earlier filaments ruptured with the application of only 22 volts. An additional 9 volts may be passed through the 5-volt observation filament during photography for even greater brightness. With this method and the use of high-speed Ektachrome film (ASA 500), shutter speeds as brief as 1/15 second may be utilized and field diameters as large as 20 mm can be included. ASA 125 film may be used with exposure times of 1/15 to 1/4 second, if the film is developed by forced processing (higher speed than ASA 125). Bulb burn-out is the main disadvantage of this system, but with

modern technology this has become rare. This method permits a larger angle of illumination than does a fiberoptic source because of the phase problem inherent in fiberoptic light systems. With fiberoptic bundles uneven light exposures may result when the distance between the lens and the light source is either too close to or too far from the adequate phase of the fiberoptic bundle. With proper arrangement of the fibers around the lens this problem has been partially cirvumcented, and in our experience it is insignificant.

With these currently available methods of illumination, it is possible to obtain color transparencies or Polaroid endovesical photographs for immediate documentation in the patient's chart (Chapter 18).

Endocinephotography

By employing high-intensity xenon light sources with the conducting fiberoptic bundle, high-quality ciné photographs are obtainable for use as teaching aids or as an ultimate means of pathologic documentation. High-speed 16-mm Ektachrome film (ASA:160, daylight) is used at a rate of 16 to 24 frames per second. Excellent teaching films are now available demonstrating many endoscopic procedures (Fig. 5).

Cystoscopy and Television

Television technology has advanced so that endoscopic procedures may now be televised with amazing accuracy of both detail and color (Chapter 19). This has become a valuable teaching tool for the urologist. Urologic endoscopic surgical symposia, where large groups can visualize procedures in progress via television have become possible, thus allowing open discussion forums to take place while a procedure is in progress. With the use of a closed circuit visual system and suitable sound systems, observers may be at great distances from the surgeon, yet still conduct two-way discussions of the procedure.

Video tapes may be made for permanent documentation of the procedure, and they may later be converted to 16-mm film. Endoscopic television requires less illumination than does endoscopic ciné photography for comparable detail.

Laser

Laser light is monochromatic and therefore not suitable for illumination.

Ureteroscopy

Flexible fiber ureteroscopy has obvious applications for the visualization of ureteral and endorenal pathology. Its potential use as a means of localizing upper tract hematuria, tumors, and stones will be a major breakthrough in diagnostic urology. However, a satisfactory ureteroscope is not yet commercially available, although a promising prototype is currently being evaluated. Its high cost and relatively large diameter (9 Fr) are its present limiting factors.

Nephroscopy

Nephroscopy is already an important adjuvant to open renal surgery. Its uses—to locate and manipulate intrarenal calculi; to aid in identification of intrarenal sites of hemorrhage; and to identify, resect, and fulgurate low-grade

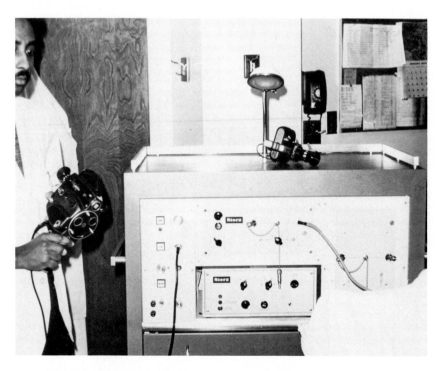

FIG. 5.   Endophotographic setup. Xenon light source with flash generator.

intrarenal transitional cell tumors—have greatly extended our ability to preserve kidney tissue, especially in instances of solitary renal surgery. Investigative work is now in progress on developing a flexible endoscope for use as a nephroscope, but the image quality is inferior to the rigid one (Chapter 6).

REFERENCES

1. Albin RJ, Soanes WA, Gonder MJ: Elution of in vivo bound anti-prostatic epithelial antibodies following multiple cryotherapies of carcinoma of the prostate. Urology 2:276, 1973
2. Angeloff A: Hydro-electrolithotripsy. J Urol 108:867, 1972
3. Berci G, Kont LA: A new optical system in endoscopy with special reference to cystoscopy. Br J Urol 41:564, 1969
4. Bottiger LE: On the distribution of tetracycline in the body. Antibiot Chemother 5:332, 1955
5. Brooks MB: Heparin in the treatment of hemorrhagic diathesis associated with prostatic carcinoma. J Urol 102:240, 1969
6. Brooks MB, Lytton B, Weiss SA: Vasectomy in the control of epididymitis after prostatectomy following urethral catheter drainage. J Urol 105:694, 1971
7. Brosman S, Hausman M, Sacks S: Immunologic alterations in patients with prostatic carcinoma. J Urol 113:841, 1975
8. Damico CF, Mebust WK, Valk WL, et al: Triamcinolone: adjuvant therapy for vesical neck contractures. J Urol 110:203, 1973
9. Dowd JA: The technique of cryosurgery of the prostate. J Urol 105:286, 1971
10. Dretler SP, Klein LA: The eradication of intraurethral condyloma accuminata with five percent 5-fluorouracil cream. J Urol 113:195, 1975
11. Drylie DM, Hahn GS: Stimulation of prostatic antibodies by cryosurgery. J Urol 110:324, 1973
12. Eaton JM, Malin JM, Glenn JF: Electrohydraulic lithotripsy. J Urol 108:865, 1972
13. Gigax JH, Robison JR: The successful treatment of intraurethral condyloma accuminata with colchicine. J Urol 105:809, 1971
14. Gonder MJ, Soanes WA, Smith V: Experimental prostate cryosurgery. Invest Urol 1:610, 1964
15. Green LF, Yalowitz PA: The advisability of concomitant transurethral excision of vesical neoplasms in prostatic hyperplasia. J Urol 107:445, 1972
16. Gursel E, Roberts M, Veenema RJ: Regression of prostatic carcinoma following sequential cryotherapy to the prostate. J Urol 108:928, 1972
17. Haralambidis G, Spinelli AN: Vasectomy: an evaluation. J Urol 89:591, 1963
18. Kendall AR: Rationale of prophylactic vasectomy. J Urol 89:712, 1963
19. Kioke R: A new apparatus with interchangeable lens groups for fluorescent cystoscopy, photography, biopsy, and coagulation. J Urol 111:31, 1974
20. Kioke R: New apparatus of cystoscopic photography with interchangeable lens groups: available for endocinematography and endotelevisionoscopy. J Urol 109:884, 1973
21. Lynn JM, Nesbitt RM: The influence of vasectomy upon the incidence of epididymitis following transurethral prostatectomy. J Urol 59:72, 1948
22. Nitze M: Kystophotographischer Atlas. Wiesbaden, 1894
23. Nitze M: Zur Photographie der menschlichen Harnblase. Klin Wochenschr 31:744, 1893
24. Nitze M: Eine neue Beobachtungs und Untersuchungsmethode für Harnrohre und Harnblase. Wien Med Wochenschr 24:650, 1879
25. Rall DP, Loo TL, Larre M, et al: Appearance and persistence of fluorescence material in tumor tissue after tetracycline administration. J Natl Cancer Inst 19:79, 1957
26. Rinker JR, Hancock CV, Henderson WD: A statistical study of unilateral prophylactic vasectomy in the prevention of epididymitis: one thousand twenty-nine cases. J Urol 104:303, 1970
27. Schmidt S, Hinman F: The effect of vasectomy upon the incidence of epididymitis after prostatectomy: an analysis of 810 operations. J Urol 63:872, 1950
28. Soanes WA, Albin RJ, Gonder WJ: Remission of metastatic lesions following cryosurgery in prostatic carcinoma: immunologic considerations. J Urol 104:154, 1970
29. Takagi T, Go T, Takayasui H, et al: Small-caliber fiberscope for visualization of the urinary tract, biliary tract, and spinal canal. Surgery 64:1033, 1968
30. Tsuchiada S, Sugawara H: A new flexible fiber cystoscope for visualization of the bladder neck. J Urol 109:830, 1973
30a. Valk V: Personal communication, 1971
31. Whitmore WF, Bush IM: Ultraviolet cystoscopy. JAMA 203:1057, 1968
32. Whitmore WF, Bush IM: Ultraviolet cystoscopy in patients with bladder cancer. J Urol 95:201, 1966

57

Pediatric Cystoscopy

Alan D. Perlmutter

Improved design of miniature endoscopes during recent years has advanced the usefulness and quality of the pediatric urologic examination at a time when improved radiographic methods have reduced the indications for endoscopic study. Pediatric cystoscopy remains an important part of the urologic armamentarium and serves as a means of extending the morphologic evaluation, studying the pathophysiology of disturbed urodynamics, and performing certain therapeutic maneuvers.

INDICATIONS AND CONTRAINDICATIONS

Cystoscopy in infants and children is often useful for the further evaluation or therapy of recurrent urinary tract infections, congenital anomalies of the upper and lower uninary tracts, intersex states, neoplasms of urinary and extraurinary origin, hypertension, urinary calculi, and renal failure.

Cystoscopic examination should always be done when required; Campbell stated that "a tender age is no contraindication."[4] However, cystoscopic manipulation should be avoided if possible in the presence of acute symptomatic urinary infection for fear of bacteremia or septicemia. Relative contraindications to cystoscopy include untreated blood dyscrasias, debilitating illnesses, or other disorders that increase the anesthesia risk.

With the increasing sophistication of uroradiographic techniques there is considerable disagreement about some of the indications

for cystoscopic study in children. Generally, however, cystoscopy is often useful for further evaluation and management of the following conditions.

Urinary Tract Infection

The most common reason for cystoscopic examination is urinary tract infection—severe or recurrent illness in girls or a single episode in boys. Many urologists including this author do not feel cystoscopy is routinely required for girls who have suffered an occasional uncomplicated urinary infection if an excretory urogram and voiding cystourethrogram are normal. However, when vesicoureteral reflux is present, one can obtain diagnostic and prognostic information regarding development of the ureteric orifices.[1,5,9,12] Also cystoscopy should be a part of the evaluation of persistent or multiple urinary infections, especially with secondary symptoms of disturbed micturition. For example, the finding of cystitis cystica (Fig. 1, Plate N)* may justify a program of more aggressive and prolonged chemotherapy to allow the mucosal lesions time to heal.

In reviews by Lyon[11] and Belman[2] cystitis cystica was characteristically found in older girls (after age 5) and was associated with a history of multiple infections dating back to early childhood and with a history of urge incontinence. Between 20 and 30 percent of these girls had vesicoureteral reflux which infrequently stopped unless antireflux surgery was

*All color plates appear at the front of the book.

performed. Both authors noted that girls with cystitis cystica required long-term treatment (6 to 12 months or more) for control of recurrent infections and for resolution of the symptoms and the inflammatory mucosal changes.

Congenital Anomalies

Endoscopy can further define a variety of congenital lesions of the upper and lower urinary tract. Retrograde catheterization of the ureter is useful with an obstructing process whenever the collecting system is incompletely visualized. For example, a megaureter poorly outlined by intravenous urography can be studied after retrograde filling, using fluoroscopy to evaluate ureteral peristalsis and emptying. Manometric recordings can be obtained by coupling the ureteral catheter to a volume displacement transducer. When the ureteral catheter does not pass easily or is tight in the orifice so that intrinsic trauma to and edema of the orifice may render physiologic studies useless, then transcutaneous nephrostogram can be done instead of or at the time of cystoscopy, and ureteral manipulation can be avoided. Using intravenous contrast material for fluoroscopic localization of the collecting system, the upper tract is punctured and pressure-flow studies can be obtained.[17]

Similarly, persistent ureterectasis after megaureter repair can be examined fluoroscopically to define or rule out a surgical obstruction. Variable ureteral dilatation occurs on occasion after ureteroneocystostomy. Retrograde ureterograms may be helpful to distinguish ureteral angulation from operative stricture. When the distal ureter has been hooked around bands or vessels the juxtavesical ureter appears flexed when the bladder is filled and straightens as the bladder is emptied, allowing the proximal ureter to drain.

The many congenital anomalies of the upper and lower urinary tract are not individually listed and described. In general, cystoscopic evaluation supplements roentgenographic data and is not required for every case. At times (e.g., ureterocele, vesical diverticulum, ureteropelvic obstruction) the endoscopic examination, as a preliminary step, is a useful adjunct to the operative procedure, thus avoiding a separate anesthesia. With ureteropelvic junction obstruction, retrograde ureterograms can be obtained to rule out additional ureteral pathology when excretory urography fails to out-

line the ureter distal to the obstruction. Operative endoscopy for treating certain lesions of the lower urinary tract is presented in a separate section.

Intersex

Endoscopic inspection of the urogenital sinus and urethra in cases of ambiguous genitalia[7] or cloacal malformation[10,13] is often required to sort out the anatomic deformities (Fig. 2, Plate N). An enlarged utriculus may be present in patients with severe hypospadias, which in some cases traps urine but which is not consistently visualized by voiding cystourethrography.

At the time of genital reconstruction and vaginoplasty in adrenogenital syndrome with severe virilization, for example, the distal vagina is small and fistulous at its entrance to the urogenital sinus.[15] Here endoscopy permits passage of a Fogarty vascular balloon catheter through the narrow connection into the vaginal cavity. Localization of this landmark is easy and precise, thus reducing the extent of surgical dissection required during the repair.

Neoplasms

Childhood urinary tract neoplasms are uncommon. Of the renal parenchymal tumors, Wilms' tumor (embryoma) is typical and renal cell carcinoma is unusual. These lesions share more diagnostic roentgenographic similarities than differences, and are usually so well delineated by excretory urography and arteriography, when indicated, that retrograde pyelography is seldom worthwhile. Because urothelial tumors are exceedingly rare before puberty, observation cystoscopy may not be needed for cases of intermittent microhematuria if the entire urinary tract has been well visualized by x-ray studies.

The botryoid form of rhabdomyosarcoma of the bladder has a characteristic radiographic appearance. Endoscopy is useful mainly for biopsy confirmation of the diagnosis.

Malignant or benign masses arising in other organ systems can sometimes be defined further by cystoscopy. Here the indications must be individualized; lesions of the retroperitoneum, internal genital ducts, or intestinal tract which appear to involve or displace portions of the urinary tract are examples.

Hypertension

The effects of general anesthesia on renal function in the anesthetized child and the difficulties of obtaining adequate renal urinary collections through small-caliber ureteral catheters limit the value of divided urinary collections for renal function studies.

Calculous Disease

Urinary calculi in children may be evaluated, bypassed, or manipulated by retrograde technique, as in the adult. In boys, however, the small caliber of the urethra may preclude introduction of a cystoscope sheath large enough to accomodate passage of a basket stone extractor used for a distal ureteral calculus. If a 14 Fr. sheath can be passed without trauma, then a 5 Fr. Dormia ureteral stone extractor can be used. In girls there are more options, as a gentle urethral dilation allows the passage of an adult-sized cystoscope sheath.

Renal Failure

Retrograde ureteropyelograms are useful to define the pyelocalyceal system whenever there is inadequate visualization by excretory study. In cases of renal failure from severe obstruction, retrograde catheterization of the ureter is one approach to drainage, although a definitive form of surgical decompression is preferred when obstruction is chronic.

METHODS OF PEDIATRIC CYSTOSCOPY

Technique

Cystoscopic technique in the infant and child is analogous to that in the adult and so is not reviewed in detail. Particular care is required to avoid urethral injury, and consistent gentleness is essential. Sterile technique is scrupulously observed. Irrigation fluid should flow at pressures not exceeding 50 to 60 cm of water.

The urethra is particularly vulnerable in the male child; forcing a sheath through a tight urethra may result in later stricture. Although there is normally a range of urethral calibers for each age group, with a particularly wide range in girls,[8] a general appreciation of maximum urethral sizes likely to be encountered may prevent unnecessary trauma from inappropriate choice of instruments during the endoscopic examination.

In the female the elasticity and distensibility of the urethra, even in the neonate, allows for flexibility in the choice among variously sized endoscopes; urethral dilation to allow accomodation of a larger sheath can precede examination whenever necessary. However, if the urethra itself is the site of pathology, preliminary dilation may obscure the findings. In such cases a sufficiently small sheath should be chosen to allow urethroscopy as the initial instrumentation.

In the male child the range of urethral sizes is more limited. The urethra of the male neonate generally does not admit an instrument larger than 8 or 10 Fr. An available 8 Fr. cystoscope (Fig. 3) is a marvel of optical precision but because of its small size is designed to serve only as a diagnostic tool with no capabilities for endoscopic manipulation. Fortunately, improved radiographic techniques now available for neonates have increased the yield of such noninvasive diagnostic studies; therefore although this 8 Fr. infant cystoscope is an important part of my armamentarium, I have found it to be of limited use.

During midchildhood the male urethra generally admits a 13 or 14 Fr. sheath without difficulty, and during late prepuberty some male urethras may calibrate at more than 16

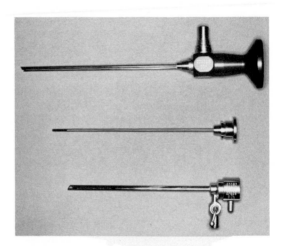

FIG. 3. Infant (8 Fr.) cystoscope. Sheath has an irrigating valve. This instrument is used for diagnostic purposes only.

Fr. The narrowest portion of the male urethra is generally the external meatus (more so in circumcised boys[3]), and meatotomy is frequently required before endoscopy. A simple technique of crush meatotomy is depicted in Figure 4. When, from voiding cystourethrography, a stricture or other narrowing is suspected, a graduated metal bougie à boule can be passed into the deep bulb to demonstrate and calibrate the area before proceeding with endoscopy.

Endoscopic Equipment

Several manufacturers produce pediatric cystoscopes, and there are many similarities among these different lines. The listed French (Fr.) sizes are approximate for sheaths with an oval cross section. The basic features of a miniature cystoscope set include interchangeable lenses (direct-vision and forward-oblique), operating and examining bridges, and assorted sizes of operating sheaths. Depicted in Figure 5 is a typical miniature cystoscope set with sufficient accessories to meet most needs. The infant 8 Fr. diagnostic cystoscope is shown in Figure 3.

A pediatric resectoscope (13 Fr.) with a transversely oriented cutting loop electrode and a longitudinal cutting loop electrode is shown in Figure 6. This instrument requires use of a direct-vision lens. A rigid biopsy and foreign body forceps (Fig. 7), also used with a direct-vision lens, fits through the 13 Fr. resectoscope sheath.

Cystoscopy Room

Because cystoscopic procedures in children almost always require some form of anesthesia, a fully equipped room within an operating or anesthesia suite is safest. I have emphasized (*Indications and Contraindications*) the importance of dynamic factors when evaluating certain urologic disorders of childhood. Accordingly, I have an image intensifier[18] mounted on the cystoscopy table in my unit (Figs. 8 and 9). Customized clamps modify the table to accommodate small knee rests for younger children. The table is hydraulically operated, including the movable tabletop. The size of the radiation field is accurately controlled by a variable collimator which has separate vertical and lateral

shutter adjustments plus a swivel mount to rotate the axis of the field.

This elaborate equipment capability is required only for selected cystoscopic examinations, and to justify the investment our service shares the fluoroscopic system with other pediatric surgical disciplines for monitoring bronchography, removing foreign bodies, and positioning central venous hyperalimentation catheters. Arrangements of a typical sterile table for pediatric cystoscopy are shown in Figure 10.

OPERATIVE CYSTOSCOPY

Endoscopic manipulation of the urinary tract of the child includes treatment of simple ureterocele, vesical neck obstruction, posterior and anterior urethral valves, spastic external urethral sphincter, lower ureteral calculi, and foreign bodies.

Ureterocele

While most authors agree that ectopic ureteroceles in infants and children are best treated by open surgery, this approach is not always required for treatment of simple ureteroceles, which are generally smaller lesions. Those who favor open repair of simple ureteroceles point out a significant incidence of vesicoureteral reflux following transurethral resection for decompression. However, the smaller simple ureteroceles may be adequately treated by cystoscopic incision. Excision of the ureterocele wall by loop electrode may cause reflux; a 2- or 3-mm incision of the stenotic meatus using a fine-tip flexible electrode or flexible endoscopic scissors should provide adequate drainage while preserving the roof of the intravesical ureter. If significant reflux results, later ureteral reimplantation is an elective option.

Bladder Neck Obstruction

Bladder neck obstruction now is seldom diagnosed in children, and I rarely have had indications to perform transurethral surgery for this diagnosis. When indications exist, however, electroincision or resection is easily accomplished using a 13 Fr. pediatric resecto-

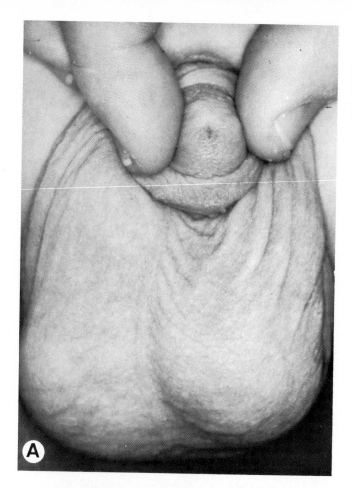

FIG. 4. Meatotomy in a circumcised preadolescent boy. **A.** Stenotic meatus. **B.** Crushing clamp applied to stenotic ventral meatal web. (Continued on facing page.)

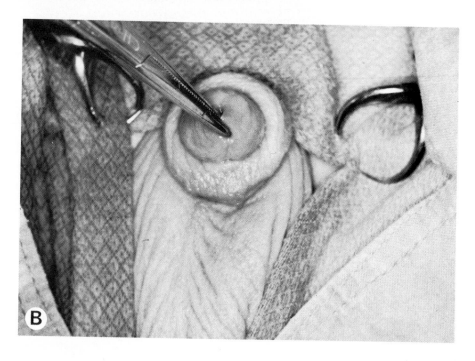

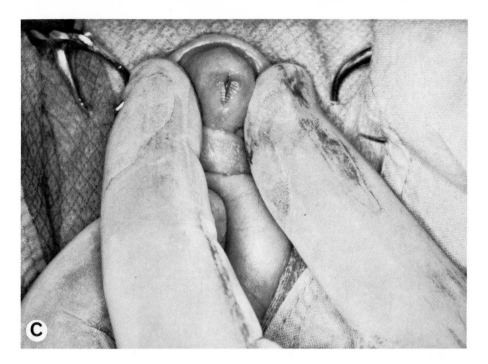

FIG. 4 (cont.). **C.** Meatotomy in a circumcised preadolescent boy. Appearance after incising crushed area. (From Gonzales and Perlmutter. In Shirkey (ed): Pediatric Therapy, 1975. Courtesy of C.V. Mosby Co.)

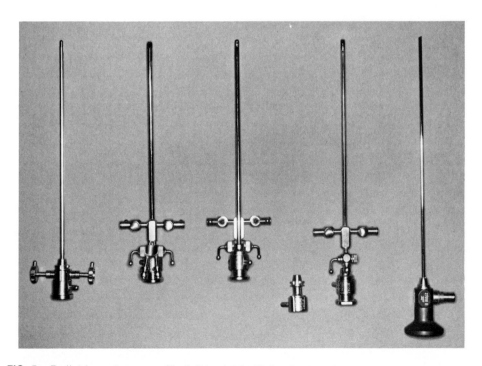

FIG. 5. Pediatric cystoscope with (left to right): 10 Fr. single catheterizing sheath, 13 and 14 Fr. double catheterizing sheaths, and optional operating bridge with adjustable deflector blade. Small bridge on right without variable deflector allows for use of one size larger catheter with the 13 and 14 Fr. sheaths. Forward-oblique telescope (far right) is interchangeable with a direct-vision telescope.

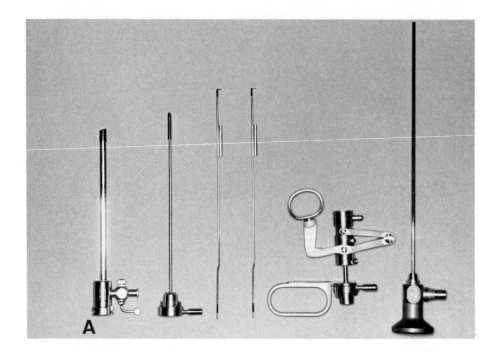

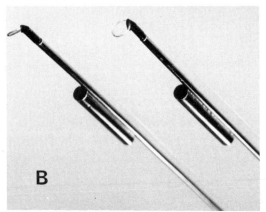

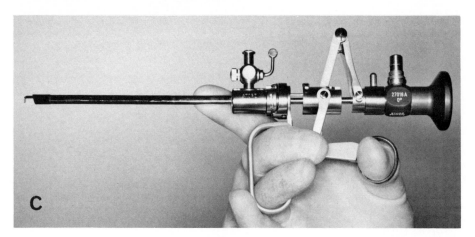

FIG. 6. **A.** Components of a 13 Fr. resectoscope. Cord is not shown. **B.** Close-up of resectoscope electrodes with longitudinal cutting blade (left) and transverse resecting blade (right). **C.** Assembled instrument with electrode partially extended.

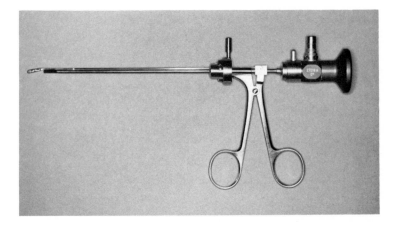

FIG. 7. Rigid miniature biopsy and foreign body forceps. Sheath is not shown.

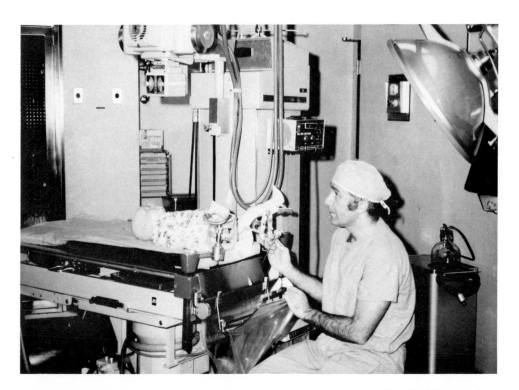

FIG. 8. Author's pediatric cystoscopy unit. Power-operated table is as described. Note under-table image-intensifier unit which includes cine camera, variable collimator, and custom clamp for small knee rests. During the actual procedure full sterile technique prevails, with the surgeon appropriately masked, gowned, and gloved.

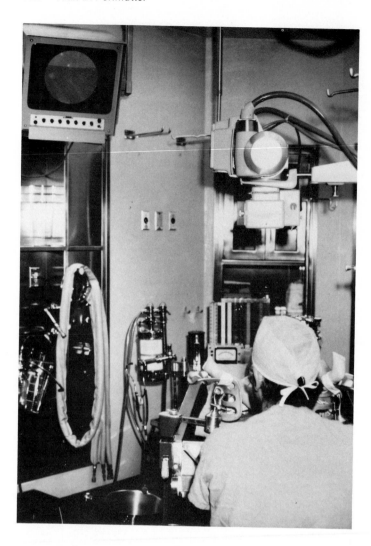

FIG. 9. View from foot of the table, showing convenient location of the television monitor.

scope and the longitudinal loop for incision or the transverse loop for excision.

Posterior and Anterior Urethral Valves

Posterior urethral valves, found in males, actually represent obstruction from a diaphragm with an eccentric annulus distal to the verumontanum.[14] The posterior portion of the diaphragm attaches proximally to the crista urethralis, below the verumontanum; the anterior portion attaches more distally. The proximal portion resembles cusps of leaflets (Fig. 11, Plate N), hence the description "valves." The degree of obstructive uropathy varies and can be of a severity incompatible with survival.

There is an extensive bibliography in the urologic literature regarding the overall management of posterior urethral valves and its associated problems.

Transurethral treatment of obstructing posterior urethral valves is the preferred approach. A 10 Fr. cystoscopic sheath usually passes in infants. A direct-view or forward-oblique telescope can be used depending on the surgeon's preference. A 3 Fr. ureteral catheter fits through the catheterization element and can be converted to a satisfactory electrode by reversing the catheter, which becomes an insulating sheath, and advancing the wire stylet 1 to 2 mm beyond the end of the catheter[6] (Fig. 12). The wire can be used as a 1- to 2-mm straight electrode or can be fastened into a

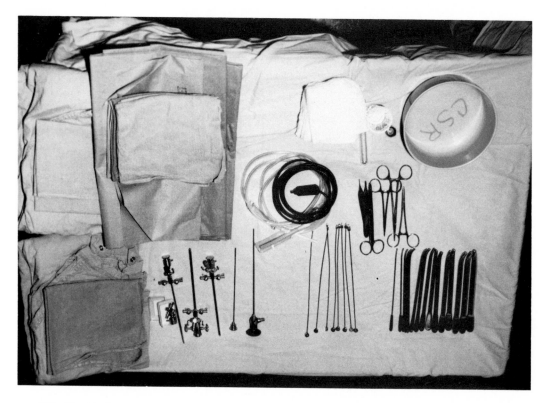

FIG. 10. Typical sterile table for pediatric cystoscopic examination and adequate for calibration, dilatation or meatotomy, and cystoscopy. Less frequently used supplies (e.g., ureteral catheters) are added as needed.

tiny, smooth loop. The electrosurgical unit should be calibrated in advance for the cleanest cut with the selected electrode. I use a cutting current to disrupt the leaflets cleanly in one or more places posterolaterally, distal to the verumontanum on each side without injuring the more distal striated sphincter.

When a 10 Fr. instrument does not pass a small urethral lumen in neonates, perineal urethrotomy can be done, placing traction sutures in the urethral edges. As the proximal bulbous urethra is more capacious, secondary traumatic urethral stricture is less likely to result. Alternatively a small midline cystotomy with a pursestring suture around the cystoscopic sheath permits endoscopic treatment of the valve from above.

In the older infant or young boy a 13 or 14 Fr. sheath most often passes, allowing use of a 4 Fr. flexible loop electrode, which when turned vertically can be used as a smooth hook to engage the valve cusps (Fig. 13). In infants and very young boys I prefer a flexible electrode to

the resectoscope loop because of the ease and safety of leaflet incision by this technique; accidental resection of a segment of the external sphincter should not occur, and incision into the sphincter is unlikely. It is not necessary to remove a segment of the valve, which is generally thin and diaphanous; simple incision usually suffices to allow the leaflets to flatten against the urethral wall with voiding, and the incisions can easily be done on a later occasion if residual leaflets are demonstrated on one or both sides. The incision should extend into the annulus or base of the valve. I reserve the resectoscope for patients with thick and fibrous valves, sometimes encountered in older boys; such valves do not yield cleanly to simple electroincision.

Anterior urethral valves may be synonymous with anterior urethral diverticulum—a fusion defect of the urethral floor. The mucosal edges of the diverticular orifice act as valve cusps during voiding, flapping up against the urethral roof to obstruct urinary outflow. Open re-

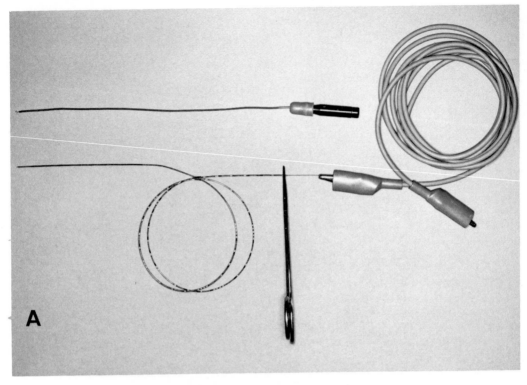

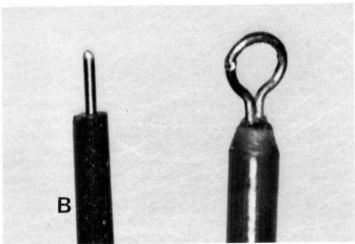

FIG. 12. A. Ureteral catheter (3 Fr.) modified as an electrode. Hemostat keeps stylet in proper position. Shown for comparison is 4 Fr. pediatric loop electrode. **B.** Close-up of stylet electrode and loop electrode.

pair is indicated for large diverticula, but when the diverticulum is shallow or abortive with no extensive urethral undermining, the obstructing mucosal flap is easily treated by transurethral incision or resection.

Spastic External Urethral Sphincter

External urethral sphincter spasm or dyssynergia, encountered in some forms of reflex neurogenic vesical dysfunction, can interfere

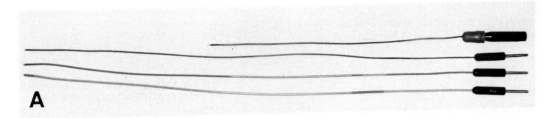

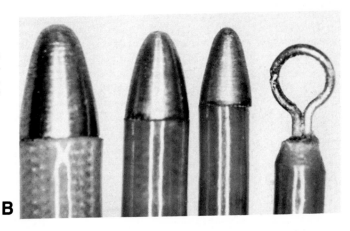

FIG. 13. A. Flexible pediatric loop electrode (4 Fr.) compared with variously sized Bugbee electrodes. **B.** Close-up to compare pediatric loop tip with Bugbee tips.

with vesical emptying, thus causing functional outflow obstruction. One form of treatment is internal sphincterotomy. The longitudinal resectoscope blade (Fig. 6B) can be used to incise the sphincter ventrally in the midline, at the 12 o'clock position. Incisions in other planes can also be used, but excessive bleeding sometimes occurs.[16]

Ureteral Calculus

Techniques for cystoscopic extraction of lower ureteral calculi are well described in standard urologic texts, and their applicability to children was briefly presented ("Indications and Contraindications," above).

Foreign Bodies

Miniature flexible or rigid alligator forceps or biopsy forceps (Fig. 7) can be used to retrieve small objects from the urethra or bladder.

COMPLICATIONS OF PEDIATRIC CYSTOSCOPY

As in the adult, complications—aside from anesthetic problems and positioning—are those directly related to instrumentation. Perforation of the renal parenchyma or ureter can result from forceful ureteral catheterization. Tearing of the bladder mucosa or rupture of the bladder wall can result from direct trauma with the cystoscope beak or rarely from hydraulic overdistention. Similarly mechanical injury to the urethra can occur, with laceration or perforation from rough handling. Even without overt trauma, stricture of the male urethra—months or years later—can follow instrumentation using a tightly fitting sheath. When urethroscopic examination is difficult or complicated, careful long-term follow-up is essential to rule out late stricture.

Aggressive treatment of valves may result in incontinence or membranous urethral stricture. Deep transurethral resection of the female bladder neck has caused vesicovaginal fistula.

With the use of careful sterile technique urinary infection following instrumentation of the normal or near-normal urinary tract is uncommon. Septic reactions are most apt to follow vigorous or prolonged manipulations of an anomalous, infected urinary tract with poor emptying dynamics.

The complications of pediatric cystoscopy can be avoided or minimized by using exquisitely gentle technique and by keeping the procedure relatively brief. When an obstructed and infected urinary tract has been instrumented, immediate establishment of adequate drainage following the study reduces the likelihood of a septic course.

SUMMARY

Cystoscopy continues to play an important role in the evaluation and management of urologic problems during infancy and childhood. The indications and specialized equipment for pediatric cystoscopy are reviewed. Meticulous technique is emphasized. The author's cystoscopy room is described in detail, and the place of urodynamic study as part of the cystoscopic procedure is discussed.

REFERENCES

1. Ambrose SS, Nicolson WP III: The causes of vesicoureteral reflux in children. J Urol 87:688, 1962
2. Belman AB: Clinical significance and long term therapy of cystitis cystica in children. Presented at the North Central Section, American Urological Association Meeting, November 1973
3. Berry CD, Cross RR: Urethral meatal caliber in circumcised and uncircumcised males. Am J Dis Child 92:152, 1956
4. Campbell M: Clinical Pediatric Urology. Philadelphia, Saunders, 1951, p 77
5. Cass AS, Ireland GW: Significance of ureteral submucosal tunnel length, orifice configuration and position in vesicoureteral reflux. J Urol 107:963, 1972
6. Hendren WH: Posterior urethral valves in boys: a broad clinical spectrum. J Urol 106:298, 1971
7. Hendren WH, Crawford JD: Adrenogenital syndrome: the anatomy of the anomaly and its repair: some new concepts. J Pediatr Surg 4:49, 1969
8. Immergut M, Culp D, Flocks RH: The urethral caliber in normal female children. J Urol 97:693, 1967
9. Ireland GW, Cass AS: The clinical measurement of the ureteral submucosal tunnel. J Urol 107:564, 1972
10. Johnson RJ, Palken M, Derrick W, et al: The embryology of high anorectal and associated genitourinary anomalies in the female. Surg Gynecol Obstet 135:759, 1972
11. Lyon RP: Cystitis cystica in girls with urinary tract infections. Presented at the Section on Urology, American Academy of Pediatrics Meeting, October 1972
12. Lyon RP, Marshall S, Tanagho EA: The ureteral orifice: its configuration and competency. J Urol 102:504, 1969
13. Palken M, Johnson R, Derrick W, et al: Clinical aspects of female patients with high anorectal agenesis. Surg Gynecol Obstet 135:411, 1972
14. Robertson WB, Hayes JA: Congenital diaphragmatic obstruction of the male posterior urethra. Br J Urol 41:592, 1969
15. Rosenberg B, Hendren WH, Crawford JD: Posterior urethrovaginal communication in apparent males with congenital adrenocortical hyperplasia. N Engl J Med 280:131, 1969
16. Rossier AB, Ott R: Urinary manometry in spinal cord injury: a follow-up study; value of cystosphinctero metrography as an indication for sphincterotomy. Br J Urol 46:439, 1974
17. Whitaker RE: Methods of assessing obstruction in dilated ureters. Br J Urol 45:15, 1973
18. Woodrow SI, Marshall VF, Evans JH: A newly assembled cystoscopic table with television-fluoroscopy and cine-fluoroscopy. J Urol 99:829, 1968

58

Cisternoscopy of the Cerebellopontine Angle

Werner Prott

Intracranial endoscopy has been performed by neurosurgeons for more than 60 years. In 1910 Lespinasse[14] was the first to introduce an endoscope into an enlarged lateral ventricle. In 1913 Dandy[6] primarily viewed the third ventricle.

In 1963 Guiot et al.[10] succeeded in visualizing endoscopically the interpeduncular cistern following ventriculoscopy by perforating the floor of the third ventricle. However, they were not yet able to observe the cerebellopontine angle, as the bridge did not allow them a view of this interesting, extracerebral space.

In 1970 I began to study whether it would be possible to reach the cerebellopontine angle endoscopically by otosurgical routes via the pyramids. We measured 135 preparations of human (adult) petromastoid bones in the temporal bone laboratory of our ENT department. We found that the transpyramidal, retrolabyrinthine approach via Trautmann's triangle is the best way to introduce an endoscope into the cerebellopontine angle.

ANATOMY

Trautmann's triangle is situated between the sigmoidal sinus, superior petrosal sinus, posterior semicircular canal, and endolymphatic sac. In this region a bone flap of at most 1×1 cm can be resected without damaging any functional structure of the inner ear or cerebellum (Fig. 1).

Thus an endoscope of up to 5 mm diameter may be introduced into the cerebellopontine angle after mastoidotomy and after opening the dura mater parallel to the superior petrosal sinus (Fig. 1). If necessary the bone covering the sigmoidal sinus may be resected, and by temporarily retracting the sinus itself the endoscope may be inserted more parallel to the posterior wall of the pyramid (Fig. 2). During the preantibiotic era many otosurgeons drained abscesses of the posterior skull base via the retrolabyrinthine approach.[2,3,15,16,22]

The anatomic situation for cisternoscopy of the cerebellopontine angle via Trautmann's triangle is advantageous. On one side the lateral pontine cistern extends often to the sigmoidal sinus so one reaches this fluid-filled space in a depth of 5 mm or more (Fig. 2). On the other side all interesting anatomic structures (e.g., the cranial nerves) are close together for only a few centimeters.

The lateral pontine cistern is 30 mm long, 18 to 20 mm wide,[13] and 15 to 20 mm deep.[20] Distances of bony structures of the posterior wall of the pyramid are illustrated in Figure 3, and those of the entrances of the cranial nerves into the dura of the pyramid in Figure 4. The lateral pontine cistern is situated 4 to 5 cm deep to the mastooccipital bone, the interpeduncular cistern 6.5 cm, and the pontocerebellar cistern 5.5 to 6 cm.[15,18,19,22]

INSTRUMENTS

For cisternoscopy ventriculoscopes* of either 3 or 5 mm diameter may be used. The latter

*Manufacturer: K. Storz Endoscopy K.G., 7200 Tuttlingen, PO Box 400, Tuttlingen, West Germany.

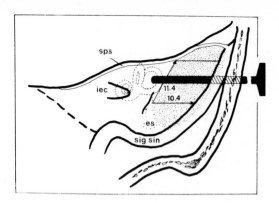

FIG. 1. Posterior wall of the pyramid. The endoscope is introduced by the mastoid via Trautmann's triangle (shaded area). **sig sin**, sigmoidal sinus. **sps**, superior petrosal sinus. **iec**, inner ear canal. **es**, endolymphatic sac. Measurements are in millimeters.

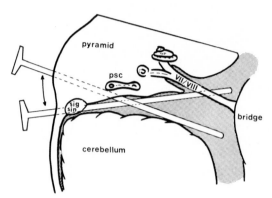

FIG. 2. Horizontal view on the cerebellopontine angle with the lateral pontine cistern (shaded area). The cisternoscope is introduced by Trautmann's triangle. The sigmoidal sinus (**sig sin**) is temporarily retracted by the endoscope. **psc**, posterior semicircular canal.

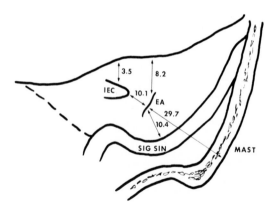

FIG. 3. Distances of bony structures (millimeters) of the posterior wall of the pyramid (average measurements in 135 human temporal bone preparations). **SIG SIN**, sigmoidal sinus. **EA**, external aperture of the vestibular aqueduct. **IEC**, inner ear canal. **MAST**, lateral bone of the mastoid.

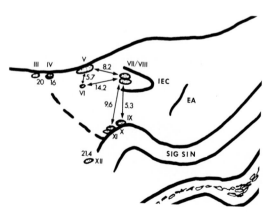

FIG. 4. Posterior wall of the pyramid with the entrances of the cranial nerves III through XII into the dura mater. Average measurements (millimeters) in 135 human petrosal bone preparations. **SIG SIN**, sigmoidal sinus. **IEC**, inner ear canal. **EA**, external aperture of the vestibular aqueduct.

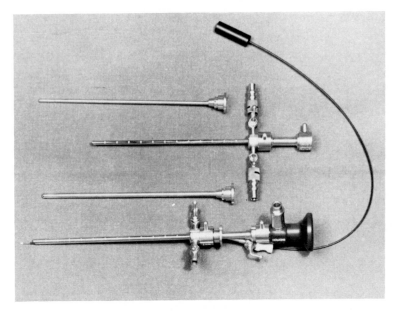

FIG. 5. Universal arthroscope-sinoscope-ventriculoscope with a Hopkins telescope. Top, Smaller instrument (diameter 3 mm). Bottom, Larger instrument (diameter 5 mm) with an electrode introduced.

has an instrument channel for electrodes or catheters. Cisternoscopes may be introduced with a blunt trocar (Fig. 5).

The Hopkins optics* are the same as those used in rhinoscopy, with a length of 20 cm and a diameter of 2.7 or 3.8 mm. Optics of 30, 70, and 120 degrees of direction of views may be used.

Still photographs have been made with an Ikarex Med. camera, zoom lens, and electronic flash.* The film used in Kodak Ektachrome (Kodak) high speed (160 ASA, daylight).

Fixation of the endoscope is made possible by a self-holding spatula. Cisternoscopy can be performed in either fluid or air after draining the cistern through the endoscope. The best position of the patient for cisternoscopy is supine, with the neck slightly extended and the head slightly flexed posteriorly.

CISTERNOSCOPIC FINDINGS

All of the photographs in the following figures were prepared from wet specimens at the Institute of Pathology of the University of Wurzburg, West Germany.

Manufacturer: K. Storz Endoscopy K.G., 7200 Tuttlingen, PO Box 400, Tuttlingen, West Germany.

Lateral Pontine Cistern

A general view on the left lateral pontine cistern is seen in Figure 6 (Plate N).* The tip of the cisternoscope lies in the subarcuate fossa. On the left side is the posterior wall of the pyramid with the posterior lip of the porus of the inner ear canal. On the right side is the typical surface of the cerebellum, which obscures the pons. Superiorly the cerebellar tentorium inserts into the upper margin of the pyramid.

The facial nerve (VII), nervus intermedius (between VII and VIII), and statoacoustic nerve (VIII) enter the inner ear canal. On the right the trigeminal nerve (V) follows an upward course. The abducens nerve (VI) is diagonal to VII/VIII and V.

The porus of the right inner ear canal with the facial (VII), intermedius, and statoacoustic (VIII) nerves are also seen in Figure 7 (Plate N). Medially and in front of these nerves is a loop of the anterior inferior cerebellar artery. A small labyrinthine artery leaves this loop and runs into the inner ear canal. Behind the nerves a small superior petrosal artery surrounds the porus.

This photograph (Plate P) demonstrates very

All color plates appear at the front of the book.

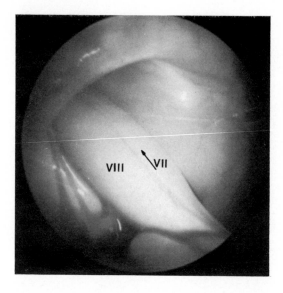

FIG. 8. Left porus of the inner ear canal with nerves VII, intermedius (arrow), and VIII.

well the distortion of the cranial nerves caused by the embryonal rotation of the pyramid. After the pons is found the facial nerve, in front of the statoacoustic nerve. In the fundus of the inner ear canal the facial nerve is situated in front of the superior vestibular nerve and above the cochlear nerve.

Figure 8 shows the left porus with the facial (VII), intermedius, and statoacoustic (VIII) nerves. Using a 120-degree angulated optic, one may be able to see several millimeters deeper into the inner ear canal. This would be applicable for early diagnosis of small acoustic tumors.

In Figure 9 the trigeminal nerve (V) enters the lateral pontine cistern, leaving the medial peduncle of the cerebellum. An arachnoidal web extends from the trigeminal nerve to the posterior wall of the pyramid. Some blood vessels are in the web. On the right and below, the abducens nerve (VI) runs into the abducens cistern, Dorello's canal.[7]

Figure 10 is a view of the right trigeminal cistern, Meckel's cave. The trigeminal nerve (V) runs below the tentorium of the cerebellum and above the upper margin of the pyramid into the cistern. This photograph was made with a 70-degree optic.

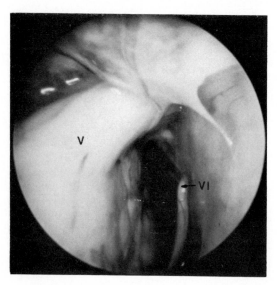

FIG. 9. Right lateral cistern of the bridge with nerves V and VI. At the top is an arachnoidal web with small vessels inside. At left is the medial peduncle of the cerebellum, and at right the posterior wall of the pyramid.

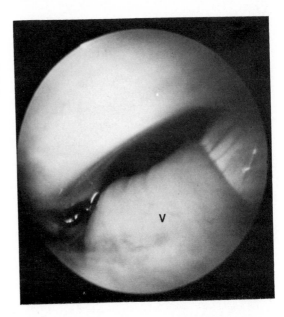

FIG. 10. View on Meckel's cavum of the right side with the trigeminal nerve (V) running in. Above the nerve is the tentorium of the cerebellum, and below it is the upper margin of the pyramid.

Figure 11 demonstrates the anatomic relationship between the trigeminal and the abducens nerves. The latter (VI) may be observed going subdurally several millimeters into Dorello's canal. Some small arteries extend from the posterior wall of the pyramid near the trigeminal nerve to the pons. They arise from the superior petrosal artery (Fig. 7). By cisternoscopy one is able to watch complete arterial circuits of the cerebellopontine angle.

The abducens nerve (VI) is the smallest and longest cranial nerve. Unlike all other cranial nerves it runs in a craniocaudal direction. It may be followed by cisternoscopy from the point of its entry to the lateral pontine cistern near the spinal bulb to the cistern of the abducens (Figs. 12 and 13).

Sometimes the abducens nerve is perforated by a labyrinthine artery, coming directly off the basilar artery (Fig. 14). This rare anomaly was described by Cushing in 1910.[4]

The endolymphatic sac is situated in the lateral part of the lateral cistern of the bridge (Fig. 15). The endolymphatic sac(s) lies subdural in the external aperture of the vestibular aqueduct.

FIG. 11. Right lateral cistern of the bridge with nerves V and VI. The abducens nerve runs into Dorellos's canal. At right is the pyramid, and at left the pons. Between the pons and the pyramid are some arteries.

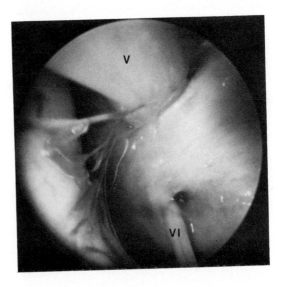

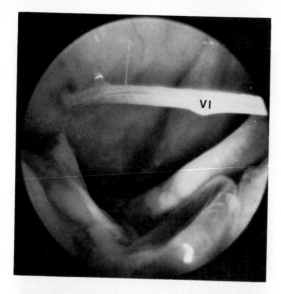

FIG. 12. Left cerebellopontine angle. Abducens nerve (VI) runs into Dorellos's canal. At bottom is the anterior inferior cerebellar artery.

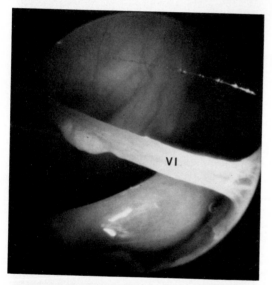

FIG. 13. Same situation as in Figure 12. The abducens nerve (VI) insertion into the pons.

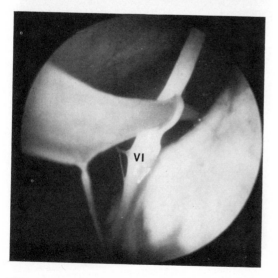

FIG. 14. Same situation as in Figure 1. The abducens nerve is perforated by a small labyrinthine artery.

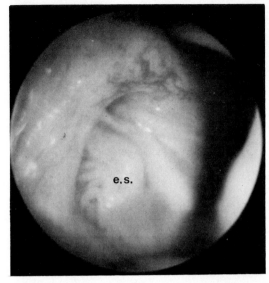

FIG. 15. Lower part of the left lateral pontine cistern. The endolymphatic sac (e.s.) is situated subdurally in the external aperture of the vestibular aqueduct.

Cisterna Ambiens and Interpeduncular Cistern

Medial to the apex of the pyramid one may observe the motor eye nerves as the oculomotor (III) and the trochlear (IV) nerves (Fig. 16). On the right side, the trochlear nerve (IV) inserts into the frontal part of the hiatus of the tentorium of the cerebellum. This happens in 65 percent of all cases.[13] The mamillary corpus can be located between the motor eye nerves. Some arachnoidal fibers extend from the corpus to the pons.

Pontocerebellar Cistern

The pontocerebellar cistern is caudal to the lateral pontine cistern. A general view of the caudal part of the lateral pontine cistern and the beginning of the pontocerebellar cistern can be seen in Figure 17 (Plate N). The cisternoscope has been introduced below the statoacoustic and facial nerves. At the top of the photograph is the trigeminal nerve (V). In the middle is the abducens nerve, which seems divided into two parts. The glossopharyngeal (IX), vagus (X), and accessory (XI) nerves run at the bottom of the picture. These three nerves separately enter special cisterns in the medial part of the jugular foramen.

Nearly the same situation prevails in another photograph (Fig. 18, Plate N). In addition, an inferior petrosal vein instead of an inferior petrosal sinus is present. This anatomic anomaly was first described by Englisch in 1863.[8]

Figure 19 demonstrates the cisternal roots of nerves IX through XII. The oliva is between the vagus nerve and the hypoglossal nerve. Even in these nerves the embryonally caused distortion of the cranial nerves is evident.

The external aperture of the fourth ventrical (Luschka's foramen) is situated near the roots of the vagus nerve. In Figure 20 the pyramid lies on the right, and the pedunculus of the cerebellar flocculus on the left. A hyperplastic lateral recess of the fourth ventricle is ballooning out of Luschka's foramen. Alexander published a monograph on this subject in 1935.[1]

INDICATIONS FOR CISTERNOSCOPY IN HUMANS

Cisternoscopy in living persons is possible and indeed has already been performed on six patients. The evaluation and follow-up of the procedure is in progress and results will be published in due time. Indications for cisternoscopy include small lesions of the inner ear canal and the cerebellopontine angle. The procedure may be useful too in early diagnosis of small acoustic neuromas and in cases of arachnoiditis and hyperplasia of the lateral recess of the fourth ventricle. Electrical recordings of the facial and the statoacoustic nerves can be obtained using cisternoscopy. Perhaps it will be useful in localization of facial palsy, in

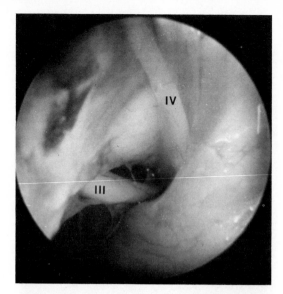

FIG. 16. Hiatus of the tentorium of the cerebellum. At right is the trochlear nerve (IV), and at left the oculomotor nerve (III). The mamillary corpus lies between the nerves.

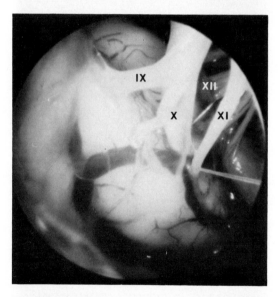

FIG. 19. Cisternal origin of nerves IX through XII of the right side. The oliva is between nerves IX, X, XI, and XII.

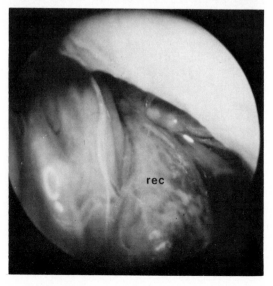

FIG. 20. External aperture of the fourth ventricle of the right side with a hyperplastic lateral recess (rec). At right is the posterior wall of the pyramid, and at left the peduncle of the cerebellar flocculus.

Ménière's disease, and in neurosensoric hearing loss.

Cisternoscopy by the retrolabyrinthine approach is a new method to observe the cerebellopontine angle *without damaging the functional structures of the ear or of the cerebellum.* It is currently the only way to observe the inner ear canal via the porus. Electrosurgery may be beneficial to the trigeminal nerve in cases of *neuralgia*, the acoustic nerve in cases of *tinnitus*, and the vestibular nerves in cases of *vertigo*.

As an adjunct to operations of the inner ear canal by the transtemporal,[9,11] transtentorial,[9] and suboccipital[12] routes cisternoscopic visualization can be useful in the diagnosis and may help to prove if it would be better to operate by only the translabyrinthine route or the suboccipital route, or by a combination of both. The experience gained during the next few years will prove the clinical value of this new endoscopic method.

REFERENCES

1. Alexander L: Zur Anatomie der Seitentaschen der IV Hirnkammer. Z Anat Entw Ges 95:531, 1931
2. Barany: Cited by Link[15]
3. Blohmke A, Link R: Die transmastoidale Cisternendrainage und ihre Bedeutung bei schwerer otogener Meningitis. Acta Otolaryngol (Stockh) 44:312, 1954
4. Cushing H: Strangulation of the nervi abducentes by lateral branches of the basilar artery in cases of brain tumor. Brain 33:204, 1910
5. Cushing H: Über eine constante Verbindung des Sinus cavernosus mit dem hinteren Ende des Sinus petrosus inferior äusserhalb des Schadels. Sitzungsbericht Kaiserl Acad Wiss Wien 48:1, 1963
6. Dandy WE: Cerebral ventriculoscopy. Bull Hopkins Hosp 33:189, 1922
7. Dorello P: Über die Ursache der transitorischen Abducenslahmung bei Mittelohrentzundungen. Zentralbl Ohrenheilk 4:418, 1906
8. Englisch: Cited by Cushing[5]
9. Fisch U: Die transtemporale, extralabyrinthare Chirurgie des inneren Gehörganges. Arch Ohr Nas Kehlk Heilk 194:232, 1969
9. Gerstler: Cited by Pool et al[17]
10. Guiot G, Rougerie M, Fourestier M, et al: Une nouvelle technique endoscopique: explorations endoscopiques intracraniennes. Presse Med 71:1225, 1963
11. House WF: Evolution of transtemporal bone removal of acoustic tumors. Arch Otolaryngol 80:731, 1964
12. Krause F: Zur Freilegung der hinteren Felsenbeinflache und des Kleinhirns. Bruns Beitr Klin Chir 37:734, 1903
13. Lang J: Die ausseren Liquorraume des Gehirns. Acta Anat (Basel) 86:267, 1973
14. Lespinasse: Cited by Walker[21]
15. Link R: Die herdnahe Behandlung der otogenen Meningitis durch Basalzisternendrainage. Arch Ohr Nas Kehlk Heilk 158:453, 1950
16. Moser F: Uber ortlich cysternale Penicillinanwendung bei otorhinogener Meningitis. HNO 3:250, 1950
17. Pool JL, Pava AA, Greenfield EC: Acoustic Nerve Tumors, 2nd ed. Springfield, Ill, Charles C Thomas, 1970
18. Prott W: Moglichkeiten einer Endoskopie des Kleinhirnbruckenwinkels auf transpyramidalem, retrolabyrintharem Zugangsweg—Cisternoskopie. HNO, in press.
19. Prott W: Untersuchungen zur Endoskopierbarkeit des Inneren Gehörganges und des Kleinhirnbruckenwinkels auf otochirurgischen Zugangsweg-Cisternoskopie. University of Wurzburg, Habil. Schrift, 1974
20. Tondury G: Angewandte und topographische Anatomie. Stuttgart, Thieme, 1951
21. Walker AE: A History of Neurological Surgery. Baltimore, Williams & Wilkins, 1951
22. Zollner F: Verfahren zum Aufsuchen und Entleeren tiefer subduraler Eiterherde an der Schadelbasis. Z Hals Nasen Ohrenheilk 49:409, 1944

59

Stereoencephaloscopy

Johannes H. Iizuka

In 1913 Dandy had already called the simple metal tube through which he could emit light reflected from his head mirror a "ventriculoscope"; he used it to observe the intraventricular space and to evacuate choroid plexus or tumors by means of a forceps. As technology advanced, tiny electric bulbs and precisely made lenses became available.

Between the first and second world wars a ventriculoscope became available with electric illumination and a telescope as reported by Fay et al.,[9] Feld,[10] Guiot et al.,[13] Putnam,[31] Scarff,[35] and Semenov et al.[38] The diameter of the endoscope was eventually reduced from 8 to 3 mm following introduction of the fiberoptic endoscope.

In 1964 the first endoscope guided by a stereotaxic aiming apparatus was designed by the author and manufactured by Richard Wolf GmbH, Knittlingen, Germany, and its clinical result was first reported at the 4th International Congress of Neurosurgery and 9th International Congress of Neurology jointly held in New York in 1969.[34] This endoscopic procedure is a new approach, compared with conventional ventriculoscopy, since:

1. The intracranial endoscopy is performed according to preliminary pneumoencephalographic findings and in association with contrast ventriculography, i.e., the foremost neuroradiologic examinations for previous selection and localization of the endoscopic target.
2. The endoscope is introduced into the intraventricular space guided stereotaxically (aiming and fixation), which has been thoroughly proved in newly developed stereotaxic neurosurgery, i.e., stereoencephalotomy.

The intracranial structures (i.e., brain tissues) are highly sensitive to surgical trauma with their postoperative functional disorders. Intracranial endoscopy is one of the oldest of the endoscopic examinations. The term ventriculoscopy was reserved for inspection of the cerebral ventricles; ventriculus ("a little belly") was named gastroscopy later; and ventriculus cordis became cardioscopy.

Ventriculoscopy has had one of the most disastrous histories in the development of endoscopy. While endoscopic techniques advanced in almost every branch of medicine and surgery, particularly following introduction of the flexible fiberoptic system after the Second World War, neurologists and neurosurgeons have not recovered from this disastrous endoscopic experience and are not willing to reintroduce this once often fatal procedure ventriculoscopy, despite the unique idea of Dandy.[6] Even today the intraventricular lesions, particularly those in the third ventricle, are often considered unapproachable.

INSTRUMENTATION

Stereoencephaloscopy is a combination of stereotaxic microsurgery and endoscopic neurosurgery. Thanks to recent developments in optics and fiberoptic illumination, there is an extremely thin endoscope (diameter 3 mm) —the size of a normal ventricular needle. With this size endoscope and a telescope with a diameter of 2.5 mm, the endoscopic examination can be performed without difficulty. The quality of a documentary film is, however, inferior, even by means of the newly developed electronic flash-fiber system with its powerful source of 800 watts/second and/or the extremely long exposure of 5 minutes performed by stereotaxic fixation (Fig. 1).

According to neurosurgical experience, this size ventricular needle, electrode for electrocauterization, probe for thermocoagulation, and cannula for cryosurgery are regarded as entirely safe from producing traumatic injury to the brain if they are not sharp, but blunt and gently inserted; we have experienced this to be true from observations in stereoencephalotomies. Incidentally, this size endoscope has an additional advantage in that it exactly corresponds or is adaptable to the usual stereotaxic apparatus.

We developed an endoscope with an external diameter of 4.5 mm as well. In this size the stereoencephaloscope incorporates an electrode

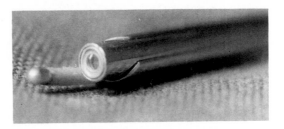

FIG. 2. Endoscope with a diameter of 4.5 mm is able to electrocauterize intraventricular tissue under endoscopic control, while an endoscope with a diameter of 3 mm is replaced with an electrode for cauterization.

for electrocauterization under an aspirating mechanism (Fig. 2). A self-acting and self-controlled aspirator on a rubber balloon enables extremely gentle (contact) suction (or "kiss") of an intraventricular pinpointed target for electrocauterization; for example, a choroid artery is selectively cauterized in a case of internal hydrocephalus and/or an afferent vessel of an intraventricular tumor (Fig. 3).

An irrigation system of the intraventricular space introduced by Scarff[36] into ventriculoscopy is, however, not adopted in stereotaxic endoscopy—not because such a system requires a greater-diameter endoscope for continuous supply with physiologic saline solution, but because it proved to be unnecessary unless the visual field is clouded by an intraventricular hemorrhage.

A detailed description of the stereotaxic instruments is not necessary here since a number of aiming apparatus for intracranial targets have been presented since the introduction of stereoencephalotomy by Spiegel and Wycis.[39] It should be mentioned that Rossolimo[33] successfully used a similar aiming apparatus (cerebral topograph) in intracranial surgery much earlier (1895) than the well known original stereotaxic apparatus of Horsley and Clarke (1908).[17] As far as the historical development of stereotaxic surgery is concerned, I suggested in 1973 at the 6th Symposium on Stereoencephalotomy[26] that even the "kephalograph" described by Harting in 1861 seemed to be not the earliest description of this method. In the meantime, I found two aiming and fixation apparatus in the literature: one described by Blasius[2] in 1833 and the another by Heister[14] in 1750 (Fig. 4).

We use three different types of aiming and fixation apparatus among many stereotaxic in-

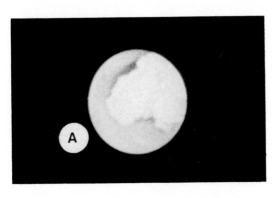

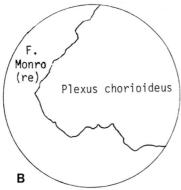

FIG. 1. One of the early films of a normal intraventricular foramen of Monro taken through an endoscope with a diameter of 2.5 mm by a Minox camera B with normal black and white film after a prolonged exposure (5 minutes). The quality of the film is inferior in spite of adequate stereotaxic fixation during the exposure.

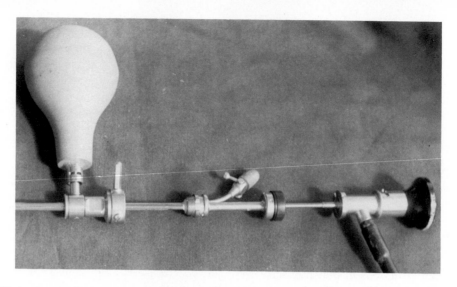

FIG. 3. For circumscribed cauterization of an endoscopic target, an aspirating mechanism is maintained by means of a rubber balloon; it does not aspirate cerebral tissue or rupture capillary vessels, in contrast to the usual aspiration used in neurosurgery.

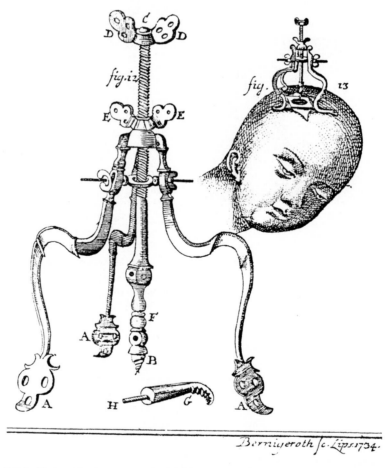

Bernigeroth fc. Lips.1734.

FIG. 4. Heister[14] described current surgical instruments in 1750 in his textbook of surgery. Among them was an aiming and fixation apparatus for trepanation of the skull.

struments, depending on the degree of ventricular dilatation and the purpose (i.e., the accuracy of aiming and stability of fixation that is required): (1) a modification of a self-acting brain spatula, which is set on the skull; (2) a handy microstereotaxic apparatus originally introduced by Woringer et al.[43] and later modified for endoscopy; and (3) a huge and stable stereotaxic apparatus designed by Riechert and Mundinger[32] initially also for surgical intervention at nuclei of the brainstem.[25,26]

TECHNIQUE

Similar to instrumental variations, we use three types of stereotaxic apparatus in endoscopy. Our intracranial approaches in endoscopic technique may be summarized by saying that no rigid rules are made whatsoever.

Since the cranial and cerebral structures differ among individuals, they must be considered from case to case. The cranial structures of adults and children, particularly infants and neonates, are completely different from the viewpoint of surgical techniques. A newborn's skull is still elastic for a few millimeters, and it has open fontanelles through which ventricular puncture is commonly practiced in pediatrics. The similar technique of cerebral puncture for air-filling (ventriculography) is adopted also for endoscopy (ventriculoscopy) without any incision of the scalp or trepanation of the skull. Occasionally we use a wound adhesive (butylcyanoacrylate; Histoacryl*)—a chemical compound similar to methylcyanoacrylate (in the United States and England) and aethylcyanoacrylate (in Japan)—to seal the tiny wound following a percutaneous puncture.

The thin skull in children older than 18 months (i.e., after ossification of the fontanelle) requires attention during trepanation in that it tends not only to deform on pressure but also to bleed because of its stronger blood supply during infancy than in adolescence, while the grown-up skull bears direct nailing of 5 mm depth for fixation of the stereotaxic instrument. This was the reason we designed two types of microstereotaxic fixations (Iizuka, 1971). Further considerations in endoscopic approach are due to the individual growth of cerebral cor-

Manufactured by B. Braun Melsungen AG, D-3508 Melsungen, West Germany.

tex as well. If our approach is mainly provided in cases of normal intracranial condition without any ventricular dilatation, why should the most sophisticated technique be performed routinely in any case? In a case of anencephaly or advanced hydrocephalus with extremely thin cerebral cortex, we certainly have definitely less risk of damaging brain tissue and/or its capillary vessels than in a normal brain during endoscopy. Even the use of endoscopy itself may well be questioned in such a case when a close look is obtainable directly through a burr-hole without any optics at all.

If we, however, leave from such a limited technical approach of conventional ventriculoscopy which was once practised only in selected cases of advanced hydrocephalus, and if we are going so far as to perform intracranial endoscopy in every optional brain, a previous pneumographic study of the ventricular system is a sine qua non in addition to the stereotaxic method of aiming and fixation (Fig. 5).

An irreversible injury to the brain tissue, and particularly a fatal intracranial hemorrhage, can be prevented only if the endoscope is inserted into an intracerebral cavity only once at a time and pin-pointed directly at the endoscopic target with complete accuracy guided by a satisfactory pneumoencephalogram and, if necessary, in association with a direct ventriculography with water soluble contrast medium.

MORPHOLOGY OF INTRACRANIAL CAVITIES

There are two different intracranial cavities subject to endoscopic procedures: the ventricular and the subarachnoid systems. The subarachnoid system is usually regarded as a cerebellomedullary and a basal cisterna; it is then divided into a pontine, ambient, vallecular, lateral, intercrural, and chiasmatic cisternae.

The ventricular system usually consists of four ventricles (i.e., two lateral and a third and a fourth ventricle) with their communicating passage (i.e., an intraventricular foramen of Monro) between the lateral and third ventricles, a mesencephalic aqueduct of Sylvius between the third and fourth ventricles, and a medial rhombencephalic foramen of Magendie as well as two lateral rhombencephalic foram-

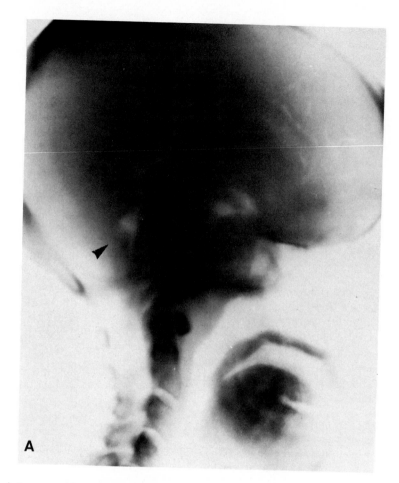

FIG. 5. A tomographic pneumoencephalogram projects air filling in different x-ray dimensions. **A.** The fourth ventricle (arrow) is seen at the midline. (Continued)

ina of Luschka; the last three openings in the roof of the fourth ventricle provide a communication between the ventricle and the subarachnoid space.

From the topographic viewpoint of endoscopy, it is important to realize that the ventricular system is not only multilocular, with their four ventricles, but also polymorphous, with an anterior, a posterior, and an inferior horn of the lateral ventricle; optic, infundibular, triangular, suprapineal, and infrapineal recesses of the third ventricle; as well as both lateral recesses and a fastigium of the fourth ventricle.

Among these, the third ventricle draws particular attention because of its deep and mainly diencephalic location in the brain, its variable configuration partly due to the recess-

es and partly to the intermediate mass, which, connecting gray matters of thalamic fibers in the midst of the ventricle, makes endoscopic inspection difficult.

In contrast to the usual endoscopic performance, intracranial endoscopy has to overcome specific problems in addition to the polymorphocellular nature of the ventricular system, i.e., the topographic and physical structures of the endoscopic object. While endoscopy is normally concerned with targets of inspection in cavities and/or ducts with external openings, there is no orifice for the ventricular system of the brain. It is true that laparoscopy requires an incision of the abdominal wall with its peritoneum, and thoracoscopy that of the thoracic wall with its pleura; it is, however, the sine qua non for intracranial endoscopy to

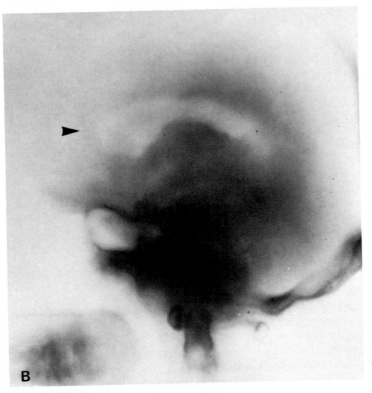

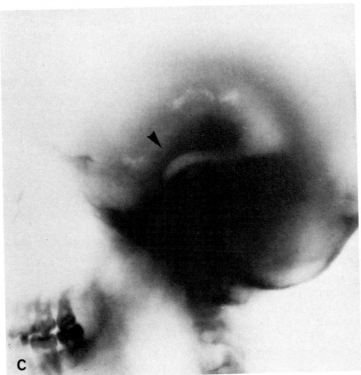

FIG. 5 (cont.). **B.** The anterior horn of the lateral ventricle 8 mm lateral to the midline. **C.** The inferior horn about 12 mm laterally. The ventricle is indicated by an arrow in each of the views (normal ventricular system).

make not only an incision in the scalp and a burr hole of the skull but also a puncture of the gray and white matter of the brain; it also introduces the endoscope into the intraventricular space, a procedure technically complicated and more hazardous for the patient than other endoscopic procedures.[19]

The cerebral cortex is frail and tender to both pressure and traction, and it is well supplied with blood by rich capillary vessels that are torn at the slightest amount of compression or traction—not only the cortical structures but also the ventricular wall (the ependymal layer is frail and bleeds easily). Once the brain tissue is damaged, there is no hope for regeneration of cerebral fibers. If it begins to bleed it is much more difficult to arrest arterial bleeding from the scarcely recognizable capillary vessels of the brain than bleeding we see in the scalp or in any other connective tissues. It was indeed this troublesome hemorrhage that delayed further progress of intracranial endoscopy.

An intraventricular hemorrhage is followed by a slightly sanguinolent, opaque cerebrospinal fluid (CSF) in the endoscopic field of the intraventricular space. Continuous irrigation with physiologic saline solution to correct this was tried by Scarff[36] without success; in fact, it sometimes resulted in fatal intraventricular hemorrhage. The mortality rate was estimated at 10 to 30 percent of cases in ventriculoscopy, a rate high enough to cause abandonment of the method.[20]

Another idea in cases where the CSF is cloudy following slight leakage of blood into the intraventricular space is to substitute air for CSF. This practice, however, is applicable only in those organs (e.g., laparoscopy) which are not as sensitive as the brain to sudden alteration of pressure; every neurologist and neurosurgeon is familiar from pneumoencephalographic experience how far changes in intracranial pressure alone can affect the cerebral circulation. Diencephalic disturbance may arise even on irrigation of the intraventricular space with saline solution if this is not exactly both biochemically and physically (e.g., temperature) physiologic. This is why the brain does not easily tolerate gaseous or liquid substitution of the CSF.

Since even a fiberscope[11] with its extremely flexible shaft has not been able to avoid the risk of perforation at the fragile ventricular wall, the usual maneuver of inserting the ventriculoscope (Fig. 6) followed by an intraven-

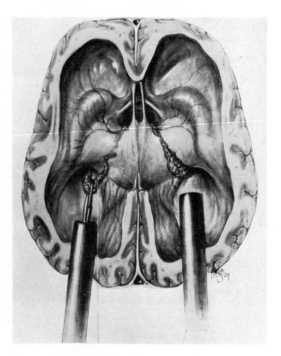

FIG. 6.   The first ventriculoscope was introduced by Dandy in 1913 and consisted of a tube through which an intraventricular tumor was removed by a forceps. (From Lewis: Practice of Surgery. Courtesy of Harper & Row)

tricular manipulation was replaced by aimed introduction of a miniature metal endoscope followed by visualization of the suspected part of the ventricle. Progress was achieved only with the combination of endoscopy and the stereotaxic approach.[21-23]

PHYSIOLOGY OF CEREBROSPINAL FLUID

While biochemical analysis of the CSF is already established, as is the cytologic examination, its function is not yet clearly explored. Schaltenbrand et al.[37] stated that the most important function of the CSF is a "stationary" one—to fill the empty intracranial space, both subarachnoid and intraventricular. Brain[3] referred to the function of CSF as "somewhat speculative."

If the function of CSF is nothing more than just being present, and only as much as is required to fill the empty subarachnoid and intraventricular space is produced, its balance, production, and resorption may be disturbed under abnormal conditions. Insufficient production—or more precisely a deficiency—of CSF, either spontaneously or temporarily by sudden loss (e.g., following lumbar puncture) may cause headaches, which in turn may well be a result of intracranial hypotension. A serious disturbance of this balance is caused by either hypersecretion or hyporesorption followed by intracranial hypertension, with fatal compression of the brainstem possibly being the final outcome. This condition arises if CSF production is abnormally stimulated by an acute inflammatory lesion of the choroid plexus, overwhelming the capacity of resorption. The resorption can also be disturbed by postinflammatory degeneration of the arachnoid membranes without adequate arrest. These antagonistic functions of the controlling mechanisms are not yet completely understood.

A similar serious condition may occur if the pathway of the CSF circulation is blocked. This can occur, for example, at the mesencephalic aqueduct, either morphologically by postinflammatory adhesions of the ependymal layer followed by obstruction of the passage or mechanically, caused by a space-occupying lesion (e.g., a tumor) in this region if the CSF production does not stop at once.[29]

If there is an accumulation of CSF in the extracortical space (i.e., an "external hydrocephalus"), we become very concerned with the dilated ventricular system (in this case the "internal hydrocephalus"). A description of hypersecretory hydrocephalus or malresorptive hydrocephalus is nothing but a hypothetical matter of comparison, and that of communicating hydrocephalus and occlusive hydrocephalus is a morphologic consideration. These findings do not at all indicate the dynamic function of the CSF. A clinical diagnosis of hypertensive or normotensive hydrocephalus is, on the contrary, a therapeutic concern, so far as the medical and surgical treatments are aimed at relieving the fatal cerebral compression caused by excessive CSF, usually in the intraventricular space.[42] A direct observation of the intraventricular condition in vivo is urgently needed to obtain further information in respect to treatment.

TOPOMETRY OF CEREBRAL VENTRICLES

To have some idea about the physiologic as well as the pathologic conditions in the in-

traventricular space, clear visualization of the ventricular system is necessary preliminary to intracranial endoscopy. A gross pattern of the voluminous lateral ventricles is sufficiently defined by injecting air via the lumbar or suboccipital route (Fig. 7A). Air filling by means of suboccipital puncture is preferred to the lumbar route because prolonged leakage of CSF from the spinal canal to the peridural tissue frequently occurs after a lumbar puncture, resulting in headaches as a consequence of intracranial hypotension. Precaution should be taken—and is often neglected—that a pneumoencephalogram is obtained at the moment directly after air injection (i.e., when the intracranial pressure is slightly elevated rather than when there is hypotension with a tendency toward cortical collapse) in order to obtain a pneumographic film of superior quality.

If intracranial hypertension due to an obstruction of the CSF pathway is suspected (e.g., on the evidence of papilledema), a lumbar or a suboccipital puncture should be avoided because of the risk of a fatal tentorial herniation, even after premedication with dehydrating agents. If an intrathecal injection of air fails to replace CSF from the intracranial space, intracranial decompression by means of direct and surgical puncture of the cerebral ventricle follows in order to rescue the medulla oblongata from subsequent fatal compression. This grave incident during pneumoencephalography can be prevented if the air is injected into the spinal subarachnoid space in association with intracranial endoscopy. An endoscopic approach provides not only safety against this complication in cases of the involved CSF circulation, but also the direct evidence of air bubbles appearing at an orifice of the mesencephalic aqueduct or the interventricular foramen in cases of a nonobstructed ventricular system.

Pneumographic visualization of minor cerebral ventricles (i.e., the third and fourth ventricles) as well as their accessory passages is technically often of poor quality, so that a special contrast medium is required. Water-soluble contrast material (Conray or Dimer-X*), compared with oily contrast medium (Myodil or Pantopaque), has the advantage of filling the tiniest and narrowest furrow of a

---

Dimer-X is manufactured by Byk Gulden GmbH, D-7750 Konstanz, West Germany.

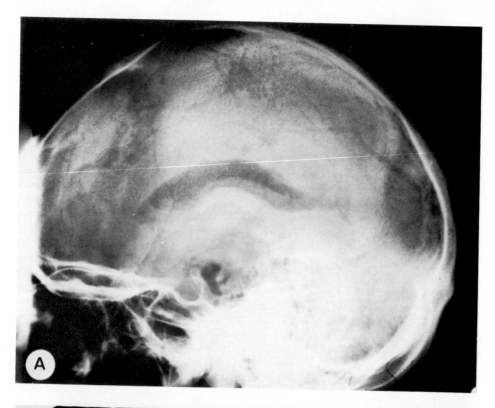

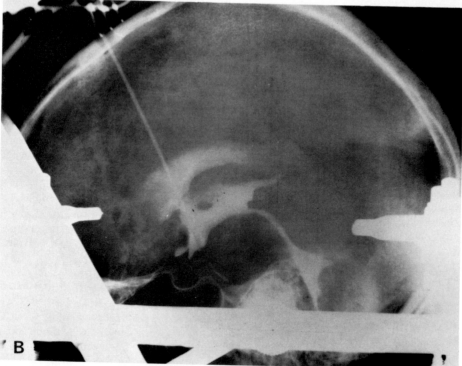

FIG. 7.   **A.** The cerebral air filling for x-ray visualization of ventricular system is sufficient only for grossly outlining the voluminous lateral ventricles. **B.** A water-soluble contrast medium is required for the accurate localization of circumscribed intraventricular lesions or precise configuration of the minor ventricles (i.e., the third and fourth ventricles with the communicating CSF pathways). (Continued)

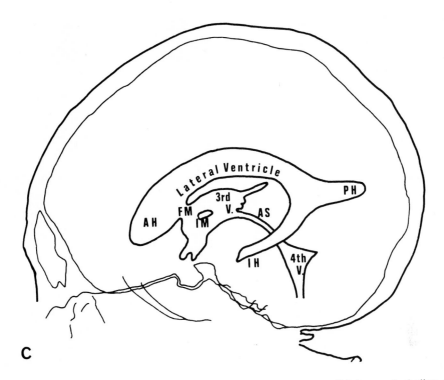

FIG. 7 (cont.).   **C.** The anterior (AH), posterior (PH), and inferior (IH) horns, including the interventricular foramen (FM), are adequately visualized by air filling, while the recesses of the minor ventricles with the intermediate mass (IM) and the mesencephalic aqueduct (AS) are shown on the ventriculogram.

ventricle by permeation, thus sharply defining the contour of a circumscribed intraventricular lesion, e.g., tumor.[22] The water-soluble contrast medium usually disappears from the intraventricular space entirely within 15 minutes depending on the injected volume. While both lateral ventricles require more than 50 ml of air on pneumography, both minor ventricles need less than 5 ml of contrast medium (Fig. 7 B, C).

If the medium is prepared in an adequate dilution (30 to 50 percent) using CSF or physiologic saline solution at 37 C (98.5 F) and is introduced directly into the third ventricle, precisely aimed and guided by a stereotaxic apparatus, neither disencephalic reactions nor epileptic seizures are observed even in patients without general anesthesia or premedication with sedative agents. Pyrexia and nausea, however, may be experienced if the dilution is not adequate or particularly if its temperature is not taken into consideration (it is often low compared with the normal body temperature). Epileptic seizures and even persistent motor or sensory disturbances can occur if the contrast

medium is injected into the cerebral tissue (e.g., the pyramidal tract) by error without endoscopic control.[22]

In advanced hydrocephalus in children with an open anterior fontanelle, a stereoencephaloscope may be introduced similarly to a ventricular puncture without any incision in the scalp. Stereoencephaloscopy is performed by means of stereotaxic aiming and fixation following topographic orientation of the lateral ventricles with the foramen of Monro in the pneumoencephalogram (Figs. 8, 9).

Endoscopic control thus provides a hazardless introduction of the water-soluble contrast medium and facilitates an accurate ventriculogram of the minor (third and fourth) ventricles. Stereoencephaloscopy has distinct advantages over conventional ventriculoscopy in association with pneumoencephalography and ventriculography (Fig. 10). The clinical advantages of the stereoencephaloscope are as follows:

1. The instrument is extremely small in diameter (normal ventricular needle or the size of an electrode for stereoencephalotomy).

2. Stereotaxic aiming renders repeated punctures of brain tissue superfluous.
3. Stereotaxic fixation prevents unexpected rupture of the arterial capillaries of the brain following undesirable movements of the endoscope.
4. Permanent (film) records of superior quality are possible.
5. In our own experience there have been no complications following stereoencephaloscopy.

TRAUMATIC LESIONS

An acute traumatic injury with cerebral contusion or a spontaneous subarachnoid hemorrhage is by no means the main indication of endoscopy. In such cases the intraventricular CSF may be stained with blood, and the endoscopic field is usually completely involved. No method is successful in replacing intraventricular blood with physiologic saline solution if the entire ventricular system is filled with blood clots as is found in aneurysmal bleeding inside the skull. Foreign bodies (e.g., a bullet or a fragment of a shell) may be better localized by an x-ray film.

Traumatic lesions following surgical intervention in the ventricular system were not recognized until recently when stereoencephaloscopy was introduced, although such lesions at the ventricular wall are not at all rare (e.g., following repeated ventricular punctures in treatment of hydrocephalus). A surgical perforation of the terminal lamina of the hypothalamus was described by Stookey and Scarff[40] during ventriculocisternostomy to establish a communication between the third ventricle and the interpeduncular cisterna in cases of an obstructed CSF pathway. The same can be achieved by stereoencephaloscopy without major surgery (Fig. 11).

INFLAMMATORY LESIONS

Intracranial infection should be considered at various stages (i.e., the initial stage of generalized inflammation and the following stage of localized inflammation). If the inflammation involves the dura mater, according to Dorland's terminology, the disease is called pachymeningitis.[8] When the arachnoid and pia mater are involved, leptomeningitis or meningitis proper is a generally accepted term. This morphologic definition hardly explains the clinical features of the acute inflammatory disease.

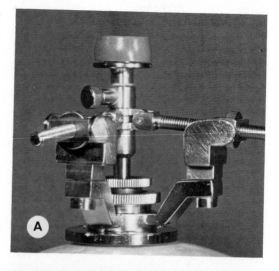

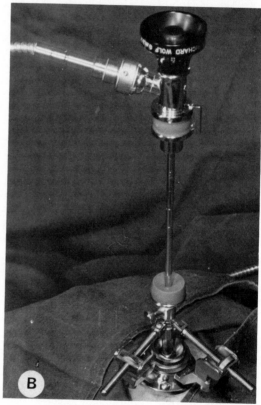

FIG. 8. **A.** This small aiming and fixation apparatus was originally introduced for microsurgical intervention of the basal ganglions in parkinsonism and was then adopted (with modifications) for intracranial endoscopy. **B.** As the shaft of the stereoencephaloscope is not larger than 1/8 inch in diameter, the small endoscope passes precisely through the aiming apparatus. (Instruments are manufactured by Richard Wolf GmbH, D-7134 Knittlingen, West Germany.)

FIG. 9. A. This stereotaxic apparatus is useful for sophisticated aiming in intracranial targets of endoscopy. Stereoencephaloscopy is performed following preliminary aiming and measurement by means of a surgical model in accordance with the ventriculographic finings. **B.** A burr hole is made with a trepan that is incorporated in the heavy stereotaxic apparatus. Then endoscope is introduced directly into the intraventricular space by usual stereotaxic technique. (Continued on p. 750)

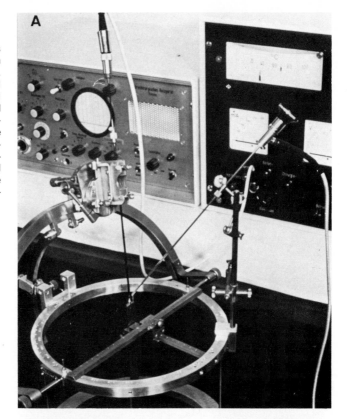

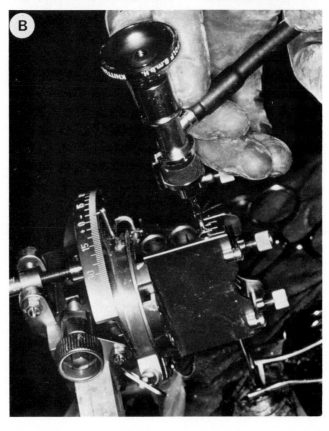

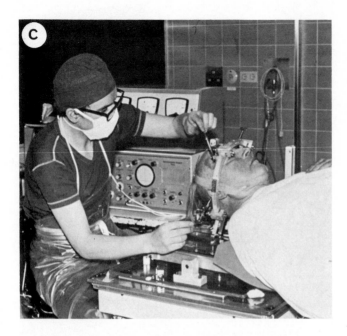

FIG. 9 (cont.). **C.** The patient's head is placed on a solid and self-contained surgical table, which holds the heavy apparatus and fixes the intracerebrally introduced endoscope, thus taking every possible precaution against undesirable movements and traumatic injuries to the brain. (Apparatus is manufactured by F.L. Fischer MT, D-7800 Freiburg, West Germany.)

From the clinical viewpoint we refer to all diseases that produce a pleocytosis (considerable increase of white cells in the CSF) as meningitis, regardless of the etiology: bacteria, virus, drugs (e.g., streptomycin), tumors (e.g., cholesteatoma), or even blood (also referred to as an internal pachymeningitis, which is, however, morphologically nothing but a subdural hematoma). Recently some clinicians have preferred "ventriculitis" to "meningitis" to indicate the septic condition following ventriculoatriostomy, thereby avoiding the expression of a postoperative meningitis.

Neither the meninges nor the CSF causes the clinical symptoms of the so-called meningitis, but they do produce disordered diencephalic and other cerebral functions (somnolence, pyrexia, etc.). On the other hand, we learned to suspect an "encephalitis" if the diencephalic symptoms are evident, the meningeal reactions (neck stiffness, pleocytosis, etc.) are less pronounced, and bacteriologic findings in the CSF are absent.

A generalized inflammation of brain tissue without inflammatory changes of the CSF is scarcely possible during the initial inflammatory stage. It is therefore suggested that the terminology "panencephalitis" is justified in such cases of meningitis, ventriculitis, or encephalitis associated with diffuse inflammation of both brain and its membranes.

An inflammatory lesion may, however, be more and more isolated later, developing into an empyema in an extracortical space, a cyst in an intraventricular space and an abscess in the cerebral tissue demarcated with a capsule (Fig. 12).

If the purlent or sanguinolent CSF does not permit endoscopic findings, cystic formations with fibrous deposit as membranes are common features in the intraventricular space, particularly in hydrocephalic ventricles, during the postinflammatory course and can be detected with stereoencephaloscopy. Such a cyst may well be a source of focal infection in an intracranial cavity; at the same time it can be a serious (temporary or permanent) obstacle to CSF circulation, producing a clinical picture of intermittent or continuous intracranial hypertension. The use of stereoencephaloscopy suggests that "arachnoiditis" or "ependymitis" is actually nothing more than a postinflammatory degeneration of the arachnoidea or ependyma and not an active inflammatory lesion.

DEVELOPMENTAL ANOMALIES

A congenital defect of the scalp or the skull (occult cranium bifidum) is not an intracranial malformation if these are definitely devel-

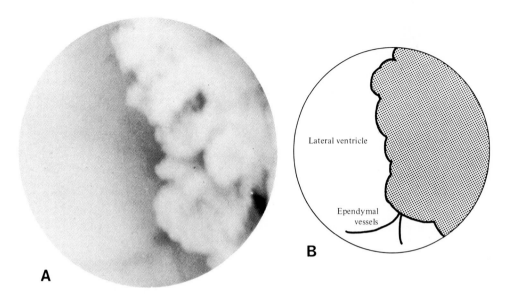

A

B

FIG. 10.   A. The choroid plexus is seen on the floor of the lateral ventricle as well as under the roof of the third ventricle. It varies from light orange to dark violet depending on its state of blood circulation. The trophic condition is variable too, and there is no direct correlation detectable on stereoencephaloscopy between the trophic development of the choroid plexus and its function. (Telescope: Lumina-Optik 180 degrees. Camera: Exakta-Varex II b. Film: Agfafilm DD 135, 32 ASA. Exposure: 1/30 second with electronic flash. Generator: type 5004, 800 watts/second.)   **B.** Schematic of photo depicted in **A.**

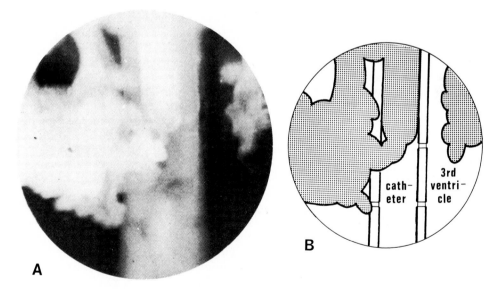

A

B

Fig. 11.   A. If a catheter of a ventriculoatrial shunt is implanted too deeply into the third ventricle, the catheter may be obstructed with aspirated tissue from the choroid plexus. It is therefore recommended that there be a stereoencephaloscopic view of the opening of the catheter in situ during its surgical insertion. (Telescope: Lumina-Optik 90 degrees. Camera: Minox 144. Film: Minox KB 14, 20 ASA. Exposure: 3 seconds at 150 watts with a continuous examining light source.)   **B.** Schematic of photo depicted in **A.**

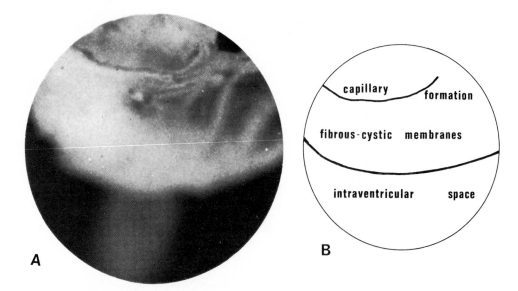

FIG. 12.   A. Following an intraventricular inflammation or surgical procedure, there may be either adhesion of the ependymal layer or formation of fibrous membranes, as is clearly seen here with capillary vessels in it. Later a cyst, often a multilocular one, may arise in the intraventricular space, particularly in the lateral ventricle. In such cases a pneumographic study does not demonstrate the polymorphous cyst. (Telescope: Lumina-Optik 90 degrees. Camera: Minox 144. Film: Minox-Isopan FF, 25 ASA. Exposure: 3 seconds at 150 watts with a continuous examining light source.)   **B.** Schematic of photo in **A**.

opmental anomalies. Intracranial congenital anomalies of the CNS include a cephalocele, an Arnold-Chiari malformation,[1] a Dandy-Walker cyst,[7] and hydrocephalus; the latter may not neccessarily be prenatal but could be a postnatal or secondary development.

There are three types of cephalocele: a simple cranial meningocele, an encephalocele or encephalomeningocele, and a cystocele or cystoencephalomeningocele, depending on involvement of the meninges, the cerebral tissue, and/or the lateral ventricle. Most cephaloceles are found in the suboccipital region on the midline and much less frequently in the parietal or frontonasal region.[23,24] A cerebral herniation into the sac of the cephalocele is evident rather frequently (45 to 75 percent of cases). An endoscopic examination is required only if there is evidence of further intracranial malformations on neuroradiologic examination.

An Arnold-Chiari malformation is a cerebellar herniation into the spinal canal and is seldom subjected to an endoscopic examination or surgical treatment.[29] Only when intracranial hypertension associated with an obstructive hydrocephalus develops is intracranial decompression required—either by surgery or by an anastomosis performed endoscopically.

A similar blockage of CSF circulation is occasionally found in cases of congenital atresia of the foramina of Magendie and Luschka, when it is called the Dandy-Walker syndrome.[7] Obstruction of the outlets of the fourth ventricle followed by dilation of the ventricular system (particularly the fourth ventricle) causes significant enlargement of the posterior cranial fossa associated with a posterior bulging of the occipital bone.

As long as the Dandy-Walker cyst is not artificially perforated, lumbar pneumoencephalography cannot demonstrate the ventricular system; such a procedure may even be hazardous in cases of intracranial hypertension because of the possible fatal compression of the medulla oblongata. An endoscopic examination, preferably stereoencephaloscopy following ventriculography, is then the procedure of choice, both diagnostically and therapeutically.

Prenatal stenosis or atresia of the mesencephalic aqueduct is much more frequently observed in hydrocephalic children; it is generally referred to as obstructive hydrocephalus. If CSF production subsequently ceases in the choroid plexus of the lateral and third ventricles, the disorder is sometimes called arrested hydrocephalus. This term should be replaced with "normotensive hydrocephalus" if intracranial hypertension is no longer present and surgical treatment is not needed.

Neuroradiologic finding of a blocked CSF pathway, marked atrophy of the cerebral cortex visible in a pneumogram, or varying degrees of mental retardation are not considered indications for surgical intervention. On the other hand, further examination and treatment are urgently required, regardless of evidence or degrees of hydrocephalus, if there is evidence of constant intracranial hypertension.

It is not easy to make an accurate diagnosis of an involved CSF circulation because there are two types of blockage: organic and functional. It is generally accepted that failed air filling of the cerebral ventricles via intrathecal puncture may be due to malpositioning of the patient for pneumography. In other words, there are constitutional variations of the rhombencephalic foramina, and a morphologic block cannot be demonstrated with certainty by the failed air filling.

A complete obstruction is accepted only if congenital atresia is present or if a morphologic adhesion of the ependymal layer, especially at the narrow mesencephalic aqueduct, develops during the postinflammatory course, seen by stereoencephaloscopy. On the other hand, an obstruction of one of the foramina of Magendie or Luschka still does not necessarily affect the entire fluid circulation since there are three outlets for the fourth ventricle.

The mesencephalic aqueduct of Sylvius, on the other hand, is definitely longer; and what is even worse, no other passages communicate between the third and fourth ventricles so that the aqueduct is vulnerable in most cases of obstructive hydrocephalus. Each of the right and left intraventricular foramina of Monro is responsible for the CSF flow for one of the lateral ventricles. It is much wider than all other intracranial foramina in spite of its considerably variable configurations.[20-22]

While an agenetic or postinflammatory aqueduct is often blocked permanently, mechanical kinking of the aqueduct is an intermittent or temporary obstruction and can usually be traced back to a space-occupying lesion in a neighboring structure (i.e., the pons, lamina quadrigemina, cerebral peduncle, or even the cerebellar tissue). In such cases of intermittent block, an air study cannot always provide evidence (not to mention the site and etiology); thus the performance of stereoen-.

cephaloscopy is eventually inevitable to establish the precise diagnosis. An internal hydrocephalus is a sequence of complexities of subacute or chronic diseases of the brain: congenital atrophy or cerebral malformation, a postinflammatory and/or posttraumatic dystrophy of the brain tissue in cases of hydrocephalus ex vacuo due to loss of the cerebral parenchyma primarily or secondarily to intracranial hypertension following obstruction of the CSF circulation or a compressive, space-occupying lesion (i.e., a tumor). An etiologic diagnosis of this internal hydrocephalus is not always simple—by either neurologic examination or neuroradiologic visualization of the ventricular system—and sometimes is difficult even at autopsy.

During stereoencephaloscopy one of the most significant criteria seems to be the "coating" of the intraventricular structures, particularly that of the choroid plexus. The ependymal layer shows a typical white or light gray granulomatous feature for a prolonged period both in postinflammatory and posthemorrhagic ventricles. The latter is rather light-colored or dark brown depending on the resolved hemosiderin in the ependyma during the first 2 to 3 weeks. A fibrous coating over the choroid plexus in the lateral ventricle is more significant in postinflammatory ventricles, if not directly proportional to the degree of severity of intraventricular infection.

In some cases with extensive fibrous and cystic formation in the intraventricular space, there is no history of an intracranial infection. Yet there are a considerable number of cases in which no significant postinflammatory reactions of the ependymal layer are apparent on stereoencephaloscopy, even if a severe and purulent infection has taken place in the intraventricular space according to the case history.

These endoscopic findings suggest that: (1) the ependymal layers react differently to an inflammatory lesion that was previously recorded on cytologic examinations of the CSF, varying from patient to patient; (2) an intracranial inflammation, either bacteriogenic or virogenic, may be overlooked if the neurologic symptoms are scarce, particularly during infancy and childhood when the meningeal excitation (e.g., meningism) is much less pronounced than in adults by comparison with the diencephalic depression (i.e., somnolence).

In cases of secondary hydrocephalus due to a

space-occupying lesion (e.g., tumor) there is no marked evidence of an ependymal reaction apparent on stereoencephaloscopy. A colored ependymal layer which is definitely seen on the films made through the endoscope is often nothing but a xanthochromia of the CSF following its obstructed circulation.

One of the most equivocal statements to be made may well be an admission of the developmental recovery of cerebral tissue in cases of congenital hydrocephalus (particularly a communicating, normotensive one) during a course of medical treatment with a neurotrophic agent and/or following surgery, e.g., ventriculoatriostomy.

It is common practice to report success after inserting a ventriculoatrial shunt—demonstrated by a pneumoencephalogram, which occasionally shows some diminution of the intraventricular space, usually in the area where an intraventricular catheter was previously implanted. A fibrous deposit soon forms a membrane in the intraventricular space after this intervention and later may even form an intraventricular cyst when the communication to the CSF is eventually closed down. Intrathecally introduced air cannot fill an encysted space that has fibrous membranes (which used to develop following insertion of the catheter owing to the moderate posthemorrhagic or postinflammatory serofibrosis); this defective air filling in a pneumogram is then often erroneously interpreted as further regeneration of cerebral tissue.

The diagnosis of parenchymatous regeneration of brain tissue or cystic formation in the intraventricular space can now be made with some degree of accuracy only with the help of stereoencephaloscopy. Cystic formation is not always complete, and it is usually not solitary but rather polymorphocellular. Generally speaking, a proportional decrease of the entire ventricular system following an arrested obstructive hydrocephalus is encouraging even if the cortical growth is moderate. On the contrary, a rapidly progressing regional defect of the air filling makes one suspicious of cystic formations, especially during the postoperative course of hydrocephalus ex vacuo.

A striking fact, proved by stereoencephaloscopy for the first time, is the discrepancy between angiographic and endoscopic findings. All three main branches of the cerebral arteries normally run in the cortical surface or ependymal layer at the ventricular wall. As the dilatation of the ventricular system advances following loss of cerebral tissue, the cerebral vessels are shifted in accordance with the degree of ventricular dilatation; this is apparent in the angiogram. The vessels on the cerebral convexity (e.g., the middle cerebral artery with its branches) stand fairly firm in the position even if the cortical tissue is as thin as a few millimeters. Cortical collapse (i.e., an external hydrocephalus) is seldom observed; when it does occur it is usually the result of a surgical procedure.

The central vessels of the brain (e.g., the anterior cerebral artery and its major branches) are displaced as the ventricular system dilates, and the artery appears to be loosely attached to the ventricular wall; eventually they are separated from the ependymal structure, as soon as the extremely stretched artery reaches its threshold of traction by the disappearing cerebral tissue. In this case the vessels run freely through the intraventricular space, more or less independent of the ventricular wall, and are well visible on stereoencephaloscopy. According to our observations, angiographic localization of the vessels does not necessarily correspond to the true trophic conditions of the cerebral tissue in advanced cases of hydrocephalus. A freely running artery in the intraventricular space is usually more or less degenerated, partly by fibrous coating around the vascular wall; it looks like a thin string in a fibrous membrane without any pulsations.

DEGENERATIVE ALTERATIONS

The endoscopic finding of degenerative alterations in senile patients, in contrast to infants, is completely different, and it may be considered a benign condition; it is often found among senile patients with Parkinson's tremor[30] during the fifth or the sixth decade of life.

On stereoencephaloscopy arteriosclerotically altered vessels show definitely impaired pulsation compared with the dynamic pulsation of a lustrous choroid artery during infancy and childhood. An atheromatous pallid artery, with its vessels of irregular caliber in the choroid plexus, constitutes one of the characteristic features of senile cerebral vessels.

As far as the choroid plexus is concerned, there is no significant correlation between its trophic condition and the age of the patient. A solitary, small cyst is more frequently found in senile patients. Such a cyst with a yellowish tint is not pathologic provided it does not obstruct the intraventricular foramen. The color of the choroid plexus, as seen on stereoencephaloscopy, is not dependent on age, but rather on the intracranial pressure (i.e., blood flow in the choroid plexus itself).

Among senile patients suffering from Parkinson's disease, a circumscribed pale area with the appearance of leukoplakia is occasionally seen on the ventricular wall (i.e., in the ependymal layer); but this too does not indicate the presence of a disease of the limbic system. It produces no clinical symptoms, and its etiology is not known.

INTRAVENTRICULAR TUMORS

Tumors of the CNS are considered according to their sites from the viewpoint of surgical approach. The results of surgical management, however, depend mainly on the histologic nature of the tumors or to some extent on the age of the patient.

While tumors of the cerebral parenchyma (i.e., gliomas) are indeed regarded as malignant in most cases, intraventricular tumors are generally benign. The surgical approach is

often difficult technically because of the deep intracerebral location.

A colloid cyst or a papilloma of the choroid plexus is seldom pathologic unless the CSF circulation is involved. The papilloma is usually seen in the atrium of the lateral ventricle (most frequently on the left side) and in the third ventricle; direct surgical intervention is performed mainly on the tumor of the fourth ventricle because of the technical problem of the approach. The tumor is coated with fibrous, smooth membranes and is rather friable; it has an insignificant blood supply so that it may well be a favorable target for both diagnosis and treatment by stereoencephaloscopy (Fig. 13).

A similar benign neoplastic transformation is the hamartoma of the ventricular system; it can be angiomatous, neuronal, or glial. The hereditary disease of Sturge-Weber[41] or Hippel-Lindau[15] is a neoplastic malformation closely related to the angiomatous hamartoma. These tumors are not necessarily solitary and are often associated with other benign tumors (e.g., astrocytoma).[5]

A typical space-occupying cyst of Hippel-Lindau (hemangioblastoma)—with an angiomatous conglomerate and cystic wall commonly in the posterior cranial fossa—produces

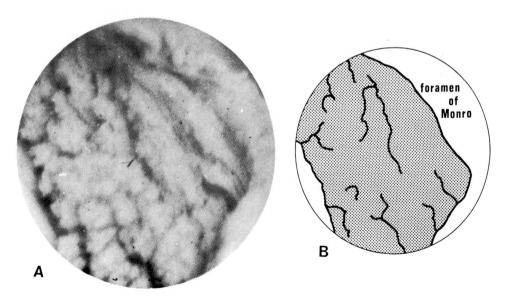

FIG. 13. A. A cystic tumor is often observed in the intraventricular space on stereoencephaloscopy, even if it is not obstructing the CSF circulation. A normotensive hydrocephalus in adults may well have such an intermittent disturbance of the CSF circulation, either at the orifice of the aqueduct or, more frequently, at the interventricular foramen. (Telescope: Lumina-Optik 180 degrees. Camera: Minox 144. Film: Minox-Adox KB, 20 ASA. Exposure: 4 seconds at 150 watts with a continuous light source.) **B.** Schematic of photo in **A.**

neurogenic disturbances due to intracranial hypertension if intervention at the hemangioblastic nucleus is eventually required.[18] Schwannomas arising from the peripherial nerve sheath and astrocytomas of the chiasma and optic nerves around the third ventricle are other lesions that can be stereoencephaloscopically diagnosed and treated. In contrast to degenerative choroid cysts, the congenital malformations (even if space-occupying) are more frequently found in young male patients (e.g., pineal tumors). The most common intraventricular tumor in adults, however, is the ependymoma, a benign tumor arising from the ependymal tissue of each cerebral ventricle. In exceptional cases their calcification may be apparent on plain x-ray films of the skull, and they are usually suspected on a ventriculogram, having the pattern of an occlusive hydrocephalus. The diagnosis may be made by stereoencephaloscopy or eventually at autopsy. In the third ventricle itself there are pineal tumors which often are deemed unapproachable by conventional neurosurgical techniques because of the associated high mortality rate, although there are a few reported isolated cases of successful surgical treatment.

Tumors in this region have long been regarded by neuropathologists as being of more morphologic than therapeutic concern since pineal tumors (both teratoma and pinealoma) have statistically comprised less than 1 percent of intracranial tumors in neurosurgical practice. The occurrence was reviewed in the literature[28] from Japan, where neurosurgeons are becoming more aware of deep-seated intracerebral tumors and are much more concerned with progress in the approach to those in the third ventricle. According to their statistics a clinical diagnosis of teratoma was made in 1.8 percent and of pinealomas in 8.4 percent of 997 patients with cerebral tumors; these figures may be compared with the clinical frequency of pinealoma reported by Grant[12] (1.1 percent of 1,169 tumors) and Cushing[4] (1.6 percent of 862), while the pinealoma was found in 12.8 percent of 404 brain tumors of autopsy. Hori et al.[16] stressed the similarity of these pineal tumors of the third ventricle found by precise and aimed ventriculography and by intracranial endoscopy (Figs. 14, 15).

RESULTS AND COMPLICATIONS

It is rather presumptuous to summarize the clinical value of this new method of intracranial microsurgery before sufficient data are available, and our experience does not yet exceed 100 cases. It is worthwhile, however, to

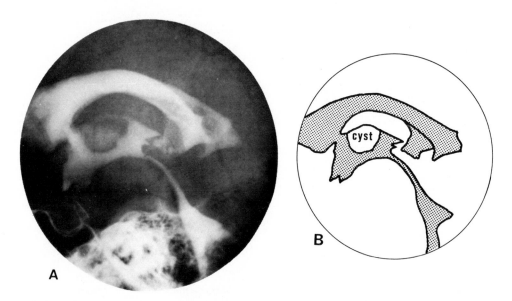

FIG. 14.   A. Fibrous formation of membranes in the intraventricular space may result in amputation of the horns of the lateral ventricles (e.g., the posterior and inferior horns): or it may form a cyst in the third ventricle, obstructing the upper half of this ventricle from its floor down to the intermediate mass. (Contrast: Dimer-X. Dilution: 30 percent, 2 ml.)   **B.** Schematic of the photo **A.**

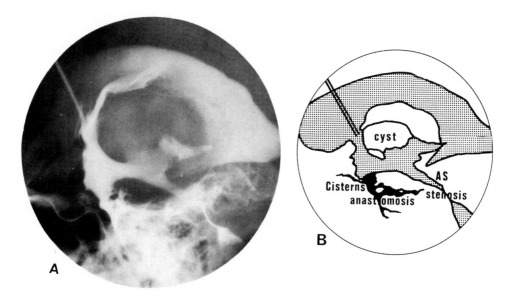

FIG. 15. **A.** Intermittent obstruction of the CSF pathway (e.g., aqueduct of Sylvius) is followed by dilatation of the ventricular system proximal to the stenosis. A ventriculocisternostomy may be performed with the help of stereoencephaloscopy without a surgical approach. (Contrast: Dimer-X. Dilution: 40 percent, 3 ml.) **B.** Schematic of photo in **A**.

analyze the main complications following stereoencephaloscopy.

Not a single postoperative infection has been seen so far, as we were careful to observe the elementary prerequisites of sterile technique. While the usual ventricular puncture for air filling in newborns was carried out in the pediatric ward, the same ventricular puncture—percutaneously via the anterior fontanelle—for endoscopy was performed primarily in an aseptic operating room. Intraventricular hemorrhage never occurred in our patients, as confirmed on endoscopy. We believe that this was because the endoscope was introduced intracerebrally following an incision of the scalp and a careful trepanation of the skull with a rounded stylet; the brain tissue thus gave way gently for the small endoscope without rupturing cortical capillary vessels.

In spite of these precautions we did experience some complications in 38 cases in which we used water-soluble contrast media (Conray 60 or Dimer-X). It is generally accepted that Dimer-X is better tolerated than Conray 60, although we found no significant difference. The more important facts may be that: (1) The contrast medium must be injected properly at physiologic temperature (37 C). (2) It must be diluted with the patient's CSF or physiologic saline solution in 30 to 45 percent for good permeation. (3) It must be restricted to 2 to 3 ml.

Kandel[27] observed headache, pyrexia (noninflammatory up to 38 C), nausea, and/or vomiting in 7 percent of 320 patients following a Conray ventriculography. Our experience corresponds with his as far as these reactions of the autonomous nervous system are concerned. He further noted epileptic seizures in 3.7 percent of his cases with Conray ventriculography, and he attributed this to erroneous injection of the contrast medium into the subarachnoid space in direct contact with the cerebral cortex. We may presume that direct contact of Conray with an injured cortex may well produce seizures, and an inadequate and blind injection of the medium into the cerebral tissue (i.e., into the capsula interna instead of intraventricular space) may well produce motor or sensory disturbances; these may be either temporary or permanent, as described in the literature and as we have seen with stereoencephalotomy.

A spinal form of epileptic seizure may be observed following suboccipital injection of the contrast medium if the spinal cord is injured at the level of the medulla oblongata with the needle; this can occur during myelography with a water-soluble contrast medium via suboccipital puncture. We have seen neither jacksonian seizures nor neurogenic disturbances during stereotaxic endoscopy of the ventricular system; it may perhaps be presumed that the endoscopic control of the position of a ventricular needle has contributed to the technical perfection of ventriculography with water-soluble contrast media.

Comparing the generally accepted fact that diencephalic dysregulation of the autonomous nervous system is frequently observed—again, according to Kandel, in about 70 to 80 percent following a pneumoventriculography and in 25 to 30 percent following a Myodil ventriculography—the rate of 7 percent following a Conray ventriculography may be regarded as rather low.

Thus the rate of complications is rather low in stereoencephaloscopy if a water-soluble contrast medium is used. A previous air study of the ventricular system may cause some undesirable diencephalic reactions for a day or two following the procedure.

Various conditions as seen by endoscopy are illustrated Figures 16–21, at Plate O.*

REFERENCES

1. Arnold J: Myelocyste, Transposition von Gewebskeimen und Sympodie. Beitr Pathol Anat 16:1, 1894
2. Blasius E: Chirurgische Abbildungen oder Darstellung der blutigen chirurgischen Operationen und der für dieselben erfundenen Werkzeuge, Berlin, 1833
3. Brain WR: Diseases of the Nervous System. London, Oxford University Press 1962
4. Cushing H: Intracranial Tumours. Springfield, Ill, Charles C Thomas, 1932
5. Dandy WE: Benign Tumors in the Third Ventricle of the Brain. Springfield, Ill, Charles C Thomas, 1933
6. Dandy WE: Extirpation of the choroid plexuses of the lateral ventricle in communicating hydrocephalus. Ann Surg 68:569, 1918
7. Dandy WE: The diagnosis and treatment of hydrocephalus due to occlusion of the foramina of Magendie and Luschka. Surg Gynecol Obstet 32:112, 1921
8. Dorland WAN: Illustrated Medical Dictionary. Philadelphia, Saunders, 1965
9. Fay T, Grant FC: Ventriculoscopy and intraventricular photography in internal hydrocephalus. JAMA 80:461, 1923
10. Feld M: Ventriculoscope coagulant utilisé dans les hydrocephalies communicantes. Presse Med 64:632, 1956
11. Fukushima T, Ishijima B, Hirakawa K, et al: Ventriculofiberscope. J Neurosurg 38:251, 1973
12. Grant FC: A study of the results of surgical treatment in 2326 consecutive patients with brain tumor. J Neurosurg 13:479, 1956

13. Guiot G, Rougerie J, Fourestier M, et al: Une novelle technique endoscopique. Presse Med 71:1225, 1963
14. Heister L: Institutiones Chirurgicae, Part 1. Amsterdam, Waesberg, 1750
15. Hippel EV: Über eine sehr seltene Erkrankung der Netzhaut. Graefes Arch Ophthalmol 59:83, 1904
16. Hori T, Fukushima T, Sekino H, et al: Tumors of the pineal region. Brain Nerve 24:973, 1972 (Japanese)
17. Horsley V, Clarke R: The structure and functions of the cerebellum examined by a new method. Brain 31:45, 1908
18. Iizuka JH: Rückfälle bei Lindautumoren. Acta Neurochir (Wien) 20:281, 1969
19. Iizuka JH: Zerebraldiagnostik im Kindesalter mittels Stereoenzephaloskopie. Z Kinderchir 10:2, 1971
20. Iizuka JH: Stereoencephaloscopic findings in internal hydrocephalus. Endoscopy 4:141, 1972
21. Iizuka JH: Stereoenzephaloskopie. Fortschr Endosk 4:209, 1973
22. Iizuka JH: Zerebraldiagnostik und Zerebraltopometrie—Isolierte Darstellung des 3. und 4. Ventrikels mittels Conray 60. Fortschr Med 90:1109, 1972
23. Iizuka JH: Die technische Entwicklung der stereotaktischen Neurochirurgie. Med Technik 93:136, 1973
24. Iizuka JH: Dysgenetische Nebenbefunde bei den Zephalozelen. Z Kinderchir 12:16, 1973
25. Iizuka JH: Stereoencephaloscopic techniques in pediatric neurosurgery. In Proceedings of the 3rd European Congress of Pediatric Neurosurgery (Göttingen, September 3–7, 1972). Stuttgart, Hippokrates, 1974
26. Iizuka JH: Development of a stereotaxic endoscopy of the ventricular system. In Proceedings of the 6th Symposium of the International Society for Research in Stereoencephalotomy (Tokyo, October 13, 1973). Basel, Karger, 1974
27. Kandel E, Chebotaryova M: Conray ventriculography in stereotaxic surgery—experience with 320 operations. Confin Neurol 34:34, 1972
28. Katsura S, Suzuki J, Wada T: A statistical study of brain tumors in the neurosurgical clinics in Japan. J Neurosurg 16:570, 1959
29. Matson DD: Neurosurgery of Infancy and Childhood. Springfield, Ill, Charles C Thomas, 1969
30. Parkinson J: An Essay on the Shaking Palsy. London, Sherwood, 1817
31. Putnam TJ: Treatment of hydrocephalus by endoscopic coagulation of the choroid plexus. N Engl J Med 210:1373, 1934
32. Riechert T, Mundinger F: Beschreibung und Anwendung eines Zielgerätes für stereotaktische Hirnoperationen (2. Modell). Acta Neurochir (Wien) (Suppl) 3:308, 1955
33. Rossolimo G: Zur Symptomatologie und chirurgische Behandlung einer eigenthümlichen Grosshirncyste. Dtsch Z Nervenheilkd 6:76, 1895

All color plates appear at the front of the book.

34. Röttgen P, Iizuka JH: Stereoencephaloscopy. Excerpta Med 193:108, 1969

35. Scarff JE: Endoscopic treatment of hydrocephalus. Arch Neurol Psychiatry 35:853, 1936

36. Scarff JE: The treatment of nonobstructive hydrocephalus by endoscopic cauterization of the choroid plexuses. J Neurosurg 33:1, 1970

37. Schaltenbrand G, Wolff H: Die Produktion und Zirkulation des Liquors und ihre Störungen. Handbuch der Neurochir, Vol 1, Part 1. Heidelberg, Springer, 1959, p 91

38. Semenov VN, Burkhanov AM: Ventriculoscope with a system for electrocoagulation of the choroid plexuses. 5:57, 1972

39. Spiegel EA, Wycis HT: Stereoencephalotomy, Part 1. New York, Grune & Stratton, 1952

40. Stookey B, Scarff JE: Occlusion of aqueduct of Sylvius by neoplastic and nonneoplastic processes with rational surgical treatment for relief of resultant obstructive hydrocephalus. Bull Neurol Inst NY 5:348, 1936

41. Sturge WA: A case of partial epilepsy apparently due to a lesion of one of the vasomotor centers of the brain. Clin Soc Lond Trans 12:162, 1879

42. Torkildsen A: Ventriculocisternostomy. Oslo, Tanun, 1947

43. Woringer E, Chambon P, Brain J: A stereotaxic apparatus with optic aiming. J Neurol Neurosurg Psychiatry 23:352, 1960

EDITORIAL COMMENT

H. B. Griffith, Department of Neurological Surgery, Frenchay Hospital, Bristol, England, also did some pioneer work in endoneurosurgery in hydrocephalic children in the form of diagnosis and treatment.

THE EDITOR

60

Retroperitoneoscopy: A Preliminary Report

R. Wittmoser

Retroperitoneoscopy is a recently developed endoscopic method that provides a relatively simple and safe approach for a retroperitoneal lumbar sympathicotomy. In common with retropleuroscopy this method occupies a special position among endoscopic techniques, because it involves the creation of a large (not preformed) cavity by means of gas insufflation into an area that consists chiefly of soft connective tissues (the retroperitoneal space). A reliably gas-tight endoscopic instrumentarium and the maintenance of an adequate gas (CO_2) pressure—in general between 10 and 30 mm Hg—are the technical requirements for efficient endo-operative work.

Through a stab incision (15–20 mm) a specially designed retroperitoneoscope (similar to a rigid rectosigmoidoscope) is inserted through the layers of the abdominal wall in an oblique dorsolateral direction. After the transverse fascia have been perforated, CO_2 is insufflated with an average pressure of 20 mm Hg, while the unfolding of the peritoneal cavity is supported by blunt preparation with the tip of the endoscope shaft.

Positioning the patient laterally and with slight angulation is important. It causes the medial displacement of the visceral sac due to gravidity and additional gas pressure, allowing one to reach the psoas without difficulties. The genitofemoralis muscle and the nerve are always visible as a landmark. At the medial margin of the psoas the dissection is performed on the right side up to the vena cava to the left of the aorta. Further exposure of these vessels is not necessary.

The operation field *sensu strictu* is situated between the large vessels and the medial margin of the psoas. On the right side of the field the lumbar lymphatic trunk is located near the vena cava. Between two dissections one can take sufficient tissue samples of the paraaortic lymph nodes for histologic examination—in itself an important indication for retroperitoneoscopy. The sympathetic trunk is located near, possibly below, the margin of the psoas and close to the vertebral bodies, which are easily visible and palpable. In general it is crossed by the vasa lumbalia. In every region between L2 and L5 an interganglionic sympathicotomy, a sympathectomy, or a division of the rami communicantes can be performed. Depending on the indication, we generally perform an interganglionic sympathicotomy at L3/4 and take out some tissue for histologic verification. The situation on the left side corresponds to that on the right, except for the limitation by the aorta of the operative field toward the midline. The ureter is easily recognized by its tubular structure and peristalsis.

The postoperative period is characterized by a short hospitalization. The patient is allowed out of bed on the day of operation and can be discharged on the first or the second day after operation. In my series I have not experienced serious complications. The gas pressure is tolerated well under general anesthesia.

In cases of hyperhidrosis of the lower extremities the procedure results in the elimination of the pathologic perspiration or secretion, according to its localization, from the knee to the buttock. In cases of functional or organic arterial obliterations an improvement of blood circulation was observed, depending of course on the basic underlying disease.

The indications for retroperitoneoscopy are similar to those of lumbar sympathectomies. Because there is only a minimal morbidity involved, in the case of hyperhidrosis of the lower extremities, functional circulatory disturbances (Raynaud's syndrome), and the lighter stage-III obliteration diseases with resting pain an endoscopic method using a small incision ("mini-approach") can be indicated. More serious stages, such as III and IV, or poor-risk patients can be considered. Cases with sympathalgic pain syndromes and posttraumatic vasopathia (Sudeck's syndrome) of the lower extremities can be attempted.

The exploration of retroperitoneal space provides access to the lymph nodes, which can be of help in staging, especially in cases of cancer of the colon, tumors of the genital apparatus, and malignancies of the lower extremities,

among others. A similar importance might be in the diagnostic and therapeutic accessibility to pancreas, kidneys, and ureter.

This chapter gives only a brief introduction to the subject. For details and results, see the references that follow.

REFERENCES

Wittmoser R: Neurochirurgie der Funktionsstörungen des Mägens und des Zwölffingerdarms. Hippokrates 36:714, 1965

————: Transthorakale-intrathorakale Möglichkeiten der endoskopischen Vagotomie beim Ulcus pepticum. Visum 98, 1967

————: Möglichkeiten der thorakoskopischen Vagotomie beim Ulcus pepticum. In Endoskopie, Methoden und Ergebnisse. First Congress of the German Society for Endoscopy in Erlangen, 1967, München-Gräfelfing, Banaschewski, 1969

————: Die Retroperitoneoskopie als neue Methode der lumbalen Sympathicotomie aus "Fortschritte der Endoskopie." Schattauer, Stuttgart, New York, Ottenjann, 1973

EDITORIAL COMMENT

This procedure is new to us. Dr. Wittmoser's description is very brief and mentions only the idea and major steps. It is unfortunate that the references mentioned are so difficult to obtain in this country. It would be an elegant "mini-approach" for the vascular surgeon to perform via endoscopy, e.g., a lumbar sympathectomy, or for the oncologist to obtain lymph nodes from this area.

The future will show whether this approach will gain wider acceptance, and whether the results by others can confirm Dr. Wittmoser's enthusiasm.

THE EDITOR

Author Index

763

Subject Index